	metoclopramide HCl	midazolam HCl	morphine sulfate	nalbuphine HCl	pentazocine lactate	pentobarbital Na	perphenazine	phenobarbital Na	prochlorperazine edisylate	promazine HCl	promethazine HCl	ranitidine HCl	scopolamine HBr	secobarbital Na	sodium bicarbonate	thiethylperazine maleate	thiopental Na
atropine sulfate	P	Y	P	Y	P	P	Y		P	P	P	Y	P				
benzquinamide HCl		Y	Y		Y	N		N					Y	N			N
butorphanol tartrate		Y	Y		Y	N	Y		Y		Y		Y			Y	
chlorpromazine HCl	P	Y	P		P	N	Y		Y	P	P	Y	P				N
cimetidine HCl		Y	Y	Y	Y	N	Y		Y	Y	Y		Y	N			
codeine phosphate																	
dimenhydrinate	P	N	P		P	N	Y		N	N	N	Y	P				N
diphenhydramine HCl	Y	Y	P		P	N	Y		P	P	P	Y	P				N
droperidol	P	Y	P	Y	P	N	Y		P	P	P		P				
fentanyl citrate	P	Y	P		P	N	Y		P	P	P	Y	P				
glycopyrrolate		Y	Y		N	N			Y	Y	Y	Y	Y	N	N		N
heparin Na	P(5)		N*		N			P(5)			N						
hydromorphone HCl		Y			Y	Y			N*		Y	Y	Y			Y	
hydroxyzine HCl	P	Y	Y	Y	Y	N			P	P	P	N	Y				
meperidine HCl	P	Y	N		P	N	P		P	P	Y	Y	P				N
metoclopramide HCl	■	Y	P		P		P		P	P	P	Y	P		N		
midazolam HCl	Y	■	Y	Y		N	N		N	Y	Y	N	Y			Y	
morphine sulfate	P	Y	■		P	N*	Y		P*	P	P*	Y	P				N
nalbuphine HCl		Y		■		N			Y		Y	Y	Y			Y	
pentazocine lactate	P		P		■	N	Y		P	Y	Y	Y	P				
pentobarbital Na		N	N*	N	N	■	N		N	N	N		Y		Y		Y
perphenazine	P	N	Y		Y	N	■		Y			Y					
phenobarbital Na								■				N					
prochlorperazine edisylate	P	N	P*	Y	P	N	Y		■	P	P	Y	P				N
promazine HCl	P	Y	P		Y	N			P	■	P	P					
promethazine HCl	P	Y	P*	Y	Y	N			P	P	■	Y	[illegible]	[illegible]	[illegible]	[illegible]	[illegible]
[illegible]	Y	N	Y	Y	Y		Y	N	Y	P	Y	■	[illegible]	[illegible]	[illegible]	[illegible]	[illegible]
[illegible]	P	Y	P	Y	P	Y			P		P	Y	[illegible]	[illegible]	[illegible]	[illegible]	[illegible]
[illegible]												[illegible]	[illegible]	[illegible]	[illegible]	[illegible]	[illegible]
[illegible]	N					Y						[illegible]	[illegible]	[illegible]	[illegible]	[illegible]	[illegible]
thiethylperazine maleate		Y		Y								Y	[illegible]	[illegible]	[illegible]	[illegible]	[illegible]
thiopental Na			N			Y			N		N	[illegible]	[illegible]	[illegible]	[illegible]	[illegible]	[illegible]

Nursing95 DRUG HANDBOOK

NURSING95 BOOKS™
SPRINGHOUSE CORPORATION
SPRINGHOUSE, PENNSYLVANIA

STAFF

The clinical procedures described and recommended in this publication are based on research and consultation with nursing, medical, and legal authorities. To the best of our knowledge, these procedures reflect currently accepted practice; nevertheless, they can't be considered absolute and universal recommendations. For individual application, all recommendations must be considered in light of the patient's clinical condition and, before administration of new or infrequently used drugs, in light of the latest package-insert information. The authors and the publisher disclaim responsibility for any adverse effects resulting directly or indirectly from the suggested procedures, from any undetected errors, or from the reader's misunderstanding of the text.

A member of the Reed Elsevier plc group

NDH-020195
ISSN 0273-320X
ISBN 0-87434-706-8

CONTENTS

Consultants, Reviewers, and Advisors vii

General Information

1. How to use *Nursing95 Drug Handbook* 1
2. Drug actions, reactions, and interactions explained 6
3. Drug therapy in children 13
4. Drug therapy in elderly patients 18
5. Drug therapy and the nursing process 21

Antimicrobial and Antiparasitic Agents

6. Amebicides and antiprotozoals 25
7. Anthelmintics 31
8. Antifungals 37
9. Antimalarials 47
10. Antituberculars and antileprotics 55
11. Aminoglycosides 65
12. Penicillins 75
13. Cephalosporins 100
14. Tetracyclines 129
15. Sulfonamides 138
16. Quinolones 145
17. Antivirals 154
18. Miscellaneous anti-infectives 167

Cardiovascular System Drugs

19. Inotropics 187
20. Antiarrhythmics 193
21. Antianginals 215
22. Antihypertensives 232
23. Vasodilators 278
24. Antilipemics 285

Central Nervous System Drugs

25. Nonnarcotic analgesics and antipyretics 296
26. Nonsteroidal anti-inflammatory drugs 311
27. Narcotic and opioid analgesics 335
28. Sedative-hypnotics 360
29. Anticonvulsants 380
30. Antidepressants 402
31. Antianxiety agents 427

32. Antipsychotics 440
33. Cerebral stimulants 467
34. Antiparkinsonian agents 481
35. Miscellaneous CNS agents 492

Autonomic Nervous System Drugs

36. Cholinergics (parasympathomimetics) 501
37. Anticholinergics 510
38. Adrenergics (sympathomimetics) 527
39. Adrenergic blockers (sympatholytics) 537
40. Skeletal muscle relaxants 541
41. Neuromuscular blockers 550

Respiratory Tract Drugs

42. Antihistamines 568
43. Bronchodilators 584
44. Expectorants and antitussives 608
45. Miscellaneous respiratory agents 613

Gastrointestinal Tract Drugs

46. Antacids, adsorbents, and antiflatulents 624
47. Digestants 632
48. Antidiarrheals 638
49. Laxatives 645
50. Antiemetics 660
51. Antiulcer agents 672

Hormonal Agents

52. Corticosteroids 680
53. Androgens and anabolic steroids 700
54. Estrogens and progestins 714
55. Gonadotropins 743
56. Antidiabetic agents and glucagon 750
57. Thyroid hormones 764
58. Thyroid hormone antagonists 772
59. Pituitary hormones 778
60. Parathyroid-like agents 786

Agents for Fluid and Electrolyte Balance

61. Diuretics 792

62. Electrolytes and replacement solutions 822
63. Acidifier and alkalinizers 836

Hematologic Agents

64. Hematinics 840
65. Anticoagulants 845
66. Hemostatics 853
67. Blood derivatives 856
68. Thrombolytic enzymes 863

Antineoplastic Agents

69. Alkylating agents 870
70. Antimetabolites 890
71. Antibiotic antineoplastic agents 903
72. Antineoplastics that alter hormone balance 914
73. Miscellaneous antineoplastic agents 923

Immunomodulation Agents

74. Immunosuppressants 937
75. Vaccines and toxoids 943
76. Antitoxins and antivenins 966
77. Immune serums 970
78. Biological response modifiers 977

Eye, Ear, Nose, and Throat Drugs

79. Ophthalmic anti-infectives 991
80. Ophthalmic anti-inflammatory agents 1006
81. Miotics 1012
82. Mydriatics 1021
83. Ophthalmic vasoconstrictors 1028
84. Miscellaneous ophthalmics 1031
85. Otics 1044
86. Nasal agents 1047

Dermatomucosal Agents

87. Local anti-infectives 1056
88. Scabicides and pediculicides 1080
89. Topical corticosteroids 1085

Nutritional Agents

90. Vitamins and minerals 1106
91. Calorics 1127

Miscellaneous Drug Categories

92. Antigout agents 1135
93. Enzymes 1141
94. Oxytocics 1144
95. Spasmolytics 1150
96. Gold salts 1152
97. Diagnostic skin tests 1155
98. Miscellaneous antagonists and antidotes 1160
99. Uncategorized drugs 1181
100. Investigational drugs 1209

Appendices and Index

Anesthetics: Local, general, and topical ophthalmic 1224
Topical agents 1238
Cancer chemotherapy: Acronyms and protocols 1244
Orphan drugs and biologicals 1262
Index 1277

CONSULTANTS, REVIEWERS, AND ADVISORS

At the time of publication, the clinical consultants, pharmacy reviewers, and advisors held the following positions.

Clinical Consultants

Mary Ann Cali-Ascani, RNC, MSN, OCN, Oncology Nurse Manager, Easton (Pa.) Hospital
Nancy G. Evans, RN, BSN, CGRN, Nurse Manager, Gastroenterology Department, Daniel Freeman Memorial and Marina Hospitals, Inglewood, Calif.
Walter Carl Faubion, RN, MHSA, Clinical Manager, Home Medicine, University of Michigan Medical Center, Ann Arbor
Terry Matthew Foster, RN, BSN, CCRN, CEN, Emergency Nursing Consultant, Staff Nurse, Emergency Department, Saint Elizabeth Medical Center, Covington, Ky.
Shirley A. Grieshaber, RN, Advanced Clinical Nurse, National Institutes of Health, Bethesda, Md.
Roseann Hendrickson, RN, Nursing Consultant, Emergency Physician Associates, Woodbury, N.J.
Karen Landis, RN, MS, CCRN, Pulmonary Clinical Nurse Specialist, Lehigh Valley Hospital Center, The Allentown (Pa.) Hospital
Rosemarie Marinaro, RN,C, MSN, Perinatal Clinical Nurse Specialist, Frankford Hospital-Perinatal Center, Philadelphia
Chris Platt Moldovanyi, RN, MSN, Nursing Consultant, Cleveland, Ohio
Nancy V. Runta, RN, BSN, CCRN, Infection Control Practitioner, North Penn Hospital, Lansdale, Pa.
Debra L. Ryan, RN, MN, CCRN, Critical Care Clinical Nurse Specialist, Memorial Medical Center, Springfield, Ill.

Pharmacy Reviewers

Douglas R. Allington, RPh, PharmD, Assistant Professor, University of Montana, Missoula
Alan D. Barreuther, RPh, PharmD, Administrator, Pharmacy Partners Health Plan (HMO), Tucson, Ariz.
Terri L. Craig, RPh, PharmD, Clinical Pharmacy Specialist, Veterans Administration Medical Center, Iowa City
Joel Glucroft, PhD, Pharmaceutical and Managed Healthcare Consultant, J. Glucroft & Associates, Canoga Park, Calif.
Sandra Hardee Hak, PharmD, Assistant Professor, East Carolina University, Greenville, N.C.
James R. Hildebrand, RPh, PharmD, Director, Drug Information Center and Associate Professor of Clinical Pharmacy, Philadelphia College of Pharmacy and Science
Laurel M. Janney, PharmD, Clinical Pharmacy Specialist, Veterans Administration Medical Center, Iowa City
Cary E. Johnson, RPh, PharmD, Associate Professor, University of Michigan College of Pharmacy; Clinical Pharmacist, University of Michigan Medical Center, Ann Arbor
Mark S. Luer, PharmD, Assistant Professor, College of Pharmacy, Department of Pharmacy Practice, University of Illinois at Chicago
David R. Pipher, RPh, PharmD, Assistant Director, Clinical Services, Forbes Regional Hospital, Monroeville, Pa.
Denise H. Rhoney, PharmD, Drug Development Fellow, University of North Carolina at Chapel Hill
Marc S. Roth, RPh, MS, Clinical Coordinator for Intravenous Nutrition, New York Hospital-Cornell Medical Center
J. Michael Spivey, RPh, PharmD, BCPS, Assistant Professor of Family Medicine, East Carolina University School of Medicine, Greenville, N.C.
Joseph F. Steiner, RPh, PharmD, Professor of Clinical Pharmacy, University of Wyoming, Schools of Human Medicine and Pharmacy, Casper
Daya R. Varma, MD PhD, Professor of Pharmacology and Therapeutics, McGill University, Montreal
Christy W. Whitley, MA, PharmD, Clinical Assistant Professor of Family Medicine, East Carolina University School of Medicine, Greenville, N.C.

Allison P. Winecoff, PharmD, Assistant Professor, Department of Pharmacy Practice, University of Georgia, Augusta

Special thanks to the following, who have made major contributions or have contributed to recent past editions: Michael J. Booth, RN, MA, CRNA; Heather Boyd-Monk, SRN, RN, BSN; Karen E. Burgess, RN, MSN; Nancy Burns, RN, PhD; Carla J. Burton, RN, BS; Bruce D. Clayton RPh, PharmD; Michael Cohen, RPh, MS, FASHP; Charmaine J. Cummings, RN, MSN; Doyle M. Cummings, RPh, PharmD; Judith Hopfer Deglin, RPh, PharmD; Mark J. Ellison, RPh, PharmD; Bruce M. Frey, RPh, PharmD; Larry N. Gever, RPh, PharmD; Jimmi Hatton, RPh, PharmD; David W. Hawkins, RPh, PharmD; Marcia Jo Hill, RN, MSN; Alan Hopefl, RPh, PharmD; Arthur I. Jacknowitz, RPh, PharmD; Nina E. Jakobowski, RPh, PharmD; Meredith Ann McCord, RN, MS; Susanne P. Mulligan, RPh, BS; Helene K. Nawrocki, RN, MSN; Sandra L. Nettina, RN,C, MSN, CRNP; Lea Anne O'Brien, RPh, PharmD; Andrew T. Pennell, RPh, PharmD; Joanne M. Sica, RPh, MHA; Margaret Smellie-Belfield, RN, BSN, CCRN; Marilyn Sawyer Sommers, RN, PhD, CCRN; Julie Tackenberg, RN, MA, CNRN; Kerri J. Vandel, RPh, PharmD; Paul J. Vitale, RPh, PharmD, FASCP.

Advisory Board

Lillian S. Brunner, RN, MSN, ScD, FAAN, Nurse-Author, Berwyn, Pa.
Luther P. Christman, RN, PhD, Nurse Consultant, Chapel Hill, Tenn.
Kathleen A. Dracup, RN, DNSc, Editor, *American Journal of Critical Care;* Professor, University of California School of Nursing, Los Angeles
Stanley J. Dudrick, MD, FACS, Surgeon-in-Chief, Hermann Hospital, Houston; Clinical Professor of Surgery, University of Texas Houston Health Science Center
Halbert E. Fillinger, MD, Forensic Pathologist, Assistant Medical Examiner, Office of the Medical Examiner, Philadelphia
M. Josephine Flaherty, RN, PhD, Principal Nursing Officer, Department of National Health and Welfare, Ottawa
Joyce LeFever Kee, RN, MSN, Associate Professor, College of Nursing, University of Delaware, Newark
Dennis E. Leavelle, MD, Associate Professor, Mayo Medical Laboratories, Mayo Clinic, Rochester, Minn.
Ara G. Paul, PhD, Dean, College of Pharmacy; Professor of Pharmacognosy, University of Michigan, Ann Arbor
Rose Pinneo, RN, MS, Professor Emeritus, University of Rochester (N.Y.) School of Nursing
Thomas E. Rubbert, JD, LLB, BSL, Attorney-at-Law, Pasadena, Calif.
Maryanne Schreiber, RN, BA, Product Manager, Patient Monitoring, Hewlett-Packard Co., Waltham (Mass.) Division
Frances Storlie, RN, PhD, Adult Nurse Practitioner (C); Director, Personal Health Services, Southwest Washington Health District, Vancouver
Claire L. Watson, RN, Clinical Documentation Associate, IVAC Corporation, San Diego

1

How to use *Nursing95 Drug Handbook*

Nursing95 Drug Handbook is meant to fill a very special need. It represents a joint effort by pharmacists and nurses to provide the nursing profession with drug information that focuses on what nurses need to know. With this in mind, it emphasizes clinical aspects and does not attempt to replace detailed pharmacology texts. Also, the information is arranged in a format designed to make it readily accessible.

Introductory information

Following this chapter, Chapter 2 explains, in a general way, how drugs work. It also tells about side effects and adverse reactions and gives general guidelines about drug use in pregnancy and the presence of drugs in breast milk. Chapters 3 and 4 discuss the unique problems of administering drugs to children and elderly patients and offer guidelines to minimize problems in these areas. Chapter 5 discusses drug therapy as it relates to the nursing process.

In the remaining chapters, all drugs are classified according to their approved therapeutic uses. Drugs that have multiple therapeutic uses are classified according to their most common use; they are also listed (with a cross-reference to the major drug entry) in drug groups that share their secondary applications. For example, nadolol, a beta-adrenergic blocker, is described in the chapter that covers antianginals because its major therapeutic application is the management of angina pectoris; because it is less commonly used to treat hypertension, it is listed among the generic drugs grouped as antihypertensives with a cross-reference to Chapter 21, Antianginals.

Such classification by therapeutic use offers several advantages. It helps the reader identify an unknown drug by its clinical application alone. At the same time, it automatically identifies all other drugs that share the same use and provides easy comparison of their dosages and effects. Thereby, it quickly identifies potential pharmacotherapeutic alternatives for patients who cannot tolerate or fail to respond to a particular drug.

Drug information

Each chapter, representing a major therapeutic use, begins with an alphabetically arranged list of the generic names of drugs described in that chapter. This is followed by a list of selected combination products in which these drugs are found. Specific information on each drug is arranged under the following headings: *How Supplied, Action, Indications & Dosage, Adverse Reactions, Interactions, Contraindications* and *Nursing Considerations.*

In each drug entry, the drug's generic name is immediately followed by an alphabetized list of its brand names. A trade name followed by an open diamond indicates a drug that is available in preparations that do not require a prescription (◇). Brands available *only* in Canada are designated with a dagger (†); those available *only* in Australia, with a double dagger (‡). A brand name with no symbol after it is available in the United States, Canada, and possibly Australia. The mention of a brand name in no way implies endorsement of that product or guarantees its legality. If a drug is a controlled substance, that is indicated (example: Controlled Substance Schedule II). Drugs regulated under the jurisdiction of the

Controlled Substances Act of 1970 are divided into the following groups, or schedules.

- Schedule I (C-I): High abuse potential and no accepted medical use – for example, heroin, marijuana, and LSD.
- Schedule II (C-II): High abuse potential with severe dependence liability – for example, narcotics, amphetamines, dronabinol, and some barbiturates.
- Schedule III (C-III): Less abuse potential than schedule II drugs and moderate dependence liability – for example, nonbarbiturate sedatives, nonamphetamine stimulants, and limited amounts of certain narcotics.
- Schedule IV (C-IV): Less abuse potential than schedule III drugs and limited dependence liability – for example, some sedatives, antianxiety agents, nonnarcotic analgesics.
- Schedule V (C-V): Limited abuse potential. Primarily small amounts of narcotics, such as codeine, used as antitussives or antidiarrheals. Under federal law, limited quantities of certain C-V drugs may be purchased without a prescription directly from a pharmacist if allowed under specific state statutes. The purchaser must be at least age 18 and must furnish suitable identification. All such transactions must be recorded by the dispensing pharmacist.

Each systemically absorbed drug has been assigned a pregnancy risk category based upon available clinical and preclinical information. The Pregnancy Risk Category parallels the five Pregnancy Categories (A, B, C, D, and X) assigned by the Food and Drug Administration to reflect a drug's potential to cause birth defects. Although drugs are best avoided during pregnancy, this rating system permits rapid assessment of the risk-benefit ratio should drug administration to a pregnant woman become necessary. Drugs in category A are generally considered safe to use in pregnancy; drugs in category X are generally contraindicated.

- A: Adequate studies in pregnant women have failed to show a risk to the fetus in the first trimester of pregnancy or in later trimesters.
- B: Animal studies have not shown a risk to the fetus, but controlled studies have not been conducted in pregnant women; or animal studies have shown an adverse effect on the fetus, but adequate studies in pregnant women have not shown a risk to the fetus during the first trimester of pregnancy or in later trimesters.
- C: Animal studies have shown an adverse effect on the fetus, but adequate studies have not been conducted in humans. The benefits from use in pregnant women may be acceptable despite potential risks; or, because of insufficient studies, pregnancy risk is unknown.
- D: The drug may cause risk to the human fetus, but the potential benefits of use in pregnant women may be acceptable despite the risks.
- X: Studies in animals or humans show fetal abnormalities, or adverse reaction reports indicate evidence of fetal risk. The risks involved clearly outweigh potential benefits.
- NR: Not rated.

In this volume, the Pregnancy Risk Category has been omitted if the drug is not rated and if such rating is not applicable.

The section titled *How Supplied* lists the preparations available for each drug (for example, tablets, capsules, solutions for injection), specifying available dosage forms and strengths. Dosage strengths available *only* in Canada are designated with a dagger (†); those available *only* in Australia, with a double dagger (‡). Preparations that do not require a prescription are marked with an open diamond (◇).

The section titled *Action* succinctly

describes the mechanism of action – that is, how the drug provides its therapeutic effect. For example, although all antihypertensives lower blood pressure, they don't all do so by the same pharmacologic process. This section also includes the onset, peak (described in terms of effect or peak blood level), and duration of drug action for each route of administration, if data are available or applicable. Values listed for onset, peak, and duration are for patients with normal renal function, unless specified otherwise.

The section titled *Indications & Dosage* lists general dosage information for adults (including recommended geriatric dosages, when available) and children, as applicable. Children's dosages are usually indicated in terms of mg/kg daily. Dosage instructions reflect current clinical trends in therapeutics and can't be considered as absolute and universal recommendations. For individual application, dosage instructions must be considered in light of the patient's clinical condition.

The section titled *Adverse Reactions* lists each drug's commonly observed adverse reactions (and selected rare ones if life-threatening). The most common adverse reactions are in *italic* type; life-threatening reactions are in ***bold italic*** type. An exception to this rule is an adverse reaction that, although normally considered hazardous, has been reported to be mild and reversible with the drug in question. For example, thrombocytopenia is considered a life-threatening adverse reaction to plicamycin but a mild and reversible reaction to methyldopa. Hence, thrombocytopenia listed as an adverse reaction to plicamycin is in bold italics, whereas the same reaction under methyldopa is not. Adverse reactions are grouped according to the body system in which they appear.

The next section, *Interactions,* lists each drug's confirmed, *clinically significant* interactions with other drugs (additive effects, potentiated effects, and antagonistic effects) or foods, with specific suggestions for avoiding dangerous drug or food interactions (for example, by reducing doses or monitoring food intake). Drug interactions are listed under the drug that is adversely affected. For example, magnesium trisilicate, an ingredient in antacids, interacts with tetracycline to cause decreased absorption of tetracycline. Therefore, this interaction is listed under tetracycline. To check on the possible effects of using two or more drugs simultaneously, refer to the interaction entry for *each* of the drugs in question.

The section titled *Contraindications* lists any conditions, especially diseases, in which the use of the drug is undesirable. Also included are recommendations for cautious use.

The final section, *Nursing Considerations,* lists other useful information, such as monitoring techniques and suggestions for prevention and treatment of adverse reactions. Also included are suggestions for patient comfort, for patient teaching, and for preparing, administering, and storing each drug. Recommendations for I.V. use are highlighted by **boldface** type.

Alcohol and tartrazine content

Many liquid drug preparations for oral use contain alcohol. Although the slight sedative effect that alcohol produces is not harmful in most patients – and can sometimes be beneficial – alcohol ingestion can be undesirable and even dangerous in some circumstances. Alcohol-containing oral drugs should be given very cautiously, if at all, to patients who are:

- concomitantly taking potent CNS depressants, such as barbiturates
- taking drugs that may produce a disulfiram-type reaction (such as chlor-

propamide, metronidazole, and furazolidone)

• taking disulfiram as part of a treatment program for their alcoholism. Such patients, upon ingestion of alcohol, will exhibit severe symptoms that may include blurred vision, confusion, dyspnea, flushing, sweating, and tachycardia.

To help prevent inadvertent exposure to alcohol, this volume signals alcohol content with a single asterisk (*) after each brand of a liquid preparation that may contain it. In many of the preparations so marked, the alcohol content is small. Nevertheless, these drugs should be avoided in patients who are susceptible to adverse effects upon exposure to alcohol.

Tartrazine dye, also known as FD&C Yellow No. 5, is a common coloring agent in some foods and drugs. Usually harmless, it can provoke a severe allergic reaction in susceptible persons. For this reason, most drug manufacturers have begun to eliminate tartrazine from their products, but many drugs still contain it.

The incidence of tartrazine sensitivity is estimated at approximately 1 in 10,000 in the general population but somewhat higher in persons with asthma and/or sensitivity to aspirin. Why this is so is unknown. The most common symptoms of tartrazine sensitivity are urticaria, rhinorrhea, asthma, and angioedema. Acutely sensitive persons may develop allergic vascular purpura, tachycardia, dyspnea, and chest pain. These allergic symptoms typically subside spontaneously upon discontinuation of the tartrazine-containing drug but may require treatment with antihistamines or epinephrine.

Avoiding exposure to tartrazine is not simply a matter of avoiding yellow-colored drugs because this substance may be present in many other color blends, such as turquoise, green, and maroon. This volume signals tartrazine content with a double asterisk (**) after each brand that may contain it. If you suspect tartrazine sensitivity in a patient receiving such a drug, inform the doctor and contact the manufacturer to determine which dosage forms contain tartrazine.

A guide to abbreviations

ACE angiotensin-converting enzyme
ADH antidiuretic hormone
AIDS acquired immunodeficiency syndrome
ALT alanine aminotransferase
AST aspartate aminotransferase
AV atrioventricular
b.i.d. twice daily
BUN blood urea nitrogen
cAMP cyclic 3′, 5′ adenosine monophosphate
CBC complete blood count
CHF congestive heart failure
CK creatine kinase
CMV cytomegalovirus
CNS central nervous system
COPD chronic obstructive pulmonary disease
CSF cerebrospinal fluid
CV cardiovascular
CVA cerebrovascular accident
D_5W dextrose 5% in water
DNA deoxyribonucleic acid
ECG electrocardiogram
EENT eyes, ears, nose, throat
FDA Food and Drug Administration
g gram
G gauge
GFR glomerular filtration rate
GI gastrointestinal
GU genitourinary
G6PD glucose-6-phosphate dehydrogenase
HIV human immunodeficiency virus
h.s. at bedtime
ID intradermal

I.M.	intramuscular
IND	investigational new drug
IPPB	intermittent positive-pressure breathing
IU	international unit
I.V.	intravenous
kg	kilogram
M	molar
m²	square meter
MAO	monoamine oxidase
mcg	microgram
mEq	milliequivalent
mg	milligram
MI	myocardial infarction
ml	milliliter
mm³	cubic millimeter
Na	sodium
NaCl	sodium chloride
NSAID	nonsteroidal anti-inflammatory drug
OTC	over the counter
PABA	para-aminobenzoic acid
P.O.	by mouth
P.R.	by rectum
p.r.n.	as needed
PT	prothrombin time
PTT	partial thromboplastin time
PVCs	premature ventricular contractions
q	every
q.d.	every day
q.i.d.	four times daily
q.o.d.	every other day
RBC	red blood cell
RDA	recommended daily allowance
REM	rapid eye movement
RNA	ribonucleic acid
RSV	respiratory syncytial virus
SA	sinoatrial
S.C.	subcutaneous
SIADH	syndrome of inappropriate antidiuretic hormone
S.L.	sublingual
t.i.d.	three times daily
UCE	urea cycle enzymopathy
USP	United States Pharmacopeia
WBC	white blood cell

2

Drug actions, reactions, and interactions explained

Administration of any drug provokes a series of physicochemical events within the body. The first event, when a drug combines with cellular drug receptors, is known as the drug action. What follows as a result of this action of the drug is known as the drug effect. Depending on the number of different cellular drug receptors affected by a given drug, a drug effect can be local, systemic, or both. Obviously, a local effect follows application to the skin; however, transdermal absorption can produce systemic effects. Moreover, local effects can follow systemic absorption. For example, the antipeptic ulcer drug cimetidine acts solely by blocking histamine receptor cells in the parietal cells of the stomach. This is known as a local drug effect because the drug action is sharply limited to one area and does not spread to other parts of the body. On the other hand, diphenhydramine produces a systemic effect in that it blocks histamine receptors in widespread areas of the body. In other words, local drug effects are specific to a limited number of organ systems, whereas systemic drug effects are generalized and affect different and diverse organ systems.

Three factors modify drug action

1. Absorption

Before a drug can act within the body, it must be absorbed into the bloodstream – usually after oral administration, the most frequently used route. Before a drug contained in a tablet or capsule can be absorbed, the dosage form must disintegrate – that is, break into smaller particles. Then, these smaller particles can dissolve in gastric juices. Only after so dissolving can a drug be absorbed into the bloodstream. Once absorbed and circulated in the bloodstream, it is bioavailable, or ready to produce a drug effect. Whether such absorption is complete or partial depends on several factors: the drug's physicochemical effects, its dosage form, its route of administration, its interactions with other substances in the GI tract, and various patient characteristics. These same factors also determine the speed of absorption. Thus, oral solutions and elixirs, which bypass the need for disintegration and dissolution, are usually absorbed more rapidly. Some tablets have enteric coatings that prevent disintegration in the acidic environment of the stomach; others may have coatings of varying thickness that delay release of the drug.

Drugs administered intramuscularly must first be absorbed through the muscle into the bloodstream. Rectal suppositories must dissolve to be absorbed through the rectal mucosa. Drugs administered intravenously, which are injected directly into the bloodstream, are completely and immediately bioavailable.

2. Distribution

After absorption, a drug moves from the bloodstream into various fluids and tissues within the body; this is distribution. Individual patient variations can greatly alter the amount of drug that is distributed throughout the body. For example, in an edematous patient, a given dose must be distributed to a larger volume than in a nonedematous patient; the amount of drug must sometimes be increased to account for this. Remember, the dose should be decreased when the edema is corrected. Conversely, in an extremely dehydrated patient, the drug will be distributed to a much smaller volume, so the dose must then be decreased. The total area to which a drug is distributed is known as volume of distribution. Patients who are particularly obese may present another problem when considering drug distribution. Some drugs – such as digoxin, gentamicin, and tobramycin – are not well distributed to fatty tissue. Therefore, dosing based on actual body weight may lead to overdose and serious toxicity. In some cases, dosing must be based on lean body weight, which may be estimated from actuarial tables that give average weight range for height.

3. Metabolism and excretion (drug elimination)

Most drugs are metabolized in the liver and excreted by the kidneys. Hepatic diseases may affect one or more of the metabolic functions of the liver. Therefore, in patients with hepatic disease, the metabolism of a drug may be increased, decreased, or unchanged. Clearly, all patients with hepatic disease must be monitored closely for drug effect and toxicity. Some drugs (digoxin, gentamicin) are eliminated almost unchanged by the kidneys. For safe use of such drugs, renal function must be adequate or the drug will accumulate, producing toxic effects. Some drugs can alter the effect and excretion of other drugs. For example, they can stimulate or inhibit hepatic-metabolizing enzymes to alter the rate of metabolism and change the drug effect. Or they can block or promote renal excretion of other drugs, causing them to accumulate and enhancing their effects, or cause rapid excretion, thereby diminishing their effects. Some slight elimination takes place by way of perspiration, saliva, breast milk, and so on. Certain volatile anesthetics, however – halothane, for instance – are eliminated primarily by exhalation.

The rate at which a drug is metabolized varies with the individual. In some patients, drugs are metabolized so quickly that their blood and tissue levels prove therapeutically inadequate. In others, the rate of metabolism is so slow that ordinary doses can produce toxic results.

Other modifying factors

An important factor that influences a drug's action and effect is its *binding to plasma proteins,* especially albumin, and other tissue components. Because only a free, unbound drug can act in the body, such binding greatly influences effectiveness and duration of effect.

The *patient's age* is another important factor. Elderly patients usually have decreased hepatic function, less muscle mass, and diminished renal function. Consequently, they need lower doses and sometimes longer dosage intervals to avoid toxicity. With similar consequences, neonates have underdeveloped metabolic enzyme systems and inadequate renal function. They need highly individualized dosage and careful monitoring.

Underlying disease can also markedly affect drug action and effect. For example, acidosis may cause insulin resistance. Genetic diseases, such as G6PD deficiency and hepatic porphyria, may turn drugs into toxins with serious consequences. Patients with G6PD deficiency may develop hemolytic anemia when given sulfonamides or a number of other drugs. A genetically susceptible patient can develop an acute porphyria attack if given a barbiturate. Also, patients who have highly active hepatic enzyme systems (for example, rapid acetylators), when treated with isoniazid, can develop hepatitis from the rapid intrahepatic buildup of a toxic metabolite.

Things to consider about administration

• *Dosage forms do matter.* Some tablets and capsules are too large to be easily swallowed by very ill patients. You may then request an oral solution or elixir of the same drug, but bear in mind that because a liquid is more easily and completely absorbed, it produces higher blood levels than a tablet. When a potentially toxic drug (such as digoxin) is given, the increased amount absorbed could cause toxicity. Sometimes a change in dosage form requires a change in dosage.

• *Routes of administration are not therapeutically interchangeable.* For example, phenytoin is readily absorbed orally but is slowly and erratically absorbed intramuscularly. On the other hand, gentamicin must be given parenterally because oral administration yields inadequate blood levels to treat systemic infections.

• *Improper storage can alter a drug's potency.* Most drugs should be stored in tight containers protected from direct sunlight and extremes in temperature and humidity that can cause them to deteriorate. Some may require special storage conditions, such as refrigeration.

• *The timing of drug administration can be important.* Sometimes, giving an oral drug during or shortly after mealtime decreases the amount of drug absorbed. This is not clinically significant with most drugs and may in fact be desirable with irritating drugs such as aspirin or phenylbutazone. But penicillins and tetracyclines should not be scheduled for administration at mealtimes because certain foods can inactivate them. If in doubt about the effect of food on a certain drug, check with the pharmacist.

• *Consider the patient's age, height, and weight.* The doctor will need this information when calculating the dosage for many drugs. It should be accurately recorded on the patient's chart. This chart should also include current laboratory data, especially renal and liver function studies, so the doctor can adjust the dosage as needed.

• *Watch for metabolic changes.* Monitor for any physiologic change (depressed respiratory function, acidosis or alkalosis) that might alter drug effect.

• *Know the patient's history.* Whenever possible, obtain a comprehensive family history from the patient or his family. Ask about past reactions to drugs, possible genetic traits that might alter drug response, and the current use of other drugs. Multiple drug therapy can cause drug interactions that can dramatically change the effects of many drugs.

Drug interactions

When one drug administered in combination with or shortly after another drug alters the effect of one or both drugs, this is known as a drug interaction. Usually, the effect of one drug is increased or decreased. For instance, one drug may inhibit or stimulate the metabolism or excretion of the other; or it may release another from plasma protein-binding sites, freeing it for further action.

Combination therapy is based on drug interaction. One drug, for example, may be given to potentiate another. Probenecid, which blocks the excretion of penicillin, is sometimes given with penicillin to maintain adequate blood levels of penicillin for a longer period. Often, two drugs with similar actions are given together precisely because of the additive effect that results. For instance, aspirin and codeine, both analgesics, are often given in combination because together they provide greater pain relief than either alone.

Drug interactions are sometimes used to prevent or antagonize certain adverse reactions. Hydrochlorothiazide and spironolactone, both diuretics, are often administered in combination because the former is potassium-depleting, whereas the latter is potassium-sparing.

But not all drug interactions are beneficial. Multiple drugs can interact to produce effects that are often undesirable and sometimes hazardous. Harmful drug interactions decrease efficacy or increase toxicity. A hypertensive patient well controlled with guanethidine may see his blood pressure rise to its former high level if he takes the antidepressant amitriptyline at the same time. Such a drug effect is known as antagonism. Drug combinations that produce these effects should be avoided if possible. Another kind of inhibiting effect occurs when a tetracycline drug is administered with calcium- or magnesium-containing drugs or foods (such as antacids or milk). These combine with tetracycline in the GI tract and cause inadequate absorption of tetracycline.

Adverse reactions

Any drug effect other than what is therapeutically intended can be called an adverse reaction. It may be expected and benign, or unexpected and potentially harmful. Mild, but *predictable,* adverse reactions are sometimes called side effects. Drowsiness caused by antihistamines is an example of this. During hay fever season, a patient may have to contend with this drowsiness to get relief from hay fever symptoms. In such a case, the dosage may be adjusted up or down to balance therapeutic effects with side effects.

An adverse reaction may be tolerated for a necessary therapeutic effect, or it may be hazardous and unacceptable and require discontinuation of the drug. Some adverse reactions subside with continued use. As an example, the drowsiness associated with methyldopa and the orthostatic hypotension associated with prazosin usually subside after several days, as the patient develops a tolerance to these effects. But many adverse reactions are dosage-related and lessen or disappear only if the dosage is reduced. Although most adverse reactions are not therapeutically desirable, an occasional one can be put to clinical use. An outstanding example of this is the drowsiness associated with diphenhydramine, which makes it clinically useful as a mild hypnotic.

Hypersensitivity, a term sometimes used interchangeably with drug allergy, is the result of an antigen-antibody immune reaction that occurs in the body when a drug is given to a susceptible patient. One of the most dangerous of all drug hypersensitivities is penicillin allergy. In its severest form, penicillin anaphylaxis can rapidly become fatal.

Rarely, idiosyncratic reactions occur. These are highly unpredictable, individual, and unusual. Probably the best known idiosyncratic drug reaction is the aplastic anemia caused by the antibiotic chloramphenicol. This reaction appears in only 1 out of 40,000 patients, but when it does, it can be fatal. A more common idiosyncratic reaction is extreme sensitivity to very low doses of a drug, or insensitivity to higher-than-normal doses.

To deal with adverse reactions correctly, you need to be alert to even minor changes in the patient's clinical status. Such minor changes may be an early warning of pending toxicity. Listen to the patient's complaints about his reactions to a drug, and consider each complaint objectively. You may be able to reduce adverse reactions in several ways. Obviously, dosage reduction often helps. But often so does a simple rescheduling of the same dose. For example, pseudoephedrine may produce stimulation that will be no problem if it's given early in the day; similarly, the drowsiness that occurs with antihistamines or tranquilizers can be totally harmless if the dose is given at bedtime. Most important, your patient needs to be told what adverse reactions to expect so he won't become worried or even stop taking the drug on his own. Of course, the patient should report any unusual or unexpected adverse reactions to the doctor.

Recognizing drug allergies or serious idiosyncratic reactions can sometimes be lifesaving. Ask each patient about drugs he is taking or has taken in the past and what, if any, unusual reactions he experienced from taking them. If a patient claims to be allergic to a drug, ask him to tell you exactly what happens when he takes it. He may be calling a harmless side effect such as upset stomach an allergic reaction, or he may have a true tendency toward anaphylaxis. In either case, you and the doctor need to know this. Of course, you must record and report any clinical changes throughout the patient's hospital stay. If you suspect a severe adverse reaction, withhold the drug until you can check with the pharmacist and the doctor.

Toxic reactions

Chronic drug toxicities are generally caused by the cumulative effect and resulting buildup of the drug in the body. These effects may be extensions of the desired therapeutic effect. For example, guanethidine-induced norepinephrine depletion produces a desired antihypertensive effect, but in larger doses, this action often produces orthostatic hypotension.

Drug toxicities typically occur when drug blood levels rise due to impaired metabolism or excretion. For example, blood levels of theophylline rise when hepatic dysfunction impairs metabolism of the drug. Similarly, digoxin toxicity can follow impaired renal function because digoxin is eliminated from the body almost exclusively by the kidneys (via glomerular filtration). Of course, toxic blood levels also follow excessive dosage. Aspirin tinnitus is usually a sign that the safe dose has been exceeded.

Most drug toxicities are predictable and dosage-related; fortunately, most are also readily reversible upon dosage adjustment. So be sure to monitor patients carefully for physiologic changes that might alter drug effect. Watch especially for impaired hepatic and renal function. Warn the patient about signs of pending toxicity, and tell him what to do if a toxic reaction occurs. Also, be sure to emphasize the importance of taking a drug exactly as prescribed. Warn the patient about serious problems that could arise if he changes the dose or the schedule for taking it.

Drugs and pregnancy

Ever since the thalidomide tragedy of the late 1950s – when thousands of malformed infants were born after their mothers used this mild sedative-hypnotic during pregnancy – use of drugs during pregnancy has been a source of serious medical concern and controversy. To identify drugs that may cause such teratogenic effects, preclinical drug studies always include tests on pregnant laboratory animals. These tests point out gross teratogenicity but do not clearly establish safety. Because different species react to drugs in different ways, animal studies do not rule out possible teratogenic effects in humans. For example, the preliminary studies on thalidomide gave no warning of teratogenic effects, and it was subsequently released for general use in Europe.

What about the placental barrier? Once thought to protect the fetus from drug effects, the placenta isn't actually much of a barrier at all. Except for drugs with exceptionally large molecular structure, almost every drug administered to a pregnant woman crosses the placenta and enters the fetal circulation. An example of a drug with a large molecular size is heparin, the injectable anticoagulant. Theoretically, then, heparin could be used in a pregnant woman without fear of harming the fetus – but even heparin carries a warning for cautious use in pregnancy. Conversely, just because a drug crosses the placenta doesn't necessarily mean it's harmful to the fetus.

Actually, only one factor – stage of fetal development – seems clearly related to exaggerated risk during pregnancy. During two stages of pregnancy – the first and the third trimesters – the fetus is especially vulnerable to damage from maternal use of drugs. During these times, *all* drugs should be given with extreme caution.

The most sensitive period for drug-induced fetal malformation is the first trimester, when fetal organs are differentiating (organogenesis). During this time, *all* drugs should be withheld unless doing so would jeopardize the mother's health. Theoretically, during this sensitive time, even aspirin could harm the fetus. So, strongly advise your patient to avoid *all* self-prescribed drugs during early pregnancy. The other time of special fetal sensitivity to drugs is the last trimester. The reason? At birth, when separated from his mother, the neonate must rely on his own metabolism to eliminate any remaining drug. Because his detoxifying systems are not fully developed, any residual drug may take a long time to be metabolized – and thus may induce prolonged toxic reactions. Consequently, drugs should be used only when absolutely necessary during the last 3 months of pregnancy.

Of course, in many circumstances, pregnant women must continue to take certain drugs. For example, a woman with a seizure disorder that is well controlled with an anticonvulsant should continue to take the drug even during pregnancy. Similarly, a pregnant woman with a bacterial infection must receive antibiotics. In such cases, the potential risk to the fetus is outweighed by the mother's need. The relative risk to the fetus is expressed by the drug's pregnancy risk category (see Chapter 1).

Following these general guidelines can prevent indiscriminate and potentially harmful use of drugs in pregnancy:

- Before a drug is prescribed for a woman of childbearing age, she should be asked the date of her last menstrual period and whether she may be pregnant. If a drug is a known teratogen (for example, isotretinoin), some manufacturers may recommend special precautions to ensure that the drug not be given to a female of childbearing age until pregnancy is ruled out.
- Especially during the first and the third trimesters, a pregnant patient should avoid *all* drugs except those *essential* to maintain the pregnancy or maternal health.
- Topical drugs are not exempt from the warning against indiscriminate use during pregnancy. Many topically applied drugs can be absorbed in large enough amounts to be harmful to the fetus.
- When a pregnant patient needs *any* drug, the doctor should prescribe the *safest* possible drug in the *lowest* possible dose to minimize any harmful effect to the fetus.
- Every pregnant patient should check with her doctor before taking *any* drug.

Drugs and lactation

Most drugs a mother takes appear in breast milk. Drug levels in breast milk tend to be high when blood levels are high – generally, shortly after taking each dose. Therefore, the mother should be advised to breast-feed *before* taking medication, not *after*.

Nevertheless, with very few exceptions, a mother who wishes to breast-feed may continue to do so with her doctor's permission. However, breast-feeding should be temporarily interrupted and replaced with bottle-feeding when the mother must take tetracyclines, chloramphenicol, sulfonamides (during first 2 weeks postpartum), oral anticoagulants, iodine-containing drugs, or antineoplastics.

To protect her infant, a breast-feeding mother should avoid taking drugs indiscriminately. If she needs to take a drug, she should first check with her doctor to be sure of taking the safest drug at the lowest dose.

What to teach patients about proper use of drugs

The following general guidelines will help to ensure that the patient gets maximal therapeutic benefits and avoids adverse reactions, accidental overdose, or potentially harmful changes in effectiveness:

- Store drugs in their original containers, at room temperature (unless directed otherwise), in places that are not accessible to children or exposed to sunlight. Avoid storage in the bathroom medicine cabinet or the glove compartment or trunk of an automobile, where extremes of temperature and humidity will cause them to deteriorate.
- Learn the trade name and generic name of any drug you are taking. Be sure to tell doctors, dentists, or other health care professionals you see regularly that you are taking it. Before taking any drug, be sure you have informed your doctor, nurse, or pharmacist about any unusual reactions you've had to drugs in the past and about your allergies to foods and other substances, any special medical problems, and any drugs you've taken over the last few weeks, including any OTC drugs.
- Always read the label before taking any drug, and take the drug exactly as prescribed at the recommended dosage and for the duration of treatment. Never share prescription drugs.
- When using a drug prescribed for occasional or prolonged use, check the container for an expiration date.
- To avoid potentially harmful changes in effectiveness, do not change brands of a drug without medical approval. Certain generic preparations are not precisely equivalent in effect to brand-name preparations of the same drug.
- Never mix different drugs in a single container, and don't remove any drug from its original container or remove the label. Relying on your memory to identify a drug and specific directions for its use is hazardous.
- Discard any drugs that are outdated or no longer needed.
- Before you have any surgery (including dental surgery), tell the doctor about all the drugs that you have been taking.
- Be sure to tell the doctor, nurse, or pharmacist about any side effects you've experienced while taking a drug.
- If you or someone else has taken an overdose, call your doctor, poison control center, or pharmacist immediately. Keep syrup of ipecac in your home to induce vomiting, but induce vomiting only if one of these professionals advises you to do so.
- Try to have all your prescriptions filled at the same pharmacy so that the pharmacist can identify and warn against potentially harmful drug interactions. Inform the pharmacist of any OTC drugs you're taking.

3

Drug therapy in children

A child's absorption, distribution, metabolism, and excretion processes undergo profound changes that affect drug dosage. To ensure optimal drug effect and minimal toxicity, consider these factors when administering drugs to a child.

Absorption

Drug absorption in children depends on the form of the drug; its physical properties; other drugs or substances, such as food, taken simultaneously; physiologic changes; and concurrent disease.

- The pH of neonatal gastric fluid is neutral or slightly acidic and becomes more acidic as the infant matures. This affects drug absorption. For example, nafcillin and penicillin G are better absorbed in an infant than in an adult because of low gastric acidity.
- Various infant formulas or milk products may increase gastric pH and impede absorption of acidic drugs. So, if possible, give a child oral medications on an empty stomach.
- Gastric emptying time and transit time through the small intestine – which is longer in children than in adults – can affect absorption. Also, intestinal hypermotility (as in diarrhea) can diminish the drug's absorption.
- A child's comparatively thin epidermis allows increased absorption of topical drugs.

Distribution

As with absorption, changes in body weight and physiology during childhood can significantly influence a drug's distribution and effects. In a premature infant, body fluid makes up about 85% of total body weight; in a full-term infant, 55% to 70%; and in an adult, 50% to 55%. Extracellular fluid (mostly blood) constitutes 40% of a neonate's body weight, compared with 20% in an adult. Intracellular fluid remains fairly constant throughout life and has little effect on drug dosage.

Extracellular fluid volume influences a water-soluble drug's concentration and effect because most drugs travel through extracellular fluid to reach their receptors. Children have a larger proportion of fluid to solid body weight, so their distribution area is proportionately greater.

Because the proportion of fat to lean body mass increases with age, the distribution of fat-soluble drugs is more limited in children than adults. As a result, a drug's lipid- or water-solubility affects the dosage for a child.

Binding to plasma proteins

As the result of a decrease in albumin concentration or intermolecular attraction between drug and plasma protein, many drugs are less bound to plasma proteins in infants than in adults.

Furthermore, preparations that bind plasma proteins may displace endogenous compounds, such as bilirubin or free fatty acids. Conversely, an endogenous compound may displace a weakly bound drug. For example, displacement of bound bilirubin can cause a rise in unbound bilirubin, which can lead to increased risk of kernicterus at normal bilirubin levels.

Since only an unbound, or free, drug has a pharmacologic effect, any alteration in ratio of a protein-bound to an unbound active drug can greatly influence its effect.

Several diseases and disorders,

such as nephrotic syndrome and malnutrition, can also decrease plasma protein and increase the concentration of an unbound drug, intensifying the drug's effect or producing toxicity.

Metabolism

A neonate's ability to metabolize a drug depends on the integrity of the hepatic enzyme system, the intrauterine exposure to the drug, and the nature of the drug itself.

Certain metabolic mechanisms are underdeveloped in neonates. Glucuronidation is a metabolic process that renders most drugs more water soluble, thereby facilitating renal excretion. This process is insufficiently developed to permit full pediatric doses until the infant is 1 month old. Because of this, the use of chloramphenicol in a neonate may cause gray syndrome, illustrating the infant's inability to metabolize the drug. Use of chloramphenicol in neonates, therefore, requires decreased dosage (25 mg/kg/day) and monitoring of blood levels.

Conversely, intrauterine exposure to drugs may induce precocious development of hepatic enzyme mechanisms, increasing the infant's capacity to metabolize potentially harmful substances.

Older children can metabolize some drugs (theophylline, for example) more rapidly than adults. This ability may come from their increased hepatic metabolic activity. Larger doses than those recommended for adults may be required.

Also, preparations given concurrently to a child may alter hepatic metabolism and induce production of hepatic enzymes. Phenobarbital, for example, can induce hepatic enzyme production and accelerate metabolism of drugs given concurrently.

Excretion

Renal excretion of a drug is the net effect of glomerular filtration, active tubular secretion, and passive tubular reabsorption. Because so many drugs are excreted in the urine, the degree of renal development or presence of renal disease can profoundly affect a child's dosage requirements.

If a child is unable to excrete a drug renally, drug accumulation and possible toxicity may result unless the dosage is reduced.

Physiologically, an infant's kidneys differ from an adult's in that they have:

- high resistance to blood flow and receive a smaller proportion of cardiac output
- incomplete glomerular and tubular development and short, incomplete loops of Henle (A child's glomerular filtration reaches adult values by ages 2½ to 5 months; his tubular secretion may reach adult values by ages 7 to 12 months.)
- low glomerular filtration rate (Penicillins are eliminated by this route.)
- decreased ability to concentrate urine or reabsorb various filtered compounds
- reduced ability of the proximal tubules to secrete organic acids.

Both children and adults have diurnal variations in urine pH that correlate with sleep-awake patterns.

Calculating and monitoring pediatric dosages

When calculating pediatric dosages, don't use formulas that modify adult dosages: a child is not a scaled-down version of an adult. Pediatric dosages should be calculated on the basis of either body weight (mg/kg) or body surface area (mg/m^2).

- Reevaluate dosages at regular intervals to ensure necessary adjustments as the child develops.
- Although body surface area provides a useful standard for adults and

older children, don't use it in premature or full-term infants. Use the body weight method instead.

- Don't exceed the maximum adult dosage when calculating amounts per kilogram of body weight (except with certain drugs, such as theophylline, if indicated).
- Obtain an accurate maternal drug history – prescription and nonprescription drugs, vitamins, and herbs or other health foods taken during pregnancy.
- Drugs passed through breast milk can also have adverse effects on the breast-feeding infant. Before a drug is prescribed for a breast-feeding mother, the potential effects on the infant should be investigated. For example, sulfonamides given to a breast-feeding mother for a urinary tract infection appear in breast milk and may cause kernicterus at lower-than-normal levels of unconjugated bilirubin. Also, high concentrations of isoniazid appear in breast milk. Since this drug is metabolized by the liver, an infant's immature hepatic enzyme mechanisms cannot metabolize the drug, and the infant may suffer CNS toxicity.

Oral medications

- *When giving oral medication to an infant,* administer it in liquid form if possible. For accuracy, measure and give the preparation by syringe; never use a vial or cup.
- Lift the patient's head to prevent aspiration of the medication, and press down on his chin to prevent choking.
- You may also place the drug in a nipple and allow the infant to suck the contents.
- *If the patient is a toddler,* explain how you're going to give him the medication. If possible, have the parents enlist the child's cooperation.
- Don't mix medication with food or call it "candy" even if it has a pleasant taste.
- Let the child drink liquid medication from a calibrated medication cup rather than from a spoon: it's easier and more accurate. If the preparation is available only in tablet form, crush it and mix it with a compatible syrup. (Check with the pharmacist to verify that the tablet can be crushed without compromising its effectiveness.)
- *If the patient is an older child* who can swallow a tablet or capsule by himself, have him place the medication on the back of his tongue and swallow it with water or fruit juice. Remember, milk or milk products may interfere with drug absorption.

I.V. infusions

When administering I.V. infusions to children, note the following special considerations.

Protecting the insertion site

In infants, use a peripheral vein or a scalp vein in the temporal region for I.V. infusions. The scalp vein is safest in that the needle is not likely to be dislodged; however, the head must be shaved around the site. Temporary disfigurement may also result from the needle and infiltrated fluids. For these reasons, the scalp veins are not used as frequently today as they were in the past.

The extremities are the most accessible insertion sites; however, since patients tend to move about, take these precautions:

- Protect the insertion site to prevent catheter or needle dislodgment.
- Use a padded arm board to minimize dislodgment. Remove the arm board during range-of-motion exercises.
- Place the clamp out of the child's reach; if extension tubing is used to allow the child greater mobility, securely tape the connection.
- Restrain the child only when necessary.
- To allay anxiety, give a simple ex-

planation to the child who must be restrained while asleep.

Maintaining flow rate and fluid balance
While administering a continuous I.V. infusion to a child, monitor flow rate and check the patient's condition and insertion site at least hourly – more frequently when giving a drug intermittently.

Adjust the flow rate only while the patient is composed; crying and emotional upset can constrict blood vessels. Flow rate may vary if a pump isn't used. Flow should be adequate because some drugs (calcium, for example) can be very irritating at low flow rates.

Making dilutions
Some drugs are hyperosmolar; in infants, these drugs must be diluted to prevent radical changes in fluid that might induce CNS hemorrhage. Sodium bicarbonate, for example, must be diluted to half-strength to lower osmolality and lessen the risk of CNS bleeding.

In general, however, use the minimum amount of compatible fluid over the shortest recommended time. Remember also to check the total daily fluid intake and the amount allotted to medication.

I.M. injections
I.M. injections are preferred when the drug cannot be given by other parenteral routes and rapid absorption is necessary.

- In children under age 2, the vastus lateralis muscle is the preferred injection site; in older children, either the ventrogluteal area or the gluteus medius muscle can be used.
- To determine correct needle size, consider the patient's age, muscle mass, and nutritional status and the drug's viscosity; record and rotate injection sites.
- Explain to the patient that the injection will hurt, but that the medication will help him. Restrain him during the injection, if needed, and comfort him afterward.

Topical medications and inhalants
- Use ear drops warmed to room temperature; cold drops can cause considerable pain and possibly vertigo.
- To administer drops, turn the patient on his side, with the affected ear up. If he is under age 3, pull the pinna down and back; if he is over age 3, pull the pinna up and back.
- Avoid using inhalants in very young children: obtaining their cooperation is difficult.
- Before attempting to administer medication through a metered-dose nebulizer to an older child, explain the inhaler to him. Then have him hold the nebulizer upside down and close his lips around the mouthpiece. Have him exhale; pinch his nostrils shut; and when he starts to inhale, release one dose of medication into his mouth. Tell the patient to continue inhaling until his lungs feel full.
- Most inhaled agents are not useful if taken orally; therefore, if you doubt the patient's ability to use the inhalant correctly, don't use it.
- Use topical corticosteroids with caution because chronic steroid use in children has been associated with delayed growth. When topical corticosteroids are used on the diaper area of infants, avoid covering this area with plastic or rubber pants, which will act as an occlusive dressing and enhance systemic absorption.

Parenteral nutrition
I.V. nutrition is given to patients who can't or won't take adequate food orally and patients with hypermetabolic conditions who need supplementation. The latter group includes premature infants and children who have burns or other major trauma, intracta-

ble diarrhea, malabsorption syndromes, GI abnormalities, emotional disorders (such as anorexia nervosa), and congenital abnormalities.

Before fat emulsions are administered to infants and children, however, potential benefits must be weighed against possible risks.

Fats – supplied as 10% or 20% emulsions – are administered both peripherally and centrally. Their use is limited by the child's ability to metabolize them. An infant or a child with a diseased liver cannot efficiently metabolize fats, for example.

Some fats, however, must be supplied both to prevent essential fatty acid deficiency and to permit normal growth and development. A minimum of calories (2% to 4%) must be supplied as linoleic acid – an essential fatty acid found in lipids. In infants, fats are essential for normal neurologic development.

Nevertheless, fat solutions may decrease oxygen perfusion and may adversely affect children with pulmonary disease. This risk can be minimized by supplying only the minimum fat needed for essential fatty acid requirements and not the usual intake of 40% to 50% of the child's total calories.

Fatty acids can also displace bilirubin bound to serum albumin, causing a rise in free, unconjugated bilirubin and an increased risk of kernicterus. However, fat solutions may interfere with some bilirubin assays and cause falsely elevated levels. To avoid this complication, a blood sample should be drawn 4 hours after infusion of the lipid emulsion; or if the emulsion is introduced over 24 hours, the blood sample should be centrifuged before the assay is performed.

4

Drug therapy in elderly patients

If you're providing drug therapy for elderly patients, you'll want to understand physiologic and pharmacokinetic changes that may alter appropriate drug dosage or cause common adverse reactions or compliance problems in elderly patients.

Physiologic changes affecting drug action

As a person ages, gradual physiologic changes occur. Some of these age-related changes may alter the therapeutic and toxic effects of medications.

Body composition

Proportions of fat, lean tissue, and water in the body change with age. Total body mass and lean body mass tend to decrease; the proportion of body fat tends to increase.

Varying from person to person, these changes in body composition affect the relationship between a drug's concentration and distribution in the body.

For example, a water-soluble drug, such as gentamicin, is not distributed to fat. Since there's relatively less lean tissue in an elderly person, more drug remains in the blood.

GI function

In elderly patients, decreases in gastric acid secretion and GI motility slow the emptying of stomach contents and the movement of intestinal contents through the entire tract. Furthermore, research suggests that elderly patients may have more difficulty absorbing medications. This is a particularly significant problem with drugs having a narrow therapeutic range, such as digoxin, in which any change in absorption can be crucial.

Hepatic function

The liver's ability to metabolize certain drugs decreases with age. This is caused by diminished blood flow to the liver, which results from the age-related decrease in cardiac output and from the diminished activity of certain liver enzymes. When an elderly patient takes certain sleep medications, such as secobarbital, the liver's reduced ability to metabolize the drug may produce a hangover effect the next morning.

Decreased hepatic function may cause:

- more intense drug effects due to higher blood levels
- longer-lasting drug effects due to prolonged blood concentrations
- greater incidence of drug toxicity.

Renal function

Although an elderly person's renal function is usually sufficient to eliminate excess body fluid and waste, the ability to eliminate some medications may be reduced by 50% or more.

Many medications commonly used by elderly patients, such as digoxin, are excreted primarily through the kidneys. If the kidneys' ability to excrete the drug is decreased, high blood concentrations may result. Digoxin toxicity, therefore, is relatively common in elderly patients who are not receiving a reduced digoxin dosage that accommodates decreased renal function.

Drug dosages can be modified to compensate for age-related decreases in renal function. Aided by laboratory tests, such as blood urea nitrogen and serum creatinine, doctors may adjust medication dosages so the patient receives the expected therapeutic benefits without the risk of toxicity. Observe your patient for signs of toxicity. A patient taking digoxin, for example, may experience anorexia, nausea, vomiting, or confusion.

Adverse drug reactions

As compared with younger people, elderly patients experience twice as many adverse drug reactions relating to greater drug consumption, poor compliance, and physiologic changes.

Signs and symptoms of adverse drug reactions – confusion, weakness, and lethargy – are often mistakenly attributed to senility or disease. If the adverse reaction isn't identified, the patient may continue to receive the drug. Furthermore, he may receive unnecessary additional medication to treat complications caused by the original medication. This can sometimes result in a pattern of inappropriate and excessive medication use.

Although any medication can cause adverse reactions, most of the serious reactions in the elderly are caused by relatively few medications. Be particularly alert for toxicities resulting from diuretics, antihypertensives, digoxin, corticosteroids, sleeping aids, and nonprescription drugs.

Diuretic toxicity

Because total body water content decreases with age, normal dosages of potassium-wasting diuretics, such as hydrochlorothiazide and furosemide, may result in fluid loss and even dehydration in an elderly patient.

These diuretics may deplete serum potassium, causing weakness in the patient; and they may raise blood uric acid and glucose levels, complicating preexisting gout and diabetes mellitus.

Antihypertensive toxicity

Many elderly people experience lightheadedness or fainting when using antihypertensive medications, partly in response to atherosclerosis and decreased elasticity of the blood vessels. Antihypertensive drugs lower blood pressure too rapidly, resulting in insufficient blood flow to the brain. This may cause dizziness, fainting, or even stroke.

Consequently, dosages of antihypertensive drugs must be carefully individualized. In elderly patients, too aggressive treatment of high blood pressure may do more harm than good, so treatment goals should be reasonable. Although bringing blood pressure down to 120/85 mm Hg may be appropriate in a young hypertensive patient, a more reasonable goal for an elderly hypertensive patient might be 150/95 mm Hg.

Digoxin toxicity

As the body's renal function and rate of excretion decline, digoxin concentrations in the blood may build to toxic levels, causing nausea, vomiting, diarrhea, and – most serious – cardiac arrhythmias. Try to prevent severe toxicity by observing your patient for early signs, such as appetite loss, confusion, or depression.

Corticosteroid toxicity

Elderly patients on corticosteroids may experience short-term effects, including fluid retention and psychological manifestations ranging from mild euphoria to acute psychotic reactions. Long-term toxic effects, such as osteoporosis, can be especially severe in elderly patients who have been taking prednisone or related steroidal compounds for months or even years. To prevent serious toxicity, carefully monitor patients on long-term regimens. Observe them for subtle changes in appearance, mood, and mobility, as well as for signs of impaired healing and fluid and electrolyte disturbances.

Sleeping aid toxicity

Sedatives or sleeping aids, such as

flurazepam, may cause excessive sedation or residual drowsiness. Keep in mind that ingestion of alcohol may exaggerate such depressant effects, even if the sleeping aid was taken the previous evening.

Nonprescription drug toxicity
When aspirin and aspirin-containing analgesics are used in moderation, toxicity is minimal, but prolonged ingestion may cause GI irritation and gradual blood loss resulting in severe anemia. Although anemia from chronic aspirin consumption can affect all age groups, elderly patients may be less able to compensate because of their already reduced iron stores.

Laxatives may cause diarrhea in elderly patients who are extremely sensitive to drugs such as bisacodyl. Chronic oral use of mineral oil as a lubricating laxative may result in lipid pneumonia from aspiration of small residual oil droplets in the patient's mouth.

Patient noncompliance
Poor compliance can be a problem with patients of any age. However, in elderly patients, specific factors linked to aging – such as diminished visual acuity, hearing loss, forgetfulness, the common need for multiple drug therapy, and various socioeconomic factors – can combine to make compliance a special problem. Approximately one-third of elderly patients fail to comply with their prescribed drug therapy. They may fail to take prescribed doses or to follow the correct schedule; they may take medications prescribed for previous disorders, discontinue medications prematurely, or use p.r.n. medications indiscriminately.

Review your patient's medication regimen with him. Be sure he understands the medication amount and the time and frequency of doses. Also, explain how he should take each medication – that is, with food or water or by itself.

Give your patient whatever help you can to avoid drug therapy problems, and refer him to the doctor or pharmacist if he needs further information.

5

Drug therapy and the nursing process

The nursing process guides nursing decisions about drug administration to ensure the patient's safety and meet medical and legal standards. This five-step process provides thorough assessment, appropriate nursing diagnosis, effective planning, correct interventions, and constant evaluation.

First step: Assessment

During assessment, the nurse focuses on direct data collection by:

- obtaining a drug history from the patient, parent, spouse, or significant other
- reviewing the patient's medical history
- performing a physical examination
- obtaining and interpreting relevant laboratory or diagnostic test results.

Drug history

Data collection begins at admission to the hospital or in an outpatient setting with specific questions about the patient's background, including allergies, medical history, habits, socioeconomic status, lifestyle and beliefs, and sensory deficits. These aspects of the patient's background can significantly influence drug therapy.

Allergies

The patient's allergy profile includes reactions to both drugs and food. Information about allergic reactions must specify the drug; a description of the reaction; its situation, time, and setting; and any contributing factors. Examples of contributing factors include concurrent use of stimulants, tobacco, alcohol, or illegal drugs, or a significant change in nutritional patterns. Asking the patient to describe his allergic reaction is especially important to help determine whether the patient reacts adversely or simply dislikes taking the drug.

Allergies to foods can also affect drug therapy. For example, allergies to shellfish can contraindicate use of drugs that contain iodine or are byproducts of shellfish. Allergies to eggs are significant in patients who are to receive vaccines, which are commonly derived from chick embryos.

Prescription drugs

The patient's drug history should explore the following:

- the reason for using the drug
- the patient's knowledge of the appropriate dosage
- the patient's knowledge about determining effectiveness of the drug (if appropriate), potential adverse effects, what to do about adverse effects, and when to contact the doctor
- route of administration
- the pattern of administration at home
- use of OTC drugs
- cognitive status.

Note any special monitoring the patient must perform, such as blood glucose monitoring before insulin administration or checking radial pulse rate before taking digoxin. Make sure the patient is performing such procedures correctly and that the results are within acceptable limits.

Discuss the effects of drug therapy with the patient and determine if new symptoms or unpredicted adverse reactions have developed. Noting the patient's pattern of administration may provide insight into why a particular drug regimen succeeds or fails.

OTC drugs

A comprehensive drug history should

also list any OTC drugs the patient is taking. Many OTC drugs can inhibit or potentiate the effects of a prescribed drug. For example, aspirin potentiates the anticoagulant effects of warfarin.

OTC drugs include a wide range of products from common aspirin and nutritional supplements to various sprays and cleansing agents. The patient may not think of these as drugs, so the nurse may have to name types of products to get an accurate response.

Dosage and frequency of use are just as important as the type of OTC product. One aspirin tablet taken once a day may have no effect on concomitant drug therapy; however, a higher dosage (such as that used for arthritis) could profoundly influence therapy.

Medical history

In gathering the medical history, note any chronic diseases or disorders the patient may have and record the following information for each:

- date of diagnosis
- initial prescribed treatment
- current treatment
- the doctor in charge.

Careful attention to this part of the medical history can uncover one of the most important problems with drug therapy – conflicting and incompatible drug regimens. The patient who does not have a family physician to oversee and coordinate all care may seek the care of several specialists who may prescribe drug treatment without knowing what other drugs the patient is taking. A carefully detailed medical history can uncover such problems. The nurse who identifies such conflicting or overlapping drug therapy must call them to the appropriate doctor's attention and then teach the patient about the importance of informing caregivers about all drugs he is taking.

Habits

Carefully consider dietary habits and the nontherapeutic use of drugs.

Certain foods can directly affect the effectiveness of many drugs. For example, a person who is taking the anticoagulant warfarin should not increase his intake of green leafy vegetables because they contain levels of vitamin K that can antagonize the drug's anticoagulant effect.

Nontherapeutic use of drugs can profoundly affect a patient's health and impair the effectiveness of drug therapy. Consider the possible use of alcohol, tobacco, caffeine, and illegal drugs, such as marijuana, cocaine, and heroin. For example, if the patient uses alcohol, note the frequency of use, the amount, and the type of alcohol consumed. Carefully document the intake of stimulants, such as caffeine, because they significantly affect a patient's cardiovascular status and nervous system. Record the type of stimulant, the frequency of intake, and the amount consumed.

For the patient who smokes, document the following information:

- the number of years the patient has smoked
- the kind of tobacco the patient smokes (cigarettes, cigar, or pipe) or chews
- how many cigarettes or cigars the patient smokes per day, or how much and how long he chews tobacco daily
- the brand of tobacco the patient smokes or chews.

Defining the patient's use of illegal drugs may be difficult. However, the nurse who suspects such use should encourage the patient to discuss it honestly, emphasizing that these drugs have profound effects that may cause serious drug interactions. If the patient admits using illegal drugs, document the drug, the amount and frequency of use, and the route of administration.

Socioeconomic status

Note the patient's age, educational level, occupation, and insurance coverage. These factors may be significant to compliance and to an effective plan of care. The patient's age, for example, can determine whom to include in the care (parents or other family members) and the level of information that is appropriate for teaching the patient.

Knowing the patient's educational background and occupation helps you select interventions at an appropriate level, plan a drug regimen that fits the patient's daily routine, and encourage compliance. Knowing the patient's insurance status may help you anticipate the need for financial assistance and counseling. Remember that noncompliance commonly results from inability to afford medications.

Lifestyle and beliefs

Support systems, marital status, childbearing status, attitudes toward health and health care, use of the health care system, and daily patterns of activities all affect the plan of care and patient compliance. For example, an 18-year-old single parent who is a high-school dropout on medical assistance and has no family support will probably require more teaching and support to gain a commitment and compliance than a 40-year-old affluent professional who has family support, can understand why she needs the drug, and can readily pay for it.

Sensory deficits

Any sensory deficit can significantly shape an appropriate plan of care. For example, impaired vision, paralysis of one or more extremities, loss of a limb, or loss of sensation in an extremity can impair the patient's ability to administer a subcutaneous injection, break a scored tablet, or open a medication container. Color blindness may cause difficulty in distinguishing between two medications. Hearing impairment can complicate effective patient instruction. Any sensory deficit requires careful consideration in any plan of prescribed drug therapy.

Clinical status

Two other factors can profoundly influence drug therapy: the patient's cognitive status and the systemic effects of the prescribed drugs. A patient's intact cognitive abilities ensure that he can understand and implement the actions necessary for compliance. During the interview, note if the patient is alert and oriented, if he is able to interact appropriately with people, and if his conversation is appropriate. Consider whether the patient can think clearly and express his thoughts coherently. Finally, check both short-term and long-term memory because the patient needs both to follow a specified drug regimen. If such evaluation identifies a cognitive deficit, determine the probable cause, which can range from a transient drug-related effect to permanent neurologic impairment, and then determine whether or not the patient can carry out the prescribed drug regimen. If not, the nurse must find another way to ensure that the patient receives the prescribed therapy.

After completing the drug history, perform a physical examination to assess those body systems that may be affected by a particular drug the patient is taking or that may be prescribed. Every drug has a desired effect on a body system, but it may have an undesired effect on another. For example, chemotherapeutic agents destroy cancerous cells, but they also affect normal cells and typically cause the patient to experience hair loss, diarrhea, or nausea. Therefore, examine the patient for expected drug effects; also closely monitor the patient for potentially harmful adverse effects.

Second step: Formulating a nursing diagnosis
Using information gathered during assessment, define any potential or actual drug-related problems by formulating each in a relevant nursing diagnosis. The most common problem statements related to drug therapy are *Knowledge deficit, Noncompliance,* and *Altered Health Maintenance*.

Third step: Planning
Nursing diagnoses provide the framework for planning interventions and outcome criteria (patient goals).

Outcome criteria
Outcome criteria state the desired patient behaviors or responses that should result from nursing care. Such criteria should be measurable and objective, concise, realistic for the patient, and attainable by nursing management; they should express patient behavior in terms of expectations and specify a time frame. A typical outcome statement is "Before discharge, the patient verbalizes major adverse effects related to his chemotherapy."

Fourth step: Intervention
After developing the outcome criteria, the nurse determines the interventions needed to help the patient reach the desired behavior or goals. Drug-related interventions may focus on patient teaching for a drug's action, adverse effects, scheduling, steps to avoid or treat a drug reaction, or drug administration techniques.

Appropriate interventions related to drug therapy will also include administration procedures and techniques, legal and ethical concerns, patient teaching, and any concerns related to special groups of patients (geriatric, pediatric, pregnant, or breast-feeding patients). Such interventions may be independent nursing actions, such as turning a bedridden patient every 2 hours, or may be nursing actions that require a doctor's order.

Fifth step: Evaluation
The final component of the nursing process, evaluation, is a formal and systematic process for determining the effectiveness of nursing care. This process enables the nurse to determine whether outcome criteria were met and thereby make informed decisions about subsequent interventions. For example, if the patient experienced relief of headache within 1 hour after the nurse administered a p.r.n. analgesic, the outcome criterion was met. If the headache was the same or worse, the outcome criterion was not met and requires a new assessment, which may result in a new plan of care or may yield new data that invalidate the nursing diagnosis or suggest new nursing interventions that are more specific or more acceptable to the patient. This assessment could lead to a higher dosage, a different analgesic, or a reevaluation of the cause.

Evaluation enables the nurse to design and implement a revised plan of care, to continuously reevaluate outcome criteria, and to plan again until each nursing diagnosis is successfully completed.

Amebicides and antiprotozoals

chloroquine hydrochloride
(See Chapter 9, ANTIMALARIALS.)
chloroquine phosphate
(See Chapter 9, ANTIMALARIALS.)
eflornithine hydrochloride
iodoquinol
metronidazole
metronidazole hydrochloride
paromomycin sulfate
pentamidine isethionate

COMBINATION PRODUCTS
None.

eflornithine hydrochloride (DFMO)
Ornidyl
Pregnancy Risk Category: C

HOW SUPPLIED
Injection (concentrate): 200 mg/ml

ACTION
Mechanism: Specifically and irreversibly inhibits the enzyme ornithine decarboxylase and limits the availability of substrate for certain amines necessary for cell differentiation and division.
Peak: Serum levels peak immediately following I.V. infusion. **Duration:** elimination half-life, 3 to 4 hours.

INDICATIONS & DOSAGE
Meningoencephalitic stage of Trypanosoma brucei gambiense *(sleeping sickness)* –
Adults: 100 mg/kg by I.V. infusion q 6 hours for 14 days.

ADVERSE REACTIONS
CNS: ***seizures, hearing impairment,*** *dizziness, headache, asthenia.*
GI: diarrhea, vomiting, abdominal pain, anorexia.
Hematologic: ***anemia, leukopenia, thrombocytopenia, myelosuppression,*** eosinophilia.
Other: facial edema, alopecia.

INTERACTIONS
None significant.

CONTRAINDICATIONS
- Contraindicated in patients with hypersensitivity to the drug.
- Use cautiously in patients with impaired renal function because most (about 80%) of the drug is excreted unchanged in the urine.
- Impose antiseizure precautions because seizures occurred in about 8% of patients receiving the drug during clinical trials.

NURSING CONSIDERATIONS
- Myelosuppression is a common and serious adverse reaction that is reversible when therapy is discontinued. Close patient monitoring is essential. Perform CBC and platelet counts before initiation of therapy, twice weekly during therapy, and weekly after the drug is discontinued until hematologic parameters return to pretreatment levels.
- Some patients have experienced hearing impairment. Obtain serial audiograms when feasible.
- The patient should be monitored for at least 24 months after treatment.
- **I.V. use:** The infusion concentrate is hypertonic and must be diluted before administration. Dilute with sterile water for injection and follow strict aseptic technique. To prepare infusion, dilute one part drug to four parts sterile water for injection by adding 25 ml (5,000 mg or 5 g) of the concentrate to each of four bags containing 100 ml of sterile water. After dilu-

tion, the final concentration of each bag will be 5,000 mg/125 ml or 40 mg/ml. Use within 24 hours.
- Administer infusion over 45 minutes. Do not administer other drugs with the infusion.
- To minimize the risk of microbial growth, store diluted drug in refrigerator (39° F [4° C]).
- The undiluted concentrate may be stored at room temperature (below 86° F [30° C]), but protect from light and freezing.

iodoquinol (diiodohydroxyquin)

Diodoquin†, Diquinol, Yodoxin

Pregnancy Risk Category: C

HOW SUPPLIED
Tablets: 210 mg, 650 mg

ACTION
Mechanism: An iodine derivative with amebicidal activity in the intestinal lumen; precise mechanism of action is unknown.
Peak: Although most of an oral dose remains in the GI tract, some iodine is absorbed.

INDICATIONS & DOSAGE
Intestinal amebiasis–
Adults: 630 to 650 mg P.O. t.i.d. after meals for 20 days. Total daily dosage should not exceed 2 g.
Children: usual dosage is 30 to 40 mg/kg of body weight daily in two to three divided doses for 20 days.

Additional doses should not be repeated before a resting interval of 2 to 3 weeks.

ADVERSE REACTIONS
CNS: neurotoxicity (dose-related), dysesthesia, weakness, vertigo, malaise, headache, agitation, retrograde amnesia, ataxia, *peripheral neuropathy.*
EENT: *optic neuritis,* optic atrophy, loss of vision.
GI: anorexia, nausea, vomiting, abdominal cramps, diarrhea, increased motility, constipation, epigastric burning and pain, gastritis, anal irritation and itching.
Hematologic: ***agranulocytosis.***
Skin: pruritus, hives, papular and pustular eruptions, urticaria, discoloration of hair and nails.
Other: thyroid enlargement, fever, chills, generalized furunculosis, alopecia.

INTERACTIONS
None significant.

CONTRAINDICATIONS
- Contraindicated in patients with hypersensitivity to 8-hydroxyquinoline derivatives or iodine-containing preparations. Iodoquinol causes liver damage in such patients. Also contraindicated in patients with hepatic or renal disease or preexisting optic neuropathy.

NURSING CONSIDERATIONS
- Patient should have periodic ophthalmic examinations during treatment.
- If the patient has difficulty swallowing, crush tablets and mix with applesauce or chocolate syrup.
- Record fluid intake and output, and color and amount of stool. Send warm specimens to laboratory for analysis.
- Watch for diarrhea during the first 2 or 3 days; notify the doctor if diarrhea continues.
- Advise the patient not to discontinue the drug prematurely. Tell him to notify the doctor if skin rash occurs.
- Iodoquinol may interfere with thyroid function tests for up to 6 months after drug discontinuation.
- To help prevent reinfestation, teach the patient about the need for personal hygiene, especially hand-washing

technique. The patient should not prepare food for others until stools are negative.

metronidazole

Apo-Metronidazole†, Flagyl, Metric-21, Metrogyl‡, Metrozine‡, Neo-Metric†, Novonidazol†, PMS Metronidazole†, Protostat, Trikoside†

metronidazole hydrochloride

Flagyl I.V. RTU, Metro I.V., Novonidazol†

Pregnancy Risk Category: B

HOW SUPPLIED
Tablets: 200 mg‡, 250 mg, 400 mg‡, 500 mg
Oral suspension (benzoyl metronidazole): 200 mg/5 ml‡
Injection: 500 mg/100 ml ready to use
Powder for injection: 500-mg single-dose vials

ACTION
Mechanism: A direct-acting trichomonacide and amebicide that works at both intestinal and extraintestinal sites.
Peak: Peak plasma levels occur immediately after I.V. infusion, within 1 to 3 hours of oral administration.
Duration: elimination half-life, 6 to 8 hours.

INDICATIONS & DOSAGE
Amebic hepatic abscess –
Adults: 500 to 750 mg P.O. t.i.d. for 5 to 10 days.
Children: 35 to 50 mg/kg daily (in three doses) for 10 days.
Intestinal amebiasis –
Adults: 750 mg P.O. t.i.d. for 5 to 10 days.
Children: 35 to 50 mg/kg daily (in three doses) for 10 days. Follow this therapy with oral iodoquinol.
Trichomoniasis –
Adults: 250 mg P.O. t.i.d. for 7 days or 2 g P.O. in single dose; 4 to 6 weeks should elapse between courses of therapy.
Refractory trichomoniasis –
Adults: 250 mg P.O. b.i.d. for 10 days.
Bacterial infections caused by anaerobic microorganisms –
Adults: loading dose is 15 mg/kg I.V. infused over 1 hour (approximately 1 g for a 70-kg adult). Maintenance dose is 7.5 mg/kg I.V. or P.O. q 6 hours (approximately 500 mg for a 70-kg adult). The first maintenance dose should be administered 6 hours after the loading dose. Maximum dosage not to exceed 4 g daily.
Giardiasis –
Adults: 250 mg P.O. t.i.d. for 5 days.
Children: 5 mg/kg P.O. t.i.d. for 5 days.
Prevention of postoperative infection in contaminated or potentially contaminated colorectal surgery –
Adults: 15 mg/kg infused over 30 to 60 minutes and completed approximately 1 hour before surgery. Then, 7.5 mg/kg infused over 30 to 60 minutes at 6 and 12 hours after the initial dose.

ADVERSE REACTIONS
CNS: vertigo, headache, ataxia, incoordination, confusion, irritability, depression, restlessness, weakness, fatigue, drowsiness, insomnia, sensory neuropathy, paresthesia of extremities, psychic stimulation, ***seizures,*** neuropathy.
CV: ECG change (flattened T wave), edema (with I.V. RTU preparation).
GI: abdominal cramping, stomatitis, *nausea, vomiting, anorexia,* diarrhea, constipation, proctitis, dry mouth.
GU: darkened urine, polyuria, dysuria, pyuria, incontinence, cystitis, decreased libido, dyspareunia, dryness of vagina and vulva, sense of pelvic pressure.

Hematologic: transient leukopenia, neutropenia.
Skin: pruritus, flushing, rash.
Other: overgrowth of nonsusceptible organisms, especially *Candida* (glossitis, furry tongue), metallic taste, fever, gynecomastia, thrombophlebitis after I.V. infusion.

INTERACTIONS
Cimetidine: increased risk of metronidazole toxicity because of inhibited hepatic metabolism. Monitor closely.
Disulfiram: acute psychoses and confusional states. Don't use together.
Ethanol: disulfiram-like reaction (nausea, vomiting, headache, cramps, flushing). Don't use together.
Oral anticoagulants: increased anticoagulant effects. Monitor closely.
Phenytoin, phenobarbital: decreased metronidazole effectiveness because of increased hepatic clearance. Monitor closely.

CONTRAINDICATIONS
- *Warning:* This drug has been shown to be carcinogenic in mice and possibly rats. Unnecessary use should be avoided.
- Use cautiously in patients with a history of blood dyscrasia or CNS disorder and in patients with retinal or visual field changes. Also use cautiously in patients with hepatic disease or alcoholism and in conjunction with known hepatotoxic drugs.

NURSING CONSIDERATIONS
- If indicated during pregnancy for trichomoniasis, the 7-day regimen is preferred over the 2-g single-dose regimen.
- Tell the patient to avoid alcohol or alcohol-containing medications during therapy and for at least 48 hours after therapy is completed.
- Tell the patient metallic taste and dark or red-brown urine may occur.
- Record number and character of stools when used in the treatment of amebiasis. Metronidazole should be used only after *Trichomonas vaginalis* has been confirmed by wet smear or culture or *Entamoeba histolytica* has been identified. Asymptomatic sexual partners of patients being treated for *T. vaginalis* infection should be treated simultaneously to avoid reinfection. Instruct the patient in proper hygiene.
- Give oral form with meals to minimize GI distress.
- **I.V. use:** No preparation is necessary for RTU (ready to use). To prepare lyophilized vials of metronidazole, add 4.4 ml of sterile water for injection, bacteriostatic water for injection, sterile 0.9% sodium chloride injection, or bacteriostatic 0.9% sodium chloride injection. The reconstituted drug contains 100 mg/ml. Add the contents of the vial to 100 ml of D_5W, lactated Ringer's injection, or 0.9% sodium chloride for a final concentration of 5 mg/ml. The resulting highly acidic solution must be neutralized before administering. Carefully add 5 mEq sodium bicarbonate for each 500 mg metronidazole; carbon dioxide gas will form that may need to be vented.
- Infuse drug over at least 1 hour. Don't give I.V. push.
- Don't refrigerate the neutralized diluted solution. Precipitation may occur. If Flagyl I.V. RTU is refrigerated, crystals may form. These will disappear after the solution is gently warmed to room temperature.
- Flagyl I.V. RTU may cause sodium retention. Observe carefully for edema, especially in patients also receiving corticosteroids.

paromomycin sulfate
Humatin
Pregnancy Risk Category: C

HOW SUPPLIED
Capsules: 250 mg

ACTION

Mechanism: Acts as an intestinal amebicide. Its specific mechanism of action is unknown.
Peak: Very little drug is absorbed; most remains within the GI tract.
Duration: appears in feces in about 8 hours.

INDICATIONS & DOSAGE

Intestinal amebiasis, acute and chronic –
Adults and children: 25 to 35 mg/kg daily P.O. in three doses for 5 to 10 days after meals.
Tapeworms (fish, beef, pork, dog) –
Adults: 1 g P.O. q 15 minutes for four doses.
Children: 11 mg/kg P.O. q 15 minutes for four doses.

ADVERSE REACTIONS

CNS: headache, vertigo.
EENT: ototoxicity.
GI: anorexia, *nausea, vomiting, epigastric pain and burning, abdominal cramps,* diarrhea, constipation, increased motility, steatorrhea, pruritus ani, malabsorption syndrome.
GU: hematuria, nephrotoxicity.
Hematologic: eosinophilia.
Skin: rash, exanthema, pruritus.
Other: overgrowth of nonsusceptible organisms.

INTERACTIONS

None significant.

CONTRAINDICATIONS

- Contraindicated in patients with impaired renal function or intestinal obstruction.
- Use cautiously in patients with ulcerative lesions of the bowel to avoid inadvertent absorption and resulting renal toxicity. Poorly absorbed orally, but will accumulate in patients with renal impairment or ulcerative lesions.

NURSING CONSIDERATIONS

- Ask about history of sensitivity to drug before giving first dose.
- Administer with or after meals.
- To help prevent reinfestation, teach patient about the need for personal hygiene, especially hand-washing technique. Patient should refrain from preparing food for others until stools are negative.
- Criterion of cure is absence of amebae in stools examined weekly for 6 weeks after treatment and thereafter at monthly intervals for 2 years. Examine feces of family members or suspected contacts.
- Avoid high doses or prolonged therapy.
- Watch for signs of superinfection (continued fever and other signs of new infections, especially monilial infections).

pentamidine isethionate

NebuPent, Pentacarinat†‡, Pentam 300, Pneumopent

Pregnancy Risk Category: C

HOW SUPPLIED

Injection: 300-mg vial
Aerosol: 300-mg vial

ACTION

Mechanism: Interferes with biosynthesis of DNA, RNA, phospholipids, and proteins in susceptible organisms.
Peak: Peak serum levels occur 1 hour after I.M. injection, immediately after I.V. infusion. Little drug is absorbed after inhalation. **Duration:** extensively tissue bound; drug appears in urine for 6 to 8 weeks after therapy.

INDICATIONS & DOSAGE

Pneumocystis carinii *pneumonia –*
Adults and children: 4 mg/kg I.V. or I.M. once daily for 14 days.
Prevention of Pneumocystis carinii *pneumonia in high-risk individuals –*
Adults: 300 mg by inhalation (using a

Respirgard II nebulizer) once every 4 weeks.

ADVERSE REACTIONS

CNS: confusion, hallucinations.
CV: ***hypotension,*** tachycardia.
GI: nausea, anorexia, metallic taste.
GU: *elevated serum creatinine,* renal toxicity.
Hematologic: *leukopenia,* thrombocytopenia, anemia.
Hepatic: elevated liver enzymes.
Skin: rash, facial flushing, pruritus.
Other: fever, ***hypoglycemia,*** hyperglycemia, hypocalcemia, *sterile abscess, pain or induration at injection site.*

INTERACTIONS

Aminoglycosides, amphotericin B, cisplatin, vancomycin, zidovudine: increased risk of nephrotoxicity.

CONTRAINDICATIONS

• Use cautiously in patients with hypertension, hypotension, hypoglycemia, hypocalcemia, leukopenia, thrombocytopenia, anemia, or hepatic or renal dysfunction.

NURSING CONSIDERATIONS

• In patients with AIDS, pentamidine may produce less severe adverse reactions than co-trimoxazole, the alternative treatment, and may be the treatment of choice.
• Monitor blood glucose, serum calcium, serum creatinine, and BUN levels daily. After parenteral administration, blood glucose level may decrease initially; hypoglycemia may be severe in 5% to 10% of patients. This may be followed by hyperglycemia and insulin-dependent diabetes mellitus, which may be permanent.
• The aerosol form should be administered only by the Respirgard II nebulizer manufactured by Marquest. Dosage recommendations are based on the particle size and delivery rate of this device. To administer aerosol, mix the contents of one vial in 6 ml of sterile water for injection. *Do not* use 0.9% sodium chloride solution because it will cause precipitation. Do not mix with other drugs.
• Do not use low-pressure (< 20 psi) compressors. The flow rate should be 5 to 7 liters/minute from a 40- to 50-psi air or oxygen source.
• Instruct the patient to use the aerosol device until the chamber is empty, which may take up to 45 minutes.
• **I.V. use:** Reconstitute drug with 3 ml of sterile water for injection. Then dilute in 50 to 250 ml of D_5W. Inject over at least 60 minutes.
• To minimize risk of hypotension, infuse drug slowly with the patient lying down. Closely monitor blood pressure.
• For I.M. injection, reconstitute drug with 3 ml of sterile water for a solution containing 100 mg/ml; administer deeply. Expect pain and induration to occur.

7

Anthelmintics

mebendazole
niclosamide
oxamniquine
piperazine adipate
piperazine citrate
praziquantel
pyrantel embonate
pyrantel pamoate
thiabendazole

COMBINATION PRODUCTS
None.

mebendazole

Mebendacin, Mebutar, Nemasole, Vermox

Pregnancy Risk Category: C

HOW SUPPLIED
Tablets (chewable): 100 mg
Oral suspension: 100 mg/5 ml‡

ACTION
Mechanism: Selectively and irreversibly inhibits uptake of glucose and other nutrients in susceptible helminths.
Peak: Only small amounts of mebendazole are absorbed; plasma levels peak within 1 hour. **Duration:** most remains in the intestinal tract; duration varies with GI transit time; elimination half-life, about 1 hour.

INDICATIONS & DOSAGE
Pinworm –
Adults and children over 2 years: 100 mg P.O. as a single dose. If infection persists 3 weeks later, repeat treatment.
Roundworm, whipworm, hookworm –
Adults and children over 2 years: 100 mg P.O. b.i.d. for 3 days. If infection persists 3 weeks later, repeat treatment.

ADVERSE REACTIONS
GI: occasional, transient abdominal pain and diarrhea in massive infection and expulsion of worms.

INTERACTIONS
None significant.

CONTRAINDICATIONS
- Contraindicated in patients with hypersensitivity to the drug.

NURSING CONSIDERATIONS
- No dietary restrictions, laxatives, or enemas are necessary.
- Treat all family members.
- Teach the patient about personal hygiene, especially hand-washing technique. To avoid reinfection, teach the patient to wash perianal area daily, to change undergarments and bedclothes daily, and to wash hands and clean fingernails before meals and after bowel movements. Advise the patient to refrain from preparing food for others during infestation.
- Tablets may be chewed, swallowed whole, or crushed and mixed with food.

niclosamide

Niclocide, Yomesan‡

Pregnancy Risk Category: B

HOW SUPPLIED
Tablets (chewable): 500 mg

ACTION
Mechanism: Inhibits oxidative phosphorylation in tapeworms.
Onset: within ½ to 2 hours of administration. **Peak:** Drug is not absorbed from the GI tract. **Duration:** varies with GI transit time.

INDICATIONS & DOSAGE
Tapeworms (fish, beef, and pork) –
Adults: 4 tablets (2 g) chewed thoroughly as a single dose.
Children more than 34 kg: 3 tablets (1.5 g) chewed thoroughly as a single dose.
Children 11 to 34 kg: 2 tablets (1 g) chewed thoroughly as a single dose.
Dwarf tapeworm –
Adults: 4 tablets chewed thoroughly, daily for 7 days.
Children over 2 years more than 34 kg: 3 tablets chewed thoroughly on the first day, then 2 tablets daily for the next 6 days.
Children over 2 years 11 to 34 kg: 2 tablets chewed thoroughly on the first day, then 1 tablet daily for the next 6 days.

ADVERSE REACTIONS
CNS: drowsiness, dizziness, headache.
EENT: oral irritation, bad taste in mouth.
GI: *nausea, vomiting, anorexia,* diarrhea.
Skin: rash, pruritus ani.

INTERACTIONS
None significant.

CONTRAINDICATIONS
• Contraindicated in patients with hypersensitivity to the drug.

NURSING CONSIDERATIONS
• Instruct the patient to chew tablets thoroughly and to wash down with water; for children, the tablets can be crushed and mixed with water or applesauce.
• Tablets should be taken as a single dose after breakfast.
• Expect to administer an antiemetic before treatment. Many clinicians also give a laxative 2 hours after a dose to expel the killed worms and prevent migration of ova into the stomach.
• When treating dwarf tapeworms, urge the patient to drink fruit juices. This helps to eliminate the accumulated intestinal mucus under which the tapeworms lodge.
• Teach the patient about personal hygiene, especially good hand-washing technique. Advise the patient to refrain from preparing food for others during infestation.
• The patient is not considered cured until the stool has been negative for tapeworms for at least 3 months.

oxamniquine
Vansil

Pregnancy Risk Category: C

HOW SUPPLIED
Capsules: 250 mg

ACTION
Mechanism: Reduces the egg load of *Schistosoma mansoni,* but its exact mechanism of action is unknown.
Peak: Plasma levels peak within 1 to 3 hours of oral dose. **Duration:** elimination half-life, 1 to 2½ hours. From 40% to 75% of a dose appears in the urine within 24 hours.

INDICATIONS & DOSAGE
Schistosomiasis caused by S. mansoni, *Western Hemisphere strains* –
Adults and children over 30 kg: 15 mg/kg given as a single oral dose.
Children under 30 kg: 10 mg/kg P.O., followed by 10 mg/kg P.O. 2 to 8 hours later.
Schistosomiasis caused by S. mansoni, *East and Central African strains* –
Adults and children: 30 mg/kg given as a single oral dose or in two equally divided doses over 1 to 2 days.
Schistosomiasis caused by S. mansoni, *in Sudan, Uganda, and Zaire* –
Adults and children: 40 mg/kg given as a single oral dose or in two equally divided doses over 1 to 2 days.
Schistosomiasis caused by S. mansoni,

in Egypt, South Africa, and Zimbabwe –
Adults and children: 60 mg/kg given as 15 mg/kg b.i.d. for 2 days or 20 mg/kg b.i.d. for 3 days.

ADVERSE REACTIONS
CNS: seizures, *dizziness, drowsiness, headache.*
GI: nausea, vomiting, abdominal pain, anorexia.
Skin: urticaria.

INTERACTIONS
None significant.

CONTRAINDICATIONS
- Contraindicated in patients with hypersensitivity to the drug.
- Use cautiously in patients with a history of epilepsy because, in rare cases, seizures have been observed within the first few hours after ingestion.

NURSING CONSIDERATIONS
- Instruct the patient to avoid driving and other hazardous activities during treatment.
- GI tolerance is improved if the drug is given after meals.
- Oxamniquine may cause a reddish discoloration of the urine.
- Although *S. mansoni* infection is rare in the United States and Canada, travelers or immigrants from such areas as Puerto Rico, Latin America, and Africa may have contracted the infection from contaminated water.

piperazine adipate
Entacyl†

piperazine citrate
Pregnancy Risk Category: B

HOW SUPPLIED
adipate
Oral suspension: 600 mg/5 ml
Granules: 2 g/packet
citrate
Tablets: 250 mg
Syrup: 500 mg/5 ml

ACTION
Mechanism: Blocks neuromuscular action, paralyzing the worm and causing its expulsion by normal peristalsis.
Onset: varies with GI transit time.
Duration: highly variable.

INDICATIONS & DOSAGE
Enterobiasis (pinworm) –
Adults and children: 65 mg/kg P.O. daily for 7 to 8 days. Maximum daily dosage is 2.5 g. Alternatively, give adults 2 g P.O. daily for 7 days, and give children 1 g/m² P.O. daily for 7 days. Some clinicians order according to body weight:
Children under 7 kg: 250 mg P.O. daily for 7 days.
Children 7 to 14 kg: 500 mg P.O. daily for 7 days.
Children 14 to 27 kg: 1 g P.O. daily for 7 days.
Children over 27 kg and adults: 2 g P.O. daily for 7 days.
Ascariasis (roundworm) –
Adults: 3.5 g P.O. in single doses for 2 consecutive days.
Children: 75 mg/kg or 2 g/m² P.O. daily for 2 consecutive days. Maximum daily dosage is 3.5 g.
Alternatively, give according to body weight:
Children under 14 kg: 1 g P.O. daily for 2 days.
Children 14 to 23 kg: 2 g P.O. daily for 2 days.
Children 23 to 45 kg: 3 g P.O. daily for 2 days.
Children over 45 kg and adults: 3.5 g P.O. daily for 2 days.
Some clinicians continue treatment for 4 days in patients with massive infestation. May repeat in 1 week if necessary.

ADVERSE REACTIONS
CNS: ataxia, tremors, choreiform movements, muscular weakness, myoclonus, hyporeflexia, paresthesia, seizures, sense of detachment, EEG abnormalities, memory defect, *headache, vertigo.*
EENT: nystagmus, blurred vision, paralytic strabismus, cataracts with visual impairment, lacrimation, difficulty in focusing, rhinorrhea.
GI: *nausea, vomiting,* diarrhea, abdominal cramps.
Skin: urticaria, photodermatitis, ***erythema multiforme,*** purpura, eczematous skin reactions.
Other: arthralgia, fever, bronchospasm, ***hemolytic anemia.***

INTERACTIONS
Pyrantel pamoate: possible antagonism. Don't administer together.

CONTRAINDICATIONS
- Contraindicated in patients with hepatic or renal impairment or seizure disorders.
- Use cautiously in patients with severe malnutrition or anemia.
- Discontinue if CNS or significant GI reactions occur.

NURSING CONSIDERATIONS
- Because of potential neurotoxicity, avoid prolonged or repeated treatment, especially in children.
- No dietary restrictions, laxatives, or enemas are necessary.
- Piperazine may be taken with food; but, for best absorption, tell the patient to take on empty stomach.
- Mix powder for oral suspension in 57 ml of water, milk, or fruit juice.
- Treat all family members.
- Teach the patient about personal hygiene, especially hand-washing technique. To avoid reinfection, teach the patient to wash perianal area, to change undergarments and bedclothes daily, and to wash hands and clean fingernails before meals and after bowel movements. Advise the patient to refrain from preparing food for others during infestation.

praziquantel
Biltricide
Pregnancy Risk Category: B

HOW SUPPLIED
Tablets: 600 mg

ACTION
Mechanism: Causes a contraction of schistosomes by a specific effect on the permeability of the cell membrane.
Peak: Serum levels peak 1 to 3 hours after oral dose. **Duration:** serum half-life, less than 1½ hours for parent drug; 4 to 6 hours for metabolites.

INDICATIONS & DOSAGE
Schistosomiasis caused by S. mekongi, S. japonicum, S. mansoni, *and* S. haematobium –
Adults and children 4 years and older: 20 mg/kg P.O. t.i.d. as a 1-day treatment. The interval between doses should be 4 to 6 hours.

ADVERSE REACTIONS
CNS: *drowsiness, malaise,* headache, dizziness.
GI: abdominal discomfort, nausea.
Hepatic: minimal increase in liver enzymes.
Skin: urticaria.
Other: fever.

INTERACTIONS
None significant.

CONTRAINDICATIONS
- Contraindicated in patients with ocular cysticercosis because destruction of the eye parasite may cause permanent eye damage.

NURSING CONSIDERATIONS

- Praziquantel may produce drowsiness. Tell the patient to avoid hazardous activities on the day of treatment and the day after.
- Adverse reactions may be more frequent or serious in patients with a heavy worm burden.
- For overdose, give a fast-acting laxative.
- Advise the patient to take the tablet during meals and to wash down the unchewed tablet.
- Tablets taste bitter. Keeping them in the mouth may cause gagging or vomiting.
- Praziquantel is effective for several different species of *Schistosoma*.
- Praziquantel may also be effective against liver flukes.

---

pyrantel embonate

Anthel‡, Combantrin‡, Early Bird‡

pyrantel pamoate

Antiminth, Combantrin†, Reese's Pinworm Medicine

Pregnancy Risk Category: C

HOW SUPPLIED

embonate
Tablets: 125 mg‡, 250 mg‡
Oral suspension: 50 mg/ml‡
Granules: 100 mg/g‡
Squares (chocolate-flavored): 100 mg‡
pamoate
Tablets: 125 mg†
Oral suspension: 50 mg/ml

ACTION

Mechanism: Blocks neuromuscular action, paralyzing the worm and causing its expulsion by normal peristalsis.
Onset: highly variable. **Peak:** Only small amounts of drug are absorbed. Plasma levels peak within 1 to 3 hours. **Duration:** varies with GI transit time and extent of infestation.

INDICATIONS & DOSAGE

Roundworm and pinworm –
Adults and children over 2 years: single dose of 11 mg/kg P.O. Maximum dosage is 1 g. For pinworm, dosage should be repeated in 2 weeks.

ADVERSE REACTIONS

CNS: headache, dizziness, drowsiness, insomnia.
GI: anorexia, nausea, vomiting, gastralgia, cramps, diarrhea, tenesmus.
Hepatic: transient elevation of AST.
Skin: rash.
Other: fever, weakness.

INTERACTIONS

Piperazine salts: possible antagonism; don't give together.

CONTRAINDICATIONS

- Contraindicated in patients with hypersensitivity to the drug.
- Use cautiously in patients with severe malnutrition or anemia or in patients with hepatic dysfunction.

NURSING CONSIDERATIONS

- No dietary restrictions, laxatives, or enemas are necessary.
- Pyrantel may be taken with food, milk, or fruit juices. Shake suspension well.
- Treat all family members.
- Teach the patient about personal hygiene, especially hand-washing technique. To avoid reinfection, teach the patient to wash perianal area daily, to change undergarments and bedclothes daily, and to wash hands and clean fingernails before meals and after bowel movements. Advise the patient to refrain from preparing food for others during infestation.

---

thiabendazole

Foldan, Mintezol, Minzolum, Triasox

Pregnancy Risk Category: C

HOW SUPPLIED
Tablets (chewable): 500 mg
Oral suspension: 500 mg/5 ml

ACTION
Mechanism: Unknown.
Peak: Plasma levels peak within 1 to 2 hours of oral dose. **Duration:** eliminated from plasma within 8 hours.

INDICATIONS & DOSAGE
Cutaneous infestations with larva migrans (creeping eruption) –
Adults and children: 25 mg/kg P.O. b.i.d. for 2 to 5 days. Maximum dosage is 3 g daily. If lesions persist after 2 days, repeat course.
Pinworm –
Adults and children: 25 mg/kg P.O. in 2 doses daily for 1 day; repeat in 7 days.
Roundworm, threadworm, whipworm –
Adults and children: 25 mg/kg P.O. in 2 doses daily for 2 successive days.
Trichinosis –
Adults and children: 25 mg/kg P.O. in 2 doses daily for 2 to 4 successive days.

ADVERSE REACTIONS
CNS: impaired mental alertness, impaired physical coordination, *drowsiness, fatigue,* giddiness, *headache,* dizziness.
CV: *hypotension.*
GI: *anorexia, nausea, vomiting,* diarrhea, epigastric distress.
Skin: *rash, pruritus,* ***erythema multiforme.***
Other: lymphadenopathy, fever, flushing, chills.

INTERACTIONS
Theophylline: may impair the hepatic metabolism of theophylline, increasing the risk of toxicity. Monitor the patient closely.

CONTRAINDICATIONS
- Use cautiously in patients with hepatic or renal dysfunction, severe malnutrition, and anemia and in patients who are vomiting. Supportive therapy indicated for anemic, dehydrated, or malnourished patients. In children under 15 kg, weigh benefits against risks.

NURSING CONSIDERATIONS
- Administer after meals. For oral suspension, shake before measuring dosage. For tablets, advise the patient to chew before swallowing.
- May cause drowsiness. Advise the patient to avoid hazardous activities such as driving.
- No dietary restrictions, laxatives, or enemas are necessary.
- Treat all family members.
- Teach the patient about personal hygiene, especially good hand-washing technique. To avoid reinfection, teach the patient to wash perianal area daily, to change undergarments and bedclothes daily, and to wash hands and clean fingernails before meals and after bowel movements. Advise the patient not to prepare food for others during infestation.

8

Antifungals

amphotericin B
fluconazole
flucytosine
griseofulvin microsize
griseofulvin ultramicrosize
itraconazole
ketoconazole
miconazole
nystatin

COMBINATION PRODUCTS
None.

amphotericin B

Fungilin Oral‡, Fungizone Intravenous

Pregnancy Risk Category: B

HOW SUPPLIED
Tablets: 100 mg‡
Oral suspension: 100 mg/ml‡
Lozenges: 10 mg‡
Injection: 50-mg lyophilized cake

ACTION
Mechanism: Probably acts by binding to sterol in the fungal cell membrane, altering cell permeability and allowing leakage of intracellular components.
Peak: Serum levels peak immediately after I.V. infusion; poorly absorbed after oral administration. **Duration:** elimination half-life, about 24 hours.

INDICATIONS & DOSAGE
Systemic fungal infections (histoplasmosis, coccidioidomycosis, blastomycosis, cryptococcosis, disseminated moniliasis, aspergillosis, phycomycosis), meningitis –
Adults: initially, 1 mg in 250 ml of D_5W infused over 2 to 4 hours; or 0.25 mg/kg daily by slow infusion over 6 hours. Increase daily dosage gradually as patient tolerance develops, to maximum 1 mg/kg daily. Therapy must not exceed 1.5 mg/kg. If drug is discontinued for 1 week or more, resume with initial dose and increase gradually.
Intrathecal: 25 mcg/0.1 ml of the reconstituted injection diluted with 10 to 20 ml of CSF and administered by barbotage two or three times weekly. Initial dose should not exceed 100 mcg.
Infections of the GI tract caused by Candida albicans –
Adults: 100 mg P.O. q.i.d. for 2 weeks.
Oral and perioral candidal infections –
Adults: 1 lozenge q.i.d. for 7 to 14 days. Lozenge should be allowed to dissolve slowly.

ADVERSE REACTIONS
CNS: headache, peripheral neuropathy; with intrathecal administration – peripheral nerve pain, paresthesia.
CV: hypotension, ***cardiac arrhythmias, asystole.***
GI: *anorexia, weight loss, nausea,* vomiting, dyspepsia, diarrhea, epigastric cramps.
GU: abnormal renal function with hypokalemia, azotemia, hyposthenuria, hypomagnesemia, renal tubular acidosis, nephrocalcinosis; with large doses – permanent renal impairment, anuria, oliguria.
Hematologic: normochromic, normocytic anemia.
Other: arthralgia, burning, stinging, irritation, tissue damage with extravasation, phlebitis, thrombophlebitis, pain at injection site, myalgia, muscle weakness secondary to hypokalemia, *fever, chills,* malaise, generalized pain.

INTERACTIONS

Corticosteroids: enhanced potassium depletion. Monitor serum potassium levels.

Digitalis glycosides: increased risk of digitalis toxicity in potassium-depleted patients. Monitor closely.

Other nephrotoxic drugs, such as antibiotics or antineoplastic agents: may cause additive renal toxicity. Administer cautiously.

CONTRAINDICATIONS

- Contraindicated in patients with hypersensitivity to the drug.
- Use cautiously in patients with impaired renal function.
- Give parenterally only in hospitalized patients, under close supervision, when diagnosis of potentially fatal fungal infection has been confirmed.

NURSING CONSIDERATIONS

- Monitor fluid intake and output; report change in urine appearance or volume. Monitor BUN and serum creatinine (or creatinine clearance) at least weekly. Kidney damage typically reversible if drug is stopped at first sign of dysfunction.
- Obtain liver and renal function studies weekly. If BUN exceeds 40 mg/100 ml, or if serum creatinine exceeds 3 mg/100 ml, doctor may reduce or stop drug until renal function improves. Monitor CBC weekly. Stop drug if alkaline phosphatase or bilirubin levels increase.
- Monitor potassium levels closely, and report signs of hypokalemia. Check calcium and magnesium levels twice weekly.
- Oral form is not available in the United States.
- Store the dry form at 2° to 8° C (35.6° to 46.4° F). Protect from light. Reconstitute with 10 ml of sterile water only. To avoid precipitation, do not mix with solutions containing sodium chloride, other electrolytes, or bacteriostatic agents such as benzyl alcohol. Do not use if solution contains precipitate or foreign matter.
- To reduce severe adverse reactions, consider premedication with antipyretics, antihistamines, antiemetics, or small doses of corticosteroids; addition of phosphate buffer and heparin to the solution; and alternate-day schedule. For severe reactions, discontinue the drug and notify the doctor.
- Amphotericin B appears to be compatible with limited amounts of heparin sodium, hydrocortisone sodium succinate, and methylprednisolone sodium succinate.
- Reconstituted solution is stable for 1 week under refrigeration or 24 hours at room temperature. It has 8-hour stability in room light.
- **I.V. use:** An initial test dose may be prescribed. 1 mg is added to 50 to 250 ml of D_5W and infused over 20 to 30 minutes; the patient's pulse, respiratory rate, temperature, and blood pressure are monitored for at least 4 hours. Some clinicians give this test dose more slowly, over a 4-hour period.
- Use an infusion pump and in-line filter with mean pore diameter larger than 1 micron. Infuse over 6 hours; rapid infusion may cause cardiovascular collapse. Warn patient of possible discomfort at the site and of other potential adverse reactions that may occur during the several months of probable therapy.
- Administer in distal veins. If veins become thrombosed, alternate administration sites.
- Give antibiotics separately; don't mix or piggyback with amphotericin B.
- Monitor vital signs every 30 minutes; fever, shaking chills, and hypotension may appear 1 to 2 hours after start of I.V. infusion and should subside within 4 hours of discontinuation.

fluconazole

Diflucan

Pregnancy Risk Category: C

HOW SUPPLIED

Tablets: 50 mg, 100 mg, 200 mg
Injection: 200 mg/100 ml, 400 mg/200 ml

ACTION

Mechanism: Inhibits fungal cytochrome P-450, an enzyme responsible for fungal sterol synthesis, and weakens fungal cell walls.
Peak: Peak serum levels occur immediately following I.V. infusion, 1 to 2 hours after oral administration. **Duration:** elimination half-life, about 30 hours.

INDICATIONS & DOSAGE

Oropharyngeal candidiasis –
Adults: 200 mg P.O. or I.V. on the first day, followed by 100 mg once daily. Therapy should continue for 2 weeks.
Esophageal candidiasis –
Adults: 200 mg P.O. or I.V. on the first day, followed by 100 mg once daily. Higher doses (up to 400 mg daily) have been used, depending on the patient's condition and tolerance of treatment. Patients should receive the drug for at least 3 weeks and for 2 weeks after symptoms resolve.
Systemic candidiasis –
Adults: 400 mg P.O. or I.V. on the first day, followed by 200 mg once daily. Treatment should continue for at least 4 weeks or for 2 weeks after symptoms resolve.
Cryptococcal meningitis –
Adults: 400 mg P.O. or I.V. on the first day, followed by 200 mg once daily. Higher doses (up to 400 mg daily) may be used. Treatment should continue for 10 to 12 weeks after CSF cultures are negative.
Suppression of relapse of cryptococcal meningitis in patients with AIDS –
Adults: 200 mg P.O. or I.V. daily.

In patients with renal failure: If creatinine clearance is 21 to 50 ml/minute, reduce dosage by 50%. If creatinine clearance is 11 to 20 ml/minute, reduce dosage by 75%. Patients receiving regular hemodialysis treatment should receive the usual dose after each dialysis session.

ADVERSE REACTIONS

CNS: headache, dizziness.
GI: *nausea,* vomiting, abdominal pain, diarrhea.
Hepatic: hepatotoxicity (rare), elevated enzymes.
Skin: rash, ***Stevens-Johnson syndrome (rare).***

INTERACTIONS

Cyclosporine, phenytoin: may increase plasma concentrations of these drugs. Monitor serum cyclosporine or phenytoin levels.
Isoniazid, phenytoin, rifampin, valproic acid, oral sulfonylureas: increased incidence of abnormally elevated hepatic transaminases. Monitor closely.
Oral antidiabetic agents (tolbutamide, glyburide, glipizide): may increase plasma concentrations of these drugs. Monitor for enhanced hypoglycemic effect.
Rifampin: enhanced metabolism of fluconazole. Monitor for lack of response.
Warfarin: increased risk of bleeding. Monitor PT.

CONTRAINDICATIONS

• Contraindicated in patients with hypersensitivity to the drug.
• As a safeguard, use cautiously in patients with hypersensitivity to other antifungal azole compounds, although no information exists regarding cross-sensitivity.

NURSING CONSIDERATIONS

- The incidence of adverse reactions appears to be greater in HIV-infected patients.
- Oral bioavailability of fluconazole is greater than 90% and is unaffected by gastric pH. Dosage is the same for oral or I.V. use.
- Periodically monitor liver function during prolonged therapy. Although adverse hepatic effects are rare, they can be serious.
- If the patient develops mild rash, monitor closely. Discontinue drug if lesions progress.
- **I.V. use:** May be administered by continuous infusion at a rate not to exceed 200 mg/hour. Use an infusion pump. To prevent air embolism, do not connect in series with other infusions. Do not add any other drugs to the solution.
- I.V. bags of fluconazole are shipped with a protective overwrap that should not be removed until just before use, to ensure product sterility. The plastic container may show some opacity from moisture absorbed during sterilization. This is normal, will not affect the drug, and will diminish over time.
- Safety and effectiveness in children have not been established, but a few children age 3 to 13 have received 3 to 6 mg/kg/day.

flucytosine (5-fluorocytosine, 5-FC)

Ancobon, Ancotil†

Pregnancy Risk Category: C

HOW SUPPLIED

Capsules: 250 mg, 500 mg

ACTION

Mechanism: Appears to penetrate fungal cells – where it is converted to fluorouracil, a known metabolic antagonist – and cause defective protein synthesis.

Peak: Serum levels peak within 6 hours of oral dose. **Duration:** elimination half-life, 2½ to 6 hours.

INDICATIONS & DOSAGE

Severe fungal infections caused by susceptible strains of Candida *(including septicemia, endocarditis, urinary tract and pulmonary infections) and* Cryptococcus *(meningitis, pulmonary infection, and possible urinary tract infections)* –

Adults and children over 50 kg: 50 to 150 mg/kg daily P.O. q 6 hours.

Adults and children under 50 kg: 1.5 to 4.5 g/m^2/day P.O. in four divided doses.

Severe infections, such as meningitis, may require doses up to 250 mg/kg.

ADVERSE REACTIONS

CNS: dizziness, drowsiness, confusion, headache, vertigo.

GI: *nausea, vomiting, diarrhea,* abdominal bloating.

Hematologic: anemia, ***leukopenia, bone marrow suppression, thrombocytopenia.***

Hepatic: elevated liver enzymes (ALT, AST); elevated serum alkaline phosphatase, BUN, or creatinine.

Skin: occasional rash.

INTERACTIONS

Amphotericin B: synergistic effects and possibly enhanced toxicity when used together. Monitor patient closely.

CONTRAINDICATIONS

- Contraindicated in patients with hypersensitivity to the drug.
- Use with extreme caution in patients with impaired hepatic or renal function or bone marrow suppression. Patients with renal dysfunction should have dosage based on plasma flucytosine levels.

NURSING CONSIDERATIONS

- Hematologic tests and renal and liver function studies should precede therapy and should be repeated at frequent intervals thereafter. Before treatment, susceptibility tests should establish that organism is flucytosine-sensitive. Tests should be repeated weekly to monitor drug resistance.
- GI adverse reactions are reduced if capsules are given over a 15-minute period.
- Monitor fluid intake and output; report any marked change.
- If possible, blood level assays of drug should be performed regularly to maintain flucytosine at therapeutic level (25 to 120 mcg/ml). Higher blood levels may be toxic.
- Inform the patient that adequate therapeutic response may take weeks or months.

griseofulvin microsize

Fulcin‡, Fulvicin-U/F, Grifulvin V, Grisactin, Grisovin‡, Grisovin 500‡, Grisovin-FP

griseofulvin ultramicrosize

Fulvicin P/G, Grisactin Ultra, Griseostatin‡, Gris-PEG

Pregnancy Risk Category: X

HOW SUPPLIED

microsize
Tablets: 250 mg, 500 mg
Capsules: 125 mg, 250 mg
Oral suspension: 125 mg/5ml
ultramicrosize
Tablets: 125 mg, 165 mg, 250 mg, 330 mg

ACTION

Mechanism: An antifungal antibiotic derived from *Penicillium* that arrests fungal cell activity by disrupting its mitotic spindle structure.
Peak: Serum levels peak within 4 to 8 hours. **Duration:** elimination half-life, 9 to 24 hours. After 5 days, about 50% of a dose appears in urine; 33%, in feces.

INDICATIONS & DOSAGE

Ringworm infections of skin, hair, nails (tinea corporis, tinea capitis) when caused by Trichophyton, Microsporum, *or* Epidermophyton –
Adults: 500 mg (microsize) P.O. daily in single or divided doses. Severe infections may require up to 1 g daily. Alternatively, may give 330 to 375 mg ultramicrosize in single or divided doses.
Tinea pedis and tinea unguium –
Adults: 0.75 to 1 g (microsize) P.O. daily. Alternatively, may give 660 to 750 mg ultramicrosize P.O. daily.
Children: 11 mg/kg/day (microsize) P.O. Alternatively, may give 7.3 mg/kg/day of the ultramicrosize.

ADVERSE REACTIONS

CNS: headache (in early stages of treatment), transient decrease in hearing, fatigue with large doses, occasional mental confusion, impaired performance of routine activities, psychotic symptoms, dizziness, insomnia.
GI: nausea, vomiting, excessive thirst, flatulence, diarrhea.
Hematologic: leukopenia, ***granulocytopenia*** (requires discontinuation of drug), porphyria.
Skin: rash, urticaria, photosensitivity, ***toxic epidermal necrolysis*** (rare).
Other: estrogen-like effects in children, oral thrush, hypersensitivity reactions (rash, ***angioedema, serum sickness-like reactions***), lupuslike syndrome or exacerbation of existing lupus erythematosus.

INTERACTIONS

Coumarin anticoagulants: decreased effectiveness. Monitor PT when used concurrently.
Ethanol: may cause tachycardia, diaphoresis, and flushing. Avoid ethanol.
Oral contraceptives: decreased effec-

tiveness. Suggest alternative methods of contraception.

Phenobarbital: decreased griseofulvin blood levels due to decreased absorption or increased metabolism. Avoid using together or administer griseofulvin t.i.d.

CONTRAINDICATIONS

- Contraindicated in patients with porphyria or hepatocellular failure.
- Also contraindicated in pregnant patients or women who intend to become pregnant during therapy. Because the drug decreases the effectiveness of oral contraceptives, a nonhormonal form of contraception should be employed.
- Use cautiously in penicillin-sensitive patients because griseofulvin is a penicillin derivative.
- Because of potential toxicity, use only when topical treatment fails to arrest mycotic disease.

NURSING CONSIDERATIONS

- Assess hematologic, renal, and hepatic function periodically during prolonged therapy.
- Advise the patient that prolonged treatment may be needed to control infection and prevent relapse, even if symptoms abate in first few days of therapy. Tell the patient to keep skin clean and dry and to maintain good hygiene.
- Caution the patient to avoid intense sunlight.
- Griseofulvin is most effectively absorbed and causes least GI distress when given after a high-fat meal.
- Effective treatment of tinea pedis may require concomitant use of a topical agent.
- Diagnosis of infecting organism should be verified in laboratory. Continue drug until clinical and laboratory examinations confirm complete eradication.
- Because griseofulvin ultramicrosize is dispersed in polyethylene glycol, it is absorbed more rapidly and completely than microsize preparations and is effective at one-half to two-thirds the usual griseofulvin dose.

itraconazole

Sporanox

Pregnancy Risk Category: C

HOW SUPPLIED

Capsules: 100 mg

ACTION

Mechanism: Interferes with fungal cell-wall synthesis by inhibiting the formation of ergosterol, a vital component, and increasing cell-wall permeability that makes the fungus susceptible to osmotic instability.

Peak: Plasma levels peak 3 to 4 hours after oral dose. Steady-state levels are reached within 15 days of daily administration. **Duration:** half-life, about 64 hours; drug is highly bound to plasma proteins and tissues.

INDICATIONS & DOSAGE

Pulmonary and extrapulmonary blastomycosis; histoplasmosis –

Adults: 200 mg P.O. daily. Increase dosage as needed and tolerated in 100-mg increments to a maximum of 400 mg daily. Dosages that exceed 200 mg daily should be given in two divided doses. Treatment should continue for a minimum of 3 months. In life-threatening illness, administer a loading dose of 200 mg t.i.d. for 3 days.

ADVERSE REACTIONS

GI: nausea, vomiting, diarrhea, abdominal pain, anorexia.

Skin: rash, pruritus.

Other: edema, fatigue, fever, malaise.

INTERACTIONS

Cyclosporine, digoxin: possible increased plasma levels of these drugs. Monitor plasma levels closely.
H_2-receptor antagonists, antacids, rifampin, phenytoin: possible lowered itraconazole plasma levels. Avoid concomitant use.
Isoniazid: may decrease plasma levels of itraconazole. Monitor closely.
Oral anticoagulants: possible enhanced anticoagulant effects. Monitor PT closely.
Oral antidiabetic agents: similar antifungals have caused hypoglycemia. Monitor blood glucose levels closely.
Terfenadine, astemizole: inhibited metabolism of these antihistamines, resulting in elevated blood levels and risk of serious cardiac toxicity. Never administer together.

CONTRAINDICATIONS

- Contraindicated in patients with hypersensitivity to the drug and in patients receiving terfenadine or astemizole. Because drug is excreted in breast milk, don't use in breast-feeding patients.
- Use cautiously in patients with hypochlorhydria because they may not absorb the drug as readily as patients with normal gastric acidity. Because hypochlorhydria can accompany HIV infection, also use cautiously in HIV-infected patients.
- Itraconazole and its metabolite are more than 99% bound to plasma proteins. Use cautiously in patients receiving other highly bound medications.

NURSING CONSIDERATIONS

- Tell the patient to take drug with food to ensure maximal absorption.
- Perform baseline liver function tests, and monitor periodically. Patients should recognize and report the signs and symptoms of liver disease (anorexia, dark urine, pale stools, unusual fatigue, or jaundice).

ketoconazole

Nizoral

Pregnancy Risk Category: C

HOW SUPPLIED

Tablets: 200 mg
Oral suspension: 100 mg/5 ml†

ACTION

Mechanism: Inhibits purine transport and DNA, RNA, and protein synthesis; increases cell-wall permeability, making the fungus more susceptible to osmotic pressure.
Peak: Serum levels peak within 1 to 2 hours after oral administration. **Duration:** terminal elimination half-life, about 8 hours.

INDICATIONS & DOSAGE

Systemic candidiasis, chronic mucocandidiasis, oral thrush, candiduria, coccidioidomycosis, histoplasmosis, chromomycosis, and paracoccidioidomycosis; severe cutaneous dermatophyte infections resistant to therapy with topical or oral griseofulvin –
Adults and children over 40 kg: initially, 200 mg P.O. daily in a single dose. Dosage may be increased to 400 mg once daily in patients who don't respond to lower dosage.
Children 2 years and over: 3.3 to 6.6 mg/kg P.O. daily.

ADVERSE REACTIONS

CNS: headache, nervousness, dizziness.
GI: *nausea, vomiting,* abdominal pain, diarrhea, constipation.
Hepatic: elevated liver enzymes, or ***fatal hepatotoxicity.***
Skin: itching.
Other: gynecomastia with tenderness.

INTERACTIONS

Antacids, anticholinergics, H_2 blockers: decreased absorption of ketoconazole. Wait at least 2 hours after keto-

conazole dose before administering these drugs.
Rifampin, isoniazid: increased ketoconazole metabolism. Monitor for decreased antifungal effect.

CONTRAINDICATIONS

- Contraindicated in patients with hypersensitivity to the drug.
- Use cautiously in patients with hepatic disease and those who are taking other hepatotoxic drugs.
- Because of the potential for serious hepatotoxicity, ketoconazole should not be used for less serious conditions, such as fungus infections of the skin or nails.

NURSING CONSIDERATIONS

- Ketoconazole requires gastric acidity for dissolution and absorption; decreased bioavailability has been reported in patients with conditions associated with hypochlorhydria, such as AIDS. Instruct the patient to dissolve each tablet in 4 ml aqueous solution of 0.2 N hydrochloric acid, to sip the mixture through a glass or plastic straw (to avoid contact with teeth), and to end the procedure with a glass of water.
- Make sure the patient understands that treatment should be continued until all clinical and laboratory tests indicate that active fungal infection has subsided. If drug is discontinued too soon, infection will recur. Minimum treatment for candidiasis is 7 to 14 days. Minimum treatment for other systemic fungal infections is 6 months. Minimum treatment for resistant dermatophyte infections is at least 4 weeks.
- Reassure the patient that, although nausea is common early in therapy, it will subside. To minimize nausea, divide the daily dosage into two doses. Taking with meals also helps to decrease nausea.
- Monitor for elevated liver enzymes and nausea that does not subside, as well as for unusual fatigue, jaundice, dark urine, or pale stools – all signs of possible hepatotoxicity.
- Much larger doses (up to 800 mg/day) can be used to treat fungal meningitis and intracerebral fungal lesions. Because CSF levels are unpredictable after oral administration, the drug should not be used alone to treat fungal meningitis.

miconazole

Monistat I.V.

Pregnancy Risk Category: C

HOW SUPPLIED

Injection: 10 mg/ml

ACTION

Mechanism: Inhibits purine transport and DNA, RNA, and protein synthesis; increases cell-wall permeability, making the fungus more susceptible to osmotic pressure.
Peak: Plasma levels peak immediately after I.V. infusion. **Duration:** terminal half-life, about 24 hours.

INDICATIONS & DOSAGE

Systemic fungal infections (coccidioidomycosis, candidiasis, cryptococcosis, paracoccidioidomycosis), chronic mucocutaneous candidiasis –
Adults: 200 to 3,600 mg/day. Dosages may vary with diagnosis and with infective agent. May divide daily dosage over 3 infusions, 200 to 1,200 mg per infusion. Dilute in at least 200 ml of 0.9% sodium chloride. Repeated courses may be needed because of relapse or reinfection.
Children 1 year and over: 20 to 40 mg/kg/day. Do not exceed 15 mg/kg per infusion.
Fungal meningitis –
Adults: 20 mg intrathecally as an adjunct to I.V. administration, q 3 to 7 days.

ADVERSE REACTIONS

CNS: dizziness, drowsiness.
GI: *nausea, vomiting,* diarrhea.
Hematologic: transient decreases in hematocrit, thrombocytopenia.
Skin: *pruritic rash.*
Other: ***anaphylactoid reactions,*** fever, chills, transient decrease in serum sodium, phlebitis at injection site.

INTERACTIONS

Oral anticoagulants: enhanced anticoagulant effect. Monitor closely.

CONTRAINDICATIONS

- Contraindicated in patients with hypersensitivity to the drug.
- Use cautiously because the drug is dissolved in a vehicle containing polyoxyl 35 castor oil, a substance known to cause anaphylactoid reactions. Give the first dose under continuous medical supervision with emergency resuscitative equipment immediately available. Subsequent doses may be administered on an outpatient basis in selected patients.

NURSING CONSIDERATIONS

- Premedication with an antiemetic may lessen nausea and vomiting.
- To lessen GI adverse reactions, do not administer at mealtimes.
- Pruritic rash may persist for weeks after drug is discontinued. Pruritus may be controlled with oral or I.V. diphenhydramine.
- Inform the patient that adequate therapeutic response may take weeks or months.
- Monitor levels of hemoglobin, hematocrit, electrolytes, and lipids regularly. Transient elevations in serum cholesterol and triglycerides may be caused by castor oil vehicle.
- In treatment of fungal meningitis and urinary bladder infections, supplement with intrathecal administration and bladder irrigation, respectively.
- **I.V. use:** Use of I.V. miconazole has been replaced largely by newer drugs that are better tolerated.
- Rapid I.V. injection of undiluted miconazole may produce arrhythmias. Dilute infusion with at least 200 ml of 0.9% sodium chloride solution and infuse over 30 to 60 minutes.
- For intrathecal use, drug may be given undiluted using a subcutaneous intrathecal (Ommaya) reservoir. Alternatively, the drug may be given by lumbar or cisternal puncture.

nystatin

Mycostatin*, Nadostine†, Nilstat, Nystex*

Pregnancy Risk Category: B

HOW SUPPLIED

Tablets: 500,000 units
Oral suspension: 100,000 units/ml
Vaginal suppositories: 100,000 units

ACTION

Mechanism: Probably acts by binding to sterols in the fungal cell membrane, altering cell permeability and allowing leakage of intracellular components.
Peak: Serum levels are not detectable after oral administration because the drug is poorly absorbed from the GI tract.

INDICATIONS & DOSAGE

GI infections –
Adults: 500,000 to 1 million units as oral tablets t.i.d.
Oral, vaginal, and intestinal infections caused by Candida albicans (Monilia) *and other* Candida *species –*
Adults: 400,000 to 600,000 units oral suspension q.i.d. for oral candidiasis.
Children and infants over 3 months: 250,000 to 500,000 units oral suspension q.i.d.
Neonates and premature infants: 100,000 units oral suspension q.i.d.

Vaginal infections –
Adults: 100,000 units, as vaginal tablets, inserted high into vagina, daily or b.i.d. for 14 days.

ADVERSE REACTIONS

GI: transient nausea, vomiting, diarrhea (usually with large oral dosage).

INTERACTIONS

None significant.

CONTRAINDICATIONS

- Contraindicated in patients with hypersensitivity to the drug.
- Nystatin is virtually nontoxic and nonsensitizing when used orally, vaginally, or topically, but advise the patient to report redness, swelling, or irritation.

NURSING CONSIDERATIONS

- Advise the patient to continue medication for at least 2 days after symptoms disappear to ensure against reinfection. Consult the doctor for exact length of therapy.
- Instruct the patient in careful hygiene for affected areas, including cleansing perineal area from front to back after defecation.
- Not effective against systemic infections.
- Vaginal tablets can be used by pregnant patients up to 6 weeks before term to treat maternal infection that may cause thrush in neonates.
- Continue therapy during menstruation.
- Instruct the patient to wash applicator thoroughly after each use.
- Explain that predisposing factors of vaginal infection include use of antibiotics, oral contraceptives, and corticosteroids; diabetes; reinfection by sexual partner; and tight-fitting panty hose. Encourage the patient to use cotton (not synthetic) underpants.
- For treatment of oral candidiasis (thrush): After the mouth is clean of food debris, have the patient hold suspension in mouth for several minutes before swallowing. When treating infants, swab medication on oral mucosa. Instruct the patient in good oral hygiene techniques. Tell the patient overuse of mouthwash or having poorly fitting dentures, especially in older patients, may alter flora and promote infection.
- For treatment of oral candidiasis, immunosuppressed patients sometimes suck on vaginal tablets (100,000 units) because this provides prolonged contact with oral mucosa.

*Liquid form contains alcohol. *Common* reactions are in italics; ***life-threatening,*** in bold italics.
**May contain tartrazine.

9

Antimalarials

chloroquine hydrochloride
chloroquine phosphate
chloroquine sulphate
hydroxychloroquine sulfate
mefloquine hydrochloride
primaquine phosphate
pyrimethamine
pyrimethamine with sulfadoxine
quinine bisulfate
quinine sulfate

COMBINATION PRODUCTS

ARALEN PHOSPHATE WITH PRIMAQUINE PHOSPHATE: chloroquine phosphate 500 mg (300 mg base) and primaquine phosphate 79 mg (45 mg base).

M-KYA, Q-VEL: quinine sulfate 64.8 mg and vitamin E 400 U (as dl-alpha-tocopheryl acetate) and lecithin.

---

chloroquine hydrochloride

Aralen HCl, Chlorquin‡

chloroquine phosphate

Aralen Phosphate, Chlorquin‡

chloroquine sulphate

Nivaquine‡

Pregnancy Risk Category: C

HOW SUPPLIED

hydrochloride

Injection: 50 mg/ml (40-mg/ml base)

phosphate

Tablets: 250 mg (150-mg base), 500 mg (300-mg base)

sulphate

Tablets: 200 mg (150-mg base)

Syrup: 68 mg (50-mg base)/5 ml

ACTION

Mechanism: As an antimalarial, chloroquine may bind to and alter the properties of DNA in susceptible parasites. As an amebicide, its mechanism of action is unknown.

Peak: Peak levels occur within 1 to 2 hours of oral dose. **Duration:** plasma half-life, 3 to 5 days.

INDICATIONS & DOSAGE

Acute malarial attacks caused by Plasmodium vivax, P. malariae, P. ovale, *and susceptible strains of* P. falciparum –

Adults: initially, 600 mg (base) P.O., then 300 mg at 6, 24, and 48 hours. Or 160 to 200 mg (base) I.M. initially; repeat in 6 hours p.r.n. Switch to oral therapy as soon as possible.

Children: initially, 10 mg (base)/kg P.O., then 5 mg (base)/kg at 6, 24, and 48 hours (do not exceed adult dose). Or 5 mg (base)/kg I.M. initially; repeat in 6 hours p.r.n. Switch to oral therapy as soon as possible.

Malaria prophylaxis –

Adults and children: 5 mg (base)/kg P.O. (not to exceed 300 mg) weekly on the same day (begin 2 weeks before probable exposure and continue for 8 weeks afterward). If treatment begins after exposure, double the initial dose (600 mg for adults, 10 mg/kg for children) in 2 divided doses P.O. 6 hours apart.

Extraintestinal amebiasis –

Adults: 1 g (600-mg base) chloroquine phosphate P.O. daily for 2 days; then 500 mg (300-mg base) daily for at least 2 to 3 weeks. Treatment is usually combined with an intestinal amebicide.

Children: 16 mg/kg chloroquine phosphate (10 mg/kg base) P.O. once daily for 2 to 3 weeks. Maximum dosage is 500 mg chloroquine phosphate (300-mg base) daily.

Rheumatoid arthritis and lupus erythematosus –

†Available in Canada only. ‡Available in Australia only. ◊Available OTC.

Adults: 250 mg chloroquine phosphate P.O. daily with evening meal.

ADVERSE REACTIONS

CNS: mild and transient headache, neuromyopathy, psychic stimulation, fatigue, irritability, nightmares, seizures, dizziness.
CV: hypotension, ECG changes.
EENT: *visual disturbances* (blurred vision; difficulty in focusing; reversible corneal changes; typically irreversible, sometimes progressive or delayed retinal changes, such as narrowing of arterioles; macular lesions; pallor of optic disk; optic atrophy; patchy retinal pigmentation, typically leading to blindness); ototoxicity (nerve deafness, vertigo, tinnitus).
GI: anorexia, abdominal cramps, diarrhea, nausea, vomiting, stomatitis.
Hematologic: ***agranulocytosis, aplastic anemia,*** hemolytic anemia, thrombocytopenia.
Skin: pruritus, lichen planus eruptions, skin and mucosal pigmentary changes, pleomorphic skin eruptions.

INTERACTIONS

Cimetidine: decreased hepatic metabolism of chloroquine. Monitor for toxicity.
Magnesium and aluminum salts, kaolin: decreased GI absorption. Separate administration times.

CONTRAINDICATIONS

- Contraindicated in patients with retinal or visual field changes or porphyria.
- Use with extreme caution in patients with severe GI, neurologic, or blood disorders.
- Use cautiously in patients with hepatic disease or alcoholism because drug concentrates in liver, and in those with G6PD deficiency or psoriasis because drug may exacerbate these conditions.

NURSING CONSIDERATIONS

- CBCs and liver function studies should be performed periodically during long-term therapy; if a severe blood disorder not attributable to the disease develops, drug may need to be discontinued.
- Overdose can quickly lead to toxic symptoms: headache, drowsiness, visual disturbances, cardiovascular collapse, and seizures, followed by cardiopulmonary arrest. Children are extremely susceptible to toxicity; avoid long-term treatment.
- Baseline and periodic ophthalmic examinations needed. Tell the patient to report blurred vision, increased sensitivity to light, or muscle weakness. Check periodically for ocular muscle weakness after long-term use. Audiometric examinations recommended before, during, and after therapy, especially if long-term.
- To enhance compliance for prophylaxis, the patient should take drug immediately before or after meals on same day each week.
- To avoid exacerbated drug-induced dermatoses, the patient should avoid excessive sun exposure.

hydroxychloroquine sulfate

Plaquenil

Pregnancy Risk Category: C

HOW SUPPLIED

Tablets: 200 mg (150-mg base)

ACTION

Mechanism: May bind to and alter the properties of DNA in susceptible organisms.
Peak: Plasma levels peak within 1 to 2 hours. **Duration:** elimination half-life, 3 to 5 days.

INDICATIONS & DOSAGE

Suppressive prophylaxis of malaria attacks caused by Plasmodium vivax,

P. malariae, P. ovale, *and susceptible strains of* P. falciparum –
Adults and children: for suppression – 5 mg (base)/kg P.O. (not to exceed 310 mg) weekly on same day of the week (begin 2 weeks before entering and continue for 8 weeks after leaving endemic area). If not started before exposure, double initial dose (620 mg for adults, 10 mg/kg for children) in 2 divided doses P.O. 6 hours apart.
Acute malarial attacks –
Adults and children over 15 years: initially, 800 mg (sulfate) P.O., then 400 mg after 6 to 8 hours, then 400 mg daily for 2 days (total 2 g sulfate salt).
Children 11 to 15 years: 600 mg (sulfate) P.O. immediately, then 200 mg 8 hours later, and 200 mg 24 hours later (total 1 g sulfate salt).
Children 6 to 10 years: 400 mg (sulfate) P.O. immediately, then 2 doses of 200 mg at 8-hour intervals (total 800 mg sulfate salt).
Children 2 to 5 years: 400 mg (sulfate) P.O. immediately, then 200 mg 8 hours later (total 600 mg sulfate salt).
Children under 2 years: 100 mg (sulfate) P.O. immediately; then 3 doses of 100 mg 6 to 9 hours apart (total 400 mg sulfate salt).
Lupus erythematosus (chronic discoid and systemic) –
Adults: 400 mg P.O. daily or b.i.d., continued for several weeks or months, depending on response. Prolonged maintenance dosage – 200 to 400 mg P.O. daily.
Rheumatoid arthritis –
Adults: initially, 400 to 600 mg P.O. daily. When good response occurs (usually in 4 to 12 weeks), cut dosage in half.

ADVERSE REACTIONS

CNS: irritability, nightmares, ataxia, seizures, psychic stimulation, toxic psychosis, vertigo, nystagmus, lassitude, fatigue, dizziness, hypoactive deep tendon reflexes, skeletal muscle weakness.
EENT: visual disturbances (blurred vision; difficulty in focusing; reversible corneal changes; typically irreversible, sometimes progressive or delayed retinal changes, such as narrowing of arterioles; macular lesions; pallor of optic disk; optic atrophy; visual field defects; patchy retinal pigmentation, commonly leading to blindness), ototoxicity (irreversible nerve deafness, tinnitus, labyrinthitis).
GI: anorexia, abdominal cramps, diarrhea, nausea, vomiting.
Hematologic: ***agranulocytosis, leukopenia,*** thrombocytopenia, ***hemolysis in patients with G6PD deficiency, aplastic anemia.***
Skin: pruritus, lichen planus eruptions, skin and mucosal pigmentary changes, pleomorphic skin eruptions.
Other: weight loss, alopecia, bleaching of hair.

INTERACTIONS

Cimetidine: decreased hepatic metabolism of hydroxychloroquine. Monitor for toxicity.
Magnesium and aluminum salts, kaolin: decreased GI absorption. Separate administration times.

CONTRAINDICATIONS

- Contraindicated in patients with retinal or visual field changes or porphyria.
- *Use with extreme caution* in patients with severe GI, neurologic, or blood disorders.
- Use cautiously in patients with hepatic disease or alcoholism because drug concentrates in liver, and in those with G6PD deficiency or psoriasis because drug may exacerbate these conditions.

NURSING CONSIDERATIONS

- CBCs and liver function studies should be performed periodically during long-term therapy; if severe blood disorder not attributable to disease develops, drug may need to be discontinued.

- Overdose can quickly lead to toxic symptoms: headache, drowsiness, visual disturbances, cardiovascular collapse, and seizures, followed by cardiopulmonary arrest. Children are extremely susceptible to toxicity; avoid long-term treatment.
- Baseline and periodic ophthalmic examinations needed. Tell the patient to report blurred vision, increased sensitivity to light, or muscle weakness. Check periodically for ocular muscle weakness after long-term use. Audiometric examinations recommended before, during, and after therapy, especially if long-term.
- To enhance compliance for prophylaxis, the patient should take hydroxychloroquine immediately before or after meals on same day each week.

mefloquine hydrochloride

Lariam, Mephaquin

Pregnancy Risk Category: C

HOW SUPPLIED

Tablets: 250 mg

ACTION

Mechanism: Exact mechanism unknown. Mefloquine is a structural analogue of quinine. Antimalarial activity may be related to its ability to form complexes with hemin.

Peak: Drug is absorbed slowly; peak levels and time to peak are not known.

Duration: mean elimination half-life, about 3 weeks.

INDICATIONS & DOSAGE

Acute malaria infections caused by mefloquine-sensitive strains of Plasmodium falciparum *or* P. vivax –

Adults: 1,250 mg P.O. as a single dose. Patients with *P. vivax* infections should receive subsequent therapy with primaquine or other 8-aminoquinolines to avoid relapse after treatment of the initial infection.

Malaria prophylaxis –

Adults: 250 mg P.O. once weekly. Initiate prophylaxis 1 week before entering endemic area, and continue for 4 weeks after return from such areas. After the patient returns to an area without malaria after a prolonged stay in an endemic area, prophylaxis ends after three doses.

ADVERSE REACTIONS

CNS: dizziness, syncope, headache, transient emotional disturbances (rare).

CV: extrasystoles.

EENT: tinnitus.

GI: loss of appetite, vomiting, *nausea,* loose stools, diarrhea, GI discomfort.

Skin: rash.

Other: fatigue, fever, chills.

INTERACTIONS

Quinine, chloroquine: increased risk of seizures.

Quinine, quinidine, beta-adrenergic blocking agents: ECG abnormalities and cardiac arrest may occur. Avoid concomitant use.

Valproic acid: decreased valproic acid blood levels and loss of seizure control at start of mefloquine therapy. Monitor anticonvulsant blood levels.

CONTRAINDICATIONS

- Contraindicated in patients with hypersensitivity to mefloquine or related compounds.
- Use cautiously in patients with cardiac disease.

NURSING CONSIDERATIONS

- Advise the patient to take the drug on the same day of the week when using it for prophylaxis.
- Tell the patient not to take the drug on an empty stomach and always to take it with a full glass (at least 8 oz [240 ml]) of water.

• Because the health risks from concomitant administration of quinine and mefloquine are great, mefloquine therapy should not begin sooner than 12 hours after the last dose of quinine or quinidine.
• Advise patients to use caution when performing hazardous activities that require alertness and coordination because dizziness, disturbed sense of balance, and neuropsychiatric reactions may occur.
• In cases of suspected overdose, induce vomiting and seek medical advice immediately because of potential for cardiotoxicity. Animal studies reveal that mefloquine has cardiac actions similar to quinidine and quinine.
• Patients taking mefloquine prophylaxis should discontinue the drug if they notice signs or symptoms of impending toxicity, such as unexplained anxiety, depression, confusion, or restlessness.
• Periodic ophthalmic examinations are recommended in patients undergoing long-term therapy because ocular lesions have been noted in laboratory animals.
• Periodic liver function tests are recommended.
• Patients with infections caused by *P. vivax* are at high risk for relapse because the drug does not eliminate the hepatic phase (exoerythrocytic parasites). Follow-up therapy is advisable.

primaquine phosphate

Pregnancy Risk Category: D

HOW SUPPLIED
Tablets: 7.5 mg (base)‡, 15 mg (base)

ACTION
Mechanism: A gametocidal drug that destroys exoerythrocytic forms and prevents delayed primary attack. Its precise mechanism of action is unknown.
Peak: Plasma levels peak about 6 hours after oral dose. **Duration:** elimination half-life, 4 to 10 hours. Plasma levels are negligible after 24 hours.

INDICATIONS & DOSAGE
Radical cure of relapsing Plasmodium vivax *malaria, eliminating symptoms and infection completely; prevention of relapse –*
Adults: 15 mg (base) P.O. daily for 14 days. (26.3-mg tablet = 15 mg of base.)

ADVERSE REACTIONS
CNS: headache.
EENT: disturbances of visual accommodation.
GI: nausea, vomiting, epigastric distress, abdominal cramps.
Hematologic: leukopenia, ***hemolytic anemia in G6PD deficiency,*** methemoglobinemia in NADH methemoglobin reductase deficiency, leukocytosis, mild anemia, ***granulocytopenia, agranulocytosis.***
Skin: urticaria.

INTERACTIONS
Magnesium and aluminum salts: decreased GI absorption. Separate administration times.
Quinacrine: enhanced toxicity of primaquine. Don't use together.

CONTRAINDICATIONS
• Contraindicated in patients with systemic diseases in which granulocytopenia may develop (such as lupus erythematosus or rheumatoid arthritis) and in those taking bone marrow suppressants and potentially hemolytic drugs.
• Use cautiously in patients with previous idiosyncratic reaction (manifested by hemolytic anemia, methemoglobinemia, or leukopenia); in those with a family or personal history of favism; and in those with erythrocytic G6PD deficiency or

NADH methemoglobin reductase deficiency.

NURSING CONSIDERATIONS

- Use with a fast-acting antimalarial, such as chloroquine. Use full dose to reduce possibility of drug-resistant strains.
- Light-skinned patients taking more than 30 mg (base) daily, dark-skinned patients taking more than 15 mg (base) daily, and patients with severe anemia or suspected sensitivity should have frequent blood studies and urine examinations.
- Sudden fall in hemoglobin concentration, erythrocyte or leukocyte count, or marked darkening of the urine suggests impending hemolytic reactions. Discontinue drug immediately and notify the doctor.
- Administer drug with meals.

---

pyrimethamine

Daraprim

pyrimethamine with sulfadoxine

Fansidar

Pregnancy Risk Category: C

HOW SUPPLIED

pyrimethamine

Tablets: 25 mg

pyrimethamine with sulfadoxine

Tablets: pyrimethamine 25 mg, sulfadoxine 500 mg

ACTION

Mechanism: Inhibits the enzyme dihydrofolate reductase, thereby impeding reduction of dihydrofolic acid to tetrahydrofolic acid. Sulfadoxine competitively inhibits use of PABA.

Peak: When administered alone, pyrimethamine serum levels peak 2 to 6 hours after oral dose. When given as the combination product, pyrimethamine levels peak 1½ to 8 hours and sulfadoxine levels peak 2½ to 6 hours after oral dose. **Duration:** plasma half-life of pyrimethamine, about 4½ days; of sulfadoxine, about 7 days.

INDICATIONS & DOSAGE

Malaria prophylaxis and transmission control (pyrimethamine) –
Adults and children over 10 years: 25 mg P.O. weekly.
Children 4 to 10 years: 12.5 mg P.O. weekly.
Children under 4 years: 6.25 mg P.O. weekly.

Continue in all age-groups at least 10 weeks after leaving endemic areas.

Acute attacks of malaria (Fansidar) –
Adults: 2 to 3 tablets as a single dose, either alone or in sequence with quinine or primaquine.
Children 9 to 14 years: 2 tablets.
Children 4 to 8 years: 1 tablet.
Children under 4 years: ½ tablet.

Malaria prophylaxis (Fansidar) –
Adults: 1 tablet weekly, or 2 tablets q 2 weeks.
Children 9 to 14 years: ¾ tablet weekly, or 1½ tablets q 2 weeks.
Children 4 to 8 years: ½ tablet weekly, or 1 tablet q 2 weeks.
Children under 4 years: ¼ tablet weekly, or ½ tablet q 2 weeks.

Acute attacks of malaria (pyrimethamine) –
Adults and children over 15 years: 25 mg P.O. daily for 2 days.
Children under 15 years: 12.5 mg P.O. daily for 2 days.
Not recommended alone in nonimmune patients; use with faster-acting antimalarials, such as chloroquine, for 2 days to initiate transmission control and suppressive cure.

Toxoplasmosis (pyrimethamine) –
Adults: initially, 100 mg P.O., then 25 mg P.O. daily for 4 to 5 weeks; at the same time give 1 g sulfadiazine P.O. q 6 hours.
Children: initially, 1 mg/kg P.O. (not to exceed 100 mg) in two equally divided doses for 2 to 4 days, then 0.5 mg/kg daily for 4 weeks, along with

100 mg sulfadiazine/kg P.O. daily, divided q 6 hours.

ADVERSE REACTIONS

CNS: stimulation and seizures (acute toxicity).
GI: anorexia, vomiting, diarrhea, atrophic glossitis.
Hematologic: ***agranulocytosis, aplastic anemia,*** megaloblastic anemia, bone marrow suppression, leukopenia, thrombocytopenia, pancytopenia.
Skin: rash, ***erythema multiforme (Stevens-Johnson syndrome), toxic epidermal necrolysis.***

INTERACTIONS

Folic acid and PABA: decreased antitoxoplasmic effects. May require dosage adjustment.
Sulfonamides, co-trimoxazole, methotrexate: additive adverse effects. Don't use together.

CONTRAINDICATIONS

- Pyrimethamine is contraindicated in patients with hypersensitivity to the drug, and in patients with megaloblastic anemia caused by folic acid deficiency. Fansidar is contraindicated in patients with porphyria because it contains sulfadoxine, a sulfonamide.
- Use cautiously in patients with impaired hepatic or renal function, severe allergy or bronchial asthma, or G6PD deficiency.
- Pyrimethamine alone is not useful in chloroquine-resistant malaria; use the combination drug with sulfadoxine (Fansidar). Use cautiously in patients with seizure disorders; smaller doses may be needed. Also use cautiously after treatment with chloroquine.

NURSING CONSIDERATIONS

- Warn patients taking Fansidar to stop drug and notify doctor at first sign of skin rash.
- Give with meals to minimize GI distress.
- Dosages required to treat toxoplasmosis approach toxic levels. Twice-weekly blood counts, including platelets, are required. If signs of folic acid or folinic acid deficiency develop, dosage should be reduced or discontinued while the patient receives parenteral folinic acid (leucovorin) until blood counts become normal.
- When used to treat toxoplasmosis in patients with AIDS, therapy may need to be continued for several months. Chronic suppressive therapy for the lifetime of the patient may also be necessary.
- The first prophylactic dose of Fansidar should be taken 1 to 2 days before traveling to an endemic area.
- Because of the possibility of severe skin reactions, Fansidar should be used only in regions where chloroquine-resistant malaria is prevalent and only when the traveler plans to stay in the region longer than 3 weeks.

quinine bisulfate (quinine bisulphate)

Bi-Chinine‡, Biquinate‡, Myoquin‡, Quinbisul‡

quinine sulfate (quinine sulphate)

Chinine‡, Legatrin, Novoquinine†, Quin-260, Quin-amino, Quinamm, Quinate‡, Quindan, Quinoctal‡, Quiphile, Q-vel, Sulquin‡

Pregnancy Risk Category: X

HOW SUPPLIED

bisulfate
Tablets: 100 mg, 300 mg
sulfate
Tablets: 260 mg, 325 mg◇
Capsules: 65 mg◇, 130 mg◇, 195 mg◇, 200 mg◇, 260 mg, 300 mg◇, 325 mg◇

ACTION

Mechanism: Mechanism of antiprotozoal action is unknown, but the drug is referred to as a generalized protoplasmic poison. As a muscle relaxant, quinine appears to have a direct effect on muscle fibers that decreases their response to repetitive stimulation.
Peak: Serum levels peak 1 to 3 hours after oral dose. **Duration:** plasma elimination half-life, 7 to 12 hours in healthy adults; 8 to 21 hours in adults with malaria (malaria may impair hepatic function).

INDICATIONS & DOSAGE

Malaria caused by Plasmodium falciparum *(chloroquine-resistant)*–
Adults: 650 mg P.O. q 8 hours for 10 days, with 25 mg pyrimethamine P.O. q 12 hours for 3 days and 500 mg sulfadiazine P.O. q.i.d. for 5 days.
Nocturnal leg cramps–
Adults: 260 to 300 mg P.O. h.s. or after the evening meal.

ADVERSE REACTIONS

CNS: severe headache, apprehension, excitement, confusion, delirium, syncope, hypothermia, seizures (with toxic doses).
CV: hypotension, ***CV collapse*** with overdose or rapid I.V. administration.
EENT: altered color perception, photophobia, blurred vision, night blindness, amblyopia, scotoma, diplopia, mydriasis, optic atrophy, tinnitus, impaired hearing.
GI: epigastric distress, diarrhea, nausea, vomiting.
GU: renal tubular damage, anuria.
Hematologic: hemolytic anemia, thrombocytopenia, ***agranulocytosis,*** hypoprothrombinemia.
Skin: rash, pruritus, thrombosis at infusion site.
Other: asthma, flushing.

INTERACTIONS

Antacids containing aluminum: decreased quinine absorption. Separate administration times by at least 2 hours.
Cimetidine: decreased hepatic metabolism of quinine. Monitor for toxicity.
Digoxin: serum digoxin levels may be increased. Monitor for toxicity.
Mefloquine: risk of seizures, ECG changes, and cardiac arrest. Don't use together.
Neuromuscular blockers: prolonged muscle paralysis. Monitor for respiratory distress or excessive weakness.
Oral anticoagulants: enhanced anticoagulant effect. Monitor for bleeding.
Sodium bicarbonate: elevated quinine levels caused by decreasing quinine excretion. Use together cautiously.

CONTRAINDICATIONS

- Contraindicated in patients with G6PD deficiency.
- Use cautiously in patients with cardiovascular disease.

NURSING CONSIDERATIONS

- Discontinue if any signs of idiosyncratic reaction or toxicity occur.
- Warn the patient to avoid food products (such as tonic water) that may contain the drug and to check with the doctor or pharmacist before taking any OTC medications.
- Quinine is no longer used for acute attacks of malaria caused by *P. vivax* or for suppression of malaria due to organism resistance.
- Administer after meals to minimize GI distress. Do not crush tablets because the drug is irritating to gastric mucosa.
- When parenteral therapy is necessary or when oral therapy is not feasible, quinidine gluconate may be used to treat severe *P. falciparum* malaria. Parenteral quinine is no longer commercially available.

10

Antituberculars and antileprotics

aminosalicylate sodium
capreomycin sulfate
clofazimine
cycloserine
dapsone
ethambutol hydrochloride
ethionamide
isoniazid
pyrazinamide
rifampin
streptomycin sulfate
(See Chapter 11, AMINOGLYCOSIDES.)

COMBINATION PRODUCTS
RIFAMATE: isoniazid 150 mg and rifampin 300 mg.
RIMACTANE/INH DUAL PACK: thirty 300-mg isoniazid tablets and sixty 300-mg rifampin capsules.

aminosalicylate sodium (para-amino salicylate, PAS)

Nemasol Sodium†, Sodium P.A.S., Tubasal
Pregnancy Risk Category: C

HOW SUPPLIED
Tablets: 500 mg

ACTION
Mechanism: Competitively inhibits the formation of folic acid by blocking the action of PABA.
Peak: Serum levels peak within 1 to 2 hours. **Duration:** half-life, about 1 hour.

INDICATIONS & DOSAGE
Adjunctive treatment of tuberculosis –
Adults: 3.3 to 4 g P.O. q 8 hours, or 5 to 6 g every 12 hours. Maximum daily dosage is 20 g. Must be taken with other antitubercular agents.
Children: 50 to 75 mg/kg P.O. q 6 hours or 66.7 to 100 mg/kg q 12 hours. Maximum daily dosage is 12 g. Must be taken with other antitubercular agents.

ADVERSE REACTIONS
GI: abdominal pain, nausea, vomiting, diarrhea, anorexia.
GU: crystalluria.
Hematologic: ***hemolytic anemia.***
Hepatic: ***hepatitis.***
Skin: rash.
Other: hypersensitivity reactions (eosinophilia, joint pain, fever), mononucleosis-like syndrome, goiter or myxedema (with long-term therapy).

INTERACTIONS
Aminobenzoate derivatives: decreased absorption of aminosalicylate sodium from the GI tract. Avoid concomitant use.
Cyanocobalamin (vitamin B_{12}): decreased absorption of vitamin B_{12} from the GI tract. Provide parenteral supplement as ordered.
Rifampin: may impair the absorption of rifampin. Separate administration times by at least 6 hours.
Probenecid, sulfinpyrazone: decreased excretion of aminosalicylate sodium, resulting in toxicity. Monitor closely.
Warfarin, other anticoagulants: enhanced anticoagulant effect. Monitor for bleeding.

CONTRAINDICATIONS
• Contraindicated in patients with hypersensitivity to the drug, other salicylates, or sulfonamides.
• Use cautiously in patients with peptic ulcer or other GI disease, and in patients with CHF. Also use cautiously in patients who may become pregnant because the drug may be te-

ratogenic. Aminosalicylate is excreted in breast milk.

NURSING CONSIDERATIONS

- Advise the patient to take the drug with meals or antacids to minimize GI adverse effects. Children may tolerate this drug better than adults.
- Tell the patient to report back pain; pain during urination; unusual bruising or bleeding; fever or sore throat; yellow eyes, sclera, or skin; or severe joint pain.
- Store away from heat, humidity, or direct sunlight. Tell the patient not to take tablets that are discolored.
- Encourage the patient to comply with therapy, which may last several months.
- Urine glucose determinations may be false-positive with copper sulfate tests (Benedict's solution, Clinitest); glucose enzymatic tests (Clinistix, Tes-Tape) are not affected.

capreomycin sulfate

Capastat Sulfate

Pregnancy Risk Category: C

HOW SUPPLIED

Injection: 1 g/vial

ACTION

Mechanism: Unknown (bacteriostatic).
Peak: Plasma levels peak 1 to 2 hours after I.M. injection. **Duration:** plasma half-life, 4 to 6 hours.

INDICATIONS & DOSAGE

Adjunctive treatment of tuberculosis – **Adults:** 15 mg/kg/day up to 1 g I.M. daily injected deeply into large muscle mass for 60 to 120 days; then 1 g two to three times weekly for 18 to 24 months. Maximum dosage should not exceed 20 mg/kg/day. Must be given in conjunction with another antitubercular drug.

ADVERSE REACTIONS

CNS: headache, ***neuromuscular blockade.***
EENT: *ototoxicity* (tinnitus, vertigo, hearing loss).
GU: *nephrotoxicity* (elevated BUN and nonprotein nitrogen levels, casts, RBC counts, leukocytes; tubular necrosis; proteinuria; decreased creatinine clearance).
Hematologic: eosinophilia, leukocytosis, leukopenia.
Other: hypokalemia; alkalosis; hepatotoxicity; pain, induration, excessive bleeding, and sterile abscesses at injection site.

INTERACTIONS

Nephrotoxic or ototoxic drugs such as aminoglycosides, colistin, polymyxin B, or vancomycin: increased risk of additive toxicity. Avoid concomitant use.

CONTRAINDICATIONS

- Contraindicated in patients receiving other ototoxic or nephrotoxic drugs. Drug is never given I.V. because this use may cause neuromuscular blockade.
- Use cautiously in patients with impaired renal function, history of allergies, or hearing impairment.

NURSING CONSIDERATIONS

- Considered a "second-line" drug in the treatment of tuberculosis, capreomycin should always be administered with other antitubercular agents to prevent the development of resistant organisms.
- Give deep I.M. to minimize local reactions. Apply ice to injection site p.r.n. for pain.
- Evaluate patient's hearing before begining therapy and every 1 to 2 weeks thereafter. Notify the doctor if the patient complains of tinnitus, vertigo, or hearing impairment.
- Monitor renal function before and during therapy; notify the doctor if

function decreases. In renal impairment, dosage must be reduced.
• Straw- or dark-colored solution does not indicate a loss in potency. Do not administer solutions that contain a precipitate.

clofazimine

Lamprene

Pregnancy Risk Category: C

HOW SUPPLIED
Capsules: 50 mg, 100 mg

ACTION
Mechanism: Inhibits mycobacterial growth by binding preferentially to mycobacterial DNA. Also has anti-inflammatory effects that suppress skin reactions of erythema nodosum leprosum.
Peak: Plasma levels peak 4 to 12 hours after oral dose. **Duration:** elimination half-life, about 8 days.

INDICATIONS & DOSAGE
Dapsone-resistant leprosy (Hansen's disease) –
Adults: 100 mg P.O. daily in combination with other antileprotics for 3 years. Then, clofazimine *alone,* 100 mg daily.
Erythema nodosum leprosum –
Adults: 100 to 200 mg P.O. daily for up to 3 months. Taper dosage to 100 mg daily as soon as possible. Dosages above 200 mg daily are not recommended.

ADVERSE REACTIONS
EENT: conjunctival and corneal pigmentation.
GI: *epigastric pain, diarrhea, nausea, vomiting, GI intolerance, bowel obstruction, GI bleeding.*
Skin: *pink to brownish black pigmentation, ichthyosis and dryness,* rash, itching.
Other: ***splenic infarction,*** discolored body fluids and excrement.

INTERACTIONS
Dapsone: impaired anti-inflammatory effects of clofazimine; no intervention appears necessary.
Isoniazid: may decrease skin levels and increase serum and urine levels of clofazimine. Monitor for decreased effectiveness.
Rifampin: decreased rifampin bioavailability. Monitor for decreased effectiveness.

CONTRAINDICATIONS
• Use cautiously in patients with GI dysfunction, such as abdominal pain and diarrhea.

NURSING CONSIDERATIONS
• Advise the patient to take the drug with meals.
• Doses that exceed 100 mg daily should be given for as short a period as possible and only under close medical supervision.
• If the patient complains of colic, burning abdominal pain, or any other GI symptom, report this to the doctor, who may reduce the dose or increase the interval between doses.
• Warn the patient that clofazimine may discolor skin, body fluids, and excrement. The color ranges from red to brownish black. Reassure the patient that the unsightly skin discoloration is reversible but may not disappear until several months or years after drug treatment ends.
• Recommend application of skin oil or cream to help reverse skin dryness or ichthyosis.

cycloserine

Seromycin

Pregnancy Risk Category: C

HOW SUPPLIED
Capsules: 250 mg

ACTION

Mechanism: Inhibits cell-wall biosynthesis by interfering with the bacterial use of amino acids (bacteriostatic).

Peak: Serum levels peak 3 to 4 hours after oral dose. **Duration:** elimination half-life, about 10 hours.

INDICATIONS & DOSAGE

Adjunctive treatment in pulmonary or extrapulmonary tuberculosis –

Adults: initially, 250 mg P.O. q 12 hours for 2 weeks; then, if blood levels are below 25 to 30 mcg/ml and no toxicity has developed, dose is increased to 250 mg q 8 hours for 2 weeks. If optimum blood levels are still not achieved, and no toxicity has developed, then dose is increased to 250 mg q 6 hours. Maximum dosage is 1 g/day. If CNS toxicity occurs, drug is discontinued for 1 week, then resumed at 250 mg daily for 2 weeks. If no serious toxic effects occur, dosage is increased by 250-mg increments q 10 days until blood level of 25 to 30 mcg/ml is obtained.

ADVERSE REACTIONS

CNS: ***seizures,*** drowsiness, headache, tremor, dysarthria, vertigo, confusion, loss of memory, ***possible suicidal tendencies*** and other psychotic symptoms, *nervousness, hallucinations, depression,* hyperirritability, paresthesia, paresis, hyperreflexia.

Other: hypersensitivity reactions (allergic dermatitis).

INTERACTIONS

Ethanol or ethionamide: increased risk of CNS toxicity (seizures).

Isoniazid: monitor for CNS toxicity (dizziness or drowsiness).

CONTRAINDICATIONS

- Contraindicated in patients with hypersensitivity to the drug and in those with seizure disorders, depression or severe anxiety, psychosis, severe renal insufficiency, or chronic alcoholism.
- Use cautiously in patients with impaired renal function; reduced dosage is required.

NURSING CONSIDERATIONS

- Considered a "second-line" drug in the treatment of tuberculosis, cycloserine should always be administered with other antitubercular agents to prevent the development of resistant organisms.
- Obtain specimen for culture and sensitivity tests before therapy begins and periodically thereafter to detect possible resistance.
- Warn the patient to avoid alcohol, which may cause serious neurologic reactions.
- Toxic reactions may occur with blood levels above 30 mcg/ml. Patients receiving high doses (more than 500 mg daily) should have periodic serum cycloserine level determinations.
- Pyridoxine, anticonvulsants, tranquilizers, or sedatives may help to relieve adverse reactions.
- Observe for psychotic symptoms, hallucinations, and possible suicidal tendencies.
- Monitor results of hematologic tests and renal and liver function studies.

dapsone

Avlosulfon†, Dapsone 100‡

Pregnancy Risk Category: C

HOW SUPPLIED

Tablets: 25 mg, 100 mg

ACTION

Mechanism: Unknown. May inhibit folic acid biosynthesis in susceptible organisms (bacteriostatic).

Peak: Plasma levels peak 4 to 12 hours after oral dose. **Duration:** elimination half-life, about 8 days.

INDICATIONS & DOSAGE
All forms of leprosy (Hansen's disease) –
Adults: 100 mg P.O. daily, indefinitely; give with rifampin 600 mg daily for 6 months.
Children: 1.4 mg/kg P.O. daily.
Dermatitis herpetiformis –
Adults: 50 mg P.O. daily; may increase to 400 mg daily.
Malaria suppression or prophylaxis for chloroquine-resistant Plasmodium falciparum *when other drugs aren't available* –
Adults: 100 mg P.O. weekly; usually given with pyrimethamine 12.5 mg P.O. weekly.
Children: 2 mg/kg P.O. weekly, with pyrimethamine 0.25 mg/kg P.O. weekly.

Continue prophylaxis during exposure and for 6 weeks afterward.
Pneumocystis carinii *pneumonia in patients with AIDS* –
Adults: 100 mg P.O. daily, with trimethoprim 20 mg/kg P.O. daily (usually divided q.i.d.).
Actinomycotic mycetoma –
Adults: 100 mg P.O. b.i.d. Treatment is usually continued for months after clinical symptoms abate.

ADVERSE REACTIONS
CNS: insomnia, psychosis, headache, dizziness, lethargy, severe malaise, paresthesia, peripheral neuropathy (with loss of motor function).
EENT: tinnitus, allergic rhinitis.
GI: anorexia, abdominal pain, nausea, vomiting.
Hematologic: ***aplastic anemia, agranulocytosis, hemolytic anemia,*** methemoglobinemia, possible leukopenia.
Hepatic: hepatitis, cholestatic jaundice.
Skin: allergic dermatitis (generalized or fixed maculopapular rash).

INTERACTIONS
Folic acid antagonists, such as methotrexate: increased risk of adverse hematologic reactions. Avoid concomitant use.
Probenecid: elevated levels of dapsone. Use together with extreme caution.
Rifampin: increased hepatic metabolism of dapsone. Monitor for lack of efficacy.

CONTRAINDICATIONS
- Contraindicated in patients with hypersensitivity to the drug.
- Use cautiously in patients with chronic renal, hepatic, or CV disease; refractory types of anemia; and G6PD deficiency.

NURSING CONSIDERATIONS
- Therapy should be interrupted if generalized, diffuse dermatitis occurs.
- Dapsone dosage should be reduced or temporarily discontinued if hemoglobin falls below 9 g/dl; if WBC count falls below 5,000/mm³; or if RBC count falls below 2.5 million/mm³ or remains low.
- Antihistamines may help to combat dapsone-induced allergic dermatitis.
- Erythema nodosum reaction may occur during therapy as a result of *Mycobacterium leprae* bacilli (malaise, fever, painful inflammatory induration in the skin and mucosa, iritis, and neuritis). In severe cases, therapy should be stopped and glucocorticoids given cautiously.
- Obtain CBC before therapy and monitor weekly for the first month, monthly for 6 months, and semiannually thereafter.
- Dapsone is also used investigationally to treat rheumatoid arthritis, allergic vasculitis, and pustular and inflammatory dermatoses.
- Instruct breast-feeding patients to report cyanosis in infants, which indicates high sulfone level.

ethambutol hydrochloride

Etibi†, Myambutol

Pregnancy Risk Category: B

HOW SUPPLIED

Tablets: 100 mg, 400 mg

ACTION

Mechanism: Interferes with the synthesis of one or more metabolites of susceptible bacteria, altering cellular metabolism during cell division (bacteriostatic).
Peak: Plasma levels peak within 3 hours of oral dose. **Duration:** elimination half-life, about 3 hours.

INDICATIONS & DOSAGE

Adjunctive treatment in pulmonary tuberculosis –
Adults and children over 13 years: for patients who have not received previous antitubercular therapy, 15 mg/kg P.O. daily in a single dose.
Re-treatment: 25 mg/kg P.O. daily in a single dose for 60 days with at least one other antitubercular drug; then decrease to 15 mg/kg/day in a single dose.

ADVERSE REACTIONS

CNS: headache, dizziness, mental confusion, possible hallucinations, peripheral neuritis (numbness and tingling of extremities).
EENT: optic neuritis (vision loss and loss of color discrimination, especially red and green).
GI: anorexia, nausea, vomiting, abdominal pain.
Other: ***anaphylactoid reactions,*** fever, malaise, bloody sputum, *elevated uric acid level.*

INTERACTIONS

None significant.

CONTRAINDICATIONS

- Contraindicated in patients with optic neuritis and in children under 13 years. Also contraindicated in patients with severe hepatic impairment and in patients with hypersensitivity to the drug.
- Use cautiously in patients with impaired renal function, cataracts, recurrent eye inflammations, gout, and diabetic retinopathy.

NURSING CONSIDERATIONS

- Reduce dosage in patients with impaired renal function.
- Ethambutol should always be administered with other antitubercular agents to prevent the development of resistant organisms.
- Monitor AST and ALT levels before therapy and every 2 to 4 weeks during treatment.
- Always monitor serum uric acid level; observe the patient for symptoms of gout.
- Perform visual acuity and color discrimination tests before and during therapy.
- Reassure the patient that visual disturbances will disappear several weeks to months after drug is stopped.

ethionamide

Trecator-SC

Pregnancy Risk Category: D

HOW SUPPLIED

Tablets: 250 mg

ACTION

Mechanism: Unknown. Probably inhibits peptide synthesis.
Peak: Plasma levels peak within 3 hours of oral dose. **Duration:** elimination half-life, 3 hours.

INDICATIONS & DOSAGE

Adjunctive treatment in pulmonary or extrapulmonary tuberculosis (when primary therapy with streptomycin or isoniazid cannot be used or has failed) –

Adults: 500 mg to 1 g P.O. daily in divided doses. Concomitant administration of other antitubercular drugs and pyridoxine recommended.
Children: 15 to 20 mg/kg P.O. daily in three to four doses. Maximum dosage is 1 g daily.
Adjunctive treatment of borderline or lepromatous leprosy –
Adults: 250 to 500 mg P.O. daily.
Children: 4 to 5 mg/kg P.O. daily.

ADVERSE REACTIONS

CNS: asthenia, drowsiness, *peripheral neuritis,* psychic disturbances (especially mental depression).
CV: postural hypotension.
GI: *anorexia,* metallic taste, nausea, vomiting, sialorrhea, *epigastric distress,* diarrhea, stomatitis, weight loss.
Hematologic: thrombocytopenia.
Hepatic: jaundice, hepatitis, elevated AST and ALT.
Skin: rash, ***exfoliative dermatitis.***

INTERACTIONS

None significant.

CONTRAINDICATIONS

- Contraindicated in patients with severe liver damage.
- Use cautiously in patients with diabetes mellitus.

NURSING CONSIDERATIONS

- Ethionamide should always be administered with other antitubercular agents to prevent the development of resistant organisms.
- Culture and sensitivity tests should be performed before starting therapy.
- Withhold drug if skin rash occurs; may progress to exfoliative dermatitis.
- Monitor hepatic function every 2 to 4 weeks.
- Give with meals or antacids to minimize GI effects. The patient may require an antiemetic.
- Pyridoxine may be ordered to prevent neuropathy.
- Instruct the patient to take this drug exactly as prescribed; warn against discontinuing drug without the doctor's consent.
- Warn against excess alcohol ingestion, which may make the patient more vulnerable to liver damage.

isoniazid (isonicotinic acid hydride, INH)

Isotamine†, Laniazid, Nydrazid**, PMS-Isoniazid†, Tubizid

Pregnancy Risk Category: C

HOW SUPPLIED

Tablets: 50 mg, 100 mg, 300 mg
Oral solution: 50 mg/5 ml
Injection: 100 mg/ml

ACTION

Mechanism: Inhibits cell-wall biosynthesis by interfering with lipid and DNA synthesis (bactericidal).
Peak: Plasma levels peak within 1 to 2 hours of oral or I.M. administration. **Duration:** plasma half-life, 1 to 4 hours, depending on individual metabolism.

INDICATIONS & DOSAGE

Actively growing tubercle bacilli –
Adults: 5 mg/kg P.O. or I.M. daily in a single dose, up to 300 mg/day, continued for 6 months to 2 years.
Infants and children: 10 to 20 mg/kg P.O. or I.M. daily in a single dose, up to 300 to 500 mg/day, continued for 18 months to 2 years. Concomitant administration of at least one other antitubercular drug is recommended.
Prevention of tubercle bacilli in those closely exposed to tuberculosis or those with positive skin test whose chest X-rays and bacteriologic studies are consistent with nonprogressive tuberculosis –
Adults: 300 mg P.O. daily in a single dose, continued for 1 year.

Infants and children: 10 mg/kg P.O. daily in a single dose, up to 300 mg/day, continued for 1 year.

ADVERSE REACTIONS

CNS: *peripheral neuropathy* (especially in patients who are malnourished, alcoholic, diabetic, or slow acetylators), usually preceded by paresthesia of hands and feet; psychosis.
GI: nausea, vomiting, epigastric distress, constipation, mouth dryness.
Hematologic: ***agranulocytosis, hemolytic anemia, aplastic anemia,*** eosinophilia, leukopenia, neutropenia, thrombocytopenia, methemoglobinemia, pyridoxine-responsive hypochromic anemia.
Hepatic: hepatitis, occasionally severe and sometimes fatal, especially in elderly patients.
Other: rheumatic syndrome and lupuslike syndrome, hypersensitivity reactions (fever, rash, lymphadenopathy, vasculitis), hyperglycemia, metabolic acidosis, irritation at I.M. injection site.

INTERACTIONS

Aluminum-containing antacids and laxatives: may decrease the rate and amount of isoniazid absorbed. Give isoniazid at least 1 hour before antacid or laxative.
Carbamazepine: increased risk of isoniazid hepatotoxicity. Use together cautiously.
Corticosteroids: may decrease therapeutic effectiveness of isoniazid. Monitor need for larger isoniazid dose.
Disulfiram: may cause neurologic symptoms, including changes in behavior and coordination. Avoid concomitant use.
Ethanol: may be associated with increased incidence of isoniazid-related hepatitis. Avoid concomitant use.
Phenytoin, carbamazepine: increased plasma levels of these anticonvulsants. Monitor closely.

CONTRAINDICATIONS

- Contraindicated in patients with acute hepatic disease or isoniazid-associated liver damage.
- Use cautiously in patients with chronic non-isoniazid-associated liver disease, seizure disorders (especially in those taking phenytoin), severe renal impairment, and chronic alcoholism and in elderly patients.

NURSING CONSIDERATIONS

- Isoniazid should always be administered with other antitubercular agents to prevent the development of resistant organisms.
- Isoniazid pharmacokinetics may vary among patients because its metabolism occurs in the liver by genetically controlled acetylation. Fast acetylators metabolize the drug up to five times as fast as slow acetylators. About 50% of blacks and whites are slow acetylators; over 80% of Chinese, Japanese, and Eskimos are fast acetylators.
- Monitor hepatic function. Tell the patient to notify the doctor immediately if symptoms of liver impairment occur (loss of appetite, fatigue, malaise, jaundice, dark urine).
- Advise the patient to avoid alcoholic beverages while taking this drug.
- Pyridoxine should be given to prevent peripheral neuropathy, especially in malnourished patients.
- Instruct the patient to take this drug exactly as prescribed; warn against discontinuing drug without the doctor's consent.
- Encourage the patient to fully comply with treatment, which may take months or years.
- Advise the patient to take with food if GI irritation occurs.
- Isoniazid is reportedly effective when used investigationally to treat arthritis and action tremor in multiple sclerosis.

*Liquid form contains alcohol.
**May contain tartrazine.

Common reactions are in italics; ***life-threatening,*** in bold italics.

pyrazinamide

PMS Pyrazinamide†, Tebrazid†, Zinamide‡

Pregnancy Risk Category: C

HOW SUPPLIED

Tablets: 500 mg

ACTION

Mechanism: Unknown (bacteriostatic).

Peak: Serum levels peak within 2 hours of oral dose. **Duration:** elimination half-life, 9 to 10 hours.

INDICATIONS & DOSAGE

Adjunctive treatment of tuberculosis (when primary and secondary antitubercular drugs cannot be used or have failed) –

Adults: 20 to 35 mg/kg P.O. daily, divided in three to four doses. Maximum dosage is 3 g daily.

ADVERSE REACTIONS

GI: anorexia, nausea, vomiting, diarrhea.

GU: dysuria.

Hematologic: sideroblastic anemia, possible bleeding tendency due to thrombocytopenia.

Other: malaise, fever, arthralgia, hepatitis, interference with control in diabetes mellitus, *hyperuricemia.*

INTERACTIONS

None significant.

CONTRAINDICATIONS

- Contraindicated in patients with severe hepatic disease.
- Use cautiously in patients with diabetes mellitus or gout.

NURSING CONSIDERATIONS

- Pyrazinamide should always be administered with other antitubercular agents to prevent the development of resistant organisms.
- Nearly 100% excreted in urine; reduced dose needed in patients with renal impairment.
- Monitor liver function studies; examine for jaundice and liver tenderness or enlargement before and frequently during therapy.
- Watch closely for signs of gout and of liver impairment (loss of appetite, fatigue, malaise, jaundice, dark urine, and liver tenderness). Notify the doctor at once.
- Question doses that exceed 35 mg/kg because they may cause liver damage.
- Monitor hematopoietic studies and serum uric acid.
- When used with surgical management of tuberculosis, start pyrazinamide 1 to 2 weeks before surgery and continue for 4 to 6 weeks postoperatively.

rifampin (rifampicin)

Rifadin, Rifadin IV, Rimactane, Rimycin‡, Rofact†

Pregnancy Risk Category: C

HOW SUPPLIED

Capsules: 150 mg, 300 mg

Injection: 600 mg

ACTION

Mechanism: Inhibits DNA-dependent RNA polymerase, thus impairing RNA synthesis (bactericidal).

Peak: Serum levels peak 2 to 4 hours after oral dose. **Duration:** plasma half-life, about 3 hours.

INDICATIONS & DOSAGE

Pulmonary tuberculosis –

Adults: 600 mg P.O. or I.V. daily in single dose 1 hour before or 2 hours after meals.

Children over 5 years: 10 to 20 mg/kg P.O. or I.V. daily in single dose 1 hour before or 2 hours after meals. Maximum dosage is 600 mg daily. Concomitant administration with other antitubercular agents is recommended.

Meningococcal carriers –

Adults: 600 mg P.O. or I.V. b.i.d. for 2 days.

Children 1 month to 12 years: 10 mg/kg P.O. or I.V. b.i.d. for 2 days, not to exceed 600 mg/day.

Neonates: 5 mg/kg P.O. or I.V. b.i.d. for 2 days.

Prophylaxis of Haemophilus influenzae *type b* –

Adults and children: 20 mg/kg P.O. daily for 4 days. Do not exceed 600 mg/day.

ADVERSE REACTIONS

CNS: headache, fatigue, *drowsiness,* ataxia, dizziness, mental confusion, generalized numbness.

GI: epigastric distress, anorexia, nausea, vomiting, abdominal pain, diarrhea, flatulence, sore mouth and tongue.

Hematologic: eosinophilia, thrombocytopenia, transient leukopenia, ***hemolytic anemia.***

Hepatic: ***serious hepatotoxicity*** as well as *transient abnormalities in liver function tests.*

Skin: pruritus, urticaria, rash.

Other: flulike syndrome, discoloration of body fluids, hyperuricemia.

INTERACTIONS

Ethanol: may increase risk of hepatotoxicity. Avoid use.

Ketoconazole, para-aminosalicylate sodium: may interfere with absorption of rifampin. Give these drugs 8 to 12 hours apart.

Probenecid: may increase rifampin levels. Use cautiously.

CONTRAINDICATIONS

- Contraindicated in patients with clinically active hepatitis.
- Use cautiously in patients with liver disease or those receiving other hepatotoxic drugs.

NURSING CONSIDERATIONS

- Concomitant treatment with at least one other antitubercular agent is recommended.
- Give 1 hour before or 2 hours after meals for optimal absorption; however, if GI irritation occurs, the patient may take rifampin with meals.
- Monitor hepatic function, hematopoietic studies, and serum uric acid.
- Watch closely for signs of hepatic impairment (loss of appetite, fatigue, malaise, jaundice, dark urine, liver tenderness). Notify the doctor if these occur.
- Rifampin is not considered a teratogen. However, it may cause hemorrhage in neonates of rifampin-treated mothers.
- Warn the patient about drowsiness and possible red-orange discoloration of urine, feces, saliva, sweat, sputum, and tears. Soft contact lenses may be permanently stained.
- Advise the patient to avoid alcoholic beverages while taking this drug because they may increase risk of hepatotoxicity.
- Rifampin increases enzyme activity in the liver; may require increased doses of warfarin, corticosteroids, oral contraceptives, and oral antidiabetic drugs. See each drug entry for specific drug interactions.
- **I.V. use:** Reconstitute vial with 10 ml of sterile water for injection to make a solution containing 60 mg/ml. Add to 100 ml of D_5W and infuse over 30 minutes, or add to 500 ml of D_5W and infuse over 3 hours. When dextrose is contraindicated, drug may be diluted with 0.9% sodium chloride injection. Do not use other I.V. solutions.

*Liver form contains alcohol. *Common* reactions are in italics; ***life-threatening,*** in bold italics.
**May contain tartrazine.

11

Aminoglycosides

amikacin sulfate
gentamicin sulfate
kanamycin sulfate
neomycin sulfate
netilmicin sulfate
streptomycin sulfate
tobramycin sulfate

COMBINATION PRODUCTS
NEOSPORIN G.U. IRRIGANT: 40 mg neomycin sulfate and 200,000 units polymixin B sulfate/ml.

amikacin sulfate

Amikin
Pregnancy Risk Category: C

HOW SUPPLIED
Injection: 50 mg/ml, 250 mg/ml

ACTION
Mechanism: Inhibits protein synthesis by binding directly to the 30S ribosomal subunit. Generally bactericidal.
Peak: Peak serum levels occur immediately after I.V. infusion, 45 minutes to 2 hours after I.M. injection. **Duration:** elimination half-life, about 3 hours; measurable serum levels persist for 8 to 12 hours.

INDICATIONS & DOSAGE
Serious infections caused by sensitive strains of Pseudomonas aeruginosa, Escherichia coli, Proteus, Klebsiella, Serratia, Enterobacter, Acinetobacter, Providencia, Citrobacter, Staphylococcus –
Adults and children: 15 mg/kg/day divided q 8 to 12 hours I.M. or I.V. infusion (in 100 to 200 ml of D_5W run in over 30 to 60 minutes). May be given by direct I.V. push if necessary.
Neonates: initially, 10 mg/kg I.M. or I.V. infusion (in D_5W run in over 1 to 2 hours), then 7.5 mg/kg q 12 hours I.M. or I.V. infusion.
Meningitis –
Adults: systemic therapy as above; may also use up to 20 mg intrathecally or intraventricularly daily.
Children: systemic therapy as above; may also use 1 to 2 mg intrathecally daily.
Uncomplicated urinary tract infections –
Adults: 250 mg I.M. or I.V. b.i.d.
In impaired renal function –
Adults: initially, 7.5 mg/kg. Subsequent doses and frequency determined by blood amikacin levels and renal function studies.

ADVERSE REACTIONS
CNS: headache, lethargy, ***neuromuscular blockade.***
EENT: *ototoxicity (tinnitus, vertigo, hearing loss).*
GU: *nephrotoxicity (cells or casts in urine, oliguria, proteinuria, decreased creatinine clearance, increased BUN and serum creatinine levels).*
Other: hypersensitivity reactions ***(anaphylaxis), hepatic necrosis.***

INTERACTIONS
Cephalothin: increased nephrotoxicity. Use together cautiously.
Dimenhydrinate: may mask symptoms of ototoxicity. Use with caution.
General anesthetics, neuromuscular blocking agents: may potentiate neuromuscular blockade.
I.V. loop diuretics (such as furosemide): increased ototoxicity. Use cautiously.
Other aminoglycosides, acyclovir, amphotericin B, cisplatin, methoxy-

flurane, vancomycin: increased nephrotoxicity. Use together cautiously. *Parenteral penicillins (such as ticarcillin):* amikacin inactivation in vitro. Don't mix together.

CONTRAINDICATIONS

• Contraindicated in patients with hypersensitivity to the drug or other aminoglycosides.
• Use cautiously in patients with impaired renal function, in neonates and infants, and in elderly patients.

NURSING CONSIDERATIONS

• Obtain specimen for culture and sensitivity tests before first dose. Therapy may begin pending results.
• Watch for superinfection (continued fever and other signs of new infections, especially of upper respiratory tract).
• If no response after 3 to 5 days, therapy may be stopped and new specimens obtained for culture and sensitivity testing.
• Peak blood levels that are above 35 mcg/ml and trough levels that are above 10 mcg/ml may be associated with higher incidence of toxicity.
• Draw blood for peak amikacin level 1 hour after I.M. injection and 30 minutes to 1 hour after infusion ends; for trough levels, draw blood just before next dose. Don't collect blood in a heparinized tube because heparin is incompatible with aminoglycosides.
• Weigh the patient and review baseline renal function studies before therapy begins.
• Monitor renal function (output, specific gravity, urinalysis, BUN and creatinine levels, and creatinine clearance). Notify the doctor of signs of decreasing renal function.
• Patient should be well hydrated while taking drug to minimize chemical irritation of the renal tubules.
• Evaluate the patient's hearing before and during therapy. Notify the doctor if the patient complains of tinnitus, vertigo, or hearing loss.
• Potency of drug is not affected if solution turns light yellow.
• **I.V. use:** After I.V. infusion, flush line with 0.9% sodium chloride solution or D_5W.
• Use preservative-free amikacin for intrathecal or intraventricular use.

gentamicin sulfate

Cidomycin†‡, Garamycin, Gentafair, Jenamicin

Pregnancy Risk Category: C

HOW SUPPLIED

Injection: 40 mg/ml (adult), 10 mg/ml (pediatric), 2 mg/ml (intrathecal)

ACTION

Mechanism: Inhibits protein synthesis by binding directly to the 30S ribosomal subunit. Usually bactericidal.
Peak: Peak serum levels occur 30 to 90 minutes after I.M. injection, immediately after I.V. infusion. **Duration:** elimination half-life, 2 to 3 hours.

INDICATIONS & DOSAGE

Serious infections caused by sensitive strains of Pseudomonas aeruginosa, Escherichia coli, Proteus, Klebsiella, Serratia, Enterobacter, Citrobacter, Staphylococcus –
Adults: 3 mg/kg daily in divided doses I.M. or I.V. infusion q 8 hours (in 50 to 200 ml of 0.9% sodium chloride solution or D_5W infused over 30 minutes to 2 hours). May be given by direct I.V. push if necessary. For life-threatening infections, the patient may receive up to 5 mg/kg daily in three to four divided doses.
Children: 2 to 2.5 mg/kg q 8 hours I.M. or by I.V. infusion.
Neonates over 1 week or infants: 2.5 mg/kg I.M. or by I.V. infusion q 8 hours.
Neonates under 1 week: 2.5 mg/kg

I.V. q 12 hours. For I.V. infusion, dilute in 0.9% sodium chloride solution or D_5W and infuse over 30 minutes to 2 hours.
Meningitis –
Adults: systemic therapy as above; may also use 4 to 8 mg intrathecally daily.
Children: systemic therapy as above; may also use 1 to 2 mg intrathecally daily.
Endocarditis prophylaxis for GI or GU procedure or surgery –
Adults: 1.5 mg/kg I.M. or I.V. 30 minutes before procedure or surgery. Maximum dosage is 80 mg. Given with ampicillin (vancomycin in penicillin-allergic patients). Repeat in 8 hours.
Children: 2 mg/kg I.M. or I.V. 30 minutes before procedure or surgery. Maximum dosage is 80 mg. Given with ampicillin (vancomycin in penicillin-allergic patients). After 8 hours, give half the initial dose.
Posthemodialysis to maintain therapeutic blood levels –
Adults: 1 to 1.7 mg/kg I.M. or by I.V. infusion after each dialysis.
Children: 2 to 2.5 mg/kg I.M. or by I.V. infusion after each dialysis.

ADVERSE REACTIONS
CNS: headache, lethargy, ***neuromuscular blockade.***
EENT: *ototoxicity (tinnitus, vertigo, hearing loss).*
GU: *nephrotoxicity (cells or casts in the urine; oliguria; proteinuria; decreased creatinine clearance; increased BUN, nonprotein nitrogen, and serum creatinine levels).*
Other: hypersensitivity reactions.

INTERACTIONS
Cephalothin: increased nephrotoxicity. Use together cautiously.
Dimenhydrinate: may mask symptoms of ototoxicity. Use with caution.
General anesthetics, neuromuscular blockers: may potentiate neuromuscular blockade.
I.V. loop diuretics (such as furosemide): increased ototoxicity. Use cautiously.
Other aminoglycosides, amphotericin B, acyclovir, cisplatin, methoxyflurane, vancomycin: increased ototoxicity and nephrotoxicity. Use together cautiously.
Parenteral penicillins (such as ampicillin and ticarcillin): gentamicin inactivation in vitro. Don't mix together.

CONTRAINDICATIONS
- Contraindicated in patients with hypersensitivity to the drug.
- Use cautiously in neonates, infants, elderly patients, and patients with impaired renal function.

NURSING CONSIDERATIONS
- Obtain specimen for culture and sensitivity tests before giving first dose.
- Watch for superinfection (continued fever and other signs of new infections, especially of upper respiratory tract).
- Therapy usually continues for 7 to 10 days. If no response occurs in 3 to 5 days, therapy may be stopped and new specimens obtained for culture and sensitivity testing.
- Peak blood levels above 12 mcg/ml and trough levels above 2 mcg/ml may be associated with higher incidence of toxicity.
- Draw blood for peak gentamicin level 1 hour after I.M. injection and 30 minutes to 1 hour after I.V. infusion; for trough levels, draw blood just before next dose. Don't collect blood in a heparinized tube because heparin is incompatible with aminoglycosides.
- Weigh the patient and review baseline renal function studies before therapy begins.
- Monitor renal function (output, spe-

cific gravity, urinalysis, BUN and creatinine levels, and creatinine clearance). Notify the doctor of signs of decreasing renal function.
• Patient should be well hydrated while taking drug to minimize chemical irritation of the renal tubules.
• Evaluate the patient's hearing before and during therapy. Notify the doctor if the patient complains of tinnitus, vertigo, or hearing loss.
• Hemodialysis (8 hours) removes up to 50% of drug from blood.
• **I.V. use:** When giving by intermittent I.V. infusion, dilute with 50 to 200 ml of D_5W or 0.9% sodium chloride injection and infuse over 30 minutes to 2 hours. After completing I.V. infusion, flush the line with 0.9% sodium chloride solution or D_5W.
• Use preservative-free formulations of gentamicin when intrathecal route is ordered.

kanamycin sulfate

Kanasig‡, Kantrex

Pregnancy Risk Category: D

HOW SUPPLIED

Capsules: 500 mg
Injection: 37.5 mg/ml (pediatric), 250 mg/ml, 333 mg/ml

ACTION

Mechanism: Inhibits protein synthesis by binding directly to the 30S ribosomal subunit. Generally bactericidal.
Peak: Peak serum levels occur immediately after I.V. infusion, 45 minutes to 2 hours after I.M. injection. Orally administered kanamycin is not absorbed. **Duration:** elimination half-life, 2 to 4 hours; measurable serum levels persist for 8 to 12 hours.

INDICATIONS & DOSAGE

Serious infections caused by sensitive strains of Escherichia coli, Proteus, Enterobacter aerogenes, Klebsiella pneumoniae, Serratia marcescens, Acinetobacter –
Adults and children with normal renal function: 15 mg/kg/day divided q 8 to 12 hours I.M. or I.V. Maximum daily dosage is 1.5 g.
Neonates: 15 mg/kg/day divided q 12 hours I.M. or I.V..
Adjunctive treatment in hepatic coma –
Adults: 8 to 12 g P.O. daily in divided doses.
Preoperative bowel sterilization –
Adults: 1 g P.O. q 1 hour for four doses, then q 4 hours for four doses; or 1 g P.O. q 1 hour for four doses, then q 6 hours for 36 to 72 hours.
Intraperitoneal irrigation –
500 mg in 20 ml sterile distilled water instilled via catheter into wound after patient has recovered from anesthesia and neuromuscular blocker effects.
Wound irrigation –
Up to 2.5 mg/ml in 0.9% sodium chloride solution.

ADVERSE REACTIONS

CNS: headache, lethargy, ***neuromuscular blockade.***
EENT: *ototoxicity (tinnitus, vertigo, hearing loss).*
GU: *nephrotoxicity (cells or casts in the urine, oliguria, proteinuria, decreased creatinine clearance, increased BUN and serum creatinine levels).*
Other: hypersensitivity reactions ***(anaphylaxis).***

INTERACTIONS

Cephalothin: increased nephrotoxicity. Use together cautiously.
Dimenhydrinate: may mask symptoms of ototoxicity. Use with caution.
General anesthetics, neuromuscular blocking agents: may potentiate neuromuscular blockade.
I.V. loop diuretics (such as furosemide): increased ototoxicity. Use cautiously.
Other aminoglycosides, acyclovir,

amphotericin B, cisplatin, methoxyflurane, vancomycin: increased nephrotoxicity. Don't use together.
Parenteral penicillins (such as ticarcillin): kanamycin inactivation in vitro. Don't mix together.

CONTRAINDICATIONS
• Contraindicated for oral use in patients with intestinal obstruction and in treatment of systemic infection. Also contraindicated in patients with hypersensitivity to the drug or other aminoglycosides.
• Use cautiously in patients with impaired renal function and in elderly patients.

NURSING CONSIDERATIONS
• Obtain specimen for culture and sensitivity tests before first dose. Therapy may begin pending results.
• Watch for superinfection (continued fever and other signs of new infection, especially of upper respiratory tract).
• If no response in 3 to 5 days, therapy may be stopped and new specimens obtained for culture and sensitivity testing.
• Peak blood levels over 30 mcg/ml and trough levels over 10 mcg/ml may be associated with increased incidence of toxicity.
• Weigh the patient and review baseline renal function studies before therapy.
• Monitor renal function (output, specific gravity, urinalysis, BUN and creatinine levels, and creatinine clearance). Notify the doctor of signs of decreasing renal function.
• Patient should be well hydrated while taking drug to minimize chemical irritation of the renal tubules.
• Evaluate the patient's hearing before and during therapy. Notify the doctor if the patient complains of tinnitus, vertigo, or hearing loss.
• **I.V. use:** Dilute 500 mg of the drug per 200 ml of 0.9% sodium chloride solution or D_5W and infuse over 30 to 60 minutes.
• For I.M. administration, inject deeply into upper outer quadrant of buttocks. Rotate injection sites.

neomycin sulfate

Mycifradin, Neosulf‡

Pregnancy Risk Category: C

HOW SUPPLIED
Tablets: 500 mg
Oral solution: 125 mg/5 ml

ACTION
Mechanism: Inhibits protein synthesis by binding directly to the 30S ribosomal subunit. Generally bactericidal.
Peak: Only small amounts are absorbed after oral administration; peak plasma levels occur in 1 to 4 hours.
Duration: elimination half-life, 2 to 3 hours; usually detectable in plasma for about 8 hours.

INDICATIONS & DOSAGE
Infectious diarrhea caused by enteropathogenic Escherichia coli –
Adults: 50 mg/kg daily P.O. in four divided doses for 2 to 3 days.
Children: 50 to 100 mg/kg daily P.O. divided q 4 to 6 hours for 2 to 3 days.
Suppression of intestinal bacteria preoperatively –
Adults: 1 g P.O. q 1 hour for four doses, then 1 g q 4 hours for the balance of the 24 hours. A saline cathartic should precede therapy.
Children: 40 to 100 mg/kg daily P.O. divided q 4 to 6 hours. First dose should follow saline cathartic.
Adjunctive treatment in hepatic coma –
Adults: 1 to 3 g P.O. q.i.d. for 5 to 6 days; or 200 ml of 1% solution or 100 ml of 2% solution as enema retained for 20 to 60 minutes q 6 hours.

ADVERSE REACTIONS
CNS: headache, lethargy.
EENT: *ototoxicity (tinnitus, vertigo, hearing loss).*
GI: nausea, vomiting.
GU: *nephrotoxicity (cells or casts in the urine, oliguria, proteinuria, decreased creatinine clearance, increased BUN and serum creatinine levels).*
Skin: rash, urticaria.
Other: hypersensitivity reactions ***(anaphylaxis).***

INTERACTIONS
Cephalothin: increased nephrotoxicity. Use together cautiously.
Dimenhydrinate: may mask symptoms of ototoxicity. Use with caution.
I.V. loop diuretics (such as furosemide): increased ototoxicity. Use cautiously.
Oral anticoagulants: inhibited vitamin K-producing bacteria; may potentiate anticoagulant effect.
Other aminoglycosides, acyclovir, amphotericin B, cisplatin, methoxyflurane, vancomycin: increased nephrotoxicity. Use together cautiously.

CONTRAINDICATIONS
- Contraindicated in patients with intestinal obstruction. Also contraindicated with patients with hypersensitivity to other aminoglycosides.
- Use cautiously in patients with impaired renal function or ulcerative bowel lesions, and in elderly patients. Never administer parenterally.

NURSING CONSIDERATIONS
- The ototoxic and nephrotoxic properties of neomycin limit its usefulness. Limited absorption prevents substantial systemic effects.
- Neomycin is nonabsorbable at recommended dosage. However, more than 4 g/day may be systemically absorbed and lead to nephrotoxicity.
- Watch for superinfection (fever or other signs of new infection).
- Monitor renal function (output, specific gravity, urinalysis, BUN and creatinine levels, and creatinine clearance). Notify the doctor of signs of decreasing renal function.
- Patient should be well hydrated while taking drug to minimize chemical irritation of the renal tubules.
- Watch for respiratory depression in patients with renal disease, hypocalcemia, or neuromuscular diseases such as myasthenia gravis.
- Evaluate hearing of the patient with hepatic or renal disease before and during prolonged therapy. Notify the doctor if the patient complains of tinnitus, vertigo, or hearing loss. Onset of deafness may occur several weeks after drug is stopped.
- As adjunctive treatment of hepatic coma, neomycin is used to decrease ammonia-producing flora in the GI tract. During such treatment, decrease the patient's dietary protein and assess neurologic status frequently.
- For preoperative disinfection, provide a low-residue diet and a cathartic immediately before oral administration of neomycin.
- Available in combination with polymyxin B as a urinary bladder irrigant.

netilmicin sulfate
Netromycin
Pregnancy Risk Category: C

HOW SUPPLIED
Injection: 10 mg/ml, 25 mg/ml, 100 mg/ml

ACTION
Mechanism: Inhibits protein synthesis by binding directly to the 30S ribosomal subunit. Generally bactericidal.
Peak: Peak serum levels occur immediately after I.V. infusion, 30 minutes to 1 hour after I.M. injection. **Duration:** elimination half-life, 2 to 2½

hours; measurable serum levels persist for 8 to 12 hours.

INDICATIONS & DOSAGE

Serious infections caused by sensitive strains of Pseudomonas aeruginosa, Escherichia coli, Proteus, Klebsiella, Serratia, Enterobacter, Citrobacter, Staphylococcus –

Adults and children over age 12: 3 to 6.5 mg/kg/day by I.M. injection or I.V. infusion. May be given q 12 hours to treat serious urinary tract infections and q 8 to 12 hours to treat serious systemic infections.

Infants and children age 6 weeks to 12: 5.5 to 8 mg/kg/day by I.M. injection or I.V. infusion given either as 1.8 to 2.7 mg/kg q 8 hours or as 2.7 to 4 mg/kg q 12 hours.

Neonates under age 6 weeks: 4 to 6.5 mg/kg/day by I.M. injection or I.V. infusion given as 2 to 3.25 mg/kg q 12 hours.

ADVERSE REACTIONS

CNS: headache, lethargy, ***neuromuscular blockade.***

EENT: *ototoxicity (tinnitus, vertigo, hearing loss).*

GU: *nephrotoxicity (cells or casts in the urine; oliguria; proteinuria; decreased creatinine clearance; increased BUN, nonprotein nitrogen, and serum creatinine levels).*

Other: hypersensitivity reactions ***(anaphylaxis).***

INTERACTIONS

Cephalothin: increased nephrotoxicity. Use together cautiously.

Dimenhydrinate: may mask symptoms of ototoxicity. Use cautiously.

General anesthetics, neuromuscular blocking agents: may potentiate neuromuscular blockade.

I.V. loop diuretics (such as furosemide): increased ototoxicity. Use cautiously.

Other aminoglycosides, acyclovir, amphotericin B, cisplatin, methoxyflurane, vancomycin: increased nephrotoxicity. Use together cautiously.

Parenteral penicillins (such as ticarcillin): netilmicin inactivation. Don't mix together.

CONTRAINDICATIONS

- Contraindicated in patients with hypersensitivity to the drug or other aminoglycosides.
- Use cautiously in patients with impaired renal function and in neonates, infants, and elderly patients. Commercially available form contains sulfites, which may cause an allergic reaction in certain individuals.

NURSING CONSIDERATIONS

- Obtain specimen for culture and sensitivity tests before first dose. Therapy may begin pending results.
- Watch for superinfection (continued fever and other signs of new infections, especially of upper respiratory tract).
- Therapy usually continues for 7 to 10 days. If no response occurs in 3 to 5 days, therapy may be stopped and new specimens obtained for culture and sensitivity testing.
- Peak blood levels above 16 mcg/ml and trough levels above 4 mcg/ml may be associated with higher incidence of toxicity.
- Draw blood for peak netilmicin level 1 hour after I.M. injection and 30 minutes to 1 hour after infusion ends; for trough levels, draw blood just before next dose. Don't draw blood in a heparinized tube because heparin is incompatible with aminoglycosides.
- Weigh the patient and review baseline renal function studies before therapy begins.
- Monitor renal function (output, specific gravity, urinalysis, BUN and creatinine levels, and creatinine clearance). Notify the doctor of signs of decreasing renal function.
- Patient should be well hydrated

while taking drug to minimize chemical irritation of the renal tubules.
• Evaluate the patient's hearing before and during therapy. Notify the doctor if the patient complains of tinnitus, vertigo, or hearing loss. However, some studies show that this drug is less ototoxic than other aminoglycosides.
• **I.V. use:** After completing I.V. infusion, flush the line with 0.9% sodium chloride solution or D_5W.

streptomycin sulfate

Pregnancy Risk Category: D

HOW SUPPLIED
Injection: 400 mg/ml, 500 mg/ml, 1-g vial, 5-g vial

ACTION
Mechanism: Inhibits protein synthesis by binding directly to the 30S ribosomal subunit. Generally bactericidal.
Peak: Serum levels peak 1 to 2 hours after I.M. injection. **Duration:** elimination half-life, about 2 to 3 hours. Most of the drug is excreted in the urine within 12 hours.

INDICATIONS & DOSAGE
Streptococcal endocarditis –
Adults: 10 mg/kg I.M. (maximum 0.5 g) q 12 hours for 2 weeks, given with penicillin.
Primary and adjunctive treatment in tuberculosis –
Adults: 1 to 1.5 g I.M. daily for 2 to 3 months, then 1 g 2 or 3 times a week.
Children: 20 to 40 mg/kg I.M. daily in divided doses injected deeply into large muscle mass. Give concurrently with other antitubercular agents, but *not* with capreomycin. Continue until sputum specimen becomes negative.
Enterococcal endocarditis –
Adults: 1 g I.M. q 12 hours for 2 weeks, then 500 mg I.M. q 12 hours for 4 weeks, given with penicillin.
Tularemia –
Adults: 1 to 2 g I.M. daily in divided doses injected deep into upper outer quadrant of buttocks. Continue until patient is afebrile for 5 to 7 days.

ADVERSE REACTIONS
CNS: headache, ***neuromuscular blockade.***
EENT: *ototoxicity (tinnitus, vertigo, hearing loss).*
GU: some nephrotoxicity (not nearly as frequent as with other aminoglycosides).
Skin: ***exfoliative dermatitis.***
Other: pain, irritation, and sterile abscesses at injection site; hypersensitivity reactions (rash, fever, urticaria, and angioedema); ***transient agranulocytosis.***

INTERACTIONS
Cephalothin: increased nephrotoxicity. Use together cautiously.
Dimenhydrinate: may mask symptoms of streptomycin-induced ototoxicity. Use together cautiously.
General anesthetics, neuromuscular blockers: may potentiate neuromuscular blockade.
I.V. loop diuretics (such as furosemide): increased ototoxicity. Use together cautiously.
Other aminoglycosides, acyclovir, amphotericin B, cisplatin, methoxyflurane, vancomycin: increased nephrotoxicity. Use together cautiously.

CONTRAINDICATIONS
• Contraindicated in patients with hypersensitivity to the drug or other aminoglycosides, and in patients with labyrinthine disease. Never administer I.V.
• Use cautiously in patients with impaired renal function and in elderly patients.

NURSING CONSIDERATIONS

- Obtain specimen for culture and sensitivity tests before first dose except when treating tuberculosis. Therapy may begin pending results.
- Patient should be well hydrated while taking drug to minimize chemical irritation of the renal tubules.
- Evaluate the patient's hearing before, during, and 6 months after therapy. Notify the doctor if the patient complains of hearing loss, roaring noises, or fullness in ears.
- Watch for signs of superinfection (continued fever and other signs of new infections).
- Endocarditis prophylaxis is recommended for all patients with rheumatic or congenital heart disease or with prosthetic heart valve. Patients should receive prophylactic antibiotics during GI or GU procedures or surgery.
- In primary treatment of tuberculosis, streptomycin is discontinued when sputum becomes negative.
- Protect hands when preparing because drug is irritating.
- Draw blood for peak streptomycin level 1 to 2 hours after I.M. injection; for trough levels, draw blood just before next dose. Don't use a heparinized tube because heparin is incompatible with aminoglycosides.
- For I.M. administration, inject deeply into upper outer quadrant of buttocks. Rotate injection sites.

tobramycin sulfate

Nebcin

Pregnancy Risk Category: D

HOW SUPPLIED

Injection: 40 mg/ml, 10 mg/ml (pediatric)

ACTION

Mechanism: Inhibits protein synthesis by binding directly to the 30S ribosomal subunit. Generally bactericidal.

Peak: Peak serum levels occur immediately after I.V. infusion, 30 to 90 minutes after I.M. injection. **Duration:** elimination half-life, 3 hours; measurable serum levels persist for about 8 hours.

INDICATIONS & DOSAGE

Serious infections caused by sensitive strains of Escherichia coli, Proteus, Klebsiella, Enterobacter, Serratia, Staphylococcus aureus, Pseudomonas, Citrobacter, Providencia –

Adults and children: 3 mg/kg I.M. or I.V. daily divided q 8 hours. Up to 5 mg/kg daily divided q 6 to 8 hours for life-threatening infections.

Neonates under 1 week: up to 4 mg/kg I.M. or I.V. daily divided q 12 hours.

For I.V. use, dilute in 50 to 100 ml of 0.9% sodium chloride solution or D_5W for adults and in less volume for children. Infuse over 20 to 60 minutes.

ADVERSE REACTIONS

CNS: headache, lethargy, ***neuromuscular blockade.***

EENT: *ototoxicity (tinnitus, vertigo, hearing loss).*

GU: *nephrotoxicity (cells or casts in the urine, oliguria, proteinuria, decreased creatinine clearance, increased BUN and serum creatinine levels).*

Other: hypersensitivity reactions ***(anaphylaxis).***

INTERACTIONS

Cephalothin: increased nephrotoxicity. Use together cautiously.

Dimenhydrinate: may mask symptoms of ototoxicity. Use with caution.

General anesthetics, neuromuscular blocking agents: may potentiate neuromuscular blockade.

I.V. loop diuretics (such as furose-

mide): increased ototoxicity. Use together cautiously.
Other aminoglycosides, acyclovir, amphotericin B, cisplatin, methoxyflurane, vancomycin: increased nephrotoxicity. Use together cautiously.
Parenteral penicillins (such as ticarcillin): tobramycin inactivation in vitro. Don't mix together.

CONTRAINDICATIONS

- Contraindicated in patients with hypersensitivity to the drug or other aminoglycosides.
- Use cautiously in patients with impaired renal function and in elderly patients.

NURSING CONSIDERATIONS

- Obtain specimen for culture and sensitivity tests before first dose. Therapy may begin pending results.
- Weigh the patient and review baseline renal function studies before starting therapy.
- If no response occurs in 3 to 5 days, therapy may be stopped and new specimens obtained for culture and sensitivity testing.
- Monitor renal function (output, specific gravity, urinalysis, BUN and creatinine levels, and creatinine clearance). Notify the doctor of signs of decreasing renal function.
- Patient should be well hydrated while taking drug to minimize chemical irritation of the renal tubules.
- Evaluate the patient's hearing before and during therapy. Notify the doctor if the patient complains of tinnitus, vertigo, or hearing loss.
- Watch for signs of superinfection (continued fever and other signs of new infections).
- Peak blood levels over 12 mcg/ml and trough levels above 2 mcg/ml may be associated with increased incidence of toxicity.
- Draw blood for peak tobramycin level 1 hour after I.M. injection and 30 minutes to 1 hour after infusion ends; draw blood for trough level just before next dose. Don't collect blood in a heparinized tube because heparin is incompatible with aminoglycosides.
- **I.V. use:** Dilute in 50 to 100 ml of 0.9% sodium chloride solution or D_5W for adults and in less volume for children. Infuse over 20 to 60 minutes. After I.V. infusion, flush line with 0.9% sodium chloride solution or D_5W.

*Liquid form contains alcohol.
**May contain tartrazine.

Common reactions are in italics; ***life-threatening,*** in bold italics.

12

Penicillins

amoxicillin/clavulanate potassium
amoxicillin trihydrate
ampicillin
ampicillin sodium
ampicillin trihydrate
ampicillin sodium/sulbactam sodium
bacampicillin hydrochloride
carbenicillin indanyl sodium
cloxacillin sodium
dicloxacillin sodium
methicillin sodium
mezlocillin sodium
nafcillin sodium
oxacillin sodium
penicillin G benzathine
penicillin G potassium
penicillin G procaine
penicillin G sodium
penicillin V
penicillin V potassium
piperacillin sodium
piperacillin sodium and tazobactam sodium
ticarcillin disodium
ticarcillin disodium/clavulanate potassium

COMBINATION PRODUCTS

AUGMENTIN, CLAVULIN†: amoxicillin 250 mg and clavulanate potassium 125 mg per tablet; amoxicillin 500 mg and clavulanate potassium 125 mg per tablet; amoxicillin 125 mg and clavulanate potassium 31.5 mg per 5 ml oral suspension; amoxicillin 250 mg and clavulanate potassium 62.5 mg per 5 ml oral suspension; amoxicillin 125 mg and clavulanate potassium 31.5 mg per chewable tablet; amoxicillin 250 mg and clavulanate potassium 62.5 mg per chewable tablet.

POLYCILLIN-PRB: ampicillin trihydrate 3.5 g and probenecid 1 g per bottle.

PRINCIPEN WITH PROBENECID: ampicillin trihydrate 3.5 g and probenecid 1 g per 9-capsule regimen.

TIMENTIN INJECTION: ticarcillin disodium 3 g and clavulanate potassium 100 mg per vial.

UNASYN INJECTION: ampicillin sodium 1 g and sulbactam sodium 500 mg per vial; ampicillin sodium 2 g and sulbactam sodium 1 g per vial.

amoxicillin/clavulanate potassium (amoxycillin/ clavulanate potassium)

Augmentin, Clavulin†

Pregnancy Risk Category: B

HOW SUPPLIED

Tablets (chewable): 125 mg amoxicillin trihydrate, 31.25 mg clavulanic acid; 250 mg amoxicillin trihydrate, 62.5 mg clavulanic acid

Tablets (film-coated): 250 mg amoxicillin trihydrate, 125 mg clavulanic acid; 500 mg amoxicillin trihydrate, 125 mg clavulanic acid

Oral suspension: 125 mg amoxicillin trihydrate and 31.25 mg clavulanic acid/5 ml (after reconstitution); 250 mg amoxicillin trihydrate and 62.5 mg clavulanic acid/5 ml (after reconstitution)

ACTION

Mechanism: An aminopenicillin that prevents bacterial cell-wall synthesis during replication. Clavulanic acid increases amoxicillin effectiveness by inactivating beta lactamases, which destroy amoxicillin.

Peak: Serum levels of both components peak in 1 to 2½ hours. **Duration:** elimination half-life for amoxicillin, 60 to 90 minutes; for clavulanate potassium, 45 to 80 minutes.

INDICATIONS & DOSAGE
Lower respiratory infections, otitis media, sinusitis, skin and skin structure infections, and urinary tract infections caused by susceptible strains of gram-positive and gram-negative organisms –
Adults: 250 mg (based on the amoxicillin component) P.O. q 8 hours. For more severe infections, 500 mg q 8 hours.
Children: 20 to 40 mg/kg (based on the amoxicillin component) P.O. daily in divided doses q 8 hours.

ADVERSE REACTIONS
GI: *nausea,* vomiting, *diarrhea.*
Hematologic: anemia, thrombocytopenia, thrombocytopenic purpura, eosinophilia, leukopenia.
Other: hypersensitivity reactions (erythematous maculopapular rash, urticaria, ***anaphylaxis***), overgrowth of nonsusceptible organisms.

INTERACTIONS
Allopurinol: increased incidence of skin rash.
Probenecid: increased blood levels of amoxicillin and other penicillins. Probenecid may be used for this purpose.

CONTRAINDICATIONS
- Contraindicated in patients with hypersensitivity to the drug or other penicillins.
- Use cautiously in patients with other drug allergies, especially to cephalosporins (possible cross-sensitivity), and in those with mononucleosis (high incidence of maculopapular rash).

NURSING CONSIDERATIONS
- Ask the patient about any allergic reactions to penicillin. However, a negative history of penicillin allergy is no guarantee against an allergic reaction.
- Obtain specimen for culture and sensitivity tests before first dose. Therapy may begin pending results.
- Tell the patient to take entire quantity of drug exactly as prescribed, even after he feels better.
- Give with food to prevent GI distress. Incidence of adverse GI effects, especially diarrhea, is greater than with amoxicillin alone.
- With large doses and prolonged therapy, bacterial or fungal superinfection may occur, especially in elderly, debilitated, or immunosuppressed patients. Observe closely.
- Both the "250" and "500" tablets contain the same amount of clavulanic acid (125 mg). Therefore, two "250" tablets are not equivalent to one "500" tablet.
- This drug combination is particularly useful in clinical settings with high prevalence of amoxicillin-resistant organisms.
- Give drug at least 1 hour before bacteriostatic antibiotics.
- Urine glucose determinations may be false-positive with copper sulfate tests (Benedict's solution, Clinitest); glucose enzymatic tests (Clinistix, Tes-Tape) are not affected.

amoxicillin trihydrate (amoxycillin trihydrate)

Alphamox‡, Amoxil, Apo-Amoxi†, Axicillin†, Cilamox‡, Ibiamox‡, Larotid, Moxacin‡, Novamoxin†, Nu-Amoxil, Polymox, Trimox, Wymox

Pregnancy Risk Category: B

HOW SUPPLIED
Tablets (chewable): 125 mg, 250 mg
Capsules: 250 mg, 500 mg
Oral suspension: 50 mg/ml (pediatric drops), 125 mg/5 ml, 250 mg/5 ml (after reconstitution)

ACTION
Mechanism: An aminopenicillin that inhibits cell-wall synthesis during

bacterial multiplication; bacteria resist amoxicillin by producing penicillinases – enzymes that hydrolyze amoxicillin.
Peak: Serum levels peak within 1 to 2½ hours. **Duration:** plasma half-life, 60 to 90 minutes.

INDICATIONS & DOSAGE

Systemic infections, acute and chronic urinary tract infections caused by susceptible strains of gram-positive and gram-negative organisms –
Adults: 750 mg to 1.5 g P.O. daily in divided doses q 8 hours.
Children: 20 to 40 mg/kg P.O. daily in divided doses q 8 hours.
Uncomplicated gonorrhea –
Adults: 3 g P.O. with 1 g probenecid given as a single dose.
Uncomplicated urinary tract infections caused by susceptible organisms –
Adults: 3 g P.O. given as a single dose.
Endocarditis prophylaxis for dental procedures –
Adults: initially, 3 g P.O. 1 hour before procedure; then 1.5 g 6 hours later.
Children: initially, 50 mg/kg P.O. 1 hour before procedure; then half the initial dose 6 hours later.

ADVERSE REACTIONS

GI: *nausea,* vomiting, *diarrhea.*
Hematologic: anemia, thrombocytopenia, thrombocytopenic purpura, eosinophilia, leukopenia.
Other: hypersensitivity reactions (erythematous maculopapular rash, urticaria, ***anaphylaxis***), overgrowth of nonsusceptible organisms.

INTERACTIONS

Allopurinol: increased incidence of skin rash.
Probenecid: increased blood levels of amoxicillin and other penicillins. Probenecid may be used for this purpose.

CONTRAINDICATIONS

- Contraindicated in patients with hypersensitivity to the drug or other penicillins.
- Use cautiously in patients with other drug allergies, especially to cephalosporins (possible cross-sensitivity), and in those with mononucleosis (high incidence of maculopapular rash).

NURSING CONSIDERATIONS

- Ask the patient about any allergic reactions to penicillin. However, a negative history of penicillin allergy is no guarantee against an allergic reaction.
- Obtain specimen for culture and sensitivity tests before first dose. Therapy may begin pending results.
- Tell the patient to take entire quantity of medication exactly as prescribed, even after he feels better.
- Give with food to prevent GI distress.
- With large doses and prolonged therapy, bacterial or fungal superinfection may occur, especially in elderly, debilitated, or immunosuppressed patients. Observe closely.
- Warn the patient never to use leftover amoxicillin for a new illness or to share it with family and friends.
- Trimox oral suspension may be stored at room temperature for up to 2 weeks. Be sure to check individual product labels for storage information.
- Tell the patient to call the doctor if rash, fever, or chills develop. A rash is the most common allergic reaction, especially when the patient is taking allopurinol.
- Urine glucose determinations may be false-positive with copper sulfate tests (Benedict's solution, Clinitest); glucose enzymatic tests (Clinistix, Tes-Tape) are not affected.
- Give amoxicillin at least 1 hour before bacteriostatic antibiotics.

ampicillin

Ampicin†, Apo-Ampi†, Novo Ampicillin†, Nu-Ampi†, Omnipen, Penbritin†, Principen

ampicillin sodium

Ampicyn Injection‡, Omnipen-N, Polycillin-N, Totacillin-N

ampicillin trihydrate

Amcill, Ampicyn Oral‡, D-Amp, Omnipen, Penamp-250, Penamp-500, Penbritin‡, Polycillin, Principen-250, Principen-500, Totacillin

Pregnancy Risk Category: B

HOW SUPPLIED

Capsules: 250 mg, 500 mg
Oral suspension: 100 mg/ml (pediatric drops), 125 mg/5 ml, 250 mg/5 ml, 500 mg/5 ml (after reconstitution)
Injection: 125 mg, 250 mg, 500 mg, 1 g, 2 g
Infusion: 500 mg, 1 g, 2 g
Pharmacy bulk package: 10-g vial

ACTION

Mechanism: An aminopenicillin that inhibits cell-wall synthesis during microorganism multiplication; bacteria resist ampicillin by producing penicillinases – enzymes that hydrolyze ampicillin.
Peak: Peak plasma levels occur immediately after I.V. administration, within 2 hours of an oral dose. **Duration:** elimination half-life, about 1 hour.

INDICATIONS & DOSAGE

Systemic infections and acute and chronic urinary tract infections caused by susceptible strains of gram-positive and gram-negative organisms –
Adults: 1 to 4 g P.O. daily, in divided doses q 6 hours; or 2 to 12 g I.M. or I.V. daily, in divided doses q 4 to 6 hours.
Children: 50 to 100 mg/kg P.O. daily, in divided doses q 6 hours; or 100 to 200 mg/kg I.M. or I.V. daily, in divided doses q 6 hours.
Meningitis –
Adults: 8 to 14 g I.V. daily in divided doses q 3 to 4 hours.
Children: up to 300 mg/kg I.V. daily in divided doses q 3 to 4 hours.
Uncomplicated gonorrhea –
Adults: 3.5 g P.O. with 1 g probenecid given as a single dose.

ADVERSE REACTIONS

GI: *nausea,* vomiting, *diarrhea,* glossitis, stomatitis.
Hematologic: anemia, thrombocytopenia, thrombocytopenic purpura, eosinophilia, leukopenia.
Other: hypersensitivity reactions (erythematous maculopapular rash, urticaria, ***anaphylaxis***), overgrowth of nonsusceptible organisms, pain at injection site, vein irritation, thrombophlebitis.

INTERACTIONS

Allopurinol: increased incidence of skin rash.
Probenecid: increased blood levels of ampicillin and other penicillins. Probenecid may be used for this purpose.

CONTRAINDICATIONS

- Contraindicated in patients with hypersensitivity to the drug or other penicillins.
- Use cautiously in patients with other drug allergies, especially to cephalosporins (possible cross-sensitivity), or in those with mononucleosis (high incidence of maculopapular rash).

NURSING CONSIDERATIONS

- Before giving, ask the patient about any allergic reactions to penicillin. However, a negative history of penicillin allergy is no guarantee against a future allergic reaction.
- Obtain specimen for culture and

sensitivity tests before first dose. Therapy may begin pending results.
• Tell the patient to take entire quantity of medication exactly as prescribed, even after he feels better.
• Tell the patient to call the doctor if rash, fever, or chills develop. A rash is the most common allergic reaction, especially if the patient is also taking allopurinol.
• When given orally, drug may cause GI disturbances. Food may interfere with absorption; therefore, give 1 to 2 hours before or 2 to 3 hours after meals.
• Dosage should be altered in patients with impaired renal function.
• With large doses or prolonged therapy, bacterial or fungal superinfection may occur, especially in elderly, debilitated, or immunosuppressed patients. Observe closely.
• In pediatric meningitis, ampicillin may be given concurrently with parenteral chloramphenicol for 24 hours pending cultures.
• Urine glucose determinations may be false-positive with copper sulfate tests (Benedict's solution, Clinitest); glucose enzymatic tests (Clinistix, Tes-Tape) are not affected.
• Give ampicillin at least 1 hour before bacteriostatic antibiotics.
• Warn the patient never to use leftover ampicillin for a new illness or to share it with family and friends.
• **I.V. use:** For I.V. injection, reconstitute using bacteriostatic water for injection. Use 5 ml for the 125-mg, 250-mg, or 500-mg vials, 7.4 ml for the 1-g vials, or 14.8 ml for the 2-g vials. Give direct I.V. injections over 3 to 5 minutes for doses of 500 mg or less; over 10 to 15 minutes for larger doses. Don't exceed a rate of 100 mg/minute. Alternatively, dilute in 50 to 100 ml of 0.9% sodium chloride injection and give by intermittent infusion over 15 to 30 minutes. Don't mix with solutions containing dextrose or fructose because these solutions promote rapid breakdown of ampicillin.
• Initial dilution in vial is stable for 1 hour. Follow manufacturer's directions for stability data when ampicillin is further diluted for I.V. infusion.
• Give I.V. intermittently to prevent vein irritation. Change site every 48 hours.
• Don't give I.M. or I.V. unless infection is severe or patient can't take oral dose.

ampicillin sodium/ sulbactam sodium

Unasyn

Pregnancy Risk Category: C

HOW SUPPLIED

Injection: vials and piggyback vials containing 1.5 g (1 g ampicillin sodium with 0.5 g sulbactam sodium) and 3 g (2 g ampicillin sodium with 1 g sulbactam sodium)

ACTION

Mechanism: Ampicillin (an aminopenicillin) inhibits cell-wall synthesis during microorganism multiplication; sulbactam inactivates bacterial betalactamase, the enzyme that inactivates ampicillin and provides bacterial resistance to it.
Peak: Peak serum levels of both drugs occur immediately after I.V. infusion. **Duration:** elimination half-life for both drugs, about 1 hour.

INDICATIONS & DOSAGE

Intra-abdominal, gynecologic, and skin structure infections caused by susceptible strains –
Adults: dosage expressed as total drug (each 1.5-g vial contains 1 g ampicillin sodium and 0.5 g sulbactam sodium) – 1.5 to 3 g I.M. or I.V. q 6 hours. Maximum daily dosage is 4 g sulbactam (12 g of the combined drugs).

ADVERSE REACTIONS

GI: *nausea,* vomiting, *diarrhea,* glossitis, stomatitis.
Hematologic: anemia, thrombocytopenia, thrombocytopenic purpura, eosinophilia, leukopenia.
Other: hypersensitivity reactions (erythematous maculopapular rash, urticaria, ***anaphylaxis***), overgrowth of nonsusceptible organisms, pain at injection site, vein irritation, thrombophlebitis.

INTERACTIONS

Allopurinol: increased incidence of skin rash.
Probenecid: increased levels of ampicillin. Probenecid may be used for this purpose.

CONTRAINDICATIONS

- Contraindicated in patients with hypersensitivity to the drug or other penicillins.
- Use cautiously in patients with other drug allergies, especially to cephalosporins (possible cross-sensitivity), or in those with mononucleosis (high incidence of maculopapular rash).

NURSING CONSIDERATIONS

- Before giving, ask the patient about any allergic reactions to penicillin. However, a negative history of penicillin allergy is no guarantee against a future allergic reaction.
- Obtain specimen for culture and sensitivity tests before first dose. Therapy may begin pending results.
- Dosage should be altered in patients with impaired renal function.
- With large doses and prolonged therapy, bacterial or fungal superinfection may occur, especially in elderly, debilitated, or immunosuppressed patients. Observe closely.
- Urine glucose determinations may be false-positive with copper sulfate tests (Benedict's solution, Clinitest); glucose enzymatic tests (Clinistix, Tes-Tape) are not affected.
- Give drug at least 1 hour before bacteriostatic antibiotics.
- Tell the patient to call the doctor if rash, fever, or chills develop. A rash is the most common allergic reaction.
- **I.V. use:** When preparing I.V. injection, reconstitute powder with any of the following diluents: 0.9% sodium chloride solution, D_5W, lactated Ringer's injection, 1/6 M sodium lactate, dextrose 5% and 0.45% saline injection, and 10% invert sugar. Stability varies with diluent, temperature, and concentration of solution.
- After reconstitution, allow vials to stand for a few minutes for foam to dissipate. This will permit visual inspection of contents for particles.
- Give I.V. dose by slow injection (over 10 to 15 minutes), or dilute in 50 to 100 ml of a compatible diluent and infuse over 15 to 30 minutes. If permitted, give intermittently to prevent vein irritation. Change site every 48 hours.
- When giving I.V., don't add or mix with other drugs because they might prove physically or chemically incompatible.
- For I.M. injection, reconstitute with sterile water for injection or 0.5% or 2% lidocaine hydrochloride injection. Add 3.2 ml to a 1.5-g vial (or 6.4 ml to a 3-g vial) to yield a concentration of 375 mg/ml. Administer deeply.

bacampicillin hydrochloride

Penglobe†, Spectrobid

Pregnancy Risk Category: B

HOW SUPPLIED

Tablets: 400 mg
Oral suspension: 125 mg/5 ml (after reconstitution)

*Liquid form contains alcohol.
**May contain tartrazine.

Common reactions are in italics; ***life-threatening,*** in bold italics.

ACTION

Mechanism: An aminopenicillin that inhibits cell-wall synthesis during microorganism multiplication; bacteria resist bacampicillin by producing penicillinases – enzymes that hydrolyze its active form (ampicillin).
Peak: Plasma ampicillin levels peak within 30 to 90 minutes. **Duration:** elimination half-life, about 1 hour.

INDICATIONS & DOSAGE

Upper respiratory tract infections and otitis media caused by streptococci, pneumococci, staphylococci, and Haemophilus influenzae; *urinary tract infections caused by* Escherichia coli, Proteus mirabilis, *and* Enterococcus faecalis; *skin infections caused by streptococci and susceptible staphylococci –*
Adults: 400 mg P.O. q 12 hours.
Children over 25 kg: 25 mg/kg/day P.O. in divided doses q 12 hours.
Lower respiratory tract infections; other severe infections –
Adults: 800 mg P.O. q 12 hours.
Children over 25 kg: 50 mg/kg/day P.O. in divided doses q 12 hours.
Gonorrhea –
Adults: 1.6 g P.O. plus 1 g probenecid given as a single dose.

ADVERSE REACTIONS

GI: *nausea,* vomiting, *diarrhea,* glossitis, stomatitis.
Hematologic: anemia, thrombocytopenia, thrombocytopenic purpura, eosinophilia, leukopenia.
Other: hypersensitivity reactions (erythematous maculopapular rash, urticaria, ***anaphylaxis***), overgrowth of nonsusceptible organisms.

INTERACTIONS

Allopurinol: increased incidence of skin rash.
Probenecid: increased blood levels of bacampicillin or other penicillins. Probenecid may be used for this purpose.

CONTRAINDICATIONS

- Contraindicated in patients with hypersensitivity to the drug or other penicillins.
- Use cautiously in patients with other drug allergies, especially to cephalosporins (possible cross-sensitivity), or in those with mononucleosis (high incidence of maculopapular rash).

NURSING CONSIDERATIONS

- Before giving, ask the patient about any allergic reactions to penicillin. However, a negative history of penicillin allergy is no guarantee against an allergic reaction.
- Obtain specimen for culture and sensitivity tests before first dose. Therapy may begin pending results.
- Bacampicillin is especially formulated to produce high blood levels of antibiotic when administered twice daily.
- Diarrhea may occur less frequently with bacampicillin than with ampicillin.
- Tell the patient to take entire quantity of medication as prescribed, even after he feels better.
- Tell the patient to call the doctor if rash, fever, or chills develop. A rash is the most common allergic reaction.
- With large doses and prolonged therapy, bacterial or fungal superinfection may occur, especially in elderly, debilitated, or immunosuppressed patients. Observe closely.
- Warn the patient never to use leftover bacampicillin for a new illness or to share it with family and friends.
- Unlike ampicillin, bacampicillin may be taken with meals without fear of diminished drug absorption.
- Give bacampicillin at least 1 hour before bacteriostatic antibiotics.
- Urine glucose determinations may be false-positive with copper sulfate tests (Benedict's solution, Clinitest); glucose enzymatic tests (Clinistix, Tes-Tape) are not affected.

carbenicillin indanyl sodium

Geocillin, Geopen Oral†

Pregnancy Risk Category: B

HOW SUPPLIED

Tablets: 382 mg

ACTION

Mechanism: An extended-spectrum penicillin that inhibits cell-wall synthesis during microorganism multiplication; bacteria resist carbenicillin by producing penicillinases – enzymes that hydrolyze its active form.
Peak: Serum levels peak within 30 minutes; drug is undetectable in serum after 6 hours. **Duration:** elimination half-life, 45 minutes to 1 hour.

INDICATIONS & DOSAGE

Urinary tract infection and prostatitis caused by susceptible strains of gram-negative organisms –
Adults: 382 to 764 mg P.O. q.i.d.
Not recommended for children.

ADVERSE REACTIONS

GI: *nausea,* vomiting, *diarrhea, flatulence, abdominal cramps, unpleasant taste.*
Hematologic: leukopenia, neutropenia, eosinophilia, ***hemolytic anemia,*** thrombocytopenia.
Other: hypersensitivity reactions (rash, chills, fever, urticaria, pruritus, ***anaphylaxis***), overgrowth of nonsusceptible organisms.

INTERACTIONS

None significant.

CONTRAINDICATIONS

- Contraindicated in patients with hypersensitivity to the drug or other penicillins.
- Use cautiously in patients with other drug allergies, especially to cephalosporins (possible cross-sensitivity).

NURSING CONSIDERATIONS

- Before giving, ask the patient about any allergic reactions to penicillin. However, a negative history of penicillin allergy is no guarantee against a future allergic reaction.
- Obtain specimen for culture and sensitivity tests before first dose. Therapy may begin pending results.
- Use only in patients whose creatinine clearance values are 10 ml/minute or more.
- Excellent treatment for *Pseudomonas* urinary tract infections in ambulatory patients.
- May be useful in treatment of cystitis, but not pyelonephritis.
- With large doses or prolonged therapy, bacterial or fungal superinfection may occur, especially in elderly, debilitated, or immunosuppressed patients. Observe closely.
- Tell the patient to take all of the medication exactly as prescribed, even after he feels better.
- Give 1 to 2 hours before or 2 to 3 hours after meals because food may interfere with absorption.
- Tell the patient to call the doctor if rash, fever, or chills develop. A rash is the most common allergic reaction.
- Warn the patient never to use leftover carbenicillin for a new illness or to share it with family and friends.
- Urine glucose determinations may be false-positive with copper sulfate tests (Benedict's solution, Clinitest); glucose enzymatic tests (Clinistix, Tes-Tape) are not affected.
- Carbenicillin may also interfere with the direct results of Coombs' test and certain tests for serum uric acid.

cloxacillin sodium

Alclox‡, Apo-Cloxi†, Austrastaph‡, Cloxapen, Novocloxin†, Nu-Cloxi†, Orbenin†, Orbenin Injection‡, Tegopen

Pregnancy Risk Category: B

HOW SUPPLIED

Capsules: 250 mg, 500 mg
Oral solution: 125 mg/5 ml (after reconstitution)

ACTION

Mechanism: A penicillinase-resistant penicillin that inhibits cell-wall synthesis during microorganism multiplication; bacteria resist penicillins by producing penicillinases – enzymes that convert penicillins to inactive penicilloic acid. Cloxacillin resists these enzymes.
Peak: Plasma levels peak within ½ to 2 hours. **Duration:** serum half-life, 25 to 50 minutes.

INDICATIONS & DOSAGE

Systemic infections caused by penicillinase-producing staphylococci –
Adults: 1 to 2 g P.O. daily, in divided doses q 6 hours.
Children: 50 to 100 mg/kg P.O. daily, in divided doses q 6 hours.

ADVERSE REACTIONS

GI: *nausea,* vomiting, *epigastric distress, diarrhea.*
Hematologic: eosinophilia.
Other: hypersensitivity reactions (rash, urticaria, chills, fever, sneezing, wheezing, ***anaphylaxis***), intrahepatic cholestasis, overgrowth of nonsusceptible organisms.

INTERACTIONS

Probenecid: increased blood levels of cloxacillin and other penicillins. Probenecid may be used for this purpose.

CONTRAINDICATIONS

- Contraindicated in patients with hypersensitivity to the drug or other penicillins.
- Use cautiously in patients with other drug allergies, especially to cephalosporins (possible cross-sensitivity), or in those with mononucleosis (high incidence of maculopapular rash).

NURSING CONSIDERATIONS

- Before giving, ask the patient about any allergic reactions to penicillin. However, a negative history of penicillin allergy is no guarantee against a future allergic reaction.
- Obtain specimen for culture and sensitivity tests before first dose. Therapy may begin pending results.
- Tell the patient to take entire quantity of medication exactly as prescribed, even after he feels better.
- Tell the patient to call the doctor if rash, fever, or chills develop. A rash is the most common allergic reaction.
- Drug may cause GI disturbances. Food may interfere with its absorption; therefore, give 1 to 2 hours before or 2 to 3 hours after meals.
- Patient should take each dose with a full glass of water, not with fruit juice or carbonated beverage, because their acid will inactivate the drug.
- With large doses and prolonged therapy, bacterial or fungal superinfection may occur, especially in elderly, debilitated, or immunosuppressed patients. Observe closely.
- Periodically assess renal, hepatic, and hematopoietic function in patients receiving long-term therapy.
- Warn the patient never to use leftover cloxacillin for a new illness or to share it with family and friends.
- Give cloxacillin at least 1 hour before bacteriostatic antibiotics.
- Cloxacillin may falsely elevate or cause false-positive results with certain tests for urine or serum proteins.

dicloxacillin sodium

Dycill, Dynapen, Pathocil
Pregnancy Risk Category: B

HOW SUPPLIED

Capsules: 125 mg, 250 mg, 500 mg
Oral suspension: 62.5 mg/5 ml (after reconstitution)

ACTION

Mechanism: A penicillinase-resistant penicillin that inhibits cell-wall synthesis during microorganism multiplication; bacteria resist penicillins by producing penicillinases – enzymes that convert penicillins to inactive penicilloic acid. Dicloxacillin resists these enzymes.

Peak: Plasma levels peak within ½ to 2 hours. **Duration:** elimination half-life, 30 to 50 minutes.

INDICATIONS & DOSAGE

Systemic infections caused by penicillinase-producing staphylococci –

Adults: 1 to 2 g P.O. daily, in divided doses q 6 hours.

Children: 25 to 50 mg/kg P.O. daily, in divided doses q 6 hours.

ADVERSE REACTIONS

CNS: neuromuscular irritability, seizures.

GI: *nausea,* vomiting, *epigastric distress,* flatulence, *diarrhea.*

Hematologic: eosinophilia.

Other: hypersensitivity reactions (pruritus, urticaria, rash, ***anaphylaxis***), overgrowth of nonsusceptible organisms.

INTERACTIONS

Probenecid: increased blood levels of dicloxacillin and other penicillins. Probenecid may be used for this purpose.

CONTRAINDICATIONS

- Contraindicated in patients with hypersensitivity to the drug or other penicillins.
- Use cautiously in patients with other drug allergies, especially to cephalosporins (possible cross-sensitivity), or in those with mononucleosis (high incidence of maculopapular rash).

NURSING CONSIDERATIONS

- Before giving, ask the patient about any allergic reactions to penicillin. However, a negative history of penicillin allergy is no guarantee against a future allergic reaction.
- Obtain specimen for culture and sensitivity tests before first dose. Therapy may begin pending results.
- Tell the patient to take entire quantity of medication exactly as prescribed, even after he feels better.
- Tell the patient to call the doctor if rash, fever, or chills develop. A rash is the most common allergic reaction.
- Drug may cause GI disturbances. Food may interfere with absorption; therefore, give 1 to 2 hours before or 2 to 3 hours after meals.
- With large doses and prolonged therapy, bacterial or fungal superinfection may occur, especially in elderly, debilitated, or immunosuppressed patients. Observe closely.
- Periodically assess renal, hepatic, and hematopoietic function in patients receiving long-term therapy.
- Warn the patient never to use leftover dicloxacillin for a new illness or to share it with family and friends.
- Give dicloxacillin at least 1 hour before bacteriostatic antibiotics.

methicillin sodium

Metin‡, Staphcillin

Pregnancy Risk Category: B

HOW SUPPLIED

Injection: 1 g, 4 g, 6 g

I.V. infusion piggyback: 1 g, 4 g

Pharmacy bulk package: 10 g

ACTION

Mechanism: A penicillinase-resistant penicillin that inhibits cell-wall synthesis during microorganism multiplication; bacteria resist penicillins by producing penicillinases – enzymes that convert penicillins to inactive

penicilloic acid. Methicillin resists these enzymes.
Peak: Peak serum levels occur immediately after I.V. infusion, within 30 to 60 minutes of I.M. injection.
Duration: elimination half-life, 25 to 30 minutes.

INDICATIONS & DOSAGE
Systemic infections caused by penicillinase-producing staphylococci –
Adults: 4 to 12 g I.M. or I.V. daily, in divided doses q 4 to 6 hours.
Children: 100 to 300 mg/kg I.M. or I.V. daily, in divided doses q 4 to 6 hours.

ADVERSE REACTIONS
CNS: neuropathy, ***seizures with high doses***.
GI: glossitis, stomatitis.
Hematologic: ***agranulocytosis***, *eosinophilia*, hemolytic anemia, transient neutropenia.
GU: interstitial nephritis.
Other: hypersensitivity reactions (chills, fever, edema, rash, urticaria, ***anaphylaxis***), overgrowth of nonsusceptible organisms, vein irritation, thrombophlebitis.

INTERACTIONS
Probenecid: increased blood levels of methicillin and other penicillins. Probenecid may be used for this purpose.

CONTRAINDICATIONS
- Contraindicated in patients with hypersensitivity to the drug or other penicillins.
- Use cautiously in patients with other drug allergies, especially to cephalosporins (possible cross-sensitivity), and in infants.

NURSING CONSIDERATIONS
- Before giving, ask the patient about any allergic reactions to penicillin. However, a negative history of penicillin allergy is no guarantee against a future allergic reaction.
- Obtain specimen for culture and sensitivity tests before first dose. Therapy may begin pending results.
- Methicillin-resistant strains of staphylococci should be treated with vancomycin.
- Closely monitor renal function. Urinalysis should be done frequently to detect interstitial nephritis.
- Patients with high blood level of this drug may develop seizures. Institute seizure precautions.
- With large doses and prolonged therapy, bacterial or fungal superinfection may occur, especially in elderly, debilitated, or immunosuppressed patients. Observe closely.
- Periodically assess hepatic, renal, and hematopoietic function in patients receiving long-term therapy.
- Give methicillin at least 1 hour before bacteriostatic antibiotics.
- **I.V. use:** Reconstitute vials using sterile water for injection or 0.9% sodium chloride injection. For 1-g vials, use 1.5 ml of diluent; for 4-g vials, 5.7 ml of diluent; and for 6-g vials, 8.6 ml of diluent. For direct injection, further dilute each 500 mg drug with 35 ml of 0.9% sodium chloride injection and inject at a rate of 10 ml/minute into the tubing of a free-flowing compatible I.V. solution. For intermittent infusion, dilute to a maximum concentration of 2 to 20 mg/ml and infuse over 20 to 30 minutes.
- Give I.V. intermittently to prevent vein irritation. Change site every 48 hours.
- For I.M. administration, inject reconstituted drug deeply into the gluteus maximus.

mezlocillin sodium
Mezlin

Pregnancy Risk Category: B

HOW SUPPLIED
Injection: 1 g, 2 g, 3 g, 4 g

ACTION

Mechanism: An extended-spectrum penicillin that inhibits cell-wall synthesis during microorganism multiplication; bacteria resist mezlocillin by producing penicillinases – enzymes that hydrolyze mezlocillin.

Peak: Peak serum levels occur immediately after I.V. injection, within 45 to 90 minutes after I.M. injection.

Duration: elimination half-life, 40 to 80 minutes.

INDICATIONS & DOSAGE

Systemic infections caused by susceptible strains of gram-positive and especially gram-negative organisms (including Proteus *and* Pseudomonas aeruginosa*)* –

Adults: 200 to 300 mg/kg daily I.V. or I.M. in four to six divided doses. Usual dose is 3 g q 4 hours or 4 g q 6 hours. For very serious infections, administer up to 24 g daily.

Children up to 12 years: 50 mg/kg q 4 hours by I.V. infusion or direct I.V. injection.

ADVERSE REACTIONS

CNS: neuromuscular irritability.

GI: nausea, diarrhea.

Hematologic: ***bleeding with high doses,*** neutropenia, thrombocytopenia, eosinophilia, leukopenia, ***hemolytic anemia.***

Other: hypersensitivity reactions (***anaphylaxis,*** edema, fever, chills, rash, pruritus, urticaria), overgrowth of nonsusceptible organisms, *hypokalemia,* pain at injection site, vein irritation, phlebitis.

INTERACTIONS

Aminoglycoside antibiotics (such as gentamicin and tobramycin): chemically incompatible. Don't mix together in I.V. solution. Give 1 hour apart, especially in patients with renal insufficiency.

Probenecid: increased blood levels of mezlocillin. Probenecid may be used for this purpose.

CONTRAINDICATIONS

- Contraindicated in patients with hypersensitivity to the drug or other penicillins.
- Use cautiously in patients with other drug allergies, especially to cephalosporins (possible cross-sensitivity), or in those with bleeding tendencies, uremia, or hypokalemia.

NURSING CONSIDERATIONS

- Before giving, ask the patient about any allergic reactions to penicillin. A negative history of penicillin allergy, however, is no guarantee against future allergic reaction.
- Obtain specimen for culture and sensitivity tests before first dose. Therapy may begin pending results.
- Dosage should be altered in patients with impaired renal function.
- Check CBC and platelet counts frequently. Drug may cause thrombocytopenia.
- Monitor serum potassium level.
- Patients with high serum level of this drug may have seizures. Institute seizure precautions.
- Almost always used with another antibiotic, such as gentamicin.
- With large doses and prolonged therapy, bacterial or fungal superinfection may occur, especially in elderly, debilitated, or immunosuppressed patients. Observe closely.
- Compared with similar antibiotics, such as piperacillin or ticarcillin, mezlocillin is less likely to cause hypokalemia.
- Drug may be better suited for patients on sodium-free diets than is ticarcillin (contains 1.85 mEq Na/g of mezlocillin).
- Give mezlocillin at least 1 hour before bacteriostatic antibiotics.
- **I.V. use:** Reconstitute vials with at least 10 ml/g of drug using sterile water for injection, D_5W, or 0.9% so-

*Liquid form contains alcohol.
**May contain tartrazine.

Common reactions are in italics; ***life-threatening,*** in bold italics.

dium chloride injection. Solutions with a concentration not exceeding 10% may be given by direct injection over 3 to 5 minutes. Alternatively, dilute in about 50 to 100 ml of suitable I.V. solution and give by intermittent infusion over 30 minutes.

- Give I.V. intermittently to prevent vein irritation. Change site every 48 hours.
- When giving I.M., don't give more than 2 g per injection. Inject deeply and slowly (12 to 15 seconds) into the body of a large muscle.
- Mezlocillin may interfere with positive direct antiglobulin (Coomb's) test results. Drug may also interfere with certain tests for serum and urine proteins; tests that use bromphenol blue (Albustix, Albutest) are not affected.

nafcillin sodium

Nafcil, Nallpen, Unipen

Pregnancy Risk Category: B

HOW SUPPLIED

Tablets: 500 mg
Capsules: 250 mg
Oral solution: 250 mg/5 ml (after reconstitution)
Injection: 500 mg, 1 g, 2 g
I.V. infusion piggyback: 1 g, 1.5 g, 2 g, 4 g
Pharmacy bulk package: 10 g

ACTION

Mechanism: A penicillinase-resistant penicillin that inhibits cell-wall synthesis during microorganism multiplication; bacteria resist penicillins by producing penicillinases – enzymes that hydrolyze penicillins. Nafcillin resists these enzymes.
Peak: Peak serum levels occur immediately after I.V. infusion, within 30 to 60 minutes after I.M. injection, ½ to 2 hours after oral administration.
Duration: serum half-life, 30 to 90 minutes.

INDICATIONS & DOSAGE

Systemic infections caused by penicillinase-producing staphylococci –
Adults: 2 to 4 g P.O. daily, in divided doses q 6 hours; 2 to 12 g I.M. or I.V. daily, in divided doses q 4 to 6 hours.
Children: 50 to 100 mg/kg P.O. daily, in divided doses q 4 to 6 hours; 100 to 200 mg/kg I.M. or I.V. daily, in divided doses q 4 to 6 hours.

ADVERSE REACTIONS

GI: *nausea,* vomiting, diarrhea.
Hematologic: transient leukopenia, neutropenia, granulocytopenia, ***thrombocytopenia*** with high doses.
Other: hypersensitivity reactions (chills, fever, rash, pruritus, urticaria, ***anaphylaxis***), vein irritation, thrombophlebitis.

INTERACTIONS

None significant.

CONTRAINDICATIONS

- Contraindicated in patients with hypersensitivity to the drug or other penicillins.
- Use cautiously in patients with other drug allergies, especially to cephalosporins (possible cross-sensitivity), or in those with GI distress.

NURSING CONSIDERATIONS

- Before giving, ask the patient about any allergic reactions to penicillin. However, a negative history of penicillin allergy is no guarantee against a future allergic reaction.
- Obtain specimen for culture and sensitivity tests before first dose. Therapy may begin pending results.
- Tell the patient to take entire quantity of medication exactly as prescribed, even after he feels better.
- Tell the patient to call the doctor if rash, fever, or chills develop. A rash is the most common allergic reaction.
- When given orally, drug may cause GI disturbances. Food may interfere with absorption; therefore, give 1 to 2

hours before or 2 to 3 hours after meals.

• With large doses and prolonged therapy, bacterial or fungal superinfection may occur, especially in elderly, debilitated, or immunosuppressed patients. Observe closely.

• Give nafcillin at least 1 hour before bacteriostatic antibiotics.

• Nafcillin may falsely elevate or cause false-positive results with certain tests for urine or serum proteins.

• **I.V. use:** Reconstitute piggyback containers according to manufacturer's instructions. Reconstitute 500-mg, 1-g, or 2-g vials using sterile water for injection, D_5W, or 0.9% sodium chloride injection. Add 1.7 ml for each 500 mg of drug. Reconstituted drug may be given I.M. Alternatively, dilute with 15 to 30 ml of sterile water for injection or 0.45% or 0.9% sodium chloride injection, and give by direct injection into a vein or into the tubing of a free-flowing I.V. solution over 5 to 10 minutes. Or dilute drug to a concentration of 2 to 40 mg/ml and give by intermittent I.V. infusion over 30 to 60 minutes.

• Avoid continuous I.V. infusions to prevent vein irritation. Change site every 48 hours.

oxacillin sodium

Bactocill, Prostaphlin

Pregnancy Risk Category: B

HOW SUPPLIED

Capsules: 250 mg, 500 mg
Oral solution: 250 mg/5 ml (after reconstitution)
Injection: 250 mg, 500 mg, 1 g, 2 g, 4 g, 10 g
I.V. infusion: 1 g, 2 g, 4 g
Pharmacy bulk package: 4 g, 10 g

ACTION

Mechanism: A penicillinase-resistant penicillin that inhibits cell-wall synthesis during microrganism multiplication; bacteria resist penicillins by producing penicillinases – enzymes that convert penicillins to inactive penicilloic acid. Oxacillin resists these enzymes.
Peak: Peak serum levels occur immediately after I.V. infusion, within ½ to 2 hours of oral dose. **Duration:** elimination half-life, 20 to 50 minutes.

INDICATIONS & DOSAGE

Systemic infections caused by penicillinase-producing staphylococci –
Adults: 2 to 4 g P.O. daily, in divided doses q 6 hours; or 2 to 12 g I.M. or I.V. daily, in divided doses q 4 to 6 hours.
Children: 50 to 100 mg/kg P.O. daily, in divided doses q 6 hours; or 100 to 200 mg/kg I.M. or I.V. daily, in divided doses q 4 to 6 hours.

ADVERSE REACTIONS

CNS: neuropathy, neuromuscular irritability, ***seizures***.
GI: oral lesions.
GU: interstitial nephritis, transient hematuria, proteinuria.
Hematologic: granulocytopenia, thrombocytopenia, eosinophilia, ***hemolytic anemia,*** transient neutropenia.
Other: hypersensitivity reactions (fever, chills, rash, urticaria, ***anaphylaxis***), overgrowth of nonsusceptible organisms, hepatitis, elevated liver enzymes, *thrombophlebitis.*

INTERACTIONS

Probenecid: increased blood levels of oxacillin and other penicillins. Probenecid may be used for this purpose.

CONTRAINDICATIONS

• Contraindicated in patients with hypersensitivity to the drug or other penicillins.

• Use cautiously in patients with other drug allergies, especially to cephalosporins (possible cross-sensi-

*Liquid form contains alcohol. *Common* reactions are in italics; ***life-threatening,*** in bold italics.
**May contain tartrazine.

tivity), in premature neonates, and in infants.

NURSING CONSIDERATIONS

- Before giving, ask the patient about any allergic reactions to penicillin. However, a negative history of penicillin allergy is no guarantee against a future allergic reaction.
- Obtain specimen for culture and sensitivity tests before first dose. Therapy may begin pending results.
- Tell the patient to take entire quantity of medication exactly as prescribed, even after he feels better.
- Tell the patient to call the doctor if rash, fever, or chills develop. A rash is the most common allergic reaction.
- When given orally, drug may cause GI disturbances. Food may interfere with absorption; therefore, give 1 to 2 hours before or 2 to 3 hours after meals.
- Periodic liver function studies are indicated; watch for elevated AST and ALT levels.
- With large doses and prolonged therapy, bacterial or fungal superinfection may occur, especially in elderly, debilitated, or immunosuppressed patients. Observe closely.
- Give oxacillin at least 1 hour before bacteriostatic antibiotics.
- Oxacillin may falsely elevate or cause false-positive results with certain tests for urine or serum proteins.
- **I.V. use:** For direct I.V. injection, reconstitute vials with sterile water for injection or 0.9% sodium chloride injection. Use 5 ml of diluent for a 250-mg or 500-mg vial, 10 ml of diluent for a 1-g vial, 20 ml of diluent for a 2-g vial, or 40 ml of diluent for a 4-g vial. When the solution is clear, withdraw the ordered dose and inject over 10 minutes. When giving by piggyback injection, reconstitute the 1-g piggyback vial with 20 to 100 ml of diluent; reconstitute the 2-g vial with 19 to 99 ml of diluent. For intermittent infusion, further dilute the drug to a concentration of 5 to 40 mg/ml.
- To prevent vein irritation, avoid continuous infusions. Change site every 48 hours.
- Don't give I.M. or I.V. unless infection is severe or the patient can't take oral dose.

penicillin G benzathine (benzylpenicillin benzathine)

Bicillin L-A, Megacillin

Pregnancy Risk Category: B

HOW SUPPLIED

Injection: 300,000 units/ml, 600,000 units/ml

ACTION

Mechanism: A natural penicillin that inhibits cell-wall synthesis during microorganism multiplication; bacteria resist penicillins by producing penicillinases – enzymes that convert penicillins to inactive penicilloic acid.
Peak: Serum levels peak 13 to 14 hours after I.M. injection. **Duration:** detectable in serum 1 to 4 weeks after injection.

INDICATIONS & DOSAGE

Congenital syphilis –
Children under 2 years: 50,000 units/kg I.M. as a single dose.
Group A streptococcal upper respiratory infections –
Adults: 1.2 million units I.M. as a single injection.
Children over 27 kg: 900,000 units I.M. as a single injection.
Children under 27 kg: 300,000 to 600,000 units I.M. as a single injection.
Prophylaxis of poststreptococcal rheumatic fever –
Adults and children: 1.2 million units I.M. once monthly or 600,000 units twice monthly.

Syphilis of less than 1 year's duration –
Adults: 2.4 million units I.M. as a single dose.
Syphilis of more than 1 year's duration –
Adults: 2.4 million units I.M. weekly for 3 successive weeks.

ADVERSE REACTIONS
CNS: neuropathy, ***seizures*** with high doses.
Hematologic: eosinophilia, hemolytic anemia, thrombocytopenia, leukopenia.
Other: hypersensitivity reactions (maculopapular and ***exfoliative dermatitis,*** chills, fever, edema, ***anaphylaxis***), pain and sterile abscess at injection site.

INTERACTIONS
Probenecid: increased blood levels of penicillin. Probenecid may be used for this purpose.

CONTRAINDICATIONS
- Contraindicated in patients with hypersensitivity to the drug or other penicillins.
- Use cautiously in patients with other drug allergies, especially to cephalosporins (possible cross-sensitivity).

NURSING CONSIDERATIONS
- Before giving, ask the patient about any allergic reactions to penicillin. However, a negative history of penicillin allergy is no guarantee against a future allergic reaction.
- Obtain specimen for culture and sensitivity tests before first dose. Therapy may begin pending results.
- Tell the patient to call the doctor if rash, fever, or chills develop. Fever and eosinophilia are the most common allergic reactions.
- With large doses and prolonged therapy, bacterial or fungal superinfection may occur, especially in elderly, debilitated, or immunosuppressed patients. Observe closely.
- Shake medication well before injection.
- Never give I.V. – inadvertent I.V. administration has caused cardiac arrest and death.
- Very slow absorption time makes allergic reactions difficult to treat.
- Inject deeply into upper outer quadrant of buttocks in adults; in midlateral thigh in infants and small children. Avoid injection into or near major nerves or blood vessels to prevent permanent neurovascular damage.
- Give penicillin G benzathine at least 1 hour before bacteriostatic antibiotics.

penicillin G potassium (benzylpenicillin potassium)

Megacillin†, Pfizerpen

Pregnancy Risk Category: B

HOW SUPPLIED
Tablets: 200,000 units, 250,000 units, 400,000 units, 500,000 units, 800,000 units
Oral suspension: 200,000 units/5 ml, 250,000 units/5 ml, 400,000 units/5 ml (after reconstitution)
Injection: 200,000 units, 500,000 units, 1 million units, 5 million units, 10 million units, 20 million units

ACTION
Mechanism: A natural penicillin that inhibits cell-wall synthesis during microorganism multiplication; bacteria resist penicillins by producing penicillinases – enzymes that convert penicillins to inactive penicilloic acid.
Peak: Peak serum levels occur immediately after I.V. infusion, within 15 to 30 minutes of I.M. injection, within ½ to 1 hour of oral dose.
Duration: elimination half-life, 20 to 60 minutes.

INDICATIONS & DOSAGE

Moderate to severe systemic infections –

Adults: 1.6 to 3.2 million units P.O. daily in divided doses q 6 hours (1 mg = 1,600 units); 1.2 to 24 million units I.M. or I.V. daily in divided doses q 4 hours.

Children: 25,000 to 100,000 units/kg P.O. daily in divided doses q 6 hours; or 25,000 to 300,000 units/kg I.M. or I.V. daily in divided doses q 4 hours.

ADVERSE REACTIONS

CNS: neuropathy, ***seizures*** with high doses.

Hematologic: ***hemolytic anemia,*** leukopenia, thrombocytopenia.

Other: hypersensitivity reactions (rash, urticaria, maculopapular eruptions, ***exfoliative dermatitis,*** chills, fever, edema, ***anaphylaxis***), overgrowth of nonsusceptible organisms, possible severe potassium poisoning with high doses (hyperreflexia, ***seizures, coma***), thrombophlebitis, pain at injection site.

INTERACTIONS

Probenecid: increased blood levels of penicillin. Probenecid may be used for this purpose.

CONTRAINDICATIONS

- Contraindicated in patients with hypersensitivity to the drug or other penicillins.
- Use cautiously in patients with other drug allergies, especially to cephalosporins (possible cross-sensitivity).

NURSING CONSIDERATIONS

- Before giving, ask the patient about any allergic reactions to penicillin. However, a negative history of penicillin allergy is no guarantee against a future allergic reaction.
- Obtain specimen for culture and sensitivity tests before first dose. Therapy may begin pending results.
- Tell the patient to take entire amount of medication exactly as prescribed, even after he feels better.
- Tell the patient to call the doctor if rash, fever, or chills develop. A rash is the most common allergic reaction.
- When given orally, drug may cause GI disturbances. Food may interfere with absorption; therefore, give 1 to 2 hours before or 2 to 3 hours after meals.
- Patients with poor renal function are predisposed to high blood levels. Monitor renal function closely.
- Patients with high blood level of this drug may develop seizures. Institute seizure precautions.
- With large doses and prolonged therapy, bacterial or fungal superinfection may occur, especially in elderly, debilitated, or immunosuppressed patients. Observe closely.
- Warn the patient never to use leftover penicillin for a new illness or to share penicillin with family and friends.
- Give penicillin G potassium at least 1 hour before bacteriostatic antibiotics.
- **I.V. use:** Reconstitute vials with sterile water for injection, D_5W, or 0.9% sodium chloride injection. Volume of diluent varies with manufacturer.
- Avoid continuous infusions to prevent vein irritation. Change site every 48 hours.
- For I.M. injection, administer deeply into large muscle; may be extremely painful.

penicillin G procaine (benzylpenicillin procaine)

Ayercillin†, Crysticillin-300 A.S., Pfizerpen-AS, Wycillin

Pregnancy Risk Category: B

HOW SUPPLIED

Injection: 300,000 units/ml, 500,000 units/ml, 600,000 units/ml

ACTION

Mechanism: A natural penicillin that inhibits cell-wall synthesis during microorganism multiplication; bacteria resist penicillins by producing penicillinases – enzymes that convert penicillins to inactive penicilloic acid.
Peak: Serum levels peak 1 to 4 hours after I.M. dose. **Duration:** drug persists in serum for 1 to 2 days; after high doses, for 5 days.

INDICATIONS & DOSAGE

Moderate to severe systemic infections –
Adults: 600,000 to 1.2 million units I.M. daily in a single dose.
Children over 1 month: 25,000 to 50,000 units/kg I.M. daily in a single dose.
Uncomplicated gonorrhea –
Adults and children over age 12: 1 g probenecid; after 30 minutes, 4.8 million units of penicillin G procaine I.M., divided between two injection sites.
Pneumococcal pneumonia –
Adults and children over age 12: 600,000 units to 1.2 million units I.M. daily for 7 to 10 days.

ADVERSE REACTIONS

CNS: ***seizures.***
Hematologic: thrombocytopenia, ***hemolytic anemia,*** leukopenia.
Other: arthralgia, hypersensitivity reactions (rash, urticaria, chills, fever, edema, prostration, ***anaphylaxis***), overgrowth of nonsusceptible organisms.

INTERACTIONS

Probenecid: increased blood levels of penicillin. Probenecid may be used for this purpose.

CONTRAINDICATIONS

- Contraindicated in patients with hypersensitivity to the drug or other penicillins.
- Use cautiously in patients with other drug allergies, especially to cephalosporins (possible cross-sensitivity). Some formulations contain sulfites, which may cause allergic reactions in sensitive persons.

NURSING CONSIDERATIONS

- Before giving, ask the patient about any allergic reactions to penicillin. However, a negative history of penicillin allergy is no guarantee against a future allergic reaction.
- Obtain specimen for culture and sensitivity tests before first dose. Therapy may begin pending results.
- Tell the patient to call the doctor if rash, fever, or chills develop. A rash is the most common allergic reaction.
- Because of drug's slow absorption rate, allergic reactions are hard to treat.
- With large doses and prolonged therapy, bacterial or fungal superinfection may occur, especially in elderly, debilitated, or immunosuppressed patients. Observe closely.
- Periodic evaluations of renal and hematopoietic function are recommended.
- Give penicillin G procaine at least 1 hour before bacteriostatic antibiotics.
- Give deep I.M. in upper outer quadrant of buttocks in adults; in midlateral thigh in small children. Do not give subcutaneously. Don't massage injection site. Avoid injection near major nerves or blood vessels to prevent permanent neurovascular damage.
- Never give I.V. – inadvertent I.V. administration has caused death from CNS toxicity caused by procaine.

penicillin G sodium (benzylpenicillin sodium)

Crystapen†

Pregnancy Risk Category: B

*Liquid form contains alcohol. *Common* reactions are in italics; ***life-threatening,*** in bold italics.
**May contain tartrazine.

HOW SUPPLIED
Injection: 5 million-units vial

ACTION
Mechanism: A natural penicillin that inhibits cell-wall synthesis during active multiplication; bacteria resist penicillins by producing penicillinases – enzymes that convert penicillins to inactive penicilloic acid.
Peak: Peak serum levels occur 15 to 30 minutes after I.M. injection, immediately after I.V. infusion. **Duration:** serum half-life, about 30 minutes to 1 hour.

INDICATIONS & DOSAGE
Moderate to severe systemic infections –
Adults: 1.2 to 24 million units daily I.M. or I.V. in divided doses q 4 to 6 hours.
Children: 25,000 to 300,000 units/kg daily I.M. or I.V. in divided doses q 4 to 6 hours.
Endocarditis prophylaxis for dental surgery –
Adults and children over 27 kg: 2 million units I.V. or I.M. 30 to 60 minutes before procedure; then 1 million units 6 hours later.

ADVERSE REACTIONS
CNS: neuropathy, ***seizures***.
CV: ***CHF*** with high doses.
Hematologic: hemolytic anemia, leukopenia, thrombocytopenia.
Other: arthralgia, hypersensitivity reactions (***exfoliative dermatitis,*** urticaria, ***anaphylaxis***), overgrowth of nonsusceptible organisms, vein irritation, pain at injection site, thrombophlebitis.

INTERACTIONS
Probenecid: increased blood levels of penicillin. Probenecid may be used for this purpose.

CONTRAINDICATIONS
- Contraindicated in patients on sodium-restricted diets.
- Use cautiously in patients with other drug allergies, especially to cephalosporins (possible cross-allergenicity).

NURSING CONSIDERATIONS
- Before giving, ask the patient about any allergic reactions to penicillin. However, a negative history of penicillin allergy is no guarantee against a future allergic reaction.
- Obtain specimen for culture and sensitivity tests before first dose. Therapy may begin pending results.
- Patients with high blood level of this drug may develop seizures. Institute seizure precautions.
- With large doses and prolonged therapy, bacterial or fungal superinfection may occur, especially in elderly, debilitated, or immunosuppressed patients. Observe closely.
- Give penicillin G sodium at least 1 hour before bacteriostatic antibiotics.
- **I.V. use:** Reconstitute vials with sterile water for injection, 0.9% sodium chloride injection, or D_5W. Check manufacturer's instructions for volume of diluent necessary to produce desired drug concentration.
- For patients receiving 10 million units of drug or more daily, dilute in 1 to 2 liters of compatible solution and administer over 24 hours. Otherwise, give by intermittent I.V. infusion: Dilute drug in 50 to 100 ml and give over 1 to 2 hours q 4 to 6 hours.
- In neonates and children, divided doses are usually given over 15 to 30 minutes.

penicillin V (phenoxymethyl penicillin)

penicillin V potassium (phenoxymethylpenicillin potassium)

Abbocillin VK‡, Apo-Pen-VK†, Beepen-VK, Betapen-VK, Cilicane VK‡, Ledercillin VK, Nadopen-V-200†, Nadopen-V-400†, Nadopen-VK†, NovoPen-VK†, Nu-Pen VK†, PVK‡, Pen Vee, Pen Vee K, PVF K†, Robicillin VK, V-Cillin K, VC-K, Veetids**

Pregnancy Risk Category: B

HOW SUPPLIED

penicillin V
Tablets: 250 mg, 500 mg
Oral suspension: 125 mg/5 ml, 250 mg/5 ml (after reconstitution)
penicillin V potassium
Tablets: 125 mg, 250 mg, 500 mg
Tablets (film-coated): 250 mg, 500 mg
Capsules: 250 mg‡
Oral suspension: 125 mg/5 ml, 250 mg/5 ml (after reconstitution)

ACTION

Mechanism: A natural penicillin that inhibits cell-wall synthesis during microorganism multiplication; bacteria resist penicillins by producing penicillinases – enzymes that convert penicillins to inactive penicilloic acid.
Peak: Serum levels peak within ½ hour. **Duration:** elimination half-life, about 30 minutes.

INDICATIONS & DOSAGE

Mild to moderate systemic infections –
Adults: 250 to 500 mg (400,000 to 800,000 units) P.O. q 6 hours.
Children: 15 to 50 mg/kg (25,000 to 90,000 units/kg) P.O. daily, in divided doses q 6 to 8 hours.
Endocarditis prophylaxis for dental surgery –
Adults: 2 g P.O. 30 to 60 minutes before procedure; then 1 g 6 hours afterward.
Children under 30 kg: half of the adult dose.

ADVERSE REACTIONS

CNS: neuropathy.
GI: *epigastric distress,* vomiting, diarrhea, *nausea.*
Hematologic: eosinophilia, hemolytic anemia, leukopenia, thrombocytopenia.
Other: hypersensitivity reactions (rash, urticaria, chills, fever, edema, ***anaphylaxis***), overgrowth of nonsusceptible organisms.

INTERACTIONS

Neomycin: decreased absorption of penicillin. Give penicillin by injection.
Probenecid: increased blood levels of penicillin. Probenecid may be used for this purpose.

CONTRAINDICATIONS

- Contraindicated in patients with hypersensitivity to the drug or other penicillins.
- Use cautiously in patients with other drug allergies, especially to cephalosporins (possible cross-sensitivity), or in those with GI disturbances.

NURSING CONSIDERATIONS

- Before giving, ask the patient about any allergic reactions to penicillins. However, a negative history of penicillin allergy is no guarantee against a future allergic reaction.
- Obtain specimen for culture and sensitivity tests before first dose. Therapy may begin pending results.
- Tell the patient to take entire quantity of medication exactly as prescribed, even after he feels better.
- Tell the patient to call the doctor if rash, fever, or chills develop. A rash is the most common allergic reaction.
- May cause GI disturbances. Food may interfere with absorption; therefore, give 1 to 2 hours before or 2 to 3 hours after meals.
- The patient should take each dose with a full glass of water only because

*Liquid form contains alcohol.
**May contain tartrazine.

Common reactions are in italics; ***life-threatening,*** in bold italics.

the acid in fruit juice or a carbonated beverage will inactivate the drug.
- With large doses and prolonged therapy, bacterial or fungal superinfection may occur, especially in elderly, debilitated, or immunosuppressed patients. Observe closely.
- Periodically assess renal and hematopoietic function in patients receiving long-term therapy.
- Warn the patient never to use leftover penicillin for a new illness or to share penicillin with family and friends.
- Give penicillin V at least 1 hour before bacteriostatic antibiotics.
- The American Heart Association considers amoxicillin the preferred agent for endocarditis prophylaxis because GI absorption is better and serum levels are sustained longer. Penicillin V is considered an alternative agent.

piperacillin sodium

Pipracil, Pipril‡

Pregnancy Risk Category: B

HOW SUPPLIED

Injection: 2 g, 3 g, 4 g
Pharmacy bulk package: 40 g

ACTION

Mechanism: Inhibits cell-wall synthesis during microorganism multiplication; bacteria resist penicillins by producing penicillinases – enzymes that convert penicillins to inactive penicilloic acid.
Peak: Peak serum levels occur immediately after I.V. infusion, within 30 to 50 minutes of I.M. dose. **Duration:** elimination half-life, 30 to 90 minutes.

INDICATIONS & DOSAGE

Systemic infections caused by susceptible strains of gram-positive and especially gram-negative organisms (including Proteus *and* Pseudomonas aeruginosa*)* –
Adults and children over 12 years: 100 to 300 mg/kg daily in divided doses q 4 to 6 hours I.V. or I.M. Doses for children under 12 years not established.
Prophylaxis of surgical infections –
Adults: 2 g I.V., given 30 to 60 minutes before surgery. Dose may be repeated during surgery and once or twice more after surgery.

ADVERSE REACTIONS

CNS: neuromuscular irritability, ***seizures,*** headache, dizziness.
GI: nausea, diarrhea.
Hematologic: *bleeding with high doses,* neutropenia, eosinophilia, leukopenia, *thrombocytopenia.*
Other: *hypokalemia,* hypersensitivity reactions (edema, fever, chills, rash, pruritus, urticaria, ***anaphylaxis***), overgrowth of nonsusceptible organisms, pain at injection site, vein irritation, phlebitis.

INTERACTIONS

Aminoglycoside antibiotics (such as gentamicin and tobramycin): chemically incompatible. Don't mix in the same I.V. container.
Probenecid: increased blood levels of piperacillin. Probenecid may be used for this purpose.

CONTRAINDICATIONS

- Contraindicated in patients with hypersensitivity to the drug or other penicillins.
- Use cautiously in patients with other drug allergies, especially to cephalosporins (possible cross-sensitivity), or in those with bleeding tendencies, uremia, and hypokalemia.

NURSING CONSIDERATIONS

- Before giving, ask the patient about any allergic reactions to penicillin. However, a negative history of peni-

cillin allergy is no guarantee against a future allergic reaction.
• Obtain specimen for culture and sensitivity tests before first dose. Therapy may begin pending results.
• Cystic fibrosis patients tend to be most susceptible to fever or rash.
• Dosage should be altered in patients with impaired renal function.
• Check CBC and platelet counts frequently. Drug may cause thrombocytopenia.
• Monitor serum potassium level.
• Patients with high serum level of this drug may have seizures. Institute seizure precautions.
• Piperacillin is typically used with another antibiotic, such as gentamicin.
• With large doses and prolonged therapy, bacterial or fungal superinfection may occur, especially in elderly, debilitated, or immunosuppressed patients. Observe closely.
• Drug may be better suited for patients on sodium-free diets than ticarcillin (contains 1.85 mEq sodium/g of piperacillin).
• Piperacillin has shown greater activity against *Pseudomonas aeruginosa* than carbenicillin, ticarcillin, or mezlocillin.
• Give piperacillin at least 1 hour before bacteriostatic antibiotics.
• **I.V. use:** Reconstitute each gram of drug with 5 ml of diluent, such as sterile or bacteriostatic water for injection, 0.9% sodium chloride injection (with or without preservative), D_5W, or dextrose 5% in 0.9% sodium chloride injection. Shake until dissolved. Inject reconstituted solution directly into a vein or into the tubing of a free-flowing I.V. solution over 3 to 5 minutes. Alternatively, dilute with at least 50 ml of a compatible I.V. solution and give by intermittent infusion over 30 minutes.
• Avoid continuous infusions to prevent vein irritation. Change site every 48 hours.
• For I.M. injection, vials may be reconstituted with sterile or bacteriostatic water for injection, 0.9% sodium chloride injection (with or without preservative), or 0.5% to 1% lidocaine hydrochloride. Add 2 ml of diluent for each gram of drug. Final solution will contain 1 g/2.5 ml.

piperacillin sodium and tazobactam sodium

Zosyn

Pregnancy Risk Category: C

HOW SUPPLIED

Powder for injection: 2 g piperacillin and 0.25 g tazobactam per vial, 3 g piperacillin and 0.375 g tazobactam per vial, 4 g piperacillin and 0.5 g tazobactam per vial

ACTION

Mechanism: Piperacillin is an extended-spectrum penicillin that inhibits cell-wall synthesis during microorganism multiplication; tazobactam increases piperacillin effectiveness by inactivating beta lactamases, which destroy penicillins.
Peak: Plasma levels peak immediately after I.V. infusion. **Duration:** plasma half-life, 45 to 75 minutes.

INDICATIONS & DOSAGE

Appendicitis (complicated by rupture or abscess) and peritonitis caused by Escherichia coli, Bacteroides fragilis, B. ovatus, B. thetaiotaomicron, *or* B. vulgatus; *skin and skin structure infections caused by* Staphylococcus aureus; *postpartum endometritis or pelvic inflammatory disease caused by* E. coli; *moderately severe community-acquired pneumonia caused by* Haemophilus influenzae –
Adults: 3 g piperacillin and 0.375 g tazobactam I.V. q 6 hours.
In patients with renal impairment –
Adults: if creatinine clearance is 20 to 40 ml/minute, give 2 g piperacillin

and 0.25 g tazobactam I.V. q 6 hours. If creatinine clearance is below 20 ml/minute, give 2 g piperacillin and 0.25 g tazobactam I.V. q 8 hours.

ADVERSE REACTIONS

CNS: *headache, insomnia,* agitation, dizziness, anxiety.
CV: hypertension, chest pain, edema.
EENT: rhinitis.
GI: *diarrhea, nausea, constipation,* vomiting, dyspepsia, stool changes, abdominal pain.
Respiratory: dyspnea.
Skin: rash (including maculopapular, bullous, urticarial, and eczematoid), pruritus.
Other: fever, pain, moniliasis.

INTERACTIONS

Aminoglycoside antibiotics (such as gentamicin and tobramycin): chemically incompatible. Don't mix in the same I.V. container.
Probenecid: increased blood levels of piperacillin. Probenecid may be used for this purpose.

CONTRAINDICATIONS

• Contraindicated in patients with hypersensitivity to the drug or other penicillins.
• Use cautiously in patients with other drug allergies, especially to cephalosporins (possible cross-sensitivity), or in those with bleeding tendencies, uremia, and hypokalemia.

NURSING CONSIDERATIONS

• Obtain specimen for culture and sensitivity tests before first dose. Therapy may begin pending results.
• With large doses and prolonged therapy, bacterial and fungal superinfection may occur, especially in elderly, debilitated, or immunosuppressed patients. Observe closely.
• **I.V. use:** Reconstitute each gram of piperacillin with 5 ml of diluent, such as sterile or bacteriostatic water for injection, 0.9% sodium chloride injection, bacteriostatic 0.9% sodium chloride injection, D_5W, dextrose 5% in 0.9% sodium chloride injection, or dextran 6% in 0.9% sodium chloride injection. Don't use lactated Ringer's injection. Shake until dissolved. Further dilute to a final volume of 50 ml before infusion.
• Infuse over at least 30 minutes. Discontinue any primary infusion during administration if possible. Don't mix with other drugs.
• Use drug immediately after reconstitution. Discard unused drug after 24 hours if held at room temperature; 48 hours if refrigerated. Once diluted, drug is stable in I.V. bags for 24 hours at room temperature or 1 week if refrigerated.
• Change I.V. site every 48 hours.
• Because hemodialysis removes 6% of the piperacillin dose and 21% of the tazobactam dose, supplemental doses may be needed after hemodialysis.

ticarcillin disodium

Ticar, Ticillin‡

Pregnancy Risk Category: B

HOW SUPPLIED

Injection: 1 g, 3 g, 6 g
I.V. infusion: 3 g
Pharmacy bulk package: 20 g, 30 g

ACTION

Mechanism: An extended-spectrum penicillin that inhibits cell-wall synthesis during microorganism multiplication; bacteria resist penicillins by producing penicillinases – enzymes that convert penicillins to inactive penicilloic acid.
Peak: Peak serum levels occur immediately after I.V. infusion, within 30 to 50 minutes after I.M. injection.
Duration: elimination half-life, 1 to 1½ hours.

INDICATIONS & DOSAGE
Severe systemic infections caused by susceptible strains of gram-positive and especially gram-negative organisms (including Pseudomonas *and* Proteus*)* –
Adults: 18 g I.V. or I.M. daily, in divided doses q 4 to 6 hours.
Children: 50 to 300 mg/kg I.V. or I.M. daily, in divided doses q 4 to 6 hours.

ADVERSE REACTIONS
CNS: *seizures,* neuromuscular excitability.
GI: nausea, diarrhea.
Hematologic: leukopenia, neutropenia, eosinophilia, *thrombocytopenia,* hemolytic anemia.
Other: hypersensitivity reactions (rash, pruritus, urticaria, chills, fever, edema, ***anaphylaxis***), overgrowth of nonsusceptible organisms, hypokalemia, pain at injection site, vein irritation, phlebitis.

INTERACTIONS
Aminoglycoside antibiotics (such as gentamicin and tobramycin): chemically incompatible. Don't mix in the same I.V. container.
Probenecid: increased blood levels of ticarcillin and other penicillins. Probenecid may be used for this purpose.

CONTRAINDICATIONS
- Contraindicated in patients with hypersensitivity to the drug or other penicillins.
- Use cautiously in patients with other drug allergies, especially to cephalosporins (possible cross-sensitivity), or in those with impaired renal function, hemorrhagic conditions, hypokalemia, or sodium restrictions (contains 5.2 to 6.5 mEq sodium/g).

NURSING CONSIDERATIONS
- Before giving, ask the patient about any allergic reactions to penicillin. However, a negative history of penicillin allergy is no guarantee against a future allergic reaction.
- Obtain specimen for culture and sensitivity tests before first dose. Therapy may begin pending results.
- Dosage should be decreased in patients with impaired renal function.
- Check CBC and platelet counts frequently. Drug may cause thrombocytopenia.
- Patients with high blood level of ticarcillin may develop seizures. Institute seizure precautions.
- Ticarcillin is typically used with another antibiotic, such as gentamicin.
- With large doses and prolonged therapy, bacterial or fungal superinfection may occur, especially in elderly, debilitated, or immunosuppressed patients. Observe closely.
- Monitor serum potassium.
- Give ticarcillin at least 1 hour before bacteriostatic antibiotics.
- **I.V. use:** Reconstitute vials using D_5W, 0.9% sodium chloride injection, sterile water for injection, or other compatible solution. Add 4 ml of diluent for each gram of drug. Further dilute to a maximum concentration of 50 mg/ml and inject slowly directly into a vein or into the tubing of a free-flowing I.V. solution. Alternatively, dilute to a concentration of 10 to 100 mg/ml and give by intermittent infusion over 30 to 120 minutes in adults or 10 to 20 minutes in neonates.
- Avoid continuous infusion to prevent vein irritation. Change site every 48 hours.
- For I.M. injection, reconstitute vials using sterile water for injection, 0.9% sodium chloride injection, or lidocaine 1% (without epinephrine). Use 2 ml diluent for each gram of drug. Administer deep I.M. into large muscle. Don't exceed 2 g per injection.

ticarcillin disodium/ clavulanate potassium

Timentin

Pregnancy Risk Category: B

HOW SUPPLIED

Injection: 3 g ticarcillin and 100 mg clavulanic acid

ACTION

Mechanism: Ticarcillin is an extended-spectrum penicillin that inhibits cell-wall synthesis during microorganism replication; clavulanic acid increases ticarcillin's effectiveness by inactivating beta lactamases, which destroy ticarcillin.

Peak: Peak serum levels occur immediately after I.V. infusion. **Duration:** serum half-life of both drugs, about 1 hour.

INDICATIONS & DOSAGE

Lower respiratory tract, urinary tract, bone and joint, and skin and skin structure infections and septicemia when caused by beta-lactamase-producing strains of bacteria or by ticarcillin-susceptible organisms –
Adults: 1 vial (ticarcillin 3 g and clavulanate potassium 0.1 g) administered by I.V. infusion q 4 to 6 hours.

ADVERSE REACTIONS

CNS: ***seizures,*** neuromuscular excitability.

GI: nausea, diarrhea.

Hematologic: leukopenia, neutropenia, eosinophilia, *thrombocytopenia,* hemolytic anemia.

Other: hypersensitivity reactions (rash, pruritus, urticaria, chills, fever, edema, ***anaphylaxis***), overgrowth of nonsusceptible organisms, hypokalemia, pain at injection site, vein irritation, phlebitis.

INTERACTIONS

Aminoglycoside antibiotics (such as gentamicin and tobramycin): chemically incompatible. Don't mix in the same I.V. container.

Probenecid: increased blood levels of ticarcillin. Probenecid may be used for this purpose.

CONTRAINDICATIONS

- Contraindicated in patients with hypersensitivity to the drug or other penicillins.
- Use cautiously in patients with other drug allergies, especially to cephalosporins (possible cross-sensitivity), and in those with impaired renal function, hemorrhagic condition, hypokalemia, or sodium restrictions (contains 4.5 mEq sodium/g).

NURSING CONSIDERATIONS

- Before giving, ask the patient about any allergic reactions to penicillin. However, a negative history of penicillin allergy is no guarantee against a future allergic reaction.
- Obtain specimen for culture and sensitivity tests before first dose. Therapy may begin pending results.
- Dosage should be decreased in patients with impaired renal function.
- With large doses and prolonged therapy, bacterial or fungal superinfection may occur, especially in elderly, debilitated, or immunosuppressed patients. Observe closely.
- Check CBC and platelet counts frequently. Drug may cause thrombocytopenia.
- Give drug at least 1 hour before bacteriostatic antibiotics.
- **I.V. use:** Reconstitute drug with 13 ml of sterile water for injection or 0.9% sodium chloride injection. Further dilute to a maximum of 10 to 100 mg/ml (based on ticarcillin component) and administer by I.V. infusion over 30 minutes. In fluid-restricted patients, dilute to a maximum of 48 mg/ml if using D_5W, 43 mg/ml if using 0.9% sodium chloride injection, or 86 mg/ml if using sterile water for injection.

Cephalosporins

cefaclor
cefadroxil monohydrate
cefamandole nafate
cefazolin sodium
cefixime
cefmetazole sodium
cefonicid sodium
cefoperazone sodium
cefotaxime sodium
cefotetan disodium
cefoxitin sodium
cefpodoxime proxetil
cefprozil
ceftazidime
ceftizoxime sodium
ceftriaxone sodium
cefuroxime axetil
cefuroxime sodium
cephalexin hydrochloride
cephalexin monohydrate
cephalothin sodium
cephapirin sodium
cephradine
loracarbef

COMBINATION PRODUCTS
None.

cefaclor

Ceclor

Pregnancy Risk Category: B

HOW SUPPLIED
Capsules: 250 mg, 500 mg
Oral suspension: 125 mg/5 ml, 250 mg/5 ml, 375 mg/5 ml

ACTION
Mechanism: A second-generation cephalosporin that inhibits cell-wall synthesis, promoting osmotic instability; usually bactericidal.
Peak: Peak levels occur within 30 to 60 minutes. **Duration:** elimination half-life, 30 to 60 minutes.

INDICATIONS & DOSAGE
Respiratory or urinary tract, skin, and soft-tissue infections and otitis media caused by Haemophilus influenzae, Streptococcus pneumoniae, S. pyogenes, Escherichia coli, Proteus mirabilis, Klebsiella *species, and staphylococci –*
Adults: 250 to 500 mg P.O. q 8 hours. For pharyngitis or otitis media, daily dosage may be given in two equally divided doses q 12 hours.
Children: 20 mg/kg daily P.O. in divided doses q 8 hours. For pharyngitis or otitis media, daily dosage may be given in two equally divided doses q 12 hours. In more serious infections, 40 mg/kg daily are recommended, not to exceed 1 g daily.

ADVERSE REACTIONS
CNS: dizziness, headache, somnolence.
GI: *nausea,* vomiting, *diarrhea,* anorexia, pseudomembranous colitis.
GU: red and white cells in urine, vaginal moniliasis, vaginitis.
Hematologic: transient leukopenia, lymphocytosis, anemia, eosinophilia.
Skin: *maculopapular rash,* dermatitis.
Other: hypersensitivity reactions (serum sickness, ***anaphylaxis***), fever.

INTERACTIONS
Probenecid: may inhibit excretion and increase blood levels of cefaclor.

CONTRAINDICATIONS
- Contraindicated in patients hypersensitive to other cephalosporins.
- Use cautiously in patients with impaired renal function or a history of sensitivity to penicillin.

*Liquid form contains alcohol.
**May contain tartrazine.

Common reactions are in italics; ***life-threatening,*** in bold italics.

NURSING CONSIDERATIONS

- Obtain specimen for culture and sensitivity tests before first dose. Therapy may begin pending test results.
- Tell the patient to take entire amount of medication exactly as prescribed, even after he feels better.
- Call the doctor if skin rash develops.
- With large doses or prolonged therapy, monitor for superinfection, especially in high-risk patients.
- Store reconstituted suspension in refrigerator. Stable for 14 days if refrigerated. Shake well before using.
- Drug may be taken with meals.
- Cefaclor is a relatively expensive antibiotic and should be used only when the organism is resistant to other agents.
- From 40% to 75% of patients receiving cephalosporins show a false-positive direct Coombs' test.
- Urine glucose determinations may be false-positive with copper sulfate tests (Clinitest); glucose enzymatic tests (Clinistix, Tes-Tape) are not affected.

---

cefadroxil monohydrate

Duricef, Ultracef

Pregnancy Risk Category: B

HOW SUPPLIED

Tablets: 1 g
Capsules: 500 mg
Oral suspension: 125 mg/5 ml, 250 mg/5 ml, 500 mg/5 ml

ACTION

Mechanism: A first-generation cephalosporin that inhibits cell-wall synthesis, promoting osmotic instability; usually bactericidal.
Peak: Serum levels peak within 1 to 2 hours after an oral dose. **Duration:** elimination half-life, 1 to 2 hours.

INDICATIONS & DOSAGE

Urinary tract infections caused by Escherichia coli, Proteus mirabilis, *and* Klebsiella *species; skin and soft-tissue infections; and streptococcal pharyngitis –*
Adults: 500 mg to 2 g P.O. daily, depending on infection being treated. Usually given once daily or b.i.d.
Children: 30 mg/kg P.O. daily in two divided doses.

ADVERSE REACTIONS

CNS: dizziness, headache, malaise, paresthesia.
GI: pseudomembranous colitis, *nausea,* anorexia, vomiting, *diarrhea,* glossitis, *dyspepsia,* abdominal cramps, anal pruritus, tenesmus, oral candidiasis.
GU: genital pruritus, moniliasis.
Hematologic: transient neutropenia, eosinophilia, leukopenia, anemia.
Skin: *maculopapular and erythematous rashes.*
Other: hypersensitivity reactions (serum sickness, ***anaphylaxis***), dyspnea.

INTERACTIONS

Probenecid: may inhibit excretion and increase blood levels of cefadroxil.

CONTRAINDICATIONS

- Contraindicated in patients with hypersensitivity to the drug or other cephalosporins.
- Use cautiously in patients with a history of sensitivity to penicillin. Also use cautiously in patients with impaired renal function; dosage adjustments may be necessary.

NURSING CONSIDERATIONS

- Obtain specimen for culture and sensitivity tests before first dose. Therapy may begin pending test results.
- If creatinine clearance is below 50 ml/minute, dosage interval should be

lengthened so drug doesn't accumulate.

- Tell the patient to take entire amount of medication exactly as prescribed, even after he feels better.
- Call the doctor if skin rash develops.
- With large doses or prolonged therapy, monitor for superinfection, especially in high-risk patients.
- Because absorption is not delayed by presence of food, tell the patient to take with food or milk to lessen GI discomfort.
- Longer half-life permits once- or twice-daily dosing.
- From 40% to 75% of patients receiving cephalosporins show a false-positive direct Coombs' test.
- Urine glucose determinations may be false-positive with copper sulfate tests (Clinitest); glucose enzymatic tests (Clinistix, Tes-Tape) are not affected.

cefamandole nafate

Mandol

Pregnancy Risk Category: B

HOW SUPPLIED

Injection: 1 g, 2 g, 10 g
Pharmacy bulk package: 10 g

ACTION

Mechanism: A second-generation cephalosporin that inhibits cell-wall synthesis, promoting osmotic instability; usually bactericidal.
Peak: Peak serum levels occur 30 minutes to 2 hours after I.M. injection, immediately after I.V. infusion.
Duration: elimination half-life, 30 minutes to 2 hours.

INDICATIONS & DOSAGE

Perioperative prophylaxis in contaminated surgery –
Adults: 1 to 2 g I.M. or I.V. 30 to 60 minutes before surgery; then 1 to 2 g I.M. or I.V. q 6 hours for 24 hours.
Children 3 months and older: 12.5 to 25 mg/kg I.M. or I.V. 30 to 60 minutes before surgery; then 12.5 to 25 mg/kg I.M. or I.V. q 6 hours for 24 hours.

Note: In cases where infection could be devastating, prophylaxis may be continued for 3 days.

Serious infections of respiratory and GU tracts; skin, soft-tissue, bone, and joint infections; septicemia; and peritonitis caused by Escherichia coli *and other coliform bacteria,* Staphylococcus aureus *(penicillinase- and non-penicillinase-producing),* S. epidermidis, *group A beta-hemolytic streptococci,* Klebsiella, Haemophilus influenzae, Proteus mirabilis, *and* Enterobacter –
Adults: 500 mg to 1 g q 4 to 8 hours. In life-threatening infections, up to 2 g q 4 hours may be needed.
Infants and children: 50 to 100 mg/kg daily in equally divided doses q 4 to 8 hours. May be increased to total daily dosage of 150 mg/kg, not to exceed maximum adult dosage.

ADVERSE REACTIONS

CNS: headache, malaise, paresthesia, dizziness.
GI: pseudomembranous colitis, nausea, anorexia, vomiting, *diarrhea,* glossitis, dyspepsia, abdominal cramps, tenesmus, anal pruritus, oral candidiasis.
GU: genital pruritus and moniliasis.
Hematologic: transient neutropenia, eosinophilia, hemolytic anemia, *hypoprothrombinemia,* bleeding.
Skin: *maculopapular and erythematous rashes, urticaria.*
Other: hypersensitivity reactions (serum sickness, ***anaphylaxis***), dyspnea, at injection site – *pain, induration, sterile abscesses,* temperature elevation, tissue sloughing; with I.V. injection – *phlebitis and thrombophlebitis.*

INTERACTIONS

Aminoglycosides: incompatible when mixed together. Administer at a different site.
Aspirin, oral anticoagulants: increased risk of bleeding. Monitor for bleeding.
Ethanol: possible disulfiram-like reaction. Warn patient not to drink alcohol for several days after discontinuing cefamandole.
Probenecid: may inhibit excretion and increase serum levels of cefamandole. Sometimes used for this effect.

CONTRAINDICATIONS

- Contraindicated in patients with hypersensitivity to the drug or other cephalosporins.
- Use cautiously in patients with a history of sensitivity to penicillin. Also use cautiously and with dosage adjustments in patients with renal failure.

NURSING CONSIDERATIONS

- Obtain specimen for culture and sensitivity tests before first dose. Therapy may begin pending test results.
- Not as effective as cefoxitin in treating anaerobic infections. Cefamandole offers little advantage over previously available drugs.
- With large doses or prolonged therapy, monitor for superinfection, especially in high-risk patients.
- The chemical structure of this drug includes the methylthiotetrazole side chain that has been associated with bleeding disorders. Vitamin K can be administered to promptly reverse bleeding if it occurs.
- From 40% to 75% of patients receiving cephalosporins show a false-positive direct Coombs' test.
- Urine glucose determinations may be false-positive with copper sulfate tests (Clinitest); glucose enzymatic tests (Clinistix, Tes-Tape) are not affected.
- **I.V. use:** Reconstitute 1 g with 10 ml of sterile water for injection, D_5W, or 0.9% sodium chloride for injection. To give by direct injection, inject into a large vein or into the tubing of a free-flowing I.V. solution over 3 to 5 minutes. If using sterile water, dilute to 20 ml to avoid giving a hypertonic solution.
- After reconstitution, drug is stable for 24 hours at room temperature; for 96 hours under refrigeration.
- For intermittent injection, dilute to 100 ml using a compatible solution.
- Don't mix with I.V. infusions containing calcium ions (chemically incompatible).
- For I.M. administration, inject deeply into a large muscle mass, such as the gluteus maximus or the lateral aspect of the thigh. I.M. cefamandole is not as painful as I.M. cefoxitin and doesn't require addition of lidocaine.

cefazolin sodium

Ancef, Kefzol, Zolicef

Pregnancy Risk Category: B

HOW SUPPLIED

Injection (parenteral): 500 mg, 5 g, 10 g
Infusion: 500 mg/50 ml vial, 500 mg/100 ml vial

ACTION

Mechanism: A first-generation cephalosporin that inhibits cell-wall synthesis, promoting osmotic instability; usually bactericidal.
Peak: Plasma levels peak within 1 to 2 hours after I.M. injection, immediately after I.V. infusion. **Duration:** elimination half-life, 1 to 2 hours.

INDICATIONS & DOSAGE

Perioperative prophylaxis in contaminated surgery –
Adults: 1 g I.M. or I.V. 30 to 60 minutes before surgery; then 0.5 to 1 g I.M. or I.V. q 6 to 8 hours for 24

hours. In long operations (> 2 hours), another 0.5 to 1 g dose may be administered intraoperatively.

Note: In cases where infection would be devastating, prophylaxis may be continued for 3 to 5 days.

Serious infections of respiratory, biliary, and GU tracts; skin, soft-tissue, bone, and joint infections; septicemia; and endocarditis caused by Escherichia coli, *Enterobacteriaceae, gonococci,* Haemophilus influenzae, Klebsiella, Proteus mirabilis, Staphylococcus aureus, Streptococcus pneumoniae, *and group A beta-hemolytic streptococci –*

Adults: 250 mg I.M. or I.V. q 8 hours to 1.5 g q 6 hours. Maximum 12 g/day in life-threatening situations.

Children over 1 month: 25 to 50 mg/kg or 1.25 g/m² daily I.M. or I.V. in three or four divided doses. In severe infections, dosage may be increased to 100 mg/kg/day.

ADVERSE REACTIONS

CNS: dizziness, headache, malaise, paresthesia.

GI: pseudomembranous colitis, nausea, anorexia, vomiting, *diarrhea,* glossitis, dyspepsia, abdominal cramps, anal pruritus, tenesmus, oral candidiasis.

GU: genital pruritus and moniliasis, vaginitis.

Hematologic: transient neutropenia, leukopenia, eosinophilia, anemia.

Skin: *maculopapular and erythematous rashes, urticaria.*

Other: hypersensitivity reactions (serum sickness, ***anaphylaxis***), dyspnea; at injection site – *pain, induration, sterile abscesses, tissue sloughing;* with I.V. injection – *phlebitis and thrombophlebitis.*

INTERACTIONS

Probenecid: may inhibit excretion and increase blood levels of cefazolin.

CONTRAINDICATIONS

- Contraindicated in patients hypersensitive to other cephalosporins.
- Use cautiously in patients with a history of sensitivity to penicillin. Also use cautiously and with dosage adjustments in patients with renal failure.

NURSING CONSIDERATIONS

- Obtain specimen for culture and sensitivity tests before first dose. Therapy may begin pending test results.
- Because of long duration of effect, most infections can be treated with a dose q 8 hour.
- With large doses or prolonged therapy, monitor for superinfection, especially in high-risk patients.
- From 40% to 75% of patients receiving cephalosporins show a false-positive direct Coombs' test.
- Urine glucose determinations may be false-positive with copper sulfate tests (Clinitest); glucose enzymatic tests (Clinistix, Tes-Tape) are not affected.
- **I.V. use:** Reconstitute with sterile water, bacteriostatic water, or 0.9% sodium chloride solution as follows: 2 ml to 500-mg vial; 2.5 ml to 1-g vial. Shake well until dissolved. Resultant concentration: 225 mg/ml or 330 mg/ml, respectively.
- Reconstituted cefazolin is stable for 24 hours at room temperature or 96 hours under refrigeration.
- For direct injection, further dilute Ancef with 5 ml, or Kefzol with 10 ml, of sterile water for injection. Inject into a large vein or into the tubing of a free-flowing I.V. solution over 3 to 5 minutes. For intermittent infusion, add reconstituted drug to 50 to 100 ml of compatible solution or use premixed solution. Commercially available frozen solutions of cefazolin in D_5W should be given only by intermittent or continuous I.V. infusion.
- Alternate injection sites if I.V. ther-

apy lasts longer than 3 days. Use of small I.V. needles in the larger available veins may be preferable.

- After reconstitution, drug may be injected I.M. without further dilution. Not as painful as other cephalosporins. Injection should be given deeply into a large muscle mass, such as the gluteus maximus or the lateral aspect of the thigh.

cefixime

Suprax

Pregnancy Risk Category: B

HOW SUPPLIED

Tablets: 200 mg, 400 mg
Oral suspension: 100 mg/5 ml (after reconstitution)

ACTION

Mechanism: A third-generation cephalosporin that inhibits cell-wall synthesis, promoting osmotic instability; usually bactericidal.
Peak: Serum levels peak within 3.1 to 4.4 hours after an oral dose. **Duration:** elimination half-life averages 2½ to 4 hours.

INDICATIONS & DOSAGE

Uncomplicated urinary tract infections caused by Escherichia coli *and* Proteus mirabilis; *otitis media caused by* Haemophilus influenzae *(beta-lactamase positive and negative strains),* Moraxella (Branhamella) catarrhalis, *and* Streptococcus pyogenes; *pharyngitis and tonsillitis caused by* S. pyogenes; *acute bronchitis and acute exacerbations of chronic bronchitis caused by* S. pneumoniae *and* H. influenzae *(beta-lactamase positive and negative strains)* –
Adults: 400 mg/day P.O. as a single 400-mg tablet or 200 mg q 12 hours.
Children: 8 mg/kg/day suspension P.O. as a single daily dose or 4 mg/kg q 12 hours.

Treat children over age 12 and those over 50 kg with the recommended adult dose.
Gonorrhea –
Adults: 400 mg P.O. as a single dose.

ADVERSE REACTIONS

CNS: headaches, dizziness.
GI: *diarrhea,* loose stools, abdominal pain, nausea, vomiting, dyspepsia, flatulence, pseudomembranous colitis.
GU: genital pruritus, vaginitis, genital candidiasis.
Hematologic: thrombocytopenia, leukopenia, eosinophilia.
Skin: pruritus, rash, urticaria.
Other: drug fever, hypersensitivity reactions (serum sickness, ***anaphylaxis***).

INTERACTIONS

Probenecid: may inhibit excretion and increase blood levels of cefixime.
Salicylates: may displace cefixime from plasma protein-binding sites. Clinical significance is unknown.

CONTRAINDICATIONS

- Contraindicated in patients with hypersensitivity to the drug or other cephalosporins.
- Use cautiously and with reduced dosage in patients with renal dysfunction; reduced dosage is necessary in patients with creatinine clearance below 60 ml/minute. Also use cautiously in patients with a history of sensitivity to penicillin.

NURSING CONSIDERATIONS

- Obtain specimen for culture and sensitivity tests before first dose. Therapy may begin pending test results.
- Call the doctor if skin rash develops.
- Preparation of oral suspension: add required amount of water to powder in two portions. Shake well after each addition. After mixing, suspension is stable for 14 days. No need to refrig-

erate, but keep tightly closed. Shake well before using.
• With large doses or prolonged therapy, monitor for superinfection, especially in high-risk patients.
• Tell the patient to take all of the medication prescribed, even after he feels better.
• From 40% to 75% of patients receiving cephalosporins show a false-positive direct Coombs' test.
• Urine glucose determinations may be false-positive with copper sulfate tests (Clinitest); glucose enzymatic tests (Clinistix, Tes-Tape) are not affected.

cefmetazole sodium (cefmetazone)

Zefazone

Pregnancy Risk Category: B

HOW SUPPLIED

Injection: 1 g, 2 g

ACTION

Mechanism: A semisynthetic cephamycin antibiotic pharmacologically similar to second-generation cephalosporins that inhibits cell-wall synthesis, promoting osmotic instability; usually bactericidal.

Peak: Plasma levels peak immediately after I.V. infusion. **Duration:** elimination half-life, about 1 hour.

INDICATIONS & DOSAGE

Lower respiratory tract infections caused by Streptococcus pneumoniae, Staphylococcus aureus *(penicillinase- and non-penicillinase-producing strains),* Escherichia coli, *and* Haemophilus influenzae *(non-penicillinase-producing strains); intra-abdominal infections caused by* E. coli *or* Bacteroides fragilis; *skin and skin-structure infections caused by* S. aureus *(penicillinase- and non-penicillinase-producing strains),* S. epidermidis, Streptococcus pyogenes, S. agalactiae, E. coli, Proteus mirabilis, Klebsiella pneumoniae, *and* B. fragilis –

Adults: 2 g I.V. q 6 to 12 hours for 5 to 14 days.

Urinary tract infections caused by E. coli –

Adults: 2 g I.V. q 12 hours.

Prophylaxis in patients undergoing vaginal hysterectomy –

Adults: 2 g I.V. 30 to 90 minutes before surgery as a single dose; or 1 g I.V. 30 to 90 minutes before surgery, repeated in 8 and 16 hours.

Prophylaxis in patients undergoing abdominal hysterectomy –

Adults: 1 g I.V. 30 to 90 minutes before surgery, repeated in 8 and 16 hours.

Prophylaxis in patients undergoing cesarean section –

Adults: 2 g I.V. as a single dose after clamping cord; or 1 g I.V. after clamping cord, repeated in 8 and 16 hours.

Prophylaxis in patients undergoing colorectal surgery –

Adults: 2 g I.V. as a single dose 30 to 90 minutes before surgery. Some clinicians follow with additional 2-g doses in 8 and 16 hours.

Prophylaxis in patients undergoing cholecystectomy (high risk) –

Adults: 1 g I.V. 30 to 90 minutes before surgery, repeated in 8 and 16 hours.

ADVERSE REACTIONS

CNS: headache.
CV: ***shock,*** hypotension.
EENT: epistaxis.
GI: nausea, vomiting, *diarrhea,* epigastric pain, pseudomembranous colitis.
GU: vaginitis.
Respiratory: pleural effusion, dyspnea, respiratory distress.
Skin: rash, pruritus, generalized erythema.
Other: fever, bacterial or fungal superinfection, hypersensitivity reac-

tions (serum sickness, ***anaphylaxis***), altered color perception, pain at injection site, phlebitis.

INTERACTIONS
Ethanol: possible disulfiram-like reaction. Should be avoided for 24 hours before and after administration of cefmetazole.
Probenecid: may inhibit excretion and increase blood levels of cefmetazole. Sometimes used for this effect.

CONTRAINDICATIONS
- Contraindicated in patients with hypersensitivity to the drug or other cephalosporins.
- Use cautiously in patients with a history of sensitivity to penicillin.

NURSING CONSIDERATIONS
- Obtain specimen for culture and sensitivity tests before first dose. Therapy may begin pending test results.
- Prolonged use may result in overgrowth of nonsusceptible organisms. Monitor patient for bacterial and fungal superinfections.
- The chemical structure of this drug includes the methylthiotetrazole side chain that has been associated with bleeding disorders. However, such bleeding has not been reported with this drug. Monitor PT and administer vitamin K as ordered.
- From 40% to 75% of patients receiving cephalosporins show a false-positive direct Coombs' test.
- Urine glucose determinations may be false-positive with copper sulfate tests (Clinitest); glucose enzymatic tests (Clinistix, Tes-Tape) are not affected.
- **I.V. use:** Reconstitute with bacteriostatic water for injection, sterile water for injection, or 0.9% sodium chloride injection. After reconstitution, drug may be further diluted to concentrations ranging from 1 to 20 mg/ml by adding it to 0.9% sodium chloride injection, D_5W, or lactated Ringer's injection. Reconstituted or dilute solutions are stable for 24 hours at room temperature (77° F [25° C]) or 1 week if refrigerated at 46° F (8° C).

cefonicid sodium
Monocid

Pregnancy Risk Category: B

HOW SUPPLIED
Injection: 500 mg, 1 g
Infusion: 1 g/100 ml
Pharmacy bulk package: 10 g

ACTION
Mechanism: A second-generation cephalosporin that inhibits cell-wall synthesis, promoting osmotic instability; usually bactericidal.
Peak: Plasma levels peak within 1 to 2 hours after I.M. dose, immediately after I.V. injection. **Duration:** serum half-life, 3½ to 6 hours.

INDICATIONS & DOSAGE
Perioperative prophylaxis in contaminated surgery –
Adults: 1 g I.M. or I.V. 30 to 60 minutes before surgery; then 1 g I.M. or I.V. daily for 2 days after surgery.
Uncomplicated gonorrhea caused by Neisseria gonorrhoeae –
Adults: 1 g I.M. as a single dose. May be given with or without probenecid 1 g P.O.
Children 3 months and over: 12.5 to 25 mg/kg I.M. or I.V. 30 to 60 minutes before surgery; then 12.5 to 25 mg/kg I.M. or I.V. q 6 hours for 24 hours.

Note: In cases where infection would be life-threatening, prophylaxis may be continued for 3 days.
Serious infections of the lower respiratory and urinary tracts, skin and skin-structure infections, septicemia, bone and joint infections, and perioperative prophylaxis. Susceptible microorgan-

isms include Streptococcus pneumoniae, Klebsiella pneumoniae, Escherichia coli, Haemophilus influenzae, Proteus mirabilis, Staphylococcus aureus, S. epidermidis, *and* Streptococcus pyogenes –
Adults: usual dosage is 1 g I.V. or I.M. q 24 hours. In life-threatening infections, 2 g q 24 hours.

ADVERSE REACTIONS
CNS: dizziness, headache, malaise, paresthesia.
GI: pseudomembranous colitis, nausea, anorexia, vomiting, diarrhea, glossitis, dyspepsia, abdominal cramps, anal pruritus, tenesmus, oral candidiasis.
GU: genital pruritus and moniliasis, vaginitis.
Hematologic: transient neutropenia, leukopenia, eosinophilia, anemia.
Skin: *maculopapular and erythematous rashes, urticaria.*
Other: dyspnea, hypersensitivity reactions (serum sickness, ***anaphylaxis***); at injection site – *pain, induration, sterile abscesses, tissue sloughing;* with I.V. injection – *phlebitis and thrombophlebitis.*

INTERACTIONS
Probenecid: may inhibit excretion and increase blood levels of cefonicid.

CONTRAINDICATIONS
- Contraindicated in patients with hypersensitivity to the drug or other cephalosporins.
- Use cautiously in patients with a history of sensitivity to penicillin. Also use cautiously and with dosage adjustments in patients with renal failure.

NURSING CONSIDERATIONS
- Obtain specimen for culture and sensitivity tests before first dose. Therapy may begin pending test results.
- With large doses or prolonged therapy, monitor for superinfection, especially in high-risk patients.
- The chemical structure of this drug includes the methylthiotetrazole side chain that has been associated with bleeding disorders. However, such bleeding has not been reported with this drug.
- From 40% to 75% of patients receiving cephalosporins show a false-positive direct Coombs' test.
- Urine glucose determinations may be false-positive with copper sulfate tests (Clinitest); glucose enzymatic tests (Clinistix, Tes-Tape) are not affected.
- **I.V. use:** Reconstitute 500-mg vial with 2 ml of sterile water for injection (yields a concentration of 220 mg/ml) and 1-g vial with 2.5 ml of sterile water for injection (yields a concentration of 325 mg/ml). Shake well. Reconstitute piggyback vials with 50 to 100 ml of sterile water for injection, bacteriostatic water for injection, or 0.9% sodium chloride.
- For I.M. use, when administering 2-g I.M. doses once daily, divide the dose equally and inject deeply into large muscle masses, such as the gluteus maximus or the lateral aspect of the thigh.

cefoperazone sodium
Cefobid

Pregnancy Risk Category: B

HOW SUPPLIED
Infusion: 1 g, 2 g piggyback
Parenteral: 1 g, 2 g

ACTION
Mechanism: A third-generation cephalosporin that inhibits cell-wall synthesis, promoting osmotic instability; usually bactericidal.
Peak: Serum levels peak 1 to 2 hours after I.M. injection, immediately after I.V. infusion. **Duration:** elimination half-life, 1½ to 2½ hours.

INDICATIONS & DOSAGE

Serious infections of the respiratory tract; intra-abdominal, gynecologic, and skin infections; bacteremia; and septicemia. Susceptible microorganisms include Streptococcus pneumoniae *and* S. pyogenes; Staphylococcus aureus *(penicillinase- and non-penicillinase-producing) and* S. epidermidis; *enterococci;* Escherichia coli; Klebsiella; Haemophilus influenzae; Enterobacter; Citrobacter; Proteus; *some* Pseudomonas, *including* P. aeruginosa; *and* Bacteroides fragilis – **Adults:** usual dosage is 1 to 2 g q 12 hours I.M. or I.V. In severe infections or in infections caused by less sensitive organisms, the total daily dosage or frequency may be increased up to 16 g/day in certain situations.

Neonates and children: 25 to 100 mg/kg I.V. q 12 hours.

No dosage adjustment is usually necessary in patients with renal impairment. However, doses of 4 g/day should be given cautiously to patients with hepatic disease or biliary obstruction. Higher dosages require monitoring of serum levels.

ADVERSE REACTIONS

CNS: headache, malaise, paresthesia, dizziness.

GI: pseudomembranous colitis, nausea, anorexia, vomiting, *diarrhea,* glossitis, dyspepsia, abdominal cramps, tenesmus, anal pruritus, oral candidiasis.

GU: genital pruritus and moniliasis.

Hematologic: transient neutropenia, eosinophilia, hemolytic anemia, hypoprothrombinemia, bleeding.

Hepatic: mildly elevated liver enzymes.

Skin: *maculopapular and erythematous rashes, urticaria.*

Other: dyspnea, hypersensitivity reactions (serum sickness, ***anaphylaxis***); at injection site – *pain, induration, sterile abscesses, temperature elevation, tissue sloughing;* with I.V. injection – *phlebitis and thrombophlebitis.*

INTERACTIONS

Aspirin, oral anticoagulants: increased risk of bleeding. Monitor for bleeding.

Ethanol: possible disulfiram-like reaction. Warn patients not to drink alcohol for several days after discontinuing cefoperazone.

Probenecid: may inhibit excretion and increase blood levels of cefoperazone.

CONTRAINDICATIONS

- Contraindicated in patients with hypersensitivity to the drug or other cephalosporins.
- Use cautiously in patients with impaired renal function or with a history of sensitivity to penicillin.

NURSING CONSIDERATIONS

- Obtain specimen for culture and sensitivity tests before first dose. Therapy may begin pending test results.
- Because of high degree of biliary excretion, cefoperazone may increase the risk of diarrhea over other cephalosporins.
- With large doses or prolonged therapy, monitor for superinfection, especially in high-risk patients.
- The chemical structure of this drug includes the methylthiotetrazole side chain that has been associated with bleeding disorders. Vitamin K can be administered to promptly reverse bleeding if it occurs. Monitor PT regularly.
- From 40% to 75% of patients receiving cephalosporins show a false-positive direct Coombs' test.
- Urine glucose determinations may be false-positive with copper sulfate tests (Clinitest); glucose enzymatic tests (Clinistix, Tes-Tape) are not affected.
- **I.V. use:** Reconstitute 1- or 2-g vial with a minimum of 2.8 ml of compat-

ible I.V. solution; the manufacturer recommends using 5 ml/g. Give by direct injection into a large vein or into the tubing of a free-flowing I.V. solution over 3 to 5 minutes. When giving by intermittent infusion, add reconstituted drug to 20 to 40 ml of a compatible I.V. solution and infuse over 15 to 30 minutes.

- To prepare drug for I.M. injection: using the 1-g vial, dissolve drug with 2 ml of sterile water for injection; then add 0.6 ml of 2% lidocaine hydrochloride for a final concentration of 333 mg/ml. Alternatively, dissolve drug with 2.8 ml of sterile water for injection; then add 1 ml of 2% lidocaine hydrochloride for a final concentration of 250 mg/ml. When using the 2-g vial, dissolve drug with 3.8 ml of sterile water for injection; then add 1.2 ml of 2% lidocaine hydrochloride for a final concentration of 333 mg/ml. Alternatively, dissolve drug with 5.4 ml of sterile water for injection; then add 1.8 ml of 2% lidocaine hydrochloride for a final concentration of 250 mg/ml.
- For I.M. administration, inject deeply into a large muscle mass, such as the gluteus maximus or the lateral aspect of the thigh.

cefotaxime sodium

Claforan

Pregnancy Risk Category: B

HOW SUPPLIED

Injection: 500 mg, 1 g, 2 g
Infusion: 1 g, 2 g
Pharmacy bulk package: 10-g vial

ACTION

Mechanism: A third-generation cephalosporin that inhibits cell-wall synthesis, promoting osmotic instability; usually bactericidal.
Peak: Serum levels peak 30 minutes after I.M. injection, immediately after I.V. infusion. **Duration:** elimination is biphasic; terminal half-life, 1 to 2 hours.

INDICATIONS & DOSAGE

Perioperative prophylaxis in contaminated surgery –
Adults: 1 g I.M. or I.V. 30 to 60 minutes before surgery. Patients undergoing bowel surgery should receive preoperative mechanical cleansing and a nonabsorbable anti-infective agent such as neomycin. Patients undergoing cesarean section should receive 1 g I.M. or I.V. as soon as the umbilical cord is clamped, followed by 1 g I.M. or I.V. 6 and 12 hours later.
Serious infections of the lower respiratory and urinary tracts, CNS, skin, bone, and joints; gynecologic and intra-abdominal infections; bacteremia; and septicemia. Susceptible microorganisms include streptococci, including Streptococcus pneumoniae *and* S. pyogenes; Staphylococcus aureus *(penicillinase- and non-penicillinase-producing) and* S. epidermidis; Escherichia coli; Klebsiella; Haemophilus influenzae; Enterobacter; Proteus; *and* Peptostreptococcus –
Adults: usual dose is 1 g I.V. or I.M. q 6 to 8 hours. Up to 12 g daily can be administered in life-threatening infections.
Children 1 month to 12 years: 50 to 180 mg/kg/day I.M. or I.V. in four to six divided doses.
Neonates to 1 week: 50 mg/kg I.V. q 12 hours.
Neonates 1 to 4 weeks: 50 mg/kg I.V. q 8 hours.

ADVERSE REACTIONS

CNS: headache, malaise, paresthesia, dizziness.
GI: pseudomembranous colitis, nausea, anorexia, vomiting, *diarrhea,* glossitis, dyspepsia, abdominal cramps, tenesmus, anal pruritus, oral candidiasis.
GU: genital pruritus and moniliasis.

Hematologic: transient neutropenia, eosinophilia, hemolytic anemia.
Skin: *maculopapular and erythematous rashes, urticaria.*
Other: hypersensitivity reactions (serum sickness, ***anaphylaxis***), dyspnea, elevated temperature; at injection site—*pain, induration, sterile abscesses, temperature elevation, tissue sloughing;* with I.V. injection—*phlebitis and thrombophlebitis.*

INTERACTIONS
Probenecid: may inhibit excretion and increase blood levels of cefotaxime. Use together cautiously.

CONTRAINDICATIONS
- Contraindicated in patients with hypersensitivity to the drug or other cephalosporins.
- Use cautiously in patients with a history of sensitivity to penicillin. Also use cautiously and with dosage adjustments in patients with renal failure.

NURSING CONSIDERATIONS
- Obtain specimen for culture and sensitivity tests before first dose. Therapy may begin pending test results.
- With large doses or prolonged therapy, monitor for superinfection, especially in high-risk patients.
- Some prescribers may use cefotaxime in situations where they formerly prescribed aminoglycosides. However, this drug is usually not effective against infections caused by *Pseudomonas* organisms.
- From 40% to 75% of patients receiving cephalosporins show a false-positive direct Coomb's test.
- Urine glucose determinations may be false-positive with copper sulfate tests (Clinitest); glucose enzymatic tests (Clinistix, Tes-Tape) are not affected.
- **I.V. use:** For direct injection, reconstitute 500-mg, 1-g, or 2-g vials with 10 ml of sterile water for injection. Solutions containing 1 g/14 ml are isotonic. Inject drug into a large vein or into the tubing of a free-flowing I.V. solution over 3 to 5 minutes.
- For I.V. infusion, reconstitute infusion vials with 50 to 100 ml of D_5W or 0.9% sodium chloride solution. Infuse drug over 20 to 30 minutes. Interrupt flow of primary I.V. solution during infusion.
- For I.M. administration, inject deeply into a large muscle mass, such as the gluteus maximus or the lateral aspect of the thigh.

cefotetan disodium
Cefotan

Pregnancy Risk Category: B

HOW SUPPLIED
Injection: 1 g, 2 g
Infusion: 1 g, 2 g piggyback

ACTION
Mechanism: A semisynthetic cephamycin antibiotic that is pharmacologically similar to the second-generation cephalosporins. Inhibits cell-wall synthesis, promoting osmotic instability; usually bactericidal.
Peak: Peak serum levels occur 1½ to 3 hours after I.M. injection, immediately after I.V. infusion. **Duration:** terminal elimination half-life, 3 to 4½ hours.

INDICATIONS & DOSAGE
Serious urinary tract and lower respiratory tract infections and gynecologic, skin and skin-structure, intra-abdominal, and bone and joint infections caused by susceptible streptococci, Staphylococcus aureus *(penicillinase- and non-penicillinase-producing) and* S. epidermidis, Escherichia coli, Klebsiella, Enterobacter, Proteus, Haemophilus influenzae, Neisseria gonorrhoeae, *and* Bacteroides,

including B. fragilis; and perioperative prophylaxis –
Adults: 1 to 2 g I.V. or I.M. q 12 hours for 5 to 10 days. Up to 6 g daily in life-threatening infections.

ADVERSE REACTIONS
CNS: headache, malaise, paresthesia, dizziness.
GI: pseudomembranous colitis, nausea, anorexia, vomiting, *diarrhea,* glossitis, dyspepsia, abdominal cramps, tenesmus, anal pruritus.
GU: genital pruritus and moniliasis.
Hematologic: transient neutropenia, eosinophilia, hemolytic anemia, hypoprothrombinemia, bleeding.
Skin: *maculopapular and erythematous rashes, urticaria.*
Other: hypersensitivity reactions (serum sickness, ***anaphylaxis***), dyspnea, elevated temperature; at injection site – *pain, induration, sterile abscesses, tissue sloughing;* with I.V. injection – *phlebitis and thrombophlebitis.*

INTERACTIONS
Aspirin, oral anticoagulants: increased risk of bleeding. Monitor closely.
Ethanol: possible disulfiram-like reaction. Warn patients not to drink alcohol for several days after discontinuing cefotetan.
Probenecid: may inhibit excretion and increase blood levels of cefotetan. Sometimes used for this effect.

CONTRAINDICATIONS
- Contraindicated in patients with hypersensitivity to the drug or other cephalosporins.
- Use cautiously in patients with a history of sensitivity to penicillin. Also use cautiously and with dosage adjustments in patients with renal failure.

NURSING CONSIDERATIONS
- Obtain specimen for culture and sensitivity tests before first dose. Therapy may begin pending test results.
- With large doses or prolonged therapy, monitor for superinfection, especially in high-risk patients.
- Like cefoxitin, cefotetan is particularly useful in intra-abdominal and gynecologic infections (highly active against *B. fragilis*).
- The chemical structure of this drug includes the methylthiotetrazole side chain that has been associated with bleeding disorders. However, such bleeding has not been reported with this drug.
- From 40% to 75% of patients receiving cephalosporins show a false-positive direct Coombs' test.
- Urine glucose determinations may be false-positive with copper sulfate tests (Clinitest); glucose enzymatic tests (Clinistix, Tes-Tape) are not affected.
- **I.V. use:** Reconstitute with sterile water for injection. Then may be mixed with 50 to 100 ml of D_5W or 0.9% sodium chloride solution. Interrupt flow of primary I.V. solution during cefotetan infusion.
- I.M. injection may be reconstituted with sterile water or bacteriostatic water for injection, 0.9% sodium chloride for injection, or 0.5% or 1% lidocaine hydrochloride. Shake to dissolve and let stand until clear.
- Reconstituted solution remains stable for 24 hours at room temperature or 96 hours if refrigerated.

cefoxitin sodium
Mefoxin
Pregnancy Risk Category: B

HOW SUPPLIED
Injection: 1 g, 2 g
Infusion: 1 g, 2 g in 50-ml or 100-ml container

*Liquid form contains alcohol. *Common* reactions are in italics; ***life-threatening,*** in bold italics.
**May contain tartrazine.

Pharmacy bulk package: 10 g

ACTION

Mechanism: A semisynthetic cephamycin antibiotic that is pharmacologically similar to the second-generation cephalosporins. Inhibits cell-wall synthesis, promoting osmotic instability; usually bactericidal.
Peak: Serum levels peak within 20 to 30 minutes after I.M. injection, immediately after I.V. infusion. **Duration:** elimination half-life, 45 minutes to 1 hour.

INDICATIONS & DOSAGE

Serious infections of respiratory and GU tracts, skin, soft-tissue, bone, and joint infections, and bloodstream and intra-abdominal infections caused by susceptible Escherichia coli *and other coliform bacteria,* Staphylococcus aureus *(penicillinase- and non-penicillinase-producing) and* S. epidermidis, *streptococci,* Klebsiella, Haemophilus influenzae, *and* Bacteroides, *including* B. fragilis; and perioperative prophylaxis –
Adults: 1 to 2 g q 6 to 8 hours for uncomplicated forms of infection. Up to 12 g daily in life-threatening infections.
Children over 3 months: 80 to 160 mg/kg daily given in four to six equally divided doses.

ADVERSE REACTIONS

CNS: headache, malaise, paresthesia, dizziness.
GI: pseudomembranous colitis, nausea, anorexia, vomiting, *diarrhea,* glossitis, dyspepsia, abdominal cramps, tenesmus, anal pruritus, oral candidiasis.
GU: genital pruritus and moniliasis.
Hematologic: transient neutropenia, eosinophilia, ***hemolytic anemia.***
Skin: *maculopapular and erythematous rashes, urticaria.*
Other: hypersensitivity reactions (serum sickness, ***anaphylaxis***), dyspnea, elevated temperature; at injection site – *pain, induration, sterile abscesses, tissue sloughing;* with I.V. injection – *phlebitis and thrombophlebitis.*

INTERACTIONS

Probenecid: may inhibit excretion and increase blood levels of cefoxitin. Sometimes used for this effect.

CONTRAINDICATIONS

- Contraindicated in patients with hypersensitivity to the drug or other cephalosporins.
- Use cautiously in patients with a history of sensitivity to penicillin. Also use cautiously and with dosage adjustments in patients with renal failure.

NURSING CONSIDERATIONS

- Obtain specimen for culture and sensitivity tests before first dose. Therapy may begin pending test results.
- Cefoxitin is useful when anaerobic or mixed aerobic-anaerobic infection is suspected, especially *B. fragilis.*
- With large doses or prolonged therapy, monitor for superinfection, especially in high-risk patients.
- Associated with development of thrombophlebitis. Assess I.V. site frequently.
- From 40% to 75% of patients receiving cephalosporins show a false-positive direct Coombs' test.
- Urine glucose determinations may be false-positive with copper sulfate tests (Clinitest); glucose enzymatic tests (Clinistix, Tes-Tape) are not affected.
- **I.V. use:** Reconstitute 1 g with at least 10 ml of sterile water for injection and 2 g with 10 to 20 ml of sterile water for injection. Solutions of dextrose 5% and 0.9% sodium chloride for injection can also be used. For direct injection, inject drug into a large vein or into the tubing of a free-flow-

ing I.V. solution over 3 to 5 minutes. For intermittent infusion, add reconstituted drug to 50 or 100 ml of dextrose 5% or 10% in water or 0.9% sodium chloride injection. Interrupt flow of primary I.V. solution during infusion.

• I.M. injection can be reconstituted with 0.5% or 1% lidocaine hydrochloride (without epinephrine) to minimize pain. Inject deeply into a large muscle mass, such as the gluteus maximus or the lateral aspect of the thigh.

• After reconstitution, remains stable for 24 hours at room temperature or 1 week under refrigeration.

cefpodoxime proxetil

Vantin

Pregnancy Risk Category: B

HOW SUPPLIED

Tablets (film-coated): 100 mg, 200 mg
Oral suspension: 50 mg/5 ml, 100 mg/5 ml in 100-ml bottles

ACTION

Mechanism: A second-generation cephalosporin that inhibits cell-wall synthesis, promoting osmotic instability; usually bactericidal.
Peak: Serum levels peak 30 minutes to 1 hour after an oral dose. **Duration:** elimination half-life, about 3 hours.

INDICATIONS & DOSAGE

Acute, community-acquired pneumonia caused by non-beta-lactamase-producing strains of Haemophilus influenzae *or* Streptococcus pneumoniae –
Adults: 200 mg P.O. q 12 hours for 14 days.
Acute bacterial exacerbation of chronic bronchitis caused by S. pneumoniae, H. influenzae *(non-beta-lactamase-producing strains only), or* Moraxella (Branhamella) catarrhalis –
Adults: 200 mg P.O. q 12 hours for 10 days.
Uncomplicated gonorrhea in men and women; rectal gonococcal infections in women –
Adults: 200 mg P.O. as a single dose. Follow with doxycycline 100 mg P.O. b.i.d. for 7 days.
Uncomplicated skin and skin-structure infections caused by Staphylococcus aureus *or* Streptococcus pyogenes –
Adults: 400 mg P.O. q 12 hours for 7 to 14 days.
Acute otitis media caused by S. pneumoniae, H. influenzae, *or* M. catarrhalis –
Children 6 months and over: 5 mg/kg (not to exceed 200 mg) P.O. q 12 hours for 10 days.
Pharyngitis or tonsillitis caused by S. pyogenes –
Adults: 100 mg P.O. q 12 hours for 10 days.
Children 6 months and over: 5 mg/kg (not to exceed 100 mg) P.O. q 12 hours for 10 days.
Uncomplicated urinary tract infections caused by Escherichia coli, Klebsiella pneumoniae, Proteus mirabilis, *or* Staphylococcus saprophyticus –
Adults: 100 mg P.O. q 12 hours for 7 days.

In patients with renal failure: When creatinine clearance is below 30 ml/minute/1.73 m^2, dosage interval should be increased to q 24 hours. Patients receiving dialysis should get the drug three times weekly, after dialysis.

ADVERSE REACTIONS

CNS: headache.
GI: *diarrhea,* nausea, vomiting, abdominal pain.
GU: vaginal fungal infections.
Skin: rash.

Other: hypersensitivity reactions *(anaphylaxis)*.

INTERACTIONS

Antacids, H_2 antagonists: decreased absorption of cefpodoxime. Avoid concomitant use.
Probenecid: decreased excretion of cefpodoxime. Monitor for toxicity.

CONTRAINDICATIONS

- Contraindicated in patients with hypersensitivity to the drug or other cephalosporins. Safety and efficacy in children under age 6 months have not been established.
- Use cautiously in patients with a history of penicillin hypersensitivity because of the risk of cross-sensitivity and in patients receiving nephrotoxic drugs because other cephalosporins have been shown to have nephrotoxic potential. Because drug is excreted in human breast milk, also use cautiously in breast-feeding women.

NURSING CONSIDERATIONS

- Obtain specimen for culture and sensitivity tests before first dose. Therapy may begin pending test results.
- May cause overgrowth of nonsusceptible bacteria or fungi. Monitor for signs and symptoms of superinfection.
- Note that the drug's pharmacokinetics are unaltered in patients with hepatic impairment, including those with ascites.
- Absorption of drug is enhanced when taken with food.
- Store suspension in the refrigerator (36° to 46° F [2° to 8° C]). Shake well before using. Discard unused portion after 14 days.
- From 40% to 75% of patients receiving cephalosporins show a false-positive direct Coombs' test.
- Urine glucose determinations may be false-positive with copper sulfate tests (Clinitest); glucose enzymatic tests (Clinistix, Tes-Tape) are not affected.

cefprozil

Cefzil

Pregnancy Risk Category: B

HOW SUPPLIED

Tablets: 250 mg, 500 mg
Oral suspension: 125 mg/5 ml, 250 mg/5 ml

ACTION

Mechanism: A second-generation cephalosporin that interferes with cell-wall synthesis during microorganism replication, leading to osmotic instability and cell lysis (bactericidal).
Peak: Serum levels peak 30 minutes to 1 hour after an oral dose. **Duration:** elimination half-life, 1 hour.

INDICATIONS & DOSAGE

Pharyngitis or tonsillitis caused by Streptococcus pyogenes –
Adults: 500 mg P.O. daily for at least 10 days.
Otitis media caused by S. pneumoniae, Haemophilus influenzae, *and* Moraxella (Branhamella) catarrhalis –
Infants and children 6 months to 12 years: 15 mg/kg P.O. q 12 hours for 10 days.
Secondary bacterial infections of acute bronchitis and acute bacterial exacerbation of chronic bronchitis caused by S. pneumoniae, H. influenzae, *and* M. catarrhalis –
Adults: 500 mg P.O. q 12 hours for 10 days.
Uncomplicated skin and skin-structure infections caused by Staphylococcus aureus *and* Streptococcus pyogenes –
Adults: 250 mg P.O. b.i.d., or 500 mg daily to b.i.d.

ADVERSE REACTIONS
CNS: dizziness, hyperactivity, headache, nervousness, insomnia.
GI: *diarrhea, nausea,* vomiting, abdominal pain.
GU: elevated BUN level, elevated serum creatinine level, genital pruritus, vaginitis.
Hematologic: decreased leukocyte count, eosinophilia.
Hepatic: elevated liver enzymes, cholestatic jaundice (rare).
Skin: rash, urticaria, diaper rash.
Other: superinfection, hypersensitivity reactions (serum sickness, ***anaphylaxis***).

INTERACTIONS
Probenecid: may inhibit excretion and increase blood levels of cefprozil.

CONTRAINDICATIONS
- Contraindicated in patients with hypersensitivity to the drug or other cephalosporins.
- Use cautiously in patients with a history of sensitivity to penicillin. Also use cautiously in patients with impaired hepatic or renal function.

NURSING CONSIDERATIONS
- Obtain specimen for culture and sensitivity tests before first dose. Therapy may begin pending test results.
- May cause overgrowth of nonsusceptible bacteria or fungi. Monitor for signs and symptoms of superinfection.
- Tell the patient to shake suspension well before measuring dose.
- Tell the patient to take all of the medication as prescribed, even after he feels better.
- Oral suspensions contain the drug in a bubble-gum flavored vehicle to improve palatability and compliance in children. Reconstituted suspension should be stored in the refrigerator, and unused drug should be discarded after 14 days.
- Drug is removed by hemodialysis; administer after treatment is completed.
- From 40% to 75% of patients receiving cephalosporins show a false-positive direct Coombs' test.
- Urine glucose determinations may be false-positive with copper sulfate tests (Clinitest); glucose enzymatic tests (Clinistix, Tes-Tape) are not affected.

ceftazidime

Ceptaz, Fortaz, Magnacef†, Pentacef, Tazicef, Tazidime

Pregnancy Risk Category: B

HOW SUPPLIED
Injection (with sodium carbonate): 500 mg, 1 g, 2 g; 6 g (pharmacy bulk package)
Injection (with arginine): 1 g, 2 g; 6 g, 10 g (pharmacy bulk package)
Infusion: 1 g, 2 g in 50-ml and 100-ml vials (premixed)

ACTION
Mechanism: A third-generation cephalosporin that inhibits cell-wall synthesis, promoting osmotic instability; usually bactericidal.
Peak: Peak serum levels occur within 1 hour after I.M. injection, immediately after I.V. infusion. **Duration:** elimination half-life, about 2 hours.

INDICATIONS & DOSAGE
Serious infections of the lower respiratory and urinary tracts; gynecologic, intra-abdominal, CNS, and skin infections; bacteremia; and septicemia. Among susceptible microorganisms are streptococci, including Streptococcus pneumoniae *and* S. pyogenes; Staphylococcus aureus *(penicillinase- and non-penicillinase-producing);* Escherichia coli; Klebsiella; Proteus; Enterobacter; Haemophilus influen-

*Liquid form contains alcohol.
**May contain tartrazine.

zae; Pseudomonas; *and some strains of* Bacteroides –
Adults: 1 g I.V. or I.M. q 8 to 12 hours; up to 6 g daily in life-threatening infections.
Children 1 month to 12 years: 30 to 50 mg/kg I.V. q 8 hours.
Neonates 0 to 4 weeks: 30 mg/kg I.V. q 12 hours.

ADVERSE REACTIONS

CNS: headache, dizziness.
GI: pseudomembranous colitis, nausea, vomiting, diarrhea, dysgeusia, abdominal cramps.
GU: genital pruritus and moniliasis.
Hematologic: eosinophilia; thrombocytosis, leukopenia.
Hepatic: transient elevation in liver enzymes.
Skin: *maculopapular and erythematous rashes, urticaria.*
Other: hypersensitivity reactions (serum sickness, ***anaphylaxis***), dyspnea, elevated temperature; at injection site – *pain, induration, sterile abscesses, tissue sloughing;* with I.V. injection – *phlebitis and thrombophlebitis.*

INTERACTIONS

Sodium bicarbonate-containing solutions: make ceftazidime unstable. Don't mix together.

CONTRAINDICATIONS

• Contraindicated in patients with hypersensitivity to the drug or other cephalosporins.
• Use cautiously in patients with a history of sensitivity to penicillin. Also use cautiously and with dosage adjustments in patients with renal failure.

NURSING CONSIDERATIONS

• Obtain specimen for culture and sensitivity tests before first dose. Therapy may begin pending test results.
• Commercially available preparations contain either sodium carbonate (Fortaz, Magnicef, Tazicef, Tazidime) or arginine (Ceptaz, Pentacef) to facilitate dissolution of drug. Safety and efficacy of arginine-containing solutions in children 12 years and under have not been established; use sodium carbonate formulations in these patients.
• May be prescribed for *Pseudomonas aeruginosa* infections, especially when aminoglycosides are potentially dangerous.
• With large doses or prolonged therapy, monitor for superinfection, especially in high-risk patients.
• From 40% to 75% of patients receiving cephalosporins show a false-positive direct Coombs' test.
• Urine glucose determinations may be false-positive with copper sulfate tests (Clinitest); glucose enzymatic tests (Clinistix, Tes-Tape) are not affected.
• **I.V. use:** Reconstitute sodium carbonate-containing solutions with sterile water for injection. Add 5 ml to a 500-mg vial; 10 ml to a 1-g or 2-g vial. Shake well to dissolve drug. Carbon dioxide is released during dissolution, and a positive pressure will develop in the vial. Reconstitute arginine-containing solutions with 10 ml of sterile water for injection. This formulation won't release gas bubbles. Each brand of ceftazidime includes specific instructions for reconstitution. Read and follow these instructions carefully.
• For I.M. administration, inject deeply into a large muscle mass, such as the gluteus maximus or the lateral aspect of the thigh.

ceftizoxime sodium

Cefizox

Pregnancy Risk Category: B

HOW SUPPLIED
Injection: 1 g, 2 g, 10 g
Infusion: 1 g, 2 g in 100-mg vials or in 50 ml of D_5W

ACTION
Mechanism: A third-generation cephalosporin that inhibits cell-wall synthesis, promoting osmotic instability; usually bactericidal.
Peak: Serum levels peak 30 minutes to 1 hour after I.M. injection, immediately after I.V. infusion. **Duration:** terminal elimination half-life, 1½ to 2 hours.

INDICATIONS & DOSAGE
Serious infections of the lower respiratory and urinary tracts, gynecologic infections, bacteremia, septicemia, meningitis, intra-abdominal infections, bone and joint infections, and skin infections. Among susceptible microorganisms are streptococci, including Streptococcus pneumoniae *and* S. pyogenes; Staphylococcus aureus *(penicillinase- and non-penicillinase-producing) and* S. epidermidis; Escherichia coli; Klebsiella; Haemophilus influenzae; Enterobacter; Proteus; *some* Pseudomonas; *and* Peptostreptococcus—
Adults: usual dosage is 1 to 2 g I.V. or I.M. q 8 to 12 hours. In life-threatening infections, up to 2 g q 4 hours.
Children over 6 months: 33 to 50 mg/kg I.V. q 6 to 8 hours. For serious infections, up to 200 mg/kg/day in divided doses may be used. Don't exceed 12 g/day.

ADVERSE REACTIONS
CNS: headache, malaise, paresthesia, dizziness.
GI: pseudomembranous colitis, nausea, anorexia, vomiting, *diarrhea,* glossitis, dyspepsia, abdominal cramps, tenesmus, anal pruritus.
GU: genital pruritus and moniliasis.
Hematologic: transient neutropenia, eosinophilia, hemolytic anemia.
Skin: *maculopapular and erythematous rashes, urticaria.*
Other: hypersensitivity reactions (serum sickness, ***anaphylaxis***), dyspnea, elevated temperature; at injection site—*pain, induration, sterile abscesses, tissue sloughing;* with I.V. injection—*phlebitis and thrombophlebitis.*

INTERACTIONS
Probenecid: may inhibit excretion and increase blood levels of ceftizoxime. Sometimes used for this effect.

CONTRAINDICATIONS
- Contraindicated in patients with hypersensitivity to ceftizoxime or other cephalosporins.
- Use cautiously in patients with a history of sensitivity to penicillin. Also use cautiously and with dosage adjustments in patients with renal failure.

NURSING CONSIDERATIONS
- Obtain specimen for culture and sensitivity tests before first dose. Therapy may begin pending test results.
- With large doses or prolonged therapy, monitor for superinfection, especially in high-risk patients.
- From 40% to 75% of patients receiving cephalosporins show a false-positive direct Coombs' test.
- Urine glucose determinations may be false-positive with copper sulfate tests (Clinitest); glucose enzymatic tests (Clinistix, Tes-Tape) are not affected.
- **I.V. use:** To reconstitute powder, add 5 ml of sterile water to a 500-mg vial, 10 ml to a 1-g vial, or 20 ml to a 2-g vial. Reconstitute piggyback vials with 50 to 100 ml of 0.9% sodium chloride solution or D_5W. Shake vial well.
- For I.M. administration, inject deeply into a large muscle mass, such as the gluteus maximus or the lateral

aspect of the thigh. Larger doses (2 g) should be divided and administered at two separate sites.

ceftriaxone sodium

Rocephin

Pregnancy Risk Category: B

HOW SUPPLIED

Injection: 250 mg, 500 mg, 1 g, 2 g
Infusion: 1 g, 2 g
Pharmacy bulk package: 10 g

ACTION

Mechanism: A third-generation cephalosporin that inhibits cell-wall synthesis, promoting osmotic instability; usually bactericidal.
Peak: Peak serum levels occur 1½ to 4 hours after I.M. injection, immediately after I.V. infusion. **Duration:** terminal elimination half-life, 5½ to 10½ hours.

INDICATIONS & DOSAGE

Uncomplicated gonococcal vulvovaginitis, urethritis, proctitis, or pharyngitis –
Adults: 250 mg I.M. as a single dose. Follow with 100 mg of doxycycline P.O. q 12 hours for 7 days.
Children: 125 mg I.M. as a single dose.
Prophylaxis of gonococcal infections in neonates born to mothers with documented peripartum gonococcal infections –
Neonates: 25 to 50 mg/kg I.M. or I.V. at birth, not to exceed 125 mg.
Gonococcal ophthalmia or disseminated gonococcal infection in neonates –
Neonates: 25 to 50 mg/kg I.M or I.V. daily for 7 days. Don't exceed 125 mg/day. For meningitis, continue treatment for 14 days.
Serious infections of the lower respiratory and urinary tracts; gynecologic, bone and joint, intra-abdominal, and skin infections; bacteremia; septicemia; and Lyme disease caused by such susceptible microorganisms as streptococci, including Streptococcus pneumoniae *and* S. pyogenes; Staphylococcus aureus *(penicillinase- and non-penicillinase-producing) and* S. epidermidis; Escherichia coli; Klebsiella; Haemophilus influenzae; Neisseria meningitidis; N. gonorrhoeae; Enterobacter; Proteus; Pseudomonas; Peptostreptococcus, *and* Serratia marcescens; and preoperative prophylaxis –
Adults and children over 12 years: 1 to 2 g I.M. or I.V. daily or in equally divided doses b.i.d. Total daily dosage should not exceed 4 g.
Children 12 years and under: 50 to 75 mg/kg, not to exceed 2 g/day, given in divided doses q 12 hours.
Meningitis –
Adults and children: 100 mg/kg given in divided doses q 12 hours. May give loading dose of 75 mg/kg, not to exceed 4 g.

ADVERSE REACTIONS

CNS: headache, dizziness.
GI: pseudomembranous colitis, nausea, vomiting, diarrhea, dysgeusia, abdominal cramps.
GU: genital pruritus and moniliasis.
Hematologic: eosinophilia, thrombocytosis, leukopenia.
Skin: *maculopapular and erythematous rashes, urticaria.*
Other: hypersensitivity reactions (serum sickness, ***anaphylaxis***), dyspnea, elevated temperature; at injection site – *pain, induration, sterile abscesses, tissue sloughing;* with I.V. injection – *phlebitis and thrombophlebitis.*

INTERACTIONS

Probenecid: high doses (1 or 2 g/day) may enhance hepatic clearance of ceftriaxone and shorten half-life. Avoid concomitant use.

CONTRAINDICATIONS

- Contraindicated in patients with hypersensitivity to ceftriaxone or other cephalosporins.
- Use cautiously in patients with a history of sensitivity to penicillin.

NURSING CONSIDERATIONS

- Obtain specimen for culture and sensitivity tests before first dose. Therapy may begin pending test results.
- Dosage adjustment usually is not needed in patients with renal insufficiency.
- Commonly used in home antibiotic programs for outpatient treatment of serious infections, such as osteomyelitis.
- With large doses or prolonged therapy, monitor for superinfection, especially in high-risk patients.
- From 40% to 75% of patients receiving cephalosporins show a false-positive direct Coombs' test.
- Urine glucose determinations may be false-positive with copper sulfate tests (Clinitest); glucose enzymatic tests (Clinistix, Tes-Tape) are not affected.
- **I.V. use:** Reconstitute with sterile water for injection, 0.9% sodium chloride injection, dextrose 5% or 10% injection, or a combination of sodium chloride and dextrose injection and other compatible solutions. Reconstitute by adding 2.4 ml of diluent to the 250-mg vial, 4.8 ml to the 500-mg vial, 9.6 ml to the 1-g vial, and 19.2 ml to the 2-g vial. All reconstituted solutions yield a concentration that averages 100 mg/ml. After reconstitution, dilute further for intermittent infusion to desired concentration. I.V. dilutions are stable for 24 hours at room temperature.
- For I.M. administration, inject deeply into a large muscle mass, such as the gluteus maximus or the lateral aspect of the thigh.

cefuroxime axetil

Ceftin

cefuroxime sodium

Kefurox, Zinacef

Pregnancy Risk Category: B

HOW SUPPLIED

axetil
Tablets: 125 mg, 250 mg, 500 mg
sodium
Injection: 750 mg, 1.5 g
Infusion: 750 mg, 1.5 g premixed, frozen solution

ACTION

Mechanism: A second-generation cephalosporin that inhibits cell-wall synthesis, promoting osmotic instability; usually bactericidal.
Peak: Peak serum levels occur within 2 hours after oral administration, 15 to 60 minutes after I.M. administration, immediately after I.V. infusion.
Duration: elimination half-life, 1 to 2 hours.

INDICATIONS & DOSAGE

Injectable form is for serious infections of the lower respiratory and urinary tracts; skin and skin-structure infections; bone and joint infections; septicemia; meningitis; and gonorrhea; and for perioperative prophylaxis; oral form is used to treat otitis media, pharyngitis, tonsillitis, infections of the urinary and lower respiratory tracts, and skin and skin-structure infections. Among susceptible organisms are Streptococcus pneumoniae *and* S. pyogenes, Haemophilus influenzae, Klebsiella, Staphylococcus aureus, Escherichia coli, Enterobacter, *and* Neisseria gonorrhoeae –
Adults: usual dosage of cefuroxime sodium is 750 mg to 1.5 g I.M. or I.V. q 8 hours for 5 to 10 days. For life-threatening infections and infections caused by less susceptible organisms, 1.5 g I.M. or I.V. q 6 hours; for bacte-

rial meningitis, up to 3 g I.V. q 8 hours.

Alternatively, administer 250 mg of cefuroxime axetil P.O. q 12 hours. For severe infections, dosage may be increased to 500 mg q 12 hours.

Children and infants over 3 months: 50 to 100 mg/kg/day cefuroxime sodium I.M. or I.V. in equally divided doses q 6 to 8 hours. Higher doses are administered when treating meningitis. Alternatively, give 125 mg of cefuroxime axetil P.O. q 12 hours.

Uncomplicated urinary tract infections –

Adults: 125 to 250 mg P.O. q 12 hours.

Otitis media –

Children under age 2: 125 mg P.O. q 12 hours.

Children age 2 and over: 250 mg P.O. q 12 hours.

ADVERSE REACTIONS

CNS: headache, malaise, paresthesia, dizziness.

GI: pseudomembranous colitis, nausea, anorexia, vomiting, *diarrhea,* glossitis, dyspepsia, abdominal cramps, tenesmus, anal pruritus.

GU: genital pruritus and moniliasis.

Hematologic: transient neutropenia, eosinophilia, ***hemolytic anemia,*** decrease in hemoglobin and hematocrit.

Skin: *maculopapular and erythematous rashes, urticaria.*

Other: hypersensitivity reactions (serum sickness, ***anaphylaxis***), dyspnea; at injection site – *pain, induration, sterile abscesses, temperature elevation, tissue sloughing;* with I.V. injection – *phlebitis and thrombophlebitis.*

INTERACTIONS

Probenecid: may inhibit excretion and increase blood levels of cefuroxime. Sometimes used for this effect.

CONTRAINDICATIONS

• Contraindicated in patients with hypersensitivity to cefuroxime or other cephalosporins.

• Use cautiously in patients with history of sensitivity to penicillin. Also use cautiously and with reduced dosage in patients with impaired renal function.

NURSING CONSIDERATIONS

• Obtain specimen for culture and sensitivity tests before first dose. Therapy may begin pending test results.

• With large doses or prolonged therapy, monitor for superinfection, especially in high-risk patients.

• Absorption of cefuroxime axetil is enhanced by food.

• Cefuroxime axetil is available only in tablet form, which may be crushed for patients who cannot swallow tablets. Tablets may be allowed to dissolve in small amounts of apple, orange, or grape juice or chocolate milk. However, the drug has a bitter taste that is difficult to mask, even with food. Until a suitable liquid suspension is developed, alternative therapy may be necessary.

• Advantage over some other cephalosporins is that cefuroxime is useful in treating meningitis.

• From 40% to 75% of patients receiving cephalosporins show a false-positive direct Coombs' test.

• Urine glucose determinations may be false-positive with copper sulfate tests (Clinitest); glucose enzymatic tests (Clinistix, Tes-Tape) are not affected.

• **I.V. use:** For each 750-mg vial of Kefurox, reconstitute with 9 ml of sterile water for injection. Withdraw 8 ml from the vial for the proper dose. For each 1.5-g vial of Kefurox, reconstitute with 16 ml of sterile water for injection; withdraw entire contents of vial for a dose. For each 750-mg vial of Zinacef, reconstitute with 8 ml of sterile water for injection; for each 1.5-g vial, reconstitute with 16 ml. In each case, withdraw entire contents of vial for a dose.

- To give by direct injection, inject into a large vein or into the tubing of a free-flowing I.V. solution over 3 to 5 minutes.
- For intermittent infusion, add reconstituted drug to 100 ml D_5W, 0.9% sodium chloride injection, or other compatible I.V. solution. Infuse over 15 to 60 minutes.
- For I.M. administration, inject deeply into a large muscle mass, such as the gluteus maximus or the lateral aspect of the thigh.

---

cephalexin hydrochloride

Keftab

cephalexin monohydrate

Apo-Cephalex†, Cefanex, Ceporex†‡, C-Lexin, Keflet, Keflex, Novolexin†, Nu-Cephalex‡

Pregnancy Risk Category: B

HOW SUPPLIED

hydrochloride
Tablets: 250 mg, 500 mg
monohydrate
Tablets: 250 mg, 500 mg, 1 g
Capsules: 500 mg, 1,250 mg
Oral suspension: 100 mg/5 ml, 125 mg/5 ml, 250 mg/5 ml

ACTION

Mechanism: A first-generation cephalosporin that inhibits cell-wall synthesis, promoting osmotic instability; usually bactericidal.
Peak: Serum levels peak within 1 hour. **Duration:** elimination half-life, 30 minutes to 1 hour.

INDICATIONS & DOSAGE

Respiratory tract, GI tract, skin, soft-tissue, bone, and joint infections and otitis media caused by Escherichia coli *and other coliform bacteria, group A beta-hemolytic streptococci,* Haemophilus influenzae, Klebsiella, Moraxella (Branhamella) catarrhalis, Proteus mirabilis, Streptococcus pneumoniae, *and staphylococci*–
Adults: 250 mg to 1 g P.O. q 6 hours.
Children: 6 to 12 mg/kg P.O. q 6 hours (monohydrate only). Maximum 25 mg/kg q 6 hours.

ADVERSE REACTIONS

CNS: dizziness, headache, malaise, paresthesia.
GI: pseudomembranous colitis, *nausea, anorexia,* vomiting, *diarrhea,* glossitis, dyspepsia, abdominal cramps, anal pruritus, tenesmus, oral candidiasis.
GU: genital pruritus and moniliasis, vaginitis.
Hematologic: transient neutropenia, eosinophilia, anemia.
Skin: *maculopapular and erythematous rashes, urticaria.*
Other: hypersensitivity reactions (serum sickness, ***anaphylaxis***), dyspnea.

INTERACTIONS

Probenecid: may increase blood levels of cephalosporins. Sometimes used for this effect.

CONTRAINDICATIONS

- Use cautiously in patients with impaired renal function or with a history of sensitivity to penicillin. Ask the patient if he has had any reaction to previous cephalosporin or penicillin therapy before administering first dose.

NURSING CONSIDERATIONS

- Obtain specimen for culture and sensitivity tests before first dose. Therapy may begin pending test results.
- Group A beta-hemolytic streptococcal infections should be treated for a minimum of 10 days.
- Tell the patient to take all of the

medication exactly as prescribed, even after he feels better.
• Tell the patient to take drug with food or milk to lessen GI discomfort.
• Call the doctor if skin rash develops.
• With large doses or prolonged therapy, monitor for superinfection, especially in high-risk patients.
• Preparation of oral suspension: Add required amount of water to powder in two portions. Shake well after each addition. After mixing, store in refrigerator. The mixture will remain stable for 14 days without significant loss of potency. Keep tightly closed and shake well before using.
• From 40% to 75% of patients receiving cephalosporins show a false-positive direct Coombs' test, but only a few of these indicate hemolytic anemia.
• Urine glucose determinations may be false-positive with copper sulfate tests (Clinitest); glucose enzymatic tests (Clinistix, Tes-Tape) are not affected.

cephalothin sodium

Ceporacin†‡, Keflin

Pregnancy Risk Category: B

HOW SUPPLIED

Injection: 1 g, 2 g, 4 g
Infusion: 1 g/50 ml, 2 g/50 ml, 1 g/dl, 2 g/dl
Pharmacy bulk package: 10 g

ACTION

Mechanism: Inhibits cell-wall synthesis, promoting osmotic instability; usually bactericidal.
Peak: Serum levels peak within 30 minutes of I.M. administration, immediately after I.V. infusion. **Duration:** elimination half-life, less than 1 hour.

INDICATIONS & DOSAGE

Serious infections of respiratory, GU, or GI tract; skin and soft-tissue infections (including peritonitis); bone and joint infections; septicemia; and endocarditis caused by such susceptible organisms as Escherichia coli *and other coliform bacteria, Enterobacteriaceae, enterococci, gonococci, group A beta-hemolytic streptococci,* Haemophilus influenzae, Klebsiella, Proteus mirabilis, Salmonella, Staphylococcus aureus, Shigella, Streptococcus pneumoniae *and* S. viridans, *and staphylococci; and perioperative prophylaxis –*
Adults: 500 mg to 1 g I.M. or I.V. (or intraperitoneally) q 4 to 6 hours; in life-threatening infections, up to 2 g q 4 hours.
Children: 100 mg/kg/day I.V. in divided doses q 4 or 6 hours. Dose should be proportionately less in accordance with age, weight, and severity of infection.

Dosage schedule is determined by degree of renal impairment, severity of infection, and susceptibility of causative organism.

ADVERSE REACTIONS

CNS: headache, malaise, paresthesia, dizziness.
GI: pseudomembranous colitis, nausea, anorexia, vomiting, *diarrhea,* glossitis, dyspepsia, abdominal cramps, tenesmus, anal pruritus, oral candidiasis.
GU: nephrotoxicity, genital pruritus and moniliasis.
Hematologic: transient neutropenia, eosinophilia, ***hemolytic anemia.***
Skin: *maculopapular and erythematous rashes, urticaria.*
Other: hypersensitivity reactions (serum sickness, ***anaphylaxis***), dyspnea, fever; at injection site – *pain, induration, sterile abscesses, tissue sloughing;* with I.V. injection – *phlebitis and thrombophlebitis.*

INTERACTIONS

Probenecid: may increase blood levels of cephalosporins. Use together cautiously.

CONTRAINDICATIONS

• Contraindicated in patients with hypersensitivity to cephalothin or other cephalosporins.
• *Use cautiously* in patients with impaired renal function and in those with a history of sensitivity to penicillin.

NURSING CONSIDERATIONS

• Obtain specimen for culture and sensitivity tests before first dose. Therapy may begin pending test results.
• With large doses or prolonged therapy, monitor for superinfection, especially in high-risk patients.
• From 40% to 75% of patients receiving cephalosporins show a false-positive direct Coombs' test; only a few of these indicate hemolytic anemia.
• Urine glucose determinations may be false-positive with copper sulfate tests (Clinitest); glucose enzymatic tests (Clinistix, Tes-Tape) are not affected.
• Drug causes severe pain when administered I.M.; avoid this route if possible.
• I.V. route is preferable in severe or life-threatening infections.
• **I.V. use:** When giving this drug I.V., check frequently for vein irritation and phlebitis. Alternate injection sites if I.V. therapy lasts longer than 3 days. Use of small I.V. needles in the larger available veins may be preferable. Addition of a small concentration of heparin (100 units) or hydrocortisone (10 to 25 mg) may reduce incidence of phlebitis.
• For I.V. administration, dilute contents of 2-g vial with at least 20 ml of sterile water for injection, dextrose 5% injection, or 0.9% sodium chloride injection and add to one of following I.V. solutions: dextrose 5% injection, dextrose 5% in lactated Ringer's injection, Ionosol B in D_5W, lactated Ringer's injection, Normosol-N in D_5W, Plasma-Lyte injection, Plasma-Lyte-N injection in dextrose 5%, Ringer's injection, or Plasma-Lyte-N in 0.9% sodium chloride injection. Choose solution and fluid volume according to patient's fluid and electrolyte status.
• For I.M. administration, reconstitute each gram of cephalothin sodium with 4 ml of sterile water for injection, providing 500 mg in each 2.2 ml. If vial contents don't dissolve completely, add an additional 0.2 to 0.4 ml of diluent, and warm contents slightly. Inject deeply into a large muscle mass, such as the gluteus maximus or the lateral aspect of the thigh.

cephapirin sodium

Cefadyl

Pregnancy Risk Category: B

HOW SUPPLIED

Injection: 500-mg, 1-g, 2-g vials; 1-g, 2-g, 4-g piggyback vials
Pharmacy bulk package: 20 g

ACTION

Mechanism: Inhibits cell-wall synthesis, promoting osmotic instability; usually bactericidal.
Peak: Serum levels peak within 30 minutes of I.M. injection, immediately after I.V. infusion. **Duration:** serum half-life, 21 to 47 minutes.

INDICATIONS & DOSAGE

Perioperative prophylaxis in contaminated or potentially contaminated surgery—
Adults: 1 to 2 g I.M. or I.V. 30 to 60 minutes before surgery; then 1 to 2 g I.M. or I.V. q 6 hours for 24 hours. In procedures longer than 2 hours, addi-

tional doses may be given during surgery. In cases where infection would be devastating, prophylaxis may be continued for 3 to 5 days.
Serious infections of respiratory, GU, or GI tract; skin and soft-tissue infections; bone and joint infections (including osteomyelitis); septicemia; and endocarditis caused by Streptococcus pneumoniae, Escherichia coli, *group A beta-hemolytic streptococci,* Haemophilus influenzae, Klebsiella, Proteus mirabilis, Staphylococcus aureus, *and* Streptococcus viridans – **Adults:** 500 mg to 1 g I.M. or I.V. q 4 to 6 hours. In life-threatening infections, up to 12 g/day may be used.
Children over 3 months: 10 to 20 mg/kg I.V. or I.M. q 6 hours; dose depends on age, weight, and severity of infection.

Patients with reduced renal function: may be treated adequately with a lower dose (7.5 to 15 mg/kg q 12 hours), depending on causative organism and severity of function. Patients with severely reduced renal function who are scheduled for dialysis should receive same dose just before dialysis and q 12 hours thereafter.

ADVERSE REACTIONS
CNS: dizziness, headache, malaise, paresthesia.
GI: pseudomembranous colitis, nausea, anorexia, vomiting, *diarrhea,* glossitis, dyspepsia, abdominal cramps, tenesmus, anal pruritus, oral candidiasis.
GU: genital pruritus and moniliasis, vaginitis.
Hematologic: transient neutropenia, eosinophilia, anemia.
Skin: *maculopapular and erythematous rashes, urticaria.*
Other: hypersensitivity reactions (serum sickness, ***anaphylaxis***), dyspnea; at injection site – *pain, induration, sterile abscesses, tissue sloughing;* with I.V. injection – *phlebitis and thrombophlebitis.*

INTERACTIONS
Probenecid: may increase blood levels of cephalosporins. Sometimes used for this effect.

CONTRAINDICATIONS
- Contraindicated in patients hypersensitive to cephapirin or other cephalosporins.
- Use cautiously in patients with a history of sensitivity to penicillin.

NURSING CONSIDERATIONS
- Obtain specimen for culture and sensitivity tests before first dose. Therapy may begin pending test results.
- With large doses or prolonged therapy, monitor for superinfection, especially in high-risk patients.
- From 40% to 75% of patients receiving cephalosporins show a false-positive direct Coombs' test, but only a few indicate hemolytic anemia.
- Urine glucose determinations may be false-positive with copper sulfate tests (Clinitest); glucose enzymatic tests (Clinistix, Tes-Tape) are not affected.
- **I.V. use:** When giving this drug I.V., check frequently for vein irritation and phlebitis. Alternate injection sites if I.V. therapy lasts longer than 3 days. Use of small I.V. needles in the larger available veins may be preferable.
- Prepare I.V. infusion using dextrose injection, sodium chloride injection, or bacteriostatic water for injection as diluent: 20 ml yields 1 g/10 ml; 50 ml yields 1 g/25 ml; 100 ml yields 1 g/50 ml.
- For I.V. infusion with Y-tubing: Dilute 4-g vial with 40 ml of diluent. During infusion of cephapirin solution, stop other solution. Check volume of cephapirin solution carefully so that calculated dose is infused.
- For I.M. use, reconstitute 1-g vial with 2 ml of sterile water for injection or bacteriostatic water for injection so

that 1.2 ml contains 500 mg of cephapirin. Prepare patient for painful I.M. injection. Inject deeply into a large muscle mass, such as the gluteus maximus or the lateral aspect of the thigh.

• Reconstituted cephapirin is stable and compatible for 10 days under refrigeration and for 24 hours at room temperature.

cephradine

Anspor, Velosef**

Pregnancy Risk Category: B

HOW SUPPLIED

Capsules: 250 mg, 500 mg
Oral suspension: 125 mg/5 ml, 250 mg/5 ml

ACTION

Mechanism: Inhibits cell-wall synthesis, promoting osmotic instability; usually bactericidal.
Peak: Serum levels peak within 1 hour after an oral dose. **Duration:** elimination half-life, 45 minutes to 2 hours.

INDICATIONS & DOSAGE

Serious infections of respiratory, GU, or GI tract; skin and soft-tissue infections; bone and joint infections; septicemia; endocarditis; and otitis media caused by such susceptible organisms as Escherichia coli *and other coliform bacteria, group A beta-hemolytic streptococci,* Haemophilus influenzae, Klebsiella, Proteus mirabilis, Staphylococcus aureus, Streptococcus pneumoniae, S. viridans, *and staphylococci; and perioperative prophylaxis –*
Adults: 250 to 500 mg P.O. q 6 hours.
Children over age 1: 6 to 12 mg/kg P.O. q 6 hours.
Otitis media – 19 to 25 mg/kg P.O. q 6 hours. Don't exceed 4 g daily.

All patients, regardless of age and weight: larger doses (up to 1 g q.i.d.) may be given for severe or chronic infections.

ADVERSE REACTIONS

CNS: dizziness, headache, malaise, paresthesia.
GI: pseudomembranous colitis, *nausea, anorexia,* vomiting, heartburn, glossitis, dyspepsia, abdominal cramping, *diarrhea,* tenesmus, anal pruritus, oral candidiasis.
GU: genital pruritus and moniliasis, vaginitis.
Hematologic: transient neutropenia, eosinophilia.
Skin: *maculopapular and erythematous rashes, urticaria.*
Other: hypersensitivity reactions (serum sickness, ***anaphylaxis***), dyspnea.

INTERACTIONS

Probenecid: may increase blood levels of cephalosporins. Sometimes used for this effect.

CONTRAINDICATIONS

• Contraindicated in patients with hypersensitivity to cephradine and to other cephalosporins.
• Use cautiously in patients with impaired renal function or with a history of sensitivity to penicillin.

NURSING CONSIDERATIONS

• Obtain specimen for culture and sensitivity tests before first dose. Therapy may begin pending test results.
• Group A beta-hemolytic streptococcal infections should be treated for a minimum of 10 days.
• Tell the patient to take all of the medication exactly as prescribed, even after he feels better.
• Tell the patient to take drug with food or milk to lessen GI discomfort.
• With large doses or prolonged therapy, monitor for superinfection, especially in high-risk patients.
• From 40% to 75% of patients re-

*Liquid form contains alcohol.
**May contain tartrazine.

ceiving cephalosporins show a false-positive direct Coombs' test, but only a few indicate hemolytic anemia.

• Urine glucose determinations may be false-positive with copper sulfate tests (Clinitest); glucose enzymatic tests (Clinistix, Tes-Tape) are not affected.

loracarbef

Lorabid

Pregnancy Risk Category: B

HOW SUPPLIED

Pulvules: 200 mg

Powder for oral suspension: 100 mg/5 ml, 200 mg/5 ml in 50-ml and 100-ml bottles

ACTION

Mechanism: A synthetic beta-lactam antibiotic of the carbacephem class with actions similar to the second-generation cephalosporins. Inhibits cell-wall synthesis, promoting osmotic instability; usually bactericidal.
Peak: Serum levels peak 30 minutes to 1 hour after an oral dose. **Duration:** elimination half-life, about 1 hour.

INDICATIONS & DOSAGE

Secondary bacterial infections of acute bronchitis –
Adults: 200 to 400 mg P.O. q 12 hours for 7 days.
Acute bacterial exacerbations of chronic bronchitis –
Adults: 400 mg P.O. q 12 hours for 7 days.
Pneumonia –
Adults: 400 mg P.O. q 12 hours for 14 days.
Pharyngitis, sinusitis, or tonsillitis –
Adults: 200 to 400 mg P.O. q 12 hours for 10 days.
Children: 15 mg/kg P.O. daily in divided doses q 12 hours for 10 days.
Acute otitis media –
Children: 30 mg/kg (oral suspension) P.O. daily in divided doses q 12 hours for 10 days.
Uncomplicated skin and skin-structure infections –
Adults: 200 mg P.O. q 12 hours for 7 days.
Impetigo –
Children: 15 mg/kg P.O. daily in divided doses q 12 hours for 7 days.
Uncomplicated cystitis –
Adults: 200 mg P.O. daily for 7 days.
Uncomplicated pyelonephritis –
Adults: 400 mg P.O. q 12 hours for 7 days.

Patients with a creatinine clearance greater than or equal to 50 ml/minute/1.73 m^2 don't require dose and interval changes. Patients with a creatinine clearance of 10 to 49 ml/minute/1.73 m^2 should receive half of the usual dose at the same interval; with a creatinine clearance below 10 ml/minute/1.73 m^2, the usual dose q 3 to 5 days. Hemodialysis patients require another dose after dialysis.

ADVERSE REACTIONS

CNS: headache, somnolence, nervousness, insomnia, dizziness.
CV: vasodilation.
GI: diarrhea, nausea, vomiting, abdominal pain, anorexia, pseudomembranous colitis.
GU: vaginal candidiasis or moniliasis, transient increases in BUN and creatinine levels.
Hematologic: transient thrombocytopenia, leukopenia, eosinophilia.
Skin: rash, urticaria, pruritus, ***erythema multiforme.***
Other: hypersensitivity reactions, including ***anaphylaxis;*** transient elevations in AST, ALT, and alkaline phosphatase levels.

INTERACTIONS

Probenecid: decreased excretion of loracarbef, causing increased plasma levels. Monitor for toxicity.

CONTRAINDICATIONS

- Contraindicated in patients with hypersensitivity to the drug or other cephalosporins and in patients with diarrhea caused by pseudomembranous colitis.
- Use cautiously in pregnant or breast-feeding women. Safety and efficacy have not been established in infants under 6 months.

NURSING CONSIDERATIONS

- Obtain specimen for culture and sensitivity tests before first dose. Therapy may begin pending test results.
- May cause overgrowth of nonsusceptible bacteria or fungi. Monitor for signs and symptoms of superinfection.
- Tell the patient to take all of the medication prescribed, even after he feels better.
- Tell the patient to take drug on an empty stomach, at least 1 hour before or 2 hours after meals.
- Beta-lactam antibiotics may trigger seizures in susceptible patients, especially when given without dosage modification to those with renal impairment. If seizures occur, discontinue drug and notify the doctor. Administer anticonvulsants as ordered.
- For otitis media, use the more rapidly absorbed oral suspension, which produces higher peak plasma levels than do the capsules.
- To reconstitute powder for oral suspension, add 30 ml of water in two portions to the 50-ml bottle or 60 ml of water in two portions to the 100-ml bottle; shake after each addition.
- After reconstitution, oral suspension is stable for 14 days at room temperature (59° to 86° F [15° to 30° C]). Instruct the patient to discard unused portion after 14 days.
- From 40% to 75% of patients receiving cephalosporins show a false-positive direct Coombs' test; only a few of these indicate hemolytic anemia.

14

Tetracyclines

demeclocycline hydrochloride
doxycycline
doxycycline hyclate
doxycycline hydrochloride
minocycline hydrochloride
oxytetracycline hydrochloride
tetracycline hydrochloride

COMBINATION PRODUCTS
UROBIOTIC-250: oxytetracycline hydrochloride 250 mg, sulfamethizole 250 mg, and phenazopyridine hydrochloride 50 mg.

demeclocycline hydrochloride

Declomycin, Ledermycin‡

Pregnancy Risk Category: D

HOW SUPPLIED
Tablets: 150 mg, 300 mg
Capsules: 150 mg

ACTION
Mechanism: Exerts bacteriostatic effect by binding to the 30S ribosomal subunit of microorganisms, thus inhibiting protein synthesis.
Peak: Serum levels peak within 3 to 4 hours after an oral dose. **Duration:** elimination half-life, 10 to 17 hours.

INDICATIONS & DOSAGE
Infections caused by susceptible gram-negative and gram-positive organisms, including Haemophilus ducreyi, Rickettsiae, Mycoplasma pneumoniae, Yersinia pestis, Campylobacter fetus. *Also indicated for the organism causing psittacosis, lymphogranuloma venereum, granuloma inguinale, relapsing fever, and trachoma –*
Adults: 150 mg P.O. q 6 hours or 300 mg P.O. q 12 hours.
Children over age 8: 6 to 12 mg/kg P.O. daily, in divided doses q 6 to 12 hours.
Gonorrhea –
Adults: initially, 600 mg P.O.; then 300 mg P.O. q 12 hours for 4 days (total 3 g).
SIADH (a hyposmolar state) –
Adults: 600 to 1,200 mg P.O. daily in divided doses q 6 to 8 hours.

ADVERSE REACTIONS
CNS: pseudotumor cerebri.
CV: pericarditis.
EENT: dysphagia, glossitis.
GI: anorexia, *nausea, vomiting, diarrhea,* enterocolitis, anogenital inflammation.
Hematologic: neutropenia, eosinophilia, thrombocytopenia, ***hemolytic anemia.***
Skin: *maculopapular and erythematous rashes, photosensitivity, increased pigmentation, urticaria.*
Other: hypersensitivity reactions *(**anaphylaxis**), increased BUN level,* diabetes insipidus syndrome (polyuria, polydipsia, weakness), permanent tooth discoloration or bone growth retardation if used in children under 8 years.

INTERACTIONS
Antacids (including sodium bicarbonate) and laxatives containing aluminum, magnesium, or calcium; antidiarrheals; food, milk, or other dairy products: decreased antibiotic absorption. Give antibiotic 1 hour before or 2 hours after any of the above.
Ferrous sulfate and other iron products, zinc: decreased antibiotic absorption. Give antibiotic 3 hours after or 2 hours before iron administration.
Methoxyflurane: may cause nephrotoxicity with tetracyclines. Monitor carefully.

Oral anticoagulants: increased anticoagulant effect. Monitor PT and adjust dosage as ordered.
Oral contraceptives: decreased contraceptive effectiveness and increased risk of breakthrough bleeding. Use a nonhormonal birth control method.

CONTRAINDICATIONS
- Contraindicated in patients with hypersensitivity to the drug or other tetracyclines.
- Use cautiously in patients with impaired renal or hepatic function. Use of these drugs during last half of pregnancy and in children under age 8 may cause permanent discoloration of teeth, enamel defects, and bone growth retardation.

NURSING CONSIDERATIONS
- Obtain specimen for culture and sensitivity tests before first dose. Therapy may begin pending test results.
- Check expiration date. Outdated or deteriorated tetracyclines have been associated with reversible nephrotoxicity (Fanconi's syndrome).
- Don't expose these drugs to light or heat; store in tight container.
- With large doses or prolonged therapy, monitor for superinfection, especially in high-risk patients.
- Check the patient's tongue for signs of monilia infection. Stress good oral hygiene.
- Warn the patient to avoid direct sunlight and ultraviolet light. A sunscreen may help prevent photosensitivity reactions. Photosensitivity persists for some time after discontinuation of drug.
- Explain to the patient that drug's effectiveness is reduced when taken with milk or other dairy products, food, antacids, or iron products. Tell him to take each dose with a full glass of water on an empty stomach, at least 1 hour before or 2 hours after meals, and to remain standing for 90 seconds after ingestion. Give at least 1 hour before bedtime to prevent esophagitis.
- Instruct the patient to take entire amount of medication, exactly as prescribed, even after he feels better.
- May cause false-negative reading of glucose enzymatic tests (Clinistix, Tes-Tape).

doxycycline
Doxylin‡, Vibramycin

doxycycline hyclate
Apo-Doxy†, Doryx, Doxy-Caps, Doxycin†, Doxy-Tabs, Monodox, Novodoxylin†, Vibramycin, Vibra-Tabs

doxycycline hydrochloride
Cyclidox‡, Doryx‡, Vibramycin‡, Vibramycin IV, Vibra-Tabs 50‡

Pregnancy Risk Category: D

HOW SUPPLIED
doxycycline
Tablets: 50 mg‡, 100 mg‡
Oral suspension: 25 mg/5 ml
Syrup: 50 mg/5 ml
doxycycline hyclate
Tablets: 50 mg, 100 mg
Capsules: 50 mg, 100 mg
Capsules (coated pellets): 100 mg
Injection: 100 mg, 200 mg
doxycycline hydrochloride
Tablets: 50 mg‡, 100 mg‡
Capsules: 50 mg‡, 100 mg‡, 250 mg‡
Injection: 100 mg‡
Powder for injection: 200 mg

ACTION
Mechanism: Exerts bacteriostatic effect by binding to the 30S ribosomal subunit of microorganisms, thus inhibiting protein synthesis.
Peak: Serum levels peak within 1½ to 4 hours after an oral dose. **Duration:** elimination half-life, 14 to 17 hours.

INDICATIONS & DOSAGE
Infections caused by sensitive gram-negative and gram-positive organisms, including Rickettsiae, Chlamydia, *and* Mycoplasma, *and the organisms that cause trachoma and Lyme disease –*
Adults: 100 mg P.O. q 12 hours on first day, then 100 mg P.O. daily; or 200 mg I.V. on first day in one or two infusions, then 100 to 200 mg I.V. daily.
Children over age 8 and under 45 kg: 4.4 mg/kg P.O. or I.V. daily, in divided doses q 12 hours on first day; then 2.2 to 4.4 mg/kg daily. For children over 45 kg, dosage is same as for adults.

Give I.V. infusion slowly (minimum 1 hour). Infusion must be completed within 12 hours (within 6 hours in lactated Ringer's solution or dextrose 5% in lactated Ringer's solution).
Gonorrhea in patients allergic to penicillin –
Adults: 200 mg P.O. initially, followed by 100 mg P.O. h.s. and 100 mg P.O. b.i.d. for 3 days; or 300 mg P.O. initially and repeat dose in 1 hour.
Primary or secondary syphilis in patients allergic to penicillin –
Adults: 300 mg P.O. daily in divided doses for at least 10 days.
Uncomplicated urethral, endocervical, or rectal infections caused by Chlamydia trachomatis *or* Ureaplasma urealyticum –
Adults: 100 mg P.O. b.i.d. for at least 7 days.
Traveler's diarrhea –
Adults: 100 mg P.O. b.i.d. for 2 to 3 days.
Prophylaxis of traveler's diarrhea –
Adults: 100 mg P.O. daily during travel (up to 2 weeks) and for 2 days after returning home.

ADVERSE REACTIONS
CNS: ***intracranial hypertension.***
CV: pericarditis.
EENT: sore throat, glossitis, dysphagia.
GI: anorexia, *epigastric distress, nausea,* vomiting, *diarrhea,* oral candidiasis, enterocolitis, anogenital inflammation.
Hematologic: neutropenia, eosinophilia.
Skin: *maculopapular and erythematous rashes, photosensitivity, increased pigmentation, urticaria.*
Other: hypersensitivity reactions *(**anaphylaxis**)*; permanent discoloration of teeth, enamel defects, bone growth retardation if used in children under age 8; superinfection; thrombophlebitis.

INTERACTIONS
Antacids (including sodium bicarbonate) and laxatives containing aluminum, magnesium, or calcium; antidiarrheals; food, milk, or other dairy products: decreased antibiotic absorption. Give antibiotic 1 hour before or 2 hours after any of the above.
Ferrous sulfate and other iron products, zinc: decreased antibiotic absorption. Give drug 3 hours after or 2 hours before iron administration.
Methoxyflurane: may cause nephrotoxicity with tetracyclines. Monitor carefully.
Oral anticoagulants: increased anticoagulant effect. Monitor PT and adjust dosage as ordered.
Oral contraceptives: decreased contraceptive effectiveness and increased risk of breakthrough bleeding. Use a nonhormonal form of birth control.
Phenobarbital, carbamazepine, alcohol: decreased antibiotic effect. Avoid if possible.

CONTRAINDICATIONS
- Contraindicated in patients with hypersensitivity to the drug or other tetracyclines.

• Use cautiously in patients with impaired renal or hepatic function. Use of these drugs during last half of pregnancy and in children under age 8 may cause permanent discoloration of teeth, enamel defects, and bone growth retardation.
• Patient may develop thrombophlebitis with I.V. administration.

NURSING CONSIDERATIONS
• Obtain specimen for culture and sensitivity tests before first dose. Therapy may begin pending test results.
• Check expiration date. Outdated or deteriorated tetracyclines have been associated with reversible nephrotoxicity (Fanconi's syndrome).
• Don't expose drug to light or heat. Protect it from sunlight during infusion.
• With large doses or prolonged therapy, monitor for superinfection, especially in high-risk patients.
• Check the patient's tongue for signs of fungal infection. Stress good oral hygiene.
• May be taken with milk or food if adverse GI effects develop.
• Tell the patient to take entire amount of medication exactly as prescribed, even after he feels better.
• Doxycycline may be used in patients with renal impairment; doesn't accumulate or cause a significant rise in BUN levels.
• Oral tablets or capsules should not be taken within 1 hour of bedtime because of possible dysphagia.
• Tell the patient to use a sunscreen and avoid strong sunlight during therapy to prevent photosensitivity reactions.
• **I.V. use:** Reconstitute powder for injection with sterile water for injection. Use 10 ml in 100-mg vial and 20 ml in 200-mg vial. Dilute solution to 100 to 1,000 ml for I.V. infusion. Avoid extravasation. Don't infuse solutions that are more concentrated than 1 mg/ml.
• Reconstituted injectable solution is stable for 72 hours if refrigerated.
• Parenteral form may cause false-positive reading of copper sulfate tests (Clinitest). All forms may cause false-negative reading of glucose enzymatic tests (Clinistix, Tes-Tape).

minocycline hydrochloride

Minocin*, Minomycin‡, Minomycin IV‡

Pregnancy Risk Category: D

HOW SUPPLIED
Capsules: 50 mg, 100 mg
Oral suspension: 50 mg/5 ml
Injection: 100 mg

ACTION
Mechanism: Exerts bacteriostatic effect by binding to the 30S ribosomal subunit of microorganisms, thus inhibiting protein synthesis.
Peak: Serum levels peak immediately after I.V. infusion, within 1 to 4 hours after oral dose. **Duration:** elimination half-life, 11 to 26 hours.

INDICATIONS & DOSAGE
Infections caused by sensitive gram-negative and gram-positive organisms, trachoma, amebiasis –
Adults: 200 mg I.V.; then 100 mg I.V. q 12 hours. Don't exceed 400 mg/day. Or give 200 mg P.O. initially; then 100 mg P.O. q 12 hours. Some clinicians use 100 or 200 mg P.O. initially, followed by 50 mg q.i.d.
Children over age 8: initially, 4 mg/kg P.O. or I.V., followed by 2 mg/kg q 12 hours.

Give I.V. in 500- to 1,000-ml solution without calcium, and administer over 6 hours.

Gonorrhea in patients sensitive to penicillin –
Adults: initially, 200 mg P.O.; then 100 mg q 12 hours for at least 4 days.

Syphilis in patients sensitive to penicillin –
Adults: initially, 200 mg P.O.; then 100 mg q 12 hours for 10 to 15 days.
Meningococcal carrier state –
100 mg P.O. q 12 hours for 5 days.
Uncomplicated urethral, endocervical, or rectal infection caused by Chlamydia trachomatis *or* Ureaplasma urealyticum –
Adults: 100 mg P.O. b.i.d. for at least 7 days.
Uncomplicated gonoccocal urethritis in men –
Adults: 100 mg P.O. b.i.d. for 5 days.

ADVERSE REACTIONS

CNS: *light-headedness, dizziness from vestibular toxicity; intracranial hypertension.*
CV: pericarditis.
EENT: dysphagia, glossitis.
GI: *anorexia,* epigastric distress, oral candidiasis, *nausea,* vomiting, *diarrhea,* enterocolitis, inflammatory lesions in anogenital region.
Hematologic: neutropenia, eosinophilia.
Skin: *maculopapular and erythematous rashes, photosensitivity, increased pigmentation, urticaria.*
Other: hypersensitivity reactions ***(anaphylaxis);*** increased BUN level; permanent discoloration of teeth, enamel defects, and bone growth retardation if used in children under age 8; superinfection; *thrombophlebitis.*

INTERACTIONS

Antacids (including sodium bicarbonate) and laxatives containing aluminum, magnesium, or calcium; antidiarrheals; food, milk, or other dairy products: decreased antibiotic absorption. Give antibiotic 1 hour before or 2 hours after any of the above.
Ferrous sulfate and other iron products, zinc: decreased antibiotic absorption. Give drug 3 hours after or 2 hours before iron administration.
Methoxyflurane: may cause nephrotoxicity with tetracyclines. Monitor carefully.
Oral anticoagulants: increased anticoagulant effect. Monitor PT and adjust dosage as ordered.
Oral contraceptives: decreased contraceptive effectiveness and increased risk of breakthrough bleeding. Use a nonhormonal form of birth control.

CONTRAINDICATIONS

- Contraindicated in patients with hypersensitivity to the drug or other tetracyclines.
- Use cautiously in patients with impaired renal or hepatic function. Use of these drugs during last half of pregnancy and in children under age 8 may cause permanent discoloration of teeth, enamel defects, and bone growth retardation.

NURSING CONSIDERATIONS

- Obtain specimen for culture and sensitivity tests before first dose. Therapy may begin pending test results.
- Check expiration date. Outdated or deteriorated tetracyclines have been associated with reversible nephrotoxicity (Fanconi's syndrome).
- Don't expose these drugs to light or heat. Keep cap tightly closed.
- With large doses or prolonged therapy, monitor for superinfection, especially in high-risk patients.
- Check the patient's tongue for signs of monilia infection. Stress good oral hygiene.
- May be taken with food. Tell the patient to take entire amount of medication exactly as prescribed, even after he feels better.
- Tell the patient to take oral form of drug with a full glass of water. Don't take within 1 hour of bedtime to avoid esophagitis.
- May cause tooth discoloration in young adults. Observe for brown pigmentation, and inform the doctor if it occurs.

• Warn the patient to avoid driving or other hazardous tasks until the adverse CNS effects of the drug are known.
• Warn the patient to avoid direct sunlight and ultraviolet light. A sunscreen may help prevent photosensitivity reactions.
• **I.V. use:** Reconstitute 100-mg of powder with 5-ml of sterile water for injection, with further dilution of 500 to 1,000 ml for I.V. infusion. Stable for 24 hours at room temperature.
• Patient may develop thrombophlebitis with I.V. administration of this drug. Avoid extravasation. Switch to oral therapy as soon as possible.
• Parenteral form may cause false-positive reading of copper sulfate tests (Clinitest). All forms may cause false-negative reading of glucose enzymatic tests (Clinistix, Tes-Tape).

oxytetracycline hydrochloride

Terramycin, Tija
Pregnancy Risk Category: D

HOW SUPPLIED

Capsules: 250 mg
Injection: 50 mg/ml, 125 mg/ml (with lidocaine 2%)

ACTION

Mechanism: Exerts bacteriostatic effect by binding to the 30S ribosomal subunit of microorganisms, thus inhibiting protein synthesis.
Peak: Serum levels peak within 2 to 4 hours after oral dose. Absorption after I.M. injection is erratic. **Duration:** elimination half-life, 6 to 10 hours.

INDICATIONS & DOSAGE

Infections caused by sensitive gram-negative and gram-positive organisms, trachoma, rickettsiae –
Adults: 250 mg P.O. q 6 hours; 100 mg I.M. q 8 to 12 hours; 250 mg I.M. as a single dose.
Children over age 8: 25 to 50 mg/kg P.O. daily, in divided doses q 6 hours; 15 to 25 mg/kg I.M. daily, in divided doses q 8 to 12 hours.
Brucellosis –
Adults: 500 mg P.O. q.i.d. for 3 weeks combined with 1 g of streptomycin I.M. q 12 hours first week, once daily second week.
Syphilis in patients sensitive to penicillin –
Adults: 30 to 40 g total dosage P.O., divided equally over 10 to 15 days.
Gonorrhea in patients sensitive to penicillin –
Adults: initially, 1.5 g P.O., followed by 0.5 g q.i.d., for a total of 9 g.

ADVERSE REACTIONS

CNS: ***intracranial hypertension.***
CV: pericarditis.
EENT: dysphagia, glossitis.
GI: *anorexia, nausea,* vomiting, *diarrhea,* oral candidiasis, enterocolitis, anogenital inflammation.
Hematologic: neutropenia, eosinophilia.
Skin: *maculopapular and erythematous rashes, urticaria, photosensitivity, increased pigmentation.*
Other: hypersensitivity reactions ***(anaphylaxis);*** permanent discoloration of teeth, enamel defects, and bone growth retardation if used in children under age 8; superinfection; increased BUN levels; *irritation after I.M. injection; thrombophlebitis.*

INTERACTIONS

Antacids (including sodium bicarbonate) and laxatives containing aluminum, magnesium, or calcium; antidiarrheals; food, milk, or other dairy products: decreased antibiotic absorption. Give antibiotic 1 hour before or 2 hours after any of the above.
Ferrous sulfate and other iron products, zinc: decreased antibiotic absorption. Give antibiotic 3 hours after or 2 hours before iron administration.
Methoxyflurane: may cause nephro-

toxicity with tetracyclines. Monitor carefully.
Oral anticoagulants: increased anticoagulant effect. Monitor PT and adjust dosage as ordered.
Oral contraceptives: decreased contraceptive effectiveness and increased risk of breakthrough bleeding. Use a nonhormonal form of birth control.

CONTRAINDICATIONS
• Contraindicated in patients with hypersensitivity to the drug or other tetracyclines.
• Use cautiously in patients with impaired renal or hepatic function. Use of these drugs during last half of pregnancy and in children under age 8 may cause permanent discoloration of teeth, enamel defects, and bone growth retardation.

NURSING CONSIDERATIONS
• Obtain specimen for culture and sensitivity tests before first dose. Therapy may begin pending test results.
• Check expiration date. Outdated or deteriorated oxytetracyclines have been associated with reversible nephrotoxicity (Fanconi's syndrome).
• Don't expose these drugs to light or heat.
• With large doses or prolonged therapy, monitor for superinfection, especially in high-risk patients.
• Check the patient's tongue for signs of fungal infection. Stress good oral hygiene.
• Warn the patient to avoid direct sunlight and ultraviolet light. A sunscreen may help prevent photosensitivity reactions. Photosensitivity persists for considerable time after discontinuation of drug.
• Explain to the patient that drug's effectiveness is reduced when taken with milk or other dairy products, food, antacids, or iron products. Tell him to take each dose with a full glass of water on an empty stomach, at least 1 hour before or 2 hours after meals. Give at least 1 hour before bedtime to prevent esophagitis.
• Tell the patient to take entire amount of medication exactly as prescribed, even after he feels better.
• For I.M. administration, inject deeply into a large muscle mass. Warn the patient that it may be painful. Rotate sites. I.M. preparations contain a local anesthetic; ask the patient about hypersensitivity reactions to local anesthetics.
• Parenteral form may cause false-positive reading of copper sulfate tests (Clinitest). All forms may cause false-negative reading of glucose enzymatic tests (Clinistix, Tes-Tape).

tetracycline hydrochloride
Achromycin V, Apo-Tetra†, Austramycin V‡, Hostacycline P‡, Nor-Tet, Novotetra†, Panmycin**, Panmycin P‡, Robitet, Sumycin, Tetracap, Tetralan, Tetralean†

Pregnancy Risk Category: D

HOW SUPPLIED
Tablets: 250 mg, 500 mg
Capsules: 100 mg, 250 mg, 500 mg
Oral suspension: 125 mg/5 ml

ACTION
Mechanism: Exerts bacteriostatic effect by binding to the 30S ribosomal subunit of microorganisms, thus inhibiting protein synthesis.
Peak: Serum levels peak within 2 to 4 hours. **Duration:** elimination half-life, 6 to 12 hours.

INDICATIONS & DOSAGE
Infections caused by sensitive gram-negative and gram-positive organisms, including Rickettsiae, Chlamydia, Mycoplasma, *and organisms that cause trachoma –*
Adults: 250 to 500 mg P.O. q 6 hours.
Children over age 8: 25 to 50 mg/kg P.O. daily, in divided doses q 6 hours.

Uncomplicated urethral, endocervical, or rectal infection caused by Chlamydia trachomatis –
Adults: 500 mg P.O. q.i.d. for at least 7 days.
Brucellosis –
Adults: 500 mg P.O. q 6 hours for 3 weeks combined with 1 g of streptomycin I.M. q 12 hours first week; daily, the second week.
Gonorrhea in patients sensitive to penicillin –
Adults: initially, 1.5 g P.O.; then 500 mg q 6 hours for a total dose of 9 g.
Syphilis in patients sensitive to penicillin –
Adults: total of 30 to 40 g P.O. in equally divided doses over 10 to 15 days.
Acne –
Adults and adolescents: initially, 250 mg P.O. q 6 hours; then 125 to 500 mg daily or every other day.

ADVERSE REACTIONS
CNS: dizziness, headache, ***intracranial hypertension.***
CV: pericarditis.
EENT: sore throat, glossitis, dysphagia.
GI: anorexia, *epigastric distress, nausea,* vomiting, *diarrhea,* esophagitis, oral candidiasis, stomatitis, enterocolitis, inflammatory lesions in anogenital region.
Hematologic: neutropenia, eosinophilia.
Skin: *candidal superinfection, maculopapular and erythematous rashes, urticaria, photosensitivity, increased pigmentation.*
Other: hypersensitivity reactions, *increased BUN levels, permanent discoloration of teeth, enamel defects, and retardation of bone growth if used in children under 8 years.*

INTERACTIONS
Antacids (including sodium bicarbonate) and laxatives containing aluminum, magnesium, or calcium; antidiarrheals containing kaolin, pectin, or bismuth subsalicylate; food, milk, or other dairy products: decreased antibiotic absorption. Give antibiotic 1 hour before or 2 hours after any of the above.
Ferrous sulfate and other iron products, zinc: decreased antibiotic absorption. Give tetracyclines 3 hours after or 2 hours before iron administration.
Lithium carbonate: may alter serum lithium levels.
Methoxyflurane: may cause severe nephrotoxicity with tetracyclines. Monitor carefully.
Oral anticoagulants: potentiated anticoagulant effects. Monitor PT and adjust anticoagulant dosage as ordered.
Oral contraceptives: decreased contraceptive effectiveness and increased risk of breakthrough bleeding. Use a nonhormonal form of birth control.

CONTRAINDICATIONS
- Contraindicated during last half of pregnancy and in children under age 8 because drug may cause permanent discoloration of teeth, enamel defects, and bone growth retardation.
- Use with extreme caution in patients with impaired renal or hepatic function.

NURSING CONSIDERATIONS
- Obtain specimen for culture and sensitivity tests before giving first dose. Therapy may begin pending test results.
- Check expiration date. Outdated or deteriorated tetracyclines have been associated with reversible nephrotoxicity (Fanconi's syndrome).
- Don't expose drug to light or heat.
- With large doses or prolonged therapy, monitor for superinfection, especially in high-risk patients.
- Check the patient's tongue for signs of monilia infection. Stress good oral hygiene.
- Warn the patient to avoid direct

sunlight and ultraviolet light. A sunscreen may help prevent photosensitivity reactions. Photosensitivity persists after discontinuation of drug.

- Explain to the patient that effectiveness is reduced when taken with milk or other dairy products, food, antacids, or iron products. Tell him to take each dose with a full glass of water on an empty stomach, at least 1 hour before or 2 hours after meals. Give at least 1 hour before bedtime to prevent esophagitis.
- Tell the patient to take drug exactly as prescribed, even after he feels better, and to take entire amount prescribed.
- May cause false-negative reading with glucose enzymatic tests (Clinistix, Tes-Tape).

15

Sulfonamides

co-trimoxazole
sulfadiazine
sulfamethoxazole
sulfasalazine
sulfisoxazole

COMBINATION PRODUCTS
AZO GANTANOL, AZO SULFAMETHOXAZOLE†, URO GANTANOL†: sulfamethoxazole 500 mg and phenazopyridine hydrochloride 100 mg.
AZO GANTRISIN, AZO SULFISOXAZOLE, SULDIAZO: sulfisoxazole 500 mg and phenazopyridine hydrochloride 50 mg.
PEDIAZOLE: sulfisoxazole 600 mg and erythromycin ethylsuccinate 200 mg per 5 ml.
TRIPLE SULFA: sulfadiazine 167 mg, sulfamerazine 167 mg, and sulfamethazine 167 mg.

co-trimoxazole (sulfamethoxazole-trimethoprim)

Apo-Sulfatrim†, Apo-Sulfatrim DS†, Bactrim*, Bactrim DS, Bactrim I.V. Infusion, Cotrim, Cotrim D.S., Novotrimel†, Novotrimel DS†, Protrin†, Protrin DF†, Resprim‡, Roubac†, Roubac DS†, Septra*, Septra DS, Septra I.V. Infusion, Septrin‡, SMZ-TMP, Sulfamethoprim, Sulfamethoprim DS, Sulmeprim, Trib‡, Uroplus DS, Uroplus SS

Pregnancy Risk Category: C (D if near term)

HOW SUPPLIED
Tablets: trimethoprim 80 mg and sulfamethoxazole 400 mg; trimethoprim 160 mg and sulfamethoxazole 800 mg
Oral suspension: trimethoprim 40 mg and sulfamethoxazole 200 mg/5 ml
Injection: trimethoprim 16 mg and sulfamethoxazole 80 mg/ml (5 ml/ampule)

ACTION
Mechanism: Sulfamethoxazole component inhibits the formation of dihydrofolic acid from PABA; the trimethoprim component inhibits dihydrofolate reductase. Both decrease bacterial folic acid synthesis.
Peak: Serum levels peak 1 to 4 hours after an oral dose or immediately after an I.V. infusion. **Duration:** serum half-life of the trimethoprim component, 8 to 11 hours; half-life of the sulfamethoxazole component, 10 to 13 hours.

INDICATIONS & DOSAGE
Urinary tract infections and shigellosis –
Adults: 160 mg trimethoprim/800 mg sulfamethoxazole (double strength tablet) P.O. q 12 hours for 10 to 14 days in urinary tract infections and for 5 days in shigellosis. For simple cystitis or acute urethral syndrome, may give one to three double strength tablets as a single dose. If indicated, give by I.V. infusion 8 to 10 mg/kg/day (based on trimethoprim component) in two to four divided doses q 6, 8, or 12 hours for up to 14 days. Maximum daily dose is 960 mg trimethoprim.
Children 2 months and over: 8 mg/kg trimethoprim/40 mg/kg sulfamethoxazole P.O. per 24 hours, in two divided doses q 12 hours (10 days for urinary tract infections; 5 days, for shigellosis). If indicated, give by I.V. infusion 8 to 10 mg/kg/day (based on trimethoprim component) in two to

four divided doses q 6, 8, or 12 hours. Don't exceed the adult dose.
Otitis media in patients with penicillin allergy or penicillin-resistant infections –
Children 2 months and over: 8 mg/kg trimethoprim/40 mg/kg sulfamethoxazole P.O. per 24 hours, in two divided doses q 12 hours for 10 days.
Pneumocystis carinii *pneumonia –*
Adults and children 2 months and over: 20 mg/kg trimethoprim/100 mg/kg sulfamethoxazole P.O. per 24 hours, in equally divided doses q 6 hours for 14 days. If indicated, give by I.V. infusion 15 to 20 mg/kg/day (based on trimethoprim component) in three or four divided doses q 6 to 8 hours for up to 14 days.
Chronic bronchitis –
Adults: 160 mg trimethoprim/800 mg sulfamethoxazole P.O. q 12 hours for 10 to 14 days. Not recommended for infants under 2 months old.
Prophylaxis of traveler's diarrhea –
Adults: 160 mg trimethoprim/800 mg sulfamethoxazole P.O. once daily, beginning on the first day of travel and continuing until 2 days after returning home. Maximum duration of therapy is 2 weeks.
Traveler's diarrhea –
Adults: 160 mg trimethoprim/800 mg sulfamethoxazole P.O. b.i.d. for 3 to 5 days. Some patients may require 2 days of therapy or less.
Urinary tract infections in males with prostatitis –
Adults: 160 mg trimethoprim/800 mg sulfamethoxazole P.O. b.i.d. for 3 to 6 months.
Prophylaxis of chronic urinary tract infections –
Adults: 40 mg trimethoprim/200 mg sulfamethoxazole (½ tablet) or 80 mg trimethoprim/400 mg sulfamethoxazole P.O. daily or three times a week for 3 to 6 months.

ADVERSE REACTIONS

CNS: headache, mental depression, seizures, hallucinations.
GI: *nausea, vomiting, diarrhea,* abdominal pain, anorexia, stomatitis.
GU: ***toxic nephrosis with oliguria and anuria,*** crystalluria, hematuria.
Hematologic: ***agranulocytosis, aplastic anemia,*** megaloblastic anemia, thrombocytopenia, leukopenia, ***hemolytic anemia.***
Hepatic: jaundice.
Skin: ***erythema multiforme (Stevens-Johnson syndrome),*** *generalized skin eruption,* ***epidermal necrolysis, exfoliative dermatitis,*** photosensitivity, urticaria, pruritus.
Other: hypersensitivity reactions (*serum sickness, drug fever,* ***anaphylaxis***).

INTERACTIONS

Ammonium chloride, ascorbic acid: doses sufficient to acidify urine may cause precipitation of sulfonamide and crystalluria. Don't use together.
Oral anticoagulants: increased anticoagulant effect. Monitor for bleeding.
Oral contraceptives: decreased contraceptive effectiveness and increased risk of breakthrough bleeding. Suggest a nonhormonal form of contraception.
Oral hypoglycemic agents: increased hypoglycemic effect. Monitor blood glucose levels.

CONTRAINDICATIONS

- Contraindicated in patients with porphyria, in megaloblastic anemia caused by folate deficiency, and in pregnancy at term.
- Use cautiously and in reduced dosages in patients with impaired hepatic or renal function, severe allergy or bronchial asthma, G6PD deficiency, and blood dyscrasia.

NURSING CONSIDERATIONS

• Obtain specimen for culture and sensitivity tests before first dose. Therapy may begin pending results.

• Adverse reactions, especially hypersensitivity reactions, rash, and fever, occur much more frequently in AIDS patients.

• This combination is typically used in extremely ill immunosuppressed patients when prescribed for treatment of *Pneumocystis carinii* pneumonia.

• Note that the "DS" or" DF" product means "double strength."

• Promptly report skin rash, sore throat, fever, or mouth sores – early signs of blood dyscrasia.

• Watch for superinfection (fever or other signs of new infection).

• Tell the patient to take entire amount of medication exactly as prescribed, even if he feels better.

• **I.V. use:** I.V. infusion must be diluted in D_5W before administration. Don't mix with other drugs or solutions. Infuse slowly over 60 to 90 minutes. Don't give by rapid infusion or bolus injection. Must be used within 2 hours of mixing. Do not refrigerate.

• Never administer I.M.

---

sulfadiazine

Microsulfon

Pregnancy Risk Category: B (D if near term)

HOW SUPPLIED

Tablets: 500 mg

ACTION

Mechanism: Inhibits formation of dihydrofolic acid from PABA, decreasing bacterial folic acid synthesis.
Peak: Serum levels peak within 6 hours of an oral dose. **Duration:** about 50% of a dose appears in the urine as parent drug and metabolites within 24 hours.

INDICATIONS & DOSAGE

Urinary tract infection –
Adults: initially, 2 to 4 g P.O., then 500 mg to 1 g P.O. q 6 hours.
Children 2 months and over: initially, 75 mg/kg or 2 g/m² P.O., then 150 mg/kg or 4 g/m² P.O. in four to six divided doses daily. Maximum daily dosage is 6 g.

Rheumatic fever prophylaxis, as an alternative to penicillin –
Children over 30 kg: 1 g P.O. daily.
Children under 30 kg: 500 mg P.O. daily.

Adjunctive treatment in toxoplasmosis –
Adults: 4 g P.O. in divided doses q 6 hours for 3 to 4 weeks (longer for immunosuppressed patients). Usually given with pyrimethamine 25 mg P.O. daily.
Children: 100 mg/kg P.O. in divided doses q 6 hours for 3 to 4 weeks; given with pyrimethamine 2 mg/kg daily for 3 days, then 1 mg/kg daily for 3 to 4 weeks.

ADVERSE REACTIONS

CNS: headache, mental depression, convulsions, hallucinations.
GI: *nausea, vomiting, diarrhea,* abdominal pain, anorexia, stomatitis.
GU: ***toxic nephrosis*** with oliguria and anuria, crystalluria, hematuria.
Hematologic: ***agranulocytosis, aplastic anemia,*** megaloblastic anemia, thrombocytopenia, leukopenia, ***hemolytic anemia.***
Skin: ***erythema multiforme (Stevens-Johnson syndrome),*** *generalized skin eruption,* ***epidermal necrolysis, exfoliative dermatitis,*** photosensitivity, urticaria, pruritus.
Other: hypersensitivity reactions (*serum sickness, drug fever,* ***anaphylaxis***), jaundice, local irritation, extravasation.

INTERACTIONS

Ammonium chloride, ascorbic acid: doses sufficient to acidify urine may

---

*Liquid form contains alcohol. *Common* reactions are in italics; ***life-threatening,*** in bold italics.
**May contain tartrazine.

cause precipitation of sulfonamide and crystalluria. Don't use together.
Oral anticoagulants: increased anticoagulant effect. Monitor for bleeding.
Oral contraceptives: decreased contraceptive effectiveness and increased risk of breakthrough bleeding. Suggest a nonhormonal form of contraception.
Oral hypoglycemic agents: increased hypoglycemic effect. Monitor blood glucose levels.
PABA-containing drugs: inhibited antibacterial action. Don't use together.

CONTRAINDICATIONS

- Contraindicated in patients with porphyria or in infants under 2 months (except in congenital toxoplasmosis).
- Use cautiously and in reduced doses in patients with impaired hepatic or renal function, bronchial asthma, history of multiple allergies, G6PD deficiency, and blood dyscrasia.

NURSING CONSIDERATIONS

- Obtain specimen for culture and sensitivity tests before first dose. Therapy may begin pending results.
- Tell the patient to drink a full glass of water with each dose and to drink plenty of water throughout the day to prevent crystalluria. Monitor fluid intake and output. Intake should be sufficient to produce output of 1,500 ml daily (between 3,000 and 4,000 ml daily for adults). To prevent crystalluria, sodium bicarbonate may be administered to alkalinize urine. Monitor urine pH daily.
- Watch for superinfection (fever or other signs of new infection).
- Tell the patient to take entire amount of medication exactly as prescribed, even if he feels better.
- Warn the patient to avoid direct sunlight and ultraviolet light to prevent photosensitivity reaction.
- Give drug on schedule to maintain constant blood level.
- Monitor for signs of blood dyscrasia (purpura, ecchymosis, sore throat, fever, and pallor). Report them immediately.
- Monitor urine cultures, CBCs, and urinalyses before and during therapy.
- Folic or folinic acid may be used during rest periods in toxoplasmosis therapy to reverse hematopoietic depression or anemia associated with pyrimethamine and sulfadiazine.

sulfamethoxazole (sulphamethoxazole)

Apo-Sulfamethoxazole†, Gantanol, Gantanol DS

Pregnancy Risk Category: B (D if near term)

HOW SUPPLIED

Tablets: 500 mg, 1,000 mg
Oral suspension: 500 mg/5 ml

ACTION

Mechanism: Inhibits formation of dihydrofolic acid from PABA, decreasing bacterial folic acid synthesis.
Peak: Serum levels peak within 2 hours of an oral dose. **Duration:** elimination half-life, 7 to 12 hours.

INDICATIONS & DOSAGE

Urinary tract and systemic infections –
Adults: initially, 2 g P.O., then 1 g P.O. b.i.d. up to t.i.d. for severe infections.
Children and infants over 2 months: initially, 50 to 60 mg/kg P.O., then 25 to 30 mg/kg b.i.d. Maximum dosage should not exceed 75 mg/kg daily.
Lymphogranuloma venereum (genital, inguinal, or anorectal infection) –
Adults: 1 g P.O. daily for at least 3 weeks.

ADVERSE REACTIONS

CNS: headache, mental depression, seizures, hallucinations.
GI: *nausea, vomiting, diarrhea,* abdominal pain, anorexia, stomatitis.
GU: ***toxic nephrosis with oliguria and anuria,*** crystalluria, hematuria.
Hematologic: ***agranulocytosis, aplastic anemia,*** megaloblastic anemia, thrombocytopenia, leukopenia, ***hemolytic anemia.***
Skin: ***erythema multiforme (Stevens-Johnson syndrome),*** *generalized skin eruption,* ***epidermal necrolysis, exfoliative dermatitis,*** photosensitivity, urticaria, pruritus.
Other: hypersensitivity reactions (*serum sickness, drug fever,* ***anaphylaxis***), *jaundice.*

INTERACTIONS

Ammonium chloride, ascorbic acid: doses sufficient to acidify urine may cause precipitation of sulfonamide and crystalluria. Don't use together.
Oral anticoagulants: increased anticoagulant effect. Monitor for bleeding.
Oral contraceptives: decreased contraceptive effectiveness and increased risk of breakthrough bleeding. Suggest a nonhormonal form of contraception.
Oral hypoglycemic agents: increased hypoglycemic effect. Monitor blood glucose levels.
PABA-containing drugs: inhibited antibacterial action. Don't use together.

CONTRAINDICATIONS

- Contraindicated in patients with porphyria or in infants under 2 months (except in congenital toxoplasmosis).
- Use cautiously and in reduced dosages in patients with impaired hepatic or renal function, severe allergy or bronchial asthma, G6PD deficiency, and blood dyscrasia.

NURSING CONSIDERATIONS

- Obtain specimen for culture and sensitivity tests before first dose. Therapy may begin pending results.
- Tell the patient to drink a full glass of water with each dose and to drink plenty of water during the day to prevent crystalluria. Monitor fluid intake and output. Intake should be sufficient to produce output of 1,500 ml daily (between 3,000 and 4,000 ml daily for adults). To help prevent crystalluria, sodium bicarbonate may be administered to alkalinize urine. Monitor urine pH daily.
- Watch for superinfection (fever or other signs of new infection).
- Tell the patient to take entire amount of medication exactly as prescribed, even if he feels better.
- Warn the patient to avoid direct sunlight and ultraviolet light to prevent photosensitivity reaction.
- Monitor urine cultures, CBCs, and urinalyses before and during therapy.
- Sulfamethoxazole is also used in adjunctive therapy for treatment of toxoplasmosis.
- Instruct the patient to report early signs of blood dyscrasia (sore throat, fever, and pallor) to the doctor immediately.

sulfasalazine (salazosulfapyridine, sulphasalazine)

Azulfidine, Azulfidine EN-Tabs, PMS Sulfasalazine E.C.†, Salazopyrin†‡, Salazopyrin EN-Tabs†‡, S.A.S., S.A.S.-Enteric

Pregnancy Risk Category: B (D if near term)

HOW SUPPLIED

Tablets: 500 mg with or without enteric coating
Oral suspension: 250 mg/5 ml

*Liquid form contains alcohol.
**May contain tartrazine.

Common reactions are in italics; ***life-threatening,*** in bold italics.

ACTION

Mechanism: Inhibits formation of dihydrofolic acid from PABA, decreasing bacterial folic acid synthesis.
Peak: Poorly absorbed; peak serum levels of parent drug occur within 1½ to 6 hours; peak levels of metabolites, within 12 to 24 hours. **Duration:** elimination half-life, 7 to 12 hours.

INDICATIONS & DOSAGE

Mild to moderate ulcerative colitis, adjunctive therapy in severe ulcerative colitis, Crohn's disease –
Adults: initially, 3 to 4 g P.O. daily in evenly divided doses; usual maintenance dosage is 1.5 to 2 g P.O. daily in divided doses q 6 hours. May need to start with 1 to 2 g, with a gradual increase in dosage to minimize adverse effects.
Children over age 2: initially, 40 to 60 mg/kg P.O. daily, divided into 3 to 6 doses; then 30 mg/kg daily in 4 doses. May need to start at lower dose if GI intolerance occurs.

ADVERSE REACTIONS

CNS: headache, mental depression, ***seizures,*** hallucinations.
GI: *nausea, vomiting, diarrhea,* abdominal pain, anorexia, stomatitis.
GU: ***toxic nephrosis with oliguria and anuria,*** crystalluria, hematuria.
Hematologic: ***agranulocytosis, aplastic anemia,*** megaloblastic anemia, thrombocytopenia, leukopenia, ***hemolytic anemia.***
Hepatic: jaundice, hepatotoxicity.
Skin: ***erythema multiforme (Stevens-Johnson syndrome),*** *generalized skin eruption,* ***epidermal necrolysis,*** *exfoliative* ***dermatitis,*** photosensitivity, urticaria, pruritus.
Other: ***hypersensitivity reactions*** *(serum sickness, drug fever,* ***anaphylaxis***) oligospermia, infertility.

INTERACTIONS

Folic acid: absorption may be decreased. No intervention necessary.
Oral anticoagulants: increased anticoagulant effect. Monitor for bleeding.
Oral contraceptives: decreased contraceptive effectiveness and increased risk of breakthrough bleeding. Suggest a nonhormonal form of contraception.
Oral hypoglycemic agents: increased hypoglycemic effect. Monitor blood glucose levels.

CONTRAINDICATIONS

- Contraindicated in patients with porphyria or intestinal and urinary obstruction, and in those allergic to sulfonamides or salicylates.
- Use cautiously and in reduced dosages in patients with impaired hepatic or renal function, severe allergy, bronchial asthma, and G6PD deficiency.

NURSING CONSIDERATIONS

- Tell the patient to take entire amount of medication exactly as prescribed, even if he feels better.
- Discontinue immediately if the patient shows signs and symptoms of hypersensitivity.
- Warn the patient to avoid direct sunlight and ultraviolet light to prevent photosensitivity reaction.
- Colors alkaline urine orange-yellow.
- Adverse reactions are usually those affecting GI tract. Minimize symptoms by spacing doses evenly and administering after food intake.

---

sulfisoxazole (sulfafurazole, sulphafurazole)

Azo-Sulfisoxazole†‡, Gantrisin, Novosoxazole†

Pregnancy Risk Category: B (D if near term)

HOW SUPPLIED
Tablets: 500 mg
Liquid: 500 mg/5 ml

ACTION
Mechanism: Inhibits formation of dihydrofolic acid from PABA, decreasing bacterial folic acid synthesis.
Peak: Serum levels peak in 2 to 4 hours; urine levels within 8 hours.
Duration: serum half-life, 5 to 8 hours.

INDICATIONS & DOSAGE
Urinary tract and systemic infections –
Adults: initially, 2 to 4 g P.O., then 1 to 2 g P.O. q.i.d.
Children over 2 months: initially, 75 mg/kg P.O. daily or 2 g/m^2 P.O. daily in divided doses q 6 hours, then 150 mg/kg or 4 g/m^2 P.O. daily in divided doses q 6 hours.

ADVERSE REACTIONS
CNS: headache, mental depression, ***seizures,*** hallucinations.
GI: *nausea, vomiting, diarrhea,* abdominal pain, anorexia, stomatitis.
GU: ***toxic nephrosis with oliguria and anuria,*** crystalluria, hematuria.
Hematologic: ***agranulocytosis, aplastic anemia,*** megaloblastic anemia, thrombocytopenia, leukopenia, ***hemolytic anemia.***
Skin: ***erythema multiforme,*** *generalized skin eruption,* ***epidermal necrolysis, exfoliative dermatitis,*** photosensitivity, urticaria, pruritus.
Other: hypersensitivity reactions (*serum sickness, drug fever,* ***anaphylaxis***), jaundice.

INTERACTIONS
Ammonium chloride, ascorbic acid: doses sufficient to acidify urine may cause crystalluria. Don't use together.
Oral anticoagulants: increased anticoagulant effect. Monitor for bleeding.
Oral contraceptives: decreased contraceptive effectiveness, increased risk of breakthrough bleeding. Suggest a nonhormonal form of contraception.
Oral hypoglycemic agents: increased hypoglycemic effect. Monitor blood glucose levels.
PABA-containing drugs: inhibited antibacterial action. Don't use together.

CONTRAINDICATIONS
- Contraindicated in porphyria and in infants under 2 months (except in congenital toxoplasmosis).
- Use cautiously in patients with impaired hepatic or renal function, severe allergy or bronchial asthma, and G6PD deficiency.

NURSING CONSIDERATIONS
- Obtain specimen for culture and sensitivity tests before first dose. Therapy may begin pending results.
- Tell the patient to drink a full glass of water with each dose and to drink plenty of water each day to prevent crystalluria. Monitor fluid intake and output. Maintain intake between 3,000 and 4,000 ml daily for adults to produce output of 1,500 ml daily. Sodium bicarbonate may be administered to alkalinize urine. Monitor urine pH daily.
- Watch for superinfection (fever or other signs of new infection).
- Tell the patient to take entire amount of medication exactly as prescribed, even if he feels better.
- Warn the patient to avoid sunlight to prevent photosensitivity reaction.
- Monitor urine cultures, CBCs, PT, and urinalyses before and during therapy.
- Tell the patient to report early signs of blood dyscrasia (sore throat, fever, and pallor) immediately to the doctor.
- When drug is given preoperatively, the patient should receive a low-residue diet and a minimal number of enemas and cathartics.

16

Quinolones

cinoxacin
ciprofloxacin
enoxacin
lomefloxacin hydrochloride
nalidixic acid
norfloxacin
ofloxacin

COMBINATION PRODUCTS
None.

cinoxacin

Cinobac

Pregnancy Risk Category: B

HOW SUPPLIED
Capsules: 250 mg, 500 mg

ACTION
Mechanism: Inhibits microbial DNA synthesis.
Peak: Plasma levels peak within 2 hours of an oral dose; urine levels peak in 2 to 4 hours. **Duration:** elimination half-life, 1 to 1½ hours; however, urine levels of the drug remain sufficient for antimicrobial effect for at least 12 hours after a dose.

INDICATIONS & DOSAGE
Initial and recurrent urinary tract infections caused by susceptible strains of Escherichia coli, Klebsiella, Enterobacter, Proteus mirabilis, Proteus vulgaris, *and* Proteus morgani, Serratia, *and* Citrobacter –
Adults and children over age 12: 1 g P.O. daily, in two to four divided doses for 7 to 14 days.

Not recommended for children under age 12.

ADVERSE REACTIONS
CNS: *dizziness, headache,* drowsiness, insomnia, seizures.
EENT: tinnitus.
GI: *nausea, vomiting, abdominal pain,* diarrhea.
Skin: rash, urticaria, pruritus, photosensitivity.

INTERACTIONS
Probenecid: may decrease urine levels of cinoxacin by inhibiting renal tubular secretion. Monitor for increased toxicity and reduced antibacterial effectiveness.

CONTRAINDICATIONS
- Contraindicated in patients with hypersensitivity to nalidixic acid.
- Use cautiously in patients with impaired renal and hepatic function.

NURSING CONSIDERATIONS
- Obtain clean-catch urine specimen for culture and sensitivity tests before starting therapy and repeat p.r.n. Therapy may begin pending results. Not effective against *Pseudomonas,* enterococci, or staphylococci.
- Remind the patient to take entire amount of this drug as prescribed, even when he feels better.
- High urine levels permit twice-daily dosing.
- Report CNS adverse reactions to the doctor immediately. They indicate serious toxicity and usually mean that administration of drug should be stopped.
- Give cinoxacin with meals to help decrease GI adverse reactions.
- Warn the patient about photosensitizing effects of the drug, and advise him to avoid bright sunlight and to wear sunblock.

ciprofloxacin

Cipro, Cipro I.V., Ciproxin‡

Pregnancy Risk Category: C

HOW SUPPLIED

Tablets: 250 mg, 500 mg, 750 mg
Infusion (premixed): 200 mg in 100 ml D_5W, 400 mg in 200 ml D_5W
Injection: 200 mg, 400 mg

ACTION

Mechanism: Exact mechanism is unknown, but bactericidal effects may result from drug's inhibiting bacterial DNA gyrase and preventing replication in susceptible bacteria.
Peak: Serum levels peak 1 to 2 hours after an oral dose or immediately after I.V. infusion. **Duration:** serum elimination half-life, 3 to 5 hours.

INDICATIONS & DOSAGE

Mild to moderate urinary tract infections –
Adults: 250 mg P.O. or 200 mg I.V. q 12 hours.
Severe or complicated urinary tract infections; mild to moderate bone and joint infections; mild to moderate respiratory tract infections; mild to moderate skin and skin-structure infections; infectious diarrhea –
Adults: 500 mg P.O. or 400 mg I.V. q 12 hours.
Severe or complicated bone or joint infections; severe respiratory tract infections; severe skin and skin-structure infections –
Adults: 750 mg P.O. q 12 hours.

ADVERSE REACTIONS

CNS: headache, restlessness, tremor, light-headedness, confusion, hallucinations, ***seizures.***
GI: *nausea, diarrhea,* vomiting, abdominal pain or discomfort, oral candidiasis.
GU: crystalluria.
Other: *rash,* eosinophilia, photosensitivity; with I.V. administration – thrombophlebitis, burning, pruritus, paresthesia, erythema, swelling.

INTERACTIONS

Antacids containing magnesium hydroxide or aluminum hydroxide, sucralfate, iron supplements: decreased ciprofloxacin absorption. Separate administration by at least 2 hours.
Probenecid: may elevate serum level of ciprofloxacin. Monitor for toxicity.
Theophylline: increased plasma theophylline concentrations and prolonged theophylline half-life. Monitor blood levels of theophylline and observe for adverse effects.

CONTRAINDICATIONS

- Contraindicated in patients sensitive to quinolone antibiotics, in pregnant or breast-feeding patients, and in children under age 18. Quinolone antibiotics have caused arthropathy in young laboratory animals.
- Use with extreme caution with theophylline. Serious (even fatal) reactions have occurred in patients receiving I.V. theophylline and ciprofloxacin. If a patient must receive theophylline or aminophylline therapy with ciprofloxacin, closely monitor serum theophylline levels and adjust dosage accordingly.
- Use cautiously in patients with CNS disorders, such as severe cerebral arteriosclerosis or seizure disorders, and in those at an increased risk for seizures. May cause CNS stimulation.

NURSING CONSIDERATIONS

- Obtain specimen for culture and sensitivity tests before first dose. Therapy may begin pending results.
- The preferred time for oral dosing is 2 hours after a meal or 2 hours before or after taking antacids, sucralfate, or products that contain iron (such as vitamins with mineral supplements). Food does not affect absorption but may delay peak serum levels.

• Dosage adjustments are necessary in patients with renal dysfunction.
• Long-term therapy may result in overgrowth of organisms resistant to ciprofloxacin.
• Advise the patient that hypersensitivity reactions may occur even after first dose. If he notices a skin rash or any allergic reaction, he should stop taking the drug immediately and notify the doctor.
• Advise the patient to avoid caffeine while taking the drug because of potential for cumulative caffeine effects.
• Drug is excreted in breast milk. Patient should discontinue breast-feeding during treatment or be treated with another drug.
• May cause dizziness or light-headedness. Warn the patient to avoid hazardous tasks that require alertness, such as driving, until CNS effects of the drug are known.
• Advise the patient to drink plenty of fluids to reduce the risk of crystalluria.
• **I.V. use:** Dilute drug using D_5W or 0.9% sodium chloride injection to a final concentration of 1 to 2 mg/ml before use. Infuse slowly (over 1 hour) into a large vein.

enoxacin
Penetrex

Pregnancy Risk Category: C

HOW SUPPLIED
Tablets: 200 mg, 400 mg

ACTION
Mechanism: Inhibits bacterial DNA synthesis; mainly by inhibiting DNA gyrase. Bactericidal.
Peak: Serum levels peak in 1 to 3 hours. **Duration:** elimination half-life, 3 to 6 hours.

INDICATIONS & DOSAGE
Uncomplicated urinary tract infections –
Adults: 200 mg P.O. q 12 hours for 7 days.
Severe or complicated urinary tract infections –
Adults: 400 mg P.O. q 12 hours for 14 days.
Uncomplicated urethral or endocervical gonorrhea –
Adults: 400 mg P.O. as a single dose. Follow with doxycycline therapy to treat possible coexisting chlamydial infection.

ADVERSE REACTIONS
CNS: headache, restlessness, tremor, light-headedness, confusion, hallucinations, ***seizures.***
GI: *nausea, diarrhea,* vomiting, abdominal pain or discomfort, oral candidiasis.
GU: crystalluria.
Other: *rash,* photosensitivity.

INTERACTIONS
Aminophylline, cyclosporine, caffeine, theophylline: increased levels of these drugs because of decreased metabolism. Use together cautiously.
Antacids containing magnesium hydroxide or aluminum hydroxide, oral iron supplements, sucralfate: decreased enoxacin absorption. Separate administration times by at least 2 hours.
Cimetidine: decreased metabolism of enoxacin. Use together cautiously; dosage adjustment may be necessary.
Oral anticoagulants: increased anticoagulant effect. Use together cautiously.
Probenecid: may elevate serum level of fluoroquinolones. Monitor for adverse reactions.

CONTRAINDICATIONS
• Contraindicated in patients with hypersensitivity to the drug or other quinolone antibiotics, in pregnant or breast-feeding patients, and in children under age 18. Quinolone drugs

have produced arthropathy in young laboratory animals.
• Use with extreme caution with theophylline. Serious reactions have occurred in patients receiving I.V. theophylline and enoxacin. If patient must receive theophylline or aminophylline therapy with a quinolone antibiotic, closely monitor serum theophylline levels and adjust dosage accordingly.
• Use cautiously in patients with CNS disorders, such as severe cerebral arteriosclerosis or seizure disorders, and in those at increased risk for seizures. May cause CNS stimulation.
• Use cautiously and with dosage adjustments in patients with impaired renal or hepatic function. If creatinine clearance is 30 ml/minute/1.73 m^2 or less, start therapy with the usual initial dose. Subsequent doses should be decreased by 50%.

NURSING CONSIDERATIONS
• Obtain specimen for culture and sensitivity tests before first dose. Therapy may begin pending results.
• Warn the patient not to drink beverages containing caffeine while taking enoxacin. Drug inhibits the metabolism of caffeine and can result in toxicity.
• Patients being treated for gonorrhea should have an initial serologic test for syphilis before therapy starts. Drug has not been shown to be effective in treating syphilis and may mask signs and symptoms of infection. Repeat the serologic test in 1 to 3 months.
• Monitor closely for superinfection.
• Preferred time for dosing is 2 hours after a meal or 2 hours before or after antacids containing magnesium hydroxide or aluminum hydroxide, sucralfate, or products that contain iron (such as vitamins with mineral supplements).
• Similar drugs have been known to cause severe phototoxicity reactions. Advise the patient to avoid overexposure to direct sunlight while taking drug and to use a sunblock and wear protective clothing while outdoors.
• Advise the patient to liberally increase fluid intake while taking drug because similar drugs have caused urine microcrystal formation.
• Warn the patient that because drug can cause light-headedness or dizziness, he should avoid driving and hazardous activities until adverse CNS effects of the drug are known.

lomefloxacin hydrochloride
Maxaquin

Pregnancy Risk Category: C

HOW SUPPLIED
Tablets: 400 mg

ACTION
Mechanism: A fluoroquinolone that inhibits bacterial DNA gyrase, an enzyme necessary for bacterial replication (bactericidal).
Peak: Plasma levels peak 1 to 1½ hours after an oral dose. **Duration:** elimination half-life about 8 hours.

INDICATIONS & DOSAGE
Acute bacterial exacerbations of chronic bronchitis caused by Haemophilus influenzae *or* Moraxella (Branhamella) catarrhalis –
Adults: 400 mg P.O. daily for 10 days.
Uncomplicated urinary tract infections (cystitis) caused by Escherichia coli, Klebsiella pneumoniae, Proteus mirabilis, *or* Staphylococcus saprophyticus –
Adults: 400 mg P.O. daily for 10 days.
Complicated urinary tract infections caused by Escherichia coli, Klebsiella pneumoniae, P. mirabilis, *or* Pseudomonas aeruginosa; *possibly effective against infections caused by* Citrobacter diversus *or* Enterobacter cloacae –

Adults: 400 mg P.O. daily for 14 days.
Prophylaxis of infections after transurethral surgical procedures –
Adults: 400 mg P.O. as a single dose 2 to 6 hours before surgery.

Patients with a creatinine clearance of 10 to 40 ml/minute/1.73 m^2 should receive a loading dose of 400 mg P.O. on the first day, followed by 200 mg daily for the duration of therapy. Hemodialysis removes negligible amounts of the drug.

ADVERSE REACTIONS

CNS: *dizziness, headache,* abnormal dreams, fatigue, malaise, asthenia, agitation, anorexia, anxiety, confusion, depersonalization, depression, increased appetite, insomnia, nervousness, somnolence, ***seizures, coma,*** hyperkinesia, tremor, vertigo, paresthesia, arthralgia, myalgia, asthenia.
CV: flushing, hypotension, hypertension, edema, syncope, arrhythmia, tachycardia, bradycardia, extrasystoles, cyanosis, angina pectoris, ***MI, cardiac failure, pulmonary embolisms,*** cerebrovascular disorder, cardiomyopathy, phlebitis.
EENT: epistaxis, abnormal vision, conjunctivitis, eye pain, earache, tinnitus, tongue discoloration.
GI: *diarrhea, nausea,* dry mouth, intermenstrual bleeding, leukorrhea, vaginitis, abdominal pain, dyspepsia, vomiting, flatulence, constipation, inflammation, dysphagia, bleeding.
GU: dysuria, hematuria, anuria, epididymitis, orchitis, vaginal moniliasis, perineal pain.
Hematologic: thrombocythemia, thrombocytopenia, lymphadenopathy, increased fibrinolysis.
Respiratory: cough, dyspnea, ***bronchospasm,*** respiratory disorder, respiratory infection, increased sputum, stridor.
Skin: pruritus, skin disorder, skin exfoliation, eczema, rash, urticaria, *photosensitivity.*
Other: ***anaphylaxis,*** increased sweating, taste perversion, leg cramps, thirst, fatigue, back pain, malaise, chills, allergic reaction, facial edema, influenza-like symptoms, decreased heat tolerance, hypoglycemia, gout.

INTERACTIONS

Antacids, sucralfate: impaired absorption after binding with lomefloxacin in the GI tract. Administer no less than 4 hours before or 2 hours after a dose.
Cimetidine: increased half-life of other quinolones when administered to patients taking cimetidine; lomefloxacin has not been tested. Monitor for toxicity.
Probenecid: decreased excretion of lomefloxacin. Monitor for toxicity.
Warfarin, cyclosporine: increased effects or serum levels when combined with other quinolones; lomefloxacin has not been tested. Monitor for toxicity.

CONTRAINDICATIONS

- Contraindicated in patients with hypersensitivity to lomefloxacin or other quinolones. Also contraindicated in children and adolescents under age 18 and in pregnant and breast-feeding patients. Lomefloxacin has caused arthropathy and lameness secondary to permanently damaged cartilage when administered to juvenile animals.
- Use cautiously in patients with known or suspected CNS disorders, such as seizure disorder or cerebral arteriosclerosis, that may predispose the patient to seizures.

NURSING CONSIDERATIONS

- Although most fluoroquinolones exhibit photosensitizing effects, early studies suggest that photosensitization and phototoxicity are more common with lomefloxacin. Some animal studies suggest that prolonged use of the drug may predispose subjects to skin cancers. Advise the patient to wear protective clothing, use a sunblock, and avoid prolonged exposure to sunlight during treatment and for a few days after therapy ends. If sunburn occurs, the patient should call the doctor as soon as possible.

- Several bacterial strains have demonstrated resistance to lomefloxacin, including *Streptococcus pneumoniae,* most group A, B, D, and G streptococci, *Pseudomonas cepacia, Ureaplasma urealyticum, Mycoplasma hominis,* and anaerobes.
- Lomefloxacin should not be used for the empiric treatment of acute exacerbations of chronic bronchitis when the causative organism is probably *S. pneumoniae* because this organism demonstrates resistance to the drug. It also should not be used to treat bacteremia caused by *P. aeruginosa* because blood levels of the drug do not readily exceed the minimum inhibitory concentration against the organism. However, lomefloxacin has been used successfully to treat complicated urinary tract infections caused by *P. aeruginosa.*
- Lomefloxacin should be taken on an empty stomach.
- Obtain culture and sensitivity tests before first dose. Therapy may begin pending results.
- Prolonged use may result in overgrowth of organisms resistant to lomefloxacin.
- Advise the patient that hypersensitivity reactions may occur even after first dose. If skin rash or other allergic reaction occurs, the patient should stop taking the drug and notify the doctor.
- Drug may cause dizziness or lightheadedness. Warn patient to avoid driving and hazardous tasks until CNS effects of drug are known.

nalidixic acid

NegGram

Pregnancy Risk Category: B

HOW SUPPLIED

Tablets: 250 mg, 500 mg, 1 g
Oral suspension: 250 mg/5 ml

ACTION

Mechanism: Inhibits microbial DNA synthesis.
Peak: Serum levels peak 1 to 2 hours after an oral dose. Urine levels peak 3 to 4 hours after a dose. **Duration:** elimination half-life, 6 to 7 hours; urinary half-life, about 6 hours.

INDICATIONS & DOSAGE

Acute and chronic urinary tract infections caused by susceptible gram-negative organisms (Proteus, Klebsiella, Enterobacter, *and* Escherichia coli)—
Adults: 1 g P.O. q.i.d. for 7 to 14 days; 2 g daily for long-term use.
Children over 3 months: 55 mg/kg P.O. daily divided q.i.d. for 7 to 14 days; 33 mg/kg daily for long-term use.

ADVERSE REACTIONS

CNS: drowsiness, weakness, headache, dizziness, vertigo, ***seizures,*** confusion, hallucinations.
EENT: sensitivity to light, change in color perception, diplopia, blurred vision.
GI: *abdominal pain, nausea, vomiting,* diarrhea.
Hematologic: eosinophilia.
Skin: pruritus, photosensitivity, urticaria, rash.
Other: angioedema, fever, chills, ***increased intracranial pressure and bulging fontanelles in infants and children.***

INTERACTIONS

Oral anticoagulants: Increased anticoagulant effect. Monitor for bleeding.

*Liquid form contains alcohol.
**May contain tartrazine.
Common reactions are in italics; ***life-threatening,*** in bold italics.

CONTRAINDICATIONS
• Contraindicated in patients with seizure disorders.
• Use with extreme caution in prepubertal children; erosion of cartilage of immature animals has been reported. Contraindicated in infants under 3 months.
• Use cautiously in patients with impaired hepatic or renal function or with severe cerebral arteriosclerosis.
• Use cautiously in patients with pulmonary disease because nalidixic acid may increase respiratory depression in those with respiratory impairment.

NURSING CONSIDERATIONS
• Obtain specimen for culture and sensitivity tests before starting therapy and repeat p.r.n. Therapy may begin pending results. Not effective against *Pseudomonas* or infections outside the urinary tract.
• Tell the patient to report visual disturbances; these usually disappear with reduced dose.
• Monitor CBC, renal, and liver function studies during long-term therapy.
• Resistant bacteria may emerge within the first 48 hours of therapy.
• May cause a false-positive Clinitest reaction. Use Clinistix or Tes-Tape to monitor urine glucose. Also gives false elevations in urine vanillylmandelic acid and 17-ketosteroids. Repeat tests after therapy is completed.
• Avoid undue exposure to sunlight because of photosensitivity. The patient may continue to be photosensitive for as long as 3 months after therapy ends.

norfloxacin
Noroxin
Pregnancy Risk Category: C

HOW SUPPLIED
Tablets: 400 mg

ACTION
Mechanism: Inhibits bacterial DNA synthesis, mainly by inhibiting DNA gyrase. Bactericidal.
Peak: Plasma levels peak within 1 to 2 hours of an oral dose. **Duration:** elimination half-life, 2½ to 4 hours.

INDICATIONS & DOSAGE
Complicated or uncomplicated urinary tract infections caused by susceptible strains of Escherichia coli, Klebsiella, Enterobacter, Proteus, Pseudomonas aeruginosa, Citrobacter, Staphylococcus aureus *(and* epidermidis*), and group D streptococci* –
Adults: for uncomplicated infections, 400 mg P.O. b.i.d. for 7 to 10 days. For complicated infections, 400 mg b.i.d. for 10 to 21 days.
Cystitis caused by E. coli, K. pneumoniae, *or* P. mirabilis –
Adults: 400 mg P.O. b.i.d. for 3 days.
Acute, uncomplicated gonorrhea –
Adults: 800 mg P.O. as a single dose, followed by doxycycline therapy to treat any coexisting chlamydial infection.

ADVERSE REACTIONS
CNS: fatigue, somnolence, headache, dizziness.
GI: nausea, constipation, flatulence, heartburn, dry mouth.
Hematologic: eosinophilia.
Skin: rash, photosensitivity.
Other: ***hypersensitivity reactions*** (rash, anaphylactoid reactions), transient elevations of AST and ALT.

INTERACTIONS
Antacids, iron products, sucralfate: may hinder absorption. Separate administration times by 2 hours.
Nitrofurantoin: decreased norfloxacin effectiveness. Don't use together.
Probenecid: may increase serum levels of norfloxacin by decreasing its excretion. Monitor for toxicity.
Theophylline: possibly impaired the-

†Available in Canada only. ‡Available in Australia only. ◇Available OTC.

ophylline metabolism, resulting in increased plasma levels and risk of toxicity. Monitor closely.

CONTRAINDICATIONS

- Contraindicated in patients with hypersensitivity to quinolones and in those with seizure disorders.
- Use cautiously in patients with conditions that may predispose them to seizure disorders, such as cerebral arteriosclerosis. Also use cautiously in those with renal impairment.

NURSING CONSIDERATIONS

- Warn the patient not to exceed the recommended dosages and to drink several glasses of water throughout the day to maintain hydration and adequate urine output.
- Advise the patient to take the drug 1 hour before or 2 hours after meals because food, antacids, iron products, and sucralfate may hinder absorption.
- Because norfloxacin may cause dizziness, the patient should avoid hazardous activities that require alertness and good coordination until the CNS effects of the drug are known.

ofloxacin

Floxin

Pregnancy Risk Category: C

HOW SUPPLIED

Tablets: 200 mg, 300 mg, 400 mg
Injection: 20 mg/ml, 40 mg/ml; 4 mg/ml premixed in D_5W

ACTION

Mechanism: Inhibits bacterial DNA gyrase and prevents DNA replication in susceptible bacteria.
Peak: Plasma levels peak immediately after an I.V. infusion, or within ½ to 2 hours after oral dose. **Duration:** terminal elimination half-life, 4 to 8 hours.

INDICATIONS & DOSAGE

Lower respiratory tract infections caused by susceptible strains of Haemophilus influenzae *or* Streptococcus pneumoniae –
Adults: 400 mg I.V. or P.O. q 12 hours for 10 days.
Cervicitis or urethritis caused by Chlamydia trachomatis *or* Neisseria gonorrhoeae –
Adults: 300 mg I.V. or P.O. q 12 hours for 7 days.
Acute, uncomplicated gonorrhea –
Adults: 400 mg I.V. or P.O. as a single dose.
Mild-to-moderate skin and skin structure infections caused by susceptible strains of Staphylococcus aureus, S. epidermidis, Streptococcus pyogenes, *or* Proteus mirabilis –
Adults: 400 mg I.V. or P.O. q 12 hours for 10 days.
Cystitis caused by Escherichia coli *or* Klebsiella pneumoniae –
Adults: 200 mg I.V. or P.O. q 12 hours for 3 days.
Urinary tract infections caused by susceptible strains of Citrobacter diversus, Enterobacter aerogenes, Escherichia coli, Proteus mirabilis, *or* Pseudomonas aeruginosa –
Adults: 200 mg I.V. or P.O. q 12 hours for 7 days. Complicated infections may require therapy for 10 days.
Prostatitis caused by E. coli –
Adults: 300 mg I.V. or P.O. q 12 hours for 6 weeks.

If creatinine clearance is 10 to 50 ml/minute, decrease dosage interval to once q 24 hours. If creatinine clearance is < 10 ml/minute, give half the recommended dose q 24 hours.

ADVERSE REACTIONS

CNS: headache, dizziness, fatigue, lethargy, malaise, drowsiness, sleep disorders, nervousness, light-headedness, insomnia, ***seizures.***
CV: chest pain.
GI: nausea, anorexia, abdominal pain

or discomfort, diarrhea, vomiting, dry mouth, flatulence, dysgeusia.
GU: vaginitis, vaginal discharge, genital pruritus.
Skin: rash, pruritus, photosensitivity.
Other: hypersensitivity reactions, ***(anaphylactoid reaction),*** visual disturbances, fever.

INTERACTIONS

Antacids containing aluminum or magnesium hydroxide, iron salts, sucralfate, products containing zinc: may interfere with the GI absorption of ofloxacin. Separate administration by at least 2 hours.
Anticoagulants: increased effect. Monitor for bleeding and altered PT.
Antineoplastic agents: may lower serum levels of quinolones. Monitor for lack of effect.
Theophylline: decreased clearance of theophylline with some quinolones. Monitor theophylline levels.

CONTRAINDICATIONS

- Contraindicated in children and in breast-feeding patients because drug has caused arthropathy or osteochondrosis in young animals. Breast milk concentrations are similar to those in plasma. Use during pregnancy only when benefits outweigh fetal risks. Also contraindicated in patients with hypersensitivity to the drug or other quinolones.
- Use cautiously in patients with a history of seizure disorders or other CNS diseases, such as cerebral arteriosclerosis. If patient experiences excessive CNS stimulation (restlessness, tremor, confusion, hallucinations), discontinue medication and notify doctor. Institute seizure precautions.
- Use cautiously and with dosage adjustments in patients with renal failure because the drug is mainly eliminated by renal excretion.

NURSING CONSIDERATIONS

- Patients treated for gonorrhea should have a serologic test for syphilis. Drug is not effective against syphilis, and treatment of gonorrhea may mask or delay symptoms of syphilis.
- Advise the patient to use sunblock and protective clothing to avoid photosensitivity reactions.
- Regular blood studies and hepatic and renal function tests are recommended during prolonged therapy.
- Advise the patient to take the drug with plenty of fluids, but not with meals, and to avoid antacids, sucralfate, and products containing iron or zinc for at least 2 hours before or after each dose.
- Because the drug may cause lightheadedness, patient should avoid hazardous tasks such as driving until the adverse CNS effects are known.
- Tell the patient to stop drug and notify the doctor if a rash or other signs of hypersensitivity reactions develop.
- **I.V. use:** Concentrate for injection must be diluted before use. Single-use vials containing 20 or 40 mg/ml must be diluted to a maximum concentration of 4 mg/ml using a compatible I.V. solution, such as D_5W, 0.9% sodium chloride injection, D_5W in 0.9% sodium chloride injection, or sterile water for injection. Infuse over not less than 60 minutes.
- Because compatibility with other drugs is not known, don't mix ofloxacin with other drugs. If giving infusion at a Y-site, discontinue other solution during infusion.

17
Antivirals

acyclovir sodium
amantadine hydrochloride
didanosine
foscarnet sodium
ganciclovir
ribavirin
rimantadine
vidarabine monohydrate
zalcitabine
zidovudine

COMBINATION PRODUCTS
None.

acyclovir sodium
Zovirax
Pregnancy Risk Category: C

HOW SUPPLIED
Capsules: 200 mg
Tablets: 400 mg
Injection: 500 mg/vial, 1 g/vial

ACTION
Mechanism: Becomes incorporated into viral DNA and inhibits viral multiplication.
Peak: Serum levels peak immediately after I.V. infusion, or within 1½ to 2½ hours. **Duration:** elimination half-life, 2 to 3½ hours.

INDICATIONS & DOSAGE
Initial and recurrent episodes of mucocutaneous herpes simplex virus (HSV-1 and HSV-2) infections in immunocompromised patients; severe initial episodes of herpes genitalis in patients who are not immunocompromised –
Adults and children over age 11: 5 mg/kg, given at a constant rate over a period of 1 hour by I.V. q 8 hours for 7 days (5 days for herpes genitalis).
Children under age 12: 250 mg/m², given at a constant rate over a period of 1 hour by I.V. q 8 hours for 7 days (5 days for herpes genitalis).
Initial genital herpes –
Adults: 200 mg P.O. q 4 hours while awake (a total of 5 capsules daily). Treatment should continue for 10 days.
Intermittent therapy for recurrent genital herpes –
Adults: 200 mg P.O. q 4 hours while awake (a total of 5 capsules daily). Treatment should continue for 5 days. Initiate therapy at the first sign of recurrence.
Chronic suppressive therapy for recurrent genital herpes –
Adults: 200 mg P.O. t.i.d. or 400 mg b.i.d. for 6 to 12 months.
Chicken pox –
Adults and children: 20 mg/kg P.O. q.i.d. for 5 days. Start therapy as soon as symptoms appear.

ADVERSE REACTIONS
CNS: (associated with I.V. dosage): *headache, encephalopathic changes (lethargy, obtundation, tremor, confusion, hallucinations, agitation,* ***seizures, coma****).*
CV: hypotension.
GI: *nausea, vomiting,* diarrhea.
GU: *transient elevations of serum creatinine levels,* hematuria.
Skin: rash, itching.
Other: *inflammation, vesicular eruptions, and phlebitis at injection site.*

INTERACTIONS
Probenecid: increased acyclovir blood levels. Monitor for possible toxicity.
Zidovudine: may cause drowsiness or lethargy. Use together cautiously.

CONTRAINDICATIONS
• Contraindicated in patients with hypersensitivity to the drug.
• Use cautiously in patients with underlying neurologic problems, renal disease, dehydration, or in those receiving other nephrotoxic drugs.

NURSING CONSIDERATIONS
• Some clinicians consider acyclovir therapy of marginal benefit for chicken pox because the disease is usually self-limiting. However, acyclovir may be more beneficial in adolescents than in young children.
• Instruct the patient that drug is effective in managing herpes infection but does not eliminate or cure it. Warn the patient that acyclovir will not prevent spread of infection to others.
• Urge the patient to recognize early symptoms of herpes infection (such as tingling, itching, or pain) so he can take acyclovir before the infection fully develops.
• Notify the doctor if serum creatinine level does not return to normal within a few days. He may increase hydration, adjust dose, or discontinue acyclovir.
• Encephalopathic changes are more likely in patients with neurologic disorders or in those who have had neurologic reactions to cytotoxic drugs.
• Burroughs-Wellcome, the manufacturer, maintains an ongoing registry of women exposed to the drug during pregnancy. Follow-up studies to date have not shown an increased risk for birth defects for infants born to patients exposed to the drug during pregnancy. Health care providers are encouraged to report such exposures to the registrar at (800) 722-9292.
• **I.V. use:** Infusion must be administered over at least 1 hour to prevent renal tubular damage. Bolus injection, dehydration (decreased urine output), preexisting renal disease, and the concomitant use of other nephrotoxic drugs increase the risk of renal toxicity.
• Don't give by bolus injection or administer I.M. or S.C.
• Concentrated solutions (10 mg/ml or more) may be associated with a higher incidence of phlebitis.
• Patient must be adequately hydrated during acyclovir infusion.

---

amantadine hydrochloride
Antadine‡, Symadine, Symmetrel
Pregnancy Risk Category: C

HOW SUPPLIED
Capsules: 100 mg
Syrup: 50 mg/5 ml

ACTION
Mechanism: Interferes with influenza A virus penetration into susceptible cells. In parkinsonism, its action is unknown.
Peak: Peak plasma levels occur 1 to 4 hours after an oral dose. **Duration:** mean elimination half-life, 24 hours.

INDICATIONS & DOSAGE
Prophylaxis or symptomatic treatment of influenza type A virus, respiratory tract illnesses –
Adults to age 64 and children age 10 and over: 200 mg P.O. daily in a single dose or divided b.i.d.
Children age 1 to 9: 4.4 to 8.8 mg/kg P.O. daily, as a single dose or divided b.i.d. or t.i.d. Don't exceed 150 mg daily.
Adults over age 64: 100 mg P.O. once daily.

Treatment should continue for 24 to 48 hours after symptoms disappear. Prophylaxis should start as soon as possible after initial exposure and continue for at least 10 days after exposure. May continue prophylactic treatment up to 90 days for repeated or suspected exposures if influenza vaccine unavailable. If used with influenza vaccine, continue dose for 2

to 3 weeks until protection from vaccine develops.
Drug-induced extrapyramidal reactions –
Adults: 100 mg P.O. b.i.d., up to 300 mg daily in divided doses. Patient may benefit from as much as 400 mg daily, but dosages over 200 mg must be closely supervised.
Idiopathic parkinsonism, parkinsonian syndrome –
Adults: 100 mg P.O. b.i.d.; in patients who are seriously ill or receiving other antiparkinsonian drugs, 100 mg daily for at least 1 week, then 100 mg b.i.d., p.r.n.

ADVERSE REACTIONS
CNS: depression, fatigue, confusion, dizziness, psychosis, hallucinations, anxiety, *irritability,* ataxia, *insomnia,* weakness, headache, light-headedness, difficulty concentrating.
CV: peripheral edema, orthostatic hypotension, *CHF.*
GI: anorexia, nausea, constipation, vomiting, dry mouth.
GU: urine retention.
Skin: *livedo reticularis* (with prolonged use).

INTERACTIONS
Anticholinergics: increased adverse anticholinergic effects. Use together cautiously.
CNS stimulants: additive CNS stimulation. Use together cautiously.
Triamterene, hydrochlorothiazide: increased levels of amantadine. Use together cautiously.

CONTRAINDICATIONS
- Contraindicated in patients with hypersensitivity to the drug.
- Use cautiously in those with seizure disorders, CHF, peripheral edema, hepatic disease, mental illness, eczematoid rash, renal impairment, orthostatic hypotension, and CV disease and in elderly patients. Dosage may need to be adjusted in patients with renal failure.

NURSING CONSIDERATIONS
- Instruct the patient to report adverse reactions to the doctor, especially dizziness, depression, anxiety, nausea, and urine retention.
- Elderly patients are more susceptible to neurological adverse effects. Taking the drug in two daily doses rather than single dose may reduce their incidence.
- If orthostatic hypotension occurs, instruct the patient not to stand or change positions too quickly.
- If insomnia occurs, the patient should take the drug several hours before bedtime.
- In the patient with parkinsonism, warn against discontinuing drug abruptly to prevent precipitating a parkinsonian crisis.

didanosine (ddl)
Videx

Pregnancy Risk Category: B

HOW SUPPLIED
Tablets (chewable): 25 mg, 50 mg, 100 mg, 150 mg
Powder for oral solution (buffered): 100 mg/packet, 167 mg/packet, 250 mg/packet, 375 mg/packet
Powder for oral solution (pediatric): 10 mg/ml in 2- and 4-g bottles

ACTION
Mechanism: Inhibits replication of HIV by preventing DNA replication. In addition, ddATP inhibits the enzyme HIV-RNA dependent DNA polymerase (reverse transcriptase).
Peak: Peak levels occur within 1 hour of an oral dose. **Duration:** elimination half-life, about 1½ hours.

INDICATIONS & DOSAGE
Advanced HIV infection in patients who cannot tolerate or who no longer respond to zidovudine therapy–
Adults 75 kg and over: 300 mg (two 150-mg tablets) P.O. q 12 hours; or 375 mg buffered powder q 12 hours.
Adults 50 to 74 kg: 200 mg (two 100-mg tablets) P.O. q 12 hours; or 250 mg buffered powder q 12 hours.
Adults 35 to 49 kg: 125 mg (one 100-mg and one 25-mg tablet) P.O. q 12 hours; or 167 mg buffered powder q 12 hours.
Children: 200 mg/m^2 P.O. daily in divided doses q 12 hours.

ADVERSE REACTIONS
CNS: *headache,* insomnia, dizziness, ***seizures,*** confusion, anxiety, nervousness, hypertonia, abnormal thinking.
CV: hypertension.
GI: *diarrhea, nausea, vomiting, abdominal pain,* ***pancreatitis,*** dry mouth, dyspepsia, flatulence.
Hepatic: liver abnormalities.
Other: *peripheral neuropathy,* rash, pruritus, asthenia, pain, myalgia, arthritis, pneumonia, infection, cough, myopathy.

INTERACTIONS
Antacids containing magnesium or aluminum hydroxides: enhanced adverse effects of the antacid component (including diarrhea or constipation) when administered with didanosine tablets or pediatric suspension. Avoid concomitant use.
Dapsone, ketoconazole, drugs that require gastric acid for adequate absorption: decreased absorption from buffering action. Administer these drugs 2 hours before didanosine.
Fluoroquinolones, tetracyclines: decreased absorption from buffering agents in didanosine tablets or antacids in pediatric suspension.

CONTRAINDICATIONS
• Contraindicated in patients with a history of hypersensitivity to any component of the formulation. Tablets are buffered with dihydroxyaluminum sodium carbonate, magnesium hydroxide, and sodium citrate and are flavored with aspartame and sugar. Powder for oral solution is buffered with sodium phosphate, sodium citrate, and citric acid and is flavored with sucrose.
• Use cautiously in patients with a history of pancreatitis. In early studies, the drug caused pancreatitis in about 9% of all patients; fatalities have occurred. Also use cautiously in patients with peripheral neuropathy, renal or hepatic impairment, or hyperuricemia.

NURSING CONSIDERATIONS
• In early clinical trials, the powder for oral solution was associated with a high incidence of diarrhea. The manufacturer suggests switching to the tablet formulation if diarrhea is a problem, although no evidence suggests that other formulations may be associated with a lower incidence of diarrhea.
• Patients receiving a sodium-restricted diet should know that each two-tablet dose of didanosine contains 529 mg of sodium; each single packet of buffered powder for oral solution contains 1.38 g of sodium.
• Administer didanosine on an empty stomach, regardless of the dosage form used; administering the drug with meals can decrease absorption by 50%.
• Most patients should receive two tablets per dose.
• Because they contain buffers that raise stomach pH to levels that prevent degradation of the active drug, the tablets should be thoroughly chewed before swallowing, and the patient should drink at least 1 oz of water with each dose. If the tablets

are manually crushed, stir them thoroughly in 1 oz of water to disperse the particles uniformly, then have the patient drink the mixture immediately.

- Children over age 1 should receive a two-tablet dose, and children under age 1 may receive a one-tablet dose.
- Single-dose packets containing buffered powder for oral solution are available. To administer, pour contents into 4 oz of water. Do not use fruit juice or other beverages that may be acidic. Stir for 2 or 3 minutes until the powder dissolves completely. Administer immediately.
- Use care when preparing the powder or crushing tablets to avoid excessive dispersal of the powder into the air.
- The pediatric powder for oral solution must be prepared by a pharmacist before dispensing. It must be constituted with Purified Water, USP, then diluted with an antacid (either Mylanta Double Strength Liquid or Maalox TC Suspension) to a final concentration of 10 mg/ml. The admixture is stable for 30 days if refrigerated (at 36° to 46° F [2° to 8° C]). Shake the solution well before measuring the dose.

foscarnet sodium (phosphonoformic acid)

Foscavir

Pregnancy Risk Category: C

HOW SUPPLIED

Injection: 24 mg/ml in 250- and 500-ml bottles

ACTION

Mechanism: Inhibits all known herpes viruses in vitro by blocking the pyrophosphate binding site on DNA polymerases and reverse transcriptases.

Peak: Peak levels occur immediately after I.V. infusion. **Duration:** terminal elimination half-life, 2½ to 3½ hours.

INDICATIONS & DOSAGE

CMV retinitis in patients with AIDS–

Adults: initially, 60 mg/kg I.V. as an induction treatment in patients with normal renal function. Administer I.V. over 1 hour q 8 hours for 2 to 3 weeks, depending on clinical response. Follow with a maintenance infusion of 90 mg/kg daily administered over 2 hours; this dose may be increased as needed and tolerated to 120 mg/kg daily if the disease shows signs of progression.

In renal failure, calculate the patient's creatinine clearance from this equation as follows:

For men: Creatinine clearance = (140 – age) ÷ (serum creatinine × 72)

For women: Multiply the above value by 0.85. Then administer foscarnet as shown below.

Induction dose–

Creatinine clearance (ml/min/kg)	Dose to administer q 8 hours (mg/kg)
1.6	60
1.5	57
1.4	53
1.3	49
1.2	46
1.1	42
1	39
0.9	35
0.8	32
0.7	28
0.6	25
0.5	21
0.4	18

Maintenance dose –

Creatinine clearance (ml/min/kg)	Equivalent to 90 mg/ kg/day	Equivalent to 120 mg/kg/day
1.4	90	120
1.2 to 1.4	78	104
1 to 1.2	75	100
0.8 to 1	71	94
0.6 to 0.8	63	84
0.4 to 0.6	57	76

ADVERSE REACTIONS

CNS: *headache,* ***seizures,*** *fatigue, rigors, malaise, asthenia, paresthesia, dizziness, hypoesthesia, neuropathy,* tremor, ataxia, generalized spasms, dementia, stupor, sensory disturbances, meningitis, aphasia, abnormal coordination, EEG abnormalities, vertigo, ***coma***, encephalopathy, abnormal gait, hypertonia, visual field defects, dyskinesia, extrapyramidal reactions, speech disorders, paralysis, peripheral neuropathy, nystagmus, ***cerebral edema.***
CV: *hypertension, palpitations, ECG abnormalities, sinus tachycardia, first-degree AV block, hypotension, flushing.*
EENT: visual disturbances.
GI: *nausea, diarrhea, vomiting, abdominal pain, anorexia,* constipation, dysphagia, rectal hemorrhage, dry mouth, melena, flatulence, ulcerative stomatitis, ***pancreatitis.***
GU: ***abnormal renal function,*** *decreased creatinine clearance and increased serum creatinine levels, albuminuria, dysuria, polyuria, urethral disorder, urine retention, urinary tract infections,* ***acute renal failure.***
Hematologic: *anemia, granulocytopenia, leukopenia,* ***bone marrow suppression,*** thrombocytopenia, platelet abnormalities, thrombocytosis, WBC count abnormalities, lymphadenopathy.
Respiratory: *cough, dyspnea,* pneumonitis, sinusitis, pharyngitis, rhinitis, respiratory insufficiency, pulmonary infiltration, stridor, pneumothorax, ***bronchospasm,*** hemoptysis.
Skin: *rash, increased sweating,* pruritus, skin ulceration, erythematous rash, seborrhea, skin discoloration.
Other: fever, pain, infection, sepsis, hypokalemia, hypomagnesemia, hypophosphatemia or hyperphosphatemia, hypocalcemia, leg cramps.

INTERACTIONS

Nephrotoxic drugs such as amphotericin B, aminoglycosides: increased risk of nephrotoxicity. Avoid concomitant use.
Pentamidine: increased risk of nephrotoxicity; severe hypocalcemia has also been reported. Don't use together.
Zidovudine: possible increased incidence or severity of anemia. Monitor blood counts.

CONTRAINDICATIONS

- Contraindicated in patients with hypersensitivity to the drug.
- Use cautiously in patients with abnormal renal function because it will result in accumulation of the drug and enhanced toxicity. Because foscarnet is nephrotoxic, it has the potential to worsen renal impairment. Some degree of nephrotoxicity occurs in most patients treated with the drug.

NURSING CONSIDERATIONS

- Administration of the drug is associated with a dose-related transient decrease in ionized serum calcium, which may not always be reflected in the patient's laboratory values. Advise the patient to report perioral tingling, numbness in the extremities, and paresthesia.
- Creatinine clearance should be determined before therapy and frequently thereafter because of the drug's adverse effects on renal function. A baseline 24-hour creatinine clearance is recommended, followed

by regular determinations two to three times weekly during induction and at least once every 1 to 2 weeks during maintenance. If creatinine clearance falls below 0.4 ml/minute/kg, discontinue the drug.

• Because the drug can adversely affect important serum electrolytes such as potassium, calcium, magnesium, and phosphorus, regular determinations of these electrolytes are recommended using a schedule similar to that established for creatinine clearance. Monitor the patient for tetany and seizures associated with abnormal electrolyte levels.

• Anemia is common (in up to 33% of patients treated with the drug). It may be severe enough to require transfusions. Monitor the patient's hemoglobin and hematocrit levels.

• Do not exceed the recommended dosage, infusion rate, or frequency of administration. All doses must be individualized according to the patient's renal function.

• Because the drug is highly toxic and toxicity is probably dose-related, the lowest effective maintenance dose should be used throughout therapy.

• Unlike ganciclovir, foscarnet does not require cellular activation by thymidine kinase or other kinases. Foscarnet may be active against certain CMV strains resistant to ganciclovir.

• **I.V. use:** An infusion pump must be used to administer foscarnet. To minimize renal toxicity, the patient must be adequately hydrated before and during the infusion.

ganciclovir

Cytovene

Pregnancy Risk Category: C

HOW SUPPLIED

Injection: 500 mg/vial

ACTION

Mechanism: Inhibits viral DNA synthesis of CMV.

Peak: Peak serum levels occur immediately after I.V. infusion. **Duration:** terminal elimination half-life, 2½ to 3½ hours.

INDICATIONS & DOSAGE

CMV retinitis in immunocompromised individuals, including patients with AIDS –

Adults: induction treatment – 5 mg/kg I.V. q 12 hours for 14 to 21 days (normal renal function); maintenance treatment – 5 mg/kg I.V. daily for 7 days each week, or 6 mg/kg daily for 5 days each week.

ADVERSE REACTIONS

CNS: altered dreams, confusion, ataxia, dizziness, headache.

CV: arrhythmias, hypotension, hypertension.

GI: nausea, vomiting, diarrhea, anorexia.

GU: hematuria.

Hematologic: *granulocytopenia,* ***thrombocytopenia.***

Other: retinal detachment in CMV retinitis patients; at injection site – inflammation, pain, phlebitis.

INTERACTIONS

Cytotoxic agents: increased toxic effects, especially hematologic effects and stomatitis. Monitor closely.

Imipenem/cilastatin: heightened seizure activity with concomitant use. Monitor closely.

Immunosuppressants such as azathioprine, cyclosporine, corticosteroids: Enhanced immune and bone marrow suppression. Use together cautiously.

Probenecid: increased ganciclovir blood levels. Monitor closely.

Zidovudine: increased incidence of granulocytopenia with concurrent use. Monitor closely.

CONTRAINDICATIONS
• Contraindicated in patients with an absolute neutrophil count below 500/mm³ or a platelet count below 25,000/mm³.
• Use cautiously and in reduced dosage in patients with renal dysfunction.

NURSING CONSIDERATIONS
• Ganciclovir infusion therapy should be accompanied by adequate hydration.
• Because of the frequency of granulocytopenia and thrombocytopenia, neutrophil and platelet counts should be obtained every 2 days during twice-daily ganciclovir dosing and at least weekly thereafter.
• Use caution when preparing ganciclovir solution, which is alkaline.
• **I.V. use:** Infusion must take place over at least 1 hour. Infusions faster than 60 minutes will result in increased toxicity. Use an infusion pump. Do not administer as an I.V. bolus.
• Do not administer S.C. or I.M.

ribavirin
Virazole

Pregnancy Risk Category: X

HOW SUPPLIED
Powder to be reconstituted for inhalation: 6 g in 100-ml glass vial

ACTION
Mechanism: Inhibits viral activity by an unknown mechanism, possibly by inhibiting RNA and DNA synthesis by depleting intracellular nucleotide pools.
Peak: Peak serum levels occur immediately after an aerosol treatment; after oral ingestion (investigational), peak levels occur in 1 to 4 hours.
Duration: plasma half-life, 6½ to 11 hours after inhalation, or greater than 48 hours after ingestion.

INDICATIONS & DOSAGE
Hospitalized infants and young children infected by RSV–
Infants and young children: solution in concentration of 20 mg/ml delivered via the Viratek Small Particle Aerosol Generator (SPAG-2). Treatment is carried out for 12 to 18 hours/day for at least 3, and no more than 7 days.

ADVERSE REACTIONS
CV: ***cardiac arrest,*** hypotension.
EENT: conjunctivitis.
Hematologic: anemia, reticulocytosis.
Respiratory: worsening of respiratory state.
Other: rash or erythema of eyelids.

INTERACTIONS
None significant.

CONTRAINDICATIONS
• Contraindicated in patients who are or may become pregnant during treatment.

NURSING CONSIDERATIONS
• Ribavirin aerosol is indicated only for severe lower respiratory tract infection caused by RSV. Although treatment may be started while awaiting diagnostic test results, existence of RSV infection must be eventually documented.
• Most infants and children with RSV infection don't require treatment because the disease is commonly mild and self-limiting. Infants with underlying conditions, such as prematurity or cardiopulmonary disease, get RSV in its severest form and benefit most from treatment with ribavirin aerosol.
• This treatment must be accompanied by, and does not replace, supportive respiratory and fluid management.
• Ribavirin aerosol *must* be administered by the Viratek Small Particle Aerosol Generator (SPAG-2). Don't

use any other aerosol-generating device.
• Ribavirin may precipitate in ventilator apparatus, causing result in equipment malfunction with serious consequences. The use of ribavirin in ventilator-dependent patients is not recommended.
• Water used to reconstitute this drug must not contain any antimicrobial agent. Use sterile USP water for injection, *not* bacteriostatic water.
• Discard solutions placed in the SPAG-2 unit at least every 24 hours before adding newly reconstituted solution.
• Store reconstituted solutions at room temperature for 24 hours.

rimantadine
Flumadine

Pregnancy Risk Category:

HOW SUPPLIED
Injection: 200 mg

ACTION
Mechanism: Prevents viral uncoating, an early step in virus reproductive cycle.
Peak: Peak plasma levels occur within 6 hours of oral administration.
Duration: elimination half-life, about 25½ hours.

INDICATIONS & DOSAGE
Influenza A –
Adults and children age 10: 100 mg P.O. b.i.d.
Children under age 10: 5 mg/kg (not to exceed 150 mg) P.O. once a day.
Elderly patients, patients with severe hepatic or renal dysfunction: 100 mg P.O. daily.

ADVERSE REACTIONS
CNS: insomnia, headache, dizziness, nervousness, fatigue, asthenia.
EENT: eye pain.
GI: nausea, vomiting, anorexia, dry mouth, abdominal pain.

INTERACTIONS
None significant.

CONTRAINDICATIONS
• Contraindicated in patients with hypersensitivity to the drug or amantadine Because animal studies have demonstrated that the drug concentrates in breast milk, avoid use in breast-feeding patients.
• High doses given to animals were fetotoxic and possibly teratogenic. Pregnant patients should consider the risks compared to the benefits before taking this drug.
• Use cautiously in patients with renal or hepatic impairment, and in patients with a history of seizures.

NURSING CONSIDERATIONS
• For influenza infections, start therapy within 48 hours of onset of symptoms and continue for 7 days after the initial signs and symptoms occurred.
• Influenza A-resistant strains can emerge during therapy. Patients taking the drug may still be able to spread the disease. Consider the risk to contacts of treated patients who may be subject to morbidity from influenza A.
• To prevent insomnia, the patient should take drug several hours before bedtime.

vidarabine monohydrate (adenine arabinoside, ara-A)
Vira-A

Pregnancy Risk Category: C

HOW SUPPLIED
Concentrate for I.V. infusion: 200 mg/ml in 5-ml vial (equivalent to 187.4 mg vidarabine)

ACTION
Mechanism: Becomes incorporated into viral DNA and inhibits viral multiplication.
Peak: Peak serum levels occur immediately after I.V. infusion. **Duration:** elimination half-life of parent drug, 1½ hours and of active metabolite, about 3½ hours.

INDICATIONS & DOSAGE
Herpes simplex virus encephalitis –
Adults and children (including neonates): 15 mg/kg I.V. daily for 10 days. Slowly infuse the total daily dose at a constant rate over 12 to 24 hours. Avoid rapid or bolus injection.
Herpes zoster in immunosuppressed patients –
Adults: 10 mg/kg I.V. daily for 5 days.

ADVERSE REACTIONS
CNS: tremor, dizziness, hallucinations, confusion, psychosis, ataxia.
GI: *anorexia, nausea,* vomiting, diarrhea.
Hematologic: anemia, neutropenia, thrombocytopenia.
Skin: pruritus, rash.
Other: weight loss; elevated AST, bilirubin; pain at injection site.

INTERACTIONS
Allopurinol: reduced metabolism of vidarabine and increased risk of adverse CNS effects. Monitor closely.

CONTRAINDICATIONS
- Contraindicated in patients with hypersensitivity to the drug.
- Use cautiously in patients with impaired renal function. Dosage adjustment may be necessary.

NURSING CONSIDERATIONS
- Can reduce mortality caused by herpes simplex virus encephalitis from about 70% to 28%. Vidarabine is not effective against other viruses.
- Monitor hematologic tests, such as hemoglobin, hematocrit, WBC count, and platelet count during therapy. Also monitor renal and liver function studies.
- **I.V. use:** Use with a 0.45-micron (or smaller) I.V. filter. Any I.V. solution is suitable as a diluent.
- Must be diluted to a concentration of less than 0.5 mg/ml. Because vidarabine is not highly soluble, each milligram of drug requires 2.2 ml of I.V. solution; the maximum concentration is 450 mg/liter. Dilute just before using, and use within 48 hours.
- Don't give I.M. or S.C. because of low solubility and poor absorption. Because large volumes of solution must be administered, monitor the patient for fluid overload.

zalcitabine (dideoxycytidine, ddC)
Hivid

Pregnancy Risk Category: C

HOW SUPPLIED
Tablets: 0.375 mg, 0.75 mg

ACTION
Mechanism: Inhibits replication of HIV by blocking viral DNA synthesis.
Peak: Peak plasma levels occur ½ hour after an oral dose. **Duration:** elimination half-life, 70 to 120 minutes.

INDICATIONS & DOSAGE
Advanced HIV infection (CD4 + T cell count below 300 cells/mm³) in patients who have demonstrated significant clinical or immunologic deterioration –
Adults 30 kg and over: 0.75 mg P.O. q 8 hours. Must be taken with zidovudine 200 mg P.O. q 8 hours.

Patients with a creatinine clearance above 40 ml/minute/1.73 m² should receive the usual dose; 10 to 40 ml/minute/1.73 m², the usual dose q 12 hours; below 10 ml/minute/1.73 m^2, the usual dose q 24 hours.

ADVERSE REACTIONS

Note: Limited data regarding drug toxicity are available. Consult current literature for more details.

CNS: *peripheral neuropathy,* headache, fatigue, dizziness.

EENT: pharyngitis.

GI: nausea, vomiting, diarrhea, abdominal pain, anorexia, constipation, stomatitis.

Hematologic: anemia, neutropenia, leukopenia.

Skin: pruritus; night sweats; erythematous, maculopapular, or follicular rash.

Other: myalgia, arthralgia, fatigue, fever, rigors, chest pain, weight increase, ***pancreatitis.***

INTERACTIONS

Aminoglycosides, amphotericin B, foscarnet, and other drugs that may impair renal function: increased risk of nephrotoxicity. Avoid concomitant use.

Chloramphenicol, cisplatin, dapsone, disulfiram, ethionamide, glutethimide, gold salts, hydralazine, iodoquinol, isoniazid, metronidazole, nitrofurantoin, phenytoin, ribavirin, and vincristine as well as other drugs that can cause peripheral neuropathy: increased risk of peripheral neuropathy. Avoid concomitant use.

Pentamidine: increased risk of pancreatitis. Avoid concomitant use.

CONTRAINDICATIONS

- Contraindicated in patients with hypersensitivity to the drug or any component of the formulation.
- Use with extreme caution in patients with preexisting peripheral neuropathy. No data exist regarding toxicity of zalcitabine because those with preexisting neuropathy were excluded from clinical trials.
- Use cautiously in patients with renal impairment (creatinine clearance below 55 ml/minute/1.73 m^2) because they may be at increased risk for toxicity to the drug. Dosage adjustments are necessary in patients with moderate to severe renal failure.
- Also use cautiously in patients with hepatic failure. In clinical trials, the drug regimen (zalcitabine plus zidovudine) exacerbated hepatic dysfunction in patients with preexisting liver impairment.
- Additionally, use cautiously in patients with a history of pancreatitis. Rarely, pancreatitis has been fatal in patients receiving zalcitabine. In patients receiving zalcitabine as the only treatment, pancreatitis was rare (less than 1%).

NURSING CONSIDERATIONS

- Peripheral neuropathy, characterized by numbness and burning in the extremities, is the major toxicity resulting from the drug. In clinical trials using zalcitabine alone, peripheral neuropathy occurred in 17% to 31% of patients. If drug isn't withdrawn, peripheral neuropathy can progress to sharp shooting pain or severe continuous burning pain requiring opioid analgesics. It may or may not be reversible.
- If the patient experiences symptoms that resemble peripheral neuropathy, drug should be discontinued if symptoms are bilateral and persist beyond 72 hours. If symptoms persist or worsen beyond 1 week, drug should be permanently discontinued. However, if all findings relevant to peripheral neuropathy have resolved to minor symptoms, the drug may be reintroduced at 0.375 mg P.O. q 8 hours.
- If zalcitabine is discontinued because of toxicity, the patient should resume the recommended dose for zidovudine (100 mg q 4 hours).
- Administering the drug with food decreases the rate and extent of absorption.

• Patients of childbearing age should use an effective contraceptive while taking this drug.
• Make sure the patient understands that drug doesn't cure HIV infection and that opportunistic infections may still occur despite continued use. Review safe sex practices with the patient.
• Inform the patient that peripheral neuropathy is the major toxicity associated with this drug and that pancreatitis is the major life-threatening toxicity. Review the signs and symptoms of these adverse reactions, and instruct the patient to call the doctor promptly if any appear.

zidovudine (azidothymidine, AZT)

Apo-Zidovudine†, Novo-AZT†, Retrovir

Pregnancy Risk Category: B

HOW SUPPLIED

Capsules: 100 mg
Syrup: 50 mg/5 ml
Injection: 20 mg/ml

ACTION

Mechanism: Prevents replication of HIV by inhibiting the enzyme reverse transcriptase.
Peak: Peak plasma levels occur in ½ to 1½ hours after an oral dose or immediately after an I.V. infusion.
Duration: plasma half-life, about 1 hour.

INDICATIONS & DOSAGE

Patients with HIV infection with evidence of impaired immunity indicated by CD4+ cell count ≤500 cells/mm³–
Adults: initially, 200 mg P.O. q 4 hours around the clock for 1 month, then 100 mg P.O. q 4 hours around the clock.
Children: dosage is individualized and varies according to the investigational new drug protocol. Some early studies have used doses between 0.9 and 1.4 mg/kg/hour by continuous I.V. infusion; others have used 100 mg/m² I.V. or P.O. q 6 hours.
Patients with AIDS or advanced AIDS-related complex (ARC) who have a history of Pneumocystis carinii *pneumonia or a CD4+ lymphocyte count below 200 cells/mm³–*
Adults: 1 to 2 mg/kg I.V. q 4 hours.
Postexposure prophylaxis–
Adults: dosage will vary according to study protocol, but most studies use 200 mg P.O. q 4 hours around the clock for 6 to 8 weeks. Some investigators try to begin therapy within 1 hour of exposure.
Asymptomatic HIV infection–
Adults: 100 mg P.O. q 4 hours while awake (500 mg daily).
Children 3 months to 12 years: 180 mg/m² P.O. q 6 hours (720 mg/m²/day), not to exceed 200 mg q 6 hours.
To reduce risk of transmission of HIV from infected mother with a baseline CD4+ lymphocyte counts greater than 200 cells/mm³ to newborn–
Adults: 100 mg P.O. given initially between 14 and 34 weeks gestation and continued throughout pregnancy. During labor, administer loading dose of 2 mg/kg followed by continuous infusion of 1 mg/kg/hour until delivery.
Infants: 2 mg/kg P.O. (syrup) q 6 hours for 6 weeks beginning 8 to 12 hours after birth.

ADVERSE REACTIONS

CNS: *headache,* ***seizures,*** agitation, malaise, restlessness, insomnia, confusion, anxiety, ataxia, nystagmus.
GI: *nausea,* anorexia.
Hematologic: ***severe bone marrow suppression (resulting in anemia), granulocytopenia, thrombocytopenia.***
Skin: *rash,* itching.
Other: myalgia.

INTERACTIONS

Acetaminophen, aspirin, co-trimoxazole, indomethacin: may impair hepatic metabolism of zidovudine, increasing the drug's toxicity.
Acyclovir: possible seizures, lethargy, and fatigue. Use together cautiously.
Amphotericin B, dapsone, flucytosine, pentamidine: increased risk of nephrotoxicity and bone marrow suppression. Monitor closely.
Other cytotoxic drugs: additive adverse effects on the bone marrow. Avoid concomitant use.
Probenecid: may decrease the renal clearance of zidovudine. Avoid concomitant use.

CONTRAINDICATIONS

- Contraindicated in patients with hypersensitivity to the drug.
- Use cautiously and with close monitoring in patients with advanced symptomatic HIV infection.
- Do not use in HIV-infected pregnant patients who have received antiretroviral therapy.

NURSING CONSIDERATIONS

- Zidovudine frequently causes a low RBC count by suppressing the bone marrow. Advise patients that blood transfusions may be needed during treatment.
- Frequent monitoring of blood studies (every 2 weeks) is recommended to detect anemia or granulocytopenia. Patients may require dosage reduction or temporary discontinuation of the drug.
- Remind patients that they *must* comply with the every-4-hour dosage schedule. Suggest ways to avoid missing doses, perhaps by using alarm clocks.
- Warn patients not to take any other drugs for AIDS (especially those available on the street) unless their doctors have approved them. Some purported AIDS cures may interfere with zidovudine's effectiveness.
- Zidovudine has been shown to temporarily decrease morbidity and mortality in certain patients with AIDS or ARC.
- The optimum duration of treatment as well as the dosage for optimum effectiveness and minimum toxicity is not yet known.
- Advise pregnant, HIV-infected patients that zidovudine therapy only *reduces* the risk of HIV transmission to their newborn. Long-term risks to infants are unknown.
- Health care workers who consider zidovudine prophylaxis after occupational exposure (following needlestick injury, for example) should understand that animal and human studies have not yet proved the drug's safety or efficacy. These persons should consider the drug's potential toxicity as well as the risk of HIV. Some clinicians do not advocate such use of zidovudine.
- **I.V. use:** Dilute before administration. Remove the calculated dose from the vial; add to D_5W to achieve a concentration that does not exceed 4 mg/ml. Infuse drug over 1 hour at a constant rate; give every 4 hours around the clock. Avoid rapid infusion or bolus injection. Adding mixture to biological or colloidal fluids (for example, blood products, protein solutions) is not recommended. After drug is diluted, the solution is physically and chemically stable for 24 hours at room temperature and for 48 hours if refrigerated at 35.6° to 46.4° F (2° to 8° C) to minimize the risk of microbial contamination. Store undiluted vials at 59° to 77° F (15° to 25° C) and protect them from light.

18

Miscellaneous anti-infectives

atovaquone
azithromycin
aztreonam
bacitracin
chloramphenicol
chloramphenicol palmitate
chloramphenicol sodium succinate
clarithryomycin
clindamycin hydrochloride
clindamycin palmitate hydrochloride
clindamycin phosphate
erythromycin base
erythromycin estolate
erythromycin ethylsuccinate
erythromycin gluceptate
erythromycin lactobionate
erythromycin stearate
imipenem/cilastatin sodium
lincomycin hydrochloride
methenamine hippurate
methenamine mandelate
methylene blue
nitrofurantoin macrocrystals
nitrofurantoin microcrystals
polymyxin B sulfate
rifabutin
spectinomycin dihydrochloride
trimethoprim
vancomycin hydrochloride

COMBINATION PRODUCTS
CYSTEX: methenamine 165 mg, salicylamide 65 mg, sodium salicylate 97 mg, and benzoic acid 32 mg.
HEXALOL: methenamine 40.8 mg, phenyl salicylate 18.1 mg, atropine sulfate 0.03 mg, hyoscyamine 0.03 mg, benzoic acid 4.5 mg, and methylene blue 5.4 mg.
MACROBID: nitrofurantoin macrocrystals 25 mg and nitrofurantoin monohydrate 75 mg.
THIACIDE: methenamine mandelate 500 mg and potassium acid phosphate 250 mg.
TRAC TABS 2X: methenamine 120 mg, methylene blue 6 mg, phenyl salicylate 30 mg, atropine sulfate 0.06 mg, hyoscyamine sulfate 0.03 mg, and benzoic acid 7.5 mg.
URISEDAMINE: methenamine mandelate 500 mg and hyoscyamine 0.15 mg.
URO-PHOSPHATE: methenamine 300 mg and sodium acid phosphate 500 mg. Sugar coated.
UROQUID-ACID: methenamine mandelate 350 mg and sodium acid phosphate 200 mg.
UROQUID-ACID NO. 2: methenamine mandelate 500 mg and sodium acid phosphate 500 mg.

atovaquone

Mepron

Pregnancy Risk Category: C

HOW SUPPLIED
Tablets: 250 mg

ACTION
Mechanism: Interferes with electron transport in protozoal mitochondria, inhibiting enzymes needed for the synthesis of nucleic acids and adenosine triphosphate.
Peak: Two peak plasma levels occur after an oral dose, suggesting enterohepatic recycling. The first occurs after 1 to 8 hours; the second occurs after 1 to 4 days. **Duration:** elimination half-life, 2 to 3 days.

INDICATIONS & DOSAGE
Mild to moderate Pneumocystis carinii *pneumonia in patients who cannot tolerate co-trimoxazole –*

Adults: 750 mg P.O. t.i.d. for 21 days.

ADVERSE REACTIONS
CNS: *headache, insomnia,* asthenia, dizziness.
EENT: *cough.*
GI: *nausea, diarrhea, vomiting,* constipation, abdominal pain.
Skin: *rash,* pruritus.
Other: *fever,* oral monilia.

INTERACTIONS
None significant.

CONTRAINDICATIONS
- Contraindicated in patients with hypersensitivity to the drug.
- Use cautiously in breast-feeding patients. In animal studies, substantial amounts of drug were excreted in breast milk.
- Because drug is highly bound to plasma protein (greater than 99.9%), also use cautiously with other highly protein-bound drugs.

NURSING CONSIDERATIONS
- Instruct patient to take drug with meals because food enhances absorption significantly.
- Drug is ineffective in treating bacterial, fungal, or viral pneumonia or mycobacterial disease. Because of the risk of other concurrent pulmonary infections, patients should be closely evaluated during therapy.

azithromycin
Zithromax

Pregnancy Risk Category: B

HOW SUPPLIED
Capsules: 250 mg

ACTION
Mechanism: Binds to the 50S subunit of bacterial ribosomes, blocking protein synthesis; bacteriostatic or bactericidal, depending on concentration.
Peak: Serum levels peak within ½ to 2 hours of an oral dose. **Duration:** elimination half-life, about 68 hours.

INDICATIONS & DOSAGE
Acute bacterial exacerbations of COPD caused by Haemophilus influenzae, Moraxella (Branhamella) catarrhalis, *or* Streptococcus pneumoniae; *mild community-acquired pneumonia caused by* H. influenzae *or* S. pneumoniae; *uncomplicated skin and skin-structure infections caused by* Staphylococcus aureus, Streptococcus pyogenes, *or* S. agalactiae; *second-line therapy of pharyngitis or tonsillitis caused by* S. pyogenes – **Adults and adolescents age 16 and over:** 500 mg P.O. as a single dose on day 1, followed by 250 mg daily on days 2 through 5. Total dose is 1.5 g.
Nongonococcal urethritis or cervicitis caused by Chlamydia trachomatis – **Adults and adolescents age 16 and over:** 1 g P.O. as a single dose.

ADVERSE REACTIONS
CNS: dizziness, vertigo, headache, fatigue, somnolence.
CV: palpitations, chest pain.
GI: *nausea, vomiting, diarrhea, abdominal pain,* dyspepsia, flatulence, melena, cholestatic jaundice.
GU: monilia, vaginitis, nephritis.
Skin: rash, photosensitivity.
Other: angioedema, pseudomembranous colitis.

INTERACTIONS
Aluminum- and magnesium-containing antacids: lowered peak plasma levels of azithromycin. Separate administration times by at least 2 hours.
Theophylline: possibly increase plasma theophylline levels with other macrolides; effect of azithromycin is unknown. Monitor theophylline levels carefully.
Warfarin: possibly increased PT with other macrolides; effect of azithromycin is unknown. Monitor PT carefully.

CONTRAINDICATIONS
- Contraindicated in patients with hypersensitivity to erythromycin or other macrolides. Do not use azithromycin to treat gonorrhea or syphilis; moderate-to-severe pneumonia in patients for whom outpatient oral therapy is inappropriate; nosocomial infections; known or suspected bacteremia; conditions requiring hospitalization; elderly or debilitated patients; or immunocompromised patients (for example, those with cancer or AIDS)
- Use cautiously in patients with impaired hepatic function.

NURSING CONSIDERATIONS
- Obtain specimen for culture and sensitivity tests before first dose. Therapy may begin pending results.
- Administer 1 hour before or 2 hours after meals, and do not administer with antacids. Tell the patient that the drug should always be taken on an empty stomach because food or antacids will decrease absorption.
- May cause overgrowth of nonsusceptible bacteria or fungi. Monitor for signs and symptoms of superinfection.
- Tell the patient to take all of the medication as prescribed, even after he feels better.

aztreonam
Azactam

Pregnancy Risk Category: B

HOW SUPPLIED
Injection: 500-mg, 1-g, 2-g vials

ACTION
Mechanism: Inhibits bacterial cell-wall synthesis, ultimately causing cell-wall destruction; bactericidal.
Peak: Serum levels peak immediately after I.V. infusion or within 1 hour of I.M. administration. **Duration:** elimination half-life, 1 to 2½ hours.

INDICATIONS & DOSAGE
Urinary tract infections, lower respiratory tract infections, septicemia, skin and skin-structure infections, intra-abdominal infections, surgical infections, and gynecologic infections caused by various aerobic organisms –
Adults: 500 mg to 2 g I.V. or I.M. q 8 to 12 hours. For severe systemic or life-threatening infections, 2 g q 6 to 8 hours may be given. Maximum dosage is 8 g daily.

ADVERSE REACTIONS
CNS: ***seizures,*** headache, insomnia.
CV: hypotension.
GI: diarrhea, nausea, vomiting.
Hematologic: neutropenia, anemia.
Other: hypersensitivity reactions (rash, ***anaphylaxis***), altered taste, halitosis, rash, transient elevation of ALT and AST, thrombophlebitis at I.V. site, discomfort and swelling at I.M. injection site.

INTERACTIONS
Furosemide, probenecid: increased serum aztreonam levels. Avoid concomitant use.

CONTRAINDICATIONS
- Contraindicated in patients with hypersensitivity to the drug.
- Use cautiously in elderly patients and in those with impaired renal function.

NURSING CONSIDERATIONS
- Aztreonam is a narrow-spectrum antibiotic, effective solely against gram-negative organisms. Because it is ineffective against gram-positive and anaerobic organisms, aztreonam must be used with other antibiotics for immediate treatment of life-threatening illnesses.
- Patients who are allergic to penicillins or cephalosporins may not be allergic to aztreonam. However, close monitoring of those who have had an

immediate hypersensitivity reaction to these antibiotics is recommended.
• Obtain urine specimen for culture and sensitivity tests before first dose. Therapy may begin pending results.
• Observe the patient for signs of superinfection.
• Aztreonam's effectiveness against gram-negative organisms is comparable to that of the aminoglycoside antibiotics, without the ototoxicity or nephrotoxicity usually associated with aminoglycosides.
• **I.V. use:** To administer a bolus of aztreonam, inject drug slowly (over 3 to 5 minutes) directly into a vein or I.V. tubing. Give infusions over 20 minutes to 1 hour.
• I.M. injections should be given deep into a large muscle mass, such as the upper outer quadrant of the gluteus maximus or the lateral aspect of the thigh. Doses greater than 1 g should be given I.V.

bacitracin

Pregnancy Risk Category: C

HOW SUPPLIED
Injection: 10,000-unit, 50,000-unit vials

ACTION
Mechanism: Hinders bacterial cell-wall synthesis, damaging the bacterial plasma membrane and making the cell more vulnerable to osmotic pressure.
Peak: Plasma levels peak within 1 hour of an I.M. injection.

INDICATIONS & DOSAGE
Pneumonia or empyema caused by susceptible staphylococci–
Infants over 2.5 kg: 1,000 units/kg I.M. daily, divided q 8 to 12 hours.
Infants under 2.5 kg: 900 units/kg I.M. daily, divided q 8 to 12 hours.

Although the drug is labeled for use in infants only, adults with susceptible staphylococcal infections may receive 10,000 to 25,000 units I.M. q 6 hours (maximum 25,000 units/dose, 100,000 units daily).

ADVERSE REACTIONS
EENT: ototoxicity.
GI: nausea, vomiting, anorexia, diarrhea, rectal itching or burning.
GU: ***nephrotoxicity*** *(albuminuria,* cylindruria, oliguria, anuria, increased BUN, ***tabular and glomerular necrosis****)*.
Hematologic: blood dyscrasia, eosinophilia.
Skin: urticaria, rash.
Other: superinfection, fever, rash, ***anaphylaxis, neuromuscular blockade,*** pain at injection site.

INTERACTIONS
Nephrotoxic drugs (such as aminoglycosides): increased nephrotoxicity. Use together cautiously.
Neuromuscular blockers, inhalational anesthetics: prolonged muscle weakness. Monitor the patient for excessive muscle weakness or respiratory distress.

CONTRAINDICATIONS
• Contraindicated in patients with impaired renal function.
• Use cautiously in those with myasthenia gravis and neuromuscular disease.

NURSING CONSIDERATIONS
• Obtain urine specimen for culture and sensitivity tests before first dose. Therapy may begin pending results.
• For deep injection only; warn the patient that injection may be painful.
• Maintain adequate fluid intake, and monitor urine output closely. If fluid intake or output decreases, notify the doctor.
• Assess baseline renal function studies before starting therapy. Monitor daily during therapy. Notify the doctor of any change.

• Report adverse effects to the doctor immediately.
• Urine pH should be kept above 6.0 to reduce the risk of nephrotoxicity.
• Prolonged therapy may result in overgrowth of nonsusceptible organisms, especially *Candida albicans.*
• Concentration of bacitracin should be between 5,000 and 10,000 units/ml. Store in refrigerator. Drug is inactivated if stored at room temperature.
• May be used with neomycin as a bowel preparation or in a solution as a wound irrigant.

chloramphenicol
Chloromycetin, Novochlorocap†

chloramphenicol palmitate
Chloromycetin Palmitate

chloramphenicol sodium succinate
Chloromycetin Sodium Succinate, Pentamycetin†

Pregnancy Risk Category: C

HOW SUPPLIED
chloramphenicol
Capsules: 250 mg, 500 mg
chloramphenicol palmitate
Oral suspension: 150 mg/5 ml
chloramphenicol sodium succinate
Injection: 1-g, 10-g vials

ACTION
Mechanism: Inhibits bacterial protein synthesis by binding to the 50S subunit of the ribosome; bacteriostatic.
Peak: Serum levels peak immediately after I.V. infusion, or within 1 hour of an oral or I.M. dose. **Duration:** elimination half-life, about 4 hours.

INDICATIONS & DOSAGE
Haemophilus influenzae *meningitis, acute* Salmonella typhi *infection, and meningitis, bacteremia, or other severe infections caused by sensitive* Salmonella *species,* Rickettsia, *lymphogranuloma, psittacosis, or various sensitive gram-negative organisms –*
Adults and children: 50 to 100 mg/kg P.O. or I.V. daily, divided q 6 hours. Maximum dosage is 100 mg/kg daily.
Premature infants and neonates 2 weeks or younger: 25 mg/kg P.O. or I.V. once daily. I.V. route must be used to treat meningitis.

ADVERSE REACTIONS
CNS: headache, mild depression, confusion, delirium, peripheral neuropathy with prolonged therapy.
EENT: optic neuritis (in patients with cystic fibrosis), glossitis, decreased visual acuity.
GI: nausea, vomiting, stomatitis, diarrhea, enterocolitis.
Hematologic: ***aplastic anemia,*** hypoplastic anemia, *granulocytopenia,* thrombocytopenia.
Other: infections from nonsusceptible organisms, hypersensitivity reactions (fever, rash, urticaria, ***anaphylaxis***), jaundice, ***gray syndrome in neonates, (abdominal distention, gray cyanosis, vasomotor collapse, respiratory distress, death within a few hours of onset of symptoms).***

INTERACTIONS
Acetaminophen: elevated chloramphenicol levels. Monitor for chloramphenicol toxicity.
Chlorpropamide, dicumarol, phenobarbital, phenytoin, tolbutamide: Increased blood levels possible. Monitor for toxicity.
Iron supplements, vitamin B_{12}, folic acid: possible delayed response in patients with anemia. Monitor closely.

CONTRAINDICATIONS
• Contraindicated in patients with hypersensitivity to the drug.
• Use cautiously in patients with impaired hepatic or renal function, acute intermittent porphyria, and G6PD de-

ficiency and with other drugs that cause bone marrow suppression or blood disorders. Do *not* use for infections caused by organisms susceptible to other agents or for trivial infections; use *only* when clearly indicated for severe infection.

NURSING CONSIDERATIONS

- Obtain specimen for culture and sensitivity tests before first dose. Therapy may begin pending results.
- Monitor CBC, platelets, serum iron, and reticulocytes before and every 2 days during therapy. Stop drug immediately if anemia, reticulocytopenia, leukopenia, or thrombocytopenia develops.
- Instruct the patient to report adverse reactions to the doctor, especially nausea, vomiting, diarrhea, fever, confusion, sore throat, or mouth sores.
- Tell the patient to take medication for as long as prescribed, exactly as directed, even after he feels better.
- Monitor for evidence of superinfection by nonsusceptible organisms.
- Therapeutic plasma concentrations are 5 to 25 mcg/ml.
- **I.V. use:** Give I.V. slowly over at least 1 minute. Check injection site daily for phlebitis and irritation.
- Reconstitute 1-g vial of powder for injection with 10 ml of sterile water for injection. Concentration will be 100 mg/ml. Stable for 30 days at room temperature, but refrigeration recommended. Do not use cloudy solutions.

clarithromycin

Biaxin Filmtabs

Pregnancy Risk Category: C

HOW SUPPLIED

Tablets: 250 mg, 500 mg

ACTION

Mechanism: Binds to the 50S subunit of bacterial ribosomes, blocking protein synthesis; bacteriostatic or bactericidal, depending on concentration. **Peak:** Serum levels peak within 1 to 4 hours of an oral dose. **Duration:** elimination half-life varies with dose and duration of therapy; range is 4 to 11 hours.

INDICATIONS & DOSAGE

Pharyngitis or tonsillitis caused by Streptococcus pyogenes –
Adults: 250 mg P.O. q 12 hours for 10 days.
Acute maxillary sinusitis caused by S. pneumoniae –
Adults: 500 mg P.O. q 12 hours for 14 days.
Acute exacerbations of chronic bronchitis caused by Moraxella (Branhamella) catarrhalis *or* S. pneumoniae; *pneumonia caused by* S. pneumoniae *or* Mycoplasma pneumoniae –
Adults: 250 mg P.O. q 12 hours for 7 to 14 days.
Acute exacerbations of chronic bronchitis caused by Haemophilus influenzae –
Adults: 500 mg P.O. q 12 hours for 7 to 14 days.
Uncomplicated skin and skin-structure infections caused by Staphylococcus aureus *or* Streptococcus pyogenes –
Adults: 250 mg P.O. q 12 hours for 7 to 14 days.
AIDS and Mycobacterium-avium-intracellulare *infection*
Adults: 500 mg to 2 g P.O. daily as part of regimen, including at least two antitubercular drugs.

ADVERSE REACTIONS

CNS: headache.
GI: *diarrhea, nausea, abnormal taste,* dyspepsia, abdominal pain or discomfort.

INTERACTIONS

Carbamazepine: may increase serum levels of carbamazepine. Monitor blood levels.

*Liquid form contains alcohol.
**May contain tartrazine.

Common reactions are in italics; ***life-threatening,*** in bold italics.

Theophylline: increased plasma theophylline levels possible with other macrolides; effect of clarithromycin is unknown. Monitor theophylline levels carefully.
Warfarin: increased PT possible with other macrolides; effect of clarithromycin is unknown. Monitor PT carefully.

CONTRAINDICATIONS
- Contraindicated in patients with hypersensitivity to erythromycin or other macrolides.
- Use cautiously in patients with hepatic or renal impairment.

NURSING CONSIDERATIONS
- Obtain urine specimen for culture and sensitivity tests before first dose. Therapy may begin pending results.
- Drug may be taken without regard to meals.
- May cause overgrowth of nonsusceptible bacteria or fungi. Monitor the patient for superinfection.
- Tell the patient to take all of the medication as prescribed, even after he feels better.

---

clindamycin hydrochloride
Cleocin HCl, Dalacin C†‡

clindamycin palmitate hydrochloride
Cleocin Pediatric, Dalacin C Palmitate†‡

clindamycin phosphate
Cleocin Phosphate, Dalacin C†‡, Dalacin C Phosphate

Pregnancy Risk Category: B

HOW SUPPLIED
hydrochloride
Capsules: 75 mg, 150 mg, 300 mg
palmitate hydrochloride
Oral solution: 75 mg/5 ml
phosphate
Injection: 150 mg/ml

ACTION
Mechanism: Inhibits bacterial protein synthesis by binding to the 50S subunit of the ribosome.
Peak: Serum levels peak immediately after I.V. infusion, 3 hours after an I.M. injection, or within 45 minutes to 1 hour of an oral dose. **Duration:** elimination half-life, 2½ to 3 hours.

INDICATIONS & DOSAGE
Infections caused by sensitive staphylococci, streptococci, pneumococci, Bacteroides, Fusobacterium, Clostridium perfringens, *and other sensitive aerobic and anaerobic organisms –*
Adults: 150 to 450 mg P.O. q 6 hours; or 300 mg I.M. or I.V. q 6, 8, or 12 hours. Up to 2,700 mg I.M. or I.V. daily, in divided doses q 6, 8, or 12 hours.

May be used for severe infections.
Children over 1 month: 8 to 20 mg/kg P.O. daily, in divided doses q 6 to 8 hours; or 15 to 40 mg/kg I.M. or I.V. daily, in divided doses q 6 hours.
Endocarditis prophylaxis for dental procedures in patients allergic to penicillin –
Adults: initially, 300 mg P.O. 1 hour before procedure; then 150 mg 6 hours later.
Children: initially, 10 mg/kg P.O. 1 hour before procedure; then half the initial dose 6 hours later.

ADVERSE REACTIONS
GI: *nausea,* vomiting, abdominal pain, *diarrhea,* pseudomembranous colitis, esophagitis, flatulence, anorexia, *bloody or tarry stools, dysphagia.*
Hematologic: transient leukopenia, eosinophilia, thrombocytopenia.
Skin: maculopapular rash, urticaria.
Other: unpleasant or bitter taste; ***anaphylaxis;*** elevated alkaline phosphatase, AST, bilirubin; *pain,* induration, *sterile abscess with I.M. injec-*

tion; thrombophlebitis, erythema, and pain after I.V. administration.

INTERACTIONS
Erythromycin: may block access of clindamycin to its site of action. Don't use together.
Kaolin: decreased absorption of oral clindamycin. Separate administration times.
Neuromuscular blockers: potentiated neuromuscular blockade possible. Monitor closely.

CONTRAINDICATIONS
- Contraindicated in patients with hypersensitivity to the antibiotic congener lincomycin and in patients with history of GI disease, especially colitis.
- Use cautiously in neonates and patients with renal or hepatic disease, asthma, or significant allergies.
- Don't use in patients with meningitis. Drug does not penetrate blood-brain barrier.

NURSING CONSIDERATIONS
- Obtain urine specimen for culture and sensitivity tests before first dose. Therapy may begin pending results.
- Instruct the patient to report adverse reactions, especially diarrhea, to the doctor. Warn the patient not to treat such diarrhea himself.
- Don't give opioid antidiarrheals to treat drug-induced diarrhea. May prolong and worsen diarrhea.
- Advise the patient taking the capsule form to take with a full glass of water to prevent dysphagia.
- Observe the patient for signs of superinfection.
- Monitor renal, hepatic, and hematopoietic functions during prolonged therapy.
- Don't refrigerate reconstituted oral solution, because it will thicken. Drug is stable for 2 weeks at room temperature.
- **I.V. use:** When giving I.V., check site daily for phlebitis and irritation. For I.V. infusion, dilute each 300 mg in 50 ml solution, and give no faster than 30 mg/minute (over 10 to 60 minutes). Never give undiluted as a bolus.
- For I.M. administration, inject deeply. Rotate sites. Warn the patient that I.M. injection may be painful. Doses greater than 600 mg per injection are not recommended.
- I.M. injection may raise creatine kinase in response to muscle irritation.

---

erythromycin base
Apo-Erythro†, EMU-V‡, E-Mycin, Erybid†, ERYC, ERYC-125†, ERYC-250†, Ery-Tab, Erythromid†, Novorythro†, PCE Disperstab, Robimycin

erythromycin estolate
Erythrozone, Ilosone, Novorythro†

erythromycin ethylsuccinate
Apo-Erythro-ES†, E.E.S., EES-400‡, EEG Dulcets‡, EES granules‡, EryPed, Erythro, Erythrocin

erythromycin gluceptate
Ilotycin

erythromycin lactobionate
Erythrocin

erythromycin stearate
Apo-Erythro-S†, Erythrocin, Erythrocot, My-E, Novorythro†, Wintrocin, Wyamycin S

Pregnancy Risk Category: B

HOW SUPPLIED
base
Tablets (enteric-coated): 250 mg, 333 mg, 500 mg
Capsules (enteric-coated pellets): 250 mg

*Liquid form contains alcohol.
**May contain tartrazine.

Common reactions are in italics; ***life-threatening,*** in bold italics.

estolate
Tablets: 500 mg
Capsules: 250 mg
Oral suspension: 125 mg/5 ml, 250 mg/5 ml
ethylsuccinate
Tablets: 400 mg
Tablets (chewable): 200 mg
Oral suspension: 200 mg/5 ml, 400 mg/5 ml, 100 mg/2.5 ml
gluceptate
Injection: 1-g vials
lactobionate
Injection: 500-mg, 1-g vials
stearate
Tablets (film-coated): 250 mg, 500 mg

ACTION
Mechanism: Inhibits bacterial protein synthesis by binding to the 50S subunit of the ribosome.
Peak: Peak serum levels occur 1 to 4 hours after an oral dose or immediately after I.V. infusion. **Duration:** plasma half-life, about 1½ hours.

INDICATIONS & DOSAGE
Acute pelvic inflammatory disease caused by Neisseria gonorrhoeae –
Adults: 500 mg I.V. (erythromycin gluceptate, lactobionate) q 6 hours for 3 days, then 250 mg (erythromycin base, estolate, stearate) or 400 mg (erythromycin ethylsuccinate) P.O. q 6 hours for 7 days.
Endocarditis prophylaxis for dental procedures in patients allergic to penicillin –
Adults: initially, 800 mg (ethylsuccinate) or 1 g (stearate) P.O. 2 hours before procedure; then 400 mg (ethylsuccinate) or 500 mg (stearate) P.O. 6 hours later.
Children: initially, 20 mg/kg (ethylsuccinate or stearate) P.O. 2 hours before procedure; then give half the initial dose 6 hours later.
Intestinal amebiasis –
Adults: 250 mg (base, estolate, stearate) or 400 mg (ethylsuccinate) P.O. q 6 hours for 10 to 14 days.
Children: 30 to 50 mg/kg (base, estolate, ethylsuccinate, stearate) P.O. daily, in divided doses q 6 hours for 10 to 14 days.
Mild to moderately severe respiratory tract, skin, and soft-tissue infections caused by sensitive group A beta-hemolytic streptococci, Diplococcus pneumoniae, Mycoplasma pneumoniae, Corynebacterium diphtheriae, Bordetella pertussis, Listeria monocytogenes –
Adults: 250 to 500 mg (erythromycin base, estolate, stearate) P.O. q 6 hours; or 400 to 800 mg (erythromycin ethylsuccinate) P.O. q 6 hours; or 15 to 20 mg/kg I.V. daily, as continuous infusion or in divided doses q 6 hours.
Children: 30 mg/kg to 50 mg/kg (oral erythromycin salts) P.O. daily, in divided doses q 6 hours; or 15 to 20 mg/kg I.V. daily, in divided doses q 4 to 6 hours.
Syphilis –
Adults: 500 mg (erythromycin base, estolate, stearate) P.O. q.i.d. for 15 days.
Legionnaire's disease –
Adults: 500 mg to 1 g I.V. or P.O. (base, estolate, stearate) or 800 to 1,600 mg (ethylsuccinate) q 6 hours for 21 days.
Uncomplicated urethral, endocervical, or rectal infections when tetracyclines are contraindicated –
Adults: 500 mg (base, estolate, stearate) or 800 mg (ethylsuccinate) P.O. q.i.d. for at least 7 days.
Urogenital Chlamydia trachomatis *infections during pregnancy –*
Adults: 500 mg (base, estolate, stearate) P.O. q.i.d. for at least 7 days or 250 mg (base, estolate, stearate) or 400 mg (ethylsuccinate) P.O. q.i.d. for at least 14 days.
Conjunctivitis caused by Chlamydia trachomatis *in neonates –*
Neonates: 50 mg/kg P.O. daily in four divided doses for at least 2 weeks.

Pneumonia of infancy caused by Chlamydia trachomatis –
Infants: 50 mg/kg/day in four divided doses for at least 3 weeks.

ADVERSE REACTIONS

EENT: hearing loss with high I.V. doses.
GI: *abdominal pain and cramping, nausea, vomiting, diarrhea.*
Hepatic: cholestatic jaundice (with erythromycin estolate).
Skin: urticaria, rashes.
Other: overgrowth of nonsusceptible bacteria or fungi; ***anaphylaxis;*** fever; *venous irritation, thrombophlebitis following I.V. injection.*

INTERACTIONS

Astemizole, terfenadine: decreased metabolism, leading to increased levels of these antihistamines and cardiotoxicity. Avoid concomitant use.
Carbamazepine: increased carbamazepine blood levels and increased risk of toxicity. Monitor closely.
Clindamycin, lincomycin: may be antagonistic. Don't use together.
Oral anticoagulants: increased anticoagulant effects. Monitor PT closely.
Theophylline: decreased erythromycin blood level and increased theophylline toxicity. Use together cautiously.

CONTRAINDICATIONS

- Contraindicated in patients with hypersensitivity to the drug or other macrolides. Erythromycin estolate is contraindicated in patients with hepatic disease. Use other erythromycin salts cautiously in patients with impaired hepatic function.

NURSING CONSIDERATIONS

- Obtain urine specimen for culture and sensitivity tests before first dose. Therapy may begin pending results.
- For best absorption, instruct the patient to take oral form of drug with full glass of water 1 hour before or 2 hours after meals. Coated tablets may be taken with meals. Tell the patient not to drink fruit juice with drug. Chewable erythromycin tablets should not be swallowed whole.
- Coated tablets or encapsulated pellets have caused fewer instances of GI upset; they may be more tolerable in patients who cannot tolerate erythromycin.
- When administering suspension, be sure to note the concentration.
- May cause overgrowth of nonsusceptible bacteria or fungi. Monitor the patient for signs and symptoms of superinfection.
- Tell the patient to take entire amount of drug exactly as prescribed, even after he feels better.
- Treat streptococcal infections for 10 days.
- Report adverse reactions, especially nausea, abdominal pain, and fever.
- Erythromycin estolate may cause serious hepatotoxicity in adults (reversible cholestatic jaundice). Monitor hepatic function (increased serum levels of alkaline phosphatase, ALT, AST, and bilirubin may occur). Other erythromycin salts cause hepatotoxicity to a lesser degree. The patient who develops hepatotoxicity from estolate may react similarly to treatment with any erythromycin preparation.
- **I.V. use:** Reconstitute according to manufacturer's directions and dilute each 250 mg in at least 100 ml of 0.9% sodium chloride solution. Infuse over 1 hour.
- Do not administer erythromycin lactobionate with other drugs.

imipenem/cilastatin sodium

Primaxin

Pregnancy Risk Category: C

HOW SUPPLIED

Injection: 250-mg, 500-mg, 750-mg vials

ACTION

Mechanism: Imipenem is bactericidal and inhibits bacterial cell-wall synthesis. Cilastatin inhibits the enzymatic breakdown of imipenem in the kidneys, making it effective in the urinary tract.
Peak: Serum levels peak immediately after I.V. infusion. **Duration:** elimination half-life, 50 to 80 minutes.

INDICATIONS & DOSAGE

Serious infections of the lower respiratory and urinary tracts, intra-abdominal and gynecologic infections, bacterial septicemia, bone and joint infections, skin and soft-tissue infections, and endocarditis. Most known microorganisms are susceptible: Staphylococcus, Streptococcus, Escherichia coli, Klebsiella, Proteus, Enterobacter, Pseudomonas aeruginosa, *and* Bacteroides, *including* B. fragilis—
Adults: 250 mg to 1 g by I.V. infusion q 6 to 8 hours. Maximum daily dosage is 50 mg/kg/day or 4 g/day, whichever is less.

ADVERSE REACTIONS

CNS: ***seizures,*** dizziness.
CV: hypotension.
GI: nausea, vomiting, diarrhea, *pseudomembranous colitis.*
Skin: rash, urticaria, pruritus.
Other: ***hypersensitivity reactions (anaphylaxis);*** *thrombophlebitis, pain at injection site.*

INTERACTIONS

Ganciclovir: may cause seizures. Avoid concomitant use.

CONTRAINDICATIONS

- Contraindicated in patients with hypersensitivity to the drug.
- Use cautiously in patients allergic to penicillins or cephalosporins because this drug has similar properties.
- Also use cautiously in patients who have a history of seizure disorders, especially if they also have compromised renal function. If seizures develop and persist, despite anticonvulsant therapy, notify the doctor. The drug should then be discontinued.
- Patients with impaired renal function may need a lower dose or longer intervals between doses.

NURSING CONSIDERATIONS

- Imipenem/cilastatin has the broadest antibacterial spectrum of any available antibiotic. The drug is most valuable for empiric treatment of infections and for mixed infections that would otherwise require a combination of antibiotics, typically including an aminoglycoside.
- Obtain urine specimen for culture and sensitivity tests before first dose. Therapy may begin pending results.
- Monitor patients for bacterial or fungal superinfections and resistant infections during and after therapy.
- **I.V. use:** Don't administer by direct I.V. bolus injection. Each 250- or 500-mg dose should be given by I.V. infusion over 20 to 30 minutes. Each 1-g dose should be infused over 40 to 60 minutes. If nausea occurs, the infusion may be slowed.
- When reconstituting powder, shake until the solution is clear. Solutions may range from colorless to yellow, and variations of color within this range do not affect the drug's potency. After reconstitution, solution is stable for 10 hours at room temperature and for 48 hours when refrigerated.

lincomycin hydrochloride

Lincocin

Pregnancy Risk Category: B

HOW SUPPLIED

Capsules: 500 mg
Pediatric capsules: 250 mg
Injection: 300 mg/ml in 2-ml and 10-ml vials and 2-ml U-Ject

ACTION

Mechanism: Inhibits bacterial protein synthesis by binding to the 50S subunit of the ribosome.
Peak: Peak levels occur immediately after I.V. infusion, 30 minutes after an I.M. injection, or less than 2 hours after an oral dose. **Duration:** plasma half-life, 4 to 6 hours.

INDICATIONS & DOSAGE

Respiratory tract, skin and soft-tissue, and urinary tract infections; osteomyelitis, septicemia caused by sensitive group A beta-hemolytic streptococci, pneumococci, and staphylococci –
Adults: 500 mg P.O. q 6 to 8 hours (not to exceed 8 g daily); or 600 mg I.M. daily or q 12 hours; or 600 mg to 1 g I.V. q 8 to 12 hours (not to exceed 8 g daily).
Children over 1 month: 30 to 60 mg/kg P.O. daily, in divided doses q 6 to 8 hours; or 10 mg/kg I.M. daily or in divided doses q 12 hours; or 10 to 20 mg/kg I.V. daily, in divided doses q 6 to 8 hours.

ADVERSE REACTIONS

CNS: dizziness, headache.
CV: hypotension with rapid I.V. infusion.
EENT: glossitis, tinnitus.
GI: nausea, vomiting, *pseudomembranous colitis, persistent diarrhea,* abdominal cramps, stomatitis, pruritus ani.
GU: vaginitis.
Hematologic: *neutropenia, leukopenia,* thrombocytopenia, purpura.
Skin: rashes, urticaria.
Other: hypersensitivity reactions ***(anaphylaxis),*** angioedema, cholestatic jaundice, pain at injection site.

INTERACTIONS

Antidiarrheals (such as kaolin, pectin, and attapulgite): reduced oral absorption of lincomycin by as much as 90%. Antidiarrheals should be avoided or given at least 2 hours before lincomycin.
Neuromuscular blockers: may potentiate neuromuscular blockade. Monitor for prolonged weakness.

CONTRAINDICATIONS

- Contraindicated in patients with hypersensitivity to clindamycin.
- Use cautiously in patients with GI disorders (especially colitis), asthma or significant allergies, hepatic or renal disease, and endocrine or metabolic disorders.

NURSING CONSIDERATIONS

- Obtain specimen for culture and sensitivity tests before first dose. Therapy may begin pending results.
- For best absorption, instruct the patient to take drug with a full glass of water 1 hour before or 2 hours after meals.
- Advise the patient to take drug exactly as directed, even after he feels better, and to take entire amount prescribed.
- Tell the patient to report adverse reactions to the doctor, especially diarrhea. Warn him not to treat diarrhea himself because it may reflect the onset of antibiotic-associated pseudomembranous colitis.
- Monitor for signs of bacterial and fungal superinfection, especially when therapy exceeds 10 days.
- Monitor hepatic function (increased levels of alkaline phosphatase, ALT, AST, or bilirubin may occur).
- Monitor CBC and platelets. Stop drug immediately if neutropenia, leukopenia, or other blood disorders develop.
- **I.V. use:** When giving I.V., check site daily for phlebitis and irritation and rotate infusion sites regularly.
- For I.V. infusion, dilute to 100 ml; infuse over 1 hour. Rapid I.V. infusion may cause hypotension and syncope. Monitor blood pressure in the patient receiving the drug parenterally.

• For I.M. administration, inject deeply. Rotate injection sites. Warn patients that I.M. injection may be painful.

methenamine hippurate
Hiprex**, Hip-Rex†, Urex

methenamine mandelate
Mandameth, Mandelamine, Sterine†
Pregnancy Risk Category: C

HOW SUPPLIED
hippurate
Tablets: 1 g
mandelate
Tablets: 500 mg, 1 g
Tablets (enteric-coated): 250 mg, 500 mg, 1 g
Tablets (film-coated): 500 mg, 1 g

ACTION
Mechanism: Hydrolyzed to ammonia and to formaldehyde, causing antibacterial action against gram-positive and gram-negative organisms. Mandelic and hippuric acids, with which methenamines are combined, are also antibacterial by unknown mechanisms.
Peak: Plasma levels peak within 1 hour of administration. Urine levels of formaldehyde peak within 2 hours of administration of a film-coated tablet, or 3 to 8 hours after an enteric-coated tablet. **Duration:** up to 90% of a dose excreted within 24 hours.

INDICATIONS & DOSAGE
Long-term prophylaxis or suppression of chronic urinary tract infections –
Adults and children over age 12: 1 g (hippurate) P.O. q 12 hours.
Children age 6 to 12: 500 mg to 1 g (hippurate) P.O. q 12 hours.
Urinary tract infections, infected residual urine in patients with neurogenic bladder –
Adults: 1 g (mandelate) P.O. q.i.d. after meals.
Children age 6 to 12: 500 mg (mandelate) P.O. q.i.d. after meals.
Children under age 6: 50 mg/kg (mandelate) P.O. divided in four doses after meals.

ADVERSE REACTIONS
GI: nausea, vomiting, diarrhea.
GU: with high doses, urinary tract irritation, dysuria, frequency, albuminuria, hematuria.
Skin: rashes.
Other: elevated liver enzymes.

INTERACTIONS
Acetazolamide: antagonized methenamine effect. Use together cautiously.
Urine alkalinizing agents: inhibited methenamine action. Don't use together.

CONTRAINDICATIONS
• Contraindicated in patients with renal insufficiency, severe hepatic disease, or severe dehydration.
• Oral suspension contains vegetable oil. Administer cautiously to elderly or debilitated patients, because aspiration could cause lipid pneumonia.

NURSING CONSIDERATIONS
• Obtain a clean-catch urine specimen for culture and sensitivity tests before starting therapy, and repeat as needed. Therapy may begin pending results.
• Ineffective against *Candida* infection.
• Monitor fluid intake and output. Intake should be at least 1,500 to 2,000 ml daily.
• Limit intake of alkaline foods, such as vegetables, milk, and peanuts. Patients may drink cranberry, plum, and prune juices. These juices or ascorbic acid may be used to acidify urine.
• Warn the patient not to take antacids, including Alka-Seltzer and sodium bicarbonate.

• For best results, maintain urine pH at 5.5 or below. Use Nitrazine paper to check pH. Large doses of ascorbic acid (12 g/day) may be necessary to effectively acidify urine.
• *Proteus* and *Pseudomonas* tend to raise urine pH; urine acidifiers are usually necessary when treating these infections.
• Monitor liver function studies periodically during long-term therapy.
• Administer after meals to minimize GI upset.
• If rash appears, withhold dose and contact the doctor.

methylene blue

Urolene Blue

Pregnancy Risk Category: C (D if injected intra-amniotically)

HOW SUPPLIED

Tablets: 55 mg, 65 mg
Injection: 10 mg/ml

ACTION

Mechanism: Converts ferrous iron of reduced hemoglobin to ferric iron to form methemoglobin, an antidote in cyanide poisoning.
Peak: Levels peak immediately after I.V. infusion; oral absorption is rapid.

INDICATIONS & DOSAGE

Cystitis, urethritis–
Adults: 55 to 130 mg P.O. b.i.d. or t.i.d. after meals with glass of water.
Methemoglobinemia and cyanide poisoning–
Adults and children: 1 to 2 mg/kg of 1% sterile solution by slow infusion.

ADVERSE REACTIONS

GI: nausea, vomiting, diarrhea, blue-green stool.
GU: dysuria, bladder irritation, blue-green urine.
Hematologic: anemia (long-term use).
Other: fever (large doses).

INTERACTIONS

None significant.

CONTRAINDICATIONS

• Contraindicated in patients with renal insufficiency.

NURSING CONSIDERATIONS

• Monitor fluid intake and output carefully. Intake should be at least 2,000 ml daily.
• Monitor hemoglobin; anemia possible from accelerated destruction of erythrocytes.
• Turns urine and stool blue-green.
• Seldom used as urinary tract antiseptic.
• **I.V. use:** Use caution when handling injectable form, because the liquid can stain the skin. Avoid extravasation.
• I.V. form has been used to treat nitrite intoxication.
• S.C. injection can cause necrotic abscess formation.

nitrofurantoin macrocrystals

Macrodantin

nitrofurantoin microcrystals

Apo-Nitrofurantoin†, Furadantin, Furan, Furanite, Macrodantin, Nephronex†, Nitrofan, Novofuran†

Pregnancy Risk Category: B

HOW SUPPLIED

macrocrystals
Capsules: 25 mg, 50 mg, 100 mg
microcrystals
Tablets: 50 mg, 100 mg
Capsules: 50 mg, 100 mg
Oral suspension: 25 mg/5 ml

ACTION

Mechanism: Interferes with bacterial enzyme systems and possibly with bacterial cell-wall formation.
Peak: Plasma levels peak within 1 to

*Liquid form contains alcohol.
**May contain tartrazine.

Common reactions are in italics; ***life-threatening***, in bold italics.

4 hours of administration. **Duration:** elimination half-life, about 20 minutes.

INDICATIONS & DOSAGE

Urinary tract infections caused by susceptible Escherichia coli, Staphylococcus aureus, *enterococci; certain strains of* Klebsiella, Proteus, *and* Enterobacter –

Adults and children over age 12: 50 to 100 mg P.O. q.i.d. with milk or meals.

Children 1 month to age 12: 5 to 7 mg/kg P.O. daily, divided q.i.d.

Long-term suppression therapy –

Adults: 50 to 100 mg P.O. daily h.s.

Children: 1 to 2 mg/kg P.O. daily h.s.

ADVERSE REACTIONS

CNS: peripheral neuropathy, headache, dizziness, drowsiness, *ascending polyneuropathy with high doses or renal impairment.*

GI: *anorexia, nausea, vomiting,* abdominal pain, *diarrhea.*

Hematologic: ***hemolysis in patients with G6PD deficiency*** (reversed after stopping drug), ***agranulocytosis,*** thrombocytopenia.

Skin: maculopapular, erythematous, or eczematous eruption; pruritus; urticaria; ***exfoliative dermatitis; Stevens-Johnson syndrome***, hepatitis.

Other: ***asthmatic attacks in patients with history of asthma;*** hypersensitivity reactions ***(anaphylaxis);*** transient alopecia; drug fever; overgrowth of nonsusceptible organisms in the urinary tract; pulmonary sensitivity reactions (cough, chest pains, fever, chills, dyspnea).

INTERACTIONS

Magnesium-containing antacids: decreased nitrofurantoin absorption. Separate administration times by 1 hour.

Nalidixic acid, norfloxacin: possible decreased effectiveness. Avoid using together.

Probenecid, sulfinpyrazone: increased blood levels and decreased urine levels. May result in increased toxicity and lack of therapeutic effect. Don't use together.

CONTRAINDICATIONS

- Contraindicated in children 1 month and under and in patients with moderate to severe renal impairment, anuria, oliguria, or creatinine clearance under 40 ml/minute.
- Use cautiously in patients with G6PD deficiency.

NURSING CONSIDERATIONS

- Obtain urine specimen for culture and sensitivity tests before starting therapy and repeat p.r.n. Therapy may begin pending results.
- Hypersensitivity may develop when used for long-term therapy.
- Monitor CBC regularly.
- Give with food or milk to minimize GI distress.
- Some patients may experience fewer GI adverse effects with nitrofurantoin macrocrystals.
- Monitor fluid intake and output carefully. May turn urine brown or darker.
- Store drug in amber container. Keep away from metals other than stainless steel or aluminum to avoid precipitate formation. Warn patients not to use containers made of these materials.
- Continue treatment for 3 days after sterile urine specimens have been obtained.
- Monitor pulmonary status.
- Has no effect in blood or tissue outside the urinary tract.
- Monitor the patient for signs of superinfection. Use of nitrofurantoin may result in growth of nonsusceptible organisms, especially *Pseudomonas.*
- May cause false-positive results with urine sugar test using copper sul-

fate reduction method (Clinitest) but not with glucose oxidase tests (Tes-Tape, Diastix, Clinistix).

• Dual-release capsules (25 mg nitrofurantoin macrocrystals combined with 75 mg nitrofurantoin monohydrate) enable patients to take drug only twice daily.

polymyxin B sulfate

Aerosporin

Pregnancy Risk Category: B

HOW SUPPLIED

Powder for injection: 500,000-unit vials

ACTION

Mechanism: Hinders bacterial cell-wall synthesis, damaging the bacterial plasma membrane and making the cell more vulnerable to osmotic pressure (bactericidal).

Peak: Peak serum levels occur immediately after I.V. infusion, or within 2 hours of an I.M. injection. **Duration:** plasma half-life, 4 to 6 hours.

INDICATIONS & DOSAGE

Acute urinary tract infections or septicemia caused by sensitive Pseudomonas aeruginosa, *or when other antibiotics are ineffective or contraindicated; bacteremia caused by sensitive* Enterobacter aerogenes *and* Klebsiella pneumoniae, *or acute urinary tract infections caused by* Escherichia coli –

Adults and children: 15,000 to 25,000 units/kg daily I.V. infusion, in divided doses q 12 hours; or 25,000 to 30,000 units/kg daily, in divided doses q 4 to 8 hours.

Meningitis caused by sensitive P. aeruginosa *or* Haemophilus influenzae *when other antibiotics ineffective or contraindicated* –

Adults and children age 2: 50,000 units intrathecally once daily for 3 to 4 days, then 50,000 units every other day for at least 2 weeks after cerebrospinal fluid tests are negative and cerebrospinal fluid sugar is normal.

Children under age 2: 20,000 units intrathecally once daily for 3 to 4 days, then 25,000 units every other day for at least 2 weeks after cerebrospinal fluid tests are negative and cerebrospinal fluid sugar is normal.

ADVERSE REACTIONS

CNS: irritability, drowsiness, facial flushing, weakness, ataxia, respiratory paralysis, headache and meningeal irritation with intrathecal administration, peripheral and perioral paresthesias, ***seizures, coma.***

EENT: blurred vision.

GU: *nephrotoxicity* (albuminuria, cylindruria, hematuria, proteinuria, decreased urine output, increased BUN level).

Skin: urticaria.

Other: hypersensitivity reactions (fever, ***anaphylaxis***), pain at I.M. injection site.

INTERACTIONS

• *Aminoglycosides, amphotericin B, cisplatin, vancomycin, zidovudine:* increased risk of nephrotoxicity. Avoid concomitant use.

• *Neuromuscular blockers:* may potentiate neuromuscular blockade. Monitor closely.

CONTRAINDICATIONS

• Contraindicated in patients with hypersensitivity to the drug.

• Use cautiously in those with impaired renal function or myasthenia gravis.

NURSING CONSIDERATIONS

• Give only to a hospitalized patient under constant supervision.

• Obtain urine specimen for culture and sensitivity tests before first dose. Therapy may begin pending results.

• Notify the doctor immediately if the patient develops fever, CNS adverse

effects, rash, or symptoms of nephrotoxicity.
• Monitor renal function (BUN, serum creatinine, creatinine clearance, urine output) before and during therapy. Fluid intake should be sufficient to maintain output at 1,500 ml/day (between 3,000 and 4,000 ml/day for adults).
• For meningitis, give intrathecally to achieve adequate cerebrospinal fluid levels.
• Don't give solution containing local anesthetics I.V. or intrathecally.
• If the patient is scheduled for surgery, notify anesthesiologist of preoperative treatment with this drug because it may prolong neuromuscular blockade.
• **I.V. use:** When giving I.V., check site daily for phlebitis and irritation. Dilute each 500,000 units in 300 to 500 ml of D_5W; infuse over 60 to 90 minutes. Rotate I.V. sites regularly.
• Avoid administering by I.M. injection because of severe local pain. If I.M. route must be used, give deeply.
• Parenteral solutions should be refrigerated and used within 72 hours.

rifabutin
Mycobutin
Pregnancy Risk Category: B

HOW SUPPLIED
Capsules: 150 mg

ACTION
Mechanism: Inhibits DNA-dependent RNA polymerase in susceptible bacteria, blocking bacterial protein synthesis.
Peak: Plasma levels peak 2 to 4 hours after an oral dose. **Duration:** plasma half-life, about 2 days.

INDICATIONS & DOSAGE
Prevention of disseminated Mycobacterium avium *complex (MAC) in patients with advanced HIV infection* –
Adults: 300 mg P.O. daily as a single dose or divided b.i.d.

ADVERSE REACTIONS
EENT: uveitis.
GI: dyspepsia, eructation, flatulence, nausea, vomiting, abdominal pain.
GU: *discolored urine.*
Hematologic: neutropenia, leukopenia, thrombocytopenia, eosinophilia.
Skin: *rash.*
Other: fever, myalgia, myositis, taste perversion.

INTERACTIONS
Oral contraceptives: decreased effectiveness. Instruct patient to use nonhormonal forms of birth control.
Zidovudine, drugs metabolized by the liver: decreased serum levels of zidovudine. Because rifabutin, like rifampin, induces liver enzymes, it may lower serum levels of many other drugs as well. Although dosage adjustments may be necessary, further study is needed.

CONTRAINDICATIONS
• Contraindicated in patients with hypersensitivity to the drug or other rifamycin derivatives (such as rifampin). Also contraindicated in patients with active tuberculosis because single-agent therapy with rifabutin increases the risk of inducing bacterial resistance to both rifabutin and rifampin.
• Use cautiously in patients with preexisting neutropenia and thrombocytopenia. Perform baseline hematologic studies and repeat periodically.

NURSING CONSIDERATIONS
• Although safety and effectiveness in children have not been fully established, several studies have indicated the maximum daily dose to be 5 mg/kg.
• High-fat meals slow the rate, but not the extent of absorption.

- Mix with soft foods, such as applesauce, for patients who have difficulty swallowing.
- No evidence exists that drug will provide effective prophylaxis against *M. tuberculosis.* Patients requiring prophylaxis against both *M. tuberculosis* and MAC may require rifampin and rifabutin.
- Drug may rarely cause uveitis; tell the patient to report photophobia, excessive lacrimation, or eye pain immediately.
- Be sure the patient understands that drug or its metabolites may discolor urine, feces, sputum, saliva, tears, and skin brownish orange. Tell him to avoid wearing soft contact lenses because they may be permanently stained.

spectinomycin dihydrochloride

Trobicin

Pregnancy Risk Category: B

HOW SUPPLIED

Injection: 2-g vial with 3.2-ml diluent; 4-g vial with 6.2-ml diluent
Powder for injection: 2 g, 4 g

ACTION

Mechanism: Inhibits protein synthesis by binding to the 30S subunit of the ribosome.
Peak: Serum levels peak 1 to 2 hours after I.M. injection. **Duration:** plasma half-life, 1 to 3 hours.

INDICATIONS & DOSAGE

Gonorrhea –
Adults: 2 to 4 g I.M. single dose injected deeply into the upper outer quadrant of the buttock.

ADVERSE REACTIONS

CNS: insomnia, dizziness.
GI: nausea.
GU: decreased urine output.
Skin: urticaria.
Other: fever, chills (may mask or delay symptoms of incubating syphilis); pain at injection site.

INTERACTIONS

None significant.

CONTRAINDICATIONS

- Contraindicated in patients with hypersensitivity to the drug.

NURSING CONSIDERATIONS

- Not effective in the treatment of syphilis. Serologic test for syphilis should be done before treatment dose and 3 months afterward.
- Should be reserved for penicillin-resistant strains of gonorrhea.
- Use 20G needle to administer drug. The 4-g dose (10 ml) should be divided into two 5-ml injections – one in each buttock.
- Shake vial vigorously after reconstitution and before withdrawing dose. Store at room temperature after reconstitution and use within 24 hours.

trimethoprim

Alprin‡, Proloprim, Trimpex, Triprim‡

Pregnancy Risk Category: C

HOW SUPPLIED

Tablets: 100 mg, 200 mg

ACTION

Mechanism: Interferes with the action of dihydrofolate reductase, inhibiting bacterial synthesis of folic acid.
Peak: Plasma levels peak 1 to 4 hours after oral dose. **Duration:** plasma half-life, 8 to 11 hours.

INDICATIONS & DOSAGE

Uncomplicated urinary tract infections caused by susceptible strains of Escherichia coli, Proteus mirabilis, Klebsiella, *and* Enterobacter –
Adults: 200 mg P.O. daily as a single

dose or in divided doses q 12 hours for 10 days.

Not recommended for children under age 12.

ADVERSE REACTIONS

GI: *epigastric distress, nausea, vomiting,* glossitis.
Hematologic: thrombocytopenia, leukopenia, megaloblastic anemia, methemoglobinemia.
Skin: *rash, pruritus,* ***exfoliative dermatitis.***
Other: fever.

INTERACTIONS

Phenytoin: may decrease phenytoin metabolism and increase its serum levels. Monitor for toxicity.

CONTRAINDICATIONS

- Contraindicated in documented megaloblastic anemia caused by folate deficiency.
- Use cautiously in patients with impaired hepatic function. Dosage should be decreased in patients with severely impaired renal function.

NURSING CONSIDERATIONS

- Obtain urine specimen for culture and sensitivity tests before first dose. Therapy may begin pending results.
- Instruct the patient to take entire amount of the drug, as prescribed, even if he feels better.
- Because resistance to trimethoprim develops rapidly when administered alone, it is usually given in combination with other drugs.
- Clinical signs such as sore throat, fever, pallor, or purpura may be early indications of serious blood disorders. CBCs should be done routinely. Prolonged use of trimethoprim at high doses may cause bone marrow suppression.

vancomycin hydrochloride

Vancocin, Vancoled

Pregnancy Risk Category: C

HOW SUPPLIED

Powder for oral solution: 1-g, 10-g bottles
Powder for injection: 500-mg, 1-g vials

ACTION

Mechanism: Hinders bacterial cell-wall synthesis, damaging the bacterial plasma membrane and making the cell more vulnerable to osmotic pressure.
Peak: Serum levels peak within 2 hours of I.V. infusion; drug not well absorbed orally. **Duration:** plasma half-life, about 6 hours.

INDICATIONS & DOSAGE

Severe staphylococcal infections when other antibiotics are ineffective or contraindicated –
Adults: 500 mg I.V. q 6 hours, or 1 g q 12 hours.
Children: 40 mg/kg I.V. daily, in divided doses q 6 hours.
Neonates: 10 mg/kg I.V. daily, in divided doses q 6 to 12 hours.
Antibiotic-associated pseudomembranous and staphylococcal enterocolitis –
Adults: 125 to 500 mg P.O. q 6 hours for 7 to 10 days.
Children: 40 mg/kg P.O. daily, in divided doses q 6 hours. Maximum daily dosage is 2 g.
Endocarditis prophylaxis for dental procedures –
Adults: 1 g I.V. slowly over 1 hour, starting 1 hour before procedure.

ADVERSE REACTIONS

EENT: tinnitus, ototoxicity.
GI: nausea.
GU: nephrotoxicity.
Hematologic: transient eosinophilia, leukopenia.
Skin: "red-neck" syndrome with

rapid I.V. infusion (maculopapular rash on face, neck, trunk, and extremities).

Other: chills, fever, ***anaphylaxis,*** superinfection, pain or thrombophlebitis with I.V. administration, necrosis.

INTERACTIONS

Aminoglycosides, amphotericin B, cisplatin, pentamidine: increased risk of nephrotoxicity. Monitor closely.

CONTRAINDICATIONS

- Contraindicated in patients with hypersensitivity to the drug.
- Use cautiously in patients receiving other neurotoxic, nephrotoxic, or ototoxic drugs; in patients over age 60, and in those with impaired hepatic or renal function, preexisting hearing loss, or allergies to other antibiotics. Patients with renal dysfunction require dosage adjustment.

NURSING CONSIDERATIONS

- Obtain urine specimen for culture and sensitivity tests before first dose. Therapy may begin pending results.
- Tell the patient to take entire amount of medication exactly as directed, even after he feels better.
- Treat staphylococcal endocarditis for at least 4 weeks.
- Have the patient's hearing evaluated before and during prolonged therapy.
- Tell the patient to stop drug immediately and report adverse reactions, especially fullness or ringing in ears.
- Monitor renal function (BUN, serum creatinine, urinalysis, creatinine clearance, and urine output) before and during therapy. Also monitor for signs of superinfection.
- Oral preparation stable for 2 weeks if refrigerated.
- **I.V. use:** For I.V. infusion, dilute in 200 ml sodium chloride injection or 5% glucose solution and infuse over 60 minutes. Check site daily for phlebitis and irritation. Report pain at infusion site. Avoid extravasation. Severe irritation and necrosis can result.
- Monitor the patient carefully for red-neck syndrome, which can occur if drug is infused too rapidly. If this reaction occurs, stop infusion and report to the doctor.
- Do not give drug I.M.
- Refrigerate I.V. solution after reconstitution and use within 96 hours.

19
Inotropics

amrinone lactate
digitoxin
digoxin
milrinone lactate

COMBINATION PRODUCTS
None.

amrinone lactate
Inocor

Pregnancy Risk Category: C

HOW SUPPLIED
Injection: 5 mg/ml

ACTION
Mechanism: Produces inotropic action by increasing cellular levels of cAMP. Produces vasodilation through a direct relaxant effect on vascular smooth muscle.
Onset: 2 to 5 minutes. **Peak:** Serum levels peak in 10 minutes. **Duration:** elimination half-life, about 6 hours; effects persist ½ to 2 hours after dose.

INDICATIONS & DOSAGE
Short-term management of CHF –
Adults: initially, 0.75 mg/kg I.V. bolus over 2 to 3 minutes. Then begin maintenance infusion of 5 to 10 mcg/kg/minute. Additional bolus of 0.75 mg/kg may be given 30 minutes after start of therapy. Total daily dosage should not exceed 10 mg/kg.

ADVERSE REACTIONS
CV: *arrhythmias,* hypotension.
GI: nausea, vomiting, cramps, dyspepsia, diarrhea.
Hematologic: *thrombocytopenia* (depends on dose and duration of therapy).
Hepatic: elevated enzymes, hepatotoxicity (rare).
Other: burning at injection site, hypersensitivity reactions (pericarditis, ascites, myositis vasculitis, pleuritis).

INTERACTIONS
Digitalis glycosides: enhanced inotropic effect. Beneficial drug interaction.
Disopyramide: severe hypotension. Use together cautiously.
Furosemide: precipitation occurs when amrinone solutions are mixed with furosemide. Don't administer both drugs through the same I.V. line.

CONTRAINDICATIONS
- Contraindicated in patients with severe aortic or pulmonic valve disease. Not recommended during acute phase of MI.
- Use cautiously in patients with hypertrophic cardiomyopathy.

NURSING CONSIDERATIONS
- Amrinone is primarily prescribed for patients who have not responded to therapy with digitalis glycosides, diuretics, and vasodilators.
- Dosage should be based on clinical response, including assessment of pulmonary artery wedge pressure and cardiac output.
- Amrinone may be added to digitalis glycoside therapy in patients with atrial fibrillation and flutter because it enhances AV conduction and increases ventricular response rate.
- Monitor blood pressure and heart rate throughout the infusion. If the patient's blood pressure falls, slow or stop infusion and notify the doctor.
- Monitor platelet count. If it falls below 150,000/mm³, decrease dosage as ordered.
- **I.V. use:** Administer amrinone with an infusion pump and use as supplied, or dilute in 0.45% or 0.9% sodium

chloride to a concentration of 1 to 3 mg/ml. Use diluted solution within 24 hours.

- Don't dilute with solutions containing dextrose because a slow chemical reaction occurs over 24 hours. However, amrinone can be injected into free-flowing dextrose infusions through a Y-connector or directly into the tubing.
- Don't mix amrinone with other drugs.
- Patients with end-stage cardiac disease may receive home treatment with an amrinone drip while awaiting heart transplantation.

digitoxin

Crystodigin, Digitaline†

Pregnancy Risk Category: C

HOW SUPPLIED

Tablets: 0.1 mg

ACTION

Mechanism: Inhibits sodium-potassium activated adenosine triphosphatase, promoting movement of calcium from extracellular to intracellular cytoplasm and thereby strengthening myocardial contraction. Also acts on CNS to enhance vagal tone, slowing conduction through the AV node and providing an antiarrhythmic effect.

Onset: ½ to 2 hours. **Peak:** Serum levels peak 4 to 10 hours after oral dose. **Duration:** elimination half-life, 5 to 7 days; effects may persist for 3 to 4 weeks after last dose.

INDICATIONS & DOSAGE

CHF, paroxysmal supraventricular tachycardia, atrial fibrillation and flutter–

Adults: loading dose is 1.2 to 1.6 mg P.O. in divided doses over 24 hours; average maintenance dosage is 0.15 mg daily (range: 0.05 to 0.3 mg daily).

Premature infants, neonates, severely ill older infants: loading dose is 0.022 mg/kg or 0.3 to 0.35 mg/m^2 P.O. in divided doses over 24 hours; maintenance dosage is 0.0022 mg/kg daily. Monitor closely for toxicity.

Children 2 weeks to 1 year: loading dose is 0.045 mg/kg P.O. in divided doses over 24 hours; maintenance dosage is 0.0045 mg/kg daily. Monitor closely for toxicity.

Children 1 to 2 years: loading dose is 0.04 mg/kg P.O. in divided doses over 24 hours; maintenance dosage is 0.004 mg/kg daily. Monitor closely for toxicity.

Children 2 to 12 years: loading dose is 0.03 mg/kg or 0.75 mg/m^2 P.O. in divided doses over 24 hours; maintenance dosage is one-tenth of loading dose or 0.003 mg/kg or 0.075 mg/m^2 daily. Monitor closely for toxicity.

ADVERSE REACTIONS

The following are signs of toxicity that may occur with all digitalis glycosides:

CNS: *fatigue, generalized muscle weakness, agitation, hallucinations,* headache, malaise, dizziness, vertigo, stupor, paresthesia.

CV: ***arrhythmias*** (most commonly conduction disturbances with or without AV block, PVCs, and supraventricular arrhythmias); arrhythmias may lead to increased severity of CHF, hypotension. ***Toxic effects on heart may be life-threatening and require immediate attention.***

EENT: *yellow-green halos around visual images, blurred vision,* light flashes, photophobia, diplopia.

GI: *anorexia, nausea,* vomiting, diarrhea.

INTERACTIONS

Amiodarone, quinidine, verapamil: possible increased serum digitoxin levels. Monitor patient closely.

Amphotericin B, corticosteroids, diuretics (including loop diuretics, chlorthalidone, metolazone, and thiazides), ti-

carcillin: hypokalemia or hypomagnesemia, predisposing patient to digitalis toxicity. Monitor serum potassium and serum magnesium levels.
Antacids, kaolin-pectin, oral neomycin, sulfasalazine: decreased absorption of digitoxin. Schedule doses as far as possible from digitoxin administration.
Cholestyramine, colestipol, metoclopramide: decreased absorption of digitoxin. Monitor for decreased effect and low blood levels. Increase dosage if necessary and as ordered.
Cimetidine: decreased digitoxin metabolism. Monitor for digitalis toxicity.
Parenteral calcium, thiazides: hypercalcemia and hypomagnesemia, predisposing patient to digitalis toxicity. Monitor serum calcium and serum magnesium levels.
Phenobarbital, phenylbutazone, phenytoin, rifampin: faster metabolism and shorter duration of digitoxin. Observe for underdigitalization.

CONTRAINDICATIONS

- Contraindicated in patients with any digitalis-induced toxicity; ventricular fibrillation; and ventricular tachycardia unless caused by CHF.
- Use with extreme caution in elderly patients and in those with acute MI, incomplete AV block, sinus bradycardia, PVCs, chronic constrictive pericarditis, hypertrophic cardiomyopathy, severe pulmonary disease, and thyroid disease. Reduce dosage in patients with renal impairment.
- Hypothyroid patients are extremely sensitive to glycosides; hyperthyroid patients may need larger doses.

NURSING CONSIDERATIONS

- Before administering loading dose, obtain baseline data (heart rate and rhythm, blood pressure, and electrolytes) and question the patient about recent use of digitalis glycosides (within the previous 2 to 3 weeks).
- Before giving, take apical-radial pulse for a full minute. Record and report to the doctor any significant changes (sudden increase or decrease in the pulse rate, pulse deficit, irregular beats, and particularly regularization of a previously irregular rhythm). If any of these changes occur, check blood pressure and obtain a 12-lead ECG.
- Always divide the loading dose over first 24 hours unless the clinical situation indicates otherwise.
- Ajust dosage to the patient's clinical condition. Assess dosage by determining serum levels of digitalis glycosides, calcium, potassium, and magnesium and by monitoring ECG.
- Therapeutic blood levels of digitoxin range from 25 to 35 ng/ml.
- Monitor serum potassium level carefully. Take corrective action before hypokalemia occurs. Encourage the patient to eat potassium-rich foods.
- Because digitoxin is a long-acting drug, watch for cumulative effects and signs of toxicity, especially in children and elderly patients. Ask the patient about nausea, vomiting, anorexia, visual disturbances, and other symptoms of toxicity.
- Excessive slowing of pulse rate (60 beats/minute or less) may be a sign of digitalis toxicity. Withhold drug and notify the doctor.
- For digitalis toxicity, administer agents that bind the drug in the intestine (for example, colestipol or cholestyramine). Treat arrhythmias with phenytoin I.V. and potentially life-threatening toxicity with specific antigen-binding fragments (such as digoxin immune FAB).
- Withhold drug for 1 to 2 days before elective cardioversion. Adjust dose after cardioversion.
- Instruct the patient and a responsible family member about drug action, dosage regimen, pulse taking, reportable signs, and follow-up plans.

• Don't substitute one brand of digitoxin for another.

digoxin

Lanoxicaps, Lanoxin*, Novodigoxin†

Pregnancy Risk Category: C

HOW SUPPLIED

Tablets: 0.125 mg, 0.25 mg, 0.5 mg
Capsules: 0.05 mg, 0.1 mg, 0.2 mg
Elixir: 0.05 mg/ml
Injection: 0.05 mg/ml†, 0.1 mg/ml (pediatric), 0.25 mg/ml

ACTION

Mechanism: Inhibits sodium-potassium activated adenosine triphosphatase, thereby promoting movement of calcium from extracellular to intracellular cytoplasm and strengthening myocardial contraction. Also acts on CNS to enhance vagal tone, slowing conduction through the SA and AV nodes and providing an antiarrhythmic effect.
Onset: ½ to 2 hours after oral dose or 5 to 30 minutes after I.V. administration. **Peak:** Serum levels peak 6 to 8 hours after oral dose or 1 to 5 hours after I.V. administration. **Duration:** elimination half-life, 30 to 40 hours; effects persist 3 to 4 days after last dose.

INDICATIONS & DOSAGE

CHF, paroxysmal supraventricular tachycardia, atrial fibrillation and flutter–
Adults: loading dose is 0.5 to 1 mg I.V. or P.O. in divided doses over 24 hours; maintenance dosage is 0.125 to 0.5 mg I.V. or P.O. daily (average is 0.25 mg). Depending on patient response, larger doses may be needed for treatment of arrhythmias. Give smaller loading and maintenance doses to patients with impaired renal function.
Adults over 65 years: 0.125 mg P.O. daily as maintenance dose. Frail or underweight elderly patients may require only 0.0625 mg daily or 0.125 mg every other day.
Premature neonates: loading dose is 0.025 mg/kg I.V. in three divided doses over 24 hours; maintenance dosage is 0.01 mg/kg daily, divided q 12 hours.
Neonates: loading dose is 0.035 mg/kg P.O., divided q 8 hours over 24 hours; I.V. loading dose is 0.02 to 0.03 mg/kg; maintenance dosage is 0.01 mg/kg P.O. daily, divided q 12 hours.
Children 1 month to 2 years: loading dose is 0.035 to 0.06 mg/kg P.O. in three divided doses over 24 hours; I.V. loading dose is 0.03 to 0.05 mg/kg; maintenance dosage is 0.01 to 0.02 mg/kg P.O. daily, divided q 12 hours.
Children over 2 years: loading dose is 0.02 to 0.04 mg/kg P.O. daily, divided q 8 hours over 24 hours; I.V. loading dose is 0.015 to 0.035 mg/kg; maintenance dosage is 0.012 mg/kg P.O. daily, divided q 12 hours.

ADVERSE REACTIONS

The following are signs of toxicity that may occur with all digitalis glycosides:
CNS: *fatigue, generalized muscle weakness, agitation, hallucinations,* headache, malaise, dizziness, vertigo, stupor, paresthesia.
CV: ***arrhythmias*** (most commonly, conduction disturbances with or without AV block, PVCs, and supraventricular arrhythmias); arrythmias may lead to increased severity of CHF, hypotension. ***Toxic effects on the heart may be life-threatening and require immediate attention.***
EENT: *yellow-green halos around visual images, blurred vision,* light flashes, photophobia, diplopia.
GI: *anorexia, nausea,* vomiting, diarrhea.

*Liquid form contains alcohol. *Common* reactions are in italics; ***life-threatening,*** in bold italics.
**May contain tartrazine.

INTERACTIONS

Amiloride: inhibited and increased digoxin excretion. Monitor for altered digoxin effect.
Amiodarone, diltiazem, nifedipine, quinidine, verapamil: increased digoxin blood levels. Monitor for toxicity.
Amphotericin B, carbenicillin, corticosteroids, diuretics (including loop diuretics, chlorthalidone, metolazone, and thiazides), ticarcillin: hypokalemia, predisposing patient to digitalis toxicity. Monitor serum potassium levels.
Antacids, kaolin-pectin: decreased absorption of oral digoxin. Schedule doses as far as possible from oral digoxin administration.
Anticholinergics: may increase digoxin absorption of oral digoxin tablets. Monitor blood levels and observe for toxicity.
Cholestyramine, colestipol, metoclopramide: decreased absorption of oral digoxin. Monitor for decreased effect and low blood levels. Increase dosage if necessary and as ordered.
Parenteral calcium, thiazides: hypercalcemia and hypomagnesemia, predisposing patient to digitalis toxicity. Monitor serum calcium and serum magnesium levels.

CONTRAINDICATIONS

- Contraindicated in patients with any digitalis-induced toxicity; ventricular fibrillation; and ventricular tachycardia unless caused by CHF.
- Use with extreme caution in elderly patients and in those with acute MI, incomplete AV block, sinus bradycardia, PVCs, chronic constrictive pericarditis, hypertrophic cardiomyopathy, renal insufficiency, severe pulmonary disease, or hypothyroidism. Reduce dosage in patients with renal impairment.
- Hypothyroid patients are extremely sensitive to digitalis glycosides; hyperthyroid patients may need larger doses.

NURSING CONSIDERATIONS

- Before administering the loading dose, obtain baseline data (heart rate and rhythm, blood pressure, and electrolytes) and question the patient about recent use of digitalis glycosides (within the previous 2 to 3 weeks).
- Before giving, take apical-radial pulse for a full minute. Record and report to the doctor any significant changes (sudden increase or decrease in pulse rate, pulse deficit, irregular beats, and particularly regularization of a previously irregular rhythm). If any of these changes occurs, check blood pressure and obtain a 12-lead ECG.
- Always divide the loading dose over first 24 hours unless the clinical situation indicates otherwise.
- Adjust dosage, as ordered, to the patient's clinical condition. Assess dosage by determining serum levels of digitalis glycosides, calcium, potassium, and magnesium and by monitoring ECG. Obtain blood for digoxin levels 8 hours after last oral dose.
- Therapeutic blood levels of digoxin range from 0.5 to 2.0 ng/ml.
- Monitor serum potassium levels carefully. Take corrective action before hypokalemia occurs. Encourage the patient to eat potassium-rich foods.
- Excessive slowing of the pulse rate (60 beats/minute or less) may be a sign of digitalis toxicity. Withhold drug and notify the doctor.
- Absorption of digoxin from parenteral route and from liquid-filled capsules is superior to absorption from tablets or elixir. Expect dosage reduction of 20% to 25% when changing from tablets or elixir to liquid-filled capsules or parenteral therapy.
- Withhold drug for 1 to 2 days before elective cardioversion. Adjust dose after cardioversion.
- Instruct the patient and a responsible family member about drug action,

dosage regimen, how to take pulse, reportable signs, and follow-up care.
- Don't substitute one brand of digoxin for another.
- **I.V. use:** Infuse drug slowly over at least 5 minutes.

milrinone lactate
Primacor

Pregnancy Risk Category: C

HOW SUPPLIED
Injection: 1 mg/ml

ACTION
Mechanism: Produces inotropic action by increasing cellular levels of cAMP. Produces vasodilation by directly relaxing vascular smooth muscle.
Onset: 5 to 15 minutes. **Peak:** Serum levels peak within 1 to 2 hours. **Duration:** 1 to 3 hours after infusion.

INDICATIONS & DOSAGE
Short-term treatment of CHF –
Adults: initial loading dose is 50 mcg/kg I.V., administered slowly over 10 minutes, followed by continuous I.V. infusion of 0.375 to 0.75 mcg/kg/minute. Adjust infusion dose according to clinical and hemodynamic responses.

In patients with renal failure: if creatinine clearance is 50 ml/minute/1.73 m^2 or less, carefully titrate dosage to maximum clinical effect and don't exceed 1.13 mg/kg/day.

ADVERSE REACTIONS
CNS: headache.
CV: ***ventricular arrhythmias,*** *ventricular ectopic activity,* nonsustained ventricular tachycardia, ***sustained ventricular tachycardia.***

INTERACTIONS
Furosemide: immediate precipitation when mixed with milrinone. Don't administer through the same I.V. line.

CONTRAINDICATIONS
- Contraindicated in patients with hypersensitivity to the drug and in those with severe obstructive pulmonic or aortic valvular disease. Also avoid use during acute phase of MI because safety and efficacy of such use have not been established.
- Use cautiously in patients with atrial flutter or fibrillation because drug slightly shortens AV node conduction time and may increase ventricular response rate. Administer a digitalis glycoside, if ordered, before beginning milrinone therapy.

NURSING CONSIDERATIONS
- Milrinone is typically given with digoxin and diuretics.
- Be aware that inotropic agents may aggravate outflow tract obstruction in patients with idiopathic cardiomyopathy.
- Patients treated with milrinone have exhibited supraventricular and ventricular arrhythmias. Monitor patients closely.
- Monitor fluid and electrolyte status, blood pressure, heart rate, and renal function during therapy. Excessive decrease in blood pressure requires discontinuation or slower rate of infusion.
- Improvement of cardiac output may result in enhanced urine output. Expect dosage reduction in patient's diuretic therapy as CHF improves. Remember that potassium loss may predispose patient to digitalis toxicity.
- **I.V. use:** Prepare I.V. infusion solution using 0.45% or 0.9% sodium chloride or D_5W. Prepare the 100-mcg/ml solution by adding 180 ml of diluent per 20-mg (20-ml) vial, the 150-mcg/ml solution by adding 113 ml of diluent per 20-mg (20-ml) vial, and the 200-mcg/ml solution by adding 80 ml of diluent per 20-mg (20-ml) vial.

20 Antiarrhythmics

adenosine
amiodarone hydrochloride
atropine sulfate
bretylium tosylate
disopyramide
disopyramide phosphate
esmolol hydrochloride
flecainide acetate
lidocaine hydrochloride
mexiletine hydrochloride
moricizine hydrochloride
phenytoin
(See Chapter 29, ANTICONVULSANTS.)
phenytoin sodium
(See Chapter 29, ANTICONVULSANTS.)
procainamide hydrochloride
propafenone hydrochloride
propranolol hydrochloride
(See Chapter 21, ANTIANGINALS.)
quinidine bisulfate
quinidine gluconate
quinidine polygalacturonate
quinidine sulfate
sotalol
tocainide hydrochloride

COMBINATION PRODUCTS
None.

adenosine
Adenocard

Pregnancy Risk Category: C

HOW SUPPLIED
Injection: 3 mg/ml in 2-ml vials

ACTION
Mechanism: A naturally occurring nucleoside that acts on the AV node to slow conduction and inhibit reentry pathways. Adenosine is also useful in treating paroxysmal supraventricular tachycardia (PSVT) associated with accessory bypass tracts (Wolff-Parkinson-White syndrome).

Onset: immediate. **Peak:** Peak effects occur immediately. **Duration:** plasma half-life, less than 10 seconds.

INDICATIONS & DOSAGE
Conversion of PSVT to sinus rhythm –
Adults: 6 mg I.V. by rapid bolus injection over 1 to 2 seconds. If PSVT is not eliminated in 1 to 2 minutes, give 12 mg by rapid I.V. push. Repeat 12-mg dose if necessary. Single doses over 12 mg are not recommended.

ADVERSE REACTIONS
CNS: apprehension, back pain, blurred vision, burning sensation, dizziness, heaviness in arms, lightheadedness, neck pain, numbness, tingling in arms.
CV: chest pain, *facial flushing,* headache, hypotension, palpitations, diaphoresis.
GI: metallic taste, nausea.
Respiratory: *chest pressure, dyspnea, shortness of breath,* hyperventilation.
Other: *tightness in throat, groin pressure.*

INTERACTIONS
Carbamazepine: higher degrees of heart block may occur.
Dipyridamole: may potentiate adenosine's effects. Smaller doses may be necessary.
Methylxanthines: antagonism of adenosine's effects. Patients receiving theophylline or caffeine may require higher doses or may not respond to adenosine therapy.

CONTRAINDICATIONS
• Contraindicated in patients with hypersensitivity to the drug and in those with atrial flutter, atrial fibrillation, and ventricular tachycardia because

the drug is ineffective in treating these arrhythmias.
• Also contraindicated in patients with second- or third-degree heart block or sick sinus syndrome unless an artificial pacemaker is present because adenosine decreases conduction through the AV node and may produce transient first-, second-, or third-degree heart block. These effects are usually transient; however, patients who develop significant heart block after a dose of adenosine should not receive additional doses.
• Although asthma attacks have not been reported, inhaled adenosine will cause bronchoconstriction in asthmatic patients.
• Experimental evidence indicates that high concentrations of adenosine may induce chromosomal damage, but the clinical significance of this effect is not known.

NURSING CONSIDERATIONS

• In clinical trials, more than half of the patients exhibited new arrhythmias, including sinus bradycardia or tachycardia, atrial premature contractions, various degrees of AV block, PVCs, and skipped beats, when adenosine was used to convert to normal sinus rhythm. Such arrhythmias are usually transient.
• **I.V. use:** Rapid I.V. injection is necessary for drug action. Administer directly into a vein if possible; when giving through an I.V. line, use the most proximal port and flush immediately and rapidly with 0.9% sodium chloride solution to ensure that the drug reaches the systemic circulation quickly.
• Crystals may form if solution is cold. If crystals are visible, gently warm solution to room temperature. Don't use solutions that aren't clear.
• Because adenosine contains no preservatives, discard any unused drug.

amiodarone hydrochloride

Aratac‡, Cordarone, Cordarone X‡

Pregnancy Risk Category: C

HOW SUPPLIED

Tablets: 100 mg†‡, 200 mg
Injection: 50 mg/ml‡

ACTION

Mechanism: A class III antiarrhythmic that prolongs the refractory period and action potential duration and decreases repolarization.
Onset: usually delayed for 1 to 3 weeks because of long half-life; if loading dose is used, onset may be reduced to 2 or 3 days. **Peak:** Serum levels peak 3 to 7 hours after oral administration; effects persist for 1 to 5 months after starting therapy. **Duration:** terminal elimination half-life, 40 to 55 days; effects persist for more than a month after last dose.

INDICATIONS & DOSAGE

Ventricular and supraventricular arrhythmias, including recurrent supraventricular tachycardia (Wolff-Parkinson-White syndrome), atrial fibrillation and flutter, and ventricular tachycardia refractory to other antiarrhythmics –
Adults: give loading dose of 800 to 1,600 mg P.O. daily for 1 to 3 weeks until initial therapeutic response occurs. Maintenance dosage is 200 to 600 mg P.O. daily.

Alternatively, give loading dose of 5 to 10 mg/kg I.V. over 20 minutes to 2 hours using a central line. Then, for 3 to 5 days, give 10 mg/kg/day P.O. I.V. slow infusion.

ADVERSE REACTIONS

CNS: peripheral neuropathy, extrapyramidal symptoms, headache, muscle weakness, *malaise, fatigue.*
CV: bradycardia, hypotension, ***arrhythmias, CHF.***

EENT: *corneal microdeposits,* visual disturbances.
GI: *nausea, vomiting,* constipation.
Hepatic: *altered liver enzymes,* hepatic dysfunction.
Respiratory: ***severe pulmonary toxicity (pneumonitis, alveolitis).***
Skin: *photosensitivity,* blue-gray skin pigmentation.
Other: hypothyroidism, hyperthyroidism, gynecomastia.

INTERACTIONS

Antiarrhythmics: amiodarone may reduce the hepatic or renal clearance of certain antiarrhythmics (especially flecainide, procainamide, or quinidine); concomitant use of amiodarone with other antiarrhythmics (especially mexilitine, propafenone, quinidine, disopyramide, or procainamide) may induce torsades de pointes.
Antihypertensives: increased hypotensive effect. Use together cautiously.
Beta blockers, calcium channel blockers: increased cardiac depressant effects; may potentiate slowing of sinus node and AV conduction. Use together cautiously.
Digitalis glycosides: increased serum digoxin levels (average of 70% to 100%). Monitor digoxin levels closely and adjust dosage as ordered.
Phenytoin: may decrease phenytoin metabolism. Monitor serum phenytoin levels and adjust dosage as ordered.
Warfarin: increased PT (average of 100% within 1 to 4 weeks of therapy). Decrease warfarin dosage 33% to 50% when amiodarone is initiated. Monitor patient closely.

CONTRAINDICATIONS

- Contraindicated in patients with hypersensitivity to the drug and in those with severe sinus node disease resulting in preexisting bradycardia. Unless an artificial pacemaker is present, drug is also contraindicated in patients with second-or third-degree AV block and in those in whom bradycardia has caused syncope.
- Use with extreme caution in patients receiving class IA antiarrhythmics.
- Use cautiously in patients with pulmonary or thyroid disease.

NURSING CONSIDERATIONS

- Although amiodarone is often effective for treatment of arrhythmias resistant to other drug therapy, the high incidence of adverse reactions limits its use.
- Because of the slow onset of antiarrhythmic effect and risk of life-threatening arrhythmias, administer loading doses in a hospital setting and with continuous ECG monitoring.
- Monitor carefully for pulmonary toxicity, which can be fatal. Incidence increases in patients receiving more than 400 mg/day.
- Monitor for symptoms of pneumonitis – exertional dyspnea, nonproductive cough, and pleuritic chest pain. Monitor pulmonary function tests and chest X-ray.
- Monitor blood pressure and heart rate and rhythm frequently. Perform continuous ECG monitoring during initiation and alteration of dosage. Notify doctor of any significant change.
- Monitor liver and thyroid function tests and serum electrolytes, particularly potassium and magnesium levels.
- Amiodarone's adverse effects are more prevalent at high doses but are generally reversible when drug therapy is stopped. Resolution of adverse reactions may take up to 4 months.
- To decrease GI intolerance, divide oral loading dose into three equal doses and give with meals. Maintenance dosage may be given once daily, but may be divided into two doses taken with meals if GI intolerance occurs.
- Within 1 to 4 months after begin-

ning amiodarone therapy, most patients show corneal microdeposits upon slit-lamp ophthalmic examination. However, only 2% to 3% have actual visual disturbances. To minimize this complication, recommend instillation of methylcellulose ophthalmic solution during amiodarone therapy.

• Advise patients to use a sunscreen to prevent photosensitivity reaction. Monitor for burning or tingling skin followed by erythema and possible skin blistering.

• 10 mg/kg by I.V. infusion via a central line, followed by an I.V.

• Continuously monitor cardiac status of patient receiving I.V. amiodarone.

atropine sulfate

Pregnancy Risk Category: C

HOW SUPPLIED

Tablets: 0.4 mg, 0.6 mg
Injection: 0.05 mg/ml, 0.1 mg/ml, 0.3 mg/ml, 0.4 mg/ml, 0.5 mg/ml, 0.6 mg/ml, 0.8 mg/ml, 1 mg/ml, 1.2 mg/ml

ACTION

Mechanism: An anticholinergic that inhibits acetylcholine at the parasympathetic neuroeffector junction, blocking vagal effects on the SA node; this enhances conduction through the AV node and speeds heart rate.
Onset: 2 to 5 minutes after I.V. injection. **Peak:** Serum levels peak within 15 to 50 minutes after I.M. injection; effects, within 30 to 45 minutes. Serum levels peak immediately after I.V. administration; effects, within 5 minutes.

INDICATIONS & DOSAGE

Symptomatic bradycardia, bradyarrhythmia (junctional or escape rhythm) –
Adults: usually 0.5 to 1 mg I.V. push; repeat q 5 minutes to maximum of 2 mg. Lower doses (less than 0.5 mg) can cause bradycardia.
Children: 0.01 mg/kg I.V. up to maximum of 0.4 mg; or 0.3 mg/m^2; may repeat q 4 to 6 hours.
Antidote for anticholinesterase insecticide poisoning –
Adults: 2 to 4 mg I.V. repeated q 5 to 10 minutes until muscarinic symptoms disappear or signs of atropine toxicity appear. Severe poisoning may require up to 6 mg every hour.
Children: 1 mg I.V. or I.M., then 0.5 to 1 mg I.V. or I.M. q 5 to 10 minutes until muscarinic signs disappear or signs of atropine toxicity appear.
Preoperatively for diminishing secretions and blocking cardiac vagal reflexes –
Adults: 0.4 to 0.6 mg I.M. 45 to 60 minutes before anesthesia.
Children: 0.01 mg/kg I.M. up to maximum dose of 0.4 mg 45 to 60 minutes before anesthesia.
Adjunctive treatment of peptic ulcer disease; treatment of functional GI disorders such as irritable bowel syndrome –
Adults: 0.4 to 0.6 mg P.O. q 4 to 6 hours.
Children: 0.01 mg/kg or 0.3 mg/m^2 (not to exceed 0.4 mg) q 4 to 6 hours.

ADVERSE REACTIONS

CNS: *headache, restlessness,* ataxia, disorientation, hallucinations, delirium, ***coma,*** *insomnia, dizziness;* excitement, agitation, and confusion (especially in elderly patients).
CV: 1 to 2 mg – *tachycardia, palpitations;* greater than 2 mg – ***tachycardia, angina.***
EENT: 1 mg – *slight mydriasis,* photophobia; 2 mg – *blurred vision, mydriasis.*
GI: *dry mouth (common even at low doses),* thirst, *constipation,* nausea, vomiting.
GU: urine retention.
Hematologic: leukocytosis.

Skin: hot, flushed skin.

INTERACTIONS

Antacids: decreased absorption of anticholinergics. Separate administration times by at least 1 hour.
Anticholinergics or drugs with anticholinergic effects such as amantadine, glutethimide, meperidine, antiarrhythmics, antiparkinsonian agents, phenothiazines, and tricyclic antidepressants: additive anticholinergic effects. Use together cautiously.
Ketoconazole, levodopa: decreased absorption. Avoid concomitant use.
Methotrimeprazine: may produce extrapyramidal symptoms. Monitor patient carefully.
Potassium chloride wax-matrix tablets: increased risk of mucosal lesions. Use cautiously.

CONTRAINDICATIONS

- Contraindicated in patients with acute angle-closure glaucoma, obstructive uropathy, obstructive disease of GI tract, myasthenia gravis, paralytic ileus, intestinal atony, unstable CV status in acute hemorrhage, and toxic megacolon.
- Use cautiously in patients with Down's syndrome because they may be more sensitive to the drug.

NURSING CONSIDERATIONS

- Many of the adverse reactions (such as dry mouth and constipation) vary with the dose and should be expected. They are an extension of the drug's pharmacologic activity.
- Watch for tachycardia in cardiac patients because it may precipitate ventricular fibrillation.
- Monitor fluid intake and urine output. Drug causes urine retention and urinary hesitancy; have patient void before receiving drug.
- Monitor closely for urine retention in elderly men with benign prostatic hyperplasia.
- Antidote for atropine overdose is physostigmine salicylate.
- **I.V. use:** Administer by direct I.V. into a large vein or I.V. tubing over at least 1 to 2 minutes.
- When given I.V., atropine may cause paradoxical initial bradycardia, especially with small doses (0.4 to 0.6 mg). This is caused by a drug effect in the CNS and usually disappears within 2 minutes.

bretylium tosylate

Bretylate†‡, Bretylol, Critifib‡

Pregnancy Risk Category: C

HOW SUPPLIED

Injection: 50 mg/ml

ACTION

Mechanism: A class III antiarrhythmic that initially exerts transient adrenergic stimulation through release of norepinephrine. Subsequent depletion of norepinephrine causes adrenergic blocking actions to predominate, prolonging repolarization and increasing duration of action potential and effective refractory.
Onset: within a few minutes; suppression of ventricular tachycardia and ventricular fibrillation may not occur for 20 minutes to 6 hours.
Peak: Serum levels peak within 6 to 9 hours. **Duration:** effects may persist 6 to 24 hours.

INDICATIONS & DOSAGE

Ventricular fibrillation or hemodynamically unstable ventricular tachycardia –
Adults: 5 mg/kg by I.V. push over 1 minute. If necessary, increase dose to 10 mg/kg and repeat q 15 to 30 minutes until 30 mg/kg have been given.
Children: safety and efficacy have not been established, but some clinicians use 2 to 5 mg/kg I.M. as a single dose, or 5 mg/kg I.V. followed by 10 mg/kg I.V. if fibrillation persists.

Other ventricular arrhythmias – **Adults:** initially, 500 mg diluted to 50 ml with D_5W or 0.9% sodium chloride and infused I.V. over more than 8 minutes at 5 to 10 mg/kg. Repeat in 1 to 2 hours if needed. Thereafter, repeat q 6 to 8 hours.

For I.V. maintenance in adults, administer infuse in diluted solution of 500 ml D_5W or 0.9% sodium chloride at 1 to 2 mg/minute.

For I.M. injection in adults, administer 5 to 10 mg/kg undiluted. Repeat in 1 to 2 hours if needed. Thereafter, repeat q 6 to 8 hours.

ADVERSE REACTIONS

CNS: *vertigo, dizziness, light-headedness, syncope* (usually secondary to hypotension).
CV: ***severe hypotension*** *(especially orthostatic),* bradycardia, anginal pain, transient arrhythmias, transient hypertension.
GI: severe nausea, vomiting (with rapid infusion).
Other: muscle atrophy and tissue necrosis with repeated injections.

INTERACTIONS

All antihypertensives: may potentiate hypotension. Monitor blood pressure.
Other antiarrhythmics: additive or antagonistic antiarrhythmic effects. Monitor for additive toxicity.
Sympathomimetics: bretylium may potentiate effects of drugs given to correct hypotension.

CONTRAINDICATIONS

- Contraindicated in digitalized patients unless the arrhythmia is life-threatening, not caused by digitalis, and unresponsive to other antiarrhythmics.
- Use cautiously in patients with fixed cardiac output, aortic stenosis, and pulmonary hypertension to avoid severe and sudden drop in blood pressure.

NURSING CONSIDERATIONS

- Bretylium is used with other cardiac life support measures, such as cardiopulmonary resuscitation, countershock, epinephrine, sodium bicarbonate, and lidocaine.
- Monitor blood pressure and heart rate and rhythm continuously. Notify doctor immediately of any significant change. If supine systolic blood pressure falls below 75 mm Hg, the doctor may order norepinephrine, dopamine, or volume expanders to raise blood pressure.
- The initial release of norepinephrine caused by bretylium may induce transient hypertension and arrhythmias. Monitor the patient closely.
- Keep the patient in the supine position until tolerance to hypotension develops. Tell the patient to avoid sudden postural changes.
- To prevent nausea and vomiting in the patient, follow dosage directions carefully.
- Avoid subtherapeutic doses (< 5 mg/kg) because such doses may cause hypotension.
- Observe for increased anginal pain in susceptible patients.
- To prevent tissue damage, rotate I.M. injection sites and don't exceed 3-ml volume in any one site.
- Bretylium has been used investigationally to treat hypertension.
- **I.V. use:** Infuse in diluted solution of 500 ml D_5W or in 0.9% sodium chloride at 1 to 2 mg/minute. Administer continuous infusion at a rate of 1 to 2 mg/minute. When infusing intermittently, give ordered dose over 10 to 30 minutes. When administering as a direct I.V. injection, use a 20G to 22G needle and inject over 1 minute into a vein or I.V. line containing a free-flowing, compatible solution.

disopyramide

Rythmodan†

*Liquid form contains alcohol.
**May contain tartrazine.

Common reactions are in italics; ***life-threatening,*** in bold italics.

disopyramide phosphate

Napamide, Norpace, Norpace CR, Rythmodan LA†

Pregnancy Risk Category: C

HOW SUPPLIED

disopyramide
Capsules: 100 mg†, 150 mg†
disopyramide phosphate
Tablets (sustained-release): 250 mg†
Capsules: 100 mg, 150 mg
Capsules (controlled-release): 100 mg, 150 mg
Injection: 10 mg/ml‡

ACTION

Mechanism: A class Ia antiarrhythmic that depresses phase O and prolongs the action potential. All class I drugs have membrane-stabilizing effects.
Onset: ½ to 3½ hours after an oral dose. **Peak:** Plasma levels peak within 2 to 2½ hours after an oral dose. **Duration:** elimination half-life, 4 to 10 hours; effects persist for 1½ to 8½ hours after last dose.

INDICATIONS & DOSAGE

PVCs (unifocal, multifocal, or coupled); ventricular tachycardia not severe enough to require cardioversion; to convert atrial fibrillation or flutter to normal sinus rhythm –
Adults: usual maintenance dosage is 150 to 200 mg P.O. q 6 hours. Give sustained-release capsule q 12 hours for patients who weigh under 50 kg or those with renal, hepatic, or cardiac impairment, give 100 mg P.O. q 6 hours.
Children under 1 year: 10 to 30 mg/kg P.O. daily.
Children 1 to 4 years: 10 to 20 mg/kg P.O. daily.
Children 4 to 12 years: 10 to 15 mg/kg P.O. daily.
Children 12 to 18 years: 6 to 15 mg/kg P.O. daily.

For pediatric dosages, divide into equal amounts and give q 6 hours.

Recommended dosages in advanced renal insufficiency: if creatinine clearance is 30 to 40 ml/minute, give q 8 hours; if creatinine clearance is 15 to 30 ml/minute, give q 12 hours; if creatinine clearance is < 15 ml/minute, give q 24 hours.

For parenteral use in adults – initially, 2 mg/kg I.V. slowly (over not less than 15 minutes). Administer until arrhythmia is eliminated or patient has received 150 mg. Repeat dosage if conversion is successful but arrhythmia returns. Total I.V. dosage should not exceed 300 mg in the first hour. Follow with an I.V. infusion of 0.4 mg/kg/hour (usually 20 to 30 mg/hour) to a maximum of 800 mg/day.

ADVERSE REACTIONS

CNS: dizziness, agitation, depression, fatigue, muscle weakness, syncope.
CV: *hypotension,* ***CHF, heart block,*** edema, weight gain, ***arrhythmias.***
EENT: *blurred vision, dry eyes, dry nose.*
GI: nausea, vomiting, anorexia, bloating, abdominal pain, *constipation, dry mouth.*
GU: urine retention, urinary hesitancy.
Hepatic: cholestatic jaundice.
Skin: rash.
Other: hypoglycemia.

INTERACTIONS

Antiarrhythmics: possible additive or antagonized antiarrhythmic effects.
Phenytoin: increased metabolism of disopyramide. Monitor for decreased antiarrhythmic effect.

CONTRAINDICATIONS

- Contraindicated in patients with cardiogenic shock or second- or third-degree heart block in the absence of an artificial pacemaker. Use very cautiously and avoid, if possible, in CHF.
- Use cautiously in patients with underlying conduction abnormalities,

†Available in Canada only. ‡Available in Australia only. ◇Available OTC.

urinary tract diseases (especially prostatic hypertrophy), hepatic or renal impairment, myasthenia gravis, or acute angle-closure glaucoma.

NURSING CONSIDERATIONS

- Most doctors prefer to prescribe disopyramide for patients not in heart failure who can't tolerate quinidine or procainamide.
- Correct any underlying electrolyte abnormalities before use.
- Check apical pulse before administering drug. Notify the doctor if pulse rate is slower than 60 beats/minute or faster than 120 beats/minute.
- Watch for recurrence of arrhythmias and check for adverse reactions; notify the doctor if any occur.
- Discontinue drug if heart block develops, if QRS complex widens by more than 25%, or if QT interval lengthens by more than 25% above baseline.
- Don't give sustained-release capsule for rapid control of ventricular arrhythmias; when therapeutic blood levels must be rapidly attained; in patients with cardiomyopathy or possible cardiac decompensation; or in those with severe renal impairment.
- When transferring patients from immediate-release to sustained-release capsules, advise them to take a sustained-release capsule 6 hours after the last immediate-release capsule was taken.
- For administration to young children, pharmacist may prepare disopyramide suspension from 100-mg capsules using cherry syrup. Suspension should be dispensed in amber glass bottles and protected from light.
- Teach the patient the importance of taking drug on time and exactly as prescribed. This may require use of an alarm clock for night doses.
- Advise the patient to chew gum or hard candy to relieve dry mouth.
- Manage constipation with proper diet or bulk laxatives.

- **I.V. use:** Add 200 mg to 200 to 500 ml of a compatible solution, such as 0.9% sodium chloride or D_5W. Do not mix with other drugs; switch to oral therapy as soon as possible.

esmolol hydrochloride

Brevibloc

Pregnancy Risk Category: C

HOW SUPPLIED

Injection: 10 mg/ml in 10-ml vials; 250 mg/ml in 10-ml ampules

ACTION

Mechanism: A class II antiarrhythmic, esmolol is an ultrashort-acting $beta_1$-selective adrenergic blocker that decreases heart rate, myocardial contractility, and blood pressure.
Onset: 1 to 4 minutes. **Peak:** Peak serum levels vary with infusion rate, but typically occur in 30 minutes.
Duration: terminal elimination half-life, about 10 minutes; effects begin to subside 1 to 2 minutes after infusion ends, with complete reversal of effects within 30 minutes.

INDICATIONS & DOSAGE

Supraventricular tachycardia; to lower heart rate and blood pressure in patients with acute myocardial ischemia; to produce controlled hypotension during anesthesia –
Adults: loading dose is 500 mcg/kg/minute by I.V. infusion over 1 minute, followed by 4-minute maintenance infusion of 50 mcg/kg/minute. If adequate response does not occur within 5 minutes, repeat loading dose followed by maintenance infusion of 100 mcg/kg/minute for 4 minutes. Repeat loading dose and increase maintenance infusion in a stepwise fashion as needed. Maximum maintenance infusion for tachycardia is 200 mcg/kg/minute; for blood pressure, maximum infusion rate is 300 mcg/kg/minute.

Management of perioperative hypotension –
Adults: loading dose is 500 mcg/kg/minute by I.V. infusion over 30 seconds, followed by 4-minute maintenance infusion of 25 mcg/kg/minute. If adequate response does not occur within 5 minutes, repeat loading dose followed by maintenance infusion of 50 mcg/kg/minute for 4 minutes. Repeat loading dose and increase maintenance infusion by 50 mcg/kg/minute for 4 minutes q 5 minutes to a maximum dosage of 300 mcg/kg/minute.

ADVERSE REACTIONS
CNS: dizziness, somnolence, headache, agitation, fatigue.
CV: *hypotension* (sometimes with diaphoresis).
GI: *nausea,* vomiting.
Respiratory: ***bronchospasm.***
Other: inflammation and induration at infusion site.

INTERACTIONS
Digoxin: esmolol may increase serum digoxin levels by 10% to 20%. Monitor serum digoxin levels.
Morphine: may increase esmolol blood levels. Titrate esmolol carefully.
Reserpine (and other catecholamine-depleting drugs): may cause additive bradycardia and hypotension. Titrate esmolol carefully.
Succinylcholine: esmolol may prolong neuromuscular blockade.

CONTRAINDICATIONS
- Contraindicated in patients with sinus bradycardia, heart block greater than first-degree, cardiogenic shock, or overt heart failure.
- Use cautiously in patients with impaired renal function, diabetes, or bronchospasm.

NURSING CONSIDERATIONS
- Esmolol has advantages over other beta blockers in treating cardiac arrhythmias because it has an extremely short duration of action and can be accurately titrated.
- Esmolol is recommended only for short-term use, for no longer than 48 hours.
- When the patient's heart rate becomes stable, esmolol will be replaced by alternative (longer-acting) antiarrhythmics, such as propranolol, digoxin, or verapamil. As the replacement drug is started, the esmolol infusion should be gradually reduced over 1 hour.
- Monitor ECG and blood pressure continuously during infusion. Up to 50% of all patients treated with esmolol develop hypotension. Monitor closely, especially if patient's pretreatment blood pressure was low.
- Hypotension can usually be reversed within 30 minutes by decreasing the dose or, if necessary, by stopping the infusion.
- If a local reaction develops at the infusion site, change to another site. Avoid using butterfly needles.
- **I.V. use:** Don't give esmolol by I.V. push; use an infusion control device. The 10-mg/ml single-dose vials may be used without diluting, but the injection concentrate (250 mg/ml) must be diluted to a maximum concentration of 10 mg/ml before infusion. Add one ampule to 250 ml of D_5W, lactated Ringer's solution, or 0.45% or 0.9% sodium chloride solution.
- Esmolol solutions are incompatible with diazepam, furosemide, sodium bicarbonate, and thiopental sodium.

flecainide acetate
Tambocor

Pregnancy Risk Category: C

HOW SUPPLIED
Tablets: 50 mg, 100 mg, 150 mg
Injection: 10 mg/ml‡

ACTION

Mechanism: A class Ic antiarrhythmic that depresses phase O. Unlike class Ia and Ib agents, however, it does not prolong or shorten the action potential. All class I drugs have membrane-stabilizing effects.

Onset: within 6 hours of oral administration. **Peak:** Serum levels peak about 3 hours after an oral dose; effects, after 2 to 3 days. **Duration:** elimination half-life, about 20 hours.

INDICATIONS & DOSAGE

Paroxysmal supraventricular tachycardia, paroxysmal atrial fibrillation or flutter in patients without structural heart disease; life-threatening ventricular arrhythmias, such as sustained ventricular tachycardia –

Adults: 100 mg P.O. q 12 hours. Increase in increments of 50 mg b.i.d. q 4 days until efficacy is achieved. Maximum dosage is 400 mg daily for most patients.

Initial dosage for patients with CHF is 50 mg q 12 hours.

Where available, flecainide may be given by I.V. injection‡ –

Adults: 2 mg/kg I.V. push over not less than 10 minutes; or dilute the dose and administer as an infusion.

ADVERSE REACTIONS

CNS: *dizziness, headache,* fatigue, tremor.

CV: ***new or worsened arrhythmias,*** chest pain, ***CHF, cardiac arrest.***

EENT: *blurred vision and other visual disturbances.*

GI: nausea, constipation, abdominal pain.

Other: *dyspnea,* edema, skin rash.

INTERACTIONS

Amiodarone, cimetidine, digoxin, propranolol: altered pharmacokinetics. Monitor for toxicity.

Digitalis glycosides: flecainide may increase plasma digoxin levels by 15% to 25%. Monitor serum digoxin levels.

Propranolol, other beta blockers: both flecainide and propranolol plasma levels increase by 20% to 30%. Monitor for propranolol and flecainide toxicity.

Urine acidifying and alkalinizing agents: extremes of urine pH may substantially alter excretion of flecainide. Monitor for flecainide toxicity.

CONTRAINDICATIONS

- Contraindicated in patients with preexisting second- or third-degree AV block or right bundle branch block when associated with a left hemiblock, in the absence of an artificial pacemaker; and in those with cardiogenic shock.
- Use cautiously in patients with preexisting CHF, cardiomyopathy, severe renal or hepatic disease, prolonged QT interval, sick sinus syndrome, or blood dyscrasias. When used to prevent ventricular arrhythmias, flecainide should be reserved for patients with documented life-threatening arrhythmias. Because of the drug's proarrhythmic effects (ventricular tachycardia, PVCs), consider risks and benefits before starting therapy.

NURSING CONSIDERATIONS

- Because of flecainide's long half-life, its full therapeutic effect may take 3 to 5 days. Concomitant I.V. lidocaine may be ordered for the first several days.
- Dosage adjustments should be made only once every 3 to 4 days.
- Flecainide can alter endocardial pacing thresholds. Determine pacing threshold 1 week before and after initiating therapy in patients with pacemakers.
- Hypokalemia or hyperkalemia may alter the effect of flecainide and should be corrected before giving this drug.
- Therapeutic serum levels of flecain-

ide range from 0.2 to 1 mcg/ml. Incidence of adverse effects increases when trough blood levels exceed 1 mcg/ml. Periodically monitor blood levels, especially in patients with renal failure or CHF.

• Most patients can be adequately maintained on an every-12-hour dosing schedule, but some need to receive flecainide every 8 hours.

• Twice-daily dosing for flecainide enhances patient compliance.

• **I.V. use:** When administering by I.V. push, give over at least 10 minutes. For I.V. infusion, mix only with D_5W.

lidocaine hydrochloride (lignocaine hydrochloride)

Lido Pen Auto-Injector, Xylocaine, Xylocard†‡

Pregnancy Risk Category: B

HOW SUPPLIED

Injection (for direct I.V. use): 1% (10 mg/ml) in 5-ml (50-mg), 10-ml (100-mg) syringes; 2% (20 mg/ml) in 5-ml (100-mg) vials, syringes, and ampules
Injection (for I.M. use): 10% (100 mg/ml) in 3-ml automatic injection device or 5-ml ampules
Injection (for I.V. admixtures): 4% (40 mg/ml) in 25-ml (1-g) vials and syringes and 50-ml (2-g) vials and syringes; 10% (100 mg/ml) in 10-ml (1-g) vials; 20% (200 mg/ml) in 5-ml (1-g) vials and syringes and 10-ml (2-g) vials and syringes
Infusion (premixed): 0.2% (2 mg/ml) in 500-ml vials; 0.4% (4 mg/ml) in 250-ml, 500-ml, 1,000-ml vials; 0.8% (8 mg/ml) in 250-ml, 500-ml vials

ACTION

Mechanism: A class Ib antiarrhythmic that depresses phase O and shortens the action potential. All class I drugs have membrane-stabilizing effects.
Onset: within 90 seconds of a bolus dose. **Peak:** Without a bolus loading dose, peak serum levels occur within 30 to 60 minutes of starting an I.V. infusion. After an I.M. injection, plasma levels peak in about 10 minutes. **Duration:** effects of bolus dose, 10 to 20 minutes; effective blood levels persist for about 60 minutes after an I.M. injection.

INDICATIONS & DOSAGE

Ventricular arrhythmias from MI, cardiac manipulation, or digitalis glycosides; ventricular tachycardia –
Adults: 50 to 100 mg (1 to 1.5 mg/kg) by I.V. bolus at 25 to 50 mg/minute. Give half this amount to elderly patients or patients under 50 kg and to those with CHF or hepatic disease. Repeat bolus q 3 to 5 minutes until arrhythmias subside or adverse reactions develop. Don't exceed 300-mg total bolus during a 1-hour period. Simultaneously, begin constant infusion of 20 to 50 mcg/kg/minute (1 to 4 mg/minute). If single bolus has been given, repeat smaller bolus 15 to 20 minutes after start of infusion to maintain therapeutic serum level. After 24 hours of continuous infusion, decrease rate by half. Alternatively, give 200 to 300 mg I.M.
Children: 1 mg/kg by I.V. bolus, followed by infusion of 30 mcg/kg/minute.

ADVERSE REACTIONS

CNS: *confusion, tremor,* lethargy, somnolence, *stupor, restlessness,* slurred speech, euphoria, depression, *light-headedness,* paresthesia, muscle twitching, ***seizures.***
CV: *hypotension,* bradycardia, ***new or worsened arrhythmias.***
EENT: *tinnitus, blurred or double vision.*
Other: ***anaphylaxis,*** soreness at injection site, sensation of cold, diaphoresis.

INTERACTIONS

Beta blockers, cimetidine: decreased metabolism of lidocaine. Monitor for toxicity.

Phenytoin, procainamide, propranolol, quinidine: additive cardiac depressant effects. Monitor carefully.

CONTRAINDICATIONS

• Contraindicated in patients who are allergic to related local anesthetics of the amide type, such as Nupercaine, and with epinephrine (for local anesthesia) to treat arrhythmias. Do not use for ventricular escape beats; use atropine instead.

• Use cautiously in patients with complete or second-degree heart block or sinus bradycardia and in elderly patients, those with CHF or renal or hepatic disease, or those who weigh under 50 kg. Reduce dosage in these patients.

NURSING CONSIDERATIONS

• In many severely ill patients, seizures may be the first clinical sign of toxicity. However, severe reactions usually are preceded by somnolence, confusion, and paresthesia.

• If signs of toxicity (such as dizziness) occur, stop drug at once and notify the doctor. Continued infusion could lead to seizures and coma. Give oxygen via nasal cannula, if not contraindicated. Keep oxygen and cardiopulmonary resuscitation equipment available.

• Monitor the patient's response, especially blood pressure and serum electrolytes, BUN, and creatinine levels. Notify the doctor promptly if abnormalities develop.

• Discontinue infusion and notify the doctor if arrhythmias worsen or ECG changes, such as widening QRS complex or substantially prolonged PR interval, are evident.

• A bolus dose not followed by an infusion will have a short-lived effect.

• A patient who has received lidocaine I.M. will show a seven-fold increase in serum CK level. Such an increase originates in the skeletal muscle, not the heart. Test isoenzymes if using I.M. route.

• Therapeutic serum levels are 2 to 5 mcg/ml.

• Give I.M. injections in the deltoid muscle only.

• **I.V. use:** Patients receiving infusions must be on a cardiac monitor and must be attended *at all times.* Use an infusion control device for administering infusion precisely. Do not exceed an infusion rate of 4 mg/minute; faster rate greatly increases risk of toxicity.

• Used investigationally to treat refractory status epilepticus.

mexiletine hydrochloride

Mexitil

Pregnancy Risk Category: C

HOW SUPPLIED

Capsules: 50 mg‡, 100 mg†, 150 mg, 200 mg, 250 mg

Injection: 250 mg/10 ml‡

ACTION

Mechanism: A class Ib antiarrhythmic that depresses phase O and shortens the action potential. All class I drugs have membrane-stabilizing effects.

Onset: ½ to 2 hours. **Peak:** Serum levels peak within 2 to 3 hours. **Duration:** elimination half-life, 10 to 12 hours.

INDICATIONS & DOSAGE

Refractory ventricular arrhythmias, including ventricular tachycardia and PVCs –

Adults: 200 to 400 mg P.O. followed by 200 mg q 8 hours. Increase dose, as ordered, to 400 mg q 8 hours if satisfactory control is not obtained. Patients who respond well to an every-

12-hour schedule may be given up to 450 mg q 12 hours.

Where available, mexiletine may be given I.V.‡ –

Adults: loading dose is 200 to 250 mg I.V. at a rate of 25 mg/minute. Then prepare an infusion solution of 250 mg mexiletine in 500 ml of D_5W and administer the first 120 ml (60 mg) over 1 hour. If clinical response is inadequate, give another bolus of 200 mg over 10 to 20 minutes. Maintenance dosage is 0.5 mg/minute (1 ml/ minute of prepared solution).

ADVERSE REACTIONS

CNS: *tremor, dizziness,* blurred vision, ataxia, diplopia, confusion, nystagmus, nervousness, headache.
CV: hypotension, bradycardia, widened QRS complex, ***new or worsened arrhythmias.***
GI: nausea, vomiting.
Skin: rash.

INTERACTIONS

Antacids, atropine, narcotics: slowed mexilitine absorption. Monitor for decreased mexilitine effectiveness.
Cimetidine: increased or decreased mexiletine blood levels. Monitor carefully.
Methylxanthines such as caffeine or theophylline: reduced clearance of methylxanthines, possibly resulting in toxicity. Monitor carefully.
Metoclopramide: mexiletine absorption may be accelerated. Monitor for toxicity.
Phenobarbital, phenytoin, rifampin, urinary acidifiers: decreased mexiletine blood levels. Monitor carefully.
Urine alkalinizers: increased mexiletine blood levels. Monitor carefully.

CONTRAINDICATIONS

- Contraindicated in patients with cardiogenic shock or preexisting second- or third-degree AV block in the absence of an artifical pacemaker.
- Use cautiously in patients with preexisting first-degree heart block, a ventricular pacemaker, preexisting sinus node dysfunction, intraventricular conduction disturbances, hypotension, or CHF.

NURSING CONSIDERATIONS

- An early sign of mexiletine toxicity is tremor, usually a fine tremor of the hands. This progresses to dizziness and later to ataxia and nystagmus as the drug's blood level increases. Question patients about these symptoms.
- Monitor blood pressure and heart rate and rhythm frequently. Notify the doctor of any significant change.
- When changing from lidocaine to mexiletine, stop the lidocaine infusion when the first mexiletine dose is given. Keep the infusion line open, however, until the arrhythmia appears to be satisfactorily controlled.
- To lessen GI distress, administer oral dose with meals.
- Therapeutic levels range from 0.75 to 2 mcg/ml.
- If you feel the patient is a good candidate for every-12-hour therapy, notify the doctor. Twice-daily dosage enhances compliance.
- **I.V. use:** Mexiletine injection is compatible with 0.9% sodium chloride, D_5W, 5% sodium bicarbonate, 1/6 M sodium lactate, and 10% fructose (levulose).

moricizine hydrochloride

Ethmozine

Pregnancy Risk Category: B

HOW SUPPLIED

Tablets: 200 mg, 250 mg, 300 mg

ACTION

Mechanism: A class I antiarrhythmic that reduces the fast inward current carried by sodium ions.
Onset: within 2 hours. **Peak:** Serum levels peak within ½ to 2 hours; effects, within 10 to 14 hours. **Dura-**

tion: serum half-life, about 2 hours; effects persist 10 to 24 hours after the last dose.

INDICATIONS & DOSAGE

Life-threatening ventricular arrhythmias –

Adults: individualized dosage is based on clinical response and patient tolerance. Therapy should begin in the hospital. Most patients respond to 600 to 900 mg P.O. daily in divided doses q 8 hours. Increase daily dosage q 3 days by 150 mg until the desired clinical effect is seen.

In patients with hepatic or renal impairment, start therapy at 600 mg or less P.O. daily. Monitor closely and adjust dosage carefully.

ADVERSE REACTIONS

CNS: *dizziness, headache, fatigue,* anxiety, hypoesthesia, asthenia, nervousness, paresthesia, sleep disorders.

CV: ***proarrhythmic events (ventricular tachycardia, PVCs),*** *ECG abnormalities (including conduction defects, sinus pause, junctional rhythm, or AV block),* ***CHF,*** *palpitations,* ***sustained ventricular tachycardia,*** *chest pain, sinus bradycardia,* ***sinus arrest.***

EENT: blurred vision.

GI: *nausea, vomiting, abdominal pain, dyspepsia, diarrhea, dry mouth.*

GU: urine retention.

Respiratory: dyspnea.

Skin: rash.

Other: drug-induced fever, diaphoresis, musculoskeletal pain.

INTERACTIONS

Cimetidine: increased plasma levels of and decreased clearance of moricizine. Begin moricizine therapy at low dosage (not more than 600 mg daily) and monitor plasma levels and therapeutic effect closely.

Digoxin, propranolol: additive prolongation of the PR interval. Monitor closely.

Theophylline: increased clearance and reduced plasma levels of theophylline. Monitor plasma levels and therapeutic response; adjust theophylline dosage as needed.

CONTRAINDICATIONS

- Contraindicated in patients with hypersensitivity to the drug and in those with preexisting second- or third-degree AV block, right bundle branch block when associated with left hemiblock (bifascicular block) unless an artificial pacemaker is present; severe hepatic insufficiency; and cardiogenic shock.
- Use with extreme caution in patients with sick sinus syndrome because drug may cause sinus bradycardia or sinus arrest in these patients. Also use with extreme caution in patients with coronary artery disease and left ventricular dysfunction because these patients may be at risk for sudden death when treated with the drug.

NURSING CONSIDERATIONS

- When substituting moricizine for another antiarrhythmic, withdraw previous drug for one to two of the drug's half-lives before starting moricizine at recommended dosage. Patients who have shown a tendency to develop life-threatening arrhythmias after withdrawal of drug therapy should be hospitalized during withdrawal and adjustment to morizicine. Start moricizine therapy after:

  – disopyramide, 6 to 12 hours after the last dose.

  – mexiletine, 8 to 12 hours after the last dose.

  – procainamide, 3 to 6 hours after the last dose.

  – propafenone, 8 to 12 hours after the last dose.

  – quinidine, 6 to 12 hours after the last dose.

  – tocainide, 8 to 12 hours after the last dose.

• Hypokalemia, hyperkalemia, and hypomagnesemia may alter the effects of the drug. Determine electrolyte status and correct imbalances before therapy.
• Patients with hepatic or renal dysfunction will have decreased moricizine clearance. Administer cautiously and monitor effects closely.
• Because drug has been detected in breast milk, a decision should be made to discontinue breast-feeding or discontinue the drug, depending on drug's potential benefit to the mother.

procainamide hydrochloride

Procainamide Durules‡, Procan SR, Promine, Pronestyl**, Pronestyl-SR

Pregnancy Risk Category: C

HOW SUPPLIED

Tablets: 250 mg, 375 mg, 500 mg
Tablets (sustained-release): 250 mg, 500 mg, 750 mg, 1,000 mg
Capsules: 250 mg, 375 mg, 500 mg
Injection: 100 mg/ml, 500 mg/ml

ACTION

Mechanism: A class Ia antiarrhythmic that depresses phase O and prolongs the action potential. All class I drugs have membrane stabilizing effects.

Onset: within 2 minutes of I.V. injection, 10 to 30 minutes of I.M. injection, or 2 hours of oral dose. **Peak:** Peak serum levels occur immediately after I.V. infusion, 15 to 60 minutes after I.M. injection, or 45 minutes to 2½ hours after oral dose. **Duration:** elimination half-life, 2½ to 5 hours; half-life of its active metabolite N-acetylprocainamide (NAPA), about 7 hours.

INDICATIONS & DOSAGE

PVCs, ventricular tachycardia, atrial arrhythmias unresponsive to quinidine, paroxysmal atrial tachycardia – **Adults:** 100 mg by slow I.V. push q 5 minutes, no faster than 25 to 50 mg/minute until arrhythmias disappear, adverse reactions develop, or 1 g has been given. Usual effective dose is 500 to 600 mg. When arrhythmias disappear, give continuous infusion of 2 to 6 mg/minute. If arrhythmias recur, repeat bolus as above and increase infusion rate; give 0.5 to 1 g I.M. q 4 to 8 hours until oral therapy begins.

Loading dose for atrial fibrillation or paroxysmal atrial tachycardia is 1 to 1.25 g P.O. If arrhythmias persist after 1 hour, give additional 750 mg. If no change occurs, give 500 mg to 1 g q 2 hours until arrhythmias disappear or adverse reactions occur.

Loading dose for ventricular tachycardia is 1 g P.O. Maintenance dosage is 50 mg/kg daily q 3 hours; average is 250 to 500 mg q 3 hours.

Note: Sustained-release tablet may be used for maintenance dosing when treating ventricular tachycardia, atrial fibrillation, and paroxysmal atrial tachycardia. Dosage is 500 mg to 1 g q 6 hours.

In patients with renal or hepatic dysfunction, decrease dose and give over 6 hours.

ADVERSE REACTIONS

CNS: hallucinations, confusion, ***seizures,*** depression.
CV: ***severe hypotension,*** *bradycardia,* AV block, ***ventricular fibrillation*** (after parenteral use).
GI: with high doses – nausea, vomiting, anorexia, diarrhea, bitter taste.
Hematologic: thrombocytopenia, ***neutropenia*** (especially with sustained-release forms), ***agranulocytosis, hemolytic anemia,*** *increased antinuclear antibody (ANA) titer.*
Skin: *maculopapular rash.*

Other: *fever, lupuslike syndrome (especially after prolonged administration), myalgia.*

INTERACTIONS

Amiodarone: increased procainamide levels and toxicity; additive effects on QT and QRS intervals. Avoid concomitant use.
Anticholinergics: additive anticholinergic effects.
Anticholinesterase agents: anticholinesterase dosage may need to be increased.
Cimetidine: may increase procainamide blood levels. Monitor for toxicity.
Neuromuscular blockers: increased skeletal muscle relaxant effects. Monitor the patient closely.

CONTRAINDICATIONS

- Contraindicated in patients with hypersensitivity to procaine and related drugs; in those with complete, second-, or third-degree heart block in the absence of an artificial pacemaker; and in patients with myasthenia gravis. Also contraindicated in patients with atypical ventricular tachycardia (torsades de pointes) because procainamide may aggravate this condition.
- Use with extreme caution when treating patients with ventricular tachycardia during coronary occlusion.
- Use cautiously in patients with CHF or other conduction disturbances, such as bundle-branch heart block, sinus bradycardia, or digitalis glycoside intoxication, or with hepatic or renal insufficiency. Also use cautiously in those with preexisting blood dyscrasias or bone marrow suppression.

NURSING CONSIDERATIONS

- Hypokalemia predisposes patients to arrhythmias; therefore, monitor serum electrolytes, especially potassium level.
- Monitor plasma levels of procainamide and its active metabolite NAPA. To suppress ventricular arrhythmias, therapeutic serum concentrations of procainamide are 4 to 8 mcg/ml; therapeutic levels of NAPA are 10 to 30 mcg/ml.
- Monitor CBC frequently during first 3 months of therapy, particularly in patients taking sustained-release dosage forms.
- Monitor QT interval closely in patients with renal failure.
- Elderly patients may be more likely to develop hypotension. Monitor blood pressure carefully.
- Positive ANA titer is common in about 60% of patients who don't have symptoms of lupuslike syndrome. This response seems to be related to prolonged use, not dosage. May progress to systemic lupus erythematosus if drug is not discontinued.
- After prolonged atrial fibrillation, restoration of normal rhythm may result in thromboembolism caused by dislodgment of thrombi from atrial wall. Anticoagulation is usually advised before giving procainamide for atrial fibrillation to normalize sinus rhythm.
- Instruct patients to report fever, rash, muscle pain, diarrhea, bleeding, bruises, or pleuritic chest pain.
- Stress to patients the importance of taking the drug exactly as prescribed. This may require use of an alarm clock for night doses.
- Reassure patients who are taking the extended-release form of procainamide that a wax-matrix "ghost" from the tablet may be passed in the stool. The drug is completely absorbed before this occurs.
- **I.V. use:** Patients receiving infusions must be attended *at all times.* Use an infusion control device to administer the infusion precisely.
- Monitor blood pressure and ECG

continuously during I.V. administration. Watch for prolonged QT and QRS intervals, heart block, or increased arrhythmias. If these occur, withhold drug, obtain rhythm strip, and notify the doctor immediately.
- Keep patients in the supine position during I.V. administration. If drug is given too rapidly, hypotension can occur. Watch closely for adverse reactions during infusion and notify the doctor if they occur.
- If procainamide solution becomes discolored, check with pharmacy and prepare to discard.
- Note that the vials for I.V. injection contain 1 g of drug: 100 mg/ml (10 ml) or 500 mg/ml (2 ml).

propafenone hydrochloride

Rythmol

Pregnancy Risk Category: C

HOW SUPPLIED

Tablets: 150 mg, 300 mg

ACTION

Mechanism: A class Ic antiarrhythmic that stabilizes cardiac cell membranes, probably by decreasing sodium influx. It also has weak beta-adrenergic blocking properties.
Onset: within 2 hours. **Peak:** Plasma levels peak within 3½ hours. Steady-state levels are reached after 4 to 5 days of therapy. **Duration:** elimination half-life in most patients, 2 to 10 hours; in < 10% of patients, 10 to 32 hours.

INDICATIONS & DOSAGE

Suppression of life-threatening ventricular arrhythmias, such as sustained ventricular tachycardia –
Adults: initially, 150 mg P.O. q 8 hours. Dosage may be increased at 3- to 4-day intervals to 225 mg q 8 hours, if necessary, increase dosage to 300 mg q 8 hours. Maximum daily dosage is 900 mg.

ADVERSE REACTIONS

CNS: anorexia, anxiety, ataxia, dizziness, drowsiness, fatigue, headache, insomnia, syncope, tremor, weakness.
CV: atrial fibrillation, bradycardia, bundle-branch heart block, ***CHF,*** chest pain, edema, first-degree AV block, hypotension, increased QRS duration, intraventricular conduction delay, palpitations, ***proarrhythmic events (ventricular tachycardia, PVCs).***
EENT: blurred vision.
GI: abdominal pain or cramps, constipation, diarrhea, dyspepsia, flatulence, nausea, vomiting, dry mouth, unusual taste.
Respiratory: dyspnea.
Skin: rash.
Other: diaphoresis, joint pain.

INTERACTIONS

Antiarrhythmics: increased potential for CHF.
Cimetidine: decreased metabolism of propafenone.
Digitalis glycosides, oral anticoagulants: propafenone may increase serum levels of these agents by about 35% to 85%, resulting in toxicity.
Local anesthetics: increased risk of CNS toxicity.
Metoprolol, propranolol: propafenone slows the metabolism of these agents. Adjust dosage as necessary and as ordered.
Quinidine: slowed metabolism of propafenone. Avoid concomitant use.
Rifampin: increased clearance of propafenone. Monitor closely.

CONTRAINDICATIONS

- Contraindicated in patients with hypersensitivity to the drug and in those with severe or uncontrolled CHF; cardiogenic shock; SA, AV, or intraventricular disorders of impulse conduction; sinus node dysfunction in the absence of a pacemaker; severe bradycardia (50 beats/minute or less); marked hypotension; bronchospastic

disorders; severe obstructive pulmonary disease; severe electrolyte imbalance; and severe hepatic failure.
• Use cautiously in patients with CHF because propafenone can exert a negative inotropic effect on the heart. Also use cautiously in patients taking other cardiac depressant drugs and in those with hepatic or renal failure.

NURSING CONSIDERATIONS
• Continuous cardiac monitoring is recommended during initiation of therapy and during dosage adjustments. If PR interval or QRS duration increases by more than 25%, a reduction in dosage may be necessary.
• During concomitant use with digoxin, frequently monitor ECG and serum digoxin levels.
• To minimize adverse GI reactions, administer drug with food.

quinidine bisulfate
(66.4% quinidine base)
Biquin Durules†, Kinidin Durules‡

quinidine gluconate
(62% quinidine base)
Duraquin, Quinaglute Dura-Tabs, Quinalan, Quinate†

quinidine polygalacturonate
(60.5% quinidine base)
Cardioquin

quinidine sulfate
(83% quinidine base)
Apo-Quinidine†, Cin-Quin, Novoquindin†, Quine, Quinidex Extentabs, Quinora

Pregnancy Risk Category: C

HOW SUPPLIED
bisulfate
Tablets (extended-release): 250 mg†‡
gluconate
Tablets (extended-release): 324 mg, 325 mg†, 330 mg
Injection: 80 mg/ml
polygalacturonate
Tablets: 275 mg
sulfate
Tablets: 100 mg, 200 mg, 300 mg
Tablets (extended-release): 300 mg
Capsules: 200 mg, 300 mg
Injection: 200 mg/ml

ACTION
Mechanism: A class Ia antiarrhythmic that depresses phase O and prolongs the action potential. All class I drugs have membrane-stabilizing effects.
Onset: 1 to 3 hours after oral administration. **Peak:** Peak plasma levels occur immediately after I.V. injection, within 1 to 2 hours after oral dose. **Duration:** 6 to 8 hours after oral dose.

INDICATIONS & DOSAGE
Atrial flutter or fibrillation –
Adults: 200 mg quinidine sulfate or equivalent base P.O. q 2 to 3 hours for five to eight doses, with subsequent daily increases until sinus rhythm is restored or toxic effects develop. Administer quinidine only after digitalization to avoid increasing AV conduction. Maximum dosage is 3 to 4 g daily.
Paroxysmal supraventricular tachycardia –
Adults: 400 to 600 mg I.M. gluconate q 2 to 3 hours until toxic adverse reactions develop or arrhythmia subsides.
Premature atrial and ventricular contractions; paroxysmal AV junctional rhythm; paroxysmal atrial tachycardia; paroxysmal ventricular tachycardia; maintenance after cardioversion of atrial fibrillation or flutter –
Adults: test dose is 50 to 200 mg P.O., then monitor vital signs before beginning therapy. Quinidine sulfate or equivalent base 200 to 400 mg P.O. q 4 to 6 hours; or initially, quinidine gluconate 600 mg I.M., then up to

400 mg q 2 hours, p.r.n.; or quinidine gluconate 800 mg (10 ml of the commercially available solution) added to 40 ml of D_5W, infused I.V. at 16 mg (1 ml)/minute.
Children: test dose is 2 mg/kg; 3 to 6 mg/kg q 2 to 3 hours for five doses P.O. daily.
Severe Plasmodium falciparum *malaria* –
Adults: 10 mg/kg gluconate I.V. diluted in 250 ml of 0.9% sodium chloride and infused over 1 to 2 hours, followed by a continuous maintenance infusion of 0.02 mg/kg/minute for 72 hours or until parasitemia is reduced to less than 1%.

Patients with impaired hepatic function and those with CHF require a reduced dosage.

ADVERSE REACTIONS

CNS: *vertigo, headache, light-headedness,* confusion, restlessness, cold sweats, pallor, fainting, dementia.
CV: ***PVCs; ventricular tachycardia; atypical ventricular tachycardia (torsades de pointes); severe hypotension;*** *SA and AV block;* ***ventricular fibrillation,*** *tachycardia;* ***aggravated CHF;*** *ECG changes (particularly widening of QRS complex, notched P waves, widened QT interval, ST-segment depression).*
EENT: *tinnitus,* excessive salivation, blurred vision.
GI: *diarrhea, nausea, vomiting,* anorexia, abdominal pain.
Hematologic: ***hemolytic anemia, thrombocytopenia, agranulocytosis.***
Hepatic: ***hepatotoxicity.***
Respiratory: acute asthmatic attack, ***respiratory arrest.***
Skin: rash, petechial hemorrhage of buccal mucosa, pruritus.
Other: angioedema, *fever, cinchonism.*

INTERACTIONS

Acetazolamide, antacids, sodium bicarbonate, thiazide diuretics: may increase quinidine blood levels because of alkaline urine. Monitor for increased effect.
Amiodarone, cimetidine: increased serum quinidine levels. Monitor for increased effect.
Barbiturates, phenytoin, rifampin: may lower blood levels of quinidine. Monitor for decreased quinidine effect.
Digoxin: increased serum digoxin levels after initiating quinidine therapy. Monitor closely.
Nifedipine: may decrease quinidine blood levels. Monitor carefully.
Other antiarrhythmics, such as lidocaine, phenytoin, procainamide, and propranolol: increased risk of toxicity. Use together cautiously.
Verapamil: may result in hypotension. Monitor blood pressure.
Warfarin: increased anticoagulant effect. Monitor closely.

CONTRAINDICATIONS

- Contraindicated in patients with digitalis glycoside toxicity when AV conduction is grossly impaired and in patients with complete AV block with AV nodal or idioventricular pacemaker.
- Use cautiously in patients with myasthenia gravis. Anticholinesterase drug doses may have to be increased.
- Use cautiously in patients receiving digitalis glycosides because quinidine may increase serum digitalis levels.

NURSING CONSIDERATIONS

- Check apical pulse rate and blood pressure before starting therapy. If you detect extremes in pulse rate, withhold drug and notify the doctor at once.
- Therapeutic plasma levels for antiarrhythmic effects are 2 to 5 mcg/ml.
- Monitor liver function tests during the first 4 to 8 weeks of therapy.
- When used to treat severe malaria, patients should be hospitalized in an intensive-care setting. Continuous

monitoring is necessary. Decrease infusion rate if plasma quinidine level exceeds 6 mcg/ml, uncorrected QT interval exceeds 0.6 second, or QRS widening exceeds 25% of baseline.
• When changing route of administration, alter dosage to compensate for variations in quinidine base content.
• Lidocaine may be effective in treating quinidine-induced arrhythmias because it increases AV conduction.
• Adverse GI reactions, especially diarrhea, are signs of toxicity. Notify the doctor. Check quinidine blood levels, which are toxic when greater than 8 mcg/ml. GI symptoms may be decreased by giving drug with meals. Monitor patient response carefully.
• Anticoagulation is commonly advised before quinidine therapy in long-standing atrial fibrillation because restoration of normal sinus rhythm may result in thromboembolism caused by dislodgment of thrombi from atrial wall.
• Never use discolored (brownish) quinidine solution.
• Store away from heat and direct light.

sotalol

Betapace, Sotacor†‡

Pregnancy Risk Category: B

HOW SUPPLIED

Tablets: 80 mg, 160 mg, 240 mg

ACTION

Mechanism: A nonselective beta-adrenergic blocker that depresses sinus heart rate, slows AV conduction, decreases cardiac output, and lowers systolic and diastolic blood pressure.
Onset: within 4 hours. **Peak:** Peak plasma levels occur within 2½ to 4 hours. Steady-state levels are reached in 2 to 3 days. **Duration:** elimination half-life, 12 hours; effects persist up to 24 hours.

INDICATIONS & DOSAGE

Documented, life-threatening ventricular arrhythmias –
Adults: initially, 80 mg P.O. b.i.d. Increase dosage q 2 to 3 days as needed and tolerated; most patients respond to daily dosage of 160 to 320 mg. A few patients with refractory arrhythmias have received as much as 640 mg daily.

In patients with renal failure: If creatinine clearance is greater than 60 ml/minute/1.73 m^2, no adjustment in dosage interval is necessary. If creatinine clearance is 30 to 60 ml/minute/ 1.73 m^2, give q 24 hours; 10 to 30 ml/ minute/1.73 m^2, q 36 to 48 hours; less than 10 ml/minute/1.73 m^2, individualize dosage.

Hypertension† –
Adults: 80 mg P.O. b.i.d. Increase dosage at weekly intervals in 80-mg increments b.i.d. as needed and tolerated. Most patients respond to daily dosage of 160 to 320 mg; patients taking 320 mg or less daily may take drug as a single morning dose.

Angina† –
Adults: 80 mg P.O. b.i.d. Increase dosage at weekly intervals in 80-mg increments b.i.d. as needed and tolerated. Most patients respond to doses of 160 mg b.i.d.; maximum daily dosage is 480 mg.

ADVERSE REACTIONS

CNS: *asthenia, headache, dizziness, weakness, fatigue.*
CV: *bradycardia,* ***arrhythmias, CHF, AV block, proarrhythmic events (ventricular tachycardia, PVCs).***
GI: *nausea.*
Respiratory: *dyspnea,* ***bronchospasm.***

INTERACTIONS

Antiarrhythmics: additive effects. Avoid concomitant use.
Antihypertensives; catecholamine-depleting drugs, such as reserpine and

*Liquid form contains alcohol. *Common* reactions are in italics; ***life-threatening,*** in bold italics.
**May contain tartrazine.

guanethidine: enhanced hypotensive effects. Monitor closely.
Calcium channel antagonists: enhanced myocardial depression. Avoid concomitant use.
Clonidine: beta blockers may enhance the rebound effect seen after withdrawal of clonidine. Discontinue sotalol several days before withdrawing clonidine.
General anesthetics: may cause additional myocardial depression. Monitor closely.

CONTRAINDICATIONS
- Contraindicated in patients with severe sinus node dysfunction, sinus bradycardia, second- and third-degree AV block in the absence of an artificial pacemaker, congenital or acquired long QT syndrome, cardiogenic shock, CHF, hypokalemia, hypomagnesemia, bronchial asthma, and allergic rhinitis.
- Use cautiously in patients with renal impairment.
- Also use cautiously in patients with diabetes mellitus. Beta blockers may mask signs and symptoms of hypoglycemia.

NURSING CONSIDERATIONS
- Adjust dosage slowly, allowing 2 to 3 days between dosage increments for adequate monitoring of QT intervals and for plasma levels of drug to reach steady state.
- Because proarrhythmic events may occur at start of therapy and during dosage adjustments, patient should be hospitalized. Facilities and personnel should be available for cardiac rhythm monitoring and interpretation of ECG waveforms.
- Although patients receiving I.V. lidocaine have started sotalol therapy without ill effect, other antiarrhythmic drugs should be withdrawn before therapy with sotalol. Sotalol therapy typically is delayed until two or three half-lives of the withdrawn drug have elapsed. After withdrawal of amiodarone, sotalol shouldn't be administered until the QT interval normalizes.
- Monitor serum electrolytes regularly, especially if patient is receiving diuretics. Electrolyte imbalances, such as hypokalemia or hypomagnesemia, may enhance QT prolongation and increase risk of serious arrhythmias, such as torsades de pointes.
- Explain to patients the importance of taking this drug as prescribed, even when they are feeling well. Caution patients not to discontinue drug suddenly.
- Because food can interfere with absorption, tell patients to take this drug on an empty stomach, 1 hour before or 2 hours after meals.

tocainide hydrochloride
Tonocard

Pregnancy Risk Category: C

HOW SUPPLIED
Tablets: 400 mg, 600 mg

ACTION
Mechanism: A class Ib antiarrhythmic that depresses phase O and shortens the action potential. All class I drugs have membrane-stabilizing effects.
Onset: within 2 hours. **Peak:** Plasma levels peak ½ to 2 hours after an oral dose. **Duration:** plasma half-life, about 15 hours.

INDICATIONS & DOSAGE
Suppression of symptomatic ventricular arrhythmias, including frequent PVCs and ventricular tachycardia – **Adults:** initially, 400 mg P.O. q 8 hours. Usual dosage is between 1,200 and 1,800 mg daily in three divided doses.

ADVERSE REACTIONS
CNS: *light-headedness, tremor,* restlessness, paresthesia, confusion, dizziness.
CV: hypotension, ***new or worsened arrhythmias, CHF.***
EENT: blurred vision.
GI: *nausea, vomiting, epigastric pain,* constipation, diarrhea, anorexia.
Hematologic: ***blood dyscrasias, including aplastic anemia.***
Hepatic: hepatitis.
Respiratory: ***respiratory arrest, pulmonary fibrosis, pneumonitis, pulmonary edema.***
Skin: rash.

INTERACTIONS
Beta blockers: decreased myocardial contractility; increased CNS toxicity.

CONTRAINDICATIONS
• Contraindicated in patients with hypersensitivity to lidocaine or other amide-type local anesthetics and in those with second- or third-degree AV block in the absence of an artificial pacemaker.
• Use cautiously in patients with CHF or diminished cardiac reserve and in those with hepatic or renal impairment. These patients may often be treated effectively with a lower dose.

NURSING CONSIDERATIONS
• Considered by cardiologists as an "oral lidocaine." May ease transition from I.V. lidocaine to oral antiarrhythmic therapy. Monitor the patient carefully during this transition period.
• Therapeutic blood levels range from 4 to 10 mcg/ml.
• Agranulocytosis and bone marrow suppression have been reported in patients taking usual doses of the drug. Most cases have been reported within the first 12 weeks of therapy. Tell the patient to report immediately any unusual bruising or bleeding, or signs of infection.
• Drug has been associated with serious pulmonary toxicity. Tell the patient to report sudden onset of any pulmonary symptoms, such as coughing, wheezing, or exertional dyspnea.
• Dizziness and falling are more likely to occur in elderly patients.
• Monitor the patient for tremor, which may indicate that the maximum dose has been reached.

21

Antianginals

amlodipine besylate
bepridil hydrochloride
diltiazem hydrochloride
erythrityl tetranitrate
isosorbide dinitrate
isosorbide mononitrate
nadolol
nicardipine
nifedipine
nitroglycerin
pentaerythritol tetranitrate
propranolol hydrochloride
verapamil
verapamil hydrochloride

COMBINATION PRODUCTS

ANGIJEN NO. 1: pentaerythritol tetranitrate 20 mg and phenobarbital sodium 15 mg.
ARCOTRATE NO. 3: pentaerythritol tetranitrate 20 mg and phenobarbital sodium 8 mg.
BITRATE: pentaerythritol tetranitrate 15 mg and phenobarbital sodium 20 mg.
DIMYCOR: pentaerythritol tetranitrate 10 mg and phenobarbital sodium 15 mg.
NITROTYM-PLUS: nitroglycerin 2.5 mg and butabarbital sodium 48 mg.
PERBUZEM: pentaerythritol tetranitrate 10 mg and butabarbital sodium 15 mg.

amlodipine besylate

Norvasc

Pregnancy Risk Category: C

HOW SUPPLIED

Tablets: 2.5 mg, 5 mg, 10 mg

ACTION

Mechanism: Inhibits calcium ion influx across cardiac and smooth muscle cells, thus decreasing myocardial contractility and oxygen demand. Also dilates coronary arteries and arterioles.
Onset: 60 to 90 minutes. **Duration:** effects persist about 24 hours.

INDICATIONS & DOSAGE

Chronic stable angina; vasospastic angina (Prinzmetal's or variant angina) –
Adults: initially, 10 mg P.O. daily. Small, frail, or elderly patients or patients with hepatic insufficiency should begin therapy at 5 mg daily. Most patients require 10 mg daily for adequate therapy.
Hypertension –
Adults: initially, 5 mg P.O. daily. Small, frail, or elderly patients; patients currently receiving other antihypertensives; or patients with hepatic insufficiency should begin therapy at 2.5 mg daily. Adjust dosage according to patient response and tolerance. Maximum daily dosage is 10 mg.

ADVERSE REACTIONS

CNS: *headache,* fatigue, somnolence.
CV: *edema,* dizziness, flushing, palpitation.
GI: nausea, abdominal pain.

INTERACTIONS

None significant.

CONTRAINDICATIONS

- Contraindicated in patients with hypersensitivity to the drug.
- Use cautiously in patients receiving other peripheral vasodilators, especially those with severe aortic stenosis, and in those with CHF. Because drug is metabolized by the liver, also use cautiously and in reduced dosage in patients with severe hepatic disease.

NURSING CONSIDERATIONS

- Some patients, especially those with severe obstructive coronary artery disease, have developed increased frequency, duration, or severity of angina or even acute MI after initiation of calcium channel blocker therapy or at time of dosage increase. Monitor the patient carefully.
- Notify the doctor if signs of CHF occur, such as swelling of hands and feet or shortness of breath.
- Sublingual nitroglycerin may be taken as needed when anginal symptoms are acute. If the patient continues nitrate therapy during titration of amlodipine dosage, urge continued compliance.
- Monitor blood pressure frequently during initiation of therapy. Because drug-induced vasodilation has a gradual onset, acute hypotension is rare.
- Caution patients to continue taking the drug, even when they are feeling better.

bepridil hydrochloride

Bepadin‡, Vascor

Pregnancy Risk Category: C

HOW SUPPLIED

Tablets: 200 mg, 300 mg, 400 mg

ACTION

Mechanism: A calcium channel blocker that inhibits calcium ion influx across cardiac and smooth muscle cells.

Peak: Plasma levels peak within 2 to 3 hours. Steady-state levels are reached after 8 days. **Duration:** half-life, about 42 hours.

INDICATIONS & DOSAGE

Chronic stable angina in patients who cannot tolerate or who fail to respond to other agents –

Adults: initially, 200 mg P.O. daily. After 10 days, increase dosage based on response. Maintenance dosage in most patients is 300 mg/day. Maximum daily dosage is 400 mg.

ADVERSE REACTIONS

CNS: dizziness.

CV: edema, flushing, palpitations, tachycardia, ***ventricular arrhythmias, including torsades de pointes.***

GI: nausea, diarrhea.

Hematologic: ***agranulocytosis.***

Skin: rash.

Other: dyspnea.

INTERACTIONS

Fentanyl anesthesia: severe hypotension has been reported with concomitant use of a beta blocker and a calcium channel blocker. Inform anesthesiologist that the patient is taking a calcium channel blocker.

CONTRAINDICATIONS

- Contraindicated in patients with hypersensitivity to the drug.
- Use cautiously in patients with CHF, especially if the patient is also receiving a beta blocker.

NURSING CONSIDERATIONS

- Bepridil is not considered a primary agent because it has been associated with severe ventricular arrhythmias, including torsades de pointes; also associated with agranulocytosis.
- Elderly patients may require more frequent monitoring to prevent adverse reactions.
- Tell patients to promptly report any unusual bruising or bleeding or signs of persistent infections, including sore throat, fever, or malaise.

diltiazem hydrochloride

Cardizem, Cardizem CD, Cardizem SR, Dilacor XR, Vasocardol SR‡

Pregnancy Risk Category: C

HOW SUPPLIED

Tablets: 30 mg, 60 mg, 90 mg, 120 mg
Capsules (extended-release; Cardizem CD): 120 mg, 180 mg, 240 mg, 300 mg
Capsules (sustained-release; Cardizem SR, Dilacor XR, Vasocardol SR‡): 60 mg, 90 mg, 120 mg
Injection: 5 mg/ml

ACTION

Mechanism: A calcium channel blocker that inhibits calcium ion influx across cardiac and smooth muscle cells, decreasing myocardial contractility and oxygen demand. Also dilates coronary arteries and arterioles.
Onset: about 3 minutes, after I.V. bolus injection, 30 to 60 minutes after oral administration of regular tablets, about 2 hours after extended- or sustained-release preparations. **Peak:** Drug action peaks 2 to 7 minutes after I.V. bolus injection. Peak plasma levels occur immediately after I.V. injection, 2 to 3 hours after regular tablet, 6 to 11 hours after sustained-release capsule, or 10 to 14 hours after extended-release capsule. **Duration:** elimination half-life, about 3½ hours after I.V injection or regular tablet, 5 to 7 hours after sustained-release capsule, or 8 hours after extended-release capsules. Effects persist 1 to 3 hours after I.V. bolus, up to 10 hours after I.V. infusion, 6 to 8 hours after regular tablet, about 12 hours after sustained-release capsule, about 24 hours after extended-release capsule.

INDICATIONS & DOSAGE

Vasospastic angina (Prinzmetal's or variant angina) and classic chronic stable angina pectoris –
Adults: 30 mg P.O. t.i.d. or q.i.d. before meals and h.s. Increase dosage gradually to maximum of 360 mg/day in divided doses. Alternatively, use 120 or 180 mg (dual-release capsule). Titrate as needed and tolerated to a maximum of 480 mg daily.
Hypertension –
Adults: 60 mg P.O. b.i.d. (sustained-release capsule). Titrate dosage to effect. Maximum recommended dosage is 360 mg/day. Alternatively, use 180 to 240 mg daily (extended-release capsule) initially. Adjust dosage as necessary. Maximum effect is seen within 14 days.
Atrial fibrillation or flutter; paroxysmal supraventricular tachycardia –
Adults: 0.25 mg/kg as a bolus injection over 2 minutes. If response is inadequate, give a dose of 0.35 mg/kg after 15 minutes and follow with a continuous infusion of 10 mg/hour. Some patients respond well to infusion rates of 5 mg/hour; do not exceed the maximum dose of 15 mg/hour.

ADVERSE REACTIONS

CNS: *headache, fatigue, drowsiness,* dizziness, nervousness, depression, insomnia, confusion.
CV: *edema, **arrhythmias,*** flushing, bradycardia, hypotension, conduction abnormalities, ***CHF.***
GI: *nausea, constipation,* vomiting, diarrhea.
GU: nocturia, polyuria.
Hepatic: transient elevation of liver enzymes.
Skin: *rash,* pruritus, photosensitivity.

INTERACTIONS

Cimetidine: may inhibit diltiazem metabolism. Monitor for toxicity.
Cyclosporine: diltiazem may increase serum cyclosporine levels, possibly by decreasing its metabolism, leading to increased risk of cyclosporine toxicity. Avoid concomitant use.
Digoxin: diltiazem may increase serum levels of digoxin. Monitor for toxicity.
Furosemide: forms a precipitate when mixed with diltiazem injection. Administer through separate I.V. lines.
Propranolol, other beta blockers: may

precipitate CHF or prolong cardiac conduction time. Use together cautiously.

CONTRAINDICATIONS

- Contraindicated in patients with sick sinus syndrome in the absence of an artificial pacemaker; in those with hypotension when systolic blood pressure is below 90 mm Hg; and in patients with second- or third-degree AV block.
- Use cautiously in elderly patients because duration of action may be prolonged; in patients with impaired ventricular function or conduction abnormalities; and in those with impaired hepatic or renal function.

NURSING CONSIDERATIONS

- Monitor blood pressure during initiation of therapy and dosage adjustments. Assist patients with ambulation during initiation of diltiazem therapy because dizziness may occur.
- If systolic blood pressure is below 90 mm Hg or heart rate is below 60 beats/minute, withhold dose and notify the doctor.
- If nitrate therapy is prescribed during titration of diltiazem dosage, urge patient compliance. Sublingual nitroglycerin, especially, may be taken concomitantly as needed when anginal symptoms are acute.
- Extended-release capsules (Cardizem CD) provide therapeutic levels of the drug over 24 hours.
- Although diltiazem may cause headaches, it is used for migraine prophylaxis in some patients.
- **I.V. use:** Infusions lasting longer than 24 hours are not recommended.

erythrityl tetranitrate

Cardilate

Pregnancy Risk Category: C

HOW SUPPLIED

Tablets (chewable): 10 mg
Tablets (oral, sublingual, buccal): 5 mg, 10 mg

ACTION

Mechanism: A nitrate that reduces cardiac oxygen demand by decreasing left ventricular end-diastolic pressure (preload) and, to a lesser extent, systemic vascular resistance (afterload). Drug also increases blood flow through the collateral coronary vessels.
Onset: within 5 minutes of S.L. administration, 15 to 30 minutes after oral administration. **Peak:** Peak effects occur within 15 minutes of S.L. administation or 60 minutes of oral administration. **Duration:** effective for up to 3 hours after S.L. administration, 6 hours after oral administration.

INDICATIONS & DOSAGE

Prophylaxis and long-term management of frequent or recurrent anginal pain, reduced exercise tolerance associated with angina pectoris –
Adults: 5 mg P.O., S.L., or buccally t.i.d., increasing in 2 to 3 days if needed.

ADVERSE REACTIONS

CNS: *headache, sometimes with throbbing; dizziness;* weakness.
CV: *orthostatic hypotension, tachycardia, flushing, palpitations,* fainting.
GI: nausea, vomiting.
Skin: cutaneous vasodilation.
Other: hypersensitivity reactions, sublingual burning.

INTERACTIONS

Ethanol: may increase hypotension. Avoid concomitant use.

CONTRAINDICATIONS

- Contraindicated in patients with hypersensitivity to nitrates; in patients

with head trauma or cerebral hemorrhage; and in those with severe anemia.
• Use cautiously in patients with hypotension.

NURSING CONSIDERATIONS
• Monitor blood pressure and intensity and duration of drug response.
• To prevent development of tolerance, a nitrate-free interval of 8 to 12 hours per day has been recommended.
• May cause headaches, especially at first; dosage may need to be reduced temporarily, but tolerance usually develops. Treat headache with aspirin or acetaminophen.
• Caution patients to take medication regularly, as prescribed, and to keep it accessible at all times.
• Advise patients that abrupt discontinuation of drug causes coronary vasospasm.
• Additional dose may be taken before anticipated stress or h.s. if angina is nocturnal.
• To minimize orthostatic hypotension, patients should change to upright position slowly. Advise patients to go up and down stairs carefully and to lie down at the first sign of dizziness.
• Tell patients to take an S.L. tablet at the first sign of an attack. The tablet should be wet with saliva and placed under the tongue until completely absorbed, and the patient should sit down and rest. Dose may be repeated every 10 to 15 minutes for a maximum of three doses. If drug doesn't provide relief, medical help should be obtained promptly.
• Patients who complain of tingling sensation with drug placed S.L. may try holding tablets in the buccal pouch.
• Advise patients to take oral tablets on an empty stomach, either ½ hour before or 1 to 2 hours after meals, and to swallow oral tablets whole.
• Store drug in a cool place, in a tightly closed container, away from light. To ensure freshness, replace supply every 3 months. Remove cotton from container because it absorbs drug.

isosorbide dinitrate

Apo-ISDN†, Cedocard-SR†, Coradur†, Coronex†, Dilatrate-SR, Iso-Bid, Isonate, Isorbid, Isordil, Isotrate, Nitro-Spray‡, Novosorbide†, Sorbitrate, Sorbitrate SA

isosorbide mononitrate

Imdur, Ismo, Monoket

Pregnancy Risk Category: C

HOW SUPPLIED
dinitrate
Tablets: 5 mg, 10 mg, 20 mg, 30 mg, 40 mg
Tablets (chewable): 5 mg, 10 mg
Tablets (sublingual): 2.5 mg, 5 mg, 10 mg
Tablets (sustained-release): 40 mg
Capsules: 40 mg
Capsules (sustained-release): 40 mg
Topical spray: 10%‡, 12.5 mg/metered spray‡
mononitrate
Tablets: 10 mg, 20 mg
Tablets (extended-release): 60 mg

ACTION
Mechanism: A nitrate that reduces cardiac oxygen demand by decreasing left ventricular end-diastolic pressure (preload) and, to a lesser extent, systemic vascular resistance (afterload). Drug also increases blood flow through the collateral coronary vessels.

Most of isosorbide dinitrate's pharmacologic activity is attributed to its active metabolite, isosorbide mononitrate.

Onset: isosorbide dinitrate – within 3 minutes after administration of S.L. or chewable form, 20 to 40 minutes after oral form, up to 4 hours after extended-release form. Isosorbide mononitrate – 30 to 60 minutes. **Duration:** isosorbide dinitrate – effective for 2 hours after administration of S.L. form, 30 minutes to 2 hours after chewable form, 4 to 6 hours after oral form, 6 to 8 hours after extended-release form. Isosorbide mononitrate – not determined.

INDICATIONS & DOSAGE

Acute anginal attacks (S.L. and chewable tablets of isosorbide dinitrate only); prophylaxis in situations likely to cause anginal attacks; chronic ischemic heart disease (by preload reduction) –

Adults: *S.L. form* – 2.5 to 10 mg under the tongue for prompt relief of anginal pain, repeated q 5 to 10 minutes (maximum of three doses for each 30-minute period). For prophylaxis, 2.5 to 10 mg q 2 to 3 hours.

Chewable form – 5 to 10 mg p.r.n. for acute attack or q 2 to 3 hours for prophylaxis, but only after initial test dose of 5 mg to determine risk of severe hypotension.

Oral form (isosorbide dinitrate) – 5 to 30 mg P.O. t.i.d. or q.i.d. for prophylaxis only (use smallest effective dose); 40 mg P.O. (sustained-release form) q 6 to 12 hours.

Oral form (isosorbide mononitrate) – 20 mg P.O. b.i.d., usually 7 hours apart (the first dose upon awakening).

Topical form (where available) – initially, 2 sprays to the chest in the morning from a distance of about 8″ (20 cm). Rub solution in. Increase dosage gradually as needed to 2 to 5 sprays, daily or b.i.d. (in the morning and h.s.).

Adjunct with other vasodilators, such as hydralazine and prazosin, in treatment of severe chronic CHF –

Adults: *Oral or chewable form* – 20 to 40 mg q 4 hours.

ADVERSE REACTIONS

CNS: *headache, sometimes with throbbing; dizziness;* weakness.

CV: *orthostatic hypotension, tachycardia, palpitations, ankle edema,* fainting.

GI: nausea, vomiting.

Skin: cutaneous vasodilation, *flushing.*

Other: hypersensitivity reactions, sublingual burning.

INTERACTIONS

Antihypertensives: possibly increased hypotensive effects. Monitor closely during initial therapy.

Ethanol: may increase hypotension. Avoid concomitant use.

CONTRAINDICATIONS

- Contraindicated in patients with hypersensitivity to nitrates; in those with head trauma or cerebral hemorrhage; and in patients with severe anemia.
- Use cautiously in patients with hypotension.

NURSING CONSIDERATIONS

- Monitor blood pressure and intensity and duration of drug response.
- To prevent development of tolerance, a nitrate-free interval of 8 to 12 hours per day has been recommended. The dosage regimen for isosorbide mononitrate (one tablet upon awakening; the second dose in 7 hours) is intended to minimize nitrate tolerance by providing a substantial nitrate-free interval.
- May cause headaches, especially at first. Dosage may need to be reduced temporarily, but tolerance usually develops. Treat headache with aspirin or acetaminophen.
- Caution patients to take medication regularly, as prescribed, and to keep it accessible at all times.
- Advise patients that abrupt discontinuation of drug causes coronary vasospams.
- An additional dose may be taken be-

fore anticipated stress or h.s. if angina is nocturnal.

- To minimize orthostatic hypotension, patients should change to upright position slowly. Advise patients to go up and down stairs carefully and to lie down at the first sign of dizziness.
- Tell patients to take an S.L. tablet at the first sign of an attack. The tablet should be wet with saliva and placed under the tongue until completely absorbed, and the patient should sit down and rest until pain subsides. Dose may be repeated every 10 to 15 minutes for a maximum of three doses. If drug doesn't provide relief, medical help should be obtained promptly.
- Patients who complain of tingling sensation with the drug placed S.L. may try holding a tablet in the buccal pouch.
- Warn the patient not to confuse S.L. with oral form.
- Teach the patient taking oral form of isosorbide dinitrate to take oral tablet on an empty stomach, either ½ before or 1 to 2 hours after meals; to swallow oral tablets whole; and to chew chewable tablets thoroughly before swallowing.
- Store in a cool place, in a tightly closed container, away from light.
- Has been used investigationally to treat diffuse esophageal spasms.

nadolol

Corgard, Syn-Nadolol†

Pregnancy Risk Category: C

HOW SUPPLIED

Tablets: 20 mg, 40 mg, 80 mg, 120 mg, 160 mg

ACTION

Mechanism: A beta-adrenergic blocker that reduces cardiac oxygen demand by blocking catecholamine-induced increases in heart rate, blood pressure, and force of myocardial contraction. Depresses renin secretion.

Onset: within 2 hours. **Peak:** Plasma levels peak within 2 to 4 hours. Steady-state levels are reached in 6 to 9 days. **Duration:** plasma half-life, 10 to 24 hours; effects may persist for a few days after last dose.

INDICATIONS & DOSAGE

Angina pectoris –

Adults: 40 mg P.O. once daily, initially. Increase dosage in 40- to 80-mg increments until optimum response occurs. Usual maintenance dosage range is 40 to 240 mg once daily.

Hypertension –

Adults: 40 mg P.O. once daily, initially. Increase dosage in 40- to 80-mg increments until optimum response occurs. Usual maintenance dosage range is 40 to 320 mg once daily. Doses of 640 mg may be necessary in rare cases.

ADVERSE REACTIONS

CNS: fatigue, lethargy.

CV: *bradycardia, hypotension, CHF,* peripheral vascular disease.

GI: nausea, vomiting, diarrhea.

Respiratory: *increased airway resistance.*

Skin: rash.

Other: fever.

INTERACTIONS

Antihypertensive: enhanced antihypertensive effect.

Digitalis glycosides: excessive bradycardia and additive effects on AV conduction. Use together cautiously.

Epinephrine: severe vasoconstriction and reflex bradycardia. Monitor blood pressure and observe the patient carefully.

Indomethacin: decreased antihypertensive effect. Monitor blood pressure and adjust dosage.

Insulin, oral antidiabetic agents: can alter dosage requirements in previously stabilized diabetics patients. Observe the patient carefully.

CONTRAINDICATIONS

- Contraindicated in patients with bronchial asthma, sinus bradycardia and greater than first-degree conduction block, and cardiogenic shock.
- Use cautiously in patients with heart failure, chronic bronchitis, or emphysema. Elderly patients may experience enhanced adverse reactions. Adjust dosage as needed in patients with renal insufficiency. Also use cautiously in diabetic patients because beta-adrenergic blockers may mask certain signs and symptoms of hypoglycemia.

NURSING CONSIDERATIONS

- Always check the patient's apical pulse before giving drug. If slower than 60 beats/minute, withhold drug and call the doctor.
- Monitor blood pressure frequently. If the patient develops severe hypotension, administer a vasopressor, as prescribed.
- Abrupt discontinuation can exacerbate angina and MI. Gradually reduce dosage over 1 to 2 weeks.
- Explain to patients the importance of taking the drug as prescribed, even when they are feeling well. Caution patients not to discontinue the drug suddenly.
- Nadolol masks common signs of shock and hyperthyroidism.
- Has been used in a limited number of patients with atrial flutter or fibrillation. Also has been used for a few patients to treat migraine headaches.

---

nicardipine

Cardene, Cardene SR

Pregnancy Risk Category: C

HOW SUPPLIED

Capsules (immediate-release): 20 mg, 30 mg

Capsules (sustained-release): 30 mg, 45 mg, 60 mg

ACTION

Mechanism: A calcium-channel blocker that inhibits calcium ion influx across cardiac and smooth muscle cells, decreasing myocardial contractility and oxygen demand. Also dilates coronary arteries and arterioles.

Onset: within 1 hour for both formulations. **Peak:** Serum levels peak within ½ to 2 hours after immediate-release capsules, 1 to 4 hours after sustained-release capsule. **Duration:** terminal elimination half-life, about 8½ hours for both formulations; effects of immediate-release product persist for 6 to 8 hours; of sustained-release preparation, up to 12 hours.

INDICATIONS & DOSAGE

Chronic stable angina (used alone or in combination with beta blockers) –

Adults: initially, 20 mg P.O. t.i.d. (immediate-release only). Titrate dosage according to patient response. Usual dosage range is 20 to 40 mg t.i.d.

Hypertension –

Adults: initially, 20 to 40 mg P.O. t.i.d. (immediate-release) or 30 mg b.i.d. (sustained-release). Increase dosage according to patient response.

In patients with renal impairment, titrate dosage slowly to achieve optimal response. Begin therapy with 20 mg P.O. t.i.d.

In patients with hepatic impairment, initially give 20 mg P.O. b.i.d. Then carefully titrate dosage to reach optimal response.

ADVERSE REACTIONS

CNS: dizziness, light-headedness, headache, paresthesia, drowsiness, asthenia.

CV: peripheral edema, palpitations, angina, tachycardia.

*Liquid form contains alcohol.
**May contain tartrazine.

Common reactions are in italics; ***life-threatening,*** in bold italics.

GI: nausea, abdominal discomfort, dry mouth.
Skin: rash, flushing.

INTERACTIONS

Antihypertensive: enhanced antihypertensive effect. Monitor patient closely.
Beta blockers: may increase cardiac depressant effects. Monitor the patient closely.
Cimetidine: may decrease metabolism of calcium channel blockers. Monitor for increased pharmacologic effect.
Cyclosporine: nicardipine may increase plasma levels of cyclosporine. Monitor for toxicity.
Theophylline: pharmacologic effects of theophylline may be enhanced. Monitor for toxicity.

CONTRAINDICATIONS

- Contraindicated in patients with hypersensitivity to the drug and in those with advanced aortic stenosis.
- Use cautiously in patients with cardiac conduction disturbances, hypotension, and CHF.

NURSING CONSIDERATIONS

- Some patients may experience increased frequency, severity, or duration of chest pain at beginning of therapy or during dosage adjustments. The mechanism for this adverse reaction is not known. Advise the patient to report chest pain immediately.
- Allow at least 3 days between dosage adjustments to achieve steady plasma levels.
- Measure blood pressure frequently during initial therapy. Maximum blood pressure response occurs about 1 hour after dosing with the immediate-release form and 2 to 4 hours with the sustained-release form. Check for potential orthostatic hypotension. Because large swings in blood pressure may occur based on blood level of drug, assess adequacy of antihypertensive effect 8 hours after dosing.
- When switching patients from the immediate-release form to the sustained-release preparation, the total daily dosage of the immediate-release form may be used as a guide; however, in many patients, it isn't a useful predictor of the total daily dosage of sustained-release drug. Individualize therapy and monitor closely.

nifedipine

Adalat, Adalat CC, Adalat FT†, Adalat P.A.†, Apo-Nifed, Nu-Nifed†, Novo-Nifedin, Procardia, Procardia XL

Pregnancy Risk Category: C

HOW SUPPLIED

Tablets (extended-release): 30 mg, 60 mg, 90 mg
Capsules: 10 mg, 20 mg

ACTION

Mechanism: Inhibits calcium ion influx across cardiac and smooth muscle cells, decreasing myocardial contractility and oxygen demand. Also dilates coronary arteries and arterioles.
Peak: Serum levels peak in ½ to 2 hours after capsules. **Duration:** effects persist for 4 to 8 hours after capsules; 16 to 24 hours after extended-release formulations.

INDICATIONS & DOSAGE

Vasospastic angina (also called Prinzmetal's or variant angina) and classic chronic stable angina pectoris; Raynaud's disease –
Adults: starting dose is 10 mg P.O. t.i.d. Usual effective dose range is 10 to 20 mg t.i.d. Some patients may require up to 30 mg q.i.d. Maximum daily dosage is 180 mg.
Hypertension –
Adults: 30 or 60 mg P.O. (extended-release form only) once daily. Titrate over a 7- to 14-day period.

ADVERSE REACTIONS

CNS: *dizziness, light-headedness, flushing, headache,* weakness, syncope.
CV: peripheral edema, hypotension, palpitations.
EENT: nasal congestion.
GI: *nausea, heartburn,* diarrhea.
Respiratory: dyspnea.
Other: muscle cramps, hypokalemia.

INTERACTIONS

Cimetidine, ranitidine: decreased nifedipine metabolism.
Propranolol, other beta blockers: may cause hypotension and heart failure. Use together cautiously.

CONTRAINDICATIONS

• Use cautiously in patients with CHF or hypotension; also use cautiously in elderly patients because duration of action may be prolonged.

NURSING CONSIDERATIONS

• Monitor blood pressure regularly, especially in patients who are also taking beta blockers or antihypertensives.
• Monitor serum potassium level regularly.
• Although rebound effect hasn't been observed when drug is stopped, dosage should still be reduced slowly under doctor's supervision.
• If the patient is kept on nitrate therapy while nifedipine dosage is being titrated, urge continued compliance. S.L. nitroglycerin, especially, may be taken as needed when anginal symptoms are acute.
• Despite the widespread S.L. use of nifedipine capsules, this route of administration should be avoided. Peak serum levels are lower and it takes longer for peak levels to occur than when capsules are bitten and swallowed.
• When a rapid response to the drug is desired, instruct the patient to bite and swallow the capsule. If he is unable to chew capsules, the liquid can be withdrawn by puncturing the capsule with a needle and squeezing the contents into the mouth. When using these methods, continuous blood pressure and ECG monitoring is recommended.
• Patient may briefly develop anginal exacerbation when beginning drug therapy or when dosage is increased. Reassure him that this symptom is temporary.
• Instruct the patient to swallow extended-release tablets without breaking, crushing, or chewing.
• Procardia XL and Adalat CC are not therapeutically equivalent because of major differences in their pharmacokinetics. Warn the patient not to switch brands.
• Reassure the patient who is taking the extended-release form of the drug that a wax-matrix "ghost" from the tablet may be passed in the stool. Drug is completely absorbed before this occurs.
• Protect capsules from direct light and moisture and store at room temperature.

nitroglycerin (glyceryl trinitrate)

Anginine‡, Deponit, GTN-Pohl‡, Klavikordal, Niong, Nitradisc‡, Nitro-Bid, Nitro-Bid I.V., Nitrocap, Nitrocap T.D., Nitrocine, Nitrodisc, Nitro-Dur, Nitro-Dur II, Nitrogard, Nitrogard SR, Nitroglyn, Nitroject, Nitrol, Nitrolin, Nitrolingual, Nitronet, Nitrong, Nitrong S.R., Nitrospan, Nitrostat, Nitrostat I.V., NTS, Transderm-Nitro, Transiderm-Nitro‡, Tridil

Pregnancy Risk Category: C

HOW SUPPLIED

Tablets (buccal): 1 mg, 2 mg, 3 mg
Tablets (sublingual): 0.15 mg (1/400 gr), 0.3 mg (1/200 gr), 0.4 mg (1/150 gr), 0.6 mg (1/100 gr)

Tablets (sustained-release): 2.6 mg, 6.5 mg, 9 mg
Capsules (sustained-release): 6.5 mg, 9 mg
Aerosol (translingual): 0.4-mg metered spray
Topical: 2% ointment
Transdermal: 2.5-mg, 5-mg, 7.5-mg, 10-mg, 15-mg 24-hour systems
Injection: 0.5 mg/ml, 0.8 mg/ml, 5 mg/ml

ACTION
Mechanism: A nitrate that reduces cardiac oxygen demand by decreasing left ventricular end-diastolic pressure (preload) and, to a lesser extent, systemic vascular resistance (afterload). Also increases blood flow through the collateral coronary vessels.
Onset: within 1 to 3 minutes after I.V. form, 1 to 3 minutes after S.L. form, 2 minutes after translingual form, 1 to 2 minutes after buccal form, 20 to 45 minutes after oral form, 30 to 60 minutes after topical ointment, 30 to 60 minutes after transdermal system. **Duration:** with I.V. form, effects last 3 to 5 minutes; with S.L. form, 30 to 60 minutes; with translingual form, 30 to 60 minutes; with buccal form, 3 to 5 hours; with oral form, 3 to 8 hours; with topical ointment, 2 to 12 hours; with transdermal system, up to 24 hours with system in place (otherwise, effects last several minutes after removal).

INDICATIONS & DOSAGE
Prophylaxis against chronic anginal attacks –
Adults: 2.5 mg sustained-release (capsule) q 8 to 12 hours; or 2% ointment: Start with ½″ ointment, increasing by ½″ increments until headache occurs, then decreasing to previous dose. Range of dosage with ointment is ½″ to 5″. Usual dose is 1″ to 2″. Alternatively, apply transdermal disc or pad (Nitrodisc, Nitro-Dur, or Transderm-Nitro) to nonhairy site once daily.
Acute angina pectoris, prophylaxis to prevent or minimize anginal attacks when taken immediately before stressful events –
Adults: 1 S.L. tablet (gr 1/400, 1/200, 1/150, 1/100) dissolved under the tongue or in the buccal pouch as soon as angina begins. Repeat q 5 minutes, if needed, for 15 minutes. Or, using Nitrolingual spray, spray one or two doses into mouth, preferably onto or under the tongue. Repeat q 3 to 5 minutes if needed, to a maximum of three doses within a 15-minute period. Or, 1 to 3 mg transmucosally q 3 to 5 hours during waking hours.
Hypertension associated with surgery; CHF associated with MI; angina pectoris in acute situations; to produce controlled hypotension during surgery (by I.V. infusion) –
Adults: initial infusion rate is 5 mcg/minute. Increase, as needed, by 5 mcg/minute q 3 to 5 minutes until a response is noted. If a 20 mcg/minute rate doesn't produce a response, increase dosage by as much as 20 mcg/minute q 3 to 5 minutes. Up to 100 mcg/minute may be needed.

ADVERSE REACTIONS
CNS: *headache, sometimes with throbbing; dizziness;* weakness.
CV: *orthostatic hypotension, tachycardia, flushing, palpitations,* fainting.
GI: nausea, vomiting.
Skin: cutaneous vasodilation.
Other: hypersensitivity reactions, sublingual burning.

INTERACTIONS
Antihypertensives: possibly enhanced hypotensive effect. Monitor closely.
Ethanol: possible increased hypotension. Advise the patient to avoid use.

CONTRAINDICATIONS

- Contraindicated in patients with hypersensitivity to nitrates and in those with head trauma or cerebral hemorrhage, hypertrophic cardiomyopathy, and severe anemia.
- Use cautiously in patients with hypotension.

NURSING CONSIDERATIONS

- Monitor blood pressure and intensity and duration of drug response.
- May cause headaches, especially at first. Dosage may need to be reduced temporarily, but tolerance usually develops. Treat headache with aspirin or acetaminophen.
- Tolerance to the drug can be minimized with a 10- to 12-hour nitrate-free interval. To achieve this, remove transdermal system in the early evening and apply a new system the next morning or omit the last daily dose of a buccal, sustained-release, or ointment form. Check with the doctor for alterations in dosage regimen if tolerance is suspected.
- Caution the patient to take nitroglycerin regularly, as prescribed, and to have it accessible at all times.
- Advise the patient that abrupt discontinuation of drug causes coronary vasospams.
- An additional dose may be taken before anticipated stress or h.s. if angina is nocturnal.
- Advise the patient to avoid alcoholic beverages.
- To minimize orthostatic hypotension, the patient should change to upright position slowly. Advise him to go up and down stairs carefully and to lie down at the first sign of dizziness.
- Tell the patient to take an S.L. tablet at the first sign of an attack. The tablet should be wet with saliva and placed under the tongue until completely absorbed and the patient should sit down and rest until pain subsides. Dose may be repeated every 10 to 15 minutes for a maximum of three doses. If drug doesn't provide relief, medical help should be obtained promptly.
- Patient who complains of a tingling sensation with the drug placed S.L. may try holding a tablet in the buccal pouch.
- Tell the patient to take oral tablets on an empty stomach, either 30 minutes before or 1 to 2 hours after meals; to swallow oral tablets whole; and not to chew tablets.
- To apply ointment, measure the prescribed amount on the application paper; then place the paper on any nonhairy area. Do not rub in. Cover with plastic film to aid absorption and to protect clothing. If using Tape-Surrounded Appli-Ruler (TSAR) system, keep the TSAR on skin to protect patient's clothing and to ensure that ointment remains in place. Remove all excess ointment from previous site before applying the next dose. Avoid getting ointment on fingers.
- Transdermal dosage forms can be applied to any nonhairy part of the skin except distal parts of the arms or legs (absorption will not be maximal at from distal sites).
- Be sure to remove transdermal patch before defibrillation. Because of its aluminum backing, the electric current may cause the patch to explode.
- When stopping transdermal treatment of angina, gradually reduce the dose and frequency of application over 4 to 6 weeks.
- Instruct the patient to use caution when wearing transdermal patch near microwave oven. Leaking radiation may heat patch's metallic backing and cause burns.
- The various brands of transdermal nitroglycerin products can be interchanged to achieve the prescribed dose. Now, standardized labels specify the amount of nitroglycerin released over 24 hours.
- Remind the patient who is using

translingual aerosol form that he should *not* inhale the spray, but should release it onto or under the tongue. Also tell him to wait about 10 seconds or so before swallowing.

- Tell the patient to place the transmucosal tablet between the lip and gum above the incisors, or between the cheek and gum. Tablets should be be swallowed or chewed.
- **I.V. use:** Dilute with D_5W or 0.9% sodium chloride injection. Concentration should not exceed 400 mcg/ml. Always administer with an infusion control device and titrate to desired response. Also, always mix in glass bottles and avoid use of I.V. filters because drug binds to plastic. Regular polyvinyl chloride (PVC) tubing can bind up to 80% of the drug, making it necessary to infuse higher dosages. A special nonabsorbent (non-PVC) tubing is available from the manufacturer; patients receive more drug when these infusion sets are used. Always use the same type of infusion set when changing I.V. lines.
- When changing the concentration of nitroglycerin infusion, flush the I.V. administration set with 15 to 20 ml of the new concentration before use. This will clear the line of the old drug solution.
- Closely monitor vital signs during infusion. Be particularly aware of blood pressure, especially if the drug is being used in a patient with an MI. Excessive hypotension may worsen the MI.
- Store drug in cool, dark place in a tightly closed container. To ensure freshness, replace supply of S.L. tablets every 3 months. Remove cotton from container because it absorbs drug.
- Tell the patient to store S.L.tablets in original container or other container specifically approved for this use and to carry the container in a jacket pocket or purse, not in a pocket close to the body.

pentaerythritol tetranitrate

Dilar, Duotrate, Naptrate, Pentritol, Pentylan, Peritrate, Peritrate Forte†, Peritrate SA, PETN

Pregnancy Risk Category: C

HOW SUPPLIED

Tablets: 10 mg, 20 mg, 40 mg, 80 mg
Tablets (sustained-release): 80 mg
Capsules (sustained-release): 30 mg, 45 mg, 80 mg

ACTION

Reduces cardiac oxygen demand by decreasing left ventricular end-diastolic pressure (preload) and, to a lesser extent, systemic vascular resistance (afterload). Also increases blood flow through the collateral coronary vessels.
Onset: 30 minutes after oral tablets, 1 hour or more after extended-release forms. **Duration:** 4 to 5 hours after oral tablets; 12 hours after extended-release forms.

INDICATIONS & DOSAGE

Prophylaxis against angina pectoris – **Adults:** 10 to 20 mg P.O. q.i.d.; titrate upward as needed to 40 mg P.O. q.i.d. ½ before or 1 hour after meals and h.s.; or 30 to 80 mg sustained-release preparation P.O. b.i.d.

ADVERSE REACTIONS

CNS: *headache, sometimes with throbbing; dizziness;* weakness.
CV: *orthostatic hypotension, tachycardia, flushing, palpitations,* fainting.
GI: nausea, vomiting.
Skin: cutaneous vasodilation.
Other: hypersensitivity reactions.

INTERACTIONS

Ethanol: may increase hypotension. Avoid concomitant use.

CONTRAINDICATIONS

• Contraindicated in patients with head trauma or cerebral hemorrhage and in those with severe anemia.
• Use cautiously in patients with hypotension or glaucoma.

NURSING CONSIDERATIONS

• Monitor blood pressure and intensity and duration of drug response.
• May cause headaches, especially at first. Dosage may need to be reduced temporarily, but tolerance usually develops. Treat headache with aspirin or acetaminophen.
• Not to be used for relief of acute anginal attacks.
• Caution the patient to take medication regularly, as prescribed, and to have it accessible at all times.
• Advise the patient that abrupt discontinuation of drug causes coronary vasospasm.
• Additional doses may be taken before anticipated stress or h.s. for nocturnal angina.
• To minimize orthostatic hypotension, the patients should change to upright position slowly. Advise him to go up and down stairs carefully and to lie down at the first sign of dizziness.
• Store in a cool place, in a tightly covered container away from light.

propranolol hydrochloride

Apo-Propranolol†, Betachron E-R, Deralin‡, Detensol†, Inderal, Inderal LA, Novopranol†, pms-Propranolol†

Pregnancy Risk Category: C

HOW SUPPLIED

Tablets: 10 mg, 20 mg, 40 mg, 60 mg, 80 mg, 90 mg
Capsules (extended-release): 60 mg, 80 mg, 120 mg, 160 mg
Oral solution: 4 mg/ml, 8 mg/ml, 80 mg/ml (concentrate)
Injection: 1 mg/ml

ACTION

Mechanism: A beta-adrenergic blocker that reduces cardiac oxygen demand by blocking catecholamine-induced increases in heart rate, blood pressure, and force of myocardial contraction. Depresses renin secretion and prevents vasodilation of cerebral arteries.
Onset: 1 minute after I.V. injection, 30 minutes after oral administration.
Peak: Peak plasma levels occur 60 to 90 minutes after oral administration or immediately after I.V. injection.
Duration: plasma half-life, 2 to 3 hours after a single dose, 3 to 6 hours in patients receiving long-term therapy.

INDICATIONS & DOSAGE

Angina pectoris –
Adults: 10 to 20 mg P.O. t.i.d. or q.i.d. Or one 80-mg extended-release capsule daily. Increase dosage at 7- to 10-day intervals. The average optimum dosage is 160 mg daily.
Mortality reduction after MI –
Adults: 180 to 240 mg P.O. daily in divided doses. Usually administered t.i.d. to q.i.d.
Supraventricular, ventricular, and atrial arrhythmias; tachyarrhythmias caused by excessive catecholamine action during anesthesia, hyperthyroidism, and pheochromocytoma –
Adults: 1 to 3 mg by slow I.V. push, not to exceed 1 mg/minute. After 3 mg have been given, another dose may be given in 2 minutes; subsequent doses, no sooner than q 4 hours. May be diluted and infused slowly. Usual maintenance dosage is 10 to 80 mg P.O. t.i.d. to q.i.d.
Hypertension –
Adults: initially, 80 mg P.O. daily in two to four divided doses or the extended-release form once daily. Increase at 3- to 7-day intervals to maximum daily dosage of 640 mg. Usual maintenance dosage is 160 to 480 mg daily.

Prevention of frequent, severe, uncontrollable, or disabling migraine or vascular headache –
Adults: initially, 80 mg P.O. daily in divided doses or 1 extended-release capsule daily. Usual maintenance dosage is 160 to 240 mg daily, t.i.d. or q.i.d.

ADVERSE REACTIONS
CNS: *fatigue, lethargy,* vivid dreams, hallucinations, mental depression.
CV: *bradycardia, hypotension,* ***CHF,*** intermittent claudication.
GI: nausea, vomiting, diarrhea.
Respiratory: *increased airway resistance.*
Skin: rash.
Other: fever, arthralgia.

INTERACTIONS
Aminophylline: antagonized beta-blocking effects of propranolol. Use together cautiously.
Cimetidine: inhibits propranolol's metabolism. Monitor for greater beta-blocking effect.
Digitalis glycosides, diltiazem, verapamil: hypotension, bradycardia, and increased depressant effect on myocardium. Use together cautiously.
Epinephrine: severe vasoconstriction. Monitor blood pressure and observe the patient carefully.
Glucagon, isoproterenol: antagonized propranolol effect. May be used therapeutically and in emergencies.
Insulin, oral antidiabetic agents: can alter requirements for these drugs in previously stabilized diabetics. Monitor for hypoglycemia.

CONTRAINDICATIONS
- Contraindicated in patients with asthma or allergic rhinitis, during ethyl ether anesthesia, in patients with sinus bradycardia and heart block greater than first-degree, in those with cardiogenic shock, and in patients with right ventricular failure secondary to pulmonary hypertension.
- Use cautiously in patients with CHF, respiratory, or hepatic disease and in those taking other antihypertensives. Because drug blocks some symptoms of hypoglycemia, use with caution in patients with diabetes mellitus. Also use cautiously in patients with thyrotoxicosis because drug may mask some signs of that disorder. Elderly patients may experience enhanced adverse reactions and may need dosage adjustment.
- Double-check dose and route. I.V. doses are much smaller than P.O.

NURSING CONSIDERATIONS
- Always check patient's apical pulse before giving drug. If you detect extremes in pulse rates, withhold drug and call the doctor immediately.
- Monitor blood pressure, ECG, and heart rate and rhythm frequently, especially during I.V. administration. If the patient develops severe hypotension, notify the doctor; a vasopressor may be prescribed.
- Caution the patient to continue taking this drug as prescribed, even when he is feeling well. Tell the patients not to discontinue the drug suddenly because this can exacerbate angina and MI.
- This drug masks common signs of shock and hypoglycemia.
- Food may increase absorption propranolol. Give consistently with meals.
- Compliance may be improved by administering drug twice daily or as extended-release capsule. Check with the doctor.
- Propranolol has also been used to treat aggression and rage, stage fright, recurrent GI bleeding, and menopausal symptoms.
- *Don't discontinue drug before surgery for pheochromocytoma.* Before any surgical procedure, notify anes-

thesiologist that the patient is receiving propranolol.

- **I.V. use:** Give by direct injection into a large vessel or into the tubing of a free-flowing, compatible I.V. solution; continuous I.V. infusion is generally not recommended. Alternatively, dilute drug with 0.9% sodium chloride and give by intermittent infusion over 10 to 15 minutes in 0.1- to 0.2-mg increments. Drug is compatible with D_5W, 0.45% and 0.9% sodium chloride, and lactated Ringer's solution.
- For overdose, give I.V. isoproterenol, I.V. atropine, or glucagon; refractory cases may require a pacemaker.

verapamil

Apo-Verap†, Calan, Isoptin, Novo-Veramil†, Nu-Verap†

verapamil hydrochloride

Anpec‡, Calan, Calan SR, Cordilox‡, Cordilox SR‡, Isoptin, Isoptin SR, Veracaps SR‡, Verelan

Pregnancy Risk Category: C

HOW SUPPLIED

verapamil
Tablets: 40 mg, 80 mg, 120 mg
verapamil hydrochloride
Tablets: 40 mg‡, 80 mg‡, 120 mg‡, 160 mg‡
Tablets (extended-release): 120 mg, 180 mg, 240 mg
Capsules (extended-release): 120 mg, 160 mg‡, 180 mg, 240 mg
Injection: 2.5 mg/ml

ACTION

Mechanism: A calcium channel blocker that inhibits calcium ion influx across cardiac and smooth-muscle cells, thus decreasing myocardial contractility and oxygen demand. Also dilates coronary arteries and arterioles.
Peak: 5 minutes after I.V. administration, 2 hours after immediate-release oral form, 6 hours after extended-release oral form. **Duration:** elimination half-life, 2 to 8 hours; effects persist 1 to 6 hours with I.V. form, about 8 hours with immediate-release oral form, about 24 hours with extended-release oral form.

INDICATIONS & DOSAGE

Vasospastic angina (also called Prinzmetal's or variant angina) and classic chronic, stable angina pectoris; chronic atrial fibrillation –
Adults: starting dose is 80 mg P.O. t.i.d. or q.i.d. Increase dosage at weekly intervals. Some patients may require up to 480 mg daily.
Supraventricular arrhythmias –
Adults: 0.075 to 0.15 mg/kg (5 to 10 mg) by I.V. push over 2 minutes with ECG and blood pressure monitoring. Repeat dose in 30 minutes if no response occurs.
Children under 1 year: 0.1 to 0.2 mg/kg as I.V. bolus over 2 minutes with continuous ECG monitoring. Repeat dose in 30 minutes if no response.
Children 1 to 15 years: 0.1 to 0.3 mg/kg as I.V. bolus over 2 minutes.
Migraine headache prophylaxis –
Adults: 80 mg P.O. q.i.d.
Hypertension –
Adults: 240-mg extended-release tablet once daily in the morning. If response is not adequate, give an additional ½ tablet in the evening or one tablet q 12 hours. Or, give 80-mg immediate-release tablet t.i.d. or q.i.d.

ADVERSE REACTIONS

CNS: dizziness, headache, fatigue.
CV: *transient hypotension, **CHF,*** bradycardia, AV block, ***ventricular asystole,*** peripheral edema.
GI: *constipation,* nausea.
Hepatic: elevated liver enzymes.

*Liquid form contains alcohol.
**May contain tartrazine.

Common reactions are in italics; ***life-threatening,*** in bold italics.

INTERACTIONS

Antihypertensives, quinidine: may result in hypotension. Monitor blood pressure.
Carbamazepine, digitalis glycosides: may increase serum levels of these drugs. Monitor the patient for toxicity.
Disopyramide, flecainide, propranolol (and other beta blockers, including ophthalmic timolol): may cause heart failure. Use together cautiously.
Lithium: may decrease serum lithium levels. Monitor closely.
Rifampin: may decrease oral bioavailability of verapamil. Monitor the patient for lack of effect.

CONTRAINDICATIONS

- Contraindicated in patients with hypersensitivity to the drug and in those with advanced heart failure, AV block, severe left ventricular dysfunction, cardiogenic shock, sinus node disease, and severe hypotension.
- Use cautiously in elderly patients; in patients with MI, sick sinus syndrome, impaired AV conduction, or heart failure with atrial tachyarrhythmia; and in patients with hepatic or renal disease. Also use cautiously in patients with a history of CHF, especially if verapamil therapy is combined with a beta-adrenergic blocker.

NURSING CONSIDERATIONS

- Monitor blood pressure at the start of therapy and during dosage adjustments. Assist the patient with ambulation because dizziness may occur.
- If verapamil is being used to terminate supraventricular tachycardia, the doctor may have the patient perform vagal maneuvers after receiving drug.
- Notify the doctor if such signs of CHF as swelling of hands and feet or shortness of breath occur.
- If the patient is kept on nitrate therapy during titration of oral verapamil dosage, urge continued compliance. Sublingual nitroglycerin, especially, may be taken as needed when anginal symptoms are acute.
- Taking extended-release tablets with food may decrease rate and extent of absorption, but allows smaller fluctuations of peak and trough blood levels.
- Monitor liver function during prolonged treatment.
- Encourage the patient to increase fluid and fiber intake to combat constipation. Administer a stool softener as ordered.
- **I.V. use:** Give by direct injection into a vein or into the tubing of a free-flowing, compatible I.V. solution. Compatible solutions include D_5W, 0.45% and 0.9% sodium chloride, and Ringer's and lactated Ringer's solutions. Administer I.V. doses over at least 3 minutes to minimize the risk of adverse reactions.
- All patients receiving I.V. verapamil should be on a cardiac monitor. Monitor the R-R interval.
- Patients with severely compromised cardiac function or those receiving beta blockers should receive lower doses of verapamil. Monitor these patients closely. Do not administer I.V. beta blockers at the same time as I.V. verapamil.

22

Antihypertensives

acebutolol
amlodipine besylate
(See Chapter 21, ANTIANGINALS.)
atenolol
benazepril hydrochloride
betaxolol hydrochloride
bisoprolol fumarate
captopril
carteolol
clonidine hydrochloride
diazoxide
diltiazem hydrochloride
(See Chapter 21, ANTIANGINALS.)
doxazosin mesylate
enalaprilat
enalapril maleate
felodipine
fosinopril sodium
guanabenz acetate
guanadrel sulfate
guanethidine monosulfate
guanfacine hydrochloride
hydralazine hydrochloride
isradipine
labetalol hydrochloride
lisinopril
mecamylamine hydrochloride
methyldopa
methyldopate hydrochloride
metoprolol succinate
metoprolol tartrate
metyrosine
minoxidil
nadolol
(See Chapter 21, ANTIANGINALS.)
nicardipine
(See Chapter 21, ANTIANGINALS.)
nifedipine
(See Chapter 21, ANTIANGINALS.)
nitroprusside sodium
penbutolol sulfate
phenoxybenzamine hydrochloride
phentolamine mesylate
pindolol
prazosin hydrochloride
propranolol hydrochloride
(See Chapter 21, ANTIANGINALS.)
quinapril hydrochloride
ramipril
rauwolfia serpentina
rescinnamine
reserpine
terazosin hydrochloride
timolol maleate
trimethaphan camsylate
verapamil hydrochloride
(See Chapter 21, ANTIANGINALS.)

COMBINATION PRODUCTS

ALDOCLOR-150: chlorothiazide 150 mg and methyldopa 250 mg.
ALDOCLOR-250: chlorothiazide 250 mg and methyldopa 250 mg.
ALDORIL-15: hydrochlorothiazide 15 mg and methyldopa 250 mg.
ALDORIL-25: hydrochlorothiazide 25 mg and methyldopa 250 mg.
ALDORIL D30: hydrochlorothiazide 30 mg and methyldopa 500 mg.
ALDORIL D50: hydrochlorothiazide 50 mg and methyldopa 500 mg.
APRESAZIDE 25/25: hydrochlorothiazide 25 mg and hydralazine hydrochloride 25 mg.
APRESAZIDE 50/50: hydrochlorothiazide 50 mg and hydralazine hydrochloride 50 mg.
APRESAZIDE 100/50: hydrochlorothiazide 50 mg and hydralazine hydrochloride 100 mg.
APRESODEX: hydrochlorothiazide 15 mg and hydralazine hydrochloride 25 mg.
APRESOLINE-ESIDRIX: hydrochlorothiazide 15 mg and hydralazine hydrochloride 25 mg.
CAM-AP-ES: hydrochlorothiazide 15 mg, hydralazine hydrochloride 25 mg, and reserpine 0.1 mg.

CAPOZIDE 25/15: hydrochlorothiazide 15 mg and captopril 25 mg.
CAPOZIDE 25/25: hydrochlorothiazide 25 mg and captopril 25 mg.
CAPOZIDE 50/15: hydrochlorothiazide 15 mg and captopril 50 mg.
CAPOZIDE 50/25: hydrochlorothiazide 25 mg and captopril 50 mg.
CHERAPAS: hydrochlorothiazide 15 mg, hydralazine hydrochloride 25 mg, and reserpine 0.1 mg.
COMBIPRES 0.1: chlorthalidone 15 mg and clonidine hydrochloride 0.1 mg.
COMBIPRES 0.2: chlorthalidone 15 mg and clonidine hydrochloride 0.2 mg.
CORZIDE: nadolol 40 mg or 80 mg and bendroflumethiazide 5 mg.
DEMI-REGROTON: chlorthalidone 25 mg and reserpine 0.125 mg.
DIUPRES-250: chlorothiazide 250 mg and reserpine 0.125 mg.
DIUPRES-500: chlorothiazide 500 mg and reserpine 0.125 mg.
DIURESE-R: trichlormethiazide 4 mg and reserpine 0.1 mg.
DIURIGEN WITH RESERPINE: chlorothiazide 250 mg and reserpine 0.125 mg.
DIUTENSEN: methyclothiazide 2.5 mg and cryptenamine 2 mg (as tannate).
DIUTENSEN-R: methyclothiazide 2.5 mg and reserpine 0.1 mg.
ENDURONYL: methyclothiazide 5 mg and deserpidine 0.25 mg.
ENDURONYL-FORTE: methyclothiazide 5 mg and deserpidine 0.5 mg.
ESIMIL: hydrochlorothiazide 25 mg and guanethidine sulfate 10 mg.
EXNA-R TABLETS: benzthiazide 50 mg and reserpine 0.125 mg.
H.H.R.: hydrochlorothiazide 15 mg, hydralazine hydrochloride 25 mg, and reserpine 0.1 mg.
HYDROMOX-R: quinethazone 50 mg and reserpine 0.125 mg.
HYDROPINE: hydroflumethiazide 25 mg and reserpine 0.125 mg.
HYDROPINE HP: hydroflumethiazide 50 mg and reserpine 0.125 mg.
HYDROPRES-25: hydrochlorothiazide 25 mg and reserpine 0.125 mg.
HYDRO-RESERP: hydrochlorothiazide 25 or 50 mg and reserpine 0.125 mg.
HYDRO-SERP: hydrochlorothiazide 25 or 50 mg and reserpine 0.125 mg.
HYDROSERPINE: hydrochlorothiazide 25 or 50 mg and reserpine 0.125 mg.
HYDROTENSIN-25 TABLETS: hydrochlorothiazide 25 mg and reserpine 0.125 mg.
INDERIDE 40/25: propranolol hydrochloride 40 mg and hydrochlorothiazide 25 mg.
INDERIDE 80/25: propranolol hydrochloride 80 mg and hydrochlorothiazide 25 mg.
INDERIDE LA 80/50: propranolol hydrochloride 80 mg and hydrochlorothiazide 50 mg.
LOPRESSOR HCT 50/25: metoprolol tartrate 50 mg and hydrochlorothiazide 25 mg.
LOPRESSOR HCT 100/25: metoprolol tartrate 100 mg and hydrochlorothiazide 25 mg.
MAXZIDE: triamterene 75 mg and hydrochlorothiazide 50 mg.
METATENSIN TABLETS #2 or #4: trichlormethiazide 2 or 4 mg and reserpine 0.1 mg.
MINIZIDE 1: polythiazide 0.5 mg and prazosin hydrochloride 1 mg.
MINIZIDE 2: polythiazide 0.5 mg and prazosin hydrochloride 2 mg.
MINIZIDE 5: polythiazide 0.5 mg and prazosin hydrochloride 5 mg.
NAQUIVAL: trichlormethiazide 4 mg and reserpine 0.1 mg.
NATURETIN W/K 2.5 mg: bendroflumethiazide 2.5 mg and potassium chloride 500 mg.
NATURETIN W/K 5 mg: bendroflumethiazide 5 mg and potassium chloride 500 mg.
NORMOZIDE 100/25: labetalol hydrochloride 100 mg and hydrochlorothiazide 25 mg.
NORMOZIDE 200/25: labetalol hydro-

chloride 200 mg and hydrochlorothiazide 25 mg.
NORMOZIDE 300/25: labetalol hydrochloride 300 mg and hydrochlorothiazide 25 mg.
ORETICYL 25: hydrochlorothiazide 25 mg and deserpidine 0.125 mg.
ORETICYL 50: hydrochlorothiazide 50 mg and deserpidine 0.125 mg.
ORETICYL FORTE: hydrochlorothiazide 25 mg and deserpidine 0.25 mg.
RAUZIDE**: bendroflumethiazide 4 mg and powdered rauwolfia serpentina 50 mg.
REGROTON: chlorthalidone 50 mg and reserpine 0.25 mg.
RENESE-R: polythiazide 2 mg and reserpine 0.25 mg.
REZIDE: hydrochlorothiazide 15 mg, hydralazine hydrochloride 25 mg, and reserpine 0.1 mg.
R-HCTZ-H: hydrochlorothiazide 15 mg, hydralazine hydrochloride 25 mg, and reserpine 0.1 mg.
SALUTENSIN: hydroflumethiazide 50 mg and reserpine 0.125 mg.
SALUTENSIN DEMI: hydroflumethiazide 25 mg and reserpine 0.125 mg.
SER-A-GEN: hydrochlorothiazide 15 mg, hydralazine hydrochloride 25 mg, and reserpine 0.1 mg.
SERALAZIDE: hydrochlorothiazide 15 mg, hydralazine hydrochloride 25 mg, and reserpine 0.1 mg.
SER-AP-ES: hydrochlorothiazide 15 mg, reserpine 0.1 mg, and hydralazine hydrochloride 25 mg.
SERPASIL-APRESOLINE #1**: reserpine 0.1 mg and hydralazine hydrochloride 25 mg.
SERPASIL-APRESOLINE #2: reserpine 0.2 mg and hydralazine hydrochloride 50 mg.
SERPASIL-ESIDRIX #1: hydrochlorothiazide 25 mg and reserpine 0.1 mg (called Serpasil-Esidrix 25 in Canada).
SERPASIL ESIDRIX #2: hydrochlorothiazide 50 mg and reserpine 0.1 mg.
SERPAZIDE: hydrochlorothiazide 15 mg, hydralazine hydrochloride 25 mg, and reserpine 0.1 mg.
TENORETIC 50: atenolol 50 mg and chlorthalidone 25 mg.
TENORETIC 100: atenolol 100 mg and chlorthalidone 25 mg.
TIMOLIDE 10/25: timolol maleate 10 mg and hydrochlorothiazide 25 mg.
TRI-HYDROSERPINE: hydrochlorothiazide 15 mg, hydralazine hydrochloride 25 mg, and reserpine 0.1 mg.
UNIPRES: hydrochlorothiazide 15 mg, reserpine 0.1 mg, and hydralazine hydrochloride 25 mg.
VASERETIC: enalapril maleate 10 mg and hydrochlorothiazide 25 mg.
ZIAC: bisoprolol fumarate 2.5 mg, 5 mg, or 10 mg and hydrochlorothiazide 6.5 mg.

acebutolol

Monitan†, Sectral

Pregnancy Risk Category: B

HOW SUPPLIED

Capsules: 200 mg, 400 mg

ACTION

Mechanism: A $beta_1$-selective blocking agent that decreases myocardial contractility and decreases heart rate. It has mild intrinsic sympathomimetic activity.
Onset: 1 to 1½ hours. **Peak:** Peak plasma levels of parent drug occur within 2 to 2½ hours; of active metabolite, in about 4 hours. Peak effects occur within 2 to 8 hours. **Duration:** terminal elimination half-life, about 11 hours; effects persist about 24 hours.

INDICATIONS & DOSAGE

Hypertension –
Adults: 400 mg P.O. either as a single daily dosage or divided b.i.d. Patients may receive as much as 1,200 mg daily.
Supraventricular arrhythmias; suppression of PVCs –

*Liquid form contains alcohol.
**May contain tartrazine.

Common reactions are in italics; ***life-threatening,*** in bold italics.

Adults: 400 mg P.O. daily divided b.i.d. Increase dosage to provide an adequate clinical response. Usual dosage is 600 to 1,200 mg daily.

In patients with impaired renal function, reduce dosage.

Elderly patients may require lower dosage; dosage should not exceed 800 mg daily.

ADVERSE REACTIONS

CNS: *fatigue,* headache, dizziness, insomnia.
CV: chest pain, edema, bradycardia, *CHF, hypotension.*
GI: nausea, constipation, diarrhea, dyspepsia.
Respiratory: dyspnea, ***bronchospasm.***
Skin: rash.
Other: fever, positive antinuclear antibody test.

INTERACTIONS

Digitalis glycosides, diltiazem, verapamil: excessive bradycardia and increased depressant effect on myocardium. Use together cautiously.
Indomethacin: decreased antihypertensive effect. Monitor blood pressure and adjust dosage.
Insulin, oral antidiabetic agents: can alter dosage requirements in previously stabilized diabetic patients. Observe the patient carefully.

CONTRAINDICATIONS

- Contraindicated in patients with persistently severe bradycardia, second- and third-degree heart block, overt cardiac failure, and cardiogenic shock.
- Use cautiously in patients with cardiac failure. Also use cautiously in diabetic patients because beta-adrenergic blockers may potentiate insulin-induced hypoglycemia and may mask certain signs and symptoms of hypoglycemia.
- Also use cautiously in patients with bronchospastic disease because, like metoprolol, acebutolol is a cardioselective beta blocker.
- Acebutolol may mask signs of hyperthyroidism.

NURSING CONSIDERATIONS

- Always check the patient's apical pulse before giving drug; if slower than 60 beats/minute, withhold drug and call the doctor.
- Before surgery, notify the anesthesiologist that the patient is taking this drug.
- Advise the patient that abrupt discontinuation of drug can exacerbate angina and MI.

atenolol

Apo-Atenolol†, Nu-Atenol†, Noten‡, Tenormin

Pregnancy Risk Category: C

HOW SUPPLIED

Tablets: 50 mg, 100 mg
Injection: 5 mg/10 ml

ACTION

Mechanism: A beta-adrenergic blocker that selectively blocks $beta_1$-adrenergic receptors; decreases cardiac output, peripheral resistance, and cardiac oxygen consumption; and depresses renin secretion.
Onset: 5 minutes after I.V. injection, 1 hour after oral administration.
Peak: Peak effects occur 2 to 4 hours after oral dose or 5 minutes after direct I.V. injection. **Duration:** effects persist less than 12 hours after I.V. dose or 24 hours after oral dose.

INDICATIONS & DOSAGE

Hypertension –
Adults: initially, 50 mg P.O. daily as a single dose. Increase dosage to 100 mg once daily after 7 to 14 days. Dosages > 100 mg are unlikely to produce further benefit. Adjust dosage in patients with creatinine clearance below 35 ml/minute.

Angina pectoris –
Adults: 50 mg P.O. once daily. Increase as needed to 100 mg daily after 7 days for optimal effect. May give as much as 200 mg daily.
To reduce cardiovascular mortality and risk of reinfarction in patients with acute MI –
Adults: 5 mg I.V. over 5 minutes, followed by another 5 mg 10 minutes later. After an additional 10 minutes, administer 50 mg P.O., followed by 50 mg in 12 hours. Thereafter, give 100 mg P.O. daily (as a single dose or 50 mg b.i.d.) for at least 7 days.
To reduce the incidence of supraventricular tachycardia in patients undergoing coronary artery bypass –
Adults: 50 mg P.O. daily starting 3 days before surgery.

In patients with renal insufficiency: If creatinine clearance is 15 to 35 ml/min/1.73 m^2, give a maximum of 50 mg daily; if creatinine clearance is < 15 ml/min/1.73 m^2, give a maximum dosage of 50 mg every other day. Give hemodialysis patients 50 mg after each dialysis session, but supervise closely because of the risk of hypotension.

ADVERSE REACTIONS
CNS: fatigue, lethargy.
CV: *bradycardia, hypotension,* ***CHF,*** intermittent claudication.
GI: nausea, vomiting, diarrhea.
Respiratory: dyspnea, ***bronchospasm.***
Skin: rash.
Other: fever.

INTERACTIONS
Antihypertensives: enhanced hypotensive effect. Use together cautiously.
Digitalis glycosides, diltiazem, verapamil: excessive bradycardia and increased depressant effect on myocardium. Use together cautiously.
Insulin, oral antidiabetic agents: can alter dosage requirements in previously stabilized diabetic patients. Observe the patient carefully.

CONTRAINDICATIONS
- Contraindicated in patients with sinus bradycardia, greater than first-degree heart block, or cardiogenic shock.
- Use cautiously in patients with CHF.
- Atenolol can be used in patients with bronchospastic diseases such as asthma and emphysema; however, use cautiously in such patients – especially when doses of 100 mg or more are given. Twice-daily dosing may help minimize risk of respiratory effects.
- Atenolol masks common signs of shock and hypoglycemia.

NURSING CONSIDERATIONS
- Always check the patient's apical pulse before giving drug; if slower than 60 beats/minute, withhold drug and call the doctor.
- Monitor blood pressure frequently.
- Caution the patient that abrupt discontinuation of drug can exacerbate angina and MI. Drug should be withdrawn gradually over a 2-week period.
- **I.V. use:** Give by slow I.V. injection, not to exceed 1 mg/minute. I.V. doses may be mixed with D_5W, 0.9% sodium chloride, or dextrose and sodium chloride solutions. Solution is stable for 48 hours after mixing.
- Once-daily dosing encourages patient compliance. Counsel patients to take drug at the same time every day. Drug can be dispensed in a 28-day calendar pack.
- Atenolol has been prescribed effectively to treat angina pectoris and alcohol withdrawal syndrome.

benazepril hydrochloride

Lotensin

Pregnancy Risk Category: C (X in 2nd and 3rd trimesters)

HOW SUPPLIED

Tablets: 5 mg, 10 mg, 20 mg, 40 mg

ACTION

Mechanism: Benazepril and its active metabolite, benazeprilat, inhibit ACE, preventing conversion of angiotensin I to angiotensin II, a potent vasoconstrictor. Reduced formation of angiotensin II decreases peripheral arterial resistance, thus decreasing aldosterone secretion. This reduces sodium and water retention and lowers blood pressure. Benazepril also has antihypertensive activity in patients with low-renin hypertension.

Onset: within 1 hour. **Peak:** Peak effects occur within 2 to 4 hours. **Duration:** effects persist 24 hours.

INDICATIONS & DOSAGE

Hypertension –

Adults: initially, 10 mg daily. Titrate dosage as needed and tolerated; most patients take 20 to 40 mg daily in one or two doses.

ADVERSE REACTIONS

CNS: headache, dizziness, lightheadedness, anxiety, amnesia, depression, insomnia, malaise, nervousness, neuralgia, neuropathy, paresthesia, somnolence, tremor, vertigo.

CV: symptomatic hypotension, syncope, angina, arrhythmia, chest pain, palpitations, ***MI***.

EENT: epistaxis, dysphagia, increased salivation.

GI: nausea, vomiting, abdominal pain, anorexia, constipation, diarrhea, dyspepsia, gastroenteritis, dry mouth, taste disturbance.

Respiratory: dry, persistent, tickling, nonproductive cough; dyspnea.

Skin: hypersensitivity reactions, rash, dermatitis, pruritus, photosensitivity, purpura.

Other: angioedema, arthralgia, arthritis, edema, impotence, increased diaphoresis, myalgia, weight gain, asthenia, hyperkalemia.

INTERACTIONS

Diuretics, other antihypertensives: risk of excessive hypotension. Discontinue diuretic or lower dose of benazepril as needed.

Lithium: increased serum lithium levels and lithium toxicity. Avoid concomitant use.

Potassium-sparing diuretics, potassium supplements, sodium substitutes containing potassium: risk of hyperkalemia. Avoid concomitant use.

CONTRAINDICATIONS

- Contraindicated in patients with hypersensitivity to ACE inhibitors or those with a history of angioedema.
- Contraindicated during pregnancy because ACE inhibitors can cause fetal or neonatal injury or death. These problems have not been detected when fetal exposure has been limited to the first trimester. If pregnancy is detected, discontinue ACE inhibitors as soon as possible.
- Use cautiously in patients with impaired hepatic or renal function and in those with diabetes mellitus. Also use cautiously in patients taking potassium-sparing diuretics, potassium supplements, and sodium substitutes containing potassium because of risk of hyperkalemia.

NURSING CONSIDERATIONS

- Measure blood pressure when drug levels are at peak (2 to 6 hours after dosing) and at trough (just before a dose) to verify adequate blood pressure control.
- Excessive hypotension can occur when drug is given with diuretics. If possible, diuretic therapy should be discontinued 2 to 3 days before start-

ing benazepril to decrease potential for excessive hypotensive response. If benazepril does not adequately control blood pressure, diuretic may be reinstituted with care. If the diuretic cannot be discontinued, initiate benazepril therapy at 5 mg P.O. daily. Monitor for hypotension.
• Adjust dosages in patients with renal impairment, as ordered.
• Assess renal and hepatic function before and periodically throughout therapy. Monitor serum potassium levels.
• Other ACE inhibitors have been associated with granulocytosis and neutropenia. Monitor CBC with differential counts before therapy, every 2 weeks for the first 3 months of therapy, and periodically thereafter. Advise patients to report any signs of infection, such as fever and sore throat.
• Also tell patients to call the doctor if any of the following signs or symptoms occur: easy bruising or bleeding; swelling of tongue, lips, face, eyes, mucous membranes, or extremities; difficulty swallowing or breathing; and hoarseness.
• Light-headedness can occur, especially during the first few days of therapy. Tell patients to rise slowly to minimize this effect and to report symptoms to doctor. Patients who experience syncope should stop taking the drug and call the doctor immediately.
• Inadequate fluid intake, vomiting, diarrhea, and excessive perspiration can lead to light-headedness and syncope. Tell patients to use caution in hot weather and during exercise.
• Tell patients to avoid sodium substitutes; these products may contain potassium, which can cause hyperkalemia in patients taking this drug.
• Instruct patients to take this drug on an empty stomach; meals, particularly those that are high in fat, can impair absorption.

betaxolol hydrochloride

Kerlone

Pregnancy Risk Category: C

HOW SUPPLIED

Tablets: 10 mg, 20 mg

ACTION

Mechanism: A beta$_1$-selective blocking agent that decreases blood pressure, probably by slowing heart rate and decreasing cardiac output.
Onset: within 3 hours. **Peak:** Serum levels peak within 2 to 4 hours after a dose. Peak antihypertensive effects occur after 7 to 14 days of therapy.
Duration: elimination half-life, 14 to 22 hours; effects persist 24 to 48 hours.

INDICATIONS & DOSAGE

Hypertension (used alone or with other antihypertensives) –
Adults: initially, 10 mg P.O. once daily. If necessary, may double dosage to 20 mg P.O. once daily.

ADVERSE REACTIONS

CV: bradycardia, chest pain, hypotension, worsening of angina, peripheral vascular insufficiency, ***CHF,*** edema, syncope, postural hypotension, conduction disturbances.
CNS: dizziness, fatigue, headache, lethargy, anxiety.
GI: flatulence, constipation, nausea, diarrhea, vomiting, anorexia, dry mouth.
Respiratory: dyspnea, wheezing, ***bronchospasm.***
Skin: rash.

INTERACTIONS

Calcium channel blockers: increased risk of hypotension, left ventricular failure, and AV conduction disturbances. Use I.V. calcium antagonists with caution.
Catecholamine-depleting drugs, reserpine: may have an additive effect.

General anesthetics: increased hypotensive effects. Observe carefully for excessive hypotension or bradycardia, or orthostatic hypotension.
Lidocaine: may increase lidocaine's effects.

CONTRAINDICATIONS

- Contraindicated in patients with severe bradycardia, greater than first-degree heart block, cardiogenic shock, or uncontrolled CHF.
- Use cautiously in patients with CHF controlled by digitalis and diuretics because these patients may exhibit signs of cardiac decompensation with beta blocker therapy.
- Beta blockade may inhibit glycogenolysis and the signs and symptoms of hypoglycemia (such as tachycardia and blood pressure changes).
- Beta blockers may mask tachycardia associated with hyperthyroidism. In patients with suspected thyrotoxicosis, withdraw beta blocker therapy gradually to avoid thyroid storm.
- Avoid beta blockers in patients with bronchospastic disease (including asthma, chronic bronchitis, and emphysema) because some $beta_2$-receptor antagonism may be associated with cardioselective agents such as betaxolol. However, some clinicians will use cardioselective beta blockers in such patients who cannot tolerate other antihypertensives.

NURSING CONSIDERATIONS

- Withdrawal of beta blocker therapy before surgery is controversial. Some clinicians advocate withdrawal to prevent any impairment of cardiac responsiveness to reflex stimuli and decreased responsiveness to administration of catecholamines. Advise the anesthesiologist that the patient is receiving a beta blocker so that isoproterenol or dobutamine is made readily available for reversal of drug's cardiac effects.
- Advise patients that abrupt discontinuation of drug may precipitate angina pectoris in patients with unrecognized coronary artery disease.
- Emphasize the importance of promptly reporting signs of CHF, including shortness of breath or difficulty breathing, unusually fast heartbeat, cough, or fatigue with exertion.

bisoprolol fumarate

Zebeta

Pregnancy Risk Category: C

HOW SUPPLIED

Tablets: 5 mg, 10 mg

ACTION

Mechanism: A $beta_1$-selective blocking agent that decreases myocardial contractility, heart rate, and cardiac output; lowers blood pressure; and reduces myocardial oxygen consumption.
Peak: Peak effects occur within 1 to 4 hours. **Duration:** effects last about 24 hours.

INDICATIONS & DOSAGE

Hypertension (used alone or in combination with other antihypertensives) – **Adults:** initially 5 mg P.O. once daily. If response is inadequate, increase to 10 mg once daily. Maximum recommended dosage is 20 mg daily.

ADVERSE REACTIONS

CNS: asthenia, fatigue, dizziness, headache, hypoesthesia, vivid dreams, depression, insomnia.
CV: bradycardia, peripheral edema, chest pain.
EENT: pharyngitis, rhinitis, sinusitis.
GI: nausea, vomiting, diarrhea, dry mouth.
Respiratory: cough, dyspnea.
Other: sweating, arthralgia.

INTERACTIONS

Indomethacin: decreased antihypertensive effect. Monitor blood pressure and adjust dosage.

CONTRAINDICATIONS

- Contraindicated in patients with hypersensitivity to the drug and in those with cardiogenic shock, overt cardiac failure, marked sinus bradycardia, or second- or third-degree AV block.
- Use cautiously in patients with bronchospastic disease. In general, these patients should avoid beta-adrenergic blockers because blockade of pulmonary $beta_2$-receptors may result in worsening of symptoms. For patients who cannot tolerate or do not respond to other antihypertensives, give bisoprolol in low doses, starting therapy at 2.5 mg daily. Know that bisoprolol blocks $beta_2$-receptors in higher doses (20 mg daily or more).
- Also use cautiously in patients with diabetes, peripheral vascular disease, or thyroid disease and in those with a history of heart failure.

NURSING CONSIDERATIONS

- Patients with renal or hepatic dysfunction should start therapy at 2.5 mg daily.
- Beta blockers may mask some of the manifestations of hypoglycemia, such as tachycardia. Nonselective beta blockers can potentiate insulin-induced hypoglycemia and delay the recovery of serum glucose levels. Because bisoprolol is a selective agent, this problem is minimal; nevertheless, warn diabetic patients to closely monitor blood glucose levels.
- Monitor blood pressure frequently.
- Teach the patient about his disease and therapy. Explain the importance of taking drug as prescribed, even when he's feeling well. Advise the patient that abrupt discontinuation of this drug can exacerbate angina and precipitate MI. Drug must be withdrawn gradually over 1 to 2 weeks. Instruct the patient to call the doctor if unpleasant adverse reactions occur.
- Tell the patient to check with the doctor or pharmacist before taking OTC medications.

captopril

Apo-Capto†, Capoten, Novo-Captopril†, Syn-Captopril†

Pregnancy Risk Category: C (D in 2nd and 3rd trimesters)

HOW SUPPLIED

Tablets: 12.5 mg, 25 mg, 50 mg, 100 mg

ACTION

Mechanism: Inhibits ACE, preventing conversion of angiotensin I to angiotensin II, a potent vasoconstrictor. Reduced formation of angiotensin II decreases peripheral arterial resistance, thus decreasing aldosterone secretion. This reduces sodium and water retention and lowers blood pressure.

Onset: 15 to 30 minutes. **Peak:** Peak effects occur in 1 to 2 hours. **Duration:** elimination half-life, 2 hours; effects persist 6 to 12 hours.

INDICATIONS & DOSAGE

Hypertension –

Adults: 25 mg P.O. b.i.d. or t.i.d. initially. If blood pressure isn't satisfactorily controlled in 1 to 2 weeks, increase dosage to 50 mg t.i.d. If not satisfactorily controlled after another 1 to 2 weeks, expect a diuretic to be added to the regimen. If further blood pressure reduction is necessary, dosage may be raised to as high as 150 mg t.i.d. while continuing the diuretic. Maximum dosage is 450 mg daily. Daily dose may also be administered b.i.d.

CHF; to reduce risk of death and slow development of heart failure after MI –

Adults: 6.25 to 12.5 mg P.O. t.i.d.

initially. Gradually increase to 50 mg t.i.d. as needed. Maximum daily dosage is 450 mg.

ADVERSE REACTIONS

CNS: dizziness, fainting.
CV: *tachycardia, hypotension,* angina pectoris, ***CHF,*** pericarditis.
GI: anorexia, *dysgeusia.*
GU: *proteinuria, nephrotic syndrome, membranous glomerulopathy,* ***renal failure*** (in patients with preexisting renal disease or patients receiving high dosages), urinary frequency.
Hematologic: ***leukopenia, agranulocytosis, pancytopenia.***
Hepatic: transient increase in hepatic enzymes.
Respiratory: dry, persistent, tickling, nonproductive cough.
Skin: *urticarial rash, maculopapular rash,* pruritus.
Other: fever, angioedema of face and extremities, hyperkalemia.

INTERACTIONS

Antacids: decreased captopril effect. Separate administration times.
Digitalis glycosides: may increase serum digoxin concentration by 15% to 30%.
Insulin, oral antidiabetic agents: risk of hypoglycemia when captopril therapy is initiated. Monitor closely.
NSAIDs: may reduce antihypertensive effect. Monitor blood pressure.
Potassium supplements, potassium-sparing diuretics: increased risk of hyperkalemia. Avoid these agents unless hypokalemic blood levels are confirmed.

CONTRAINDICATIONS

• Contraindicated during pregnancy because ACE inhibitors can cause fetal and neonatal injury or death. These problems have not been detected when fetal exposure has been limited to the first trimester. If pregnancy is detected, discontinue ACE inhibitors as soon as possible.
• Use cautiously in patients with impaired renal function or serious autoimmune disease (particularly systemic lupus erythematosus) or in patients who have been exposed to other drugs known to affect WBC counts or immune response.

NURSING CONSIDERATIONS

• Reevaluate captopril therapy in patients who develop persistent proteinuria or proteinuria that exceeds 1 g daily.
• Monitor the patient's blood pressure and pulse rate frequently.
• Monitor WBC and differential counts before starting treatment, every 2 weeks for the first 3 months of therapy, and periodically thereafter. Advise patients to report any signs of infection, such as fever and sore throat.
• Although captopril can be used alone, its beneficial effects are increased when a thiazide diuretic is added.
• Light-headedness can occur, especially during the first few days of therapy. Tell patients to rise slowly to minimize this effect and to report symptoms to the doctor. Patients who experience syncope should stop taking the drug and call the doctor immediately.
• Inadequate fluid intake, vomiting, diarrhea, and excessive perspiration can lead to light-headedness and syncope. Tell patients to use caution in hot weather and during exercise.
• Elderly patients may be more sensitive to the drug's hypotensive effects.
• Instruct patients to take this medication 1 hour before meals; food in the GI tract may reduce absorption.
• Captopril has been prescribed to treat rheumatoid arthritis.

carteolol

Cartrol

Pregnancy Risk Category: C

HOW SUPPLIED

Tablets: 2.5 mg, 5 mg

ACTION

Mechanism: A nonselective beta-adrenergic blocker with intrinsic sympathomimetic activity. Its antihypertensive effects are probably caused by decreased sympathetic outflow from the brain and decreased cardiac output. Carteolol does not have a consistent effect on renin output.
Peak: Peak effects occur within 4 to 6 hours after a dose. **Duration:** effects persist 2 or more days and may be seen for up to 3 weeks after therapy ends.

INDICATIONS & DOSAGE

Hypertension –
Adults: initially, 2.5 mg P.O. as a single daily dose. Gradually increase dosage as required to 5 or 10 mg as a single daily dose. Dosages that exceed 10 mg daily do not produce a greater response and may actually decrease response.

In patients with substantial renal failure: If creatinine clearance is >60 ml/minute, give at 24-hour intervals; 20 to 60 ml/minute, at 48-hour intervals; <20 ml/minute, at 72-hour intervals.

ADVERSE REACTIONS

CNS: lassitude, tiredness, fatigue, somnolence, *asthenia*.
CV: conduction disturbances.
Other: *muscle cramps.*

INTERACTIONS

Calcium channel blockers: increased risk of hypotension, left ventricular failure, and AV conduction disturbances. Use I.V. calcium antagonists with caution.
Catecholamine-depleting drugs, reserpine: may have an additive effect.
Digitalis glycosides: may produce additive effects on slowing AV nodal conduction. Avoid concomitant use.
General anesthetics: increased hypotensive effects. Observe carefully for excessive hypotension or bradycardia, or orthostatic hypotension.
Insulin, oral antidiabetic agents: may alter hypoglycemic response. Adjust dosage as necessary.

CONTRAINDICATIONS

- Contraindicated in patients with bronchial asthma, severe bradycardia, greater than first-degree heart block, cardiogenic shock, or uncontrolled CHF.
- Use cautiously in patients with CHF controlled by digitalis and diuretics because these patients may exhibit signs of cardiac decompensation with beta blocker therapy.
- Beta blockade may inhibit glycogenolysis and the signs and symptoms of hypoglycemia (such as tachycardia and blood pressure changes). It may also attenuate insulin release.
- Beta blockers may mask tachycardia associated with hyperthyroidism. In patients with suspected thyrotoxicosis, withdraw beta blocker therapy gradually to avoid thyroid storm.

NURSING CONSIDERATIONS

- Patients with unrecognized coronary artery disease may exhibit signs of angina pectoris on withdrawal of drug.
- Withdrawal of beta blocker therapy before surgery is controversial. Some clinicians advocate withdrawal to prevent any impairment of cardiac responsiveness to reflex stimuli and decreased responsiveness to administration of catecholamines. However, the beta blocking effects of carteolol may persist for weeks, and discontinuing drug before surgery may be impracti-

cal. Advise the anesthesiologist that the patient is receiving a beta blocker so that isoproterenol or dobutamine is made readily available for reversal of the drug's cardiac effects.

• Emphasize the importance of reporting signs of CHF, including shortness of breath or difficulty breathing, unusually fast heartbeat, cough, or fatigue with exertion.

clonidine hydrochloride

Catapres, Catapres-TTS, Dixarit†‡

Pregnancy Risk Category: C

HOW SUPPLIED

Tablets: 0.025 mg†‡, 0.1 mg, 0.2 mg, 0.3 mg

Transdermal: TTS-1 (releases 0.1 mg/24 hours), TTS-2 (releases 0.2 mg/24 hours), TTS-3 (releases 0.3 mg/24 hours)

ACTION

Mechanism: Inhibits the central vasomotor centers, thereby decreasing sympathetic outflow.

Onset: 15 to 30 minutes after oral administration, 1 to 3 days after transdermal application. **Peak:** Peak effects occur within 3 to 5 hours after oral dose, about 3 days after transdermal application. **Duration:** plasma half-life, 6 to 20 hours. Effects persist 6 to 8 hours after an oral dose; effects gradually decline over several days after transdermal system removal.

INDICATIONS & DOSAGE

Essential, renal, and malignant hypertension –

Adults: initially, 0.1 mg P.O. b.i.d. Then increase by 0.1 to 0.2 mg daily on a weekly basis. Usual dosage range is 0.2 to 0.8 mg daily in divided doses; infrequently, dosages as high as 2.4 mg daily are used.

Or, apply transdermal patch to a nonhairy area of intact skin on the upper arm or torso, once every 7 days.

Prophylaxis of migraine –

Adults: 0.025 mg P.O. b.i.d. or q.i.d. Increase to 15 mg daily in divided doses. After 2 weeks, increase dosage to 0.05 mg b.i.d.

Menopausal flushing –

Adults: 0.025 to 0.075 mg b.i.d.

Suppression of abstinence symptoms during narcotics withdrawal –

Adults: 0.1 mg P.O. t.i.d.

ADVERSE REACTIONS

CNS: *drowsiness,* dizziness, fatigue, sedation, nervousness, headache, vivid dreams.

CV: orthostatic hypotension, bradycardia, ***severe rebound hypertension.***

GI: *constipation,* dry mouth, nausea, vomiting.

GU: urine retention, impotence.

Skin: *pruritus, dermatitis* (from transdermal patch).

Other: transient glucose intolerance (after large doses).

INTERACTIONS

CNS depressants: enhanced CNS depression. Use together cautiously.

MAO inhibitors, tricyclic antidepressants: may decrease antihypertensive effect. Use together cautiously.

Propranolol, other beta blockers: paradoxical hypertensive response. Monitor carefully.

CONTRAINDICATIONS

• Contraindicated in patients with hypersensitivity to the drug. Transdermal form is contraindicated in patients with hypersensitivity to any component of the adhesive layer of the transdermal system.

• Use cautiously in patients with severe coronary insufficiency, diabetes, MI, cerebrovascular disease, chronic renal failure, or history of depression or in those taking other antihypertensives.

NURSING CONSIDERATIONS

- Monitor blood pressure and pulse rate frequently. Dosage is usually adjusted to patient's blood pressure and tolerance.
- Clonidine may be given to rapidly lower blood pressure in some hypertensive emergency situations.
- Discontinuing clonidine for surgery is not recommended.
- Advise the patient that abrupt discontinuation of drug may cause severe rebound hypertension. Reduce dosage gradually over 2 to 4 days.
- When stopping therapy in patients receiving both clonidine and a beta blocker, gradually withdraw the beta blocker first to minimize adverse reactions.
- Observe for tolerance to drug's therapeutic effects that may require increased dosage.
- Elderly patients may be more sensitive to drug's hypotensive effects.
- Antihypertensive effects of transdermal clonidine may take 2 to 3 days to become apparent. Oral antihypertensive therapy may have to be continued in the interim.
- Remove transdermal patch before defibrillation to prevent arcing.
- Reassure the patient that the transdermal patch usually adheres despite showering and other routine daily activities. Instruct him on the use of the adhesive "overlay" to provide additional skin adherence if necessary. Also tell the patient to place the patch at a different site each week.
- Inform the patient that orthostatic hypotension can be minimized by rising slowly and avoiding sudden position changes.
- Caution the patient that drug can cause drowsiness, but that tolerance to this adverse effect will develop.
- Tell patients to take their last dose immediately before retiring.
- Clonidine has been used investigationally to treat dysmenorrhea (0.025 mg b.i.d. for 14 days before and during menses).
- May also suppress craving for nicotine in nicotine addiction.

diazoxide

Hyperstat

Pregnancy Risk Category: C

HOW SUPPLIED

Injection: 300 mg/20 ml

ACTION

Mechanism: Directly relaxes arteriolar smooth muscle.

Onset: within 2 minutes. **Peak:** Peak effects occur within 5 to 15 minutes after bolus dose. **Duration:** elimination half-life, 21 to 45 hours (probably shorter in children); effects persist 3 to 12 hours.

INDICATIONS & DOSAGE

Hypertensive crisis –

Adults and children: 1 to 3 mg/kg by I.V. bolus (up to a maximum of 150 mg) q 5 to 15 minutes until adequate response is seen. Repeat at intervals q 4 to 24 hours p.r.n.

ADVERSE REACTIONS

CNS: *headaches,* dizziness, lightheadedness, euphoria.

CV: *sodium and water retention, orthostatic hypotension,* diaphoresis, flushing, warmth, angina, myocardial ischemia, arrhythmias, ECG changes.

GI: *nausea, vomiting,* abdominal discomfort.

Other: inflammation and pain from extravasation, *hyperglycemia,* hyperuricemia.

INTERACTIONS

Hydralazine: may cause severe hypotension. Use together cautiously.

Thiazide diuretics: may increase diazoxide's effects. Use together cautiously.

CONTRAINDICATIONS

• Use cautiously in patients with impaired cerebral or cardiac function or uremia and in those taking other antihypertensives.

• Diazoxide may alter requirements for insulin, diet, or oral antidiabetic agents in previously controlled diabetic patients. Monitor blood glucose daily; watch closely for signs of severe hyperglycemia or hyperosmolar nonketotic syndrome. Insulin may be needed.

NURSING CONSIDERATIONS

• Monitor the patient's fluid intake and output carefully. If fluid or sodium retention develops, the doctor may order diuretics.

• Weigh the patient daily and notify the doctor of any weight increase.

• Check the patient's uric acid levels frequently and report abnormalities to the doctor.

• **I.V. use:** Monitor blood pressure and ECG continuously. Place the patient in the supine position or in Trendelenburg's position during and for 1 hour after infusion. Notify the doctor immediately if severe hypotension develops. Keep norepinephrine available.

• Check the patient's standing blood pressure before discontinuing close monitoring for hypotension.

• Inform the patient that orthostatic hypotension can be minimized by rising slowly and avoiding sudden position changes. Instruct the patient to remain in the supine position for 30 minutes after injection.

• Take care to avoid extravasation.

• Infusion of diazoxide has been shown to be as effective as a bolus in some patients.

• Protect I.V. solutions from light. Darkened I.V. solutions of diazoxide are subpotent and should not be used.

doxazosin mesylate

Cardura

Pregnancy Risk Category: B

HOW SUPPLIED

Tablets: 1 mg, 2 mg, 4 mg, 8 mg

ACTION

Mechanism: An alpha-adrenergic blocker that acts on the peripheral vasculature to produce vasodilation. **Peak:** Peak antihypertensive effect occurs within 4 to 8 hours. **Duration:** effects persist about 24 hours.

INDICATIONS & DOSAGE

Essential hypertension –

Adults: initiate dosage at 1 mg P.O. daily and determine effect on standing and supine blood pressure at 2 to 6 hours and 24 hours after dosing. If necessary, increase dose to 2 mg daily. To minimize adverse reactions, titrate dosage slowly (dosage typically increased only q 2 weeks). If necessary, increase dose to 4 mg daily, then 8 mg. Maximum daily dosage is 16 mg, but dosage that exceeds 4 mg daily is associated with a greater incidence of adverse reactions.

ADVERSE REACTIONS

CNS: dizziness, vertigo, headache, somnolence, drowsiness, fatigue, malaise, syncope, paresthesia.

CV: *orthostatic hypotension,* hypotension, edema, palpitations, ***arrhythmias,*** tachycardia, peripheral ischemia.

Skin: rash, pruritus.

Other: rhinitis, arthralgia, myalgia, muscle weakness.

INTERACTIONS

None significant.

CONTRAINDICATIONS

• Contraindicated in patients with hypersensitivity to the drug and quina-

zoline derivatives (including prazosin and terazosin).
- Use cautiously in patients with impaired hepatic function.

NURSING CONSIDERATIONS
- Patients taking doxazosin are susceptible to a "first-dose" effect similar to that produced by other alpha-adrenergic blockers – marked orthostatic hypotension accompanied by dizziness or syncope. Orthostatic hypotension is most common after first dose, but can also occur when therapy is interrupted for a few days and during dosage adjustment periods. Warn patients that dizziness or fainting may occur. Advise them to avoid driving and other hazardous activities or situations.
- If syncope occurs, place the patient in a recumbent position and treat supportively. A transient hypotensive response is not considered a contraindication to continued therapy.
- Warn the patient that doxazosin may cause drowsiness and to avoid driving and other hazardous activities that require alertness until drug's adverse CNS effects are known.

---

enalaprilat
Vasotec I.V.

enalapril maleate
Amprace‡, Renitec‡, Vasotec

Pregnancy Risk Category: C (D in 2nd and 3rd trimesters)

HOW SUPPLIED
Tablets: 2.5 mg, 5 mg, 10 mg, 20 mg
Injection: 1.25 mg/ml in 2-ml vials

ACTION
Mechanism: Inhibits ACE, preventing conversion of angiotensin I to angiotensin II, a potent vasoconstrictor. Reduced formation of angiotensin II decreases peripheral arterial resistance, thus decreasing aldosterone secretion. This reduces sodium and water retention and lowers blood pressure.
Onset: 5 to 15 minutes after I.V. injection, 1 hour after oral dose. **Peak:** Peak effects occur 1 to 4 hours after I.V. injection or 4 to 8 hours after oral dose. **Duration:** effects persist about 6 hours after I.V. injection or 12 to 24 hours after oral dose.

INDICATIONS & DOSAGE
Hypertension –
Adults: initially, 5 mg P.O. once daily, then adjust according to response. Usual dosage range is 10 to 40 mg daily as a single dose or two divided doses. Alternatively, give by I.V. infusion 1.25 mg q 6 hours over 5 minutes.
To convert from I.V. therapy to oral therapy –
Adults: initially, 5 mg P.O. once daily. Adjust dosage to response.
To convert from oral therapy to I.V. therapy –
Adults: 1.25 mg I.V. over 5 minutes q 6 hours. Higher doses have not demonstrated greater efficacy.
Treatment adjunct in heart failure (with diuretics and digitalis) –
Adults: initially, 2.5 mg P.O. b.i.d. Adjust dosage based on clinical or hemodynamic response. Usual range is 5 to 20 mg daily in two divided doses; maximum dosage is 40 mg/day.

ADVERSE REACTIONS
CNS: *headache, dizziness, lightheadedness, fatigue,* insomnia.
CV: *hypotension.*
GI: diarrhea, nausea.
GU: decreased renal function (in patients with bilateral renal artery stenosis or CHF).
Hematologic: ***neutropenia, agranulocytosis.***
Respiratory: dry, persistent, tickling, nonproductive cough.
Skin: rash.
Other: ***angioedema.***

INTERACTIONS

Insulin, oral antidiabetic agents: risk of hypoglycemia, especially at initiation of enalapril therapy. Monitor closely.

Lithium: lithium toxicity can occur. Monitor lithium levels.

NSAIDs: may reduce antihypertensive effect. Monitor blood pressure.

Potassium supplements, potassium-sparing diuretics: increased risk of hyperkalemia. Avoid these drugs unless hypokalemic blood levels are confirmed.

CONTRAINDICATIONS

- Contraindicated during pregnancy because ACE inhibitors can cause fetal and neonatal injury or death. These problems have not been detected when fetal exposure has been limited to the first trimester. If pregnancy is suspected, discontinue ACE inhibitors as soon as possible.
- Use cautiously in patients with preexisting renal impairment or collagen vascular disease. Diabetic patients, those with impaired renal function or CHF, and those receiving drugs that can increase serum potassium may develop hyperkalemia. Monitor potassium intake and serum potassium level.

NURSING CONSIDERATIONS

- Discontinue diuretic therapy 2 to 3 days before enalapril therapy begins. This will reduce the risk of hypotension. Then, if enalapril does not control blood pressure, diuretic therapy may be added.
- When drug is used to treat heart failure, monitor the patient closely for hypotension, especially after initial dose. Observe the patient for at least 2 hours and then for at least 1 hour after blood pressure has stabilized.
- Enalapril is similar to captopril, another ACE inhibitor, but has a longer duration of action. Many patients may get satisfactory therapeutic results by taking enalapril once daily.
- Angioedema (including laryngeal edema) may occur, especially after the first dose. Advise the patient to report any signs or symptoms, such as swelling of face, eyes, lips, or tongue or breathing difficulty.
- Monitor CBC with differential counts before therapy, every 2 weeks for the first 3 months of therapy, and periodically thereafter. Advise the patient to report any signs of infection, such as fever and sore throat.
- Light-headedness can occur, especially during the first few days of therapy. Tell the patient to rise slowly to minimize this effect and to report symptoms to the doctor. Patients who experience syncope should stop taking drug and call the doctor immediately.
- Inadequate fluid intake, vomiting, diarrhea, and excessive perspiration can lead to light-headedness and syncope. Tell the patient to use caution in hot weather and during exercise.
- Advise the patient to avoid sodium substitutes; these products may contain potassium, which can cause hyperkalemia in patients taking this drug.
- **I.V. use:** Inject drug slowly over at least 5 minutes, or dilute in 50 ml of a compatible solution and infuse over 15 minutes. Compatible solutions include D_5W, 0.9% sodium chloride injection, dextrose 5% in lactated Ringer's injection, and dextrose 5% in 0.9% sodium chloride injection.

felodipine

Agon‡, Agon SR‡, Plendil, Plendil ER‡, Renedil†

Pregnancy Risk Category: C

HOW SUPPLIED

Tablets: 5 mg‡

Tablets (extended-release): 5 mg, 10 mg

ACTION

Mechanism: A hydropyridine-derivative calcium channel blocker that prevents the entry of calcium ions into vascular smooth muscle and cardiac cells; shows some selectivity for smooth muscle as compared with cardiac muscle.
Onset: 2 to 5 hours. **Peak:** Plasma levels peak within 2½ to 5 hours.
Duration: effects persist 24 hours.

INDICATIONS & DOSAGE

Hypertension –
Adults: initially, 5 mg P.O. daily. Adjust dosage according to patient response, generally at intervals not less than 2 weeks. Usual dose is 5 to 10 mg daily; maximum recommended dosage is 20 mg daily.

In elderly patients and patients with impaired hepatic function, give 5 mg P.O. daily; adjust dosage as for adults. Maximum recommended dosage is 10 mg daily.

ADVERSE REACTIONS

CNS: headache, dizziness, paresthesia, asthenia.
CV: *peripheral edema,* chest pain, palpitations, increased heart rate.
EENT: rhinorrhea, pharyngitis.
GI: dyspepsia, abdominal pain, nausea, constipation, diarrhea.
Respiratory: upper respiratory infection, cough.
Skin: rash, *flushing.*
Other: muscle cramps, back pain, gingival hyperplasia.

INTERACTIONS

Cimetidine: decreased clearance of felodipine. Use lower doses of felodipine.
Digoxin: decreased peak levels of digoxin, but total absorbed drug is unchanged. Clinical significance is unknown.
Metoprolol: may alter pharmacokinetics of metoprolol. No dosage adjustment appears necessary; monitor for adverse effects.

CONTRAINDICATIONS

- Contraindicated in patients with hypersensitivity to the drug.
- Use cautiously in patients with heart failure, particularly those receiving beta-adrenergic blockers, and in patients with impaired hepatic function because clearance of drug from the blood is dependent on the liver. Although felodipine metabolites accumulate in the plasma of patients with renal disease, these metabolites are inactive.
- Also use cautiously in patients with angina. A reflex increase in heart rate commonly occurs during the first week of therapy. This increased rate, which may precipitate chest pain in certain patients, gradually diminishes over time, but heart rate increases of 5 to 10 beats/minute may persist with chronic dosing. Administration of beta-adrenergic blockers will attenuate this effect.

NURSING CONSIDERATIONS

- In a small study, bioavailability of drug was increased more than twofold when felodipine was taken with doubly concentrated grape juice as compared with water or orange juice.
- Because use of drug has been associated with mild gingival hyperplasia, patients should be advised to observe good oral hygiene and to see a dentist regularly.
- Peripheral edema appears to be both dose- and age-dependent: it's more common in patients taking higher doses, especially those over age 60.
- Tell the patient to swallow tablets whole and not to crush or chew them.
- Be sure the patient understands his disease. He should continue taking the drug, even when he feels better; watch his diet; and check with the doctor or pharmacist before taking

any other medications, including OTC drugs.

fosinopril sodium

Monopril

Pregnancy Risk Category: D

HOW SUPPLIED

Tablets: 10 mg, 20 mg

ACTION

Mechanism: Inhibits ACE, preventing conversion of angiotensin I to angiotensin II, a potent vasoconstrictor. Reduced formation of angiotensin II decreases peripheral arterial resistance, thus decreasing aldosterone secretion. This reduces sodium and water retention and lowers blood pressure. Fosinopril also has antihypertensive activity in patients with low-renin hypertension.

Onset: within 1 hour. **Peak:** Peak antihypertensive effects occur after 2 to 3 days of therapy. **Duration:** effects persist about 24 hours.

INDICATIONS & DOSAGE

Hypertension –

Adults: initially, 10 mg P.O. daily; adjust dose based on blood pressure response at peak and trough levels. Usual dose is 20 to 40 mg, up to 80 mg daily. Divide dose if needed.

ADVERSE REACTIONS

CNS: headache, dizziness, fatigue, light-headedness, syncope, memory disturbances, mood changes, paresthesia, sleep disturbance, drowsiness, weakness, ***CVA.***

CV: chest pain, angina, ***MI, hypertensive crisis,*** rhythm disturbances, palpitations, hypotension, flushing, claudication, orthostatic hypotension.

EENT: tinnitus, vision disturbances, eye irritation, epistaxis, pharyngitis, sinusitis, rhinitis.

GI: nausea, vomiting, diarrhea, pancreatitis, hepatitis, dysphagia, dry mouth, abdominal distention, abdominal pain, flatulence, constipation, heartburn, appetite change, weight change.

GU: sexual dysfunction, decreased libido, urinary frequency, renal insufficiency.

Respiratory: dry, persistent, tickling, nonproductive cough; ***bronchospasm,*** laryngitis, hoarseness.

Skin: urticaria, rash, photosensitivity, pruritus.

Other: ***angioedema,*** fever, arthralgia, musculoskeletal pain, myalgia, jaundice, gout, hyperkalemia.

INTERACTIONS

Antacids: may impair absorption. Separate administration times by at least 2 hours.

Diuretics, other antihypertensives: risk of excessive hypotension. Discontinue diuretic or lower dose of fosinopril as needed.

Lithium: increased serum lithium levels and lithium toxicity. Avoid concomitant use.

Potassium-sparing diuretics, potassium supplements, sodium substitutes containing potassium: risk of hyperkalemia. Avoid concomitant use.

CONTRAINDICATIONS

- Contraindicated in patients with hypersensitivity to ACE inhibitors or with a history of angioedema.
- Contraindicated during pregnancy because ACE inhibitors can cause fetal or neonatal injury or death. These problems have not been detected when fetal exposure has been limited to the first trimester. If pregnancy is detected, discontinue ACE inhibitors as soon as possible.
- Use cautiously in patients with impaired renal or hepatic function, renal insufficiency, or diabetes mellitus.
- Detectable levels of fosinopril have been found in breast milk. Avoid use of drug in patients who are breast-feeding.

NURSING CONSIDERATIONS

- Excessive hypotension can occur when drug is given with diuretics. If possible, discontinue diuretic therapy 2 to 3 days before starting fosinopril to reduce potential for excessive hypotensive response. If fosinopril does not adequately control blood pressure, diuretic may be reinstituted with care.
- Assess renal and hepatic function before and periodically throughout therapy. Monitor potassium levels.
- Other ACE inhibitors have been associated with agranulocytosis and neutropenia. Monitor CBC with differential counts before therapy, every 2 weeks for the first 3 months of therapy, and periodically thereafter. Advise the patient to report any signs of infection, such as fever and sore throat.
- Also tell the patient to call the doctor if any of the following signs or symptoms occur: easy bruising or bleeding; swelling of tongue, lips, face, eyes, mucous membranes, or extremities; difficulty swallowing or breathing; and hoarseness.
- Inadequate fluid intake, vomiting, diarrhea, and excessive perspiration can lead to light-headedness and syncope. Tell patient to use caution in hot weather and during exercise.
- Tell the patient to avoid sodium substitutes; these products may contain potassium, which can cause hyperkalemia in patients taking this drug.
- Absorption may be slowed by presence of food in the GI tract. Instruct the patient to take drug on an empty stomach, 1 hour before or 2 hours after meals.

---

guanabenz acetate
Wytensin

Pregnancy Risk Category: C

HOW SUPPLIED

Tablets: 4 mg, 8 mg

ACTION

Mechanism: A centrally acting antihypertensive that inhibits the central vasomotor centers, thereby decreasing sympathetic outflow.

Onset: within 1 hour. **Peak:** Peak effects occur within 2 to 7 hours. **Duration:** effects persist about 8 hours.

INDICATIONS & DOSAGE

Hypertension –

Adults: initially, 4 mg P.O. b.i.d. Increase dosage in increments of 4 to 8 mg/day q 1 to 2 weeks. Maximum dosage is 32 mg b.i.d. To ensure adequate overnight blood pressure control, give last dose h.s.

Treatment adjunct in opiate withdrawal –

Adults: 4 mg P.O. b.i.d. to q.i.d.

ADVERSE REACTIONS

CNS: *drowsiness, sedation, dizziness, weakness,* headache, ataxia, depression.

CV: ***severe rebound hypertension.***

GI: *dry mouth.*

GU: sexual dysfunction.

INTERACTIONS

CNS depressants: may cause increased sedation. Use together cautiously.

Tricyclic antidepressants, MAO inhibitors: may decrease antihypertensive effect.

CONTRAINDICATIONS

- Contraindicated in patients with hypersensitivity to the drug.
- Use cautiously in patients with vascular insufficiency, coronary insufficiency, recent MI, cerebrovascular disease, or severe hepatic or renal failure.
- Administration in management of opiate withdrawal is an off-label use. Consult literature for current recommendations.

NURSING CONSIDERATIONS

- Guanabenz can be used alone or in combination with a thiazide diuretic.
- Caution the patient that abrupt discontinuation of drug may cause rebound hypertension.
- Advise the patient to avoid driving and other hazardous tasks that require alertness until drug's CNS effects are known.
- Inform the patient that orthostatic hypotension can be minimized by rising slowly and avoiding sudden position changes. Dry mouth can be relieved with chewing gum, sour hard candy, or ice chips.
- Elderly patients may be more sensitive to drug's hypotensive effects.
- Warn the patient that tolerance to alcohol or other CNS depressants may be diminished.

guanadrel sulfate

Hylorel

Pregnancy Risk Category: B

HOW SUPPLIED

Tablets: 10 mg, 25 mg

ACTION

Mechanism: Acts peripherally, inhibiting norepinephrine release and depleting norepinephrine stores in adrenergic nerve endings.

Onset: ½ to 2 hours. **Peak:** Peak effects occur within 4 to 6 hours. **Duration:** effects persist 4 to 14 hours.

INDICATIONS & DOSAGE

Hypertension –

Adults: initially, 5 mg P.O. b.i.d. Adjust dosage until blood pressure is controlled. Most patients require dosages of 20 to 75 mg/day, usually given b.i.d.; however, tolerance to hypotensive effect may necessitate upward titration of dosage to 100 to 400 mg daily in three to four divided doses.

ADVERSE REACTIONS

CNS: *fatigue, dizziness,* drowsiness, faintness.

CV: *orthostatic hypotension,* edema.

GI: diarrhea, dry mouth.

GU: impotence, ejaculation disturbances.

INTERACTIONS

Amphetamines, ephedrine, methylphenidate, norepinephrine, phenothiazines, tricyclic antidepressants: may inhibit guanadrel's antihypertensive effect. Adjust dose accordingly.

MAO inhibitors: antagonized hypotensive effects of guanadrel. Don't give guanadrel concurrently or within 1 week of MAO inhibitor therapy.

CONTRAINDICATIONS

- Contraindicated in patients with known or suspected pheochromocytoma or frank CHF.
- Use cautiously in patients with peripheral vascular disease, asthma, or history of peptic ulcer disease.

NURSING CONSIDERATIONS

- Discontinue guanadrel 48 to 72 hours before surgery to minimize risk of vascular collapse during anesthesia.
- Monitor both supine and standing blood pressure, especially during dosage adjustment periods.
- Warn the patient to avoid strenuous exercise and hot showers; these may cause a hypotensive reaction. An ambient temperature that is too hot may also potentiate the hypotensive effects of guanadrel.
- Inform the patient that orthostatic hypotension can be minimized by rising slowly from a supine position and by avoiding sudden position changes. Dry mouth can be relieved with chewing gum, sour hard candy, or ice chips.
- Elderly patients may be more sensitive to drug's hypotensive effects.

guanethidine monosulfate

Apo-Guanethidine†, Ismelin
Pregnancy Risk Category: C

HOW SUPPLIED

Tablets: 10 mg, 25 mg

ACTION

Mechanism: An adrenergic neuron blocker that acts peripherally, inhibiting norepinephrine release and depleting norepinephrine stores in adrenergic nerve endings.
Onset: 1 to 3 weeks. **Duration:** terminal elimination half-life, 5 days; effects persist 3 to 4 days; blood pressure returns to pretreatment levels in 1 to 3 weeks.

INDICATIONS & DOSAGE

Moderate to severe hypertension (typically used in combination with other antihypertensives) –
Adults: initially, 10 mg P.O. daily. Increase by 10 mg at weekly to monthly intervals, p.r.n. Usual dosage is 25 to 50 mg daily. Some patients may require up to 300 mg.
Children: initially, 200 mcg/kg P.O. daily. Increase gradually q 1 to 3 weeks to maximum of eight times the initial dose.

ADVERSE REACTIONS

CNS: *dizziness, weakness, syncope.*
CV: *orthostatic hypotension, bradycardia,* ***CHF, arrhythmias.***
EENT: *nasal stuffiness*.
GI: *diarrhea,* dry mouth.
Other: *edema, weight gain, inhibition of ejaculation.*

INTERACTIONS

Ethanol, levodopa: may increase hypotensive effect of guanethidine. Use together cautiously.
Amphetamines, ephedrine, MAO inhibitors, methylphenidate, norepinephrine, phenothiazines, tricyclic antidepressants: may inhibit guanethidine's antihypertensive effect. Adjust dose accordingly.

CONTRAINDICATIONS

- Contraindicated in patients with pheochromocytoma.
- Use cautiously in patients with severe cardiac disease, recent MI, cerebrovascular disease, peptic ulceration, impaired renal function, or bronchial asthma and in those taking other antihypertensives.

NURSING CONSIDERATIONS

- Discontinue drug 2 to 3 weeks before elective surgery to reduce the possibility of vascular collapse and cardiac arrest during anesthesia.
- Warn the patient to avoid strenuous exercise and hot showers; these may cause a hypotensive reaction. An ambient temperature that is too hot may also potentiate the hypotensive effects of guanethidine.
- Patients should receive instruction on a low-sodium diet. Monitor for possible weight gain and edema.
- Inform the patient that orthostatic hypotension can be minimized by rising slowly and avoiding sudden position changes. Dry mouth can be relieved with chewing gum, sour hard candy, or ice chips.
- Elderly patients may be more sensitive to drug's hypotensive effects.
- If the patient develops diarrhea, the doctor may prescribe atropine or paregoric.

guanfacine hydrochloride

Tenex
Pregnancy Risk Category: B

HOW SUPPLIED

Tablets: 1 mg

ACTION

Mechanism: Inhibits the central vasomotor center, thereby decreasing sympathetic outflow.

Onset: 1 to 3 hours. **Peak:** Peak antihypertensive effects occur after 3 to 7 days of therapy. **Duration:** effects persist 24 hours.

INDICATIONS & DOSAGE
Mild to moderate hypertension –
Adults: initially, 0.5 to 1 mg P.O. daily h.s. Average dosage is 1 to 3 mg daily.

ADVERSE REACTIONS
CNS: *drowsiness, dizziness,* fatigue, headache, insomnia.
CV: bradycardia, orthostatic hypotension, rebound hypertension.
GI: *constipation,* diarrhea, nausea, dry mouth.
Skin: dermatitis, pruritus.

INTERACTIONS
None significant.

CONTRAINDICATIONS
- Contraindicated in patients with hypersensitivity to the drug.
- Use cautiously in patients with severe coronary insufficiency, recent MI, cerebrovascular disease, or chronic renal or hepatic insufficiency.

NURSING CONSIDERATIONS
- Guanfacine appears to be as effective as methyldopa and clonidine; long half-life permits once-daily dosing.
- Guanfacine may be used alone or with a diuretic.
- The incidence and severity of adverse reactions increase with higher dosages.
- Tell the patient not to discontinue therapy abruptly. Rebound hypertension is less common than with similar drugs, such as clonidine, but may occur.
- Because guanfacine causes drowsiness, advise the patient to avoid activities that require alertness until response to drug is established.

hydralazine hydrochloride

Alphapress‡, Apresoline**, Novo-Hylazin†

Pregnancy Risk Category: C

HOW SUPPLIED
Tablets: 10 mg, 25 mg, 50 mg, 100 mg
Injection: 20 mg/ml

ACTION
Mechanism: A direct-acting vasodilator that relaxes arteriolar smooth muscle.
Onset: within 5 minutes of I.V. injection, 20 to 30 minutes of oral dose.
Peak: Peak effects occur 10 to 80 minutes after I.V. administration or 2 hours after oral dose. **Duration:** effects persist 2 to 6 hours after I.V. administration or 2 to 4 hours after oral dose.

INDICATIONS & DOSAGE
Essential hypertension (orally, alone or in combination with other antihypertensives); to reduce afterload in severe CHF (with nitrates); severe essential hypertension (parenterally, to lower blood pressure quickly) –
Adults: initially, 10 mg P.O. q.i.d.; gradually increase to 50 mg q.i.d. Maximum recommended dosage is 200 mg daily, but some patients may require 300 to 400 mg daily. Can be given b.i.d. for CHF.
I.V. – 10 to 20 mg given slowly and repeated as necessary, generally q 4 to 6 hours. Switch to oral antihypertensives as soon as possible.
I.M. – 20 to 40 mg repeated as necessary, generally q 4 to 6 hours. Switch to oral form as soon as possible.
Children: initially, 0.75 mg/kg P.O. daily in four divided doses (25 mg/m^2 daily). If necessary, increase gradually to ten times this dosage.
I.V. – 1.7 to 3.5 mg/kg daily or 50 to 100 mg/m^2 daily given slowly in four to six divided doses.

I.M. – 1.7 to 3.5 mg/kg daily or 50 to 100 mg/m² daily in four to six divided doses.

ADVERSE REACTIONS

CNS: peripheral neuritis, *headache,* dizziness.
CV: orthostatic hypotension, *tachycardia,* arrhythmias, *angina, palpitations, sodium retention.*
GI: *nausea, vomiting, diarrhea, anorexia.*
Hematologic: neutropenia, leukopenia.
Skin: rash.
Other: *lupuslike syndrome* (especially with high doses), *weight gain.*

INTERACTIONS

Diazoxide, MAO inhibitors: may cause severe hypotension. Use together cautiously.

CONTRAINDICATIONS

- Contraindicated in patients with hypersensitivity to the drug.
- Use cautiously in patients with cardiac disease, CVA, or severe renal impairment and in those taking other antihypertensives.

NURSING CONSIDERATIONS

- Monitor CBC, lupus erythematosus cell preparation, and antinuclear antibody titer determinations before therapy and periodically during long-term therapy.
- Monitor the patient's blood pressure, pulse rate, and body weight frequently. Some clinicians combine hydralazine therapy with diuretics and beta-adrenergic blockers to decrease sodium retention and tachycardia and prevent anginal attacks.
- Watch the patient closely for signs of lupuslike syndrome (sore throat, fever, muscle and joint aches, skin rash). Call the doctor immediately if any of these develop.
- Inform the patient that orthostatic hypotension can be minimized by rising slowly and avoiding sudden position changes.
- Elderly patients may be more sensitive to drug's hypotensive effects.
- Instruct the patient to take oral form with meals to increase absorption.
- Compliance may be improved by administering drug b.i.d. Check with the doctor.
- **I.V. use:** Give slowly and repeat as necessary, generally every 4 to 6 hours. Hydralazine will undergo color changes in most infusion solutions; these color changes do not indicate loss of potency. Compatible with 0.9% sodium chloride, Ringer's and lactated Ringer's solutions, and several other common I.V. solutions. Drug may undergo a reaction with dextrose. The manufacturer does not recommend mixing the drug in infusion solutions. Check with the pharmacist for additional compatibility information.
- Hydralazine I.V. has been prescribed during pregnancy to treat eclampsia.

isradipine

DynaCirc

Pregnancy Risk Category: C

HOW SUPPLIED

Capsules: 2.5 mg, 5 mg

ACTION

Mechanism: A calcium channel blocker that inhibits calcium ion influx across cardiac and smooth muscle cells, decreasing arteriolar resistance and reducing blood pressure.
Onset: 2 to 3 hours. **Peak:** Serum levels peak within 1½ hours. **Duration:** terminal elimination half-life, 8 hours; effects persist more than 12 hours.

INDICATIONS & DOSAGE

Essential hypertension –
Adults: initially, 2.5 mg P.O. b.i.d.,

alone or with a thiazide diuretic. Adjust dosage based on tolerance and response to a maximum of 20 mg daily. Increase dosage by gradual titration. If response is inadequate after first 2 to 4 weeks, increase dosage to 5 mg b.i.d. Continue increasing at 5-mg/day intervals q 2 to 4 weeks to a maximum of 10 mg b.i.d. Most patients show no additional response at dosages over 10 mg daily (5 mg b.i.d.).

In elderly patients and patients with impaired hepatic function, bioavailability of isradipine is increased. However, the starting dosage should still be 2.5 mg b.i.d.

ADVERSE REACTIONS
CNS: dizziness.
CV: edema, flushing, palpitations, tachycardia, orthostatic hypotension.
GI: nausea, diarrhea.
GU: frequent urination.
Respiratory: dyspnea.
Skin: rash.

INTERACTIONS
Fentanyl anesthesia: severe hypotension has been reported with concomitant use of a beta blocker and a calcium channel blocker.

CONTRAINDICATIONS
- Contraindicated in patients with hypersensitivity to the drug.
- Use cautiously in patients with CHF, especially if combined with a beta blocker.

NURSING CONSIDERATIONS
- Before surgery, inform the anesthesiologist that the patient is taking a calcium channel blocker.
- Isradipine has some diuretic activity. Patients may note an increased need to void.
- Like other calcium channel blockers, isradipine is known to cause symptomatic hypotension; however, syncope and severe dizziness have not been reported. Most adverse reactions are mild and transient and related to vasodilation (dizziness, edema, flushing, palpitations, and tachycardia).

labetalol hydrochloride
Normodyne, Presolol‡, Trandate
Pregnancy Risk Category: C

HOW SUPPLIED
Tablets: 100 mg, 200 mg, 300 mg
Injection: 5 mg/ml

ACTION
Mechanism: A beta-adrenergic blocker that prevents response to alpha and beta stimulation and depresses renin secretion and that also has unique alpha-adrenergic blocking effects. Unlike other beta blockers, labetalol does not decrease heart rate or cardiac output.
Onset: 2 to 5 minutes after I.V. administration, within 20 minutes after oral dose. **Peak:** Peak effects occur within 15 minutes of I.V. administration, 2 to 4 hours of oral dose. **Duration:** plasma half-life, 6 to 8 hours; effects persist 2 to 4 hours after I.V. dose and 12 to 24 hours after oral dose.

INDICATIONS & DOSAGE
Hypertension –
Adults: 100 mg P.O. b.i.d. with or without a diuretic. If needed, increase dose to 200 mg b.i.d. after 2 days. Further dose increases may be made q 1 to 3 days until optimum response is reached. Usual maintenance dosage is 200 to 400 mg b.i.d.
Severe hypertension and hypertensive emergencies –
Adults: Dilute 200 mg to 200 ml with D_5W. Infuse at 2 mg/minute until satisfactory response is obtained, then stop infusion. May repeat q 6 to 8 hours.

Alternatively, administer by repeated I.V. injection: Initially, give 20 mg I.V. slowly over 2 minutes. May repeat injections of 40 to 80 mg q 10 minutes until maximum dosage of 300 mg is reached.

ADVERSE REACTIONS
CNS: vivid dreams, fatigue, headache, transient scalp tingling.
CV: *orthostatic hypotension and dizziness,* peripheral vascular disease, bradycardia.
EENT: nasal stuffiness.
GI: nausea, vomiting, diarrhea.
GU: sexual dysfunction, urine retention.
Respiratory: increased airway resistance.
Skin: rash.

INTERACTIONS
Cimetidine: may enhance labetalol's effect. Give together cautiously.
Halothane: additive hypotensive effect.
Insulin, oral antidiabetic agents: can alter dosage requirements in previously stabilized diabetic patients. Observe the patient carefully.

CONTRAINDICATIONS
- Contraindicated in patients with bronchial asthma.
- Use cautiously in patients with CHF, hepatic failure, chronic bronchitis, emphysema, preexisting peripheral vascular disease, and pheochromocytoma. Also use cautiously in diabetic patients because beta-adrenergic blockers may mask certain signs and symptoms of hypoglycemia.
- Labetalol also masks common signs of shock.

NURSING CONSIDERATIONS
- Monitor blood pressure frequently.
- Tell the patient that abrupt discontinuation of therapy can exacerbate angina and precipitate MI.
- Dizziness is the most troublesome adverse reaction and tends to occur in early stages of treatment, in patients also receiving diuretics, and in those receiving higher dosages. Inform the patient that this can be minimized by rising slowly and avoiding sudden position changes. Taking a dose at bedtime or taking smaller doses t.i.d. will also help minimize this adverse reaction. Discuss changes in medication schedule with the doctor.
- **I.V. use:** Administer labetalol injection with an infusion control device. Monitor blood pressure closely: every 5 minutes for 30 minutes, then every 30 minutes for 2 hours, then hourly for 6 hours. The patient should remain in a supine position for 3 hours after infusion.
- When administered I.V. for hypertensive emergencies, labetalol produces a rapid, predictable fall in blood pressure within 5 to 10 minutes.

lisinopril
Prinivil, Zestril

Pregnancy Risk Category: C (D in 2nd and 3rd trimesters)

HOW SUPPLIED
Tablets: 5 mg, 10 mg, 20 mg

ACTION
Mechanism: Inhibits ACE, preventing conversion of angiotensin I to angiotensin II, a potent vasoconstrictor. Reduced formation of angiotensin II decreases peripheral arterial resistance, thus decreasing aldosterone secretion. This reduces sodium and water retention and lowers blood pressure.
Onset: within 1 hour. **Peak:** Plasma levels peak within 7 hours; effects occur within 6 hours. **Duration:** elimination half-life, about 12 hours; effects persist 24 hours.

INDICATIONS & DOSAGE
Mild to severe hypertension –
Adults: initially, 10 mg P.O. daily. Most patients are well controlled on 20 to 40 mg daily as a single dose.

Treatment adjunct in heart failure (with diuretics and digitalis) – **Adults:** 5 to 20 mg P.O. daily.

In patients with renal impairment: If creatinine clearance is 10 to 30 ml/minute/1.73 m², give 5 mg daily; if < 10 ml/minute/1.73 m², give 2.5 mg. Maximum dosage is 40 mg daily.

ADVERSE REACTIONS

CNS: *dizziness, headache, fatigue,* depression, somnolence, paresthesia.
CV: hypotension, *orthostatic hypotension,* chest pain.
EENT: *nasal congestion.*
GI: *diarrhea,* nausea, dyspepsia, dysgeusia.
GU: impotence.
Hematologic: neutropenia.
Respiratory: *dry, persistent, tickling, nonproductive cough.*
Skin: rash.
Other: *muscle cramps,* ***angioedema,*** decreased libido, hyperkalemia.

INTERACTIONS

Diuretics: excessive hypotension.
Indomethacin: attenuated hypotensive effect.
Insulin, oral antidiabetic agents: risk of hypoglycemia, especially at initiation of lisinopril therapy. Monitor closely.
Potassium-sparing diuretics, potassium supplements, potassium-containing sodium substitutes: possible hyperkalemia.
• *Thiazide diuretics:* attenuation of potassium loss from thiazide diuretics. Discontinue diuretics 2 to 3 days before lisinopril therapy, or reduce lisinopril dosage to 5 mg once daily.

CONTRAINDICATIONS

• Contraindicated during pregnancy because ACE inhibitors can cause fetal and neonatal injury or death. These problems have not been detected when fetal exposure has been limited to the first trimester. If pregnancy is detected, discontinue ACE inhibitors as soon as possible.

NURSING CONSIDERATIONS

• If drug does not adequately control blood pressure, diuretics may be added.
• Monitor WBC with differential counts before therapy, every 2 weeks for the first 3 months of therapy, and periodically thereafter. Advise the patient to report any signs of infection, such as fever and sore throat.
• Light-headedness can occur, especially during the first few days of therapy. Tell the patient to rise slowly to minimize this effect and to report symptoms to the doctor. Patients who experience syncope should stop taking drug and call the doctor immediately.
• Angioedema (including laryngeal edema) may occur, especially after first dose. Advise the patient to report any signs or symptoms, such as swelling of face, eyes, lips, or tongue or breathing difficulty.
• Tell the patient not to discontinue drug suddenly, but to call the doctor, if unpleasant adverse reactions occur.

mecamylamine hydrochloride

Inversine

Pregnancy Risk Category: C

HOW SUPPLIED

Tablets: 2.5 mg

ACTION

Mechanism: A ganglionic blocker that competes with acetylcholine for ganglionic cholinergic receptors.
Onset: ½ to 2 hours. **Peak:** Peak effects occur within 3 to 5 hours. **Duration:** effects persist 6 to 12 hours.

INDICATIONS & DOSAGE

Moderate to severe essential hypertension and uncomplicated malignant hypertension –

Adults: initially, 2.5 mg P.O. b.i.d. Increase by 2.5 mg daily q 2 days. Average daily dosage is 25 mg in three divided doses.

ADVERSE REACTIONS

CNS: *paresthesia,* sedation, *fatigue, tremor, choreiform movements,* seizures, mood changes, dizziness, *weakness, headache.*
CV: *orthostatic hypotension.*
EENT: dilated pupils, *blurred vision.*
GI: *anorexia, nausea, vomiting, constipation, adynamic ileus, diarrhea, dry mouth,* glossitis.
GU: urine retention, impotence, decreased libido.

INTERACTIONS

Acetazolamide, sodium bicarbonate: may increase effect of mecamylamine. Use together cautiously. Watch for increased hypotensive effects and toxicity.
Bethanecol, ethanol: excessive hypotension. Don't use together.

CONTRAINDICATIONS

- Contraindicated in patients with recent MI, uremia, or chronic pyelonephritis.
- Use cautiously in patients with lower urinary tract pathology, renal insufficiency, glaucoma, pyloric stenosis, or coronary insufficiency and in those taking other antihypertensives.

NURSING CONSIDERATIONS

- Mecamylamine is typically reserved for moderate to severe hypertension that is refractory to treatment with other drugs.
- High ambient temperature, fever, stress, or severe illness can increase drug's effects.
- Advise the patient that abrupt discontinuation of drug may result in rebound hypertension.
- Frequently monitor patient's standing blood pressure.
- For more gradual absorption, drug should be taken with meals. Don't restrict sodium intake.
- The doctor may instruct patients who develop constipation from this drug to take milk of magnesia, but to avoid bulk laxatives.
- Inform the patient that orthostatic hypotension can be minimized by rising slowly and avoiding sudden position changes. Dry mouth can be relieved with chewing gum, sour hard candy, or ice chips.

---

methyldopa

Aldomet, Aldomet M‡, Apo-Methyldopa†, Dopamet†, Hydopa‡, Novomedopa†, Nu-Medopa†

methyldopate hydrochloride

Aldomet, Aldomet Ester Injection‡

Pregnancy Risk Category: B

HOW SUPPLIED

methyldopa
Tablets: 125 mg, 250 mg, 500 mg
Oral suspension: 250 mg/5 ml
methyldopate hydrochloride
Injection: 250 mg/5 ml in 5-ml vials

ACTION

Mechanism: Inhibits the central vasomotor centers, thereby decreasing sympathetic outflow.
Peak: Peak effects occur within 4 to 6 hours of oral or I.V. doses. **Duration:** elimination half-life, about 2 hours; effects persist 10 to 16 hours after I.V. dose or 12 to 24 hours after single oral dose; after repeated oral doses, effects persist 24 to 48 hours.

INDICATIONS & DOSAGE

Sustained mild to severe hypertension; should not be used for acute treatment of hypertensive emergencies –
Adults: initially, 250 mg P.O. b.i.d. to t.i.d. in first 48 hours. Then increase as needed q 2 days. May give

entire daily dosage in the evening or h.s. Adjust dosages as needed if other antihypertensives are added to or deleted from therapy. Maintenance dosage is 500 mg to 2 g daily in two to four divided doses. Maximum recommended daily dosage is 3 g.
I.V. – 250 to 500 mg q 6 hours, diluted in D_5W and administered over 30 to 60 minutes. Maximum dosage is 1 g q 6 hours. Switch to oral antihypertensives as soon as possible.
Children: initially, 10 mg/kg P.O. daily in two to three divided doses; or 20 to 40 mg/kg I.V. daily in four divided doses. Increase dose daily until desired response occurs. Maximum daily dosage is 65 mg/kg, 2 g/m^2, or 3 g, whichever is least.

ADVERSE REACTIONS
CNS: *sedation,* headache, asthenia, weakness, dizziness, *decreased mental acuity,* involuntary choreoathetotic movements, psychic disturbances, depression, nightmares.
CV: bradycardia, *orthostatic hypotension,* aggravated angina, myocarditis, *edema.*
EENT: *nasal stuffiness.*
GI: nausea, vomiting, diarrhea, pancreatitis, *dry mouth*.
Hematologic: ***hemolytic anemia,*** reversible granulocytopenia, thrombocytopenia.
Hepatic: ***hepatic necrosis.***
Other: gynecomastia, galactorrhea, skin rash, ***drug-induced fever,*** impotence, *weight gain*.

INTERACTIONS
Amphetamines, norepinephrine, phenothiazines, tricyclic antidepressants: possible hypertensive effects. Monitor carefully.
Levodopa: additive hypotensive effects; possible increased adverse CNS reactions.

CONTRAINDICATIONS
- Contraindicated in patients with hypersensitivity to the drug.
- Use cautiously in patients receiving other antihypertensives or MAO inhibitors and in patients with impaired hepatic function.

NURSING CONSIDERATIONS
- Methyldopa is frequently used to treat hypertension in pregnant women, apparently without ill effects to the fetus if the patient is closely monitored. Some clinicians recommend that therapy not begin between 16 and 20 weeks' gestation, if possible.
- After dialysis, monitor the patient for hypertension. The patient may need an extra dose of methyldopa.
- In patients who have received this drug for several months, positive reaction to direct Coombs' test indicates hemolytic anemia.
- Patients who require blood transfusions should have direct and indirect Coombs' tests to prevent crossmatching problems.
- Monitor CBC with differential before therapy, every 2 weeks for the first 3 months of therapy, and periodically thereafter. Advise the patient to report any signs of infection, such as fever and sore throat.
- Tell the patient to check his weight daily and notify the doctor of weight increases > 5 lb. Sodium and water retention may occur but can be relieved with diuretics.
- Tell the patient not to suddenly stop taking drug, but to contact the doctor, if unpleasant adverse reactions occur.
- Warn the patient that drug may impair ability to perform tasks that require mental alertness, particularly at start of therapy. Once-daily dosage at bedtime will minimize daytime drowsiness.
- Inform the patient that orthostatic hypotension can be minimized by rising slowly and avoiding sudden posi-

tion changes. Dry mouth can be relieved with chewing gum, sour hard candy, or ice chips.

- Tell the patient that urine may turn dark in toilet bowls treated with bleach.
- Elderly patients are more likely to experience sedation and hypotension.
- **I.V. use:** Observe for and report any involuntary choreoathetoid movements. The doctor may decide to discontinue drug if this occurs.

metoprolol succinate
Toprol XL

metoprolol tartrate
Apo-Metoprolol†, Apo-Metoprolol (Type L)†, Betaloc†‡, Betaloc Durules†, Lopresor†, Lopresor SR†, Lopressor, Minax‡, Novometoprol†, Nu-Metop†

Pregnancy Risk Category: B

HOW SUPPLIED
succinate
Tablets (extended-release): 50 mg, 100 mg, 200 mg
tartrate
Tablets: 50 mg, 100 mg
Tablets (extended-release): 100 mg†, 200 mg†
Injection: 1 mg/ml in 5-ml ampules or refilled syringes

ACTION
Mechanism: A $beta_1$-selective blocking agent that decreases myocardial contractility, heart rate, and cardiac output; lowers blood pressure; and reduces myocardial oxygen consumption. Also depresses renin secretion.
Onset: within 5 minutes of I.V. dose, 15 minutes of oral dose. **Peak:** Peak effects occur within 20 minutes of I.V. dose, 1 hour after regular-release tablet, or 6 to 12 hours after long-acting dosage forms. **Duration:** elimination half-life, 3 to 7 hours; effects persist 5 to 8 hours after I.V. dose, 6 to 12 hours after regular-release oral tablets, up to 24 hours after long-acting forms.

INDICATIONS & DOSAGE
Hypertension (used alone or in combination with other antihypertensives) –
Adults: initially, 50 mg b.i.d. or 100 mg once daily P.O., then give up to 200 to 400 mg daily in two to three divided doses. Alternatively, give 50 to 100 mg of extended-release tablets (tartrate) once daily. Adjust dosage as needed and tolerated at intervals of not less than 1 week to a maximum of 400 mg daily. Or, 100 to 400 mg extended-release tablets (tartrate) once daily.
Early intervention in acute MI –
Adults: three 5-mg I.V. boluses q 2 minutes. Then, beginning 15 minutes after last dose, administer 50 mg P.O. q 6 hours for 48 hours. Maintenance dosage is 100 mg P.O. b.i.d.
Angina pectoris –
Adults: initially, 100 mg P.O. daily as a single dose or in two equally divided doses. Increase dosage at weekly intervals until an adequate response or a pronounced decrease in heart rate is seen. Daily dosage beyond 400 mg has not been studied. Alternatively, give 100 mg extended-release tablets (tartrate) once daily. Adjust dosage as needed and tolerated at intervals of not less than 1 week to a maximum of 400 mg daily. Or, 100 to 400 mg extended-release tablets (tartrate) once daily.

ADVERSE REACTIONS
CNS: fatigue, lethargy, dizziness.
CV: *bradycardia, hypotension,* ***CHF,*** peripheral vascular disease.
GI: nausea, vomiting, diarrhea.
Respiratory: dyspnea, ***bronchospasm.***
Skin: rash.
Other: fever, arthralgia.

INTERACTIONS
Barbiturates, rifampin: increased metabolism of metoprolol. Monitor for decreased effect.
Chlorpromazine, cimetidine, verapamil: decreased hepatic clearance. Monitor for greater beta-blocking effect.
Digitalis glycosides, diltiazem, verapamil: excessive bradycardia and increased depressant effect on myocardium. Use together cautiously.
Indomethacin: decreased antihypertensive effect. Monitor blood pressure and adjust dosage.
Insulin, oral antidiabetic agents: can alter dosage requirements in previously stabilized diabetic patients. Observe the patient carefully.

CONTRAINDICATIONS
- Contraindicated in patients with hypersensitivity to the drug or other beta blockers and in patients with sinus bradycardia, heart block greater than first degree, cardiogenic shock, or overt cardiac failure.
- Use cautiously in patients with heart failure, diabetes, or respiratory or hepatic disease and in those taking other antihypertensives.
- Although most patients with asthma and bronchitis can take drug without fear of worsening their condition, doses over 100 mg daily should be used cautiously.
- Metoprolol masks common signs of shock and hypoglycemia.

NURSING CONSIDERATIONS
- Always check the patient's apical pulse rate before giving drug. If it's slower than 60 beats/minute, withhold drug and call the doctor immediately.
- Monitor blood pressure frequently.
- Tell the patient that abrupt discontinuation of therapy can exacerbate angina and precipitate MI. Withdraw drug gradually over 1 to 2 weeks.
- Food may increase absorption of metoprolol. Give consistently with meals.
- **I.V. use:** Give undiluted by direct injection. Although mixing with other drugs should be avoided, studies have shown that metoprolol is compatible when mixed with meperidine hydrochloride or morphine sulfate or when administered with alteplase infusions at a Y-site connection.
- Store drug at room temperature and protect from light. Discard solution if it's discolored or contains particles.

metyrosine
Demser

Pregnancy Risk Category: C

HOW SUPPLIED
Capsules: 250 mg

ACTION
Mechanism: Inhibits the enzyme tyrosine hydroxylase, thus inhibiting endogenous catecholamine synthesis.
Onset: 1 to 3 hours **Peak:** Peak effects occur after 3 to 4 days of therapy. **Duration:** plasma half-life, 3 to 7 hours; effects persist 2 to 3 days.

INDICATIONS & DOSAGE
Preoperative preparation of patients with pheochromocytoma; management of such patients when surgery is contraindicated; control or prevention of hypertension before or during pheochromocytomectomy –
Adults and children over 12 years: 250 mg P.O. q.i.d. If needed, increase by 250 to 500 mg daily in divided doses to a maximum of 4 g daily. For preoperative preparation, give optimally effective dosage for at least 5 to 7 days. In normotensive patients, adjust dosage to produce a 50% reduction in urinary metanephrines and vanillylmandelic acid.

ADVERSE REACTIONS
CNS: *sedation;* extrapyramidal symptoms, such as speech difficulty and tremor, disorientation.
GI: *diarrhea,* nausea, vomiting, abdominal pain.
GU: *crystalluria,* hematuria, impotence.
Other: hypersensitivity.

INTERACTIONS
Haloperidol, phenothiazines: increased inhibition of catecholamine synthesis may result in extrapyramidal symptoms. Use cautiously.

CONTRAINDICATIONS
- Contraindicated in patients with hypersensitivity to the drug.

NURSING CONSIDERATIONS
- During surgery, monitor blood pressure and ECG continuously. If a serious arrhythmia occurs during anesthesia and surgery, treatment with a beta blocker or lidocaine may be necessary.
- If the patient's hypertension is not adequately controlled by metyrosine, an alpha-adrenergic blocker (such as phenoxybenzamine) should be added to the regimen.
- Warn the patient that sedation almost always occurs in those treated with metyrosine. Sedation usually subsides after several days' treatment.
- Instruct the patient to increase daily fluid intake to prevent crystalluria. Daily urine volume should be 2,000 ml or more.
- Insomnia may occur when metyrosine is stopped.

minoxidil
Loniten, Minodyl
Pregnancy Risk Category: C

HOW SUPPLIED
Tablets: 2.5 mg, 10 mg, 25 mg‡

ACTION
Mechanism: Produces direct arteriolar vasodilation.
Onset: about 30 minutes. **Peak:** Peak effects occur within 2 to 8 hours.
Duration: plasma half-life, 4 to 5 hours; effects persist 2 to 5 days.

INDICATIONS & DOSAGE
Severe hypertension –
Adults: initially, 5 mg P.O. as a single dose. Effective dosage range is usually 10 to 40 mg daily. Maximum dosage is 100 mg daily.
Children under 12 years: 0.2 mg/kg (maximum 5 mg) as a single daily dose. Effective dosage range usually is 0.25 to 1 mg/kg daily. Maximum dosage is 50 mg.

ADVERSE REACTIONS
CV: *edema, tachycardia, pericardial effusion and tamponade,* ***CHF,*** ECG changes.
Skin: rash, ***Stevens-Johnson syndrome.***
Other: *hypertrichosis* (elongation, thickening, and enhanced pigmentation of fine body hair), breast tenderness, weight gain.

INTERACTIONS
Guanethidine: severe orthostatic hypotension. Advise the patient to stand up slowly.

CONTRAINDICATIONS
- Contraindicated in patients with pheochromocytoma.

NURSING CONSIDERATIONS
- Minoxidil is a potent vasodilator that should be used only when therapy with other antihypertensives has failed.
- Patients with malignant hypertension should be hospitalized during initial therapy.
- Closely monitor blood pressure and pulse at beginning of therapy.
- Teach the patient how to take his

own pulse and to report increases greater than 20 beats/minute to the doctor.

- Monitor fluid intake and urine output and check for weight gain and edema. Tell the patient to weigh himself at least weekly and to report weight gain >5 lb.
- Elderly patients may be more sensitive to drug's hypotensive effects.
- About 8 out of 10 patients will experience hypertrichosis within 3 to 6 weeks of beginning treatment. Unwanted hair can be controlled with a depilatory or shaving. Assure the patient that extra hair will disappear within 1 to 6 months of stopping minoxidil. Advise the patient, however, not to discontinue drug without the doctor's approval.
- Minoxidil is usually prescribed with a beta blocker to control tachycardia and a diuretic to counteract fluid retention. Make sure the patient understands the importance of compliance with total treatment regimen.
- Tell the patient not to suddenly stop taking the drug, but to call the doctor, if unpleasant adverse effects occur.
- Make sure the patient receives and reads the package insert prepared by the manufacturer that describes in layman's terms the drug and its adverse reactions. Provide an oral explanation also.
- Minoxidil is removed by hemodialysis. Be sure to administer dose after dialysis.
- Prescribed in various topical forms for treatment of some types of male pattern baldness.

nitroprusside sodium

Nipride, Nitropress

Pregnancy Risk Category: C

HOW SUPPLIED

Injection: 50 mg/vial in 2-ml, 5-ml vials

ACTION

Mechanism: Relaxes both arteriolar and venous smooth muscle.

Onset: within 1 minute. **Peak:** Peak effects are evident within 5 minutes.

Duration: elimination half-life, 3 to 7 days; effects dissipate within 10 minutes after infusion.

INDICATIONS & DOSAGE

To lower blood pressure quickly in hypertensive emergencies; to produce controlled hypotension during anesthesia; to reduce preload and afterload in cardiac pump failure or cardiogenic shock (may be used with or without dopamine) –

Adults: 50-mg vial diluted with 2 to 3 ml of D_5W and then added to 250, 500, or 1,000 ml of D_5W. Infuse at 0.5 to 10 mcg/kg/minute. Average dose is 3 mcg/kg/minute. Maximum infusion rate is 10 mcg/kg/minute.

Patients taking other antihypertensives along with nitroprusside are extremely sensitive to drug. Adjust dosage accordingly.

ADVERSE REACTIONS

The following adverse reactions usually indicate overdosage:

CNS: *headache, dizziness,* ataxia, loss of consciousness, ***coma,*** weak pulse, absent reflexes, widely dilated pupils, *restlessness, muscle twitching, diaphoresis.*

CV: distant heart sounds, palpitations.

GI: *vomiting, nausea, abdominal pain.*

Respiratory: dyspnea, shallow breathing.

Skin: pink color.

Other: acidosis.

INTERACTIONS

None significant.

CONTRAINDICATIONS

- Contraindicated in patients with hypersensitivity to the drug.

• Use cautiously in patients with hypothyroidism or hepatic or renal disease and in those receiving other antihypertensives.

NURSING CONSIDERATIONS

• Sometimes used with a direct-acting cardiac stimulant such as dopamine in patients with refractory heart failure.
• Keep the patient in the supine position when initiating or titrating nitroprusside therapy.
• Obtain baseline vital signs before giving drug, and find out what parameters the doctor wants to achieve.
• **I.V. use:** Infuse with a infusion pump. Drug is best run piggyback through a peripheral line with no other medication. Don't adjust rate of main I.V. line while drug is running. Even a small bolus of nitroprusside can cause severe hypotension.
• Check blood pressure every 5 minutes at start of infusion and every 15 minutes thereafter. If severe hypotension occurs, turn off I.V. nitroprusside – effects of drug quickly reverse. Notify the doctor. If possible, start an arterial pressure line. Regulate drug flow to specified level.
• Excessive doses or rapid infusion greater than 15 mcg/kg/minute can cause cyanide toxicity; therefore, check serum thiocyanate levels every 72 hours. Thiocyanate levels above 100 mcg/ml are associated with toxicity. Watch for signs of thiocyanate toxicity: profound hypotension, metabolic acidosis, dyspnea, headache, loss of consciousness, ataxia, and vomiting. If these occur, discontinue drug immediately and notify the doctor.
• Because the drug is sensitive to light, wrap I.V. solution in foil; it's not necessary to wrap the tubing. Fresh solution should have faint brownish tint. Discard after 24 hours.
• Don't use bacteriostatic water for injection or sterile sodium chloride solution for reconstitution.

penbutolol sulfate

Levatol

Pregnancy Risk Category: C

HOW SUPPLIED

Tablets: 20 mg

ACTION

Mechanism: Blocks both $beta_1$- and $beta_2$-adrenergic receptors.
Onset: within 1 hour. **Peak:** Peak effects occur within 1½ to 3 hours.
Duration: plasma half-life, 5 hours; effects persist up to 24 hours.

INDICATIONS & DOSAGE

Mild to moderate hypertension –
Adults: 20 mg P.O. once daily. Usually given with other antihypertensives, such as thiazide diuretics.

ADVERSE REACTIONS

CNS: syncope, *dizziness,* vertigo, headache, fatigue, paresthesia, hypoesthesia or hyperesthesia, lethargy, anxiety, nervousness, diminished concentration, sleep disturbances, nightmares, bizarre or frequent dreams, sedation, changes in behavior, reversible mental depression, catatonia, hallucinations, alteration of time perception, memory loss, emotional lability, light-headedness.
CV: *bradycardia,* chest pain, ***CHF,*** asymptomatic hypotension, peripheral ischemia, worsening of angina or arterial insufficiency, peripheral vascular insufficiency, claudication, edema, ***pulmonary edema,*** vasodilation, symptomatic postural hypotension, tachycardia, palpitations, conduction disturbances, first-degree and third-degree heart block, intensification of AV block.
EENT: eye discomfort, pharyngitis.
GI: gastric pain, flatulence, nausea, constipation, heartburn, vomiting, taste alteration, dry mouth.
GU: impotence, nocturia, urine retention.

Respiratory: ***laryngospasm,*** respiratory distress, shortness of breath.
Skin: pallor, flushing, rash.
Other: hypersensitivity reactions, decreased libido, hyperglycemia, hypoglycemia.

INTERACTIONS
Clonidine: may cause paradoxical hypertension. Also, beta blockers may enhance rebound hypertension when clonidine is withdrawn.
Digoxin, diltiazem, verapamil: may produce additive depressant effects on AV nodal conduction. Monitor closely.
Insulin, oral antidiabetic agents: hypoglycemic response to these drugs may be altered. Monitor patient closely.
NSAIDs: possibly decreased antihypertensive effects.
Prazosin, terazosin: "first dose" orthostatic hypotension seen with these drugs may be enhanced.
Sympathomimetics, including isoproterenol, dopamine, dobutamine, or norepinephrine: decreased hypotensive response.
Theophylline: possibly decreased bronchodilator effect.

CONTRAINDICATIONS
- Contraindicated in patients with hypersensitivity to the drug or other beta blockers and in those with sinus bradycardia, cardiogenic shock, CHF, and overt cardiac failure; greater than first-degree heart block; pheochromocytoma unless alpha-adrenergic blockers are also used; and chronic airway disease, such as chronic bronchitis or emphysema.
- Use cautiously in patients with CHF controlled by drug therapy and in those with a history of bronchospastic disease. Also use cautiously in diabetic patients because beta-adrenergic blockers may mask certain signs and symptoms of hypoglycemia.

NURSING CONSIDERATIONS
- Always check the patient's apical pulse before giving drug. If you detect extremes in pulse rates, withhold drug and call the doctor immediately.
- Monitor blood pressure, ECG, and heart rate and rhythm frequently.
- Tell the patient to avoid abrupt discontinuation of therapy; sudden withdrawal of other beta blockers has precipitated angina and MI.
- Teach the patient the signs and symptoms of CHF (edema and pulmonary congestion). Advise him to contact the doctor if these symptoms occur.

phenoxybenzamine hydrochloride
Dibenyline‡, Dibenzyline
Pregnancy Risk Category: C

HOW SUPPLIED
Capsules: 10 mg
Injection: 50 mg/ml‡

ACTION
Mechanism: An alpha-adrenergic blocker that noncompetitively blocks the effect of catecholamines on alpha-adrenergic receptors.
Onset: several hours after oral administration. **Duration:** plasma half-life, about 24 hours; effects may persist for 3 to 4 days.

INDICATIONS & DOSAGE
Control of hypertension and diaphoresis secondary to pheochromocytoma; may be used in combination with propranolol to control excessive tachycardia –
Adults: initially, 10 mg P.O. daily. Increase daily dosage by 10 mg q 4 days. Maintenance dosage is 20 to 60 mg daily.
Children: initially, 0.2 mg/kg or 6 mg/m^2 P.O. daily in a single dose. Maintenance dosage is 12 to 36 mg/

m^2 daily as a single dose or in divided doses.

Control of Raynaud's disease, frostbite, acrocyanosis –
Adults: initially, 10 mg P.O., then increase by 10 mg q 4 days to a maximum of 60 mg daily.

Treatment adjunct in severe shock‡ –
Adults: 1 mg/kg I.V.

ADVERSE REACTIONS

CNS: lethargy, drowsiness.
CV: *orthostatic hypotension, tachycardia, **shock**.*
EENT: *nasal stuffiness, miosis.*
GI: vomiting, abdominal distress, *dry mouth*.
GU: *impotence, inhibition of ejaculation.*

INTERACTIONS

Antihypertensives: excessive hypotension. Use together cautiously.

CONTRAINDICATIONS

- Contraindicated in patients with hypersensitivity to the drug.
- Use cautiously in patients with cerebrovascular or coronary insufficiency, advanced renal disease, or respiratory disease.

NURSING CONSIDERATIONS

- Watch the patient closely for adverse reactions, and call the doctor promptly if they occur. If severe hypotension develops, the patient may require norepinephrine to counteract effect.
- Patients with tachycardia may require concurrent propranolol therapy.
- Monitor the patient's heart rate and blood pressure frequently.
- Monitor respiratory status carefully. Drug may aggravate symptoms of pneumonia and asthma.
- Reassure the patient that nasal congestion, inhibition of ejaculation, and impotence usually decrease with continued therapy.
- Tell the patient to avoid abrupt discontinuation of therapy.
- Inform the patient that orthostatic hypotension can be minimized by rising slowly and avoiding sudden position changes. Dry mouth can be relieved with chewing gum, sour hard candy, or ice chips. GI distress can be relieved by taking drug in divided doses or with milk.
- Used investigationally to treat chronic urine retention.
- **I.V. use:** Calculate needed dose and add to 200 to 500 ml of plasma, blood, plasma expander, or I.V. solution. Infuse over not less than 2 hours.

phentolamine mesylate

Regitine, Rogitine†

Pregnancy Risk Category: C

HOW SUPPLIED

Injection: 5 mg/ml in 1-ml vials, 10 mg/ml‡

ACTION

Mechanism: An alpha-adrenergic blocker that competitively blocks the effects of catecholamines on alpha-adrenergic receptors.
Onset: Effects occur within 10 minutes after intracavernosal injection.
Duration: half-life, about 19 minutes with parenteral use; effects persist 1 to 6 hours after intracavernosal injection.

INDICATIONS & DOSAGE

To aid in diagnosis of pheochromocytoma; to control or prevent hypertension before or during pheochromocytomectomy –
Adults: I.V. diagnostic dose is 5 mg, with close monitoring of blood pressure.

Before surgical removal of tumor, give 2 to 5 mg I.M. or I.V. During surgery, the patient may need small I.V. doses (1 mg) or small I.M. doses (3 mg).

Children: I.V. diagnostic dose is 0.1 mg/kg or 3 mg/m² as a single dose, with close monitoring of blood pressure.

Before surgical removal of tumor, give 1 mg I.V. or 3 mg I.M. During surgery, the patient may need small I.V. doses (1 mg).

Extravasation –
Adults and children: infiltrate area with 5 to 10 mg phentolamine in 10 ml 0.9% sodium chloride solution or give half the dosage through the infiltrated I.V. and the other half around the site. Must be done within 12 hours.

Treatment adjunct in impotence –
Adults: 0.5 to 1 mg by intracavernosal injection. Usually used with papaverine 30 mg.

ADVERSE REACTIONS
CNS: *dizziness, weakness, flushing.*
CV: *hypotension,* ***shock,*** *arrhythmias,* palpitations, *tachycardia,* angina pectoris.
EENT: *nasal stuffiness.*
GI: *diarrhea,* abdominal pain, *nausea, vomiting,* hyperperistalsis.
Other: hypoglycemia.

INTERACTIONS
Epinephrine: excessive hypotension. Don't use together.
Narcotics, sedatives, rauwolfia alkaloids: false-positive test results. Don't give 24 hours before phentolamine is given as a diagnostic test. Withdraw rauwolfia alkaloids at least 4 weeks before such testing.

CONTRAINDICATIONS
- Contraindicated in patients with angina, coronary artery disease, or history of MI.
- Use cautiously in patients with gastritis or peptic ulceration and in those receiving other antihypertensives.

NURSING CONSIDERATIONS
- Don't administer epinephrine to treat phentolamine-induced hypotension. May cause additional fall in blood pressure ("epinephrine reversal"). Use norepinephrine instead.
- When drug is given as a diagnostic test for pheochromocytoma, check the patient's blood pressure first; also check blood pressure frequently during administration.
- Test is positive for pheochromocytoma if I.V. test dose causes severe hypotension.

pindolol

Barbloc‡, Novo-Pindol†, Syn-Pindolol†, Visken

Pregnancy Risk Category: B

HOW SUPPLIED
Tablets: 5 mg, 10 mg, 15 mg‡

ACTION
Mechanism: Blocks both $beta_1$- and $beta_2$-adrenergic receptors. The first commercially available beta blocker with partial beta-*agonist* activity – that is, pindolol *stimulates* beta-adrenergic receptors as well as blocks them. Therefore, it decreases cardiac output less than other beta-adrenergic blockers and may be advantageous for patients who develop bradycardia with other beta blockers.
Onset: within 1 hour. **Peak:** Peak effect occurs in 1 to 2 hours. **Duration:** plasma half-life, 3 to 4 hours; effects persist 6 to 12 hours.

INDICATIONS & DOSAGE
Hypertension –
Adults: initially, 5 mg P.O. t.i.d. Increase dosage as needed and tolerated to a maximum of 40 mg daily in three or four divided doses.
Angina –
Adults: initially, 5 mg P.O. b.i.d. Increase dosage by 10 mg daily q 2 to 3

†Available in Canada only. ‡Available in Australia only. ◇Available OTC.

weeks up to a maximum of 60 mg daily.

ADVERSE REACTIONS

CNS: *insomnia, fatigue, dizziness, nervousness,* vivid dreams, hallucinations, lethargy.
CV: *edema,* bradycardia, ***CHF,*** peripheral vascular disease, hypotension.
EENT: visual disturbances.
GI: *nausea,* vomiting, diarrhea.
Respiratory: *increased airway resistance.*
Skin: rash.
Other: hypoglycemia without tachycardia, *muscle pain, joint pain.*

INTERACTIONS

Digitalis glycosides, diltiazem, verapamil: excessive bradycardia and additive depression of AV node. Use together cautiously.
Epinephrine: severe vasoconstriction. Monitor blood pressure and observe the patient carefully.
Indomethacin: decreased antihypertensive effect. Monitor blood pressure and adjust dosage.
Insulin, oral antidiabetic agents: can alter requirements for these drugs in previously stabilized diabetic patients. Monitor the patient for hypoglycemia.

CONTRAINDICATIONS

- Contraindicated in patients with hypersensitivity to the drug and in patients with severe asthma or allergic rhinitis, sinus bradycardia and heart block greater than first degree, cardiogenic shock, or right ventricular failure secondary to pulmonary hypertension.
- Use cautiously in patients with CHF or respiratory disease and in those taking other antihypertensives. Also use cautiously in diabetic patients because beta-adrenergic blockers may mask certain signs and symptoms of hypoglycemia.

NURSING CONSIDERATIONS

- Always check the patient's apical pulse rate before giving this drug. If you detect extremes in pulse rates, withhold medication and call the doctor immediately.
- Monitor blood pressure frequently and notify the doctor if severe hypotension occurs. A vasopressor may be required.
- Withdraw drug gradually (over 1 to 2 weeks) after long-term administration.
- Tell the patient that abrupt discontinuation of drug can exacerbate angina and precipitate MI.

prazosin hydrochloride

Minipress

Pregnancy Risk Category: C

HOW SUPPLIED

Capsules: 1 mg, 2 mg, 5 mg

ACTION

Mechanism: An alpha-adrenergic blocker that relaxes both arteriolar and venous smooth muscle.
Onset: within 2 hours. **Peak:** Peak effects occur in 4 hours, but peak antihypertensive effect does not occur for 4 to 6 weeks after therapy begins.
Duration: plasma half-life, 2 to 4 hours; effects persist about 24 hours.

INDICATIONS & DOSAGE

Mild to moderate hypertension, alone or in combination with a diuretic or other antihypertensive; reduction of afterload in severe chronic CHF –
Adults: P.O. test dose is 1 mg h.s. to prevent "first-dose syncope." Initial dose is 1 mg t.i.d. Increase dosage slowly. Maximum daily dosage is 20 mg. Maintenance dosage is 3 to 20 mg daily in three divided doses. Some patients have required dosages larger than this (up to 40 mg daily). If other antihypertensives or diuretics are added to this drug, decrease prazosin

dosage to 1 to 2 mg t.i.d. and retitrate.

ADVERSE REACTIONS

CNS: *dizziness,* headache, drowsiness, weakness, *"first-dose syncope,"* depression.
CV: orthostatic hypotension, *palpitations.*
EENT: blurred vision.
GI: vomiting, diarrhea, abdominal cramps, constipation, *nausea,* dry mouth.
GU: priapism, impotence.

INTERACTIONS

Propranolol and other beta blockers: increased frequency of syncope with loss of consciousness. Advise the patient to sit or lie down if dizziness occurs.

CONTRAINDICATIONS

- Contraindicated in patients with hypersensitivity to the drug.
- Use cautiously in patients receiving other antihypertensives.

NURSING CONSIDERATIONS

- Monitor the patient's blood pressure and pulse rate frequently.
- If initial dose is greater than 1 mg, severe syncope with loss of consciousness may occur ("first-dose syncope"). Increase dosage slowly. Patients who experience dizziness should sit or lie down.
- Elderly patients may be more sensitive to hypotensive effects.
- Tell the patient not to suddenly stop taking this drug, but to call the doctor, if unpleasant adverse reactions occur.
- Advise the patient to minimize orthostatic hypotension by rising slowly and avoiding sudden position changes. Dry mouth can be relieved with chewing gum, sour hard candy, or ice chips.
- Compliance *may* be improved with once-daily dosing. Suggest this dosing change with the doctor if you suspect compliance problems.
- Prazosin has been used to treat Raynaud's disease.

quinapril hydrochloride

Accupril, Asig‡

Pregnancy Risk Category: D

HOW SUPPLIED

Tablets: 5 mg, 10 mg, 20 mg, 40 mg

ACTION

Mechanism: Quinapril and its active metabolite, quinaprilat, inhibit ACE, preventing conversion of angiotensin I to angiotensin II, a potent vasoconstrictor. Reduced formation of angiotensin II decreases peripheral arterial resistance, thus decreasing aldosterone secretion. This reduces sodium and water retention and lowers blood pressure. Quinapril also has antihypertensive activity in patients with low-renin hypertension.
Onset: within 1 hour. **Peak:** Peak serum levels of quinapril are seen in 1 hour; quinaprilat, in 2 hours. Peak effects occur within 2 to 4 hours. **Duration:** plasma half-life of quinapril, 1 to 2 hours; of quinaprilat, 3 hours. Effects persist about 24 hours.

INDICATIONS & DOSAGE

Hypertension –
Adults: initially, 10 mg daily. Adjust dosage based on patient response at intervals of about 2 weeks. Most patients are controlled at 20, 40, or 80 mg daily as a single dose or in two divided doses.

In patients with renal impairment, adjust dosage as necessary.

Heart failure –
Adults: initially, 5 mg P.O. b.i.d. Increase dosage at weekly intervals. Usual effective dose is 20 to 40 mg b.i.d. in equally divided doses.

ADVERSE REACTIONS

CNS: somnolence, vertigo, light-headedness, syncope, nervousness, depression.
CV: palpitations, vasodilation, tachycardia, ***MI, hypertensive crisis, CVA,*** angina, orthostatic hypotension, rhythm disturbances.
EENT: cough, dry throat.
GI: dry mouth, abdominal pain, constipation, GI hemorrhage, pancreatitis.
Hepatic: elevated liver enzymes.
Respiratory: dry, persistent, tickling, nonproductive cough.
Skin: pruritus, ***exfoliative dermatitis,*** *photosensitivity*.
Other: ***angioedema,*** hyperkalemia, back pain, malaise, diaphoresis.

INTERACTIONS

Diuretics, other antihypertensives: risk of excessive hypotension. Discontinue diuretic or lower dose of quinapril as needed.
Lithium: increased serum lithium levels and lithium toxicity. Avoid concomitant use.
Potassium-sparing diuretics, potassium supplements, sodium substitutes containing potassium: risk of hyperkalemia. Avoid concomitant use.

CONTRAINDICATIONS

- Contraindicated in patients with hypersensitivity to ACE inhibitors or with a history of angioedema.
- Contraindicated during pregnancy because ACE inhibitors can cause fetal and neonatal injury or death. These problems have not been detected when fetal exposure has been limited to the first trimester. If pregnancy is suspected, discontinue ACE inhibitors as soon as possible.
- Use cautiously in patients with impaired renal or hepatic function or diabetes mellitus.

NURSING CONSIDERATIONS

- Excessive hypotension can occur when drug is given with diuretics. If possible, discontinue diuretic therapy 2 to 3 days before starting quinapril to decrease potential for excessive hypotensive response. If quinapril does not adequately control blood pressure, diuretic may be reinstituted with care. If diuretic cannot be discontinued, initiate therapy with quinapril at 5 mg P.O. daily.
- Assess renal and hepatic function before and periodically throughout therapy.
- Other ACE inhibitors have been associated with agranulocytosis and neutropenia. Monitor CBC with differential counts before therapy, every 2 weeks for the first 3 months of therapy, and periodically thereafter. Advise the patient to report any signs of infection, such as fever and sore throat.
- Monitor serum potassium levels.
- Angioedema (including laryngeal edema) may occur, especially after the first dose. Advise the patient to report any signs or symptoms, such as swelling of face, eyes, lips, or tongue or breathing difficulty.
- Light-headedness can occur, especially during the first few days of therapy. Tell the patient to rise slowly to minimize effect and to report symptoms to the doctor. Patients who experience syncope should stop taking drug and call the doctor immediately.
- Inadequate fluid intake, vomiting, diarrhea, and excessive perspiration can lead to light-headedness and syncope. Tell the patient to use caution in hot weather and during exercise.
- Tell the patient to avoid sodium substitutes; these products may contain potassium, which can cause hyperkalemia in patients taking quinapril.

ramipril

Altace, Ramace‡, Tritace‡

Pregnancy Risk Category: D

HOW SUPPLIED

Capsules: 1.25 mg, 2.5 mg, 5 mg, 10 mg

ACTION

Mechanism: Inhibits ACE, preventing the conversion of angiotensin I to angiotensin II, a potent vasoconstrictor. Reduced formation of angiotensin II decreases peripheral arterial resistance, thus decreasing aldosterone secretion. This reduces sodium and water retention and lowers blood pressure.

Onset: 1 to 2 hours. **Peak:** Peak serum levels of ramipril occur within 1 hour; of ramiprilat, in 3 hours. Peak effect occurs in 3 to 6 hours. **Duration:** plasma half-life of ramipril, about 5 hours; of ramiprilat, 13 to 17 hours. Effects persist about 24 hours.

INDICATIONS & DOSAGE

Essential hypertension (alone or in combination with diuretics) –

Adults: initially, 2.5 mg P.O. once daily. Increase dosage as necessary based on patient response. Maintenance dosage is 2.5 to 20 mg daily as a single dose or in divided doses.

In patients with renal insufficiency: If creatinine clearance is < 40 ml/min/1.73 m^2, start therapy at 1.25 mg P.O. daily. Titrate dosage gradually according to response. Maximum daily dosage is 5 mg.

ADVERSE REACTIONS

CNS: headache, dizziness, fatigue, asthenia, malaise, light-headedness, anxiety, amnesia, ***seizures,*** depression, insomnia, nervousness, neuralgia, neuropathy, paresthesia, somnolence, tremor, vertigo.

CV: orthostatic hypotension, syncope, angina, ***arrhythmia,*** chest pain, palpitations, ***MI.***

EENT: epistaxis, dysphagia, increased salivation.

GI: nausea, vomiting, abdominal pain, anorexia, constipation, diarrhea, dyspepsia, dry mouth, taste disturbance, gastroenteritis.

GU: impotence.

Respiratory: dry, persistent, tickling, nonproductive cough; dyspnea.

Skin: hypersensitivity reactions, rash, dermatitis, pruritus, photosensitivity, purpura.

Other: ***angioedema,*** edema, hyperkalemia, increased diaphoresis, weight gain, arthralgia, arthritis, myalgia.

INTERACTIONS

Diuretics: excessive hypotension, especially at the start of therapy. Discontinue diuretic at least 3 days before therapy begins, increase sodium intake, or reduce starting dose of ramipril.

Insulin, oral antidiabetic agents: risk of hypoglycemia, especially at initiation of ramipril therapy. Monitor closely.

Lithium: increased serum lithium levels. Use together cautiously and monitor serum lithium levels.

Potassium-sparing diuretics, potassium supplements, sodium substitutes containing potassium: increased risk of hyperkalemia because ramipril attenuates potassium loss. Avoid concomitant use or monitor plasma potassium levels closely.

CONTRAINDICATIONS

- Contraindicated in patients with hypersensitivity to the drug or a history of angioedema.
- Contraindicated during pregnancy because ACE inhibitors can cause fetal and neonatal injury or death. These problems have not been detected when exposure has been limited to the first trimester. If pregnancy is

suspected, discontinue ACE inhibitors as soon as possible.
• Use cautiously in patients with renal insufficiency or diabetes mellitus.

NURSING CONSIDERATIONS
• Patients with severe CHF whose renal function depends on the angiotensin-aldosterone system have experienced acute renal failure during ACE inhibitor therapy. Hypertensive patients with renal artery stenosis may also show signs of worsening renal function at start of therapy. Closely assess renal function in such patients during first few weeks of therapy.
• Regular assessment of renal function (serum creatinine and BUN levels) is advisable.
• Monitor CBC with differential counts before therapy, every 2 weeks for the first 3 months of therapy, and periodically thereafter. Advise the patient to report any signs of infection, such as fever and sore throat. These effects may occur especially in patients with impaired renal function or collagen vascular diseases (systemic lupus erythematosus or scleroderma).
• Tell the patient to avoid abrupt discontinuation of therapy.
• Light-headedness can occur, especially during the first few days of therapy. Tell the patient to rise slowly to minimize this effect and to report symptoms to the doctor. Patients who experience syncope should stop taking drug and call the doctor immediately.
• Angioedema (including laryngeal edema) may occur, especially after the first dose. Advise the patient to report any signs or symptoms, such as swelling of face, eyes, lips, or tongue or breathing difficulty.
• Tell the patient to avoid sodium substitutes; these products may contain potassium, which can cause hyperkalemia in patients taking ramipril.

rauwolfia serpentina
Raudixin**, Rauval, Rauverid

Pregnancy Risk Category: D

HOW SUPPLIED
Tablets: 50 mg, 100 mg

ACTION
Mechanism: A rauwolfia alkaloid that acts peripherally, inhibiting norepinephrine release and depleting norepinephrine stores in adrenergic nerve endings.
Onset: within 2 hours. **Peak:** Peak effects vary; full antihypertensive effect does not occur for at least 2 weeks.
Duration: plasma half-life, 5 hours to 11 days; effects may persist several days to weeks after long-term therapy ends.

INDICATIONS & DOSAGE
Mild to moderate hypertension –
Adults: initially and for 1 to 3 weeks thereafter, 200 to 400 mg P.O. daily as a single dose or in two divided doses. Maintenance dosage is 50 to 300 mg daily.

ADVERSE REACTIONS
CNS: mental confusion, *depression, drowsiness, nervousness, paradoxical anxiety,* nightmares, sedation, headache, extrapyramidal symptoms.
CV: orthostatic hypotension, bradycardia, syncope.
EENT: *nasal stuffiness,* glaucoma.
GI: *hypersecretion of gastric acid, nausea, vomiting, dry mouth,* bleeding.
GU: impotence.
Skin: pruritus, rash.
Other: weight gain.

INTERACTIONS
Digitalis glycosides: rauwolfia may predispose patients to digitalis-induced arrhythmias. Use together cautiously.
MAO inhibitors: may cause excitabil-

ity and hypertension. Use together cautiously.

CONTRAINDICATIONS
- Contraindicated in patients with mental depression.
- Use cautiously in patients with severe cardiac or cerebrovascular disease, impaired renal function, peptic ulceration, ulcerative colitis, or gallstones; in those undergoing surgery; in elderly or debilitated patients; and in those taking other antihypertensives or tricyclic antidepressants.

NURSING CONSIDERATIONS
- Monitor blood pressure and pulse rate frequently.
- Tell the patient not to discontinue drug suddenly, but to call the doctor, if unpleasant adverse reactions occur.
- Warn the patient that drug can cause drowsiness. Patients should not drive or perform other activities that require alertness and good coordination until CNS effects are known.
- Watch the patient closely for signs of mental depression. Warn him to notify the doctor promptly if nightmares occur.
- Advise the patient to minimize orthostatic hypotension by rising slowly and avoiding sudden position changes. Dry mouth can be relieved with chewing gum, sour hard candy, or ice chips. Tell the patient to contact the doctor if relief is needed for nasal stuffiness.
- Drug should be taken with meals.
- Tell the patient to weigh himself daily and notify the doctor of any weight gain over 5 lb.
- Advise the patient to have periodic eye examinations.

rescinnamine
Moderil
Pregnancy Risk Category: D

HOW SUPPLIED
Tablets: 0.25 mg, 0.5 mg

ACTION
Mechanism: A rauwolfia derivitive that acts peripherally, inhibiting norepinephrine release and depleting norepinephrine stores in adrenergic nerve endings.
Onset: 24 hours or longer. **Duration:** plasma half-life, more than 30 hours.

INDICATIONS & DOSAGE
Mild to moderate hypertension (used alone or in combination with other antihypertensives) –
Adults: initially, 0.5 mg P.O. b.i.d. Maintenance dosage is 0.25 to 0.5 mg daily.

ADVERSE REACTIONS
CNS: mental confusion, *depression, drowsiness, nervousness, anxiety, nightmares,* sedation, parkinsonism.
CV: *orthostatic hypotension, bradycardia, syncope.*
EENT: *nasal stuffiness,* glaucoma.
GI: *hypersecretion of gastric acid, nausea, vomiting, dry mouth,* GI bleeding.
GU: impotence.
Skin: pruritus, rash.
Other: *weight gain.*

INTERACTIONS
MAO inhibitors: may cause excitability and hypertension. Use together cautiously.

CONTRAINDICATIONS
- Contraindicated in patients with mental depression.
- Use cautiously in patients with severe cardiac or cerebrovascular disease, peptic ulcer, ulcerative colitis, or gallstones; in those undergoing surgery; in elderly or debilitated patients, and in patients taking other antihypertensives.

NURSING CONSIDERATIONS

- Monitor blood pressure and pulse rate frequently.
- Tell the patient not to discontinue drug suddenly, but to call the doctor, if unpleasant adverse reactions occur.
- Warn the patient that drug can cause drowsiness. Patients should not drive or perform other tasks that require alertness and coordination until drug's adverse CNS effects are known.
- Watch the patient closely for signs of mental depression. Warn him to notify the doctor promptly if nightmares occur.
- Advise the patient to minimize orthostatic hypotension by rising slowly and avoiding sudden position changes. Dry mouth can be relieved with chewing gum, sour hard candy, or ice chips. Tell the patient to contact the doctor if relief is needed for nasal stuffiness.
- Drug should be taken with meals.
- Tell the patient to weigh himself daily and to notify the doctor of any weight gain over 5 lb.
- Advise the patient to have periodic eye examinations.

reserpine

Novoreserpine†, Serpalan, Serpasil†*

Pregnancy Risk Category: C

HOW SUPPLIED

Tablets: 0.1 mg, 0.25 mg, 1 mg

ACTION

Mechanism: A rauwolfia derivative that acts peripherally, inhibiting norepinephrine release and depleting norepinephrine stores in adrenergic nerve endings.
Onset: within 2 hours. **Peak:** Peak antihypertensive effect is evident after 2 to 3 weeks of therapy. **Duration:** plasma half-life, 2 to 7 days; effects may persist for several weeks.

INDICATIONS & DOSAGE

Mild to moderate essential hypertension –
Adults: 0.1 to 0.25 mg P.O. daily.
Children: 5 to 20 mcg/kg P.O. daily.

ADVERSE REACTIONS

CNS: mental confusion, *drowsiness, sedation, nervousness, paradoxical anxiety, nightmares, depression,* extrapyramidal symptoms.
CV: *orthostatic hypotension, bradycardia, syncope.*
EENT: *nasal stuffiness,* glaucoma.
GI: *hyperacidity, nausea, vomiting, dry mouth,* bleeding.
GU: *impotence.*
Skin: pruritus, rash.
Other: *weight gain.*

INTERACTIONS

MAO inhibitors: may cause excitability and hypertension. Use together cautiously.

CONTRAINDICATIONS

- Contraindicated in patients with mental depression or patients receiving electroconvulsive therapy (ECT). Also contraindicated in patients with ulcerative colitis.
- Use cautiously in patients with history of seizures or peptic ulceration, in patients undergoing surgery, and in those taking other antihypertensives.

NURSING CONSIDERATIONS

- Monitor blood pressure and pulse rate frequently.
- Tell the patient not to discontinue drug suddenly, but to call the doctor, if unpleasant adverse reactions occur.
- Warn the patient that drug can cause drowsiness. Patients should avoid hazardous activities that require alertness and coordination until drug's CNS effects are known.
- Watch the patient closely for signs of mental depression. Warn him to notify the doctor promptly if nightmares occur.

• Advise the patient to minimize orthostatic hypotension by rising slowly and avoiding sudden position changes. Dry mouth can be relieved with chewing gum, sour hard candy, or ice chips. Tell the patient to contact the doctor if relief is needed for nasal stuffiness.
• Drug should be taken with meals.
• Tell the patient to weigh himself daily and to notify the doctor of any weight gain over 5 lb.
• Advise the patient to have periodic eye examinations.

terazosin hydrochloride

Hytrin

Pregnancy Risk Category: C

HOW SUPPLIED

Tablets: 1 mg, 2 mg, 5 mg

ACTION

Mechanism: Decreases blood pressure by vasodilation produced in response to blockade of alpha$_1$-adrenergic receptors. Improves urine flow in patients with benign prostatic hyperplasia (BPH) by blocking alpha$_1$-adrenergic receptors in the smooth muscle of the bladder neck and prostate, thus relieving urethral pressure and reestablishing urine flow.
Onset: within 15 minutes. **Peak:** Peak effects on blood pressure occur within 3 hours. Steady-state levels are reached after about 6 weeks. **Duration:** half-life, about 12 hours; effects persist 24 hours.

INDICATIONS & DOSAGE

Hypertension –
Adults: initially, 1 mg P.O. h.s., not to be exceeded. Increase dosage gradually according to patient response. Usual dosage range is 1 to 5 mg daily. Maximum recommended dosage is 20 mg/day.
Symptomatic BPH –
Adults: initally, 1 mg P.O. h.s. Increase dosage in a stepwise fashion to 2 mg, 5 mg, or 10 mg once daily to achieve optimal response. Most patients require 10 mg daily for optimal response.

ADVERSE REACTIONS

CNS: asthenia, *dizziness,* headache, nervousness, paresthesia, somnolence.
CV: *palpitations,* postural hypotension, tachycardia, *peripheral edema.*
EENT: *nasal congestion,* sinusitis, blurred vision.
GI: *nausea.*
GU: impotence, decreased libido.
Respiratory: dyspnea.
Other: weight gain, back pain, muscle pain.

INTERACTIONS

Antihypertensives: excessive hypotension. Use together cautiously.

CONTRAINDICATIONS

• Contraindicated in patients with hypersensitivity to the drug.

NURSING CONSIDERATIONS

• If terazosin is discontinued for several days, the patient will need to be retitrated using initial dosing regimen (1 mg P.O. h.s.).
• Warn the patient to avoid hazardous activities that require mental alertness, such as driving or operating heavy machinery for 12 hours after the first dose.
• Tell the patient not to discontinue drug suddenly, but to call the doctor, if adverse reactions occur.

timolol maleate

Apo-Timol†, Blocadren

Pregnancy Risk Category: C

HOW SUPPLIED

Tablets: 5 mg, 10 mg, 20 mg

ACTION

Mechanism: Blocks both $beta_1$- and $beta_2$-receptors and depresses renin secretion.

Onset: 15 to 30 minutes. **Peak:** Peak effects occur in 1 to 2 hours. **Duration:** plasma half-life, about 4 hours; effects persist for 6 to 12 hours.

INDICATIONS & DOSAGE

Hypertension (alone or in combination with diuretics) –

Adults: initially, 10 mg P.O. b.i.d. Usual daily maintenance dosage is 20 to 40 mg. Maximum daily dosage is 60 mg. Allow at least 7 days to elapse between increases in dosage.

MI (long-term prophylaxis in patients who have survived acute phase) –

Adults: 10 mg P.O. b.i.d.

Migraine headache prophylaxis –

Adults: initially, 20 mg P.O. daily as a single dose or in divided doses b.i.d. Increase dosage as needed and tolerated to maximum 30 mg daily. Discontinue treatment if no response occurs after 6 to 8 weeks of therapy at maximum dosage.

Prophylaxis of angina pectoris –

Adults: highly individualized; dosages of 15 to 45 mg P.O. daily in three or four divided doses have been used. Adjust dosage to maintain clinical response and keep the patient's resting heart rate at 55 to 60 beats/minute.

ADVERSE REACTIONS

CNS: fatigue, lethargy, vivid dreams.

CV: *bradycardia, hypotension,* ***CHF,*** peripheral vascular disease.

GI: nausea, vomiting, diarrhea.

Respiratory: dyspnea, ***bronchospasm, increased airway resistance.***

Skin: rash.

Other: fever.

INTERACTIONS

Digitalis glycosides, diltiazem, verapamil: excessive bradycardia and increased depressant effect on myocardium. Use together cautiously.

Indomethacin: decreased antihypertensive effect. Monitor blood pressure and adjust dosage.

Insulin, oral antidiabetic agents: can alter requirements for these drugs in previously stabilized diabetic patients. Monitor the patient for hypoglycemia.

CONTRAINDICATIONS

- Contraindicated in patients with severe asthma or allergic rhinitis, sinus bradycardia and heart block greater than first degree, cardiogenic shock, or right ventricular failure secondary to pulmonary hypertension.
- Use cautiously in patients with CHF and hepatic, renal, or respiratory disease and in those taking other antihypertensives. Also use cautiously in diabetic patients because beta-adrenergic blockers may mask certain signs and symptoms of hypoglycemia.

NURSING CONSIDERATIONS

- Always check the patient's apical pulse rate before giving drug. If you detect extremes in pulse rates, withhold drug and call the doctor immediately.
- Monitor blood pressure frequently.
- Tell the patient that abrupt discontinuation of drug can exacerbate angina and precipitate MI. Dosage should be gradually reduced over 1 to 2 weeks.

trimethaphan camsylate

Arfonad

Pregnancy Risk Category: C

HOW SUPPLIED

Injection: 50 mg/ml in 10-ml ampules, 250 mg/vial‡

ACTION

Mechanism: A ganglionic blocker that stabilizes postsynaptic membranes.

Onset: immediate. **Peak:** Peak effects occur within 5 minutes. **Duration:** effects dissipate within 10 minutes of discontinuing drug.

INDICATIONS & DOSAGE

To lower blood pressure quickly in hypertensive emergencies; to control hypotension during surgery –

Adults: 500 mg (10 ml) diluted in 500 ml D_5W to yield concentration of 1 mg/ml I.V. Start I.V. drip at 1 to 2 mg/minute and titrate to achieve desired hypotensive response. Range is 0.3 mg to 6 mg/minute.

ADVERSE REACTIONS

CNS: dilated pupils, *extreme weakness.*

CV: *severe orthostatic hypotension, tachycardia.*

GI: anorexia, *nausea, vomiting, dry mouth.*

GU: urine retention.

Respiratory: respiratory depression.

Skin: urticaria, itching.

INTERACTIONS

Anesthetics, diuretics, procainamide: increased hypotensive effect. Monitor the patient closely.

CONTRAINDICATIONS

- Contraindicated in patients with anemia and in those with respiratory insufficiency.
- Use cautiously in patients with arteriosclerosis; cardiac, hepatic, or renal disease; degenerative CNS disorders; Addison's disease; or diabetes mellitus and in those receiving other antihypertensives or glucocorticoids.

NURSING CONSIDERATIONS

- Monitor blood pressure and vital signs continuously.
- Place the patient in the supine position during drug administration. If necessary, elevate the head of the bed for maximal effect to avoid cerebral anoxia. Do not elevate bed more than 30 degrees.
- Watch closely for respiratory distress, especially if large doses are used. Large doses have caused apnea and respiratory arrest.
- If extreme hypotension occurs, discontinue drug and call the doctor. Use phenylephrine or mephentermine to counteract hypotension.
- Discontinue drug before wound closure in surgery to allow blood pressure to return to normal.
- **I.V. use:** Refrigerate before reconstitution and prepare solution just before use. Solution is stable for 24 hours after reconstitution.
- Use infusion pump to administer drug slowly and precisely.

23
Vasodilators

amyl nitrite
cyclandelate
dipyridamole
ethaverine hydrochloride
isoxsuprine hydrochloride
nimodipine
papaverine hydrochloride
tolazoline hydrochloride

COMBINATION PRODUCTS
None.

amyl nitrite

Pregnancy Risk Category: C

HOW SUPPLIED
Ampules (crushable): 0.18 ml, 0.3 ml

ACTION
Mechanism: Reduces cardiac oxygen demand by decreasing left ventricular end-diastolic pressure (preload) and systemic vascular resistance (afterload). Also increases blood flow through the collateral coronary vessels. Converts hemoglobin to methemoglobin (which binds cyanide) to treat cyanide poisoning.
Onset: within 30 seconds. **Peak:** Peak effects occur within 1 minute.
Duration: effects persist 3 to 5 minutes.

INDICATIONS & DOSAGE
Relief of angina pectoris; relief of renal or gallbladder colic –
Adults and children: 0.2 to 0.3 ml by inhalation (one glass ampule) p.r.n.
Antidote for cyanide poisoning –
0.2 or 0.3 ml by inhalation for 30 to 60 seconds q 5 minutes until conscious.

ADVERSE REACTIONS
CNS: *headache, sometimes with throbbing;* dizziness; weakness.
CV: *orthostatic hypotension, tachycardia,* flushing, palpitations, fainting.
GI: nausea, vomiting.
Hematologic: methemoglobinemia.
Skin: cutaneous vasodilation.
Other: hypersensitivity reactions.

INTERACTIONS
None significant.

CONTRAINDICATIONS
- Contraindicated in patients with hypersensitivity to nitrites or with acute MI.
- Use cautiously in patients with head injury or cerebral hemorrhage and in those with hypotension or glaucoma.

NURSING CONSIDERATIONS
- Extinguish all cigarettes before use, or ampule may ignite.
- Wrap ampule in cloth and crush. Hold near the patient's nose and mouth so vapor is inhaled.
- Watch for orthostatic hypotension. Have the patient sit down and avoid rapid position changes while inhaling drug.
- Advise the patient that keeping the head low, deep breathing, and movement of extremities may help relieve dizziness, syncope, or weakness from orthostatic hypotension.
- Drug is often abused. Claimed to have aphrodisiac benefits. Street name is "Amy."
- Seldom, if ever, used for treatment of angina because it's expensive and inconvenient and frequently causes adverse reactions.
- Sometimes used to induce changes in heart murmurs. The patient inhales

drug until reflex tachycardia is induced, then discontinues.
• Store away from light.

cyclandelate

Cyclospasmol

Pregnancy Risk Category: C

HOW SUPPLIED
Tablets: 200 mg, 400 mg
Capsules: 200 mg, 400 mg

ACTION
Mechanism: Inhibits phosphodiesterase, directly relaxing smooth muscle and increasing concentrations of cAMP.
Peak: Peak effects occur within 1½ hours.

INDICATIONS & DOSAGE
Adjunct in intermittent claudication, arteriosclerosis obliterans, vasospasm and muscular ischemia associated with thrombophlebitis, nocturnal leg cramps, Raynaud's phenomenon, and selected cases of ischemic cerebral vascular disease –
Adults: initially, 1.2 to 1.6 g P.O. daily in divided doses before meals and h.s. For maintenance, decrease dosage by 200 mg/day to the lowest effective level. Maintenance dosage is usually 400 to 800 mg daily in two to four divided doses.

ADVERSE REACTIONS
CNS: *headache, tingling of the extremities, dizziness.*
CV: *mild flushing,* tachycardia.
GI: pyrosis, eructation, nausea, heartburn.
Other: *diaphoresis.*

INTERACTIONS
None significant.

CONTRAINDICATIONS
• Contraindicated in patients with hypersensitivity to the drug.
• Use with extreme caution in patients with severe obliterative coronary artery or cerebrovascular disease because circulation to these diseased areas may be compromised by vasodilatory effects elsewhere (coronary steal syndrome).
• Use cautiously in patients with glaucoma or hypotension.

NURSING CONSIDERATIONS
• Adverse reactions usually disappear after several weeks of therapy.
• To reduce GI distress, give with food or antacids.
• Short-term therapy is of little benefit. Instruct the patient to expect long-term treatment and to continue to take medication.

dipyridamole

Apo-Dipyridamole†, Dipridacot, I.V. Persantine, Novodipiradol†, Persantin‡, Persantin 100‡, Persantine**

Pregnancy Risk Category: C

HOW SUPPLIED
Tablets: 25 mg, 50 mg, 75 mg
Injection: 10 mg/2 ml†

ACTION
Mechanism: Inhibits platelet adhesion and the enzymes adenosine deaminase and phosphodiesterase.
Peak: Plasma levels peak 45 to 150 minutes after oral dose. **Duration:** terminal elimination half-life, 10 to 12 hours.

INDICATIONS & DOSAGE
Inhibition of platelet adhesion in prosthetic heart valves (in combination with warfarin or aspirin) –
Adults: 75 to 100 mg P.O. q.i.d.
Transient ischemic attack –
Adults: 400 to 800 mg P.O. daily in divided doses.
Alternative to exercise in evaluation of

coronary artery disease during thallium myocardial perfusion imaging–
Adults: 0.57 mg/kg as an I.V. infusion at a constant rate over 4 minutes (0.142 mg/kg/minute). Do not give more than 60 mg.
Acute coronary insufficiency‡–
Adults: 10 mg I.V. or I.M.

ADVERSE REACTIONS
CNS: *headache, dizziness,* weakness.
CV: flushing, fainting, *hypotension; chest pain,* ***ECG abnormalities,*** *blood pressure lability, hypertension* (with I.V. infusion).
GI: *nausea,* vomiting, diarrhea.
Skin: rash, irritation (with undiluted injection).

INTERACTIONS
None significant.

CONTRAINDICATIONS
- Contraindicated in patients with hypersensitivity to the drug.
- Use cautiously in patients with hypotension and in those receiving anticoagulants.

NURSING CONSIDERATIONS
- Observe for adverse reactions, especially with large doses. Monitor blood pressure.
- Observe for signs of bleeding; note prolonged bleeding time (especially with large doses or long-term therapy).
- If the patient develops GI distress, administer 1 hour before meals or with meals.
- Don't use dipyridamole alone for thromboembolism prophylaxis in postoperative prosthetic valve patients; use with oral anticoagulants.
- Dipyridamole's value as part of an antithrombosis regimen is controversial: using it may not provide significantly better results than using aspirin alone.
- **I.V. use:** If administering as a diagnostic agent, dilute in 0.45% or 0.9% sodium chloride or D_5W in at least a 1:2 ratio for a total volume of 20 to 50 ml. Inject thallium-201 within 5 minutes after completing the 4-minute dipyridamole infusion.

ethaverine hydrochloride

Ethaquin, Ethatab, Ethavex-100, Isovex

Pregnancy Risk Category: C

HOW SUPPLIED
Tablets: 100 mg
Capsules: 100 mg

ACTION
Mechanism: Inhibits phosphodiesterase, directly relaxing smooth muscle and increasing concentrations of cAMP.
Peak: Peak effects occur after 1 to 4 hours. **Duration:** effects persist 6 to 8 hours.

INDICATIONS & DOSAGE
Long-term treatment of peripheral and cerebrovascular insufficiency associated with arterial spasm; spastic conditions of GI and GU tracts–
Adults: 100 to 200 mg P.O. t.i.d.

ADVERSE REACTIONS
CNS: *headache,* drowsiness.
CV: *hypotension, flushing,* sweating, vertigo, cardiac depression, arrhythmias.
EENT: *dry throat.*
GI: *nausea, anorexia, abdominal distress,* constipation, diarrhea.
Hepatic: jaundice, altered liver function tests.
Respiratory: respiratory depression.
Skin: rash.
Other: malaise, lassitude.

INTERACTIONS
None significant.

CONTRAINDICATIONS
• Contraindicated in patients with complete AV dissociation and in those with severe hepatic disease.
• May precipitate arrhythmias. Use cautiously in women who are pregnant or of childbearing age and in patients with glaucoma or pulmonary embolismsm.

NURSING CONSIDERATIONS
• If signs of hypersensitivity reactions develop (GI symptoms, altered liver function tests, jaundice, eosinophilia), withhold dose and call the doctor.
• The FDA has announced this drug may not be effective for disease states indicated.

isoxsuprine hydrochloride
Duvadilan‡, Vasodilan

Pregnancy Risk Category: C

HOW SUPPLIED
Tablets: 10 mg, 20 mg

ACTION
Mechanism: Stimulates beta receptors and may also be a direct-acting peripheral vasodilator.
Peak: Peak effects occur within 1 hour. **Duration:** effects persist 3 to 6 hours.

INDICATIONS & DOSAGE
Adjunct for relief of symptoms associated with cerebrovascular insufficiency, peripheral vascular diseases (such as arteriosclerosis obliterans, thromboangiitis obliterans, Raynaud's disease) –
Adults: 10 to 20 mg P.O. t.i.d. or q.i.d.

ADVERSE REACTIONS
CNS: trembling, nervousness.
CV: tachycardia, hypotension.
GI: vomiting, abdominal distress, intestinal distention.
Skin: severe rash, flushing.

INTERACTIONS
None significant.

CONTRAINDICATIONS
• Contraindicated in immediate postpartum period and in patients with arterial bleeding.
• Use cautiously in patients with cardiovascular or cerebrovascular disease.
• Safe use during pregnancy and lactation has not been established, although drug has been used to inhibit contractions in premature labor.

NURSING CONSIDERATIONS
• Discontinue drug if rash develops.
• To minimize the risk of orthostasis, instruct the patient to avoid sudden position changes.
• Isoxsuprine has also been used to minimize cramping in patients with severe primary dysmenorrhea.

nimodipine
Nimotop

Pregnancy Risk Category: C

HOW SUPPLIED
Capsules: 30 mg

ACTION
Mechanism: Inhibits calcium ion influx across cardiac and smooth muscle cells, decreasing myocardial contractility and oxygen demand, and dilates coronary and cerebral arteries and arterioles. Initially thought to relieve vasospasm in patients after subarachnoid hemorrhage, its mechanism of action is not fully known; blockade of calcium influx into cerebral neurons may contribute to drug's effect.
Onset: within ½ hour. **Peak:** Peak effects occur within 1 hour. **Duration:** elimination half-life, 2 to 9 hours after oral dose, 1 to 1½ hours after I.V. use. Effects persist 3 to 4 hours.

INDICATIONS & DOSAGE
Improvement of neurologic deficits in patients after subarachnoid hemorrhage from ruptured congenital aneurysms –
Adults: 60 mg P.O. q 4 hours for 21 days. Begin therapy within 96 hours after subarachnoid hemorrhage.

In patients with hepatic failure, begin therapy with lower dosage – 30 mg P.O. q 4 hours – with close monitoring of blood pressure and heart rate.

ADVERSE REACTIONS
CNS: headache.
CV: decreased blood pressure, flushing, edema.

INTERACTIONS
Antihypertensives: possible enhanced hypotensive effect.
Calcium channel blockers: possible enhanced cardiovascular effects.

CONTRAINDICATIONS
- Nimodipine should be reserved for patients who are in good neurologic condition (for example, Hunt and Hess grades I to II).

NURSING CONSIDERATIONS
- Monitor blood pressure and heart rate in all patients, especially at start of therapy.

papaverine hydrochloride
Cerespan, Genabid, Pavabid, Pavabid HP Capsulets, Pavabid Plateau Caps, Pavacels, Pavacot, Pavagen, Pavarine Spancaps, Pavased, Pavatine, Pavatym, Paverolan Lanacaps
Pregnancy Risk Category: C

HOW SUPPLIED
Tablets: 30 mg, 60 mg, 100 mg, 150 mg, 200 mg, 300 mg
Tablets (timed-release): 200 mg
Capsules (timed-release): 150 mg
Injection: 30 mg/ml, 32.5 mg/ml†

ACTION
Mechanism: Inhibits phosphodiesterase, directly relaxing smooth muscle and increasing concentrations of cAMP.
Onset: 15 to 30 minutes. **Duration:** effects persist 3 to 6 hours.

INDICATIONS & DOSAGE
Relief of cerebral and peripheral ischemia associated with arterial spasm and myocardial ischemia; smooth muscle spasm (coronary occlusion, angina pectoris, sequelae of peripheral and pulmonary embolismsm, certain cerebral angiospastic states) and visceral spasms (biliary, ureteral, or GI colic) –
Adults: 60 to 300 mg P.O. one to five times daily, or 150- to 300-mg sustained-release preparations q 8 to 12 hours; 30 to 120 mg I.M. or I.V. q 3 hours, as indicated. Alternatively, give 30 to 40 mg by intra-arterial injection.
Treatment adjunct in impotence –
Adults: 30 mg by intracavernosal injection. Usually given with phentolamine, 0.5 to 1 mg.

ADVERSE REACTIONS
CNS: *headache,* depression.
CV: *increased heart rate, increased blood pressure* (with parenteral use), depressed AV and intraventricular conduction, hypotension, ***arrhythmias.***
GI: constipation, dry mouth, *nausea.*
Hepatic: ***liver damage.***
Respiratory: increased depth of respiration, ***apnea.***
Other: *diaphoresis, flushing,* malaise.

INTERACTIONS
Lactated Ringer's solution: precipitate forms when mixed with papaverine. Don't mix together.
Levodopa: papaverine may interfere

with levodopa's therapeutic effects in patients with Parkinson's disease.

CONTRAINDICATIONS
- Contraindicated for I.V. use in patients with Parkinson's disease or complete AV block.
- Use cautiously in patients with glaucoma.

NURSING CONSIDERATIONS
- Not often used parenterally, except when immediate effect is desired.
- Most effective when given early in the course of a disorder.
- Monitor blood pressure and heart rate and rhythm, especially in cardiac disease. Withhold dose and notify the doctor immediately if changes occur.
- Monitor for adverse hepatic reactions in patients receiving long-term therapy.
- **I.V. use:** Give by direct injection over 1 to 2 minutes. Slow administration minimizes the risk of serious adverse reactions.
- Tell the patient to take medication regularly; long-term therapy is required.
- Advise the patient to avoid tasks that require mental alertness such as driving or operating heavy machinery, until drug's CNS effects are known.
- To minimize the risk of orthostasis, instruct the patient to avoid sudden posture changes.
- The FDA has announced this drug may not be effective for disease states indicated.

tolazoline hydrochloride
Priscoline

Pregnancy Risk Category: C

HOW SUPPLIED
Injection: 25 mg/ml

ACTION
Mechanism: Direct-acting vasodilator. May have some alpha-receptor blocking effects.
Onset: 15 to 30 minutes. **Peak:** Peak effects occur within 30 to 60 minutes.
Duration: elimination half-life, 1½ to 41 hours.

INDICATIONS & DOSAGE
Persistent pulmonary hypertension of the newborn –
Neonates: initially, 1 to 2 mg/kg I.V. over 10 minutes, followed by infusion of 1 to 2 mg/kg/hour.
Peripheral vasospastic disorders –
Adults: 10 to 50 mg I.M. or I.V. q.i.d.

ADVERSE REACTIONS
CNS: weakness, paradoxical response in seriously damaged limbs, increased pilomotor activity, tingling, chilliness, apprehension.
CV: ***arrhythmias,*** anginal pain, *hypertension, flushing,* transient postural vertigo, palpitations, *orthostatic hypotension.*
GI: *nausea, vomiting, diarrhea, epigastric discomfort, exacerbation of peptic ulceration.*
Hematologic: ***agranulocytosis,*** thrombocytopenia.
Respiratory: ***pulmonary hemorrhage.***
Other: burning at injection site.

INTERACTIONS
Ethanol: possible disulfiram-like reaction (including chills and flushing) from accumulation of acetaldehyde. Use together cautiously.
Vasopressors (epinephrine, norepinephrine): may cause paradoxical fall in blood pressure.

CONTRAINDICATIONS
- Contraindicated in patients with coronary artery disease or active peptic ulceration or after CVA.
- Use cautiously in patients with a

history of peptic ulceration, gastritis, or known or suspected mitral stenosis.

NURSING CONSIDERATIONS

- Often used to distinguish between functional (vasospastic) and organic (obstructive) forms of peripheral vascular disease.
- Monitor vital signs. Watch especially for blood pressure changes and arrhythmias.
- To increase response, keep the patient warm during parenteral administration.
- **I.V. use:** Response to treatment of persistent pulmonary hypertension of the newborn should be evident within 30 minutes. Little information exists regarding infusions lasting longer than 48 hours.
- Place the patient in the supine position during infusion.
- Appearance of flushing usually indicates maximum tolerable dose.
- To minimize the risk of orthostasis, instruct the patient to avoid sudden posture changes.
- Warn the patient against exposure to cold, which can aggravate tissue damage.

Antilipemics

cholestyramine
clofibrate
colestipol hydrochloride
dextrothyroxine sodium
fluvastatin sodium
gemfibrozil
lovastatin
niacin
(See Chapter 90, VITAMINS AND MINERALS.)
pravastatin sodium
probucol
simvastatin

COMBINATION PRODUCTS
None.

cholestyramine

Cholybar, Questran**, Questran Light, Questran Lite‡

Pregnancy Risk Category: C

HOW SUPPLIED
Bar: 4 g
Powder: 378-g cans, 9-g single-dose packets. Each scoop of powder or single-dose packet contains 4 g of cholestyramine resin.

ACTION
Mechanism: A bile-acid sequestrant that combines with bile acid to form an insoluble compound that is excreted. The liver must synthesize new bile acid from cholesterol, which reduces low-density-lipoprotein cholesterol levels.
Onset: some serum cholesterol level reduction within 4 to 6 weeks. **Peak:** Peak effects vary; maximal effects are usually evident within 4 months.

INDICATIONS & DOSAGE
Primary hyperlipidemia, pruritus, and diarrhea caused by excess bile acid; adjunct for reduction of elevated serum cholesterol in patients with primary hypercholesterolemia; reduction of risks of atherosclerotic coronary artery disease (CAD) and MI–
Adults: 4 g before meals and h.s., not to exceed 32 g daily.
Children: 240 mg/kg daily P.O. in three divided doses with beverage or food. Safe dosage not established for children under 6 years.

ADVERSE REACTIONS
GI: *constipation,* fecal impaction, hemorrhoids, *abdominal discomfort,* flatulence, *nausea,* vomiting, steatorrhea.
Skin: *rash,* irritation of skin, tongue, and perianal area.
Other: *vitamin A, D, and K deficiency from decreased absorption;* hyperchloremic acidosis with long-term use or very high dosage.

INTERACTIONS
Acetaminophen, beta-adrenergic blockers, corticosteroids, digitalis glycosides, fat-soluble vitamins (A, D, E, and K), iron preparations, thiazide diuretics, thyroid hormone, warfarin and other coumarin anticoagulants: absorption may be substantially decreased by cholestyramine. Administer at least 2 hours apart.

CONTRAINDICATIONS
- Contraindicated in patients with hypersensitivity to bile-acid sequestering resins and in those with complete biliary obstruction.
- Use cautiously in patients predisposed to constipation and in those with conditions aggravated by constipation, such as severe, symptomatic CAD. Long-term use may be associated with deficiency of vitamins A, D, E, and K and folic acid.

NURSING CONSIDERATIONS

• Monitor serum cholesterol and triglyceride levels regularly during therapy.

• Monitor serum levels of digitalis glycosides in patients receiving digitalis glycosides and cholestyramine concurrently. If cholestyramine therapy is discontinued, adjust dosage of digiltalis glycosides to avoid toxicity.

• Monitor bowel habits. Encourage a diet high in fiber and fluids. If severe constipation develops, decrease dosage, add a stool softener, or discontinue drug.

• Instruct the patient never to take drug in its dry form; esophageal irritation or severe constipation may result. Using a large glass, the patient should sprinkle the powder on the surface of preferred beverage; let the mixture stand a few minutes; then stir thoroughly. The best diluents are water, milk, and juice (especially pulpy fruit juice). Mixing with carbonated beverages may result in excess foaming. After drinking this preparation, the patient should swirl a small additional amount of liquid in the same glass and then drink it to ensure ingestion of the entire dose.

• Advise the patient to take all other drugs at least 1 hour before or 4 to 6 hours after cholestyramine to avoid blocking their absorption.

• Teach the patient about proper dietary management of serum lipids (restricting total fat and cholesterol intake), as well as measures to control other cardiac disease risk factors. When appropriate, recommend weight control, exercise, and stop-smoking programs.

clofibrate

Abitrate, Arterioflexin‡, Atromid-S, Claripex†, Col‡, Novofibrate†

Pregnancy Risk Category: C

HOW SUPPLIED

Capsules: 500 mg

ACTION

Mechanism: Seems to inhibit biosynthesis of cholesterol at an early stage, but exact mechanism is unknown.
Onset: rapid. **Peak:** Peak plasma levels occur 2 to 6 hours after a dose. Peak antilipemic effects occur after 3 to 4 weeks of therapy. **Duration:** plasma half-life, 6 to 24 hours; effects persist about 3 weeks.

INDICATIONS & DOSAGE

Hyperlipidemia –
Adults: 2 g P.O. daily in two or four divided doses. Some patients may respond to lower doses as assessed by serum lipid monitoring.

ADVERSE REACTIONS

CNS: fatigue, weakness.
CV: ***arrhythmias.***
GI: *nausea, diarrhea, vomiting,* stomatitis, *dyspepsia,* flatulence.
GU: impotence and decreased libido, ***acute renal failure.***
Hematologic: leukopenia.
Hepatic: gallstones, *transient and reversible elevations of liver function tests.*
Skin: rash, urticaria, pruritus, dry skin and hair.
Other: myalgia and arthralgia, resembling a flulike syndrome; *weight gain; polyphagia;* fever.

INTERACTIONS

Furosemide, sulfonylureas: clofibrate may potentiate the clinical effects of these agents. Monitor the patient closely.
Lovastatin, simvastatin, pravastatin: risk of myositis, rhabdomyolysis, and renal failure. Avoid concomitant use.
Oral anticoagulants: clofibrate may potentiate the anticoagulant effects of warfarin or dicumarol. Decrease the anticoagulant dosage.
Oral contraceptives, rifampin: may

antagonize clofibrate's lipid-lowering effect. Monitor serum lipids.
Probenecid: increased clofibrate effect. Monitor for toxicity.

CONTRAINDICATIONS
• Contraindicated in children and patients with severe renal or hepatic disease.

NURSING CONSIDERATIONS
• Used to treat patients with high serum triglyceride levels (type IV or V hyperlipidemia). These patients typically have serum triglyceride levels over 2,000 mg/dl.
• Monitor serum cholesterol and triglyceride levels regularly during therapy.
• Monitor renal and hepatic function, blood counts, and serum electrolyte and blood glucose levels. If liver function tests show steady rise, expect discontinuation of clofibrate.
• Drug is typically discontinued if significant lipid lowering is not achieved within 3 months.
• Advise patients to report any flulike symptoms immediately because their occurrence may indicate rhabdomyolysis-induced renal failure.
• Teach patients about proper dietary management of serum lipids (restricting total fat and cholesterol intake), as well as measures to control other cardiac disease risk factors. When appropriate, recommend weight control, exercise, and stop-smoking programs.
• Clofibrate has been used investigationally to treat diabetes insipidus at doses of 1.5 to 2 g daily.

colestipol hydrochloride
Colestid

Pregnancy Risk Category: C

HOW SUPPLIED
Granules: 500-g bottles, 5-g packets

ACTION
Mechanism: Combines with bile acid to form an insoluble compound that is excreted. The liver must synthesize new bile acid from cholesterol; this leads to reduced low-density-lipoprotein cholesterol levels.
Onset: reduced plasma cholesterol levels within 1 to 2 days. **Peak:** Antilipemic effects peak after about 1 month of therapy. **Duration:** lipid levels return to pretreatment values within 1 month of discontinuing treatment.

INDICATIONS & DOSAGE
Primary hypercholesterolemia and xanthomas –
Adults: 5 to 30 g P.O. daily in two to four divided doses.

ADVERSE REACTIONS
CNS: headache, dizziness.
GI: *constipation,* fecal impaction, hemorrhoids, abdominal discomfort, flatulence, nausea, vomiting, steatorrhea.
Skin: rash; irritation, tongue, and perianal area.
Other: vitamin A, D, E, and K deficiency from decreased absorption; hyperchloremic acidosis with long-term use or high dosage.

INTERACTIONS
Oral antidiabetic agents: may antagonize response to colestipol. Monitor serum lipids.
Orally administered drugs: colestipol may decrease absorption. Separate administration times: give other drugs at least 1 hour before or 4 hours after colestipol.

CONTRAINDICATIONS
• Contraindicated in patients with hypersensitivity reactions to bile-acid sequestering resins and in those with complete biliary obstruction.
• Use cautiously in patients predisposed to constipation and in those

with conditions aggravated by constipation, such as severe, symptomatic coronary artery disease. Long-term use may be associated with deficiency of vitamins A, D, E, and K and folic acid.

NURSING CONSIDERATIONS

- Advise the patient to take all other drugs at least 1 hour before or 4 to 6 hours after colestipol to avoid blocking their absorption.
- Monitor serum levels of digitalis glycosides in patients receiving digitalis glycosides and colestipol concurrently. If colestipol therapy is discontinued, adjust dosage of digitalis glycosides to avoid toxicity.
- Monitor bowel habits; if severe constipation develops, decrease dosage or add stool softener. Encourage a diet high in fiber and fluids.
- Instruct the patient never to take drug in its dry form; esophageal irritation or severe constipation may result. Using a large glass, the patient should sprinkle the powder on the surface of the preferred beverage; let the mixture stand a few minutes; then stir thoroughly to obtain a uniform suspension.
- To prepare, instruct the patient to use a large glass containing water, milk, or juice (especially pulpy fruit juice). After drinking this preparation, the patient should swirl a small additional amount of liquid in the same glass and then drink it to ensure ingestion of the entire dose.
- To enhance palatability, mix and refrigerate the next daily dose the previous evening.
- Teach the patient about proper dietary management of serum lipids (restricting total fat and cholesterol intake), as well as measures to control other cardiac disease risk factors. When appropriate, recommend weight control, exercise, and stop-smoking programs.

dextrothyroxine sodium (d-thyroxine sodium)

Choloxin**

Pregnancy Risk Category: C

HOW SUPPLIED

Tablets: 1 mg, 2 mg, 4 mg, 6 mg

ACTION

Mechanism: Accelerates hepatic catabolism of cholesterol and increases bile secretion to lower cholesterol levels.
Peak: Peak effects on serum lipids occur after 1 to 2 months of therapy.
Duration: plasma half-life, about 18 hours; effects persist for 1½ to 3 months.

INDICATIONS & DOSAGE

Hyperlipidemia in euthyroid patients, especially when cholesterol and triglyceride levels are elevated –
Adults: initially, 1 to 2 mg P.O. daily, increased by 1 to 2 mg daily at monthly intervals to a total of 4 to 8 mg daily.
Children: initially, 0.05 mg/kg P.O. daily, increased by 0.05 mg/kg daily at monthly intervals to a maximum of 4 mg daily. Alternatively, give 1.5 mg/m^2 P.O. daily, increased by 1.5 mg/m^2 daily at monthly intervals. Maximum daily dosage is 4 mg. The usual maintenance dosage is 0.1 mg/kg or 3 mg/m^2 daily in euthyroid children.

ADVERSE REACTIONS

CV: palpitations, angina pectoris, ***arrhythmias,*** ischemic myocardial changes on ECG, ***MI.***
EENT: visual disturbances, ptosis.
GI: nausea, vomiting, diarrhea, constipation, decreased appetite.
Other: *insomnia, weight loss, diaphoresis,* flushing, hyperthermia, hyperthyroidism, hair loss, menstrual irregularities.

INTERACTIONS

Digitalis glycosides: dextrothyroxine may enhance clinical effect. Use together cautiously.
Oral anticoagulants: dextrothyroxine may potentiate anticoagulant effect of warfarin or dicumarol.
Sympathomimetics, thyroid hormones: dextrothyroxine may precipitate arrhythmias or coronary insufficiency in patients with cardiac disease.

CONTRAINDICATIONS

- Contraindicated in patients with hepatic or renal disease, or iodism.
- Use cautiously and in smaller doses in patients with a history of cardiac disease, including arrhythmias, hypertension, or angina pectoris, and in patients with diabetes mellitus.
- May increase need for insulin, diet therapy, or oral antidiabetic agents in those with diabetes.

NURSING CONSIDERATIONS

- If anticoagulants are being considered, discontinue dextrothyroxine 2 weeks before surgery to avoid possible potentiation of anticoagulant effect.
- Observe the patient for signs of hyperthyroidism, such as nervousness, insomnia, and weight loss. If these occur, decrease dosage or discontinue drug.
- Teach the patient about proper dietary management of serum lipids (restricting total fat and cholesterol intake), as well as measures to control other cardiac disease risk factors. When appropriate, recommend weight control, exercise, and stop-smoking programs.

---

fluvastatin sodium

Lescol

Pregnancy Risk Category: X

HOW SUPPLIED

Capsules: 20 mg, 40 mg

ACTION

Mechanism: Inhibits 3-hydroxy-3-methylglutaryl coenzyme A reductase. This enzyme is an early (and rate-limiting) step in the synthetic pathway of cholesterol.
Onset: antilipemic effect after several weeks. **Peak:** Plasma levels peak within 1 hour.

INDICATIONS & DOSAGE

Reduction of low-density lipoprotein and total cholesterol levels in patients with primary hypercholesterolemia (types IIa and IIb) –
Adults: initially, 20 mg P.O. h.s. Increase dosage as needed to a maximum of 40 mg daily.

ADVERSE REACTIONS

GI: dyspepsia, diarrhea, nausea.
Hematologic: thrombocytopenia, leukopenia, ***hemolytic anemia***.
Respiratory: sinusitis.
Other: arthropathy, muscle pain, hypersensitivity reactions ***(anaphylaxis, angioedema)***.

INTERACTIONS

Cholestyramine, colestipol: may bind fluvastatin in the GI tract and decrease absorption. Separate administration times by at least 4 hours.
Cimetidine, omeprazole, ranitidine: decreased fluvastatin metabolism. Monitor for enhanced effects.
Cyclosporine and other immunosuppressants, erythromycin, gemfibrozil, niacin: possible increased risk of polymyositis and rhabdomyolysis. Avoid concomitant use.
Digoxin: may alter digoxin pharmacokinetics. Monitor serum digoxin levels carefully.
Ethanol: increased risk of hepatotoxicity. Avoid concomitant use.
Rifampin: enhanced fluvastatin metabolism and decreased plasma levels. Monitor for lack of effect.

CONTRAINDICATIONS

- Contraindicated in patients with hypersensitivity to the drug, and in those with active liver disease or conditions associated with unexplained persistent elevations of serum transaminase levels; in pregnant and breast-feeding women; and in women of childbearing age unless there is no risk of pregnancy.
- Use cautiously in patients with severe renal impairment with history of liver diseaase or heavy alcohol ingestion.

NURSING CONSIDERATIONS

- Initiate fluvastatin only after diet and other nonpharmacologic therapies have proven ineffective. The patient should be on a standard low-cholesterol diet during therapy.
- May be taken without regard to meals; however, efficacy is enhanced if the drug is taken in the evening.
- Watch for signs of myositis.
- Liver function tests should be performed at the start of therapy and periodically thereafter.
- Warn the patient to restrict alcohol intake.
- Tell the patient to inform the doctor of any adverse reactions, particularly muscle aches and pains.
- Teach the patient about proper dietary management, weight control, and exercise. Explain their importance in controlling elevated serum lipids levels.

---

gemfibrozil

Lopid

Pregnancy Risk Category: B

HOW SUPPLIED

Tablets: 600 mg
Capsules: 300 mg

ACTION

Mechanism: Inhibits peripheral lipolysis and also reduces triglyceride synthesis in the liver. Lowers serum triglyceride levels and increases high-density-lipoprotein cholesterol levels.
Onset: 2 to 5 days. **Peak:** Peak effect occurs after 4 weeks of treatment.
Duration: plasma half-life, about 1½ hours.

INDICATIONS & DOSAGE

Type IV hyperlipidemia (hypertriglyceridemia) and severe hypercholesterolemia unresponsive to diet and other drugs; reduction of risk of coronary heart disease in patients who cannot tolerate or who are refractory to treatment with bile acid sequestrants or niacin –
Adults: 1,200 mg P.O. in two divided doses. Usual dosage range is 900 to 1,500 mg daily. If no beneficial effect is seen after 3 months of therapy, drug should be discontinued.

ADVERSE REACTIONS

CNS: blurred vision, headache, dizziness.
GI: *abdominal and epigastric pain, diarrhea, nausea,* vomiting, flatulence.
Hematologic: anemia, leukopenia.
Hepatic: bile duct obstruction, elevated enzymes.
Skin: rash, dermatitis, pruritus.
Other: painful extremities.

INTERACTIONS

Lovastatin: myopathy with rhabdomyolysis has been reported. Don't use together.
Oral anticoagulants: gemfibrozil may enhance the clinical effects of oral anticoagulants. Monitor the patient closely.

CONTRAINDICATIONS

- Contraindicated in patients with hepatic or severe renal dysfunction – including primary biliary cirrhosis – and preexisting gallbladder disease.

NURSING CONSIDERATIONS
- Periodic CBC and liver function tests should be performed during the first 12 months of therapy.
- Instruct the patient to take drug ½ hour before breakfast and dinner.
- Tell the patient to observe bowel movements and to report any evidence of steatorrhea or other signs of bile duct obstruction.
- Because of possible dizziness and blurred vision, advise the patient to avoid driving or other potentially hazardous activities until drug's CNS effects are known.
- Teach the patient about proper dietary management of serum lipids (restricting total fat and cholesterol intake), as well as measures to control other cardiac disease risk factors. When appropriate, recommend weight control, exercise, and stop-smoking programs.

---

lovastatin (mevinolin)
Mevacor

Pregnancy Risk Category: X

HOW SUPPLIED
Tablets: 20 mg

ACTION
Mechanism: Inhibits 3-hydroxy-3-methylglutaryl coenzyme A reductase. This enzyme is an early (and rate-limiting) step in the synthetic pathway of cholesterol.
Onset: several weeks. **Peak:** Plasma levels peak within 2 to 4 hours after a dose. **Duration:** plasma half-life, 1 to 2 hours; effects persist 4 to 6 weeks.

INDICATIONS & DOSAGE
Reduction of low-density lipoprotein and total cholesterol levels in patients with primary hypercholesterolemia (types IIa and IIb) –
Adults: initially, 20 mg P.O. once daily with the evening meal. For patients with severely elevated cholesterol levels (for example, over 300 mg/dl), give initial dose of 40 mg. Recommended dosage range is 20 to 80 mg in single or divided doses.

ADVERSE REACTIONS
CNS: headache, dizziness, peripheral neuropathy.
EENT: blurred vision.
GI: constipation, diarrhea, dyspepsia, flatulence, abdominal pain or cramps, heartburn, dysgeusia, nausea.
Skin: rash, pruritus.
Other: muscle cramps, myalgia, myositis, ***rhabdomyolysis***, elevated serum transaminase levels, abnormal liver test results.

INTERACTIONS
Cyclosporine or other immunosuppressive agents, erythromycin, gemfibrozil, niacin: possible increased risk of polymyositis and rhabdomyolysis. Maximum recommended lovastatin dosage is 20 mg daily; monitor the patient closely.
Ethanol: increased risk of hepatotoxicity. Avoid concomitant use.

CONTRAINDICATIONS
- Contraindicated in patients with hypersensitivity to the drug and in those with active liver disease or conditions associated with unexplained persistent elevations of serum transaminase levels; in pregnant and breast-feeding patients; and in women of childbearing age unless there is no risk of pregnancy.

NURSING CONSIDERATIONS
- Initiate lovastatin therapy only after diet and other nonpharmacologic therapies have proved ineffective. The patient should be on a standard low-cholesterol diet during therapy.
- Liver function tests should be performed at the start of therapy and periodically thereafter.
- Instruct the patient to take lovasta-

tin with the evening meal, when absorption is enhanced and cholesterol biosynthesis is greater.
• Advise the patient to have periodic eye examinations; related compounds have caused cataracts in laboratory animals.
• Teach the patient about proper dietary management of serum lipids (restricting total fat and cholesterol intake), as well as measures to control other cardiac disease risk factors. When appropriate, recommend weight control, exercise, and stop-smoking programs.
• Store tablets at room temperature in a light-resistant container.

pravastatin sodium

Pravachol

Pregnancy Risk Category: X

HOW SUPPLIED

Tablets: 10 mg, 20 mg

ACTION

Mechanism: Inhibits 3-hydroxy-3-methylglutaryl coenzyme A reductase. This enzyme is an early (and rate-limiting) step in the synthetic pathway of cholesterol.
Onset: 4 weeks or more. **Peak:** Plasma levels peak 1 hour after a dose.

INDICATIONS & DOSAGE

Reduction of low-density lipoprotein and total cholesterol levels in patients with primary hypercholesterolemia (types IIa and IIb) –
Adults: initially, 5 to 10 mg daily h.s. Adjust dosage q 4 weeks based on patient tolerance and response; maximum daily dosage is 40 mg. Most elderly patients respond to a daily dosage of 20 mg or less.

ADVERSE REACTIONS

CNS: headache, fatigue, dizziness.
CV: chest pain.
EENT: rhinitis.
GI: vomiting, diarrhea, heartburn, nausea.
Respiratory: cough.
Skin: rash.
Other: flulike symptoms, cough, renal failure secondary to myoglobinuria, myositis, myopathy, localized muscle pain, myalgia, ***rhabdomyolysis.***

INTERACTIONS

Cholestyramine, colestipol: concomitant administration decreases plasma levels of pravastatin. Administer pravastatin 1 hour before or 4 hours after these drugs.
Drugs that decrease levels or activity of endogenous steroids (such as cimetidine, ketoconazole, spironolactone): may increase risk of developing endocrine dysfunction. No intervention appears necessary; take complete drug history in patients who develop endocrine dysfunction.
Ethanol, hepatotoxic drugs: increased risk of hepatotoxicity. Avoid concomitant use.
Erythromycin, fibric acid derivatives (such as clofibrate or gemfibrozil), immunosuppressants (such as cyclosporine), high doses of niacin (nicotinic acid; 1 g or more daily): may increase the risk of rhabdomyolysis. Monitor the patient closely if concomitant use cannot be avoided.
Gemfibrozil: decreases protein-binding and urinary clearance of pravastatin. Avoid concomitant use.

CONTRAINDICATIONS

• Contraindicated in patients with hypersensitivity to the drug and in those with active liver disease or conditions that have unexplained persistent elevations of serum transaminase levels; in pregnant and breast-feeding patients; and in women of childbearing age unless there is no risk of pregnancy.

NURSING CONSIDERATIONS

- Initiate pravastatin therapy only after diet and other nonpharmacologic therapies have proved ineffective. Patients should continue a cholesterol-lowering diet during therapy.
- Adjust dosage about every 4 weeks. If cholesterol level falls below the target range, dosage may be reduced.
- Liver function tests should be performed at the start of therapy and periodically thereafter. A liver biopsy may be performed if enzyme elevations persist.
- Temporarily discontinue drug in any patient with an acute condition that suggests a developing myopathy or in patients with risk factors that may predispose them to renal failure secondary to rhabdomyolysis: severe acute infection; severe endocrine, metabolic, or electrolyte disorders; hypotension; major surgery; or uncontrolled seizures.
- Instruct the patient to take the recommended dosage in the evening, preferably at bedtime.
- Teach the patient about proper dietary management of serum lipids (restricting total fat and cholesterol intake), as well as measures to control other cardiac disease risk factors. When appropriate, recommend weight control, exercise, and stop-smoking programs.

probucol

Lorelco, Lurselle‡

Pregnancy Risk Category: B

HOW SUPPLIED

Tablets: 250 mg, 500 mg

ACTION

Mechanism: Inhibits cholesterol transport from the intestine, prevents oxidation of low-density lipoprotein, and may also decrease cholesterol synthesis. Appears to be more effective in patients with mild cholesterol elevations than in those with severe hypercholesterolemia.

Peak: Peak effect occurs after 20 to 50 days of therapy. Plasma levels gradually rise with continued therapy; peak levels occur after 3 to 4 months of treatment. **Duration:** plasma half-life, 12 hours to more than 500 hours.

INDICATIONS & DOSAGE

Primary hypercholesterolemia – **Adults:** 500 mg P.O. b.i.d. with morning and evening meals. Do not exceed 1 g daily.

Not recommended for children.

ADVERSE REACTIONS

CV: prolonged QT interval, arrhythmias.

GI: *diarrhea, flatulence, abdominal pain, nausea, vomiting.*

Hepatic: elevated liver enzymes.

Other: *hyperhidrosis,* fetid sweat, ***angioedema.***

INTERACTIONS

Tricyclic antidepressants, class Ia antiarrhythmics, phenothiazines, beta blockers, digitalis glycosides, calcium channel blockers: increased risk of arrhythmias.

CONTRAINDICATIONS

- Contraindicated in patients with arrhythmias. Discontinue drug in any patient whose ECG shows prolonged QT interval. Monitor ECG periodically.

NURSING CONSIDERATIONS

- Instruct the patient to take drug with food; effect is enhanced.
- Teach the patient about proper dietary management of serum lipids (restricting total fat and cholesterol intake), as well as measures to control other cardiac disease risk factors. When appropriate, recommend weight control, exercise, and stop-smoking programs.
- Because of drug's long half-life, ad-

vise women who wish to become pregnant to stop taking drug and use effective contraception for 6 months to delay pregnancy.

simvastatin (syvinolin)

Lipex‡, Zocor

Pregnancy Risk Category: X

HOW SUPPLIED

Tablets: 5 mg, 10 mg, 20 mg, 40 mg

ACTION

Mechanism: Inhibits 3-hydroxy-3-methylglutaryl coenzyme A reductase. This enzyme is an early (and rate-limiting) step in the synthetic pathway of cholesterol.

Peak: Peak plasma levels occur 1 to 2½ hours after a dose. Peak antilipemic effects occur after 4 to 8 weeks of therapy.

INDICATIONS & DOSAGE

Reduction of low-density lipoprotein and total cholesterol levels in patients with primary hypercholesterolemia (types IIa and IIb) –

Adults: initially, 5 to 10 mg daily in the evening. Adjust dosage q 4 weeks based on patient tolerance and response; maximum daily dosage is 40 mg.

ADVERSE REACTIONS

CNS: headache, asthenia.

GI: abdominal pain, constipation, diarrhea, dyspepsia, flatulence, nausea.

Hepatic: elevated liver enzymes.

Respiratory: cough.

Other: flulike symptoms, myositis, myopathy, ***rhabdomyolysis.***

INTERACTIONS

Digoxin: simvastatin may slightly elevate digoxin levels. Closely monitor plasma digoxin levels at initiation of simvastatin therapy.

Drugs that decrease levels or activity of endogenous steroids (such as cimetidine, ketoconazole, spironolactone): may increase risk of developing endocrine dysfunction. No intervention appears necessary; take complete drug history in patients who develop endocrine dysfunction.

Ethanol, hepatotoxic drugs: increased risk of hepatotoxicity. Avoid concomitant use.

Erythromycin, fibric acid derivatives (such as clofibrate or gemfibrozil), immunosuppressants (such as cyclosporine), high doses of niacin (nicotinic acid; 1 g or more daily): may increase risk of rhabdomyolysis. Monitor the patient closely if concomitant use cannot be avoided. Limit daily dosage of simvastatin to 10 mg if the patient must take cyclosporine.

Warfarin: anticoagulant effect may be slightly enhanced. Monitor the patient's PT at start of therapy and during dosage adjustments.

CONTRAINDICATIONS

- Contraindicated in patients with hypersensitivity to the drug and in those with active liver disease or conditions that have unexplained persistent elevations of serum transaminase; in pregnant and breast-feeding patients; and in women of childbearing age unless there is no risk of pregnancy.

NURSING CONSIDERATIONS

- Initiate simvastatin therapy only after diet and other nonpharmacologic therapies have proved ineffective. The patient should be on a standard low-cholesterol diet during therapy.
- Liver function tests should be performed at the start of therapy and periodically thereafter. A liver biopsy may be performed if enzyme elevations persist.
- Adjust dosage about every 4 weeks. If the cholesterol level falls below the target range, dosage may be reduced.
- Temporarily discontinue drug in any patient with an acute condition

that suggests a developing myopathy or in patients with risk factors that may predispose them to renal failure secondary to rhabdomyolysis: severe acute infection; severe endocrine, metabolic, or electrolyte disorders; hypotension; major surgery; or uncontrolled seizures.

- Tell the patient to inform the doctor of any adverse reactions, particularly muscle aches and pains.
- Instruct the patient to take simvastatin with the evening meal; absorption is enhanced and cholesterol biosynthesis is greater.
- Teach the patient about proper dietary management of serum lipids (restricting total fat and cholesterol intake), as well as measures to control other cardiac disease risk factors. When appropriate, recommend weight control, exercise, and stop-smoking programs.

25

Nonnarcotic analgesics and antipyretics

acetaminophen
aspirin
choline magnesium trisalicylate
choline salicylate
diflunisal
magnesium salicylate
methotrimeprazine hydrochloride
(See Chapter 28, SEDATIVE-HYPNOTICS.)
phenazopyridine hydrochloride
salsalate
sodium salicylate
sodium thiosalicylate

COMBINATION PRODUCTS

ALLEREST NO DROWSINESS TABLETS◇, COLDRINE◇, ORNEX NO DROWSINESS CAPLETS◇, SINUS RELIEF TABLETS, SINUTAB MAXIMUM STRENGTH WITHOUT DROWSINESS◇: acetaminophen 325 mg and pseudoephedrine hydrochloride 30 mg.

AMAPHEN, ANOQUAN, BUTACE, ENDOLOR, ESGIC, FEMCET, FIORICET, ISOPAP, MEDIGESIC, PACAPS, REPAN, ROGESIC, TENCET, TRIAD, TWO-DYNE: acetaminophen 325 mg, caffeine 40 mg, and butalbital 50 mg.

ASCRIPTIN: aspirin 325 mg, magnesium hydroxide 50 mg, aluminum hydroxide 50 mg, and calcium carbonate 50 mg.◇

ASCRIPTIN A/D: aspirin 325 mg, magnesium hydroxide 75 mg, aluminum hydroxide 75 mg, and calcium carbonate 75 mg.◇

AXOTAL: aspirin 650 mg and butalbital 50 mg.

CAMA, ARTHRITIS STRENGTH: aspirin 500 mg, magnesium oxide 150 mg, and aluminum hydroxide 150 mg.

COPE: aspirin 421 mg, caffeine 32 mg, magnesium hydroxide 50 mg, and aluminum hydroxide 25 mg.

EXCEDRIN P.M.◇: acetaminophen 500 mg and diphenhydramine citrate 38 mg.

EXCEDRIN EXTRA STRENGTH◇: aspirin 250 mg, acetaminophen 250 mg, caffeine 65 mg.

EXTRA STRENGTH DOAN'S P.M.◇: magnesium salicylate 500 mg, and diphenhydramine 25 mg.

FIORINAL, ISOLLYL IMPROVED, LANIROIF, LANORINAL, MARNAL: aspirin 325 mg, caffeine 40 mg, and butalbital 50 mg.

FIORICET WITH CODEINE: acetaminophen 325 mg, butalbital 50 mg, caffeine, 40 mg and codeine phosphate 30 mg.

PAC REVISED FORMULA◇: aspirin 400 mg and caffeine 32 mg.

MIDRIN: isometheptene mucate 65 mg, dichloralphenazone 100 mg, and acetaminophen 325 mg.

PHRENILIN: acetaminophen 325 mg and butalbital 50 mg.

PHRENILIN FORTE: acetaminophen 650 mg and butalbital 50 mg.

SINUS EXCEDRIN NO DROWSINESS◇: acetaminophen 500 mg and pseudophedrine hydrochloride 30 mg.

SINUTAB◇: acetaminophen 325 mg, chlorpheniramine 2 mg, and pseudoephedrine hydrochloride 30 mg.

SINUTAB MAXIMUM STRENGTH◇: acetaminophen 500 mg, pseudoephedrine hydrochloride 30 mg, and chlorpheniramine maleate, 2 mg.

TECNAL†: aspirin 330 mg, caffeine 40 mg, and butalbital 50 mg.

VANQUISH◇: aspirin 227 mg, acetaminophen 194 mg, caffeine 33 mg, aluminum hydroxide 25 mg, and magnesium hydroxide 50 mg.

acetaminophen (APAP, paracetamol)

Abenol†◊; Aceta Elixir*◊; Acetaminophen Uniserts◊; Aceta Tablets◊; Actamin◊; Actamin Extra◊; Actimol†◊; Aminofen◊; Aminofen Max◊; Anacin-3◊; Anacin-3 Children's Elixir*◊; Anacin-3 Children's Tablets◊; Anacin-3 Extra Strength◊; Anacin-3 Infants'◊; Anacin-3 Maximum Strength Caplets◊; Apacet Capsules◊; Apacet Elixir*◊; Apacet Extra Strength Caplets◊; Apacet Extra Strength Tablets◊; Apacet Infants'◊; Apacet Regular Strength Tablets◊; Apo-Acetaminophen†◊; Arthritis Pain Formula Aspirin Free◊; Atasol Caplets†◊; Atasol Drops†◊; Atasol Elixir*†◊; Atasol Forte Caplets†◊; Atasol Forte Tablets†◊; Atasol Tablets†◊; Banesin◊; Dapa◊; Dapa XS◊; Dolanex*◊; Dorcol Children's Fever and Pain Reducer◊; Dymadon‡◊; Dymadon P‡◊; Exdol†◊; Exdol Strong†◊; Feverall Children's‡; Feverall Junior Strength‡; Feverall Sprinkle Caps, Children's‡; Feverall Sprinkle Caps, Junior Strength‡; Genapap Children's Elixir◊; Genapap Children's Tablets◊; Genapap Extra Strength Caplets◊; Genapap Extra Strength Tablets◊; Genapap, Infants'◊; Genapap Regular Strength Tablets◊; Genebs Regular Strength Tablets◊; Genebs Extra Strength Caplets◊; Genebs X-Tra◊; Halenol Elixir*◊; Liquiprin Infants' Drops◊; Meda Cap◊; Myapap Elixir*◊; Myapap, Infants'◊; Neopap◊; Oraphen-PD◊; Panadol◊; Panadol, Children's◊; Panadol Extra Strength◊; Panadol, Infants'◊; Panadol Junior Strength Caplets◊; Panadol Maximum Strength Caplets◊; Panadol Maximum Strength Tablets◊; Panamax‡◊; Panex◊; Panex-500◊; Paralgin‡◊; Paraspen‡◊; Redutemp◊; Ridenol Caplets◊; Robigesic†◊; Rounox†◊; Setamol-500‡◊; Snaplets-FR◊; St. Joseph Aspirin-Free Fever Reducer for Children◊; Suppap-120◊; Suppap-325◊; Suppap-650◊; Tapanol Extra Strength Caplets◊; Tapanol Extra Strength Tablets◊; Tempra◊; Tempra Caplets◊; Tempra Chewable Tablets◊; Tempra Drops◊; Tempra D.S.◊; Tempra, Infants'◊; Tempra Syrup◊; Tenol◊; Tylenol Caplets◊; Tylenol Chewable Tablets◊; Tylenol Children's Elixir◊; Tylenol Children's Tablets◊; Tylenol Drops◊; Tylenol Elixir*◊; Tylenol Extra Strength Adult Liquid Pain Reliever◊; Tylenol Extra Strength Caplets◊; Tylenol Extra Strength Gelcaps◊; Tylenol Extra Strength Tablets◊; Tylenol, Infants'◊; Tylenol Junior Strength Caplets◊; Tylenol Junior Strength Tablets◊; Tylenol Regular Strength Caplets◊; Tylenol Regular Strength Tablets◊; Tylenol Tablets◊; Ty-Pap◊; Ty-Pap, Infants'◊; Ty-Pap Syrup◊; Ty-Tab Caplets◊; Ty-Tab Capsules◊; Ty-Tab, Children's◊; Ty-Tab Tablets◊; Valorin◊; Valorin Extra◊

Pregnancy Risk Category: B

HOW SUPPLIED

Tablets: 160 mg◊, 325 mg◊, 500 mg◊, 650 mg◊
Tablets (chewable): 80 mg◊, 160 mg◊
Capsules: 500 mg◊
Oral solution: 48 mg/ml◊, 100 mg/ml◊
Oral suspension: 120 mg/5 ml‡, 100 mg/ml◊, 160 mg/ml◊
Oral liquid: 160 mg/5 ml◊, 500 mg/15 ml◊
Elixir: 130 mg/5 ml*◊, 167 mg/5 ml*◊, 325 mg/5 ml*◊
Granules: 80 mg/packet◊, 325 mg/capful◊
Powder for solution: 1 g/packet

†Available in Canada only. ‡Available in Australia only. ◊Available OTC.

Sprinkles: 80 mg/capsule, 160 mg/capsule
Tablets for solution: 325 mg
Suppositories: 120 mg◊, 125 mg◊, 300 mg◊, 324 mg◊, 650 mg◊
Wafers: 120 mg◊

ACTION

Mechanism: Produces analgesia by blocking generation of pain impulses, probably by inhibiting prostaglandin synthesis in the CNS or the synthesis or action of other substances that sensitize pain receptors to mechanical or chemical stimulation. It relieves fever by central action in the hypothalamic heat-regulating center.
Onset: 10 to 60 minutes. **Peak:** Peak effects vary; average peak blood levels occur in 40 to 60 minutes. **Duration:** effects persist about 4 hours.

INDICATIONS & DOSAGE

Mild pain or fever–
Adults and children over 11 years: 325 to 650 mg P.O. q 4 to 6 hours; or 1 g P.O. t.i.d. or q.i.d., p.r.n. Maximum dosage should not exceed 4 g daily. Dosage for long-term therapy should not exceed 2.6 g daily.
Children 11 years and under: 10 mg/kg P.O. q 4 hours. Do not exceed five doses in 24 hours. Alternatively, use these guidelines.
Children 11 years: 480 mg/dose.
Children 9 to 10 years: 400 mg/dose.
Children 6 to 8 years: 320 mg/dose.
Children 4 to 5 years: 240 mg/dose.
Children 2 to 3 years: 160 mg/dose.
Children 12 to 23 months: 120 mg/dose.
Children 4 to 11 months: 80 mg/dose.
Children up to 3 months: 40 mg/dose.
Mild pain or fever in patients who can't tolerate oral medication–
Adults: 650 mg P.R. q 4 to 6 hours. Give no more than 6 suppositories in 24 hours.
Children 6 to 12 years: 325 mg P.R. q 4 to 6 hours. Give no more than 2.6 g in 24 hours.
Children 3 to 6 years: 120 mg P.R. q 4 to 6 hours. Give no more than 720 mg in 24 hours.
Children 2 years and under: consult a doctor.

ADVERSE REACTIONS

Hematologic: hemolytic anemia, neutropenia, leukopenia, pancytopenia, thrombocytopenia (rare).
Hepatic: ***severe liver damage with toxic doses,*** jaundice.
Skin: rash, urticaria.
Other: hypoglycemia.

INTERACTIONS

Barbiturates, carbamazepine, hydantoins, rifampin, sulfinpyrazone: high doses or long-term use of these drugs may reduce the therapeutic effects and enhance the hepatotoxic effects of acetaminophen. Avoid concomitant use.
Caffeine: may enhance analgesic effects of acetaminophen.
Diflunisal: increased acetaminophen blood levels. Don't use together.
Ethanol: increased risk of hepatic damage. Avoid concomitant use.
Warfarin: increased hypoprothrombinemic effect with long-term use with high doses of acetaminophen. Monitor PTs closely.
Zidovudine: may increase the incidence of bone marrow suppression because of impaired zidovudine metabolism. Monitor patient closely.

CONTRAINDICATIONS

- Contraindicated for repeated use in patients with anemia or renal or hepatic disease.
- Use cautiously in patients with history of chronic alcohol abuse because hepatotoxicity has occurred after therapeutic doses. Limit daily intake to 2 g.
- Consult a doctor before giving this drug to children under 2 years.

NURSING CONSIDERATIONS

- This drug is only for short-term use. Tell patients to consult a doctor if administering to children for more than 5 days or adults for more than 10 days.
- Acetaminophen has no significant anti-inflammatory effect.
- Don't use for self-medication of marked fever (over 103.1° F [39.5° C]), fever persisting longer than 3 days, or recurrent fever unless directed by doctor.
- For antipyretic effects, consider additional methods to help cool the patient: tepid baths, loosened clothing, and lowered ambient temperature. However, excessive cooling may cause the patient to shiver.
- Many OTC products contain acetaminophen; be aware of this when calculating total daily dosage.
- Liquid form is recommended for children and for all patients who have difficulty swallowing.
- Acetaminophen crosses the placenta but is apparently safe for short-term use at therapeutic doses during pregnancy. It is routinely used during all stages of pregnancy to treat pain and fever.
- Acetaminophen is found in breast milk in low concentrations (less than 1% of dose). Breast-feeding patients may use it safely if therapy is short-term and does not exceed recommended doses.
- Warn patient that high doses or unsupervised long-term use can cause hepatic damage. Excessive ingestion of alcoholic beverages may increase the risk of hepatotoxicity.
- Acetaminophen may interfere with certain laboratory tests for urinary 5-hydroxyindoleacetic acid. It may also produce false-positive decreases in blood glucose levels in home monitoring systems using Chemstrip bG, Dextrostix, or Visidex II.

aspirin (acetylsalicylic acid)

Ancasal†◇, Arthrinol†◇, Artria SR◇, ASA◇, ASA Enseals◇, Aspergum◇, Aspro‡, Astrin†◇, Bayer Aspirin◇, Bex‡, Coryphen†◇, Easprin◇, Ecotrin◇, Empirin◇, Entrophen†◇, Measurin◇, Norwich Aspirin Extra Strength◇, Novasen†◇, Riphen-10†◇, Sal-Adult†◇, Sal-Infant†◇, Solprin‡, Supasa†◇, Triaphen-10†◇, Vincent's Powders‡, Winsprin Capsules‡, ZORprin◇

Pregnancy Risk Category: C (D in 3rd trimester)

HOW SUPPLIED

Tablets◇: 65 mg, 75 mg, 81 mg, 300 mg, 325 mg, 500 mg, 600 mg, 650 mg
Tablets (chewable): 81 mg◇
Tablets (enteric-coated): 325 mg◇, 500 mg◇, 650 mg◇, 975 mg
Tablets (extended-release): 800 mg
Tablets (timed-release): 650 mg◇
Capsules: 325 mg◇, 500 mg◇
Powder: 500 mg
Chewing gum: 227.5 mg◇
Suppositories: 60 to 120 mg◇

ACTION

Mechanism: Produces analgesia by blocking prostaglandin synthesis (peripheral action). Aspirin and other salicylates may prevent the lowering of the pain threshold that occurs when prostaglandins sensitize pain receptors to mechanical and chemical stimulation. Exerts its anti-inflammatory effect by inhibiting prostaglandin synthesis; may also inhibit the synthesis or action of other mediators of the inflammatory response. Relieves fever by acting on the hypothalamic heat-regulating center to cause peripheral vasodilation. This increases peripheral blood supply and promotes sweating, which leads to heat loss and to cooling by evaporation. In low doses, aspirin also appears to impede clot-

ting by blocking prostaglandin synthesis, which prevents formation of the platelet-aggregating substance thromboxane A_2.
Onset: 5 to 30 minutes after an oral dose. **Peak:** With oral solution, serum aspirin levels peak in 15 to 40 minutes; peak serum levels of salicylate, its active metabolite, in ½ to 1 hour. With regular tablets, peak serum aspirin levels in 25 to 40 minutes; peak serum salicylate levels, in 1 to 2 hours. With buffered tablets, peak serum aspirin and salicylate levels occur in 1 to 2 hours. With extended-release tablets, peak aspirin levels occur in 1 to 2 hours; peak salicylate levels, in 3 to 4 hours. With enteric-coated tablets, peak aspirin and salicylate levels occur in 4 to 8 hours. With suppositories, peak aspirin and salicylate levels occur in 3 to 4 hours. **Duration:** 1 to 4 hours; serum half-life, 15 to 20 minutes.

INDICATIONS & DOSAGE

Arthritis –
Adults: 3.6 to 5.4 g P.O. daily in divided doses.
Children: 90 to 130 mg/kg P.O. daily divided q 4 to 6 hours.
Mild pain or fever –
Adults and children over 11 years: 325 to 650 mg P.O. or P.R. q 4 hours, p.r.n.
Children 2 to 11 years: 1.5 g/m^2 or 65 mg/kg P.O. or P.R. daily in 4 to 6 divided doses.
Thromboembolic disorders –
Adults: 325 to 650 mg P.O. daily or b.i.d.
Transient ischemic attacks in men –
Adults: most protocols employ doses of 650 mg P.O. b.i.d. or 325 mg q.i.d.
Reduction of risk of heart attack in patients with previous MI or unstable angina –
Adults: most protocols employ doses of 80 to 325 mg P.O. daily or 325 mg every other day.
Kawasaki syndrome (mucocutaneous lymph node syndrome) –
Adults: 80 to 100 mg/kg daily in 4 divided doses during the febrile phase. Some patients may need up to 120 mg/kg. When fever subsides, decrease dosage to 3 to 8 mg/kg once daily, adjusted according to serum salicylate concentration.

ADVERSE REACTIONS

EENT: *tinnitus and hearing loss.*
GI: *nausea, vomiting, GI distress, occult bleeding.*
Hematologic: *prolonged bleeding time.*
Hepatic: abnormal liver function studies, hepatitis.
Skin: *rash,* bruising.
Other: hypersensitivity reactions, (***anaphylaxis,*** asthma), Reye's syndrome.

INTERACTIONS

Ammonium chloride (and other urine acidifiers): increased blood levels of aspirin products. Monitor for aspirin toxicity.
Antacids in high doses (and other urine alkalinizers): decreased levels of aspirin products. Monitor for decreased aspirin effect.
Antihypertensives: decreased antihypertensive effect. Avoid long-term aspirin use if patient is taking antihypertensives.
Corticosteroids: enhanced salicylate elimination. Monitor for decreased salicylate effect.
Ethanol, NSAIDs, steroids: increased risk of GI bleeding. Avoid concomitant use.
Heparin, oral anticoagulants, valproic acid: increased risk of bleeding. Avoid using together if possible.
Methotrexate: increased risk of methotrexate toxicity. Avoid concomitant use.
NSAIDs, including diflunisal, fenoprofen, ibuprofen, indomethacin, piroxicam, meclofenamate, naproxen:

altered pharmacokinetics of these agents, leading to lowered serum levels and decreased effectiveness. Avoid concomitant use.
Oral antidiabetic agents: increased hypoglycemic effect. Monitor closely.
Probenecid, sulfinpyrazone: decreased uricosuric effect. Avoid aspirin during therapy with these agents.

CONTRAINDICATIONS

- Contraindicated in patients with GI ulcer, GI bleeding, bleeding disorders, or aspirin hypersensitivity. Also contraindicated in children or teenagers with chicken pox or influenza-like illness.
- Use cautiously in patients with hypoprothrombinemia, renal failure, or vitamin K deficiency and in asthmatics with nasal polyps (may cause severe bronchospasm).
- Aspirin should be avoided during pregnancy. It may also increase the risk of hemorrhage in both neonate and mother and may also contribute to congenital heart disease or other malformations.
- Because of epidemiologic association with Reye's syndrome, the Centers for Disease Control and Prevention recommends not giving children or teenagers with chicken pox or influenza-like illness salicylates.
- Consult a doctor before administering this drug to children under 12 years.

NURSING CONSIDERATIONS

- For inflammatory conditions, rheumatic fever, and thrombosis, aspirin is administered on a scheduled, rather than p.r.n., basis. During prolonged therapy, hematocrit, hemoglobin level, PT, and renal function should be assessed periodically.
- Advise patients receiving prolonged treatment with large doses of aspirin to watch for petechiae, bleeding gums, and signs of GI bleeding, and to maintain adequate fluid intake. Encourage the use of a soft toothbrush.
- Tell patients to consult a doctor if administering to children for more than 5 days or adults for more than 10 days.
- Febrile, dehydrated children can develop toxicity rapidly.
- Elderly patients may be more susceptible to aspirin's toxic effects.
- Therapeutic blood salicylate level in arthritis is 10 to 30 mg/100 ml. Tinnitus may occur at plasma levels of 30 mg/100 ml and above, but this is not a reliable indicator of toxicity, especially in very young patients and those over age 60. With chronic therapy, mild toxicity may occur at plasma levels of 20 mg/100 ml.
- Aspirin may increase serum levels of AST, ALT, alkaline phosphatase, and bilirubin.
- Because enteric-coated tablets are slowly absorbed, they are not suitable for rapid relief of acute pain or inflammation. They do cause less GI bleeding and may be more suited for long-term therapy, such as the treatment of arthritis.
- Evidence suggests that aspirin may prevent sunburn and inhibit sunburn pain by preventing cells from manufacturing prostaglandins.
- Aspirin irreversibly inhibits platelet aggregation. It should be discontinued 5 to 7 days before elective surgery to allow time for the production and release of new platelets.
- To reduce GI adverse reactions, advise patients to take with food, milk, antacid, or large glass of water.
- Because of the many possible drug interactions involving aspirin, warn patients taking prescription drugs to check with a doctor or pharmacist before taking aspirin or OTC combination products containing aspirin.
- For patients who cannot tolerate oral medications, use aspirin rectal suppositories. Watch for rectal mucosal irritation or bleeding.

• For patients with swallowing difficulties, crush non-enteric-coated aspirin and dissolve in soft food or liquid. Administer liquid immediately after mixing because drug will break down rapidly.
• Keep out of reach of children – aspirin is one of the leading causes of poisoning in children. Encourage the use of child-resistant containers.
• Aspirin tablets that have a strong vinegar-like odor should be discarded.

choline magnesium trisalicylate (choline salicylate and magnesium salicylate)

Tricusal, Trilisate

Pregnancy Risk Category: C

HOW SUPPLIED

Tablets: 500 mg, 750 mg, 1,000 mg of salicylate
Solution: 500 mg of salicylate/5 ml

ACTION

Mechanism: Produces analgesia by blocking prostaglandin synthesis (peripheral action). Salicylates may prevent the lowering of the pain threshold that occurs when prostaglandins sensitize pain receptors to mechanical and chemical stimulation. Exerts its anti-inflammatory effect by inhibiting prostaglandin synthesis. Relieves fever by acting on the hypothalamic heat-regulating center to produce peripheral vasodilation. This increases peripheral blood supply and promotes sweating, which leads to heat loss and to cooling by evaporation.
Peak: Serum levels peak within 1 to 2 hours. **Duration:** elimination half-life, 9 to 17 hours.

INDICATIONS & DOSAGE

Arthritis, mild –
Adults: 1 to 2 teaspoonsful or tablets P.O. b.i.d. Total daily dosage can also be given at one time (usually h.s.)
Rheumatoid arthritis and osteoarthritis –
Adults: initially, 3 g P.O. daily either as a single dose h.s. or b.i.d. Dosage is adjusted according to patient response. Dosage range is 1 to 4.5 g daily.
Juvenile rheumatoid arthritis –
Children (12 to 37 kg): 50 mg/kg/day P.O. in divided doses.
Children (more than 37 kg): 2,250 mg P.O. in divided doses.
Mild to moderate pain and fever –
Adults: 2 to 3 g P.O. daily divided b.i.d.
Children (12 to 37 kg): 50 mg/kg/day P.O. in divided doses.

ADVERSE REACTIONS

EENT: tinnitus and hearing loss.
GI: GI distress.
Skin: rash.
Other: hypersensitivity reactions, ***(anaphylaxis)***.

INTERACTIONS

Ammonium chloride (and other urine acidifiers): increased blood levels of salicylates. Monitor for salicylate toxicity.
Antacids in high doses (and other urine alkalinizers): decreased levels of salicylates. Monitor for decreased salicylate effect.
Corticosteroids: enhanced salicylate elimination. Monitor for decreased salicylate effect.
Ethanol, steroids, and other NSAIDs: enhanced risk of adverse GI effects.
Methotrexate: increased risk of methotrexate toxicity. Avoid concomitant use.
Oral anticoagulants: increased risk of bleeding. Use together cautiously.

CONTRAINDICATIONS

• Contraindicated in patients hypersensitive to the drug. Also contraindicated in children or teenagers with chicken pox or influenza-like illness.
• Use cautiously in patients with

chronic renal failure, peptic ulcer disease, and gastritis, and in those with a known allergy to salicylates.

NURSING CONSIDERATIONS

- Each 500-mg tablet or teaspoonful is equal in salicylate content to 650 mg of aspirin; each 750-mg tablet, 975 mg of aspirin; each 1,000-mg tablet, 1,300 mg of aspirin.
- Because of epidemiologic association with Reye's syndrome, the Centers for Disease Control and Prevention recommends not giving children or teenagers with chicken pox or influenza-like illness salicylates.
- Anti-inflammatory, analgesic, and antipyretic effects of salicylate salts are comparable to those of aspirin; however, platelet function is not affected. Do not substitute these agents for aspirin during antithrombotic therapy.
- Febrile, dehydrated children can develop toxicity rapidly.
- Therapeutic blood salicylate level in arthritis is 10 to 30 mg/100 ml. Tinnitus may occur at plasma levels of 30 mg/100 ml and above, but this is not a reliable indicator of toxicity, especially in very young patients and those over age 60. With chronic therapy, mild toxicity may occur at plasma levels of 20 mg/100 ml.
- Periodically monitor hemoglobin level and PT in patients receiving long-term treatment with large doses.
- Causes less GI distress than aspirin. If an antacid is needed, give it 2 hours after meals and choline magnesium trisalicylate before meals.
- Tell patients to take tablets with food or a full glass of water. Solution may be mixed with fruit juice, but not antacids.

---

choline salicylate

Arthropan, Teejel†*

Pregnancy Risk Category: C

HOW SUPPLIED

Liquid: 870 mg/5 ml◊
Gel: 87 mg/g†*

ACTION

Mechanism: Produces analgesia by blocking prostaglandin synthesis (peripheral action). Salicylates may prevent the lowering of the pain threshold that occurs when prostaglandins sensitize pain receptors to mechanical and chemical stimulation. Exerts its anti-inflammatory effect by inhibiting prostaglandin synthesis. Relieves fever by acting on the hypothalamic heat-regulating center to produce peripheral vasodilation. This increases peripheral blood supply and promotes sweating, which leads to heat loss and to cooling by evaporation.
Peak: Serum levels peak in 20 minutes.

INDICATIONS & DOSAGE

Rheumatoid arthritis, osteoarthritis, minor pain or fever –
Adults and children over 12 years: 1 teaspoonful (870 mg of choline salicylate) P.O. q 3 to 4 hours p.r.n. If tolerated and needed, dosage may be increased to 2 teaspoonsful. Do not exceed 6 teaspoonsful daily.
Relief of pain from inflamed gums –
Adults and children over 2 years: apply 1 cm of gel to affected area q 3 to 4 hours and h.s., p.r.n.

ADVERSE REACTIONS

EENT: tinnitus and hearing loss.
GI: nausea, vomiting, GI distress.
Skin: rash.
Other: hypersensitivity reactions ***(anaphylaxis)***.

INTERACTIONS

Ammonium chloride (and other urine acidifiers): increased blood levels of salicylates. Monitor for salicylate toxicity.
Antacids in high doses (and other urine alkalinizers): decreased levels

of salicylates. Monitor for decreased salicylate effect.
Corticosteroids: enhanced salicylate elimination. Monitor for decreased salicylate effect.
Ethanol, other NSAIDs, steroids: enhanced risk of adverse GI reactions.
Methotrexate: increased risk of methotrexate toxicity. Avoid concomitant use.

CONTRAINDICATIONS

- Contraindicated in patients hypersensitive to the drug. Also contraindicated in children or teenagers with chicken pox or influenza-like illness.
- Use cautiously in patients with chronic renal failure, peptic ulcer disease, and gastritis, and in those with a known allergy to salicylates.

NURSING CONSIDERATIONS

- Because of epidemiologic association with Reye's syndrome, the Centers for Disease Control and Prevention recommends not giving children or teenagers with chicken pox or influenza-like illness salicylates.
- Febrile, dehydrated children can develop toxicity rapidly.
- Therapeutic blood salicylate level in arthritis is 10 to 30 mg/100 ml. Tinnitus may occur at plasma levels of 30 mg/100 ml and above, but this is not a reliable indicator of toxicity, especially in very young patients and those over age 60. With chronic therapy, mild toxicity may occur at plasma levels of 20 mg/100 ml.
- Periodically monitor hemoglobin level and PT in patients receiving long-term treatment with large doses.
- Anti-inflammatory, analgesic, and antipyretic effects of salicylate salts are comparable to those of aspirin; however, platelet function is not affected. Do not substitute these agents for aspirin during antithrombotic therapy.
- Causes less GI distress than aspirin. If an antacid is needed, give it 2 hours after meals and choline salicylate before meals.
- Tell patients they may mix drug with water, fruit juice, or carbonated drinks, but not antacids.

---

diflunisal

Dolobid

Pregnancy Risk Category: C

HOW SUPPLIED

Tablets: 250 mg, 500 mg

ACTION

Mechanism: Mechanism of action is unknown, but probably related to inhibition of prostaglandin synthesis.
Onset: 1 to 2 hours. **Peak:** Peak plasma levels and analgesic effects occur in 2 to 3 hours. **Duration:** plasma half-life, 8 to 12 hours.

INDICATIONS & DOSAGE

Mild to moderate pain and osteoarthritis –
Adults: 500 to 1,000 mg P.O. daily in two divided doses, usually q 12 hours. Maximum dosage is 1,500 mg daily.
Adults over 65: start with one-half the usual adult dose.

ADVERSE REACTIONS

CNS: *dizziness,* somnolence, insomnia, *headache,* fatigue.
EENT: *tinnitus, visual disturbances (rare).*
GI: *nausea, dyspepsia, GI pain, diarrhea,* vomiting, constipation, flatulence.
GU: renal impairment, hematuria, interstitial nephritis.
Skin: *rash,* pruritus, sweating stomatitis, ***toxic epidermal necrolysis, Stevens-Johnson syndrome.***
Other: dry mucous membranes.

INTERACTIONS

Acetaminophen, hydrochlorothiazide, indomethacin: diflunisal may substantially increase blood levels, in-

creasing the risk of toxicity. Avoid concomitant use.
Antacids, aspirin: decreased diflunisal blood levels. Monitor for possible decreased therapeutic effect.
Cyclosporine: diflunisal may enhance the nephrotoxicity of cyclosporine. Avoid concomitant use.
Methotrexate: diflunisal may enhance the toxicity of methotrexate. Avoid concomitant use.
Oral anticoagulants, thrombolytic agents: diflunisal may enhance pharmacologic effects of these agents. Use together cautiously.
Sulindac: diflunisal decreases blood levels of sulindac's active metabolite. Monitor for decreased pharmacologic effect.

CONTRAINDICATIONS
• Contraindicated in patients for whom acute asthmatic attacks, urticaria, or rhinitis are precipitated by aspirin or other NSAIDs. Also contraindicated in children or teenagers with chicken pox or influenza-like illness.
• Use cautiously in patients with active GI bleeding or history of peptic ulcer disease, renal impairment, liver disease, and compromised cardiac function. Also use cautiously in those taking anticoagulants.

NURSING CONSIDERATIONS
• Diflunisal is a salicylic acid derivative similar to aspirin, but is metabolized differently. Anti-inflammatory, analgesic, and antipyretic effects are comparable to those of aspirin; however, platelet function is not affected. Do not substitute for aspirin during antithrombotic therapy.
• Because of the epidemiologic association with Reye's syndrome, the Centers for Disease Control and Prevention recommends not giving children and teenagers with chicken pox or influenza-like illness salicylates.
• Advise the patient to take with water, milk, or meals.

magnesium salicylate
Extra-Strength Doan's◇, Magan◇, Mobidin◇, Original Doan's◇

Pregnancy Risk Category: C

HOW SUPPLIED
Tablets: 545 mg, 600 mg
Caplets: 325 mg◇, 500 mg◇

ACTION
Mechanism: Produces analgesia by blocking prostaglandin synthesis (peripheral action). Salicylates may prevent the lowering of the pain threshold that occurs when prostaglandins sensitize pain receptors to mechanical and chemical stimulation. Exerts its anti-inflammatory effect by inhibiting prostaglandin synthesis. Relieves fever by acting on the hypothalamic heat-regulating center to produce peripheral vasodilation. This increases peripheral blood supply and promotes sweating, which leads to heat loss and to cooling by evaporation.
Onset: within 30 minutes. **Peak:** Blood levels peak within 1½ to 2 hours of a dose.

INDICATIONS & DOSAGE
Arthritis –
Adults: 545 mg to 1.2 g P.O. t.i.d. or q.i.d. not to exceed 4.8 g daily.
Mild pain or fever –
Adults: 300 to 600 mg P.O. q 4 hours, not to exceed 3.5 g/24 hours.

ADVERSE REACTIONS
EENT: *tinnitus and hearing loss.*
GI: *nausea, vomiting, GI distress.*
Hepatic: abnormal liver function studies, hepatitis.
Skin: *rash,* bruising.
Other: hypersensitivity reactions (***anaphylaxis,*** asthma).

INTERACTIONS
Ammonium chloride (and other urine acidifiers): increased blood levels of

salicylates. Monitor for salicylate toxicity.
Antacids in high doses (and other urine alkalinizers): decreased levels of salicylates. Monitor for decreased salicylate effect.
Corticosteroids: enhanced salicylate elimination. Monitor for decreased salicylate effect.
Ethanol, other NSAIDs, steroids: increased risk of GI bleeding. Avoid concomitant use.
Heparin, oral anticoagulants: increased risk of bleeding. Avoid using together if possible.
Methotrexate: increased risk of methotrexate toxicity. Avoid concomitant use.

CONTRAINDICATIONS
- Contraindicated in patients with severe chronic renal insufficiency because of risk of magnesium toxicity. Also contraindicated in patients with GI ulcer, GI bleeding, or aspirin hypersensitivity, and in children or teenagers with chicken pox or influenza-like illness.
- Use cautiously in patients with hypoprothrombinemia, vitamin K deficiency, and bleeding disorders.

NURSING CONSIDERATIONS
- Because of epidemiologic association with Reye's syndrome, the Centers for Disease Control and Prevention recommends not giving children or teenagers with chicken pox or influenza-like illness salicylates.
- Febrile, dehydrated children can develop toxicity rapidly.
- Therapeutic blood salicylate level in arthritis is 10 to 30 mg/100 ml. Tinnitus may occur at plasma levels of 30 mg/100 ml and above, but this is not a reliable indicator of toxicity, especially in very young patients and those over age 60. With chronic therapy, mild toxicity may occur at plasma levels of 20 mg/100 ml.
- Magnesium salicylate may cause increased serum levels of AST, ALT, alkaline phosphatase, and bilirubin.
- Monitor hemoglobin level and PT in patients receiving long-term treatment with large doses.
- Anti-inflammatory, analgesic, and antipyretic effects of salicylate salts are comparable to those of aspirin; however, platelet function is not affected. Do not substitute these agents for aspirin during antithrombotic therapy.
- To reduce GI adverse reactions, tell patients to take this drug with food, milk, antacid, or large glass of water.

phenazopyridine hydrochloride (phenylazo diamino pyridine hydrochloride)

Azo-Standard◊, Baridium◊, Di-Azo◊, Eridium◊, Geridium◊, Phenazo†, Phenazodine◊, Pyrazodine◊, Pyridiate◊, Pyridin◊, Pyridium, Pyronium†, Urodine◊, Urogesic◊, Viridium◊

Pregnancy Risk Category: B

HOW SUPPLIED
Tablets: 95 mg◊, 100 mg◊, 200 mg

ACTION
Mechanism: Exerts local anesthetic action on urinary mucosa through unknown mechanism.
Peak: Peak urinary excretion of drug occurs within 5 to 6 hours of a dose.
Duration: total elimination, 20½ hours (average).

INDICATIONS & DOSAGE
Pain with urinary tract irritation or infection –
Adults: 100 to 200 mg P.O. t.i.d.
Children: 12 mg/kg P.O. daily in 3 equally divided doses.

ADVERSE REACTIONS
CNS: headache, vertigo.
GI: nausea.

Skin: rash.

INTERACTIONS
None significant.

CONTRAINDICATIONS
- Contraindicated in patients with glomerulonephritis, severe hepatitis, uremia, pyelonephritis during pregnancy, or renal insufficiency.
- Also contraindicated in acute and postoperative pain and should not be used for mild or intermittent pain.

NURSING CONSIDERATIONS
- Colors urine red or orange. May stain fabrics.
- Phenazopyridine is used as an analgesic in combination with an antibiotic. It should only be used for the first 2 days of therapy.
- Advise patients that taking the drug with meals may minimize GI distress.
- May alter Clinistix or Tes-Tape results. Use Clinitest for accurate urine glucose test results.
- Caution patients to stop taking drug and to notify the doctor immediately if skin or sclera becomes yellow-tinged. These signs may indicate accumulation caused by impaired renal excretion.

---

salsalate (disalicylic acid, salicylsalicylic acid)
Amigesic, Argesic-SA, Arthra-G, Disalcid, Mono-Gesic, Salflex, Salgesic, Salsitab

Pregnancy Risk Category: C

HOW SUPPLIED
Tablets: 500 mg, 750 mg
Caplets: 750 mg
Capsules: 500 mg

ACTION
Mechanism: The salicylic ester of salicylic acid, each molecule of salsalate is hydrolyzed to two molecules of salicylate in vivo. Produces analgesia by blocking prostaglandin synthesis (peripheral action). Salicylates prevent the lowering of the pain threshold that occurs when prostaglandins sensitize pain receptors to mechanical and chemical stimulation. Drug also has an ill-defined effect on the hypothalamus. Exerts its anti-inflammatory effect by inhibiting prostaglandin synthesis; may also inhibit the synthesis or action of other mediators of the inflammatory response.
Peak: Plasma levels of salsalate peak within 1½ hours of an oral dose; of salicylate, within 2 to 4 hours. Steady state levels and peak analgesic effect may be delayed for 3 to 4 days after therapy begins. **Duration:** plasma half-life, about 1 hour.

INDICATIONS & DOSAGE
Arthritis –
Adults: 3 g P.O. daily, divided b.i.d. or t.i.d. Usual maintenance dosage is 2 to 4 g daily.

ADVERSE REACTIONS
EENT: *tinnitus and hearing loss.*
GI: *nausea, vomiting, GI distress,* occult bleeding (rare).
Hepatic: abnormal liver function studies, hepatitis.
Skin: *rash,* bruising.
Other: hypersensitivity reactions (***anaphylaxis,*** asthma).

INTERACTIONS
Ammonium chloride (and other urine acidifiers): increased blood levels of salicylates. Monitor for salicylate toxicity.
Antacids in high doses (and other urine alkalinizers): decreased levels of salicylates. Monitor for decreased salicylate effect.
Corticosteroids: enhanced salicylate excretion. Monitor for decreased salicylate effect.
Ethanol, NSAIDs, steroids: increased risk of GI bleeding. Avoid concomitant use.

Methotrexate: increased risk of methotrexate toxicity. Avoid concomitant use.
Oral anticoagulants: possible increased risk of bleeding. Avoid using together if possible.

CONTRAINDICATIONS

• Contraindicated in patients with salsalate hypersensitivity. Also contraindicated in children or teenagers with chicken pox or influenza-like illness salicylates.
• Use cautiously in patients with GI bleeding, aspirin hypersensitivity, renal insufficiency, hypoprothrombinemia, vitamin K deficiency, and bleeding disorders.

NURSING CONSIDERATIONS

• Because of epidemiologic association with Reye's syndrome, the Centers for Disease Control and Prevention recommends not giving children or teenagers with chicken pox or influenza-like illness salicylates.
• Therapeutic blood salicylate level in arthritis is 10 to 30 mg/100 ml. Tinnitus may occur at plasma levels of 30 mg/100 ml and above, but this is not a reliable indicator of toxicity, especially in very young patients and those over age 60. With long-term therapy, mild toxicity may occur at plasma levels of 20 mg/100 ml.
• Salsalate may cause increased serum levels of AST, ALT, alkaline phosphatase, and bilirubin.
• In patients on long-term therapy, obtain hemoglobin and PT tests periodically.
• Advise patients receiving long-term treatment with large doses to watch for petechiae, bleeding gums, and signs of GI bleeding, and to maintain adequate fluid intake. Encourage the use of a soft toothbrush.
• To reduce GI adverse reactions, tell patients to take this drug with food, milk, antacid, or large glass of water.

sodium salicylate

Pregnancy Risk Category: C

HOW SUPPLIED

Tablets (enteric-coated): 325 mg◊, 650 mg◊

ACTION

Mechanism: Produces analgesia by blocking prostaglandin synthesis (peripheral action). Salicylates may prevent the lowering of the pain threshold that occurs when prostaglandins sensitize pain receptors to mechanical and chemical stimulation. Exerts its anti-inflammatory effect by inhibiting prostaglandin synthesis; may also inhibit the synthesis or action of other mediators of the inflammatory response. Relieves fever by acting on the hypothalamic heat-regulating center to produce peripheral vasodilation. This increases peripheral blood supply and promotes sweating, which leads to heat loss and to cooling by evaporation.
Onset: within 45 minutes. **Peak:** Plasma levels peak within 6 hours of oral administration.

INDICATIONS & DOSAGE

Minor pain or fever –
Adults: 325 to 650 mg P.O. q 4 to 6 hours, p.r.n. Maximum dosage is 1 g daily.
Arthritis –
Adults: 3.6 to 5.4 g P.O. daily in divided doses.

ADVERSE REACTIONS

EENT: *tinnitus, hearing loss.*
GI: *nausea, vomiting, GI distress.*
Hepatic: abnormal liver function studies, hepatitis.
Skin: *rash.*
Other: hypersensitivity reactions (***anaphylaxis,*** asthma).

*Liquid form contains alcohol.
**May contain tartrazine.

Common reactions are in italics; ***life-threatening,*** in bold italics.

INTERACTIONS

Ammonium chloride (and other urine acidifiers): increased blood levels of salicylates. Monitor for salicylate toxicity.

Antacids in large doses (and other urine alkalinizers): decreased levels of salicylates. Monitor for decreased salicylate effect.

Corticosteroids: enhanced salicylate elimination. Monitor for decreased salicylate effect.

Ethanol, other NSAIDs, steroids: increased risk of GI distress. Avoid concomitant use.

Methotrexate: increased risk of methotrexate toxicity. Avoid concomitant use.

Oral anticoagulants: increased risk of bleeding. Avoid using together if possible.

CONTRAINDICATIONS

- Contraindicated in patients with GI ulcer, GI bleeding, or aspirin hypersensitivity. Also contraindicated in children or teenagers with chicken pox or influenza-like illness.
- Use cautiously in patients with hypoprothrombinemia, vitamin K deficiency, bleeding disorders, and asthmatic patients with nasal polyps (may cause severe bronchospasm). Also use cautiously in patients with CHF or hypertension because of increased sodium load.

NURSING CONSIDERATIONS

- Because of epidemiologic association with Reye's syndrome, the Centers for Disease Control and Prevention recommends not giving children or teenagers with chicken pox or influenza-like illness salicylates.
- Febrile, dehydrated children can develop toxicity rapidly.
- Therapeutic salicylate level in arthritis is 10 to 30 mg/100 ml. Tinnitus may occur at plasma levels of 30 mg/100 ml and above, but this is not a reliable indicator of toxicity, especially in very young patients and those over age 60. With long-term therapy, mild toxicity may occur at plasma levels of 20 mg/100 ml.
- Sodium salicylate may increase serum levels of AST, ALT, alkaline phosphatase, and bilirubin.
- In patients on long-term therapy, monitor hemoglobin level and PT periodically.
- Advise patients receiving long-term treatment with large doses to watch for petechiae, bleeding gums, and signs of GI bleeding, and to maintain adequate fluid intake.
- Anti-inflammatory, analgesic, and antipyretic effects of salicylate salts are comparable to those of aspirin; however, platelet function is not affected. Do not substitute these agents for aspirin therapy during antithrombotic therapy.
- To reduce GI adverse reactions, tell patients to take this drug with food, milk, antacid, or large glass of water.
- **I.V. use:** Dilute drug in 1 liter of 0.9% sodium chloride or lactated Ringer's solution and infuse over 4 to 8 hours. Avoid extravasation because the drug is highly irritating to local tissues. Rapid infusion may cause thrombophlebitis.

sodium thiosalicylate

Rexolate, Tusal

Pregnancy Risk Category: C

HOW SUPPLIED

Injection: 50 mg/ml in 2-ml ampules or 30-ml vials.

ACTION

Mechanism: Produces analgesia by blocking prostaglandin synthesis (peripheral action). Salicylates may prevent the lowering of the pain threshold that occurs when prostaglandins sensitize pain receptors to mechanical and chemical stimulation. Drug also has an ill-defined effect on the hypo-

thalamus. Relieves fever by acting on the hypothalamic heat-regulating center to produce peripheral vasodilation. This increases peripheral blood supply and promotes sweating, which leads to loss of heat and to cooling by evaporation.
Onset: effects occur within 1 hour of injection. Drug detected in plasma within 1½ hours of injection.

INDICATIONS & DOSAGE

Mild pain–
Adults: 50 to 100 mg I.M. daily or every other day.
Acute gout–
Adults: 100 mg I.M. q 3 to 4 hours for 2 days; then 100 mg daily.
Rheumatic fever–
Adults: 100 to 150 mg I.M. q 4 to 8 hours for 3 days, followed by 100 mg b.i.d. until asymptomatic.

ADVERSE REACTIONS

EENT: *tinnitus and hearing loss.*
GI: *nausea, vomiting, GI distress, occult bleeding.*
Hepatic: abnormal liver function studies, hepatitis.
Skin: *rash,* bruising.
Other: hypersensitivity reactions (***anaphylaxis,*** asthma).

INTERACTIONS

Ammonium chloride (and other urine acidifiers): increased blood levels of salicylates. Monitor for salicylate toxicity.
Antacids in large doses (and other urine alkalinizers): decreased levels of salicylates. Monitor for decreased salicylate effect.
Corticosteriods: enhance salicylate elimination. Monitor for decreased salicylate effects.
Heparin, oral anticoagulants: increased risk of bleeding. Avoid using together if possible.

CONTRAINDICATIONS

- Contraindicated in GI ulcer, GI bleeding, or aspirin sensitivity.
- Use cautiously in hypoprothrombinemia, vitamin K deficiency, bleeding disorders, and asthma with nasal polyps (may cause severe bronchospasm).

NURSING CONSIDERATIONS

- Because of epidemiologic association with Reye's syndrome, the Centers for Disease Control and Prevention recommends not giving children or teenagers with chicken pox or influenza-like illness salicylates.
- Tinnitus, headache, dizziness, confusion, fever, sweating, thirst, drowsiness, dim vision, hyperventilation, and tachycardia are signs of mild toxicity.
- Sodium thiosalicylate may increase serum levels of AST, ALT, alkaline phosphatase, and bilirubin.
- I.M. route is preferred because of increased risk of complications associated with I.V. use.

26
Nonsteroidal anti-inflammatory drugs

diclofenac sodium
etodolac
fenoprofen calcium
flurbiprofen
ibuprofen
indomethacin
indomethacin sodium trihydrate
ketoprofen
ketorolac tromethamine
meclofenamate
mefenamic acid
nabumetone
naproxen
naproxen sodium
oxaprozin
oxyphenbutazone
phenylbutazone
piroxicam
sulindac
tolmetin sodium

COMBINATION PRODUCTS
CO ADVIL SINUS◇, DRISTAN SINUS CAPLETS◇: pseudoephedrine hydrochloride 30 mg and ibuprofen 200 mg.

diclofenac sodium
Fenac‡, Voltaren, Voltaren SR†

Pregnancy Risk Category: B

HOW SUPPLIED
Tablets (enteric-coated): 25 mg, 50 mg, 75 mg
Tablets (slow-release): 100 mg†
Suppositories: 50 mg†, 100 mg†

ACTION
Mechanism: Produces anti-inflammatory, analgesic, and antipyretic effects, possibly by inhibiting prostaglandin synthesis.
Peak: Plasma levels peak within 2 to 3 hours of oral administration of enteric-coated tablets. **Duration:** terminal elimination half-life, 1 to 2 hours.

INDICATIONS AND DOSAGE
Ankylosing spondylitis –
Adults: 25 mg P.O. q.i.d. and h.s.
Osteoarthritis –
Adults: 50 mg P.O. b.i.d. or t.i.d., or 75 mg P.O. b.i.d.
Rheumatoid arthritis –
Adults: 75 to 100 mg P.O. b.i.d., or 50 to 100 mg P.R. (where available) h.s. as a substitute for the last oral dose of the day. Do not exceed 200 mg daily.

ADVERSE REACTIONS
CNS: anxiety, depression, dizziness, drowsiness, insomnia, irritability, myoclonus, migraine, *headache.*
CV: ***CHF,*** hypertension, edema, fluid retention.
EENT: *tinnitus,* laryngeal edema, swelling of the lips and tongue, blurred vision, eye pain, night blindness.
GI: *abdominal pain or cramps, constipation, diarrhea, indigestion, nausea,* abdominal distention, flatulence, peptic ulceration, ***bleeding,*** melena, bloody diarrhea, appetite change, colitis.
GU: azotemia, proteinuria, acute renal failure, oliguria, interstitial nephritis, papillary necrosis, ***nephrotic syndrome,*** *fluid retention.*
Hepatic: elevated liver enzymes, jaundice, hepatitis, ***hepatotoxicity.***
Respiratory: asthma.
Skin: rash, pruritus, urticaria, eczema, dermatitis, alopecia, photosensitivity, bullous eruption, ***Stevens-Johnson syndrome (rare),*** allergic purpura.
Other: ***anaphylaxis; anaphylactoid reactions;*** angioedema; back, leg, or

joint pain; hypoglycemia; hyperglycemia.

INTERACTIONS

Anticoagulants (including warfarin): possible increased incidence of bleeding. Monitor patient closely.
Aspirin: concomitant use not recommended by manufacturer.
Cyclosporine, digoxin, lithium, methotrexate: diclofenac may reduce renal clearance of these drugs and increase risk of toxicity. Monitor patient closely.
Diuretics: decreased effectiveness of diuretics.
Insulin, oral antidiabetic agents: diclofenac may alter requirements for antidiabetic agents. Monitor patient closely.
Potassium-sparing diuretics: enhanced potassium retention and increased serum potassium levels.

CONTRAINDICATIONS

- Contraindicated in patients with hypersensitivity to this drug, aspirin, or other NSAIDs and in patients with a history of asthma, urticaria, or other allergic reactions after taking these drugs. Not recommended for use during pregnancy or breast-feeding.
- Use cautiously in patients with a history of peptic ulcer disease, hepatic dysfunction, cardiac disease, or other conditions associated with fluid retention or impaired renal function.

NURSING CONSIDERATIONS

- Elevations of liver tests may occur during therapy. Measure serum transaminase, especially ALT levels, periodically in patients undergoing long-term therapy. Make the first serum transaminase measurement no later than 8 weeks after initiation of therapy.
- Serious GI toxicity, including peptic ulceration and bleeding, can occur in patients taking NSAIDs despite the absence of GI symptoms. Teach patients the signs and symptoms of GI bleeding, and tell them to contact the doctor immediately if any of these occurs.
- To minimize GI distress, tell patients to take diclofenac with milk or meals.
- Because NSAIDs impair the synthesis of renal prostaglandins, they can decrease renal blood flow and lead to reversible renal impairment, especially in patients with preexisting renal failure, liver dysfunction, or heart failure; in elderly patients; and in those taking diuretics. Monitor these patients closely.
- Teach patients the signs and symptoms of hepatotoxicity, including nausea, fatigue, lethargy, pruritus, jaundice, right upper quadrant tenderness, and flulike symptoms. Tell them to contact doctor immediately if these symptoms appear.
- Do not crush, break, or chew enteric-coated tablets.
- Because of their antipyretic and anti-inflammatory actions, NSAIDs may mask the signs and symptoms of infection.

etodolac (ultradol)

Lodine

Pregnancy Risk Category: C

HOW SUPPLIED

Capsules: 200 mg, 300 mg
Tablets: 400 mg

ACTION

Mechanism: Unknown, but believed related to inhibition of prostaglandin biosynthesis.
Onset: within 30 minutes. **Peak:** Plasma levels peak within 1 to 2 hours. **Duration:** plasma half-life, about 7½ hours; analgesic effects persist 4 to 12 hours.

INDICATIONS & DOSAGE

Acute and chronic management of osteoarthritis and pain –
Adults: for acute pain, give 200 to 400 mg P.O. q 6 to 8 hours p.r.n., not to exceed 1,200 mg daily. For patients weighing 132 lb (60 kg) or under, total daily dose should not exceed 20 mg/kg.

ADVERSE REACTIONS

CNS: *asthenia, malaise,* dizziness, depression, drowsiness, nervousness, insomnia, headache.
CV: anemia, hypertension, ***CHF,*** flushing, palpitations, edema, fluid retention.
EENT: blurred vision, tinnitus, photophobia, dry mouth.
GI: *dyspepsia, flatulence, abdominal pain, diarrhea, nausea,* constipation, gastritis, melena, vomiting, anorexia, peptic ulceration with or without bleeding or perforation, ulcerative stomatitis, thirst.
GU: dysuria, urinary frequency, ***renal failure.***
Hematologic: anemia (rare), leukopenia, thrombocytopenia.
Hepatic: hepatitis.
Respiratory: asthma.
Skin: pruritus, rash, photosensitivity, ***Stevens-Johnson syndrome.***
Other: chills, fever, weight gain.

INTERACTIONS

Antacids: may decrease peak levels of the drug. Monitor for decreased effect of etodolac.
Aspirin: reduced protein-binding of etodolac without altering its clearance. Clinical significance unknown.
Cyclosporine: impaired elimination and increased risk of nephrotoxicity. Avoid concomitant use.
Digoxin, lithium, methotrexate: etodolac may impair elimination of these drugs, resulting in increased levels and risk of toxicity. Monitor blood levels.
Warfarin: etodolac decreases the protein-binding of warfarin but does not change its clearance. Although no dosage adjustment is necessary, monitor PT closely and watch for bleeding.

CONTRAINDICATIONS

- Contraindicated in patients with hypersensitivity to the drug and in those with a history of NSAID-induced asthma, rhinitis, urticaria, or other allergic reactions to NSAIDs.
- Use cautiously in patients with a history of GI bleeding, ulceration, and perforation and renal or hepatic impairment.

NURSING CONSIDERATIONS

- Etodolac is not recommended for patients with rheumatoid arthritis. Other currently available NSAIDs typically are more effective.
- Serious GI toxicity, including peptic ulceration and bleeding, can occur in patients taking NSAIDs despite the absence of GI symptoms. Teach patients the signs and symptoms of GI bleeding, and tell them to contact the doctor immediately if any of these occurs. However, etodolac appears to cause fewer GI problems than most NSAIDS. Minimal GI blood loss has been reported at dosages up to 1,200 mg daily.
- To minimize GI discomfort, tell patients to take etodolac with milk or meals.
- Because NSAIDs impair the synthesis of renal prostaglandins, they can decrease renal blood flow and lead to reversible renal impairment, especially in patients with preexisting renal failure, liver dysfunction, or heart failure; in elderly patients; and in those taking diuretics. Monitor these patients closely during therapy.
- This drug has been associated with photosensitivity reactions. Advise patients to use a sunblock, wear protective clothing, and avoid prolonged exposure to sunlight.

• Metabolites of etodolac may cause a false-positive test for urinary bilirubin, decreased serum uric acid levels, and borderline elevations of one or more liver function tests.

fenoprofen calcium

Nalfon, Nalfon-200

Pregnancy Risk Category: B (D in 3rd trimester)

HOW SUPPLIED

Tablets: 600 mg
Capsules: 200 mg, 300 mg

ACTION

Mechanism: Produces anti-inflammatory, analgesic, and antipyretic effects, possibly by inhibiting prostaglandin synthesis.
Onset: 15 to 30 minutes. **Peak:** Plasma levels peak in about 2 hours.
Duration: plasma half-life, about 3 hours; analgesic effects persist 4 to 6 hours.

INDICATIONS & DOSAGE

Rheumatoid arthritis and osteoarthritis –
Adults: 300 to 600 mg P.O. q.i.d. Maximum dosage is 3.2 g daily.
Mild to moderate pain –
Adults: 200 mg P.O. q 4 to 6 hours, p.r.n.

ADVERSE REACTIONS

CNS: *headache, drowsiness, dizziness, somnolence.*
CV: peripheral edema.
EENT: auditory abnormalities.
GI: *epigastric distress, nausea,* ***GI bleeding,*** vomiting, occult blood loss, peptic ulceration, constipation, anorexia.
GU: oliguria, azotemia, interstitial nephritis, proteinuria, reversible renal failure.
Hematologic: prolonged bleeding time, anemia, ***aplastic anemia, agranulocytosis,*** thrombocytopenia.
Hepatic: elevated enzymes, hepatitis.
Respiratory: pulmonary infiltrates.
Skin: *pruritus,* rash, urticaria, ***toxic epidermal necrolysis.***

INTERACTIONS

Aspirin: decreased fenoprofen half-life; may increase GI toxicity. Avoid concomitant use.
Diuretics: decreased diuretic effectiveness. Monitor closely.
Ethanol, corticosteroids: increased risk of adverse GI reactions. Avoid concomitant use.
Oral anticoagulants, sulfonylureas: fenoprofen enhances pharmacologic effects of these drugs. Use together cautiously.
Phenobarbital: enhanced metabolism of fenoprofen. Monitor for lack of fenoprofen effectiveness.

CONTRAINDICATIONS

• Contraindicated in patients with hypersensitivity to this drug, aspirin, or other NSAIDs.
• Use cautiously in elderly patients; in patients with GI disorders, angioedema, or cardiovascular disease; and in those with a history of peptic ulcer disease.

NURSING CONSIDERATIONS

• Serious GI toxicity, including peptic ulceration and bleeding, can occur in patients taking NSAIDs despite the absence of GI symptoms. Teach patients the signs and symptoms of GI bleeding, and tell them to contact the doctor immediately if any occurs.
• Tell patients to take this drug 30 minutes before or 2 hours after meals. If adverse GI reactions occur, drug may be taken with milk or meals.
• Tell patients that full therapeutic effect for arthritis may be delayed for 2 to 4 weeks.
• Check renal, hepatic, and auditory function periodically in long-term therapy. Stop drug if abnormalities occur.

• Because NSAIDs impair the synthesis of renal prostaglandins, they can decrease renal blood flow and lead to reversible renal impairment, especially in patients with preexisting renal failure, liver dysfunction, or heart failure; in elderly patients; and in those taking diuretics. Monitor these patients closely during therapy.
• Because fenoprofen may cause somnolence, warn patients to avoid driving and other hazardous activities that require alertness until adverse CNS effects of the drug are known.
• Because of their antipyretic and anti-inflammatory actions, NSAIDs may mask the signs and symptoms of infection.
• PT may be prolonged in patients receiving coumarin-type anticoagulants. Fenoprofen decreases platelet aggregation and may prolong bleeding time.
• Fenoprofen may cause false elevations in free and total serum triiodothyronine (T_3) levels as measured by the Amerlex-T assay. Fenoprofen or its metabolite may cross-react with the antibody used in the Amerlex-M assay. Limited data suggest that drug may alter free and total T_3 concentrations determined by the Corning method.

flurbiprofen

Ansaid, Apo-Flurbiprofen†, Froben†, Froben SR†

Pregnancy Risk Category: B

HOW SUPPLIED

Tablets: 50 mg, 100 mg
Capsules (extended-release)†*:* 200 mg

ACTION

Mechanism: Interferes with prostaglandin synthesis.
Peak: Serum levels peak about 1½ hours after a dose. **Duration:** elimination half-life, about 5½ hours.

INDICATIONS AND DOSAGE

Rheumatoid arthritis and osteoarthritis –
Adults: 200 to 300 mg P.O. daily, divided b.i.d. to q.i.d. Where available, patients maintained on 200 mg daily may switch to one 200-mg extended-release capsule P.O. daily, taken in the evening after food.

ADVERSE REACTIONS

CNS: *headache,* anxiety, insomnia, increased reflexes, tremors, amnesia, asthenia, drowsiness, malaise, depression, dizziness.
CV: *edema, **CHF,*** hypertension, vasodilation.
EENT: rhinitis, tinnitus, visual changes.
GI: *dyspepsia, diarrhea, abdominal pain, nausea,* constipation, ***bleeding,*** flatulence, vomiting.
GU: *symptoms suggesting urinary tract infection,* nephrotoxicity.
Hematologic: thrombocytopenia, neutropenia, anemia, ***aplastic anemia.***
Hepatic: elevated liver enzymes, jaundice.
Respiratory: asthma.
Skin: rash.
Other: weight changes.

INTERACTIONS

Aspirin: decreased flurbiprofen levels. Concomitant use is not recommended.
Diuretics: possible decreased diuretic effect. Monitor patient closely.
Methotrexate: increased risk of methotrexate toxicity. Monitor closely.
Oral anticoagulants: increased bleeding tendencies. Monitor patient closely.

CONTRAINDICATIONS

• Contraindicated in patients with hypersensitivity, including asthma or urticaria, to aspirin or other NSAIDs.
• Use cautiously in patients with a

history of peptic ulcer disease, hepatic dysfunction, cardiac disease, or other conditions associated with fluid retention or impaired renal function.

NURSING CONSIDERATIONS

- Serious GI toxicity, including peptic ulceration and bleeding, can occur in patients taking NSAIDs despite the absence of GI symptoms. Teach patients the signs and symptoms of GI bleeding, and tell them to contact the doctor immediately if any of these occurs.
- Tell patients to take drug with food, milk, or antacid if GI upset occurs.
- Elderly or debilitated patients and those patients with hepatic or renal dysfunction should be closely monitored and probably should receive lower doses. These patients may be at risk for renal toxicity, jaundice, or toxic hepatitis. Periodically monitor renal and hepatic function.
- Because NSAIDs impair the synthesis of renal prostaglandins, they can decrease renal blood flow and lead to reversible renal impairment, especially in patients with preexisting renal failure, liver dysfunction, or heart failure; in elderly patients; and in those taking diuretics. Monitor these patients closely during therapy.
- Patients receiving long-term therapy should have periodic liver function studies, eye examinations, and hematocrit determinations.
- Advise patients to avoid hazardous activities that require mental alertness until CNS effects are known.
- Tell patients taking extended-release capsules to swallow them whole; do not crush, chew, or break open the capsules.

ibuprofen

Aches-N-Pain◇, ACT-3‡, Advil◇, Amersol†, Apo-Ibuprofen†, Brufen‡, Children's Advil, Excedrin-IB Caplets◇, Excedrin-IB Tablets◇, Genpril Caplets◇, Genpril Tablets◇, Haltran◇, Ibu-Cream‡, Ibuprin◇, Ibuprohm Caplets◇, Ibuprohm Tablets◇, Ibu-Tab◇, Inflam‡, Medipren Caplets◇, Medipren Tablets◇, Midol-200◇, Motrin, Motrin IB Caplets◇, Motrin IB Tablets◇, Novoprofen†, Nuprin Caplets◇, Nuprin Tablets◇, Nurofen‡, PediaProfen, Rafen‡, Rufen, Saleto-200, Saleto-400, Saleto-600, Saleto-800, Trendar◇

Pregnancy Risk Category: B (D in 3rd trimester)

HOW SUPPLIED

Tablets: 200 mg◇, 300 mg, 400 mg, 600 mg, 800 mg
Caplets: 200 mg◇
Oral suspension: 100 mg/5 ml
Topical cream: 10%

ACTION

Mechanism: Produces anti-inflammatory, analgesic, and antipyretic effects, possibly by inhibiting prostaglandin synthesis.
Onset: analgesic and antipyretic effects, within 30 minutes; antirheumatic effects, within 7 days. **Peak:** Plasma levels peak 2 hours after oral dose. **Duration:** effects persist 4 to 6 hours.

INDICATIONS & DOSAGE

Mild to moderate pain, arthritis, primary dysmenorrhea, gout, postextraction dental pain –
Adults: 200 to 800 mg P.O. t.i.d. or q.i.d. not to exceed 3.2 g/day.
Juvenile arthritis –
Children: 20 to 40 mg/kg P.O. daily in three or four divided doses.
Fever –
Adults: 200 to 400 mg P.O. q 4 to 6

hours. Do not exceed 1.2 g daily or give longer than 3 days.
Children 1 to 12 years: if fever is below 102.5° F (39.2° C), the recommended dose is 5 mg/kg P.O. q 6 to 8 hours. Treat higher fevers with 10 mg/kg q 6 to 8 hours. Do not exceed 40 mg/kg daily.
External treatment of joint pain; swelling of tissues adjacent to joints‡ –
Adults: apply a 4- to 10-cm strip of cream to the skin and massage briskly. Apply t.i.d.

ADVERSE REACTIONS
CNS: *headache, drowsiness, dizziness,* cognitive dysfunction, aseptic meningitis.
CV: *peripheral edema, hypertension,* ***CHF.***
EENT: visual disturbances, *tinnitus.*
GI: *epigastric distress, nausea, occult blood loss, peptic ulceration.*
GU: reversible renal failure.
Hematologic: prolonged bleeding time, anemia, neutropenia, pancytopenia, thrombocytopenia, aplastic anemia, leukopenia, agranulocytosis.
Hepatic: elevated enzymes.
Respiratory: ***bronchospasm.***
Skin: pruritus, rash, urticaria, photosensitivity, ***Stevens-Johnson syndrome.***
Other: edema.

INTERACTIONS
Antihypertensives, furosemide, thiazide diuretics: ibuprofen may decrease the effectiveness of diuretics or antihypertensives.
Aspirin: may decrease serum levels of ibuprofen. Avoid concomitant use.
Aspirin, corticosteroids, ethanol: increased risk of adverse GI reactions. Avoid concomitant use.
Lithium, oral anticoagulants: ibuprofen may increase plasma levels or effects of these drug. Monitor for toxicity.

CONTRAINDICATIONS
- Contraindicated in patients with hypersensitivity to this drug, aspirin, or other NSAIDs.
- Use cautiously in patients with GI disorders, history of peptic ulcer disease, angioedema, hepatic or renal disease, cardiac decompensation, known intrinsic coagulation defects, and in asthmatic patients with nasal polyps.

NURSING CONSIDERATIONS
- Tell patients that full therapeutic effect for arthritis may be delayed for 2 to 4 weeks. Although analgesic effect occurs at low dosage levels, anti-inflammatory effect does not occur at dosages below 400 mg q.i.d.
- Check renal and hepatic function periodically in patients on long-term therapy. Stop drug if abnormalities occur.
- Serious GI toxicity, including peptic ulceration and bleeding, can occur in patients taking NSAIDs despite the absence of GI symptoms. Teach patients the signs and symptoms of GI bleeding, and tell them to contact the doctor immediately if any occurs.
- To reduce adverse GI reactions, give with meals or milk.
- Caution patients that concomitant use with aspirin, alcohol, or corticosteroids may increase the risk of GI adverse reactions.
- Drug is available OTC in several brands (200 mg). Instruct the patient to not exceed 1.2 g daily, give to children under age 12, or self-medicate for extended periods without consulting the doctor.
- Because of their antipyretic and anti-inflammatory actions, NSAIDs may mask the signs and symptoms of infection.

indomethacin

Apo-Indomethacin†, Arthrexin‡, Indameth, Indochron E-R, Indocid†‡, Indocid SR†, Indocin, Indocin SR, Novomethacin†, Rheumacin‡

indomethacin sodium trihydrate

Apo-Indomethacin†, Indameth, Indocid PDA†, Indocin I.V., Novomethacin†

Pregnancy Risk Category: B (D in 3rd trimester)

HOW SUPPLIED

indomethacin

Capsules: 10 mg, 25 mg, 50 mg, 75 mg

Capsules (sustained-release): 75 mg

Oral suspension: 25 mg/5 ml

Suppositories: 50 mg

indomethacin sodium trihydrate

Injection: 1-mg vials

ACTION

Mechanism: Produces anti-inflammatory, analgesic, and antipyretic effects, possibly by inhibiting prostaglandin synthesis.

Onset: analgesic action, within 30 minutes; antirheumatic action, within 7 days. **Peak:** Serum levels peak within 1 to 2 hours after a dose of immediate-release capsules or oral suspension, within 2 to 4 hours of a sustained-release capsule, or immediately following an I.V. injection. Peak antirheumatic effects occur after 1 to 2 weeks of therapy. **Duration:** plasma half-life, about 4 ½ hours; analgesic effects persist 4 to 6 hours.

INDICATIONS & DOSAGE

Moderate to severe arthritis, ankylosing spondylitis –

Adults: 25 mg P.O. or P.R. b.i.d. or t.i.d. with food or antacids; may increase dosage by 25 mg daily q 7 days up to 200 mg daily. Alternatively, sustained-release capsules (75 mg) may be given: 75 mg P.O. to start, in the morning or h.s., followed, if necessary, by 75 mg b.i.d.

Acute gouty arthritis –

Adults: 50 mg P.O. t.i.d. Reduce dose as soon as possible; then discontinue. Sustained-release capsules shouldn't be used for this condition.

To close a hemodynamically significant patent ductus arteriosus in premature infants (I.V. form only) –

Neonates under 48 hours: 0.2 mg/kg I.V. followed by two doses of 0.1 mg/kg at 12- to 24-hour intervals.

Neonates 2 to 7 days: 0.2 mg/kg I.V. followed by two doses of 0.2 mg/kg at 12- to 24-hour intervals.

Neonates over 7 days: 0.2 mg/kg I.V. followed by two doses of 0.25 mg/kg at 12- to 24-hour intervals.

ADVERSE REACTIONS

Oral and rectal form:

CNS: *headache, dizziness,* depression, drowsiness, confusion, peripheral neuropathy, ***seizures,*** psychic disturbances, syncope, *vertigo.*

CV: hypertension, *edema,* ***CHF.***

EENT: *blurred vision, corneal and retinal damage,* hearing loss, tinnitus.

GI: *nausea, vomiting,* anorexia, *diarrhea, peptic ulceration,* ***GI bleeding,*** pancreatitis.

GU: hematuria, ***acute renal failure.***

Hematologic: ***hemolytic anemia, aplastic anemia, agranulocytosis,*** leukopenia, thrombocytopenic purpura, iron deficiency anemia.

Hepatic: elevated enzymes.

Skin: pruritus, urticaria, ***Stevens-Johnson syndrome.***

Other: hypersensitivity (rash, respiratory distress, ***anaphylaxis, angioedema),*** hyperkalemia.

I.V. form:

GI: ***bleeding,*** vomiting.

GU: ***renal dysfunction, azotemia.***

Hematologic: decreased platelet aggregation.

Other: ***hyponatremia, hyperkalemia,***

*Liquid form contains alcohol.
**May contain tartrazine.

Common reactions are in italics; ***life-threatening,*** in bold italics.

hypoglycemia, hypersensitivity (rash, respiratory distress, ***anaphylaxis, angioedema)***.

INTERACTIONS

Aminoglycosides, cyclosporine, methotrexate: indomethacin may enhance the toxicity of these agents. Avoid concomitant use.
Antihypertensive agents: reduced antihypertensive effect. Monitor closely.
Aspirin: decreased blood levels of indomethacin. Avoid concomitant use.
Corticosteroids, ethanol: increased risk of GI toxicity. Don't use together.
Diflunisal, probenecid: decreased indomethacin excretion; watch for increased incidence of indomethacin adverse reactions.
Digoxin: indomethacin may prolong the half-life of digoxin. Use together cautiously.
Dipyridamole: enhanced fluid retention. Avoid concomitant use.
Furosemide, thiazide diuretics: impaired response to both drugs. Avoid using together if possible.
Lithium: increased plasma lithium levels. Monitor for toxicity.
Triamterene: possible nephrotoxicity. Don't use together.

CONTRAINDICATIONS

- Contraindicated in patients with hypersensitivity to this drug, other NSAIDs, or aspirin and in those with active peptic ulcer disease. Also contraindicated in infants with untreated infection, active bleeding, coagulation defects or thrombocytopenia, necrotizing enterocolitis, or impaired renal function.
- Use cautiously in patients with seizure disorders, coagulation disorders, parkinsonism, hepatic or renal disease, cardiovascular disease, infection, and history of mental illness. Also use cautiously in elderly patients.

NURSING CONSIDERATIONS

Oral form:

- Severe headache may occur. Decrease dose if headache persists.
- Indomethacin has an antipyretic effect.
- Tell patients to notify the doctor immediately if any visual or hearing changes occurs. Patients on long-term therapy should have regular eye examinations, hearing tests, CBC, and renal function tests to monitor for toxicity.
- Serious GI toxicity, including peptic ulceration and bleeding, can occur in patients taking NSAIDs despite the absence of GI symptoms. Teach patients the signs and symptoms of GI bleeding, and tell them to contact the doctor immediately if any of these occurs.
- Tell patients to take this drug with food, milk, or antacid if GI upset occurs.
- Concomitant use with aspirin, alcohol, or corticosteroids may increase the risk of adverse GI reactions.
- Adverse CNS reactions are more common and serious in elderly patients.
- Monitor for bleeding in patients receiving anticoagulants, patients with coagulation defects, and neonates.
- Because NSAIDs impair the synthesis of renal prostaglandins, they can decrease renal blood flow and lead to reversible renal impairment, especially in patients with preexisting renal failure, liver dysfunction, or heart failure; in elderly patients; and in those taking diuretics. Monitor these patients closely during therapy.
- Causes sodium retention; monitor for weight gain (especially in elderly patients) and increased blood pressure in patients with hypertension.
- Used as prophylaxis for gout when colchicine is not well tolerated.
- Because of its high incidence of adverse effects during chronic use, indo-

methacin should not be used routinely as an analgesic or antipyretic.

• Because of their antipyretic and anti-inflammatory actions, NSAIDs may mask the signs and symptoms of infection.

I.V. form:

• **I.V. use:** Reconstitute powder for injection with sterile water for injection or 0.9% sodium chloride. For each 1-mg vial, add 1 ml of diluent for a solution containing 1 mg/ml; add 2 ml of diluent to yield a solution containing 0.5 mg/ml. Give by direct injection over 5 to 10 seconds.

• Use only preservative-free diluents to prepare I.V. injection. Never use diluents containing benzyl alcohol because this has been associated with a fatal gasping syndrome in neonates. Because the injection contains no preservatives, reconstitute immediately before administration, and discard any unused solution.

• Don't administer second or third scheduled dose if anuria or marked oliguria is evident.

• If ductus arteriosus reopens, a second course of one to three doses may be given. If ineffective, surgery may be necessary.

• Indomethacin may enhance the hypothalamic-pituitary-adrenal axis response to the dexamethasone suppression test. Inform clinical laboratory personnel that the patient is taking indomethacin.

• Monitor carefully for bleeding and for reduced urine output. Discontinue drug and notify the doctor if either occurs.

ketoprofen

Apo-Keto†, Apo-Keto-E†, Novo-Keto-EC†, Orudis, Orudis E†, Orudis SR†‡, Oruvail, Rhodis†, Rhodis-E†, Rhodis-EC†

Pregnancy Risk Category: B (D in 3rd trimester)

HOW SUPPLIED

Tablets (sustained-release): 200 mg
Tablets (enteric-coated): 50 mg†, 100 mg†
Capsules (extended-release): 200 mg
Capsules: 25 mg, 50 mg, 75 mg
Suppositories: 100 mg†

ACTION

Mechanism: Produces anti-inflammatory, analgesic, and antipyretic effects, possibly by inhibiting prostaglandin synthesis.
Peak: Serum levels peak ½ to 2 hours after immediate-release capsule, 5 to 12 hours after sustained-release preparation. **Duration:** plasma half-life, 2 to 4 hours.

INDICATIONS & DOSAGE

Rheumatoid arthritis and osteoarthritis –
Adults: 150 to 300 mg P.O. in three or four divided doses or 200 mg as a sustained- release tablet. Usual dosage is 75 mg t.i.d. Maximum dosage is 300 mg/day.

Alternatively, where suppository is available, 100 mg P.R. b.i.d.; or 1 suppository h.s. (in conjunction with oral ketoprofen during the day).

Mild to moderate pain; dysmenorrhea –
Adults: 25 to 50 mg P.O. q 6 to 8 hours p.r.n.

ADVERSE REACTIONS

CNS: *headache,* dizziness, *CNS inhibition or excitation.*
EENT: tinnitus, visual disturbances.
GI: *nausea, abdominal pain, diarrhea, constipation, flatulence,* ***peptic ulceration,*** anorexia, vomiting, stomatitis.
GU: ***nephrotoxicity,*** *elevated BUN.*
Hematologic: prolonged bleeding time, thrombocytopenia, ***agranulocytosis.***
Hepatic: elevated liver enzymes.
Respiratory: dyspnea, ***bronchospasm, laryngeal edema.***

*Liquid form contains alcohol.
**May contain tartrazine.

Common reactions are in italics; ***life-threatening,*** in bold italics.

Skin: rash, photosensitivity, ***exfoliative dermatitis.***

INTERACTIONS

Aspirin, corticosteroids, ethanol: increased risk of adverse GI reactions. Avoid concomitant use.
Aspirin, probenecid: increased plasma levels of ketoprofen. Avoid concomitant use.
Hydrochlorothiazide, other diuretics: decreased diuretic effectiveness. Monitor for lack of effect.
Lithium, methotrexate: increased levels of these drugs, leading to toxicity. Monitor closely.
Oral anticoagulants: increased risk of bleeding. Monitor closely.

CONTRAINDICATIONS

- Contraindicated in patients with hypersensitivity to this drug, aspirin, or other NSAIDs.
- Use cautiously in patients with history of peptic ulcer disease or renal dysfunction.

NURSING CONSIDERATIONS

- Serious GI toxicity, including peptic ulceration and bleeding, can occur in patients taking NSAIDs despite the absence of GI symptoms. Teach patients the signs and symptoms of GI bleeding, and tell them to contact the doctor immediately if any of these occurs.
- Concomitant use with aspirin, alcohol, or corticosteroids may increase the risk of adverse GI reactions.
- Tell patients to report visual or auditory adverse reactions immediately.
- Because NSAIDs impair the synthesis of renal prostaglandins, they can decrease renal blood flow and lead to reversible renal impairment, especially in patients with preexisting renal failure, liver dysfunction, or heart failure; in elderly patients; and in those taking diuretics. Monitor these patients closely during therapy.
- Tell patients that full therapeutic effect may be delayed for 2 to 4 weeks.
- Check renal and hepatic function every 6 months or as indicated during long-term therapy.
- Tell patients to take drug 30 minutes before or 2 hours after meals. If adverse GI reactions occur, patients may take the drug with milk or meals.
- Ketoprofen may interfere with some laboratory determinations of blood glucose and serum iron levels, depending on the testing method used.
- NSAIDs may mask the signs and symptoms of infection because of their antipyretic and anti-inflammatory actions.
- This drug has been associated with photosensitivity reactions. Advise patients to use a sunblock, wear protective clothing, and avoid prolonged exposure to sunlight.
- The sustained-release dosage form is not recommended for patients in acute pain.

ketorolac tromethamine

Toradol

Pregnancy Risk Category: B

HOW SUPPLIED

Tablets: 10 mg
Injection: 15 mg, 30 mg, 60 mg

ACTION

Mechanism: Acts by inhibiting prostaglandin synthesis.
Onset: within 10 minutes of an I.M. injection. **Peak:** Plasma levels peak in 30 minutes to 1 hour after either oral or I.M. administration. **Duration:** analgesic effects persist up to 6 hours.

INDICATIONS & DOSAGE

Short-term management of pain –
Adults: initially, give 30 or 60 mg I.M. as a loading dose, followed by half of the loading dose (15 or 30 mg) I.M. q 6 hours on a regular schedule or p.r.n. Subsequent dosage should be

based on patient response. If pain returns before 6 hours, dosage may be increased by as much as 50% (up to 60 mg); if pain relief continues for 8 to 12 hours, increase interval between doses to q 8 to 12 hours, or reduce dose. The recommended maximum dosage is 150 mg I.M. on the first day and 120 mg daily thereafter.

Alternatively, the drug may be used orally on a short-term basis. Give 10 mg P.O. q 4 to 6 hours p.r.n. Do not give more than 40 mg daily, and use the drug *only* for a short time.

ADVERSE REACTIONS

CNS: *drowsiness, sedation,* dizziness, headache, sweating.
CV: edema, hypertension, palpitations, arrhythmias.
GI: *nausea, dyspepsia, GI pain,* diarrhea, peptic ulceration.
Hematologic: decreased platelet adhesion.
Other: hyperkalemia, pain at injection site.

INTERACTIONS

Antihypertensives, diuretics: decreased effectiveness. Monitor closely.
Lithium: increased lithium levels. Monitor closely.
Methotrexate: decreased methotrexate clearance and increased toxicity. Don't use together.
Salicylates, warfarin: ketorolac may increase the levels of free (unbound) salicylates or warfarin in the blood. Clinical significance is unknown.

CONTRAINDICATIONS

- Contraindicated in patients with hypersensitivity to this drug, aspirin, or other NSAIDS.
- Use cautiously in patients with hepatic or renal impairment.
- Trace amounts of ketorolac have been detected in breast milk. Use with caution in breast-feeding patients.

NURSING CONSIDERATIONS

- This drug is intended solely for short-term management of pain. The incidence and severity of adverse reactions should be less than that observed in patients taking NSAIDs on a chronic basis.
- When switching patients from injectable to oral ketorolac, do not exceed a total dosage of 120 mg of drug on the day of transition, including a maximum of 40 mg P.O.
- Carefully observe patients with coagulopathies and those who are taking anticoagulants. Ketorolac inhibits platelet aggregation and can prolong bleeding time. This effect will disappear within 48 hours of discontinuing the drug. It will not alter platelet count, PTT, or PT.
- Serious GI toxicity, including peptic ulceration and bleeding, can occur in patients taking NSAIDs despite the absence of GI symptoms. Teach patients the signs and symptoms of GI bleeding, and tell them to contact the doctor immediately if any occurs.
- I.M. administration may cause pain at the injection site. Holding pressure over the site for 15 to 30 seconds after the injection may minimize local effects.
- Use lower initial doses in patients who are over age 65 or who weigh less than 110 lb (50 kg).
- NSAIDs may mask the signs and symptoms of infection because of their antipyretic and anti-inflammatory actions.

meclofenamate

Meclofen, Meclomen

Pregnancy Risk Category: B (D in 3rd trimester)

HOW SUPPLIED

Capsules: 50 mg, 100 mg

ACTION

Mechanism: Produces anti-inflammatory, analgesic, and antipyretic effects, possibly by inhibiting prostaglandin synthesis.

Onset: antirheumatic effects, within a few days of therapy. **Peak:** Plasma levels peak in ½ to 1 hour; peak antirheumatic activity occurs after 2 to 3 weeks of therapy. **Duration:** elimination half-life, 2 to 3½ hours.

INDICATIONS & DOSAGE

Rheumatoid arthritis and osteoarthritis –

Adults: 200 to 400 mg/day P.O. in three or four equally divided doses.

Mild to moderate pain –

Adults: 50 to 100 mg P.O. q 4 to 6 hours. Maximum dosage is 400 mg/day.

ADVERSE REACTIONS

CNS: fatigue, malaise, insomnia, *dizziness,* nervousness, *headache.*

CV: edema.

EENT: blurred vision, eye irritation.

GI: *abdominal pain, flatulence,* ***peptic ulceration,*** nausea, vomiting, *diarrhea,* hemorrhage.

GU: dysuria, hematuria, nephrotoxicity.

Hematologic: leukopenia, thrombocytopenia, ***agranulocytosis, aplastic anemia.***

Hepatic: ***hepatotoxicity.***

Skin: rash, urticaria.

INTERACTIONS

Antihypertensives, diuretics: decreased effectiveness. Monitor closely.

Aspirin: decreased plasma levels of meclofenamate.

Corticosteroids, ethanol, other NSAIDS: increased risk of GI adverse reactions. Avoid concomitant use.

Oral anticoagulants: enhanced anticoagulant effect. Monitor for toxicity.

CONTRAINDICATIONS

- Contraindicated in patients with GI ulceration or inflammation.
- Use cautiously in patients with hepatic or renal disease, cardiovascular disease, blood dyscrasia, diabetes mellitus, and in those with a history of peptic ulcer disease; and in elderly patients, who are more likely to experience adverse reactions.

NURSING CONSIDERATIONS

- Serious GI toxicity, including peptic ulceration and bleeding, can occur in patients taking NSAIDs despite the absence of GI symptoms. Teach patients the signs and symptoms of GI bleeding, and tell them to contact the doctor immediately if any of these occurs.
- To minimize adverse GI reactions, tell patients to take this drug with food.
- Caution patients that concomitant use with other NSAIDs, alcohol, or corticosteroids may increase the risk of GI adverse reactions.
- Advise patients to avoid driving or other hazardous activities that require mental alertness until CNS effects are known.
- Tell patients to stop drug and contact the doctor immediately if rash, visual disturbances, or diarrhea develops.
- Because NSAIDs impair the synthesis of renal prostaglandins, they can decrease renal blood flow and lead to reversible renal impairment, especially in patients with preexisting renal failure, liver dysfunction, or heart failure; in elderly patients; and in those taking diuretics. Monitor these patients closely during therapy.
- CBC and renal and hepatic function should be assessed every 6 months or as indicated in patients receiving long-term therapy.
- False-positive reactions for urine bilirubin using the diazo tablet test have been reported.

• NSAIDs may mask the signs and symptoms of infection because of their anti-inflammatory and antipyretic actions.

mefenamic acid

Mefic‡, Ponstan†, Ponstel

Pregnancy Risk Category: C

HOW SUPPLIED

Capsules: 250 mg

ACTION

Mechanism: Produces anti-inflammatory, analgesic, and antipyretic effects, possibly by inhibiting prostaglandin synthesis.
Peak: Serum levels peak 2 to 4 hours after a dose. **Duration:** plasma half-life, 2 to 4 hours.

INDICATIONS & DOSAGE

Mild to moderate pain, dysmenorrhea –
Adults and children over 14 years: Initially, 500 mg P.O.; then 250 mg q 6 hours, p.r.n. Maximum therapy 1 week.

ADVERSE REACTIONS

CNS: *drowsiness, dizziness,* nervousness, headache.
CV: edema.
EENT: blurred vision, eye irritation.
GI: nausea, vomiting, *diarrhea, **peptic ulceration, pancreatitis,*** hemorrhage.
GU: dysuria, hematuria, nephrotoxicity.
Hematologic: leukopenia, thrombocytopenia, ***agranulocytosis, aplastic anemia, hemolytic anemia.***
Hepatic: ***hepatotoxicity.***
Skin: rash, urticaria.

INTERACTIONS

Antihypertensives, diuretics: decreased effect. Monitor closely.
Aspirin, corticosteroids, ethanol: increased risk of GI adverse reactions. Avoid concomitant use.
Oral anticoagulants, sulfonylureas, and other drugs that are highly protein-bound: increased risk of toxicity.

CONTRAINDICATIONS

• Contraindicated in patients hypersensitive to the drug and in those with GI ulceration or inflammation.
• Use cautiously in patients with hepatic or renal disease, cardiovascular disease, blood dyscrasia, diabetes mellitus; and in those with a history of peptic ulcer disease.

NURSING CONSIDERATIONS

• Serious GI toxicity, including peptic ulceration and bleeding, can occur in patients taking NSAIDs despite the absence of GI symptoms. Teach patients the signs and symptoms of GI bleeding, and tell them to contact the doctor immediately if any of those occurs.
• To mimimize adverse GI reactions, tell patients to take this drug with food.
• Caution patients that concomitant use with aspirin, alcohol, or corticosteroids may increase the risk of GI adverse reactions.
• Because NSAIDs impair the synthesis of renal prostaglandins, they can decrease renal blood flow and lead to reversible renal impairment, especially in patients with preexisting renal failure, liver dysfunction, or heart failure; in elderly patients; and in those taking diuretics. Monitor these patients closely during therapy.
• Warn patient against hazardous activities that require alertness until CNS effects are known.
• Severe hemolytic anemia may occur with prolonged use. Monitor CBC every 4 to 6 months or as indicated.
• Tell patients to stop drug and contact the doctor immediately if rash, visual disturbances, or diarrhea develops.

- Mefenamic acid should not be administered for more than 1 week at a time because of increased risk of toxicity.
- NSAIDs may mask the signs and symptoms of infection because of their anti-inflammatory and antipyretic actions.
- False-positive reactions for urine bilirubin using the diazo tablet test have been reported.

nabumetone

Relafen

Pregnancy Risk Category: C

HOW SUPPLIED

Tablets: 500 mg, 750 mg

ACTION

Mechanism: Probably acts by inhibiting prostaglandin synthesis.
Peak: Plasma levels peak 2 to 4 hours after a dose. **Duration:** elimination half-life, 22 to 30 hours.

INDICATIONS & DOSAGE

Acute and chronic treatment of rheumatoid arthritis or osteoarthritis –
Adults: initially, 1,000 mg P.O. daily as a single dose or in divided doses b.i.d. Maximum daily dosage is 2,000 mg.

ADVERSE REACTIONS

CNS: *dizziness, headache,* fatigue, increased sweating, insomnia, nervousness, somnolence.
CV: vasculitis.
EENT: *tinnitus.*
GI: *diarrhea, dyspepsia, abdominal pain, constipation, flatulence, nausea,* dry mouth, gastritis, stomatitis, vomiting, ***bleeding,*** ulceration.
Respiratory: dyspnea, pneumonitis.
Skin: *pruritus, rash.*
Other: *edema.*

INTERACTIONS

Diuretics: NSAIDs may decrease diuretic effectiveness. Monitor patients closely during therapy.
Drugs that are highly bound to plasma proteins (such as warfarin): increased risk of adverse effects from displacement of drug by nabumetone. Use cautiously.
Ethanol: associated with an increased risk of additive GI toxicity. Concomitant use should be avoided.

CONTRAINDICATIONS

- Contraindicated in patients with hypersensitivity reactions, including asthma, urticaria, or other allergic reactions to this drug, aspirin, or other NSAIDS.
- Use cautiously in patients with renal or hepatic impairment; CHF, hypertension, or other conditions that may predispose the patient to fluid retention; and in patients with a history of peptic ulcer disease.

NURSING CONSIDERATIONS

- Instruct patients to take this drug with food, milk, or antacids. Nabumetone is absorbed more rapidly when administered with food or milk.
- Because NSAIDs impair the synthesis of renal prostaglandins, they can decrease renal blood flow and lead to reversible renal impairment, especially in patients with preexisting renal failure, liver dysfunction, or heart failure; in elderly patients; and in those taking diuretics. Monitor these patients closely during therapy.
- Serious GI toxicity, including peptic ulceration and bleeding, can occur in patients taking NSAIDs despite the absence of GI symptoms. Teach patients the signs and symptoms of GI bleeding and tell them to contact the doctor immediately if any occurs.
- During long-term therapy, periodically monitor renal and liver function, CBC, and hematocrit; assess these pa-

tients for signs and symptoms of GI bleeding.
• Advise patients to limit alcohol intake because of additive GI toxicity risk.

naproxen

Apo-Naproxen†, Inza-250‡, Inza-500‡, Naprosyn, Naprosyn-E†, Naprosyn SR†‡, Naxen†‡, Novonaprox†, Nu-Naprox†

naproxen sodium

Aleve◇, Anaprox, Anaprox DS, Apo-Napro-Na†, Naprogesic‡, Novonaprox Sodium†, Synflex†

Pregnancy Risk Category: B (D in 3rd trimester)

HOW SUPPLIED

naproxen
Tablets: 250 mg, 375 mg, 500 mg
Tablets (extended-release)†: 750 mg, 1,000 mg
Oral suspension: 125 mg/5 ml
Suppositories: 500 mg‡
naproxen sodium
Tablets (film-coated): 220 mg◇, 275 mg, 550 mg
Note: 275 mg of naproxen sodium = 250 mg of naproxen

ACTION

Mechanism: Produces anti-inflammatory, analgesic, and antipyretic effects, possibly by inhibiting prostaglandin synthesis.
Onset: analgesic effect, within 1 hour; antirheumatic effect, within 14 days. **Peak:** Peak serum levels after administration of naproxen sodium occur within 1 to 2 hours; peak levels after naproxen (base) occur in 2 to 4 hours. **Duration:** serum half-life, 12 to 15 hours; analgesic effects persist about 7 hours.

INDICATIONS & DOSAGE

Arthritis, primary dysmenorrhea (free base) –
Adults: 250 to 500 mg P.O. b.i.d. Alternatively, where suppository is available, give 500 mg P.R. h.s. with oral naproxen during the day. Maximum dosage is 1,250 mg daily.
Mild to moderate pain, primary dysmenorrhea (naproxen sodium) –
Adults: 2 tablets (275 mg each tablet) P.O. to start, followed by 275 mg q 6 to 8 hours p.r.n. Maximum daily dosage should not exceed 1,375 mg.
Minor aches and pains associated with colds; headache; toothache; backache; minor arthritis; menstrual cramps; fever –
Adults and children over age 12: 1 tablet (220 mg) P.O. q 8 to 12 hours. Some patients may obtain better relief from an initial dose of 2 tablets followed by a single tablet 12 hours later. Do not exceed 3 tablets per 24 hours.
Adults over age 65: 1 tablet (220 mg) P.O. q 12 hours.

ADVERSE REACTIONS

CNS: *headache,* drowsiness, *dizziness,* tinnitus, cognitive dysfunction, aseptic meningitis.
CV: peripheral edema, palpitations, digital vasculitis.
EENT: visual disturbances.
GI: *epigastric distress, occult blood loss, nausea,* ***peptic ulceration.***
GU: nephrotoxicity.
Hematologic: prolonged bleeding time, ***agranulocytosis,*** neutropenia.
Hepatic: elevated liver enzymes.
Respiratory: dyspnea.
Skin: *pruritus, rash,* urticaria.
Other: hyperkalemia.

INTERACTIONS

Antihypertensives, diuretics: decreased effect of these drugs. Monitor closely.
Aspirin, corticosteroids, ethanol: increased risk of adverse GI reactions. Avoid concomitant use.
Methotrexate: increased risk of toxicity. Monitor closely.
Oral anticoagulants, sulfonylureas,

*Liquid form contains alcohol. *Common* reactions are in italics; ***life-threatening,*** in bold italics.
**May contain tartrazine.

and drugs that are highly protein-bound: increased risk of toxicity. Monitor closely.
Probenecid: decreased elimination of naproxen. Monitor for toxicity.

CONTRAINDICATIONS

- Contraindicated in patients with hypersensitivity to this drug, aspirin, or other NSAIDs.
- Use cautiously in elderly patients and in patients with renal disease, cardiovascular disease, GI disorders, hepatic disease, a history of peptic ulcer disease, or angioedema.

NURSING CONSIDERATIONS

- Serious GI toxicity, including peptic ulceration and bleeding, can occur in patients taking NSAIDs despite the absence of GI symptoms. Teach patients the signs and symptoms of GI bleeding and tell them to contact the doctor immediately if any of these occurs.
- To minimize GI upset, advise patients to take drug with food or milk. A full glass of water or other liquid should be taken with each dose.
- Because NSAIDs impair the synthesis of renal prostaglandins, they can decrease renal blood flow and lead to reversible renal impairment, especially in patients with preexisting renal failure, liver dysfunction, or heart failure; in elderly patients; and in those taking diuretics. Monitor these patients closely during therapy.
- Caution patients that concomitant use with aspirin, alcohol, or corticosteroids may increase the risk of adverse GI reactions.
- Monitor CBC and renal and hepatic function every 4 to 6 months or as indicated during long-term therapy. Advise patient to have periodic eye examinations.
- Tell patients taking prescription doses of naproxen for arthritis that full therapeutic effect may be delayed 2 to 4 weeks.
- Warn patients against taking both naproxen and naproxen sodium at the same time because both circulate in the blood as the naproxen anion.
- Naproxen and naproxen sodium have also been used to manage pain of vascular headache, osteitis deformans (Paget's disease of bone), and Bartter's syndrome.
- Naproxen may interfere with certain urinary assays of 5-hydroxyindoleacetic acid and may cause false elevations of urinary 17-ketosteroid concentrations. Inform clinical laboratory personnel that patient is taking naproxen.
- Because of their antipyretic and anti-inflammatory actions, NSAIDs may mask the signs and symptoms of infection.

oxaprozin

Daypro

Pregnancy Risk Category: C

HOW SUPPLIED

Caplets: 600 mg

ACTION

Mechanism: Produces anti-inflammatory, analgesic, and antipyretic effects, possibly by inhibiting prostaglandin synthesis.
Onset: antirheumatic effects, within 7 days. **Peak:** Serum levels peak 3 to 5 hours after a dose. **Duration:** plasma half-life, 42 to 50 hours.

INDICATIONS & DOSAGE

Acute and long-term use in the management of signs and symptoms of osteoarthritis or rheumatoid arthritis – **Adults:** initially, 1,200 mg P.O. daily. Individualize to the smallest effective dosage to minimize adverse reactions. Smaller patients or those with mild symptoms may require only 600 mg daily. Maximum is 1,800 mg or 26 mg/kg, whichever is lower, in divided doses.

ADVERSE REACTIONS

CNS: depression, sedation, somnolence, confusion, sleep disturbances.
EENT: tinnitus, visual disturbances.
GI: *nausea, dyspepsia, diarrhea, constipation,* abdominal pain or distress, anorexia, flatulence, vomiting, ***hemorrhage.***
GU: dysuria, urinary frequency.
Hepatic: elevated liver function test results (with chronic use); severe hepatic dysfunction (rare).
Skin: *rash,* photosensitivity.

INTERACTIONS

Antihypertensives, diuretics: decreased effect. Monitor closely and adjust dosage as ordered.
Aspirin, corticosteroids, ethanol: increased risk of adverse GI reactions. Avoid concomitant use.
Aspirin: oxaprozin displaces salicylates from plasma protein-binding sites, increasing risk of salicylate toxicity. Avoid concomitant use.
Methotrexate: increased risk of methotrexate toxicity. Avoid concomitant use.
Oral anticoagulants: although problems haven't been reported, there is an increased risk of bleeding. Use together cautiously.

CONTRAINDICATIONS

- Contraindicated in patients with hypersensitivity to this drug, aspirin, or other NSAIDs.
- Use cautiously in patients with a history of peptic ulcer disease or hepatic or renal dysfunction.

NURSING CONSIDERATIONS

- Serious GI toxicity, including peptic ulceration and bleeding, can occur in patients taking NSAIDs despite the absence of GI symptoms. Teach patients the signs and symptoms of GI bleeding and tell them to contact the doctor immediately if any occurs.
- Tell patients to take this drug 30 minutes before or 2 hours after meals. If adverse GI reactions occur, drug may be taken with milk or meals.
- Because renal prostaglandins play a role in the maintenance of renal perfusion, patients with preexisting conditions leading to a reduction in renal blood flow may experience renal toxicity with NSAID therapy. Those at greatest risk are elderly patients, patients taking diuretics, and those with impaired renal, hepatic, or cardiac function. Closely monitor renal function in these patients, and discontinue NSAID therapy if problems develop.
- Elevations of liver function tests can occur after chronic use. These abnormal findings may persist, worsen, or resolve with continued therapy. Rarely, patients may progress to severe hepatic dysfunction. Periodically monitor liver function tests in patients receiving long-term therapy, and closely monitor patients with abnormal test results.
- Tell patients to report visual or auditory adverse reactions immediately.
- Tell patients that full therapeutic effects may be delayed for 2 to 4 weeks.
- Because of their antipyretic and anti-inflammatory actions, NSAIDs may mask the signs and symptoms of infection.
- This drug has been associated with photosensitivity reactions. Advise patients to use a sunblock, wear protective clothing, and avoid prolonged exposure to sunlight.

oxyphenbutazone

Pregnancy Risk Category: D

HOW SUPPLIED

Tablets: 100 mg

ACTION

Mechanism: Produces anti-inflammatory, analgesic, and antipyretic effects, possibly by inhibiting prostaglandin synthesis.
Peak: Plasma levels peak about 2½

*Liquid form contains alcohol.
**May contain tartrazine.

Common reactions are in italics; ***life-threatening,*** in bold italics.

hours after a dose. **Duration:** plasma half-life, about 3 days.

INDICATIONS & DOSAGE

Pain and inflammation in arthritis, bursitis, superficial venous thrombosis –

Adults: initially, 100 to 200 mg P.O. t.i.d. or q.i.d.; then 100 to 200 mg P.O. daily as a maintenance dose. Maximum daily maintenance dosage is 400 mg.

Acute gouty arthritis –

Adults: 400 mg initially as single dose; then 100 mg q 4 hours for 4 days or until relief is obtained.

ADVERSE REACTIONS

CNS: restlessness, confusion, lethargy, headache, tremors, numbness.

CV: hypertension, pericarditis, myocarditis, fluid retention, ***cardiac decompensation.***

EENT: optic neuritis, blurred vision, retinal hemorrhage or detachment, hearing loss.

GI: *nausea, vomiting, diarrhea,* ***peptic ulceration,*** *occult blood loss.*

GU: proteinuria, hematuria, glomerulonephritis, nephrotic syndrome, ***renal failure.***

Hematologic: ***bone marrow suppression (fatal aplastic anemia, agranulocytosis, thrombocytopenia), hemolytic anemia,*** leukopenia.

Hepatic: ***hepatitis.***

Skin: petechiae, pruritus, purpura, various dermatoses from rash to ***toxic necrotizing epidermolysis.***

Other: toxic and nontoxic goiter, hyperglycemia, respiratory alkalosis, metabolic acidosis.

INTERACTIONS

Antihypertensives, diuretics: decreased effect. Monitor closely.

Ethanol: increased risk of GI toxicity. Avoid concomitant use.

Insulin, oral antidiabetic agents: enhanced antidiabetic effect. Monitor patient closely.

Lithium, phenytoin: increased plasma levels after oxyphenbutazone administration.

Oral anticoagulants: enhanced risk of bleeding. Avoid concomitant use.

CONTRAINDICATIONS

- Contraindicated in children under age 14 and in patients with senility, GI ulcer, blood dyscrasia, and renal, hepatic, cardiac, and thyroid disease. Should not be used in patients receiving long-term anticoagulant therapy.
- Use cautiously in patients with a history of peptic ulcer disease, hepatic dysfunction, cardiac disease, or other conditions associated with fluid retention or impaired renal function.
- Use drug only if less toxic alternatives are ineffective or contraindicated. Limit initial therapy to 1 week. If patient does not respond or cannot tolerate medication, discontinue use. Patients over age 60 should not receive drug for longer than 1 week.

NURSING CONSIDERATIONS

- Warn patients to stop drug and notify the doctor immediately if fever, sore throat, mouth ulcers, GI discomfort, black or tarry stools, bleeding, bruising, rash, or weight gain occurs.
- Tell patients to take this drug with food, milk, or antacids.
- Because NSAIDs impair the synthesis of renal prostaglandins, they can decrease renal blood flow and lead to reversible renal impairment, especially in patients with preexisting renal failure, liver dysfunction, or heart failure; in elderly patients; and in those taking diuretics. Monitor these patients closely during therapy.
- Complete physical examination and laboratory evaluation are recommended before therapy. Warn patients to remain under close medical supervision and to keep all doctor and laboratory appointments.
- Monitor CBC before therapy and after 3 days.

• Response should be seen in 2 or 3 days. Stop drug if no response occurs within 1 week.
• NSAIDs may mask the signs and symptoms of infection because of their anti-inflammatory and antipyretic actions.

phenylbutazone

Apo-Phenylbutazone†, Azolid, Butatab, Butazolidin, Butazone, Cotylbutazone, Intrabutazone†, Novobutazone†

Pregnancy Risk Category: D

HOW SUPPLIED

Tablets: 100 mg
Capsules: 100 mg

ACTION

Mechanism: Produces anti-inflammatory, analgesic, and antipyretic effects, possibly by inhibiting prostaglandin synthesis.
Peak: Plasma levels peak in about 2½ hours after a dose.
Duration: elimination half-life, about 77 hours.

INDICATIONS & DOSAGE

Pain and inflammation in arthritis, bursitis, acute superficial thrombophlebitis –
Adults: initially, 100 to 200 mg P.O. t.i.d. or q.i.d. Maximum dosage is 600 mg daily. When improvement is obtained, decrease dosage to 100 mg t.i.d. or q.i.d. Maximum maintenance dosage is 400 mg daily.
Acute, gouty arthritis –
Adults: 400 mg P.O. initially as single dose; then 100 mg q 4 hours for 4 days or until relief is obtained.

ADVERSE REACTIONS

CNS: agitation, confusion, lethargy, headache, tremors, numbness.
CV: hypertension, edema, fluid retention, pericarditis, myocarditis, ***cardiac decompensation.***
EENT: optic neuritis, blurred vision, retinal hemorrhage or detachment, hearing loss.
GI: *nausea, vomiting, diarrhea,* ***peptic ulceration,*** *occult blood loss.*
GU: proteinuria, hematuria, glomerulonephritis, nephrotic syndrome, ***renal failure.***
Hematologic: ***bone marrow suppression (fatal aplastic anemia, agranulocytosis, thrombocytopenia), hemolytic anemia,*** leukopenia.
Hepatic: ***hepatitis.***
Skin: petechiae, pruritus, purpura, various dermatoses from rash to ***toxic necrotizing epidermolysis.***
Other: hyperglycemia, toxic and nontoxic goiter, respiratory alkalosis, metabolic acidosis.

INTERACTIONS

Antihypertensives: decreased effectiveness. Monitor blood pressure closely.
Cholestyramine: may alter phenylbutazone absorption. Give 1 hour before cholestyramine.
Ethanol: increased risk of toxicity. Avoid concomitant use.
Insulin, oral antidiabetics: enhanced antidiabetic effect. Monitor patient closely.
Lithium, phenytoin: increased plasma levels after phenylbutazone administration. Monitor for toxicity.
Oral anticoagulants: enhanced risk of bleeding. Monitor patient closely.

CONTRAINDICATIONS

• Contraindicated in patients with hypersensitivity to this drug, aspirin, or other NSAIDs; in children under age 14; and in patients with senility, GI ulcer, blood dyscrasias, or moderate to severe renal, hepatic, cardiac, or thyroid disease.
• Use cautiously in patients with mild cardiac, renal, hepatic, or thyroid disease; in those with GI disorders or a history of peptic ulcer disease; and in

patients who may be predisposed to fluid retention.
- Should not be used in patients receiving long-term anticoagulant therapy, hepatotoxic or nephrotoxic drugs, or thrombolytic therapy.
- Use this drug only if less toxic alternatives are ineffective or contraindicated. Limit initial therapy to 1 week. If patient does not respond or cannot tolerate medication, discontinue use. Patients over age 60 should not receive drug for longer than 1 week.

NURSING CONSIDERATIONS
- Warn patients to stop taking drug and notify doctor immediately if fever, sore throat, mouth ulcers, GI discomfort, black or tarry stools, bleeding, bruising, rash, or weight gain occurs.
- Because NSAIDs impair the synthesis of renal prostaglandins, they can decrease renal blood flow and lead to reversible renal impairment, especially in patients with preexisting renal failure, liver dysfunction, or heart failure; in elderly patients; and in those taking diuretics. Monitor these patients closely during therapy.
- Complete physical examination and laboratory evaluation are recommended before therapy. Warn patients to remain under close medical supervision and to keep all doctor and laboratory appointments.
- Monitor hepatic, renal, and thyroid function and CBC before therapy. Check CBC again after 3 days and assess for bleeding.
- Response occurs in 3 to 4 days. Discontinue drug if no response within 1 week.
- This drug has limited use because it produces severe adverse reactions in up to 45% of patients.
- Tell patients to take this drug with food, milk, or antacids to minimize GI upset.
- Phenylbutazone may interfere with thyroid function studies by competing for thyroxine-binding sites and blocking uptake of iodine into the thyroid.
- NSAIDs may mask the signs and symptoms of infection because of their antipyretic and anti-inflammatory actions.

piroxicam
Apo-Piroxicam†, Feldene, Novopirocam†

Pregnancy Risk Category: C

HOW SUPPLIED
Capsules: 10 mg, 20 mg

ACTION
Mechanism: Produces anti-inflammatory, analgesic, and antipyretic effects, by inhibiting prostaglandin synthesis.
Onset: analgesic action, within 1 hour; antirheumatic action, 7 to 12 days. **Peak:** Serum levels peak in 3 to 5 hours; peak rheumatic action occurs after 2 to 3 weeks of therapy. **Duration:** elimination half-life, 30 to 86 hours; analgesic effects persist 2 to 3 days.

INDICATIONS & DOSAGE
Osteoarthritis and rheumatoid arthritis –
Adults: 20 mg P.O. daily. If desired, the dosage may be divided b.i.d.

ADVERSE REACTIONS
CNS: headache, drowsiness, dizziness, paresthesia, somnolence.
CV: peripheral edema.
EENT: auditory disturbances.
GI: *epigastric distress, nausea, occult blood loss,* ***peptic ulceration, severe GI bleeding.***
GU: ***nephrotoxicity,*** elevated BUN level.
Hematologic: prolonged bleeding time, anemia, leukopenia, ***aplastic anemia, agranulocytosis.***
Hepatic: elevated liver enzymes.

Skin: pruritus, rash, urticaria, *photosensitivity*.
Other: hyperkalemia, acidosis, dilutional hypernatremia.

INTERACTIONS

Aspirin, corticosteroids, ethanol: increased risk of GI toxicity. Decreased plasma levels of piroxicam. Avoid concomitant use.
Lithium: increased plasma lithium levels. Monitor for toxicity.
Oral anticoagulants: enhanced risk of bleeding. Monitor patient closely.
Oral antidiabetic agents: enhanced antidiabetic effects. Monitor patient closely.

CONTRAINDICATIONS

- Contraindicated in patients with hypersensitivity to this drug, aspirin, or other NSAIDs.
- Use cautiously in elderly patients and in patients with angioedema, GI disorders, history of renal or peptic ulcer disease, or cardiac disease.

NURSING CONSIDERATIONS

- Serious GI toxicity, including peptic ulceration and bleeding, can occur in patients taking NSAIDs despite the absence of GI symptoms. Teach patients the signs and symptoms of GI bleeding and tell them to contact the doctor immediately if any of these occurs.
- If adverse GI reactions occur, tell patients to take this drug with milk, antacids, or meals.
- Tell patients that full therapeutic effects may be delayed for 2 to 4 weeks.
- Because NSAIDs impair the synthesis of renal prostaglandins, they can decrease renal blood flow and lead to reversible renal impairment, especially in patients with preexisting renal failure, liver dysfunction, or heart failure; in elderly patients; and in those taking diuretics. Monitor these patients closely during therapy.
- Check renal, hepatic, and auditory function and CBC periodically during prolonged therapy. Discontinue drug if abnormalities occur.
- Causes adverse skin reactions more often than other drugs in its class. Photosensitivity reactions are the most common. Advise patients to use a sunblock, wear protective clothing, and avoid prolonged exposure to sunlight.
- NSAIDs may mask the signs and symptoms of infection because of their antipyretic and anti-inflammatory actions.

sulindac

Aclin‡, Apo-Sulin†, Clinoril, Novo-Sundac†

Pregnancy Risk Category: B (D in 3rd trimester)

HOW SUPPLIED

Tablets: 100 mg‡, 150 mg, 200 mg

ACTION

Mechanism: Produces anti-inflammatory, analgesic, and antipyretic effects, possibly by inhibiting prostaglandin synthesis.
Onset: antirheumatic effects, within 7 days. **Peak:** Plasma levels peak 2 to 4 hours after a dose; peak antirheumatic effects occur in 2 to 3 weeks.

INDICATIONS & DOSAGE

Osteoarthritis, rheumatoid arthritis, ankylosing spondylitis –
Adults: initially, 150 mg P.O. b.i.d.; may increase to 200 mg b.i.d.
Acute subacromial bursitis or supraspinatus tendinitis, acute gouty arthritis –
Adults: 200 mg P.O. b.i.d. for 7 to 14 days. Dose may be reduced as symptoms subside.

ADVERSE REACTIONS

CNS: dizziness, headache, nervousness, delerium, psychosis, neuropa-

thy, extrapyramidal effects, hallucinations, aseptic meningitis.
CV: hypertension.
EENT: tinnitus, transient visual disturbances.
GI: *epigastric distress, **peptic ulceration, pancreatitis,*** occult blood loss, nausea.
GU: interstitial nephritis, ***nephrotic syndrome, renal failure.***
Hematologic: prolonged bleeding time, ***aplastic anemia,*** thrombocytopenia, neutropenia.
Hepatic: elevated liver enzymes.
Skin: rash, pruritus, ***Stevens-Johnson syndrome***
Other: edema, drug fever, ***anaphylaxis.***

INTERACTIONS

Anticoagulants: increased risk of bleeding. Monitor PT closely.
Cyclosporine: increased nephrotoxicity of cyclosporine. Avoid concomitant use.
Diflunisal, dimethyl sulfoxide: decreased metabolism of sulindac to its active metabolite, reducing its effectiveness. Don't use together.
Methotrexate: increased methotrexate toxicity. Avoid concomitant use.
Probenecid: increased plasma levels of sulindac and its active metabolite. Monitor for toxicity.
Sulfonamides, sulfonylureas, other highly protein-bound drugs: possible displacement of these drugs from plasma protein-binding sites, leading to increased toxicity. Monitor closely.

CONTRAINDICATIONS

- Contraindicated in patients with acute asthma whose conditions are exacerbated by other NSAIDs or by aspirin. Also contraindicated in patients who have active ulcers and GI bleeding.
- Use cautiously in patients with a history of ulcers and GI bleeding, renal dysfunction, compromised cardiac function, or hypertension and in those receiving oral anticoagulants or oral antidiabetic agents.

NURSING CONSIDERATIONS

- Serious GI toxicity, including peptic ulceration and bleeding, can occur in patients taking NSAIDs despite the absence of GI symptoms. Teach patients the signs and symptoms of GI bleeding and tell them to contact the doctor immediately if any of these occurs.
- To reduce adverse GI reactions, tell patients to take this drug with food, milk, or antacids.
- Patients should notify the doctor and have complete eye examinations if any visual disturbances occur.
- Periodically monitor hepatic and renal function and CBC in patients receiving long-term therapy.
- Tell patients to notify the doctor immediately if easy bruising or prolonged bleeding occurs.
- Drug causes sodium retention but is thought to have less effect on the kidneys than other NSAIDs. Patients should report edema and have blood pressure checked monthly.
- Advise patients to avoid driving or other hazardous activities that require mental alertness until CNS effects are known.
- Because of their antipyretic and anti-inflammatory actions, NSAIDs may mask the signs and symptoms of infection.

tolmetin sodium

Tolectin, Tolectin-200, Tolectin-400, Tolectin-600, Tolectin DS

Pregnancy Risk Category: B (D in 3rd trimester)

HOW SUPPLIED

Tablets: 200 mg, 600 mg
Capsules: 400 mg

ACTION

Mechanism: Produces anti-inflammatory, analgesic, and antipyretic ef-

fects, possibly by inhibiting prostaglandin synthesis.
Onset: antirheumatic action, within 7 days. **Peak:** Serum levels peak in 30 minutes to 1 hour; peak antirheumatic effect occurs 1after 1 to 2 weeks.
Duration: plasma half-life, 1 to 1½ hours.

INDICATIONS & DOSAGE

Rheumatoid arthritis, osteoarthritis, gout, dysmenorrhea, juvenile rheumatoid arthritis –
Adults: 400 mg P.O. t.i.d. or q.i.d. Maximum daily dosage is 1.8 g.
Children 2 years or over: 15 to 30 mg/kg P.O. daily in divided doses.

ADVERSE REACTIONS

CNS: headache, dizziness, drowsiness.
EENT: tinnitus, visual disturbances.
GI: *epigastric distress, **peptic ulceration,*** occult blood loss, nausea.
GU: ***nephrotoxicity,*** pseudoproteinuria.
Hematologic: prolonged bleeding time, granulocytopenia, thrombocytopenia, ***agranulocytosis.***
Skin: rash, urticaria, pruritus.
Other: sodium retention, edema, ***anaphylaxis.***

INTERACTIONS

Ethanol: increased risk of GI toxicity. Avoid concomitant use.
Oral anticoagulants: increased risk of bleeding. Monitor patient closely.

CONTRAINDICATIONS

- Contraindicated in patients with hypersensitivity to this drug, aspirin, or other NSAIDs.
- Use cautiously in patients with cardiac and renal disease, GI bleeding, and history of peptic ulcer disease.

NURSING CONSIDERATIONS

- Serious GI toxicity, including peptic ulceration and bleeding, can occur in patients taking NSAIDs despite the absence of GI symptoms. Teach patients the signs and symptoms of GI bleeding and tell them to contact the doctor immediately if any occurs.
- To reduce adverse GI reactions, tell patients to take this drug with food, milk, or antacids.
- Tell patients to notify the doctor immediately if any visual or hearing change occurs. During prolonged therapy, patients should have regular eye examinations, hearing tests, CBCs, and renal function tests to monitor for toxicity.
- Because NSAIDs impair the synthesis of renal prostaglandins, they can decrease renal blood flow and lead to reversible renal impairment, especially in patients with preexisting renal failure, liver dysfunction, or heart failure; in elderly patients; and in those taking diuretics. Monitor these patients closely during therapy.
- Tell patients that therapeutic effect begins within 1 week, but full effect may be delayed 2 to 4 weeks.
- Advise patients to avoid driving or other hazardous activities that require mental alertness until the CNS effects of the drug are known.
- Tolmetin may interfere with certain tests for urinary proteins; it does not interfere with dye-impregnated reagent strips.
- NSAIDs may mask the signs and symptoms of infection because of their antipyretic and anti-inflammatory actions.

27

Narcotic and opioid analgesics

alfentanil hydrochloride
buprenorphine hydrochloride
butorphanol tartrate
codeine phosphate
codeine sulfate
dezocine
fentanyl citrate
fentanyl transdermal system
fentanyl transmucosal
hydromorphone hydrochloride
levorphanol tartrate
meperidine hydrochloride
methadone hydrochloride
morphine hydrochloride
morphine sulfate
morphine tartrate
nalbuphine hydrochloride
oxycodone hydrochloride
oxycodone pectinate
oxymorphone hydrochloride
pentazocine hydrochloride
pentazocine hydrochloride and naloxone hydrochloride
pentazocine lactate
propoxyphene hydrochloride
propoxyphene napsylate
sufentanil citrate

COMBINATION PRODUCTS

222†: aspirin 375 mg, codeine phosphate 8 mg, and caffeine citrate 30 mg.

222 FORTE†: aspirin 500 mg, codeine phosphate 8 mg, and caffeine citrate 30 mg.

282†: aspirin 375 mg, codeine phosphate 15 mg, and caffeine citrate 30 mg.

292†: aspirin 375 mg, codeine phosphate 30 mg, and caffeine citrate 30 mg.

293†: aspirin 375 mg, codeine phosphate 30 mg, codeine phosphate (slow-release) 30 mg, and caffeine citrate 30 mg.

692†: aspirin 375 mg, propoxyphene hydrochloride 65 mg, and caffeine 30 mg.

A.C.&C.†: aspirin 375 mg, codeine phosphate 8 mg, and caffeine 30 mg.

ACETACO, ACETA WITH CODEINE, EMPRACET-30†, EMTEC-30†, M-G PYREGESIC-C, TYLAPRIN WITH CODEINE: acetaminophen 300 mg and codeine phosphate 30 mg.

ALLAY, ANOLOR DH5, BANCAP-HC, DOLACET, HYCOMED, HYCO-PAP, HYDROCET, HYDROGESIC, LORCET-HD, MEGAGESIC, POLYGESIC, PRO-PAIN-HC, ROGESIC NO. 3, SENEFEN III, ULTRAGESIC, ZYDONE: acetaminophen 500 mg and hydrocodone bitartrate 5 mg.

AMACODONE, ANEXSIA 5/500, ANODYNOS DHC, CO-GESIC, DUOCET, DURADYNE DHC, HY-5, HYCOPAP, HY-PHEN, LORTAB 5/500, NORCET, VAPOCET, VICODIN: acetaminophen 500 mg and hydrocodone bitartrate 5 mg.

ANACIN WITH CODEINE†: aspirin 325 mg, codeine phosphate 8 mg, and caffeine 32 mg.

ANCASAL 8†, C2 WITH CODEINE†: aspirin 375 mg, codeine phosphate 8 mg, and caffeine 15 mg.

ANCASAL 15†: aspirin 375 mg, codeine phosphate 15 mg, and caffeine 15 mg.

ANCASAL 30†: aspirin 375 mg, codeine phosphate 30 mg, and caffeine 15 mg.

ANEXSIA 7.5/650, LORCET PLUS, NORCET 7.5: acetaminophen 650 mg and hydrocodone bitartrate 7.5 mg.

BEXOPHENE, COTANAL-65, DARVON COMPOUND-65, DORAPHEN COMPOUND-65, DOXAPHENE COMPOUND, MARGESIC A-C, PRO POX PLUS: aspirin 389 mg, propoxyphene hydrochloride 65 mg, and caffeine 32.4 mg.

†Available in Canada only. ‡Available in Australia only. ◇Available OTC.

BUFF-A-COMP NO. 3: aspirin 325 mg, codeine phosphate 30 mg, caffeine 40 mg, and butalbital 50 mg.
CAPITAL WITH CODEINE, MYAPAP WITH CODEINE*, TYLENOL WITH CODEINE ELIXIR*, TY-PAP WITH CODEINE ELIXIR*: acetaminophen 120 mg and codeine phosphate 12 mg/5 ml.
CODALAN NO. 1: acetaminophen 500 mg, codeine phosphate 8 mg, and caffeine 30 mg.
CODALAN NO. 2: acetaminophen 500 mg, codeine phosphate 15 mg, and caffeine 30 mg.
CODALAN NO. 3: acetaminophen 500 mg, codeine phosphate 30 mg, and caffeine 30 mg.
CODAMINOPHEN†: acetaminophen 300 mg, codeine phosphate 8 mg, and caffeine 30 mg.
DARVOCET-N 50: acetaminophen 325 mg and propoxyphene napsylate 50 mg.
DARVOCET-N 100, DOXAPAP-N, PROPACET 100: acetaminophen 650 mg and propoxyphene napsylate 100 mg.
DARVON COMPOUND†: aspirin 325 mg, propoxyphene hydrochloride 32 mg, and caffeine 32.4 mg.
DARVON-N COMPOUND†: aspirin 375 mg, propoxyphene napsylate 100 mg, and caffeine 30 mg.
DARVON-N WITH ASA†: aspirin 325 mg and propoxyphene napsylate 100 mg.
DARVON WITH ASA†: aspirin 325 mg and propxyphene hydrochloride 65 mg.
DEMEROL-APAP: acetaminophen 300 mg and meperidine hydrochloride 50 mg.
DOLENE-AP-65, D-REX-65, E-LOR, GENAGESIC, PRO POX WITH APAP, WYGESIC: acetaminophen 650 mg and propoxyphene hydrochloride 65 mg.
EMCODEINE NO. 2, EMPIRIN WITH CODEINE NO. 2: aspirin 325 mg and codeine phosphate 15 mg.
EMCODEINE NO. 3, EMPIRIN WITH CODEINE NO. 3: aspirin 325 mg and codeine phosphate 30 mg.
EMCODEINE NO. 4, EMPIRIN WITH CODEINE NO. 4: aspirin 325 mg and codeine phosphate 60 mg.
EMPRACET-60†: acetaminophen 300 mg and codeine phosphate 60 mg.
ENDOCAN†, OXYCODAN†, PERCODAN†: aspirin 325 mg and oxycodone hydrochloride 5 mg.
ENDOCET†, OXYCOCET†, PERCOCET, ROXICET: acetaminophen 325 mg and oxycodone hydrochloride 5 mg.
HYCODAN: hydrocodone bitartrate 5 mg and homatropine methylbromide 1.5 mg/5 ml.
HYCOTUSS*: hydrocodone bitartrate 5 mg and guaifenesin 100 mg/5 ml.
INNOVAR INJECTION: droperidol 2.5 mg and fentanyl citrate 0.05 mg/ml.
LENOLTEC WITH CODEINE NO. 1†, NOVAGESIC C8†: acetaminophen 300 mg, codeine phosphate 8 mg, and caffeine 15 mg.
LCET 10/650: acetaminophen 650 mg and hydrocodone bitartrate 10 mg.
LORTAB 2.5/500: acetaminophen 500 mg and hydrocodone bitartrate 2.5 mg.
LORTAB 7.5/500: acetaminophen 500 mg and hydrocodone bitartrate 7.5 mg.
LORTAB ORAL SOLUTION: acetaminophen 120 mg and hydrocodone bitartrate 2.5 mg/5 ml.
NOVOPROPOXYN COMPOUND: aspirin 375 mg, propoxyphene hydrochloride 65 mg, and caffeine 30 mg.
PERCODAN-DEMI: aspirin 325 mg, oxycodone hydrochloride 2.25 mg, and oxycodone terephthalate 0.19 mg.
PERCODAN-DEMI†: aspirin 325 mg and oxycodone hydrochloride 2.5 mg.
PERCODAN, ROXIPRIN: aspirin 325 mg, oxycodone hydrochloride 4.5 mg, and oxycodone terephthalate 0.38 mg.
PHENAPHEN-650 WITH CODEINE:

acetaminophen 650 mg and codeine phosphate 30 mg.
PHENAPHEN WITH CODEINE NO. 2: acetaminophen 325 mg and codeine phosphate 15 mg.
PHENAPHEN WITH CODEINE NO. 3: acetaminophen 325 mg and codeine phosphate 30 mg.
PHENAPHEN WITH CODEINE NO. 4: acetaminophen 325 mg and codeine phosphate 60 mg.
ROUNOX AND CODEINE 15†: acetaminophen 325 mg and codeine phosphate 15 mg.
ROUNOX AND CODEINE 30†: acetaminophen 325 mg and codeine phosphate 30 mg.
ROUNOX AND CODEINE 60†: acetaminophen 325 mg and codeine phosphate 60 mg.
ROXICET 5/500: acetaminophen 500 mg and oxycodone hydrochloride 5 mg.
ROXICET ORAL SOLUTION*: acetaminophen 325 mg and oxycodone hydrochloride 5 mg/5 ml.
TALACEN: acetaminophen 650 mg and pentazocine 25 mg.
TALWIN COMPOUND: aspirin 325 mg and pentazocine 12.5 mg.
TYLENOL WITH CODEINE NO. 1: acetaminophen 300 mg and codeine phosphate 7.5 mg.
TYLENOL WITH CODEINE NO. 2, TY-TAB WITH CODEINE NO. 2: acetaminophen 300 mg and codeine phosphate 15 mg.
TYLENOL WITH CODEINE NO. 3, TY-TAB WITH CODEINE NO. 3: acetaminophen 300 mg and codeine phosphate 30 mg.
TYLENOL WITH CODEINE NO. 4, TY-TAB WITH CODEINE NO. 4: acetaminophen 300 mg and codeine phosphate 60 mg.
TYLOX: acetaminophen 500 mg and oxycodone hydrochloride 5 mg.
VICODIN: acetaminophen 500 mg and hydrocodone bitartrate 5 mg.
VICODIN ES: acetaminophen 750 mg and hydrocodone bitartrate 7.5 mg.

alfentanil hydrochloride

Alfenta
Controlled Substance Schedule II
Pregnancy Risk Category: C

HOW SUPPLIED

Injection: 500 mcg/ml

ACTION

Mechanism: Binds with opiate receptors in the CNS, altering both perception of and emotional response to pain through an unknown mechanism.
Onset: immediate. **Duration:** elimination half-life, about 1 to 2 hours.

INDICATIONS & DOSAGE

Adjunct to general anesthetic –
Adults: initially, 8 to 50 mcg/kg I.V.; then give increments of 3 to 15 mcg/kg I.V.
As a primary anesthetic –
Adults: initially, 130 to 245 mcg/kg I.V.; then give 0.5 to 1.5 mcg/kg/minute I.V.

In elderly and debilitated patients: dosage should be reduced.

ADVERSE REACTIONS

CNS: blurred vision, agitation, anxiety, headache, *confusion.*
CV: hypotension, hypertension, bradycardia, tachycardia, palpitations, headache, orthostatic hypotension.
GI: nausea, vomiting.
Respiratory: ***chest wall rigidity, bronchospasm, respiratory depression,*** hypercapnia.
Skin: itching.
Other: intraoperative muscle movement.

INTERACTIONS

CNS depressants, ethanol: additive effects. Use together cautiously.

CONTRAINDICATIONS

• Contraindicated in patients with hypersensitivity to this drug or other opiate analgesics.

• Use cautiously in patients with head injury, pulmonary disease, or decreased respiratory reserve.

NURSING CONSIDERATIONS
• Should be administered only by persons specifically trained in the use of I.V. anesthetics.
• As a primary anesthetic, alfentanil may be prescribed for induction of anesthesia for general surgery requiring endotracheal intubation and medical ventilation.
• Keep narcotic antagonist (naloxone) and resuscitation equipment available when giving drug I.V.
• Periodically monitor postoperative vital signs and bladder function. Because drug decreases both rate and depth of respirations, monitoring of arterial oxygen saturation may aid in assessing respiratory depression.
• **I.V. use:** Compatible with D_5W, D_5W in lactated Ringer's solution, and 0.9% sodium chloride. Most clinicians use infusions containing 25 to 80 mcg/ml.
• Discontinue infusion at least 10 to 15 minutes before the end of surgery.
• To administer small volumes of alfentanil accurately, use a tuberculin syringe.

buprenorphine hydrochloride

Buprenex, Temgesic Injection‡
Controlled Substance Schedule V

Pregnancy Risk Category: C (D for prolonged use or high doses at term)

HOW SUPPLIED
Injection: 0.324 mg (equivalent to 0.3 mg base/ml).

ACTION
Mechanism: Binds with opiate receptors in the CNS, altering both perception of and emotional response to pain through an unknown mechanism.
Onset: within 15 minutes. **Peak:** Analgesic effects peak within 1 hour.
Duration: half-life, 2 to 3 hours; effects persist about 6 hours.

INDICATIONS & DOSAGE
Moderate to severe pain –
Adults: 0.3 mg I.M. or slow I.V. q 6 hours, p.r.n. or around the clock. May administer up to 0.6 mg/dose if necessary.

ADVERSE REACTIONS
CNS: *dizziness, sedation, headache,* confusion, nervousness, euphoria, increased intracranial pressure.
CV: hypotension, bradycardia, tachycardia, hypertension.
EENT: *miosis,* blurred vision.
GI: *nausea,* vomiting, constipation.
GU: urine retention.
Respiratory: ***respiratory depression,*** hypoventilation.
Skin: pruritus, *sweating.*

INTERACTIONS
CNS depressants, ethanol, MAO inhibitors: additive effects. Use together cautiously.
Narcotic analgesics: possible decreased analgesic effect. Avoid concomitant use.

CONTRAINDICATIONS
• Contraindicated in patients with hypersensitivity to this drug or other opiate analgesics.
• Use cautiously in patients with head injury and increased intracranial pressure; severe respiratory, liver, and kidney impairment; CNS depression; thyroid irregularities; adrenal insufficiency; and prostatic hyperplasia.

NURSING CONSIDERATIONS
• Naloxone will not completely reverse the respiratory depression caused by buprenorphine overdose; an overdose may necessitate mechanical ventilation. Larger than customary

doses of naloxone (more than 0.4 mg) and doxapram may also be ordered.

- When used postoperatively, encourage turning, coughing, and deep breathing to prevent atelectasis.
- If dependence occurs, withdrawal symptoms may appear up to 14 days after drug is stopped.
- Drug's narcotic antagonist properties may precipitate abstinence syndrome in narcotic-dependent patients.
- S.C. administration not recommended.
- Buprenorphine 0.3 mg is equal to 10 mg of morphine and 75 mg of meperidine in analgesic potency. Has longer duration of action than morphine or meperidine.
- Caution ambulatory patients about getting out of bed or walking.
- **I.V. use:** Give by direct I.V. injection, slowly into a vein or through the tubing of a free-flowing, compatible I.V. solution over not less than 2 minutes.
- Buprenorphine has been given by continuous I.V. infusion. Dilute in 0.9% sodium chloride injection to a concentration of 15 mcg/ml and give at a rate of 25 to 250 mcg/hour.
- Buprenorphine has also been given by epidural injection. Concentrations of 6 to 30 mcg/ml have been injected every 6 hours.

butorphanol tartrate

Stadol, Stadol NS

Pregnancy Risk Category: B (D for prolonged use or high doses at term)

HOW SUPPLIED

Injection: 1 mg/ml, 2 mg/ml
Nasal spray: 10 mg/ml

ACTION

Mechanism: Binds with opiate receptors in the CNS, altering both perception of and emotional response to pain through an unknown mechanism.

Onset: immediately after an I.V. injection; within 10 to 15 minutes after I.M. injection; within 15 minutes of nasal use. **Peak:** Analgesic effects peak within 30 minutes to 1 hour of I.M. or I.V. use, within 1 to 2 hours of nasal use. **Duration:** plasma half-life, 2½ to 4 hours; analgesic effects persist 3 to 4 hours after I.M. or I.V. use, or 4 to 5 hours after nasal administration.

INDICATIONS & DOSAGE

Moderate to severe pain –
Adults: 1 to 4 mg I.M. q 3 to 4 hours, p.r.n. or around the clock; or 0.5 to 2 mg I.V. q 3 to 4 hours, p.r.n. or around the clock. Do not exceed 4 mg per dose. Alternatively, give 1 mg by nasal spray q 3 to 4 hours (1 spray in one nostril). Repeat in 60 to 90 minutes if pain relief is inadequate.

ADVERSE REACTIONS

CNS: *sedation, headache, vertigo, floating sensation,* lethargy, confusion, nervousness, unusual dreams, agitation, euphoria, hallucinations, flushing, increased intracranial pressure.
CV: palpitations, fluctuation in blood pressure.
EENT: diplopia, blurred vision, *nasal congestion (with nasal spray),* dry mouth.
GI: *nausea,* vomiting, constipation.
Respiratory: ***respiratory depression.***
Skin: rash, hives, *clamminess, excessive sweating.*

INTERACTIONS

CNS depressants, ethanol: additive effects. Use together cautiously.
Narcotic analgesics: possible decreased analgesic effect. Avoid concomitant use.

CONTRAINDICATIONS

- Contraindicated in patients with narcotic addiction; may precipitate narcotic abstinence syndrome.

• Use cautiously in patients with head injury, increased intracranial pressure, acute MI, ventricular dysfunction, coronary insufficiency, respiratory disease or depression, and renal or hepatic dysfunction.

NURSING CONSIDERATIONS

• Psychological and physical addiction may occur.
• Respiratory depression apparently does not increase with larger dosage.
• S.C. route not recommended.
• Periodically monitor postoperative vital signs and bladder function. Because drug decreases both rate and depth of respirations, monitoring of arterial oxygen saturation may aid in assessing respiratory depression.
• Also used as a preoperative medication, as the analgesic component of balanced anesthesia, and for relief of postpartum pain.
• Caution ambulatory patients about getting out of bed or walking. Warn outpatients to avoid driving and other potentially hazardous activities that require mental alertness until adverse CNS effects are known.
• **I.V. use:** Give by direct injection into a vein or into the tubing of a free-flowing I.V. solution. Compatible solutions include D_5W and 0.9% sodium chloride.

codeine phosphate

Paveral†

codeine sulfate

Controlled Substance Schedule II
Pregnancy Risk Category: C (D for prolonged use or high doses at term)

HOW SUPPLIED

phosphate
Oral solution: 15 mg/5 ml, 10 mg/ml†
Injection: 30 mg/ml, 60 mg/ml
Soluble tablets: 30 mg, 60 mg

sulfate
Tablets: 15 mg, 30 mg, 60 mg
Soluble tablets: 15 mg, 30 mg, 60 mg

ACTION

Mechanism: Binds with opiate receptors in the CNS, altering both perception of and emotional response to pain through an unknown mechanism. Also suppresses the cough reflex by direct action on the cough center in the medulla.
Onset: 10 to 30 minutes after I.M. injection, 30 to 60 minutes after oral use. **Peak:** Peak effects occur within 30 minutes to 1 hour after I.M. injection. **Duration:** effects persist 4 to 6 hours.

INDICATIONS & DOSAGE

Mild to moderate pain –
Adults: 15 to 60 mg P.O. or 15 to 60 mg (phosphate) S.C., I.M., or I.V. q 4 hours, p.r.n. or around the clock.
Children over age 2: 0.5 mg/kg P.O., S.C., or I.M. q 4 hours, p.r.n. or around the clock.
Nonproductive cough –
Adults: 10 to 20 mg P.O. q 4 to 6 hours. Maximum dosage is 120 mg/24 hours.
Children 6 to 12 years: 5 to 10 mg P.O. q 4 to 6 hours. Maximum dosage is 60 mg/24 hours.
Children 2 to 6 years: 0.25 mg/kg P.O. q 6 hours. Do not exceed 30 mg in 24 hours.

ADVERSE REACTIONS

CNS: *sedation, clouded sensorium, euphoria,* dizziness, ***seizures*** (with large doses).
CV: *hypotension,* bradycardia.
GI: *nausea, vomiting, constipation, dry mouth,* ileus.
GU: *urine retention.*
Respiratory: ***respiratory depression.***
Skin: pruritus, flushing.
Other: physical dependence.

INTERACTIONS

CNS depressants, ethanol, general anesthetics, hypnotics, MAO inhibitors, other narcotic analgesics, sedatives, tranquilizers, tricyclic antidepressants: additive effects. Use together with extreme caution. Monitor patient response.

CONTRAINDICATIONS

- Contraindicated in patients with hypersensitivity to this drug or other opiate analgesics.
- Use with extreme caution in patients with head injury, increased intracranial pressure, increased CSF pressure, hepatic or renal disease, hypothyroidism, Addison's disease, acute alcoholism, seizures, severe CNS depression, bronchial asthma, COPD, respiratory depression, and shock. Also use with extreme caution in elderly or debilitated patients.

NURSING CONSIDERATIONS

- Monitor respiratory and circulatory status.
- To mimimize GI distress caused by oral administration, advise patients to take this drug with milk or meals.
- Opiates may cause constipation. Assess bowel function and need for stool softeners or laxatives. Constipating effect makes codeine useful in the treatment of diarrhea.
- Caution ambulatory patients about getting out of bed or walking. Warn outpatients to avoid driving and other potentially hazardous activities that require mental alertness until adverse CNS effects of the drug are known.
- For full analgesic effect, take or give drug before patient has intense pain.
- Codeine and aspirin or acetaminophen are often prescribed together to provide enhanced pain relief.
- Drug is an antitussive and should not be used when cough is a valuable diagnostic sign or is beneficial (as after thoracic surgery).
- Monitor cough type and frequency.
- Codeine's abuse potential is much less than morphine's.
- **I.V. use:** Give by direct injection into a large vein. Administer very slowly. Don't mix with other solutions because codeine phosphate is incompatible with many drugs.
- Don't administer discolored injection solution.

dezocine

Dalgan

Pregnancy Risk Category: C

HOW SUPPLIED

Injection: 5 mg/ml, 10 mg/ml, 15 mg/ml

ACTION

Mechanism: Synthetic opioid agonist-antagonist that produces postoperative analgesia qualitatively similar to morphine.

Onset: within 15 minutes of I.V. injection, 30 minutes of I.M. injection. **Peak:** Peak effects occur within ½ to 2½ hours. **Duration:** plasma half-life, 1½ to 2½ hours; effects persist 2 to 4 hours, depending upon dose.

INDICATIONS & DOSAGE

Management of moderate to severe pain –

Adults: 5 to 20 mg I.M. q 3 to 6 hours or 2.5 to 10 mg I.V. q 2 to 4 hours. Maximum recommended single I.M. dose is 20 mg, with a maximum daily dosage of 120 mg. Maximum dosage for I.V. use has not been determined.

In patients with renal or hepatic failure: use with caution and in lower doses. Elimination half-life increases in these patients.

ADVERSE REACTIONS

CNS: *sedation, dizziness, vertigo,* anxiety, mood disorders, sleep distur-

bances, headache, slurred speech, sweating, chills, flushing, pallor.
CV: edema, hypotension, irregular heartbeat, hypertension, chest pain, thrombophlebitis.
EENT: dry mouth.
GI: *nausea, vomiting,* constipation, diarrhea, abdominal distress.
Hematologic: low hemoglobin.
Respiratory: respiratory depression
Skin: rash, pruritus, *irritation at injection site.*

INTERACTIONS

CNS depressants, ethanol: may increase risk of CNS depression.
Opiates: opioid-dependent patients may experience withdrawal symptoms after receiving dezocine. May increase risk of CNS depression.

CONTRAINDICATIONS

- Contraindicated in patients with hypersensitivity to the drug.
- Use with extreme caution in patients with head injury because drug's CNS depressant effects may obscure clinical signs. Related drugs have caused elevations of CSF pressure in patients with head injury.
- Use cautiously and in lower doses in patients with chronic respiratory disease and in patients undergoing biliary surgery. Related drugs have caused significant increases in pressure within the common bile duct.
- Like other potent analgesics, dezocine should be administered with caution to elderly patients.

NURSING CONSIDERATIONS

- Dezocine produces a dose-dependent respiratory depression similar to that of morphine, usually peaking within 15 minutes of administration. Use only in clinical settings where adequate respiratory support and an opiate antagonist (naloxone) is available to reverse respiratory depression.
- Use of dezocine is not recommended in patients who are opioid-dependent because it may precipitate a withdrawal syndrome. Also not recommended for patients with chronic pain because of limited experience and because drug can precipitate an abstinence syndrome in patients with substantial tolerance to opiates.
- Caution ambulatory patients about getting out of bed or walking. Warn outpatients to avoid driving and other potentially hazardous activities that require mental alertness until adverse CNS effects of the drug are known.
- Plasma concentrations higher than 45 ng/ml are associated with an increased incidence of adverse reactions.
- Although currently not a controlled substance, dezocine will replace morphine in animal drug-dependence studies. However, tolerance or physical dependance has not been reported in humans. Nevertheless, in persons with a history of opiate use or dependence, abuse of this drug is a potential risk.
- Because it is not known if dezocine is excreted in breast milk, breast-feeding is not recommended.
- **I.V. use:** Give by direct injection into a large vein. Avoid mixing with other drugs because there is little information regarding drug and solution compatibility. Infuse over at least 5 minutes. The injection contains sulfite preservatives, which may cause allergic reactions in certain sensitive patients.

fentanyl citrate

Sublimaze

fentanyl transdermal system

Duragesic-25, Duragesic-50, Duragesic-75, Duragesic-100

fentanyl transmucosal

Fentanyl Oralet

Controlled Substance Schedule II

Pregnancy Risk Category: B (D for prolonged use or high doses at term)

HOW SUPPLIED

Injection: 50 mcg/ml
Transdermal system: patches designed to release 25 mcg, 50 mcg, 75 mcg, or 100 mcg of fentanyl/hour.
Transmucosal: 200 mcg, 300 mcg, 400 mcg

ACTION

Mechanism: Binds with opiate receptors in the CNS, altering both perception of and emotional response to pain through an unknown mechanism.
Onset: immediately after I.V. use; within 7 to 8 minutes of I.M. injection; within 5 to 15 minutes of transmucosal use; onset after transdermal use may take several hours.
Peak: Peak effect after I.V. use occurs in 3 to 5 minutes; after I.M. or transmucosal use, 20 to 30 minutes; after trandermal use, 1 to 3 days. **Duration:** elimination half-life, about 3½ hours after parenteral use, 5 to 15 hours after transmucosal use, and 18 hours after transdermal use; effects persist ½ to 1 hour after I.V. use or 1 to 2 hours after I.M. use.

INDICATIONS & DOSAGE

Adjunct to general anesthetic –
Adults: for low-dose therapy, give 2 mcg/kg I.V. For moderate-dose therapy, give 2 to 20 mcg I.V.; then 25 to 100 mcg I.V. p.r.n. For high-dose therapy, give 20 to 50 mcg I.V.; then 25 mcg to one-half the initial loading dose I.V. p.r.n.
Adjunct to regional anesthesia –
Adults: 0.05 to 0.1 mg I.M. q 1 to 2 hours p.r.n.
Postoperatively –
Adults: 0.05 to 0.1 mg I.M. q 1 to 2 hours p.r.n.
Preoperatively –
Adults: 0.05 to 0.1 mg I.M. 30 to 60 minutes before surgery.
Children 2 to 12 years: 1.7 to 3.3 mcg/kg I.M.
Management of chronic pain –
Adults: apply one transdermal system to a portion of the upper torso on an area of skin that is not irritated and has not been irradiated. Initiate therapy with the 25-mcg/hour system; adjust dosage as needed and tolerated. Each system may be worn for 72 hours.

ADVERSE REACTIONS

CNS: *sedation, somnolence, clouded sensorium, euphoria,* dizziness, ***seizures*** (with large doses).
CV: *hypotension,* bradycardia.
GI: nausea, vomiting, *constipation,* ileus.
GU: *urine retention.*
Respiratory: ***respiratory depression.***
Skin: reaction at application site (erythema, papules, edema), *pruritus.*
Other: muscle rigidity, physical dependence.

INTERACTIONS

CNS depressants, ethanol, general anesthetics, hyponotics, MAO inhibitors, other narcotic analgesics, sedatives, tricyclic antidepressants: additive effects. Use together with extreme caution. Fentanyl dose should be reduced by one-quarter to one-third. Also give above drugs in reduced dosages.

CONTRAINDICATIONS

- Contraindicated in patients who have received MAO inhibitors within 14 days and in those with myasthenia gravis.
- Use with extreme caution in patients with head injury, increased CSF pressure, asthma, COPD, respiratory depression, seizures, hepatic or renal disease, hypothyroidism, Addison's disease, alcoholism, increased intracranial pressure, CNS depression, and

shock. Also use with extreme caution in elderly or debilitated patients.

NURSING CONSIDERATIONS

- Keep narcotic antagonist (naloxone) and resuscitation equipment available when giving drug I.V.
- Epidural injection or infusion has been used for postoperative analgesia, chronic pain management, or postpartum pain control. May be administered with local anesthetics such as bupivicaine to enhance analgesic effects.
- Monitor respirations of neonates exposed to drug during labor.
- Use as postoperative analgesic only in recovery room. Make sure another analgesic is ordered for later use.
- Monitor circulatory and respiratory status and urinary function carefully. Drug may cause respiratory depression, hypotension, urine retention, nausea, vomiting, ileus, or altered level of consciousness without regard to route of administration.
- Periodically monitor postoperative vital signs and bladder function. Because drug decreases both rate and depth of respirations, monitoring of arterial oxygen saturation (SaO_2) may help to assess respiratory depression. Immediately report respiratory rate below 12 breaths/minute, decreased respiratory volume, or decreased SaO_2.
- For better analgesic effect, administer drug before patient has intense pain.
- When used postoperatively, encourage turning, coughing, and deep breathing to prevent atelectasis.
- Pruritus is common, especially after intraspinal administration. Give diphenhydramine or naloxone S.C. as ordered.
- High doses can produce muscle rigidity, which can be reversed with neuromuscular blockers; however, patient must be artificially ventilated.
- **I.V. use:** Only staff trained in administrating I.V. anesthetics and managing their potential adverse effects should administer I.V. fentanyl.
- Often used I.V. with droperidol to produce neuroleptanalgesia.

Transdermal form:

- Transdermal fentanyl is not recommended for postoperative pain.
- Dosage equivalent charts are available to calculate the fentanyl transdermal dose based on the daily morphine intake – for example, for every 90 mg of oral morphine or 15 mg of I.M. morphine per 24 hours, 25 mcg/hour of transdermal fentanyl is required. Some patients will require alternative means of opiate administration when the dose exceeds 300 mcg/hour.
- Dosage adjustments in patients using the transdermal system should be made gradually. Reaching steady-state levels of a new dose may take up to 6 days; delay dose adjustment until after at least two applications.
- Monitor patients who develop adverse reactions to the transdermal system for at least 12 hours after removal. Serum levels of fentanyl drop very gradually and may take as long as 17 hours to decline by 50%.
- Most patients experience good control of pain for 3 days while wearing the transdermal system, but a few may need a new application after 48 hours. Because serum fentanyl concentration rises for the first 24 hours after application, analgesic effect cannot be evaluated for the first day. Be sure the patient has adequate supplemental analgesic to prevent breakthrough pain.
- When reducing opiate therapy or switching to a different analgesic, withdraw the transdermal system gradually. Because fentanyl's serum level drops very gradually after removal, give half of the equianalgesic dose of the new analgesic 12 to 18 hours after removal.
- Teach patients proper application of the transdermal patch. Clip hair at the

application site, but do not use a razor, which may irritate the skin. Wash area with clear water if necessary, but not with soaps, oils, lotions, alcohol or other substances that may irritate the skin or prevent adhesion. Dry the area completely before application.
• Remove the transdermal system from the package just before applying. Hold in place for 10 to 20 seconds, and be sure the edges of the patch adhere to the patient's skin.
• Teach patients to dispose of the transdermal patch by folding so the adhesive side adheres to itself and then flushing it down the toilet.
• If another patch is needed after 72 hours, apply to a new site.

hydromorphone hydrochloride (dihydromorphinone hydrochloride)

Dilaudid, Dilaudid HP
Controlled Substance Schedule II
Pregnancy Risk Category: B (D for prolonged use or use of high doses at term)

HOW SUPPLIED

Tablets: 1 mg, 2 mg, 3 mg, 4 mg
Injection: 1 mg/ml, 2 mg/ml, 3 mg/ml, 4 mg/ml, 10 mg/ml
Suppositories: 3 mg

ACTION

Mechanism: Binds with opiate receptors in the CNS, altering both perception of and emotional response to pain through an unknown mechanism. Also suppresses the cough reflex by direct action on the cough center in the medulla.
Onset: 10 to 15 minutes after I.V. injection, about 15 minutes after S.C. or I.M. administration, about 30 minutes after oral dose. **Peak:** Peak effects occur 15 to 30 minutes after I.V. injection, 30 to 60 minutes after I.M. injection, 30 to 90 minutes after S.C. administration, 1½ to 2 hours after oral administration. **Duration:** effects persist about 2 to 3 hours after I.V. injection, 4 to 5 hours after I.M. injection, 4 hours after S.C. or oral administration.

INDICATIONS & DOSAGE

Moderate to severe pain –
Adults: 1 to 6 mg P.O. q 4 to 6 hours, p.r.n. or around the clock; or 2 to 4 mg I.M., S.C., or I.V. q 4 to 6 hours p.r.n. or q 6 to 8 hours around the clock (I.V. dose should be given over 3 to 5 minutes); or 3 mg rectal suppository h.s., p.r.n., or q 6 to 8 hours around the clock.
Cough –
Adults: 1 mg P.O. q 3 to 4 hours p.r.n.
Children 6 to 12 years: 0.5 mg P.O. q 3 to 4 hours p.r.n.

ADVERSE REACTIONS

CNS: *sedation, somnolence, clouded sensorium,* dizziness, *euphoria,* ***seizures*** with large doses.
CV: *hypotension,* bradycardia.
EENT: blurred vision, diplopia, nystagmus.
GI: *nausea, vomiting, constipation,* ileus.
GU: *urine retention.*
Respiratory: ***respiratory depression, bronchospasm.***
Other: induration with repeated S.C. injections, physical dependence.

INTERACTIONS

CNS depressants, ethanol, general anesthetics, hypnotics, MAO inhibitors, other narcotic analgesics, sedatives, tranquilizers, tricyclic antidepressants: additive effects. Use together with extreme caution. Reduce hydromorphone dose and monitor patient response.

CONTRAINDICATIONS

• Contraindicated in patients with hypersensitivity to this drug or other opiate analgesics and in those with status asthmaticus.

- Use with extreme caution in patients with increased CSF pressure, respiratory depression, hepatic or renal disease, hypothyroidism, shock, Addison's disease, acute alcoholism, seizures, head injury, severe CNS depression, brain tumor, bronchial asthma, and COPD. Also use with extreme caution in elderly or debilitated patients.

NURSING CONSIDERATIONS

- Monitor respiratory and circulatory status and bowel function.
- Keep narcotic antagonist (naloxone) available.
- Commonly abused narcotic.
- Caution ambulatory patients about getting out of bed or walking. Warn outpatients to avoid driving and other potentially hazardous activities that require mental alertness until adverse CNS effects of the drug are known.
- Oral dosage form is particularly convenient for patients with chronic pain because tablets are available in 1 mg, 2 mg, 3 mg, and 4 mg. This enables these patients to titrate dosage.
- For better analgesic effect, give this drug before patient has intense pain.
- When used postoperatively, encourage turning, coughing, and deep breathing to avoid atelectasis.
- May worsen or mask gallbladder pain.
- Rotate injection sites to avoid induration with S.C. injection.
- Dilaudid HP, a highly concentrated form (10 mg/ml), may be administered in smaller volumes, preventing the discomfort associated with large-volume I.M. or S.C. injections.
- **I.V. use:** Give by direct injection over no less than 2 minutes. For infusion, drug may be mixed in D_5W, 0.9% sodium chloride, dextrose 5% in 0.9% sodium chloride, dextrose 5% in 0.45% sodium chloride, or Ringer's or lactated Ringer's solutions.
- Respiratory depression and hypotension can occur with I.V. administration. Give very slowly and monitor constantly. Keep resuscitation equipment available.
- Epidural injection or infusion has been used for management of chronic pain.

levorphanol tartrate

Levo-Dromoran

Controlled Substance Schedule II

Pregnancy Risk Category: B (D for prolonged use or high doses at term)

HOW SUPPLIED

Tablets: 2 mg
Injection: 2 mg/ml

ACTION

Mechanism: Binds with opiate receptors in the CNS, altering both perception of and emotional response to pain through an unknown mechanism.
Onset: 10 to 60 minutes following oral administration. **Peak:** Peak effect occurs within 20 minutes after I.V. administration, 60 minutes after I.M. injection, 60 to 90 minutes after S.C. injection, 1½ to 2 hours after oral administration. **Duration:** with all routes of administration, effects persist about 4 to 5 hours.

INDICATIONS & DOSAGE

Moderate to severe pain –
Adults: 2 to 3 mg P.O. or S.C. q 6 to 8 hours, p.r.n. or around the clock.

ADVERSE REACTIONS

CNS: *sedation, somnolence, clouded sensorium,* dizziness, *euphoria,* ***seizures*** (with large doses).
CV: *hypotension,* bradycardia.
GI: *nausea, vomiting, constipation,* ileus.
GU: urine retention.

*Liquid form contains alcohol.
**May contain tartrazine.

Common reactions are in italics; ***life-threatening,*** in bold italics.

Respiratory: ***respiratory depression.***
Other: physical dependence.

INTERACTIONS

CNS depressants, ethanol, general anesthetics, hypnotics, MAO inhibitors, other narcotic analgesics, sedatives, tranquilizers, tricyclic antidepressants: additive effects. Use together with extreme caution. Reduce levorphanol dose and monitor patient response.

CONTRAINDICATIONS

- Contraindicated in patients with hypersensitivity to this drug or other opiate analgesics, acute alcoholism, bronchial asthma, increased intracranial pressure, respiratory depression, and anoxia.
- Use with extreme caution in patients with hepatic or renal disease, hypothyroidism, Addison's disease, seizures, head injury, severe CNS depression, brain tumor, COPD, and shock. Also use with extreme caution in elderly or debilitated patients.

NURSING CONSIDERATIONS

- Caution ambulatory patients about getting out of bed or walking. Warn outpatients to avoid driving and other potentially hazardous activities that require mental alertness until adverse CNS effects are known.
- Monitor circulatory and respiratory status and bowel function.
- Keep narcotic antagonist (naloxone) available.
- For better analgesic effect, give this drug before patient has intense pain.
- When used postoperatively, encourage turning, coughing, and deep breathing to prevent atelectasis.
- Warn patient drug has bitter taste.
- **I.V. use:** Give by direct injection. Administer slowly.
- Protect from light.

meperidine hydrochloride (pethidine hydrochloride)

Demerol
Controlled Substance Schedule II
Pregnancy Risk Category: B (D for prolonged use or high doses at term)

HOW SUPPLIED

Tablets: 50 mg, 100 mg
Syrup: 50 mg/ml
Injection: 10 mg/ml, 25 mg/ml, 50 mg/ml, 75 mg/ml, 100 mg/ml

ACTION

Mechanism: Binds with opiate receptors in the CNS, altering both perception of and emotional response to pain through an unknown mechanism.
Onset: about 1 minute following I.V. administration; 10 to 15 minutes after S.C. or I.M. injection, about 15 minutes after oral administration. **Peak:** Peak effect occurs within 5 to 7 minutes after I.V. injection, 30 to 50 minutes after I.M. injection, 60 to 90 minutes after S.C. injection or oral administration. **Duration:** plasma half-life, about 2½ to 4 hours; with all routes of administration, effects persist 2 to 4 hours.

INDICATIONS & DOSAGE

Moderate to severe pain –
Adults: 50 to 150 mg P.O., I.M., or S.C. q 3 to 4 hours, p.r.n. or around the clock; or 15 to 35 mg/hour by continuous I.V. infusion.
Children: 1.1 to 1.76 mg/kg P.O., I.M., or S.C. q 3 to 4 hours. Maximum dosage is 100 mg q 4 hours, p.r.n. or around the clock.
Preoperatively –
Adults: 50 to 100 mg I.M. or S.C. 30 to 90 minutes before surgery.
Children: 1 to 2.2 mg/kg I.M. or S.C. 30 to 90 minutes before surgery.

ADVERSE REACTIONS

CNS: *sedation, somnolence, clouded sensorium, euphoria,* paradoxical excitement, tremor, dizziness, ***seizures*** (with large doses).
CV: *hypotension,* bradycardia, tachycardia.
GI: *nausea, vomiting, constipation,* ileus.
GU: *urine retention.*
Respiratory: ***respiratory depression.***
Skin: pain at injection site, local tissue irritation and induration after S.C. injection; phlebitis after I.V. use.
Other: physical dependence, muscle twitching.

INTERACTIONS

Barbiturates: incompatible when mixed in the same I.V. container.
CNS depressants, ethanol, general anesthetics, hypnotics, other narcotic analgesics, phenothiazines, sedatives, tricyclic antidepressants: possible respiratory depression, hypotension, profound sedation, or coma. Use together with extreme caution. Reduce meperidine dose.
MAO inhibitors: increased CNS excitation or depression that can be severe or fatal. Don't use together.
Phenytoin: decreased blood levels of meperidine. Monitor for decreased analgesia.

CONTRAINDICATIONS

- Contraindicated in patients with hypersensitivity to this drug or other opiate analgesics and in patients who have received MAO inhibitors within 14 days.
- Use with extreme caution in patients with increased intracranial pressure, increased CSF pressure, shock, CNS depression, head injury, asthma, COPD, respiratory depression, supraventricular tachycardias, seizures, acute abdominal conditions, hepatic or renal disease, hypothyroidism, Addison's disease, urethral stricture, prostatic hyperplasia, and alcoholism; in children under 12 years; and in elderly or debilitated patients.

NURSING CONSIDERATIONS

- May be used in some patients allergic to morphine.
- Meperidine and active metabolite normeperidine accumulate. Monitor for increased toxic effect, especially in patients with impaired renal function.
- Because meperidine toxicity often appears after several days of treatment, this drug is not recommended for treatment of chronic pain.
- Caution ambulatory patients about getting out of bed or walking. Warn outpatients to avoid driving and other potentially hazardous activities that require mental alertness until adverse CNS effects of the drug are known.
- Monitor respirations of neonates exposed to drug during labor. Have resuscitation equipment and naloxone available.
- P.O. dose is less than half as effective as parenteral dose. Give I.M. if possible. When changing from parenteral to P.O. route, dose should be increased.
- Syrup has local anesthetic effect. Give with full glass of water.
- Monitor respiratory and cardiovascular status carefully. Don't give if respirations are below 12 breaths/minute, if respiratory rate or depth is decreased, or if change in pupils is noted.
- Monitor bladder function in postoperative patients.
- Monitor bowel function. Patient may need a laxative or stool softener.
- Watch for withdrawal symptoms if drug is discontinued abruptly after long-term use.
- Alternating a centrally active narcotic with a more peripherally active nonnarcotic analgesic (aspirin, acetaminophen, or NSAID) may improve pain control while requiring lower narcotic doses.

• When used postoperatively, encourage turning, coughing, and deep breathing and use of an incentive spirometer to prevent atelectasis.
• S.C. injection is not recommended because it is very painful.
• **I.V. use:** Give slowly by direct I.V. injection. Meperidine may also be given by I.V. infusion. Drug is compatible with most I.V. solutions, including D_5W, 0.9% sodium chloride, and Ringer's and lactated Ringer's solutions.
• Keep narcotic antagonist (naloxone) available when giving this drug I.V.

methadone hydrochloride

Dolophine, Methadose, Physeptone‡
Controlled Substance Schedule II

Pregnancy Risk Category: B (D for prolonged use or high doses at term)

HOW SUPPLIED

Tablets: 5 mg, 10 mg
Dispersible tablets (for methadone maintenance therapy): 40 mg
Oral solution: 5 mg/5 ml, 10 mg/5 ml, 10 mg/ml (concentrate)
Injection: 10 mg/ml

ACTION

Mechanism: Binds with opiate receptors at many sites in the CNS (brain, brain stem, and spinal cord), altering both perception of and emotional response to pain through an unknown mechanism.
Onset: immediately after I.V. administration, 10 to 20 minutes after I.M. injection, 30 to 60 minutes after oral administration. **Peak:** Peak effects occur within 15 to 30 minutes after I.V injection, 1 to 2 hours after I.M. injection, 1½ to 2 hours after oral administration. **Duration:** half-life, 15 to 25 hours; effects persist 2 to 4 hours after I.V. use, 4 to 5 hours after I.M. use, 4 to 6 hours after oral use.

INDICATIONS & DOSAGE

Severe pain –
Adults: 2.5 to 10 mg P.O., I.M., or S.C. q 3 to 4 hours, p.r.n. or around the clock.
Narcotic abstinence syndrome –
Adults: 15 to 40 mg P.O. daily (highly individualized). Maintenance dosage is 20 to 120 mg P.O. daily. Adjust dose as needed. Daily dosages greater than 120 mg require special state and federal approval.

ADVERSE REACTIONS

CNS: *sedation, somnolence, clouded sensorium, euphoria,* dizziness, choreic movements, ***seizures*** (with large doses).
CV: *hypotension,* bradycardia.
EENT: visual disturbances.
GI: *nausea, vomiting, constipation,* ileus.
GU: *urine retention,* decreased libido.
Respiratory: ***respiratory depression.***
Skin: pain at injection site, tissue irritation, induration following S.C. injection, diaphoresis.
Other: physical dependence.

INTERACTIONS

Ammonium chloride and other urine acidifiers, phenytoin: may reduce methadone effect. Monitor for decreased pain control.
CNS depressants, ethanol, general anesthetics, hypnotics, MAO inhibitors, sedatives, tranquilizers, tricyclic antidepressants: possible respiratory depression, hypotension, profound sedation, or coma. Use together with extreme caution. Monitor patient response.
Rifampin: withdrawal symptoms; reduced blood levels of methadone. Use together cautiously.

CONTRAINDICATIONS

• Contraindicated in patients with hypersensitivity to this drug or other opiate analgesics.
• Use with extreme caution in pa-

tients with acute abdominal conditions, severe hepatic or renal impairment, hypothyroidism, Addison's disease, prostatic hyperplasia, urethral stricture, head injury, increased intracranial pressure, asthma, COPD, respiratory depression, and CNS depression. Also use with extreme caution in elderly or debilitated patients.

NURSING CONSIDERATIONS

• When used as an adjunct in the treatment of narcotic addiction (maintenance), withdrawal will usually be delayed and mild.
• Safe use as maintenance drug in adolescent addicts not established.
• Once-daily dosage is adequate for maintenance. No advantage to divided doses.
• Oral liquid form legally required in maintenance programs. Completely dissolve tablets in 120 ml of orange juice or powdered citrus drink.
• Patient treated for narcotic abstinence syndrome will usually require an additional analgesic if pain control is necessary.
• Oral dose is half as potent as injected dose.
• Has cumulative effect; marked sedation can occur after repeated doses.
• Monitor circulatory and respiratory status and bladder and bowel function. Patient may need a laxative.
• Caution ambulatory patients about getting out of bed or walking. Warn outpatients to avoid driving and other potentially hazardous activities that require mental alertness until adverse CNS effects of the drug are known.
• An around-the-clock regimen is necessary to manage severe, chronic pain.
• For parenteral use, I.M. injection is preferred. Rotate injection sites.
• **I.V. use:** Dilute to a maximum concentration of 10 mg/ml using 0.9% sodium chloride. Give slowly by direct injection. Alternatively, dilute to 1 mg/ml and give as a slow I.V. infusion (15 to 35 mg/hour).

morphine hydrochloride

Morphitec†, M.O.S.†, M.O.S.-S.R.†

morphine sulfate

Astramorph PF, Duramorph, Duramorph PF, Epimorph†, Infumorph 200, Infumorph 500, Morphine H.P.†, MS Contin, MSIR, Oramorph SR, RMS Uniserts, Roxanol, Roxanol 100, Roxanol Rescudose, Roxanol SR, Roxanol UD, Statex†

Controlled Substance Schedule II

morphine tartrate‡

Pregnancy Risk Category: B (D for prolonged use or high doses at term)

HOW SUPPLIED

hydrochloride

Tablets: 10 mg†, 20 mg†, 40 mg†, 60 mg†
Tablets (extended-release): 30 mg†, 60 mg†
Oral solution†*:* 1 mg/ml, 5 mg/ml, 10 mg/ml, 20 mg/ml, 50 mg/ml
Syrup: 1 mg/ml†, 5 mg/ml†, 10 mg/ml†, 20 mg/ml†, 50 mg/ml†
Suppositories: 10 mg†, 20 mg†, 30 mg†

sulfate

Tablets: 15 mg, 30 mg
Tablets (extended-release): 15 mg, 30 mg, 60 mg, 100 mg
Soluble tablets: 10 mg, 15 mg, 30 mg
Oral solution: 10 mg/5 ml, 20 mg/5 ml, 20 mg/ml (concentrate)
Syrup: 1 mg/ml, 5 mg/ml
Injection (with preservative): 500 mcg/ml, 1 mg/ml, 2 mg/ml, 3 mg/ml, 4 mg/ml, 5 mg/ml, 8 mg/ml, 10 mg/ml, 15 mg/ml, 25 mg/ml, 50 mg/ml
Injection (without preservative): 500 mcg/ml, 1 mg/ml, 10 mg/ml, 25 mg/ml

Suppositories: 5 mg, 10 mg, 20 mg, 30 mg
tartrate
Injection: 80 mg/ml‡

ACTION

Mechanism: Binds with opiate receptors in the CNS, altering both perception of and emotional response to pain through an unknown mechanism.
Onset: within 1 hour after oral dose, 20 to 60 minutes after rectal dose, 10 to 30 minutes after S.C. or I.M. dose, less than 5 minutes after I.V. dose, 15 to 60 minutes after epidural or intrathecal dose. **Peak:** Peak analgesic effect is 1 to 2 hours after oral dose, 20 to 60 minutes after rectal dose, 50 to 90 minutese after S.C. dose, 30 to 60 minutes after I.M. dose, 20 minutes after direct I.V. injection, 15 to 60 minutes after epidural injection.
Duration: effects persist 4 to 5 hours after immediate-release oral forms, 8 to 12 hours after extended-release oral forms, 4 to 5 hours after rectal, S.C., I.M., or I.V. dose, up to 24 hours after intrathecal or epidural dose.

INDICATIONS & DOSAGE

Severe pain –
Adults: 5 to 20 mg S.C. or I.M. or 2.5 to 15 mg I.V. q 4 hours p.r.n. or around the clock; or 10 to 30 mg P.O. or 10 to 20 mg rectally q 4 hours, p.r.n. or around the clock. When given by continuous I.V. infusion, a loading dose of 15 mg I.V. may be followed by a continuous infusion of 0.8 to 10 mg/hour. May also administer controlled-release tablets 30 to 60 mg P.O. q 8 to 12 hours. As an epidural injection, 5 mg by epidural catheter q 24 hours.
Children: 0.1 to 0.2 mg/kg S.C. or I.M. q 4 hours. Maximum single dose is 15 mg.

ADVERSE REACTIONS

CNS: *sedation, somnolence, clouded sensorium, euphoria,* ***seizures*** (with large doses), dizziness, *nightmares* (with long-acting oral forms).
CV: *hypotension,* bradycardia.
GI: *nausea, vomiting, constipation,* ileus.
GU: *urine retention.*
Hematologic: thrombocytopenia.
Respiratory: ***respiratory depression.***
Skin: pruritus and skin flushing (with epidural administration).
Other: *physical dependence.*

INTERACTIONS

CNS depressants, ethanol, general anesthetics, hypnotics, MAO inhibitors, other narcotic analgesics, sedatives, tranquilizers, tricyclic antidepressants: possible respiratory depression, hypotension, profound sedation, or coma. Use together with extreme caution. Reduce morphine dose and monitor patient response.

CONTRAINDICATIONS

- Contraindicated in patients with hypersensitivity to this drug or other opiate analgesics.
- Use with extreme caution in patients with head injury, increased intracranial pressure, seizures, asthma, COPD, alcoholism, prostatic hyperplasia, severe hepatic or renal disease, acute abdominal conditions, hypothyroidism, Addison's disease, increased CSF pressure, urethral stricture, cardiac arrhythmias, reduced blood volume, and toxic psychosis. Also use with extreme caution in elderly or debilitated patients.

NURSING CONSIDERATIONS

- Monitor circulatory, respiratory, bladder, and bowel functions carefully. Drug may cause respiratory depression, hypotension, urine retention, nausea, vomiting, ileus, or altered level of consciousness regardless of the route used. Withhold dose and notify doctor if respirations are below 12 breaths/minute.

- Caution ambulatory patients about getting out of bed or walking. Warn outpatients to avoid driving and other potentially hazardous activities that require mental alertness until adverse CNS effects are known.
- Constipation is often severe with maintenance dosage. Ensure that stool softener or other laxative is ordered.
- Morphine is the drug of choice in relieving pain of MI. May cause transient decrease in blood pressure.
- Keep narcotic antagonist (naloxone) and resuscitation equipment available.
- An around-the-clock regimen best manages severe, chronic pain.
- When using postoperatively, encourage turning, coughing, and deep breathing and use of the incentive spirometer to prevent atelectasis.
- Oral solutions of various concentrations are available as well as an intensified oral solution (20 mg/ml). Carefully note the strength you are administering.
- Do not crush or break extended-release tablets.
- S.L. administration may be ordered. Measure oral solution with tuberculin syringe. Administer dose a few drops at a time to allow maximal S.L. absorption and minimize swallowing.
- Refrigeration of rectal suppository is not necessary. In some patients, rectal and oral absorption may not be equivalent.
- Preservative-free preparations are available for epidural and intrathecal administration.
- When given epidurally, monitor closely for respiratory depression up to 24 hours after the injection. Check respiratory rate and depth every 30 to 60 minutes for 24 hours.
- May worsen or mask gallbladder pain.
- **I.V. use:** When given by direct injection, 2.5 to 15 mg may be diluted in 4 or 5 ml of sterile water for injection and given over 4 to 5 minutes. Alternatively, the drug may be mixed with D_5W to a concentration of 0.1 to 1 mg/ml and administered by a continuous infusion device. Morphine sulfate is compatible with most common I.V. solutions.

nalbuphine hydrochloride

Nubain

Pregnancy Risk Category: B (D for prolonged use or high doses at term)

HOW SUPPLIED

Injection: 10 mg/ml, 20 mg/ml

ACTION

Mechanism: Binds with opiate receptors in the CNS, altering both perception of and emotional response to pain through an unknown mechanism.
Onset: 2 to 3 minutes after I.V. administration, within 15 minutes of S.C. or I. M. injection. **Peak:** Peak effects occur within 30 minutes of I.V. adminstration, 60 minutes of I.M. injection. **Duration:** half-life, 5 hours; effects persist 3 to 4 hours after I.V. use, 3 to 6 hours after S.C. or I.M. injection.

INDICATIONS & DOSAGE

Moderate to severe pain –
Adults: For an average (70 kg) person, give 10 to 20 mg S.C., I.M., or I.V. q 3 to 6 hours, p.r.n. or around the clock. Maximum daily dosage is 160 mg.

ADVERSE REACTIONS

CNS: *headache, sedation,* dizziness, nervousness, depression, restlessness, crying, euphoria, hostility, unusual dreams, confusion, hallucinations, speech difficulty, delusions.
CV: hypertension, hypotension, tachycardia, bradycardia.
EENT: blurred vision.

GI: cramps, dyspepsia, bitter taste, *nausea, vomiting,* constipation.
GU: urinary urgency.
Skin: itching; burning; urticaria; *sweaty, clammy feeling.*
Respiratory: ***respiratory depression, pulmonary edema.***

INTERACTIONS

CNS depressants, ethanol, general anesthetics, hypnotics, MAO inhibitors, sedatives, tranquilizers, tricyclic antidepressants: possible respiratory depression, hypertension, profound sedation, or coma. Use together with extreme caution. Monitor patient response.
Narcotic analgesics: possible decreased analgesic effect. Avoid concomitant use.

CONTRAINDICATIONS

- Contraindicated in patients with hypersensitivity to the drug, emotional instability, history of drug abuse, head injury, or increased intracranial pressure.
- Use cautiously in patients with hepatic and renal disease. These patients may overreact to customary doses.

NURSING CONSIDERATIONS

- Causes respiratory depression, which at 10 mg is equal to the respiratory depression produced by 10 mg of morphine.
- Monitor respirations of neonates exposed to the drug during labor.
- Psychological and physical dependence may occur.
- Monitor circulatory and respiratory status and bladder and bowel function. Withhold dose and notify doctor if respirations are shallow or rate is below 12 breaths/minute.
- Constipation is often severe with maintenance therapy. Make sure stool softener or other laxative is ordered.
- Also acts as a narcotic antagonist; may precipitate abstinence syndrome. For patients who have chronically received opiates, administer 25% of the usual dose initially. Observe for signs of withdrawal.
- Caution ambulatory patients about getting out of bed or walking. Warn outpatients to avoid driving and other potentially hazardous activities that require mental alertness until adverse CNS effects are known.
- **I.V. use:** Inject slowly over at least 2 to 3 minutes into a vein or into an I.V. line containing a compatible, free-flowing I.V. solution, such as D_5W, 0.9% sodium chloride, or lactated Ringer's solution.
- Respiratory depression can be reversed with naloxone. Keep resuscitative equipment available, particularly when administering I.V.

oxycodone hydrochloride

Endone‡, Roxicodone, Roxicodone Intensol, Supeudol†
Controlled Substance Schedule II

oxycodone pectinate

Proladone‡

Pregnancy Risk Category: B (D for prolonged use or high doses at term)

HOW SUPPLIED

hydrochloride
Tablets: 5 mg
Oral solution: 5 mg/5 ml, 20 mg/ml (concentrate)
Suppositories: 10 mg, 20 mg
pectinate
Suppositories: 30 mg‡

ACTION

Mechanism: Binds with opiate receptors in the CNS, altering both perception of and emotional response to pain through an unknown mechanism.
Peak: Peak effects occur within 1 hour. **Duration:** half-life, 2 to 3 hours; effects persist 3 to 4 hours.

INDICATIONS & DOSAGE

Moderate to severe pain –

Adults: available in combination with other drugs, such as aspirin (Percodan, Percodan-Demi) or acetaminophen (Percocet, Tylox). One to 2 tablets P.O. q 6 hours, p.r.n. or around the clock. Alternatively, 5 mg of oxycodone oral solution P.O. q 6 hours, or 1 to 3 suppositories P.R. daily, p.r.n. or around the clock.

Children 6 to 12 years: (Percodan-Demi) ¼ tablet P.O. q 6 hours, p.r.n. or around the clock.

Children over 12 years: (Percodan-Demi) ½ tablet P.O. q 6 hours, p.r.n. or around the clock.

ADVERSE REACTIONS

CNS: *sedation, somnolence, clouded sensorium, euphoria,* dizziness, ***seizures*** with large doses.

CV: *hypotension,* bradycardia.

GI: *nausea, vomiting, constipation,* ileus.

GU: *urine retention.*

Respiratory: ***respiratory depression.***

Other: physical dependence.

INTERACTIONS

Anticoagulants: oxycodone hydrochloride products containing aspirin may increase anticoagulant effect. Monitor clotting times. Use together cautiously.

CNS depressants, ethanol, general anesthetics, hypnotics, MAO inhibitors, other narcotic analgesics, sedatives, tranquilizers, tricyclic antidepressants: additive effects. Use together with extreme caution. Reduce oxycodone dose and monitor patient response.

CONTRAINDICATIONS

- Contraindicated in patients with hypersensitivity to this drug or other opiate analgesics.
- Use with extreme caution in patients with head injury, increased intracranial pressure, increased CSF pressure, seizures, asthma, COPD, alcoholism, prostatic hypertrophy, severe hepatic or renal disease, acute abdominal conditions, urethral stricture, hypothyroidism, Addison's disease, cardiac arrhythmias, reduced blood volume, and toxic psychosis. Also use with extreme caution in elderly or debilitated patients.
- Don't give to children, except for Percodan-Demi and Percocet-Demi.

NURSING CONSIDERATIONS

- Caution ambulatory patients about getting out of bed or walking. Warn outpatients to avoid driving and other potentially hazardous activities that require mental alertness until adverse CNS effects are known.
- Monitor circulatory and respiratory status and bladder and bowel function. Withhold dose and notify doctor if respirations are shallow or if respiratory rate falls below 12 breaths/minute.
- Patient may require a laxative because drug has a constipating effect.
- For full analgesic effect, this drug should be taken or given before patient has intense pain.
- To minimize GI upset, tell patients to take this drug after meals or with milk.
- Single-agent oxycodone solution or tablets are especially good for patients who shouldn't take aspirin or acetaminophen.

oxymorphone hydrochloride

Numorphan, Numorphan HP

Controlled Substance Schedule II

Pregnancy Risk Category: B (D for prolonged use or high doses at term)

HOW SUPPLIED

Injection: 1 mg/ml, 1.5 mg/ml

Suppositories: 5 mg

ACTION

Mechanism: Binds with opiate receptors in the CNS, altering both perception of and emotional response to pain through an unknown mechanism.
Onset: within 5 to 10 minutes after I.V. use, 10 to 15 minutes after I.M. use, 10 to 20 minutes after S.C. use, 15 to 30 minutes after rectal use.
Peak: Peak effects occur within 15 to 30 minutes after I.V. use, 30 to 90 minutes after I.M. use, 60 to 90 minutes after S.C. use, 2 hours after rectal use. **Duration:** effects persist 3 to 4 hours after I.V. use; 3 to 6 hours after I.M., S.C., or rectal use.

INDICATIONS & DOSAGE

Moderate to severe pain –
Adults: 1 to 1.5 mg I.M. or S.C. q 4 to 6 hours, p.r.n. or around the clock; or 0.5 mg I.V. q 4 to 6 hours, p.r.n. or around the clock; or 2.5 to 5 mg P.R. q 4 to 6 hours, p.r.n. or around the clock.

ADVERSE REACTIONS

CNS: *sedation, somnolence, clouded sensorium, euphoria,* dizziness, ***seizures*** (with large doses).
CV: *hypotension,* bradycardia.
GI: *nausea, vomiting, constipation,* ileus.
GU: *urine retention.*
Respiratory: ***respiratory depression.***
Other: physical dependence.

INTERACTIONS

CNS depressants, ethanol, general anesthetics, MAO inhibitors, tricyclic antidepressants: additive effects. Use together with extreme caution.

CONTRAINDICATIONS

• Contraindicated in patients with hypersensitivity reactions to this drug or other opiate analgesics.
• Use with extreme caution in patients with head injury, increased intracranial pressure, seizures, asthma, COPD, alcoholism, increased CSF pressure, acute abdominal conditions, prostatic hyperplasia, severe hepatic or renal disease, urethral stricture, CNS depression, respiratory depression, hypothyroidism, Addison's disease, cardiac arrhythmias, reduced blood volume, and toxic psychosis. Also use with extreme caution in elderly or debilitated patients.

NURSING CONSIDERATIONS

• Caution ambulatory patients about getting out of bed or walking. Warn outpatients to avoid driving and other potentially hazardous activities that require mental alertness until adverse CNS effects of the drug are known.
• Monitor cardiovascular and respiratory status and bladder and bowel function. Withhold dose and notify doctor if respirations decrease or rate is below 12 breaths/minute.
• Patients may need laxative.
• Well absorbed rectally. Alternative to narcotics with limited dosage forms.
• Keep narcotic antagonist (naloxone) and resuscitation equipment available.
• For better analgesic effect, this drug should be taken or given before patient has intense pain.
• When used postoperatively, encourage turning, coughing, and deep breathing and use of the incentive spirometer to avoid atelectasis.
• Not intended for mild to moderate pain. May worsen gallbladder pain.
• **I.V. use:** Give by direct I.V. injection. If necessary, drug may be diluted in 0.9% sodium chloride.

pentazocine hydrochloride

Fortral†‡, Talwin†

pentazocine hydrochloride and naloxone hydrochloride

Talwin Nx
Controlled Substance Schedule IV

pentazocine lactate

Fortral‡, Talwin
Controlled Substance Schedule IV
Pregnancy Risk Category: B (D for prolonged use or high doses at term)

HOW SUPPLIED

hydrochloride
Tablets: 25 mg‡, 50 mg†‡
hydrochloride and naloxone hydrochloride
Tablets: 50 mg pentazocine hydrochloride and 500 mcg naloxone hydrochloride
lactate
Injection: 30 mg/ml

ACTION

Mechanism: Binds with opiate receptors at many sites in the CNS, altering both perception of and emotional response to pain through an unknown mechanism.
Onset: 2 to 3 minutes after I.V. use, 15 to 20 minutes after I.M. or S.C. use, 15 to 30 minutes after oral use.
Peak: Peak effects occur within 15 to 30 minutes after I.V. use, 30 to 60 minutes after I.M. or S.C. use, 60 to 90 minutes after oral use. **Duration:** half-life, 2 to 3 hours; effects persist 2 to 3 hours after parenteral use, 2 to 3 hours after oral use.

INDICATIONS & DOSAGE

Moderate to severe pain –
Adults: 50 to 100 mg P.O. q 3 to 4 hours, p.r.n. or around the clock. Maximum oral dosage is 600 mg/day. Alternatively, may give 30 mg I.M., I.V., or S.C. q 3 to 4 hours, p.r.n. or around the clock. Maximum parenteral dosage is 360 mg/day. Single doses above 30 mg I.V. or 60 mg I.M. or S.C. are not recommended.

ADVERSE REACTIONS

CNS: *sedation,* visual disturbances, *hallucinations,* drowsiness, *dizziness, light-headedness,* confusion, euphoria, headache, *psychotomimetic effects.*
CV: hypotension.
EENT: dry mouth, dysgeusia.
GI: *nausea, vomiting,* constipation.
GU: *urine retention.*
Respiratory: ***respiratory depression.***
Skin: induration, nodules, sloughing, and sclerosis of injection site.
Other: hypersensitivity reactions ***(anaphylaxis)***, physical and psychological dependence.

INTERACTIONS

CNS depressants, ethanol: additive effects. Use together cautiously.
Narcotic analgesics: possible decreased analgesic effect. Avoid concomitant use.

CONTRAINDICATIONS

- Contraindicated in patients with hypersensitivity to the drug, emotional instability, drug abuse, head injury, and increased intracranial pressure. Injectable form contains sulfites, which may precipitate allergic reactions in some patients.
- Use cautiously in patients with hepatic or renal disease and in patients with acute MI.

NURSING CONSIDERATIONS

- Tablets are not well absorbed.
- Possesses narcotic antagonist properties. May precipitate abstinence syndrome in narcotic-dependent patients.
- Psychological and physical dependence may occur.
- Respiratory depression can be reversed with naloxone.
- Caution ambulatory patients about getting out of bed or walking. Warn outpatients to avoid driving and other potentially hazardous activities that require mental alertness until adverse CNS effects of the drug are known.
- Pentazocine may interfere with certain laboratory tests for urinary 17-hydroxycorticosteroids.

• Talwin Nx, the oral pentazocine available in the U.S., contains the narcotic antagonist naloxone. This prevents illicit I.V. use.
• When giving by S.C. or I.M. injection, rotate injection sites to minimize tissue irritation. If possible, avoid giving by S.C.route.
• **I.V. use:** Give by direct I.V. injection. Administer slowly. Do not mix in same syringe with aminophylline, barbiturates, or other alkaline substances.

propoxyphene hydrochloride (dextropropoxyphene hydrochloride)

Darvon, Dolene, Doraphen, Doxaphene, Novopropoxyn†, Pro-Pox, Propoxycon, 642†

propoxyphene napsylate (dextropropoxyphene napsylate)

Darvocet-N, Darvon-N, Doloxene‡, Doloxene Co‡

Controlled Substance Schedule IV
Pregnancy Risk Category: C (D for prolonged use)

HOW SUPPLIED

hydrochloride
Capsules: 32 mg, 65 mg
napsylate
Tablets: 100 mg
Capsules: 50 mg, 100 mg
Oral suspension: 10 mg/ml

ACTION

Mechanism: Binds with opiate receptors in the CNS, altering both perception of and emotional response to pain through an unknown mechanism.
Onset: 15 to 60 minutes. **Peak:** Plasma levels peak in 2 to 2½ hours.
Duration: plasma half-life, 6 to 12 hours for the parent drug, 30 to 36 hours for its active metabolite; effects persist 4 to 6 hours.

INDICATIONS & DOSAGE

Mild to moderate pain –
Adults: 65 mg (hydrochloride) P.O. q 4 hours p.r.n. Do not exceed 390 mg/day.
Mild to moderate pain –
Adults: 100 mg (napsylate) P.O. q 4 hours p.r.n. Do not exceed 600 mg/day.

ADVERSE REACTIONS

CNS: *dizziness,* headache, sedation, euphoria, paradoxical excitement, insomnia.
GI: nausea, vomiting, constipation.
Respiratory: ***respiratory depression.***
Other: psychological and physical dependence.

INTERACTIONS

Carbamazepine: may increase carbamazepine levels. Monitor closely.
CNS depressants, ethanol: additive effects. Use together cautiously.
Warfarin: increased anticoagulant effect. Monitor PT.

CONTRAINDICATIONS

• Contraindicated in patients with hypersensitivity to this drug or other opiate analgesics.
• Use cautiously in patients with hepatic or renal disease, emotional instability, or a history of drug abuse.

NURSING CONSIDERATIONS

• Respiratory depression, hypotension, profound sedation, and coma may result if used in excessive doses or with other CNS depressants. Studies have shown that propoxyphene-containing products alone or in combination with other drugs are a major cause of drug-related overdose and death. Warn patient not to exceed recommended dosage.
• Not to be prescribed for maintenance purposes in patients with narcotic addiction.
• Caution ambulatory patients about getting out of bed or walking. Warn

outpatients to avoid driving and other hazardous activities that require mental alertness until adverse CNS effects are known.
• Do not use caffeine or amphetamines to treat overdose; may cause fatal seizures. Use naloxone instead.
• May cause false decreases in urinary steroid excretion tests.
• Remember that 65 mg of propoxyphene hydrochloride equals 100 mg of propoxyphene napsylate.
• Can be considered a mild narcotic analgesic, but pain relief is equivalent to that provided by aspirin. Tolerance and physical dependence have been observed. Typically used with aspirin or acetaminophen to maximize analgesia.
• To minimize GI upset, advise patient to take drug with food or milk.
• Advise patient to limit alcohol intake when taking this drug.

sufentanil citrate

Sufenta
Controlled Substance Schedule II
Pregnancy Risk Category: C (D for prolonged use or high doses at term)

HOW SUPPLIED
Injection: 50 mcg/ml

ACTION
Mechanism: Binds with opiate receptors in the CNS, altering both perception of and emotional response to pain through an unknown mechanism.
Onset: within 1 minute. **Duration:** analgesic effects, 5 minutes. Following high doses, patients may regain consciousness in ½ to 3 hours.

INDICATIONS & DOSAGE
Adjunct to general anesthetic –
Adults: 1 to 8 mcg/kg I.V. administered with nitrous oxide and oxygen.
As a primary anesthetic –
Adults: 8 to 30 mcg/kg I.V. administered with 100% oxygen and a muscle relaxant.

In elderly and debilitated patients: reduced dosage required.

ADVERSE REACTIONS
CNS: chills, ***seizures.***
CV: *hypotension,* hypertension, bradycardia, tachycardia.
GI: nausea, vomiting.
Respiratory: ***chest wall rigidity, respiratory depression.***
Skin: itching.
Other: intraoperative muscle movement.

INTERACTIONS
CNS depressants, ethanol: additive effects. Use together cautiously.

CONTRAINDICATIONS
• Contraindicated in patients with hypersensitivity to this drug or other opiate analgesics.
• Use with extreme caution in patients with head injury; in those with pulmonary, hepatic, or renal disease; in those with decreased respiratory reserve; and in elderly or debilitated patients.

NURSING CONSIDERATIONS
• Should be administered only by persons specifically trained in the use of I.V. anesthetics.
• When used at doses over 8 mcg/kg, postoperative mechanical ventilation and observation are essential because of prolonged respiratory depression.
• For obese patients who exceed 20% of their ideal body weight, dosage calculations should be based upon an estimate of ideal weight.
• Keep narcotic antagonist (naloxone) and resuscitation equipment available.
• Monitor respirations of neonates exposed to the drug during labor.
• Because drug decreases both rate and depth of respirations, monitoring of arterial oxygen saturation may aid in assessing respiratory depression.

Notify the doctor if respirations decrease or rate falls below 12 breaths/ minute.

- Monitor postoperative vital signs frequently, including circulatory and respiratory status and urinary function. Drug may cause respiratory depression, hypotension, urine retention, nausea, vomiting, ileus, or altered level of consciousness. Encourage turning, coughing, and deep breathing to prevent atelectasis.
- Has more rapid onset and shorter duration of action than fentanyl.
- High doses can produce muscle rigidity reversible by neuromuscular blockers; however, patient must be artificially ventilated.
- **I.V. use:** Give by direct I.V. injection. Although the drug has been given by intermittent I.V. infusion, drug compatibility and stability in I.V. solutions have not been fully investigated.

28

Sedative-hypnotics

amobarbital
amobarbital sodium
aprobarbital
butabarbital sodium
chloral hydrate
estazolam
ethchlorvynol
flurazepam hydrochloride
glutethimide
methotrimeprazine hydrochloride
midazolam hydrochloride
pentobarbital
pentobarbital sodium
phenobarbital sodium
(See Chapter 29, ANTICONVULSANTS.)
quazepam
secobarbital sodium
temazepam
triazolam
zolpidem tartrate

COMBINATION PRODUCTS
TRI-BARBS CAPSULES: phenobarbital 32 mg, butabarbital sodium 32 mg, and secobarbital sodium 32 mg.
TUINAL 200 MG PULVULES: amobarbital sodium 100 mg and secobarbital sodium 100 mg.

---

amobarbital
Amytal

amobarbital sodium
Amytal Sodium

Controlled Substance Schedule II
Pregnancy Risk Category: B

HOW SUPPLIED
amobarbital
Tablets: 50 mg
amobarbital sodium
Capsules: 200 mg
Powder for injection: 500 mg

ACTION
Mechanism: Probably interferes with transmission of impulses from the thalamus to the cortex of the brain. A barbiturate.
Onset: about 60 minutes. **Duration:** effects persist 10 to 12 hours.

INDICATIONS & DOSAGE
Sedation –
Adults: usually 50 mg P.O. b.i.d. or t.i.d.
Children: 3 to 6 mg/kg P.O. daily in four equally divided doses.
Insomnia –
Adults: 50 to 200 mg P.O. or deep I.M. h.s.; I.M. injection not to exceed 5 ml in any one site. Maximum dosage is 500 mg.
Children: 3 to 5 mg/kg deep I.M. h.s.; I.M. injection not to exceed 5 ml in any one site.
Preanesthetic sedation –
Adults and children: 200 mg P.O. or I.M. 1 to 2 hours before surgery.
Manic reactions, as an adjunct in psychotherapy, anticonvulsant –
Adults and children over 6 years: 65 to 500 mg slow I.V.; not to exceed 100 mg/minute. Maximum dosage is 1 g.
Children under 6 years: 3 to 5 mg/kg slow I.V. or I.M.

ADVERSE REACTIONS
CV: bradycardia, hypotension, syncope.
CNS: *drowsiness, lethargy, hangover,* paradoxical excitement.
GI: nausea, vomiting.
Hematologic: exacerbation of porphyria.
Respiratory: respiratory depression.
Skin: rash, urticaria, ***Stevens-Johnson syndrome;*** pain, irritation, sterile abscess at injection site.
Other: angioedema.

INTERACTIONS

Chloramphenicol, MAO inhibitors, valproic acid: inhibit metabolism of barbiturates; may cause prolonged CNS depression. Reduce barbiturate dosage.
Corticosteroids, digitoxin, doxycycline, estrogens and oral contraceptives, oral anticoagulants, tricyclic antidepressants: amobarbital may enhance the metabolism of these drugs. Monitor for decreased effect.
Ethanol or other CNS depressants, including narcotic analgesics: excessive CNS and respiratory depression. Use together cautiously.
Griseofulvin: decreased absorption of griseofulvin.
Rifampin: may decrease barbiturate levels. Monitor for decreased effect.

CONTRAINDICATIONS

- Contraindicated in patients with uncontrolled severe pain, respiratory disease with dyspnea or obstruction, hypersensitivity to barbiturates, previous addiction to sedatives, or porphyria.
- Use cautiously in patients with hepatic or renal impairment.

NURSING CONSIDERATIONS

- Elderly patients are more sensitive to the drug's adverse CNS effects. Assess mental status before and after initiating therapy.
- Because barbiturates potentiate narcotic effects, reduce dose when giving during labor. Excessive dose may cause respiratory depression in neonate.
- Long-term high dosage may cause drug dependence and severe withdrawal symptoms. Withdraw barbiturates gradually.
- Take precautions to prevent hoarding or self-overdosing by patients who are depressed, suicidal, or drug-dependent, or who have a history of drug abuse.
- Assess CBCs before and periodically during long-term therapy. Observe for signs of hematologic toxicity, such as easy bruising or bleeding, or signs of infection.
- Skin eruptions may precede potentially fatal reactions to barbiturate therapy. Discontinue drug when skin reactions occur. In some patients, high fever, stomatitis, headache, or rhinitis may precede skin reactions.
- Watch for signs of barbiturate toxicity: coma, pupillary constriction, cyanosis, clammy skin, and hypotension. Overdose can be fatal.
- Morning "hangover" common after hypnotic dose, which also suppresses REM sleep. Patients may experience increased dreaming after drug is discontinued.
- Caution patients about performing activities that require mental alertness or physical coordination. For inpatients, supervise walking and raise bed rails, particularly for elderly patients.
- Patients using oral contraceptives should consider alternate birth control methods because drug may enhance contraceptive hormone metabolism and decrease its effect.
- **I.V. use:** Reserve I.V. injection for emergency treatment. Give under close supervision. Be prepared to give artificial respiration. Administer slowly I.V.; do not exceed 100 mg/minute.
- I.V. administration of barbiturates may cause severe respiratory depression, laryngospasm, or hypotension. Have emergency resuscitation equipment available.
- Local tissue reactions and injection site pain have been noted with I.V. use. Assess patency of I.V. site before and during administration.
- To minimize deterioration, use injection solution within 30 minutes after opening container. Don't use cloudy or precipitated solution. Don't shake solution; mix with sterile water only.

• Administer I.M. injection deeply. Superficial injection may cause pain, sterile abscess, and sloughing.
• Used in psychiatric settings as an "Amytal interview" to elicit information that patient can't or won't offer when fully conscious.
• Also used in Wada testing to help determine language and memory function.

aprobarbital

Alurate*
Controlled Substance Schedule III
Pregnancy Risk Category: D

HOW SUPPLIED

Elixir: 40 mg/5 ml

ACTION

Mechanism: Probably interferes with transmission of impulses from the thalamus to the cortex of the brain. A barbiturate.
Onset: 45 to 60 minutes. **Duration:** effects persist 6 to 8 hours.

INDICATIONS & DOSAGE

Sedation –
Adults: 15 to 40 mg P.O. t.i.d. or q.i.d.; usual dose is 40 mg t.i.d.
Insomnia –
Adults: 40 to 160 mg P.O. h.s.

ADVERSE REACTIONS

CNS: *drowsiness, lethargy, hangover,* paradoxical excitement in elderly patients.
GI: nausea, vomiting.
Hematologic: exacerbation of porphyria.
Respiratory: ***respiratory depression.***
Skin: rash, urticaria, ***Stevens-Johnson syndrome.***
Other: ***angioedema***

INTERACTIONS

Chloramphenicol, MAO inhibitors, valproic acid: inhibit metabolism of barbiturates; may cause prolonged CNS depression. Reduce barbiturate dosage.
Corticosteroids, digitoxin, doxycycline, estrogens and oral contraceptives, oral anticoagulants, tricyclic antidepressants: aprobarbital may enhance the metabolism of these drugs. Monitor for decreased effectiveness.
Ethanol or other CNS depressants, including narcotic analgesics: excessive CNS and respiratory depression. Use together cautiously.
Griseofulvin: decreased absorption of griseofulvin.
Rifampin: may decrease barbiturate levels. Monitor for decreased effect.

CONTRAINDICATIONS

• Contraindicated in patients with uncontrolled severe pain, respiratory disease with dyspnea or obstruction, hypersensitivity to barbiturates, previous addiction to sedatives, or porphyria.
• Use cautiously in patients with hepatic or renal impairment and in elderly patients.

NURSING CONSIDERATIONS

• Long-term use is not recommended: drug loses its efficacy in promoting sleep after 14 days of continued use. Long-term high dosage may cause drug dependence, and patient may experience withdrawal symptoms if drug is suddenly stopped. Withdraw barbiturates gradually.
• Take precautions to prevent hoarding or self-overdosing by patients who are depressed, suicidal, or drug-dependent, or who have a history of drug abuse.
• Watch for signs of barbiturate toxicity: coma, pupillary constriction, cyanosis, clammy skin, and hypotension. Overdose can be fatal.
• Caution patients about performing activities that require mental alertness or physical coordination. For inpatients, supervise walking and raise

bed rails, particularly for elderly patients.
• Morning "hangover" common after hypnotic dose, which also suppresses REM sleep. Patients may experience increased dreaming after drug is discontinued.
• Skin eruptions may precede potentially fatal reactions to barbiturate therapy. Discontinue drug when skin reactions occur. In some patients, high fever, stomatitis, headache, or rhinitis may precede skin reactions.
• Patients using oral contraceptives should consider alternate birth control methods because drug may enhance contraceptive hormone metabolism and decrease its effect.

butabarbital sodium (butabarbitone sodium)

Busodium, Butalan*, Butisol* **, Saneryl‡, Sarisol No. 2* **
Controlled Substance Schedule III
Pregnancy Risk Category: D

HOW SUPPLIED
Tablets: 15 mg, 30 mg, 50 mg, 100 mg
Capsules: 15 mg, 30 mg
Elixir: 30 mg/5 ml, 33.3 mg/5 ml

ACTION
Mechanism: Probably interferes with transmission of impulses from the thalamus to the cortex of the brain. A barbiturate.
Onset: 45 to 60 minutes. **Duration:** effects persist 6 to 8 hours.

INDICATIONS & DOSAGE
Sedation –
Adults: 15 to 30 mg P.O. t.i.d. or q.i.d.
Children: 2 to 6 mg/kg P.O. divided t.i.d. Dosage range is 7.5 to 30 mg P.O. t.i.d.
Preoperatively –
Adults: 50 to 100 mg P.O. 60 to 90 minutes before surgery.
Insomnia –
Adults: 50 to 100 mg P.O. h.s.

ADVERSE REACTIONS
CNS: *drowsiness, lethargy, hangover,* paradoxical excitement in elderly patients.
GI: nausea, vomiting.
Hematologic: exacerbation of porphyria.
Respiratory: ***respiratory depression.***
Skin: rash, urticaria, ***Stevens-Johnson syndrome.***
Other: ***angioedema.***

INTERACTIONS
Chloramphenicol, MAO inhibitors, valproic acid: inhibited metabolism of barbiturates; may cause prolonged CNS depression. Reduce barbiturate dosage.
Corticosteroids, digitoxin, doxycycline, estrogens and oral contraceptives, oral anticoagulants, tricyclic antidepressants: barbiturates may enhance the metabolism of these drugs. Monitor for decreased effectiveness.
Ethanol or other CNS depressants, including narcotic analgesics: excessive CNS and respiratory depression. Use together cautiously.
Griseofulvin: decreased absorption of griseofulvin.
Rifampin: may decrease barbiturate levels. Monitor for decreased effect.

CONTRAINDICATIONS
• Contraindicated in patients with uncontrolled severe pain, respiratory disease with dyspnea or obstruction, hypersensitivity to barbiturates, previous addiction to sedatives, or porphyria.
• Use cautiously in patients with hepatic or renal impairment.

NURSING CONSIDERATIONS
• Elderly patients are more sensitive to drug's adverse CNS reactions. Assess mental status before and after initiating therapy.

• Long-term use is not recommended: drug loses its efficacy in promoting sleep after 14 days. A drug-free interval of at least 1 week is advised if continued treatment is appropriate. Long-term high dosage may cause drug dependence, and patients may experience withdrawal symptoms if drug is suddenly stopped. Withdraw barbiturates gradually.
• Take precautions to prevent hoarding or self-overdosing by patients who are depressed, suicidal, or drug-dependent, or who have a history of drug abuse.
• Caution patients about performing activities that require mental alertness or physical coordination. For inpatients, supervise walking and raise bed rails, particularly for elderly patients.
• Watch for signs of barbiturate toxicity: coma, pupillary constriction, cyanosis, clammy skin, and hypotension. Overdose can be fatal.
• Discontinue drug when skin reactions occur because skin eruptions may precede potentially fatal reactions to barbiturate therapy. In some patients, high fever, stomatitis, headache, or rhinitis may precede skin reactions.
• Morning "hangover" common after hypnotic dose.
• Hypnotic doses suppress REM sleep. Patients may experience increased dreaming after drug is discontinued.
• Patients using oral contraceptives should consider alternate birth control methods because drug may enhance contraceptive hormone metabolism and decrease its effect.

chloral hydrate

Aquachloral Supprettes, Dormel‡, Novochlorhydrate†
Controlled Substance Schedule IV
Pregnancy Risk Category: C

HOW SUPPLIED
Capsules: 250 mg, 500 mg
Syrup: 250 mg/5 ml, 500 mg/5 ml
Suppositories: 324 mg, 500 mg, 648 mg

ACTION
Mechanism: Unknown. Sedative effects may be caused by its primary metabolite, trichloroethanol.
Onset: within 30 minutes. **Duration:** half-life of active metabolite trichloroethanol, 7 to 10 hours; effects persist 4 to 8 hours.

INDICATIONS & DOSAGE
Sedation –
Adults: 250 mg P.O. or P.R. t.i.d. after meals.
Children: 8.3 mg/kg or 250 mg/m^2 P.O. or P.R. t.i.d. Maximum dosage is 500 mg t.i.d.
Insomnia –
Adults: 500 mg to 1 g P.O. or P.R. 15 to 30 minutes before bedtime.
Children: 50 mg/kg or 1.5 g/m^2 P.O. or P.R. 15 to 30 minutes before bedtime. Maximum single dose is 1 g.
Premedication for EEG –
Children: 20 to 25 mg/kg P.O. or P.R. Maximum single dose is 1 g.
Management of alcohol withdrawal symptoms –
Adults: 500 mg to 1 g P.O. or P.R. q 6 hours, not to exceed 2 g daily.

ADVERSE REACTIONS
CNS: *hangover, drowsiness,* nightmares, dizziness, ataxia, paradoxical excitement.
GI: *nausea,* vomiting, diarrhea, flatulence.
Hematologic: eosinophilia, leukopenia.
Skin: hypersensitivity reactions.

INTERACTIONS
Alkaline solutions: incompatible with aqueous solutions of chloral hydrate. Don't mix together.
Ethanol or other CNS depressants, in-

*Liquid form contains alcohol.
**May contain tartrazine.

Common reactions are in italics; ***life-threatening,*** in bold italics.

cluding narcotic analgesics: excessive CNS depression or vasodilation reaction. Use together cautiously.
Furosemide I.V.: sweating, flushes, variable blood pressure, and uneasiness. Use together cautiously or use a different hypnotic drug.
Oral anticoagulants: increased risk of bleeding. Monitor patient closely.
Phenytoin: decreased phenytoin levels. Monitor closely.

CONTRAINDICATIONS
• Contraindicated in patients with hepatic or renal impairment and in those with hypersensitivity to chloral hydrate or trichloroacetic acid. Oral administration contraindicated in patients with gastric disorders.
• Use cautiously in patients with severe cardiac disease, mental depression, and suicidal tendencies.

NURSING CONSIDERATIONS
• Long-term use is not recommended: drug loses its efficacy in promoting sleep after 14 days of continued use. Long-term use may cause drug dependence, and patient may experience withdrawal symptoms if drug is suddenly stopped.
• To minimize unpleasant taste and stomach irritation, dilute or administer with liquid. Drug should be taken after meals.
• Note two strengths of oral liquid form. Double-check dose, especially when administering to children. Fatal overdoses have occurred.
• Take precautions to prevent hoarding or self-overdosing by patients who are depressed, suicidal, or drug-dependent or who have a history of drug abuse.
• Caution patients about performing activities that require mental alertness or physical coordination. For inpatients, supervise walking and raise bed rails, particularly for elderly patients.
• Large dosage may raise BUN levels.
• May interfere with fluorometric tests for urine catecholamines and Reddy-Jenkins-Thorn test for urine 17-hydroxycorticosteroids. Do not administer drug for 48 hours before fluorometric test. May also cause false-positive tests for urine glucose when using copper sulfate tests. Use glucose enzymatic tests instead.
• Store in dark container; store suppositories in refrigerator.

estazolam

ProSom
Controlled Substance Schedule IV
Pregnancy Risk Category: X

HOW SUPPLIED
Tablets: 1 mg, 2 mg

ACTION
Mechanism: Acts on the limbic system and thalamus of the CNS by binding to specific benzodiazepine receptors.
Onset: 1 to 3 hours.
Duration: variable; half-life, 10 to 24 hours.

INDICATIONS & DOSAGE
Adjunctive treatment of insomnia –
Adults: 1 mg P.O. h.s. Some patients may require 2 mg.
Elderly patients: 1 mg P.O. h.s. Use higher doses with extreme care. Frail elderly or debilitated patients may take 0.5 mg, but this low dose may be only marginally effective.

ADVERSE REACTIONS
CNS: fatigue, dizziness, *daytime drowsiness, somnolence, asthenia, hypokinesia,* headache.
GI: dyspepsia.

INTERACTIONS
Cigarette smoking, rifampin: may increase metabolism and clearance and decrease plasma half-life. Monitor for decreased effectiveness.

Cimetidine, disulfiram, isoniazid, oral contraceptives: may impair the metabolism and clearance of benzodiazepines and prolong their plasma half-life. Monitor for increased CNS depression.
CNS depressants including antihistamines, opiate analgesics, and other benzodiazepines; ethanol: increased CNS depression. Avoid concomitant use.
Theophylline: pharmacologic antagonism. Monitor for decreased effectiveness.

CONTRAINDICATIONS
- Contraindicated in patients allergic to this drug or other benzodiazepines, in pregnant patients, and in patients with suspected or confirmed sleep apnea.
- Use cautiously in patients with hepatic, renal, or pulmonary disease.

NURSING CONSIDERATIONS
- Liver and renal function and CBC should be checked before and periodically during long-term therapy.
- Take precautions to prevent hoarding by depressed, suicidal, or drug-dependent patients or those who have a history of drug abuse.
- Warn patients that additive depressant effects can occur if alcohol is consumed while taking this drug or within 24 hours after use of the drug.
- Patients who receive prolonged treatment with benzodiazepines may experience withdrawal symptoms if the drug is suddenly discontinued (possibly after 6 weeks of continuous therapy).
- Caution patients about performing activities that require mental alertness or physical coordination. For inpatients, supervise walking and raise bed rails, particularly for elderly patients.
- Tell patients not to increase dosage of the drug but to inform the doctor if they feel that the drug is no longer effective.
- Patients using oral contraceptives should consider alternate birth control methods when taking this drug because drug may enhance contraceptive hormone metabolism and decrease its effect.
- If estazolam overdose occurs, flumazenil (a specific benzodiazepine antagonist) may be useful. However, flumazenil's duration is shorter than estazolam's, and resedation is possible.

ethchlorvynol

Placidyl**
Controlled Substance Schedule IV
Pregnancy Risk Category: C

HOW SUPPLIED
Capsules: 200 mg, 500 mg, 750 mg**

ACTION
Mechanism: Unknown; pharmacologic effects are similar to those produced by barbiturates.
Onset: 30 minutes to 1 hour. **Peak:** Plasma levels peak within 2 hours.
Duration: plasma half-life, about 10 to 20 hours; effects persist about 5 hours.

INDICATIONS & DOSAGE
Sedation –
Adults: 100 to 200 mg P.O. b.i.d. or t.i.d.
Insomnia –
Adults: 500 mg to 1 g P.O. h.s. May repeat 100 to 200 mg if awakened in early morning.

ADVERSE REACTIONS
CNS: facial numbness, drowsiness, fatigue, nightmares, dizziness, residual sedation, hangover, muscular weakness, syncope, ataxia.
CV: hypotension.
EENT: unpleasant aftertaste, blurred vision.

*Liquid form contains alcohol.
**May contain tartrazine.

Common reactions are in italics; ***life-threatening,*** in bold italics.

GI: distress, nausea, vomiting.
Hematologic: thrombocytopenia, exacerbation of porphyria.
Skin: rashes, urticaria.

INTERACTIONS
Ethanol or other CNS depressants, including MAO inhibitors, narcotic analgesics, and tricyclic antidepressants: excessive CNS depression. Use together cautiously.
Oral anticoagulants: ethchlorvynol may enhance the metabolism of coumarin derivatives, decreasing their effectiveness. Monitor closely.

CONTRAINDICATIONS
• Contraindicated in patients with hypersensitivity to this drug and in those with uncontrolled pain or porphyria.
• Use cautiously in hepatic or renal impairment, in elderly or debilitated patients, and in mental depression with suicidal tendencies.

NURSING CONSIDERATIONS
• Effective for short-term use only; treatment period should not exceed 1 week.
• Minimize transient dizziness or ataxia caused by rapid absorption by giving this drug with milk or food.
• May cause dependence and severe withdrawal symptoms. Withdraw gradually.
• Take precautions to prevent hoarding or self-overdosing by patients who are depressed, suicidal, or drug-dependent, or who have a history of drug abuse. Overdosage is difficult to treat and is associated with high mortality.
• Watch for signs of toxicity, such as poor muscle coordination, confusion, hypothermia, speech or vision disturbances, tremor, and weakness.
• The 750-mg strength contains tartrazine dye, which may cause allergic reactions in susceptible patients.
• Caution patients about performing activities that require mental alertness or physical coordination. For inpatients, supervise walking and raise bed rails, particularly for elderly patients.
• Slight darkening of liquid from exposure to air and light doesn't affect safety or potency, but store in tight, light-resistant container to avoid possible deterioration.

flurazepam hydrochloride

Apo-Flurazepam†, Dalmane, Durapam, Novoflupam†
Controlled Substance Schedule IV
Pregnancy Risk Category: D

HOW SUPPLIED
Capsules: 15 mg, 30 mg

ACTION
Mechanism: Acts on the limbic system, thalamus, and hypothalamus of the CNS to produce hypnotic effects. A benzodiazepine.
Onset: within 30 minutes. **Peak:** Peak effects occur in 1 to 2 hours.
Duration: for some active metabolites, 50 to 100 hours; effects persist 7 to 10 hours.

INDICATIONS & DOSAGE
Insomnia –
Adults: 15 to 30 mg P.O. h.s. May repeat dose once.
Adults over 65 years: 15 mg P.O. h.s.

ADVERSE REACTIONS
CNS: *daytime sedation, dizziness, drowsiness, disturbed coordination,* lethargy, confusion, *headache.*
GI: nausea, vomiting, heartburn.
Hepatic: elevated enzymes.
Other: physical or psychological dependence.

INTERACTIONS
Cigarette smoking, rifampin: enhanced metabolism of benzodiaze-

pines. Monitor for decreased effectiveness.
Cimetidine: increased sedation. Monitor carefully.
Disulfiram, isoniazid, oral contraceptives: decreased metabolism of benzodiazepines, leading to toxicity. Monitor closely.
Ethanol or other CNS depressants, including narcotic analgesics: excessive CNS depression. Use together cautiously.
Phenytoin: increased phenytoin levels. Monitor for toxicity.

CONTRAINDICATIONS
- Contraindicated in patients with hypersensitivity to benzodiazepines.
- Use cautiously in patients with impaired hepatic or renal function, mental depression, suicidal tendencies, or history of drug abuse.

NURSING CONSIDERATIONS
- May cause elevations in certain liver function tests (AST, ALT, total and direct bilirubin, and alkaline phosphatase). Check hepatic and renal function and CBC before and periodically during long-term therapy.
- Elderly patients are more sensitive to the drug's adverse CNS reactions. Assess mental status before initiating therapy.
- Take precautions to prevent hoarding or self-overdosing by patients who are depressed, suicidal, or drug-dependent, or who have a history of drug abuse.
- Caution patients about performing activities that require mental alertness or physical coordination. For inpatients, supervise walking and raise bed rails, particularly for elderly patients.
- Physical and psychological dependence is possible with long-term use.
- Advise patients that this drug is more effective on second, third, and fourth nights of use because active metabolite accumulates. Encourage them to continue drug, even if it doesn't relieve insomnia the first night.
- If flurazepam overdose occurs, flumazenil (a specific benzodiazepine antagonist) may be useful. However, flumazenil's duration of action is shorter than flurazepam's, and resedation is possible.

glutethimide
Doriglute
Controlled Substance Schedule II
Pregnancy Risk Category: C

HOW SUPPLIED
Tablets: 250 mg, 500 mg

ACTION
Mechanism: Unknown. Pharmacologic effects are similar to those produced by barbiturates.
Onset: within 30 minutes. **Peak:** Plasma levels peak in 1 to 6 hours.
Duration: half-life, about 10 to 12 hours; effects persist 4 to 8 hours.

INDICATIONS & DOSAGE
Insomnia –
Adults: 250 to 500 mg P.O. h.s. May be repeated, but not less than 4 hours before intended awakening. Total daily dosage should not exceed 1 g.

ADVERSE REACTIONS
CNS: *residual sedation, dizziness, ataxia,* paradoxical excitation, headache, vertigo.
CV: tachycardia.
EENT: dry mouth, blurred vision, mydriasis.
GI: irritation, nausea.
GU: bladder atony, urine retention.
Hematologic: thrombocytopenic purpura, leukopenia, ***aplastic anemia,*** exacerbation of porphyria.
Skin: rash, urticaria.

INTERACTIONS

Ethanol or other CNS depressants, including narcotic analgesics: excessive CNS depression. Use together cautiously.

Oral anticoagulants: glutethimide enhances the metabolism of coumarin derivatives. Monitor for decreased effect.

CONTRAINDICATIONS

- Contraindicated in patients with hypersensitivity to this drug and in patients with uncontrolled pain, severe renal impairment, or porphyria.
- Use cautiously in patients with mental depression, suicidal tendencies, history of drug abuse, and conditions that may be worsened by the drug's anticholinergic activity (prostatic hypertrophy, stenosing peptic ulceration, pyloroduodenal or bladder-neck obstruction, acute angle-closure glaucoma, and cardiac arrhythmias).

NURSING CONSIDERATIONS

- Drug is effective for short-term use only.
- Caution patients about performing activities that require mental alertness or physical coordination. For inpatients, supervise walking and raise bed rails, particularly for elderly patients.
- Take precautions to prevent hoarding or self-overdosing by patients who are depressed, suicidal, or drug-dependent, or who have a history of drug abuse.
- Abrupt withdrawal after long-term use may produce nausea, vomiting, nervousness, tremor, chills, fever, nightmares, insomnia, tachycardia, delirium, numbness of extremities, hallucinations, dysphagia, and seizures. Withdraw drug gradually.
- Assess patient for anticholinergic symptoms, including mydriasis, dry mouth, tachycardia, or urine retention.
- Monitor PT carefully when patient on glutethimide starts or ends anticoagulant therapy. Anticoagulant dose may need adjusting.
- Suppresses REM sleep, as do barbiturates. Patient may experience increased dreaming after discontinuation.
- May interfere with laboratory determinations of 17-hydroxycorticosteroids using the Glenn-Nelson technique.

---

methotrimeprazine hydrochloride (levomepromazine hydrochloride)

Levoprome, Nozinan Liquid†*, Nozinan Oral Drops†*

methotrimeprazine maleate

Nozinan†

Pregnancy Risk Category: C

HOW SUPPLIED

methotrimeprazine hydrochloride

Oral solution: 40 mg/ml†

Drops: 25 mg/ml†

Injection: 20 mg/ml in 10-ml vials, 25 mg/ml†

methotrimeprazine maleate

Tablets: 2 mg†, 5 mg†, 25 mg†, 50 mg†

ACTION

Mechanism: Acts on the limbic system, thalamus, and hypothalamus of the CNS to produce hypnotic effects. A phenothiazine.

Onset: 10 to 20 minutes after I.M. injection. **Peak:** Peak effects occur in 20 to 40 minutes; serum levels peak in about 60 minutes. **Duration:** effects persist about 4 hours.

INDICATIONS & DOSAGE

Postoperative analgesia –

Adults and children over 12 years: initially, 2.5 to 7.5 mg I.M. q 4 to 6 hours; then adjust dose.

Preanesthetic medication –
Adults and children over 12 years: 2 to 20 mg I.M. 45 minutes to 3 hours before surgery.
Sedation, analgesia –
Adults and children over 12 years: 10 to 20 mg deep I.M. q 4 to 6 hours as required; or 6 to 25 mg P.O. daily in three divided doses with meals. For severe pain, dosage may be increased to 50 to 75 mg daily in two or three divided doses with meals.
Adults over 65 years: 5 to 10 mg I.M. q 4 to 6 hours.
Psychosis –
Adults: 6 to 25 mg P.O. daily in three divided doses with meals. Dosage may be gradually increased as needed and tolerated to 50 to 75 mg daily in two or three divided doses.
Sedation and analgesia during labor –
Adults: 15 to 20 mg I.M.

ADVERSE REACTIONS

CNS: *fainting, weakness, dizziness,* drowsiness, excessive sedation, amnesia, disorientation, euphoria, headache, slurred speech, syncope, dystonic reaction (rare).
CV: *orthostatic hypotension,* palpitations, tachycardia.
EENT: dry mouth, nasal congestion, mydriasis.
GI: nausea, vomiting, abdominal discomfort.
GU: difficulty urinating.
Hematologic: ***agranulocytosis*** and other dyscrasias after long-term high dosage; leukocytosis (rare).
Skin: *pain, inflammation, swelling at injection site.*
Other: fever (rare).

INTERACTIONS

Antihypertensive agents: increased orthostatic hypotension. Don't use together.
Epinephrine: methotrimeprazine reverses the effect of epinephrine on blood pressure, worsening hypotension. Don't use together.
Ethanol or other CNS depressants: additive CNS depression. Avoid concomitant use.
MAO inhibitors: Additive depressant and anticholinergic effects. Don't use together.

CONTRAINDICATIONS

- Contraindicated in patients with a history of seizure disorders or of hypersensitivity to phenothiazines; in those with severe cardiac, hepatic, or renal disease; in those who have experienced previous CNS depressant overdose; and in comatose patients.
- Use with extreme caution in elderly or debilitated patients with cardiac disease or in any patient who may suffer serious consequences from a sudden blood pressure drop.
- Because the injectable form contains sulfites, use cautiously in asthmatic patients or in patients with sulfite sensitivity.

NURSING CONSIDERATIONS

- Use low initial dose in debilitated patients; increase gradually, frequently checking pulse rate, blood pressure, and circulation.
- Blood pressure drops 10 to 20 minutes after I.M. injection. May last 4 to 12 hours.
- Keep patients in bed or closely supervised for 6 to 12 hours after each of the first several injections because orthostatic hypotension may occur, particularly with high doses (> 100 mg). If hypotension is severe, combat with phenylephrine, methoxamine, or levarterenol. Don't use epinephrine because it may worsen hypotension.
- Because drowsiness and amnesia may occur, warn patients to avoid hazardous activities that require mental alertness or physical coordination.
- Assess patients for anticholinergic symptoms, including mydriasis, dry

mouth, tachycardia, or urine retention.
- Don't use for longer than 30 days except in terminal illness or when narcotics are contraindicated.
- In patients on long-term use, monitor liver function and blood studies periodically.
- Inject I.M. into large muscle masses. Rotate sites. Do not administer S.C. because of local irritation. I.V. injection not recommended.
- May be mixed in same syringe with reduced dose of atropine and scopolamine. Do not mix with other drugs. Protect solution from light.
- Rarely, may cause neuroleptic malignant syndrome, with fever, leukocytosis, and dystonic reaction. Can be fatal if untreated.
- Methotrimeprazine interferes with provocative and blocking tests for pheochromocytoma because of its alpha-adrenergic antagonist effects.

midazolam hydrochloride

Hypnovel‡, Versed
Controlled Substance Schedule IV
Pregnancy Risk Category: D

HOW SUPPLIED

Injection: 1 mg/ml, 5 mg/ml

ACTION

Mechanism: Depresses CNS at the limbic and subcortical levels of the brain by potentiating the effects of gamma amino butyric acid (GABA). **Onset:** 1½ to 5 minutes after I.V. injection, within 15 minutes of I.M. injection. **Peak:** Peak effect occurs within 15 to 60 minutes of I.M. injection. **Duration:** plasma half-life, 2½ hours (average); effects typically persist about 2 hours, but may last up to 6 hours.

INDICATIONS & DOSAGE

Preoperative sedation (to induce sleepiness or drowsiness and relieve apprehension) –
Adults: 0.07 mg to 0.08 mg/kg I.M. approximately 1 hour before surgery. May be administered with atropine or scopolamine and reduced doses of narcotics.
Conscious sedation before short diagnostic or endoscopic procedures –
Adults: initially, 0.035 mg/kg slowly I.V. (not to exceed 2.5 mg). Dose is then titrated in small amounts to a total dosage of 0.1 mg/kg.
Induction of general anesthesia –
Adults: 0.3 to 0.35 mg/kg I.V. over 20 to 30 seconds. Additional increments of 25% of the initial dose may be needed to complete induction. Up to 0.6 mg/kg total dosage may be given.

ADVERSE REACTIONS

CNS: headache, oversedation, involuntary movements, combativeness, amnesia.
CV: variations in blood pressure and pulse rate.
GI: nausea, vomiting, hiccups.
Respiratory: decreased respiratory rate, apnea.
Skin: pain and tenderness at injection site.

INTERACTIONS

Ethanol or other CNS depressants: may increase the risk of apnea. Avoid concomitant use. Prepare to adjust dosage of midazolam if used with opiates or other CNS depressants.

CONTRAINDICATIONS

- Contraindicated in patients with acute angle-closure glaucoma, shock, coma, or acute alcohol intoxication.
- Use cautiously in patients with CHF, COPD, or renal disease, and in elderly or debilitated patients.

NURSING CONSIDERATIONS

- Monitor blood pressure, heart rate and rhythm, respirations, airway integrity, and arterial oxygen saturation during procedure, especially in patients premedicated with narcotics.
- Midazolam's beneficial amnestic effect diminishes a patient's recall of perioperative events. However, this effect requires extra caution when teaching patients. Written information, family member instruction, and follow-up contact may be required to ensure that the patient has adequate information.
- Caution patients about performing activities that require mental alertness or physical coordination. For inpatients, supervise walking and raise bed rails, particularly for elderly patients.
- **I.V. use:** Administer slowly over at least 2 minutes, and wait at least 2 minutes when titrating doses to effect.
- Before administering, have oxygen and resuscitation equipment available in case of severe respiratory depression. Excessive dosage or rapid infusion has been associated with respiratory arrest, particularly in elderly or debilitated patients.
- When administering I.V., take care to avoid extravasation.
- When injecting I.M., give deep into a large muscle mass.
- May be mixed in the same syringe with morphine sulfate, meperidine, atropine sulfate, or scopolamine.
- If midazolam overdose occurs, flumazenil (a specific benzodiazepine antagonist) may be useful. However, flumazenil's duration of action is shorter than midazolam's, and resedation is possible.

pentobarbital (pentobarbitone)

Nembutal* **

pentobarbital sodium

Carbrital‡, Nembutal Sodium*, Nova Rectal†, Novopentobarb†

Controlled Substance Schedule II

Pregnancy Risk Category: D

HOW SUPPLIED

pentobarbital

Elixir: 20 mg/5 ml

pentobarbital sodium

Capsules: 50 mg, 100 mg

Injection: 50 mg/ml

Suppositories: 30 mg, 60 mg, 120 mg, 200 mg

ACTION

Mechanism: Probably interferes with transmission of impulses from the thalamus to the cortex of the brain. A barbiturate.

Onset: immediately after I.V. administration, within 15 minutes after oral administration. **Duration:** effects persist 3 to 4 hours.

INDICATIONS & DOSAGE

Sedation –

Adults: 20 to 40 mg P.O. b.i.d., t.i.d., or q.i.d.

Children: 2 to 6 mg/kg daily P.O. in divided doses. Maximum single dose is 100 mg.

Insomnia –

Adults: 100 to 200 mg P.O. h.s. or 150 to 200 mg deep I.M.; 100 mg initially I.V.; then additional doses up to 500 mg; 120 to 200 mg rectally.

Children: 3 to 5 mg/kg I.M. Maximum dosage is 100 mg. Rectal doses are: 2 months to 1 year, 30 mg; 1 to 4 years, 30 to 60 mg; 5 to 12 years, 60 mg; 12 to 14 years, 60 to 120 mg.

Preoperative sedation –

Adults: 150 to 200 mg I.M. or P.O. in two divided doses.

ADVERSE REACTIONS

CNS: *drowsiness, lethargy, hangover,* paradoxical excitement in elderly patients.

GI: nausea, vomiting.

*Liquid form contains alcohol.

**May contain tartrazine.

Common reactions are in italics; ***life-threatening,*** in bold italics.

Hematologic: exacerbation of porphyria.
Skin: rash, urticaria, ***Stevens-Johnson syndrome***.
Other: ***angioedema***.

INTERACTIONS
Corticosteroids, doxycycline, estrogens and oral contraceptives, oral anticoagulants: pentobarbital may enhance the metabolism of these drugs. Monitor for decreased effect.
Ethanol or other CNS depressants, including narcotic analgesics: excessive CNS and respiratory depression. Use together cautiously.
Griseofulvin: decreased absorption of griseofulvin.
MAO inhibitors: inhibited metabolism of barbiturates; may cause prolonged CNS depression. Reduce barbiturate dosage.
Rifampin: may decrease barbiturate levels. Monitor for decreased effect.

CONTRAINDICATIONS
• Contraindicated in patients with uncontrolled severe pain, respiratory disease with dyspnea or obstruction, hypersensitivity to barbiturates, previous addiction to sedatives, or porphyria.
• Use cautiously in patients with hepatic or renal impairment.

NURSING CONSIDERATIONS
• Elderly patients are more sensitive to the drug's adverse CNS effects. Assess mental status before initiating therapy.
• Caution patients about performing activities that require mental alertness or physical coordination. For inpatients, supervise walking and raise bed rails, particularly for elderly patients.
• Long-term use is not recommended: drug loses its efficacy in promoting sleep after 14 days of continued use. Long-term high dosage may cause drug dependence, and patient may experience withdrawal symptoms if drug is suddenly discontinued. Withdraw barbiturates gradually.
• Take precautions to prevent hoarding or self-overdosing by patients who are depressed, suicidal, or drug-dependent, or who have a history of drug abuse.
• Pentobarbital has no analgesic effect and may cause restlessness or delirium in patients with pain.
• Watch for signs of barbiturate toxicity: coma, pupillary constriction, cyanosis, clammy skin, and hypotension. Overdose can be fatal.
• Skin eruptions may precede potentially fatal reactions to barbiturate therapy. Discontinue drug when skin reactions occur. In some patients, high fever, stomatitis, headache, or rhinitis may precede skin reactions.
• To ensure accurate dosage, don't divide suppositories.
• Morning "hangover" is common after hypnotic dose, which suppresses REM sleep. Patient may experience increased dreaming after drug is discontinued.
• Patients who use oral contraceptives should consider alternate birth control methods because drug may enhance contraceptive hormone metabolism and decrease its effect.
• Hypnotic doses suppress REM sleep. Patient may experience increased dreaming after drug is discontinued.
• **I.V. use:** Reserve I.V. injection for emergency treatment, which should be given under close supervision. Administer slowly at a rate not exceeding 50 mg/minute.
• To minimize deterioration, use injection solution within 30 minutes after opening container. Don't use cloudy solution.
• I.V. administration of barbiturates may cause severe respiratory depression, laryngospasm, or hypotension. Have emergency resuscitation equipment available.

• Parenteral solution is alkaline. Local tissue reactions and injection site pain have followed I.V. use. Avoid extravasation. Assess patency of I.V. site before and during administration.
• Administer I.M. injection deeply. Superficial injection may cause pain, sterile abscess, and sloughing.
• Do not mix in syringe or I.V. with other drugs.

quazepam

Doral
Controlled Substance Schedule IV
Pregnancy Risk Category: X

HOW SUPPLIED

Tablets: 7.5 mg, 15 mg

ACTION

Mechanism: Acts on the limbic system and thalamus of CNS by binding to specific benzodiazepine receptors. **Onset:** within 1 hour. **Peak:** Plasma levels peak in about 2 hours. **Duration:** variable; some active metabolites have long half-lives (3 days).

INDICATIONS & DOSAGE

Insomnia –
Adults: 15 mg P.O. h.s. Some patients may respond to lower doses. Decrease dosage in elderly patients to 7.5 mg P.O. h.s. after 2 days of therapy.

ADVERSE REACTIONS

CNS: *fatigue, dizziness, daytime drowsiness, headache.*

INTERACTIONS

Ethanol or other CNS depressants, including antihistamines, opiate analgesics, and other benzodiazepines: increased CNS depression. Avoid concomitant use.

CONTRAINDICATIONS

• Contraindicated in patients allergic to this drug or other benzodiazepines, in pregnant patients, and in patients with suspected or established sleep apnea.
• Use cautiously in patients with hepatic, renal, or respiratory disease, and in elderly patients.

NURSING CONSIDERATIONS

• Warn patients about the possible additive depressant effects that can occur if alcohol is consumed within 24 hours of quazepam.
• Patients on long-term therapy with benzodiazepines may experience withdrawal symptoms if the drug is suddenly withdrawn (possibly after 6 weeks of continuous therapy).
• Check CBC before and periodically during long-term therapy. Observe for signs of hematologic toxicity, such as easy bruising or bleeding, or signs of infection.
• Take precautions to prevent hoarding or self-overdosing by patients who are depressed, suicidal, or drug-dependent, or who have a history of drug abuse.
• Caution patients about performing activities that require mental alertness or physical coordination. For inpatients, supervise walking and raise bed rails, particularly for elderly patients.
• Warn patients not to increase the drug dosage but to inform the doctor if they feel lack of effectiveness.
• If quazepam overdose occurs, flumazenil (a specific benzodiazepine antagonist) may be useful. However, flumazenil's duration of action is shorter than quazepam's, and resedation is possible.

secobarbital sodium

Novosecobarb†, Seconal Sodium
Controlled Substance Schedule II
Pregnancy Risk Category: D

HOW SUPPLIED
Tablets: 100 mg
Capsules: 50 mg, 100 mg
Injection: 50 mg/ml
Rectal injection: 50 mg/ml
Suppositories: 200 mg

ACTION
Mechanism: Probably interferes with transmission of impulses from the thalamus to the cortex of the brain. A barbiturate.
Onset: 10 to 15 minutes after oral administration. **Duration:** effects persist 3 to 4 hours.

INDICATIONS & DOSAGE
Sedation, preoperatively –
Adults: 200 to 300 mg P.O. 1 to 2 hours before surgery.
Children: 2 to 6 mg/kg P.O. or 4 to 5 mg/kg P.R. 1 to 2 hours before surgery. Maximum single dose is 100 mg.
Insomnia –
Adults: 100 to 200 mg P.O. or I.M.
Children: 3 to 5 mg/kg I.M., not to exceed 100 mg, with no more than 5 ml injected in any one site or 4 to 5 mg/kg P.R.
Acute tetanus seizure –
Adults and children: 5.5 mg/kg I.M. or slow I.V., repeated q 3 to 4 hours, if needed; I.V. injection rate not to exceed 50 mg/15 seconds.
Acute psychotic agitation –
Adults: 50 mg/minute I.V. up to 250 mg I.V. initially; additional doses given cautiously after 5 minutes if desired response is not obtained. Not to exceed 500 mg total.
Status epilepticus –
Adults and children: 5 to 6 mg/kg slow I.V. or I.M.

ADVERSE REACTIONS
CNS: *drowsiness, lethargy, hangover,* paradoxical excitement in elderly patients.
CV: hypotension (with I.V. use).
GI: nausea, vomiting.
Hematologic: exacerbation of porphyria.
Respiratory: ***respiratory depression.***
Skin: rash, urticaria, ***Stevens-Johnson syndrome,*** tissue reactions and injection site pain.
Other: ***angioedema.***

INTERACTIONS
Chloramphenicol, MAO inhibitors, valproic acid: inhibited metabolism of barbiturates; may cause prolonged CNS depression. Reduce barbiturate dosage.
Corticosteroids, digitoxin, doxycycline, estrogens and oral contraceptives, oral anticoagulants, tricyclic antidepressants: secobarbital may enhance the metabolism of these drugs. Monitor for decreased effect.
Ethanol or other CNS depressants, including narcotic analgesics: excessive CNS and respiratory depression. Use together cautiously.
Griseofulvin: decreased absorption of griseofulvin.
Lactated Ringer's solution, acidic solutions: incompatible with I.V. form of drug. Don't mix.
Rifampin: may decrease barbiturate levels. Monitor for decreased effect.

CONTRAINDICATIONS
- Contraindicated in patients with uncontrolled severe pain, respiratory disease with dyspnea or obstruction, hypersensitivity to barbiturates, previous addiction to sedatives, or porphyria.
- Use cautiously in patients with hepatic or renal impairment and in pregnant patients with toxemia or history of bleeding.

NURSING CONSIDERATIONS
- If used to manage seizures, appropriate precautions should be taken.
- Elderly patients are more sensitive to the drug's adverse CNS reactions. Assess mental status before initiating therapy.

• Because barbiturates potentiate the effects of narcotics, reduce dose when giving during labor. Excessive dose may cause respiratory depression in neonate.
• Caution patients about performing activities that require mental alertness or physical coordination. For inpatients, supervise walking and raise bed rails, particularly for elderly patients.
• May cause drug dependence and severe withdrawal symptoms. Withdraw barbiturates gradually.
• Take precautions to prevent hoarding or self-overdosing by patients who are depressed, suicidal, or drug-dependent, or who have a history of drug abuse.
• Watch for signs of barbiturate toxicity: coma, pupillary constriction, cyanosis, clammy skin, and hypotension. Overdose can be fatal.
• Morning "hangover" is common after hypnotic dose, which suppresses REM sleep. Patient may experience increased dreaming after drug is discontinued.
• Long-term use is not recommended: drug loses its efficacy in promoting sleep after 14 days of continued use. Long-term high dosage may cause drug dependence, and patient may experience withdrawal symptoms if drug is suddenly stopped.
• Skin eruptions may precede potentially fatal reactions to barbiturate therapy. Discontinue drug when skin reactions occur. In some patients, high fever, stomatitis, headache, or rhinitis may precede skin reactions.
• Patients who use oral contraceptives should consider alternate birth control methods because drug may enhance contraceptive hormone metabolism and decrease its effect.
• **I.V. use:** Reserve I.V. injection for emergency treatment and give under close supervision by direct injection, and administer slowly at a rate not exceeding 50 mg/15 seconds. May be administered as supplied or diluted.
• Use injection solution within 30 minutes after opening container to minimize deterioration. Don't use cloudy solution.
• Secobarbital sodium injection is not compatible with lactated Ringer's solution, but is compatible with Ringer's solution, sterile water for injection, and 0.9% sodium chloride. Don't mix with acidic solutions.
• I.V. administration of barbiturates may cause severe respiratory depression, laryngospasm, or hypotension. Have emergency resuscitation equipment readily available.
• Local tissue reactions and injection site pain have been noted with I.V. use. Assess patency of I.V. site before and during administration.
• Give I.M. injection deeply. Superficial injection may cause pain, sterile abscess, and sloughing.

temazepam

Euhypnos 10‡, Euhypnos 20‡, Razepam, Normison‡, Restoril, Temaze‡

Controlled Substance Schedule IV

Pregnancy Risk Category: X

HOW SUPPLIED

Capsules: 10 mg‡, 15 mg, 20 mg‡, 30 mg

ACTION

Mechanism: Acts on the limbic system, thalamus, and hypothalamus of CNS to produce hypnotic effects. A benzodiazepine.
Onset: typically 30 to 60 minutes, but possibly up to 2½ hours. **Peak:** Serum levels peak in 1 to 3 hours.
Duration: half-life, 10 to 17 hours.

INDICATIONS & DOSAGE

Insomnia –
Adults: 15 to 30 mg P.O. h.s.

Adults over 65 years: 15 mg P.O. h.s.

ADVERSE REACTIONS

CNS: *drowsiness, dizziness, lethargy,* disturbed coordination, daytime sedation, confusion.

GI: anorexia, diarrhea.

INTERACTIONS

Ethanol or other CNS depressants, including narcotic analgesics: increased CNS depression. Use together cautiously.

CONTRAINDICATIONS

- Contraindicated in patients hypersensitive to this drug or other benzodiazepines.
- Use cautiously in patients with impaired hepatic or renal function, mental depression, suicidal tendencies, and history of drug abuse. Also use cautiously and in low end of dosage range in elderly or debilitated patients.

NURSING CONSIDERATIONS

- Elderly patients are more sensitive to the drug's adverse CNS reactions. Assess mental status before initiating therapy.
- Take precautions to prevent hoarding or self-overdosing by patients who are depressed, suicidal, or drug-dependent, or who have a history of drug abuse.
- Caution patients about performing activities that require mental alertness or physical coordination. For inpatients, supervise walking and raise bed rails, particularly for elderly patients.
- May cause less residual sedation ("hangover") than flurazepam and diazepam. Relatively short-acting.
- Tell patients that onset of the drug's effects may take as long as 2 to 2 ½ hours.
- If temazepam overdose occurs, flumazenil (a specific benzodiazepine antagonist) may be useful. However, flumazenil's duration of action is shorter than temazepam's, and resedation is possible.

triazolam

Apo-Triazo†, Halcion, Novotriolam†, Nu-Triazo†

Controlled Substance Schedule IV

Pregnancy Risk Category: X

HOW SUPPLIED

Tablets: 0.125 mg, 0.25 mg

ACTION

Mechanism: Acts on the limbic system, thalamus, and hypothalamus of the CNS to produce hypnotic effects. A benzodiazepine.

Onset: 15 to 30 minutes. **Peak:** Serum levels peak in 1 to 2 hours.

Duration: plasma half-life, 1½ to 5½ hours.

INDICATIONS & DOSAGE

Insomnia –

Adults: 0.125 to 0.25 mg P.O. h.s.

Adults over 65: 0.125 mg P.O. h.s.; increase as needed to 0.25 mg P.O. h.s.

ADVERSE REACTIONS

CNS: *drowsiness, dizziness, headache,* rebound insomnia, amnesia, light-headedness, lack of coordination, mental confusion, depression.

GI: nausea, vomiting.

Other: physical or psychological abuse.

INTERACTIONS

Cimetidine, erythromycin: may cause prolonged triazolam blood levels. Monitor for increased sedation.

Ethanol or other CNS depressants, including narcotic analgesics: excessive CNS depression. Use together cautiously.

CONTRAINDICATIONS
- Contraindicated in patients with hypersensitivity to benzodiazepines.
- Use cautiously in patients with impaired hepatic or renal function, mental depression, suicidal tendencies, or history of drug abuse.

NURSING CONSIDERATIONS
- Elderly patients are more sensitive to the drug's adverse CNS reactions. Assess mental status before initiating therapy.
- Use drug in the lowest effective dose for only 5 to 7 days.
- Take precautions to prevent hoarding or self-overdosing by patients who are depressed, suicidal, or drug-dependent, or who have a history of drug abuse.
- Caution patients about performing activities that require mental alertness or physical coordination. For inpatients, supervise walking and raise bed rails, particularly for elderly patients.
- Physical and psychological dependence is possible with long-term use.
- Triazolam is a benzodiazepine compound with similarities to flurazepam. However, it is very short-acting and therefore has less tendency to cause morning drowsiness.
- Warn patients not to take more than the prescribed amount because overdosage can occur at a total daily dose of 2 mg (or four times the highest recommended amount).
- Tell patients that rebound insomnia may develop for one or two nights after stopping therapy.
- Because of numerous reports of adverse CNS reactions, triazolam has been withdrawn from several foreign markets. An FDA panel recently reviewed the drug's safety and efficacy; it is currently still available in the United States.
- If triazolam overdose occurs, flumazenil (a specific benzodiazepine antagonist) may be useful. However, flumazenil's duration of action is shorter than triazolam's, and resedation is possible.

zolpidem tartrate

Ambien

Controlled Substance Schedule IV

Pregnancy Risk Category: B

HOW SUPPLIED

Tablets: 5 mg, 10 mg

ACTION

Mechanism: Although zolpidem interacts with one of three identified GABA-benzodiazepine (gamma-aminobutyric acid-benzodiazepine) receptor complexes, it's not a benzodiazepine. It exhibits hypnotic activity, but no muscle relaxant or anticonvulsant properties.
Peak: Serum levels peak in 1½ hours.
Duration: serum half-life, about 2½ hours.

INDICATIONS & DOSAGE

Short-term management of insomnia – **Adults:** 10 mg P.O. immediately before bedtime.

In elderly or debilitated patients; patients with hepatic insufficiency: 5 mg P.O. immediately before bedtime. Maximum daily dosage is 10 mg.

ADVERSE REACTIONS

CNS: daytime drowsiness, light-headedness, abnormal dreams, amnesia, dizziness, headache, hangover effect, sleep disorder.
CV: palpitations.
EENT: sinusitis, pharyngitis, dry mouth.
GI: nausea, vomiting, diarrhea.
Skin: rash.
Other: back or chest pain, influenza-like symptoms, hypersensitivity reactions.

INTERACTIONS

Ethanol or other CNS depressants: enhanced CNS depression. Avoid concomitant use.

CONTRAINDICATIONS

- Contraindicated in patients with hypersensitivity to the drug.
- Use cautiously in patients with compromised respiratory status because hypnotics may depress respiratory drive. Also use cautiously in patients with depression or a history of alcohol or drug abuse.

NURSING CONSIDERATIONS

- Use hypnotics only for short-term management of insomnia, usually 7 to 10 days. Persistent insomnia may indicate a primary psychiatric or medical disorder. Reevaluate patient if drug is taken for more than 2 to 3 weeks. Typically, prescriptions for this drug provide a maximum of 1 month's supply.
- Because most adverse reactions are dose-related, use the smallest effective dose in all patients, but especially in elderly and debilitated patients.
- Caution patients about performing activities that require mental alertness or physical coordination. For inpatients, supervise walking and raise bed rails, particularly for elderly patients.
- Food decreases drug's absorption. For faster sleep onset, instruct patients not to take drug with or immediately after meals.
- Although abrupt discontinuation of hypnotics after prolonged therapy is commonly associated with withdrawal syndrome, no clear evidence of such a syndrome after abrupt termination of zolpidem therapy exists.
- Take precautions to prevent hoarding or self-overdosing by patients who are depressed, suicidal, or drug-dependent or who have a history of drug abuse.
- Zolpidem overdose may be treated with flumazenil, a specific benzodiazepine antagonist; however, because the mean elimination half-life of zolpidem (2½ hours) is longer than that of flumazenil, repeated doses of flumazenil may be necessary.

29
Anticonvulsants

acetazolamide sodium
(See Chapter 61, DIURETICS.)
carbamazepine
clonazepam
diazepam
(See Chapter 31, ANTIANXIETY AGENTS.)
ethosuximide
ethotoin
felbamate
gabapentin
magnesium sulfate
mephenytoin
mephobarbital
methsuximide
paramethadione
phenacemide
phenobarbital
phenobarbital sodium
phensuximide
phenytoin
phenytoin sodium
phenytoin sodium (extended)
primidone
trimethadione
valproate sodium
valproic acid
divalproex sodium

COMBINATION PRODUCTS
DILANTIN WITH PHENOBARBITAL: phenytoin sodium 100 mg and phenobarbital 16 mg; phenytoin sodium 100 mg and phenobarbital 32 mg.

carbamazepine
Apo-Carbamazepine†, Epitol, Mazepine†, Novocarbamaz†, PMS-Carbamazepine†, Tegretol, Tegretol Chew-Tabs, Tegretol CR†, Teril‡

Pregnancy Risk Category: C

HOW SUPPLIED
Tablets: 200 mg
Tablets (chewable): 100 mg
Tablets (extended-release)†: 200 mg, 400 mg
Oral suspension: 100 mg/5 ml

ACTION
Mechanism: Stabilizes neuronal membranes and limits seizure activity by either increasing efflux or decreasing influx of sodium ions across cell membranes in the motor cortex during generation of nerve impulses.
Onset: in trigeminal neuralgia, 8 to 72 hours; anticonvulsant effect, hours to days. **Peak:** Serum levels peak in 1 ½ hours after oral suspension, 4 to 12 hours after tablets. **Duration:** half-life, initially 25 to 65 hours; half-life, 12 to 17 hours with chronic use.

INDICATIONS & DOSAGE
Generalized tonic-clonic and complex-partial seizures, mixed seizure patterns –
Adults and children over 12 years: initially, 200 mg P.O. b.i.d. May increase at weekly intervals by 200 mg P.O. daily, in divided doses at 6- to 8-hour intervals. Adjust to minimum effective level when control is achieved. Do not exceed 1 g/day in children ages 12 to 15, or 1.2 g/day in patients over age 15.
Children under 12 years: initially 100 mg P.O. b.i.d. Increase at weekly intervals by 100 mg P.O. daily. Do not exceed 1 g/day. Alternatively, give 10 to 20 mg/kg P.O. daily in 3 to 4 divided doses.
Trigeminal neuralgia –
Adults: initially, 100 mg P.O. b.i.d. with meals. Increase by 100 mg q 12 hours until pain is relieved. Don't exceed 1.2 g/day. Maintenance dosage is 200 to 400 mg P.O. b.i.d.
Prophylaxis and treatment of bipolar disorder; psychotic disorders –

Adults: initially, 100 mg P.O. b.i.d. with meals. Increase by 100 mg q 12 hours as needed and tolerated. Don't exceed 1.6 g daily.

ADVERSE REACTIONS

CNS: dizziness, *vertigo, drowsiness,* fatigue, *ataxia,* ***worsening of seizures*** (usually in patients with mixed seizure disorders including atypical absence seizures).
CV: ***CHF,*** hypertension, hypotension, aggravation of coronary artery disease.
EENT: conjunctivitis, dry mouth and pharynx, blurred vision, diplopia, nystagmus.
GI: *nausea,* vomiting, abdominal pain, diarrhea, anorexia, *stomatitis,* glossitis.
GU: urinary frequency, urine retention, impotence, albuminuria, glycosuria, elevated BUN.
Hematologic: ***aplastic anemia, agranulocytosis,*** eosinophilia, leukocytosis, ***thrombocytopenia.***
Hepatic: abnormal liver function tests, ***hepatitis.***
Respiratory: pulmonary hypersensitivity.
Skin: *rash,* urticaria, erythema multiforme, ***Stevens-Johnson syndrome.***
Other: excessive sweating, fever, chills, water intoxication.

INTERACTIONS

Cimetidine, diltiazem, macrolides such as erythromycin, isoniazid, propoxyphene, valproic acid, verapamil: may increase carbamazepine blood levels. Use cautiously.
Doxycycline, haloperidol, phenytoin, theophyline, warfarin: carbamazepine may decrease blood levels of these drugs. Monitor for decreased effect.
Lithium: increased CNS toxicity of lithium. Avoid concomitant use.
MAO inhibitors: increased depressant and anticholinergic effects. Don't use together.
Nicotinic acid, phenobarbital, phenytoin, primidone: may decrease carbamazepine levels. Monitor for decreased effect.

CONTRAINDICATIONS

- Contraindicated in patients with bone marrow suppression or hypersensitivity to carbamazepine or tricyclic antidepressants and in patients who have taken an MAO inhibitor within 14 days of therapy.
- Use cautiously in patients with cardiac, kidney, or liver damage and in those with increased intraocular pressure. Also use cautiously in children with mixed seizure disorders because they may experience an increased incidence of seizures (usually atypical absence or generalized seizures).

NURSING CONSIDERATIONS

- When managing seizures, institute appropriate precautions.
- Shake oral suspension well before measuring dose.
- When administering by nasogastric tube, mix dose with an equal volume of water, 0.9% sodium chloride, or D_5W. Flush tube with 100 ml of diluent after administering dose.
- Not effective in treating absence seizures.
- Therapeutic carbamazepine blood level is 3 to 9 mcg/ml. Monitor blood levels and effects closely. Ask the patient when last dose of medication was taken to approximately evaluate blood levels.
- Obtain baseline determinations of urinalysis, BUN level, liver function, CBC, platelet and reticulocyte counts, and serum iron level. Monitor periodically thereafter.
- Advise patients to avoid driving or other potentially hazardous activities that require mental alertness until the CNS effects of the drug are known.
- May cause mild to moderate dizziness and drowsiness when first taken. Effect usually disappears within 3 to 4 days. Administer three times a day,

when possible, to provide consistent blood levels.
• Observe for signs of anorexia or subtle appetite changes, which may indicate excessive blood levels.
• Never discontinue suddenly when treating seizures or status epilepticus. Notify doctor immediately if adverse reactions occur.
• Periodic eye examinations are recommended.
• Tell patients to notify the doctor immediately if fever, sore throat, mouth ulcers, or easy bruising or bleeding occurs.
• When used for trigeminal neuralgia, attempt to decrease dosage or withdraw drug every 3 months.
• Adverse reactions may be minimized by increasing dosage gradually.
• An alternative to lithium in treatment of some affective disorders.
• Take carbamazepine with food to minimize GI distress.
• Tell patients to keep tablets in their original container, tightly closed, and away from moisture. Some formulations may harden when exposed to excess moisture, resulting in decreased bioavailability and loss of seizure control.

clonazepam

Klonopin, Rivotril
Controlled Substance Schedule IV
Pregnancy Risk Category: C

HOW SUPPLIED
Tablets: 0.5 mg, 1 mg, 2 mg
Drops: 2.5 mg/ml‡
Injection: 1 mg/ml‡

ACTION
Mechanism: A benzodiazepine that acts by facilitating the effects of the inhibitory neurotransmitter gamma amino butyric acid.
Onset: 20 to 30 minutes. **Peak:** Serum levels peak in 1 to 2 hours.
Duration: effects persist 6 to 12 hours.

INDICATIONS & DOSAGE
Lennox-Gastaut syndrome and atypical absence seizures; akinetic and myoclonic seizures –
Adults: initially, not to exceed 1.5 mg P.O. daily in three divided doses. May be increased by 0.5 to 1 mg q 3 days until seizures are controlled. If given in unequal doses, the largest dose should be given h.s. Maximum recommended daily dosage is 20 mg.
Children up to 10 years or 30 kg: initially, 0.01 to 0.03 mg/kg P.O. daily (not to exceed 0.05 mg/kg daily), divided q 8 hours. Increase dosage by 0.25 to 0.5 mg q third day to a maximum maintenance dosage of 0.1 to 0.2 mg/kg daily.
Status epilepticus (where parenteral form is available) –
Adults: 1 mg by slow I.V. infusion.
Children: 0.5 mg by slow I.V. infusion.

ADVERSE REACTIONS
CNS: *drowsiness, ataxia, behavioral disturbances (especially in children),* slurred speech, tremor, confusion, psychosis, agitation.
EENT: *increased salivation,* diplopia, nystagmus, abnormal eye movements, sore gums.
GI: constipation, gastritis, change in appetite, nausea, abnormal thirst.
GU: dysuria, enuresis, nocturia, urine retention.
Hematologic: leukopenia, thrombocytopenia, eosinophilia.
Respiratory: ***respiratory depression.***
Skin: rash.

INTERACTIONS
Ethanol or other CNS depressants: increased CNS depression. Monitor closely.

*Liquid form contains alcohol.
**May contain tartrazine.
Common reactions are in italics; ***life-threatening,*** in bold italics.

CONTRAINDICATIONS

- Contraindicated in patients with hepatic disease; in those with sensitivity to chlordiazepoxide, diazepam, or other benzodiazepines; or in patients with acute angle-closure glaucoma.
- Use cautiously in patients with mixed seizure types because drug may precipitate generalized tonic-clonic seizures. Also use cautiously in patients with chronic respiratory disease, impaired renal function, or open-angle glaucoma.

NURSING CONSIDERATIONS

- Therapeutic blood level is 20 to 80 ng/ml.
- Elderly patients are more sensitive to the drug's CNS effects.
- Advise patients to avoid driving or other potentially hazardous activities that require mental alertness until the CNS effects are known.
- Never withdraw suddenly because seizures may worsen. Call the doctor at once if adverse reactions develop.
- Monitor CBC and liver function tests.
- Monitor patient for oversedation.
- Withdrawal symptoms are similar to those of barbiturates.
- Instruct parents to monitor child's school performance because clonazepam may interfere with attentiveness in school.
- **I.V. use‡:** Give slowly by direct injection or by slow I.V. infusion. Drug may be diluted with D_5W, dextrose 2½% in water, 0.9% sodium chloride, or 0.45% sodium chloride.
- Mix solutions in glass bottles because the drug binds to polyvinyl chloride (PVC) plastics. If PVC infusion bags are used, administer immediately and infuse at a rate of 60 ml/hour or greater.

ethosuximide

Zarontin

Pregnancy Risk Category: C

HOW SUPPLIED

Capsules: 250 mg
Syrup: 250 mg/5 ml

ACTION

Mechanism: Increases seizure threshold. Reduces the paroxysmal spike-and-wave pattern of absence seizures by depressing nerve transmission in the motor cortex. A succinimide derivative.
Peak: Peak effect occurs in 3 to 7 hours. **Duration:** plasma half-life, 56 to 60 hours in adults, 30 to 36 hours in children.

INDICATIONS & DOSAGE

Absence seizure –
Adults and adolescents: initially, 15 to 30 mg/kg P.O. daily. Alternatively, give 250 mg P.O. b.i.d. May increase by 250 mg q 4 to 7 days up to 1.5 g daily.
Children: 15 to 40 mg/kg P.O. daily in divided doses. Alternatively, give 250 mg P.O. daily or 125 mg P.O. b.i.d. May increase by 250 mg q 4 to 7 days up to 1 g daily.
Note: The optimal dosage for most children is 20 mg/kg P.O. daily.

ADVERSE REACTIONS

CNS: *drowsiness,* headache, *fatigue, dizziness,* ataxia, irritability, hiccups, *euphoria, lethargy, depression, psychosis.*
EENT: myopia, tongue swelling, gum hypertrophy.
GI: *nausea, vomiting,* diarrhea, weight loss, cramps, *anorexia, epigastric and abdominal pain.*
GU: vaginal bleeding, urinary frequency.
Hematologic: leukopenia, eosinophilia, ***agranulocytosis,*** pancytopenia, ***aplastic anemia.***

Skin: urticaria, pruritic and erythematous rashes, hirsutism.

INTERACTIONS
None significant.

CONTRAINDICATIONS
- Contraindicated in patients with hypersensitivity to succinimide derivatives.
- Use cautiously in patients with hepatic or renal disease.

NURSING CONSIDERATIONS
- Never withdraw drug suddenly. Abrupt withdrawal may precipitate absence seizures. Call doctor immediately if adverse reactions develop.
- Advise patients to avoid driving or other potentially hazardous activities that require mental alertness until the CNS effects are known.
- Obtain CBC every 3 to 6 months.
- Therapeutic blood levels are 40 to 80 mcg/ml.
- May increase frequency of generalized tonic-clonic seizures when used alone in patients who have mixed types of seizures.
- May cause positive direct Coombs' test.
- Currently the drug of choice for treating absence seizures.
- Advise patients to take ethosuximide with food to minimize GI distress.

ethotoin
Peganone

Pregnancy Risk Category: D

HOW SUPPLIED
Tablets: 250 mg, 500 mg

ACTION
Mechanism: Stabilizes neuronal membranes and limits seizure activity by either increasing efflux or decreasing influx of sodium ions across cell membranes in the motor cortex during generation of nerve impulses. Hydantoin derivative.
Peak: Serum levels peak about 2 hours after a dose. **Duration:** half-life, 3 to 9 hours.

INDICATIONS & DOSAGE
Generalized tonic-clonic or complex-partial seizures—
Adults: initially, 250 mg P.O. q.i.d. after meals. May increase slowly over several days to 3 g daily divided q.i.d.
Children: initially, 250 mg P.O. b.i.d. May increase up to 250 mg P.O. q.i.d.

ADVERSE REACTIONS
CNS: fatigue, insomnia, dizziness, headache, numbness, slurred speech, ataxia.
CV: chest pain.
EENT: diplopia, nystagmus, gingival hyperplasia (rare).
GI: *nausea, vomiting, diarrhea.*
Hematologic: thrombocytopenia, leukopenia, ***agranulocytosis, pancytopenia,*** megaloblastic anemia.
Skin: rash.
Other: fever, lymphadenopathy.

INTERACTIONS
Antihistamines, chloramphenicol, cimetidine, diazepam, disulfiram, isoniazid, phenylbutazone, salicylates, sulfamethizole, valproate: increased ethotoin activity and toxicity; monitor closely.
Diazoxide: decreased ethotoin activity. Monitor closely.
Ethanol (chronic use), folic acid: decreased ethotoin activity; monitor closely.
Phenacemide: paranoia. Use together cautiously.

CONTRAINDICATIONS
- Contraindicated in patients with hydantoin hypersensitivity and in those with hepatic or hematologic disorders.

• Use cautiously in patients receiving other hydantoin derivatives.

NURSING CONSIDERATIONS

• Never withdraw drug suddenly because seizures may worsen. Call the doctor at once if adverse reactions develop.
• Advise patients to avoid driving or other potentially hazardous activities that require mental alertness until the CNS effects of the drug are known.
• Monitor CBC and urinalysis when therapy starts and periodically thereafter. Also, periodically monitor liver function tests on long-term use.
• Tell patients to take drug after meals. Schedule doses as evenly as possible over 24 hours.
• Discontinue if lymphadenopathy or lupuslike syndrome (fever, bruising, and sore throat) develops.
• Caution patients that heavy alcohol use may diminish drug's benefits.
• Ethotoin is the hydantoin derivative of choice for young adults prone to gingival hyperplasia caused by phenytoin. Otherwise, infrequently used to treat epilepsy.
• Ethotoin generally produces milder adverse reactions than phenytoin; however, the large doses required to maintain its therapeutic effect frequently cause GI distress.

felbamate

Felbatol

Pregnancy Risk Category: C

HOW SUPPLIED

Tablets: 400 mg, 600 mg
Oral suspension: 600 mg/5 ml

ACTION

Mechanism: A dicarbamate anticonvulsant; mechanism of action is unclear. Drug may act by elevating the seizure threshold or preventing the spread of seizure activity.

Duration: plasma elimination half-life, 20 to 23 hours.

INDICATIONS & DOSAGE

Refractory partial seizures in adults; Lennox-Gastaut syndrome –

Adults and children ages 14 and older: when used as the sole treatment, initiate therapy at 1,200 mg P.O. daily in 3 or 4 divided doses. Titrate dosage in 600-mg increments every 2 weeks to 2,400 mg/day and finally to 3,600 mg/day if needed and tolerated.

When used in patients taking other anticonvulsant drugs, initiate therapy at 1,200 mg daily in 3 or 4 divided doses while reducing the dosage of carbamazepine, phenytoin, or valproic acid by 20%. Increase felbamate dosage by 1,200 mg/day in divided doses at weekly intervals to a maximum of 3,600 mg/day; concomitant reductions in the dosage of other anticonvulsants may be necessary.

To switch to felbamate from other anticonvulsants –

Adults and children ages 14 and over: initiate therapy at 1,200 mg/day in 3 or 4 divided doses while reducing the dosage of concurrent anticonvulsants by one-third. During the second week of treatment, increase the felbamate dosage to 2,400 mg daily in 3 or 4 divided doses while cutting the dosage of the other anticonvulsant by another one-third. Increase the dosage of felbamate to 3,600 mg/day in divided doses by the third week, and continue to reduce the dosage of other anticonvulsants as needed and tolerated.

Children ages 2 to 14: initiate therapy at 15 mg/kg/day in divided doses 3 or 4 times a day while reducing the dosage of carbamazepine, phenytoin, or valproic acid by 20%. Increase dosage by 15 mg/kg/day in 3 or 4 divided doses in weekly intervals to a maximum of 45 mg/day. Reduce dosage of other anticonvulsants as needed to minimize adverse effects.

ADVERSE REACTIONS

CNS: *insomnia, headache,* fatigue, anxiety.
EENT: blurred or double vision, otitis media.
GI: *dyspepsia, vomiting, constipation, diarrhea.*
GU: urinary tract infection, intramenstrual bleeding.
Skin: acne, rash.
Other: increased ALT, *upper respiratory infection, rhinitis,* hypophosphatemia, weight loss, facial edema.

INTERACTIONS

Carbamazepine: decreased steady-state levels of carbamazepine and increased levels of its active metabolite; increased felbamate clearance, resulting in decreased plasma levels. Use together cautiously.
Phenytoin, valproic acid: increased steady-state levels of phenytoin or valproic acid; increased felbamate clearance, reducing its blood levels. Use together cautiously.

CONTRAINDICATIONS

- Contraindicated in patients hypersensitive to the drug.
- Use cautiously in patients hypersensitive to other carbamates. Because the drug has been detected in breast milk, consider risk-benefit before giving to breast-feeding patients.

NURSING CONSIDERATIONS

- Discontinue other antiepileptic drugs slowly because of a possible increase in the frequency of seizures.
- When managing seizures, institute appropriate seizure precautions.
- Shake oral suspension well before measuring dose.
- Warn patients to avoid hazardous activities that require alertness and good psychomotor coordination until CNS effects are known.
- When added to other anticonvulsants, monitor blood levels of these drugs and patient response closely because felbamate can alter pharmacokinetics of carbamazepine, phenytoin, and valproic acid. Ask the patient when last dose of medication was taken to approximately evaluate blood levels. When used alone, routine monitoring of felbamate blood levels is not necessary.
- Food does not interfere with absorption of felbamate's tablet form; food's effects on the suspension are unknown.

gabapentin

Neurontin

Pregnancy Risk Category: C

HOW SUPPLIED

Capsules: 100 mg, 300 mg, 400 mg

ACTION

Mechanism: Unknown. Although structurally related to gamma-amino butyric acid (GABA), the drug doesn't interact with GABA receptors and isn't converted metabolically into GABA or a GABA agonist.
Duration: elimination half-life, 5 to 7 hours.

INDICATIONS & DOSAGE

Adjunctive treatment of partial seizures with and without secondary generalization –
Adults: initially 300 mg P.O. h.s. on day 1. Increase to 300 mg P.O. b.i.d. on day 2, then 300 mg P.O. t.i.d. on day 3. Increase dosage as needed and tolerated to 1,800 mg daily in divided doses. The usual dosage is 300 to 600 mg P.O. t.i.d., although dosages up to 3,600 mg/day have been well tolerated.

In patients with renal failure: if creatinine clearance is > 60 ml/minute, give 400 mg P.O. t.i.d.; if creatinine clearance is 30 to 60 ml/minute, give

300 mg P.O. b.i.d.; if creatinine clearance is 15 to 30 ml/minute, give 300 mg P.O. daily; if creatinine clearance is < 15 ml/minute, give 300 mg P.O. every other day. Patients on dialysis should receive a loading dose of 300 to 400 mg P.O.; then 200 mg to 300 mg P.O. following every 4 hours of hemodialysis.

ADVERSE REACTIONS

CNS: *somnolence, dizziness, ataxia, fatigue, nystagmus, tremor,* nervousness, dysarthria, amnesia, depression, abnormal thinking, twitching, abnormal coordination.
CV: peripheral edema, vasodilation.
EENT: *diplopia,* rhinitis, pharyngitis, dry throat, coughing, amblyopia.
GI: nausea, vomiting, dyspepsia, dry mouth, constipation.
GU: impotence.
Hematologic: leukopenia, decreased WBC count.
Skin: pruritus, abrasion.
Other: dental abnormalities, increased appetite, weight gain, back pain, myalgia, fractures.

INTERACTIONS

Antacids: decreased absorption of gabapentin. Separate administration times by at least 2 hours.

CONTRAINDICATIONS

- Contraindicated in patients hypersensitive to the drug.
- Use cautiously in elderly patients and in patients with renal impairment.

NURSING CONSIDERATIONS

- Warn patients to avoid driving or operating heavy machinery until the adverse CNS effects of the drug are known.
- Give the first dose at bedtime to minimize drowsiness, dizziness, fatigue, and ataxia.
- If gabapentin therapy is discontinued or alternative medication is substituted, do so gradually over at least 1 week to minimize risk of precipitating seizures. Do not suddenly withdraw other anticonvulsant drugs in patients starting gabapentin therapy.
- Tell patients to take the drug without regard to meals.
- Routine monitoring of plasma levels of gabapentin is not necessary. The drug does not appear to alter plasma levels of other anticonvulsants.
- May cause false-positive tests for urine protein when the Ames-N-Multistix SG dipstick test is used.

magnesium sulfate

Pregnancy Risk Category: B

HOW SUPPLIED

Injection: 10% (0.8 mEq/ml), 12.5% (1 mEq/ml), 25% (2 mEq/ml), 50% (4 mEq/ml)

ACTION

Mechanism: May decrease acetylcholine released by nerve impulses, but its anticonvulsant mechanism is unknown.
Onset: 1 to 2 minutes after I.V. use; after I.M. injection, 1 hour. **Duration:** effects persist about 30 minutes after I.V. administration, 3 to 4 hours after I.M. injection.

INDICATIONS & DOSAGE

Hypomagnesemic seizures –
Adults: 1 to 2 g (as 10% solution) I.V. over 15 minutes; then 1 g I.M. q 4 to 6 hours, based on patient response and blood magnesium levels.
Seizures secondary to hypomagnesemia in acute nephritis –
Children: 0.2 ml/kg of 50% solution I.M. q 4 to 6 hours, p.r.n. or 100 mg/kg of 10% solution I.V. very slowly. Titrate dosage according to blood magnesium levels and seizure response.
Prevention or control of seizures in preeclampsia or eclampsia –
Women: initially, 4 g I.V. in 250 ml

D_5W and 4 g deep I.M. each buttock; then 4 g deep I.M. into alternate buttock q 4 hours, p.r.n. Alternatively, 4 g I.V. loading dose, followed by 1 to 4 g hourly as I.V. infusion.

Management of paroxysmal atrial tachycardia –

Adults: 3 to 4 g I.V. over 30 seconds.

Management of life-threatening ventricular arrhythmias, such as sustained ventricular tachycardia or torsades de pointes –

Adults: 2 to 6 g I.V. over several minutes, followed by a continuous infusion of 3 to 20 mg/minute for 5 to 48 hours. Dosage and duration of therapy depend on patient response and serum magnesium levels.

ADVERSE REACTIONS

CNS: drowsiness, *depressed reflexes,* flaccid paralysis, hypothermia.

CV: *hypotension, flushing,* ***circulatory collapse,*** depressed cardiac function, ***heart block.***

Other: diaphoresis, ***respiratory paralysis,*** hypocalcemia.

INTERACTIONS

Anesthetics, CNS depressants: may cause additive CNS depression. Use cautiously.

Digitalis: concomitant use may exacerbate arrhythmias. Use together cautiously.

Neuromuscular blocking agents: may cause increased neuromuscular blockade. Use cautiously.

CONTRAINDICATIONS

- Use cautiously in patients with arrhythmias, impaired renal function, myocardial damage, and heart block. Also use cautiously in women in labor.

NURSING CONSIDERATIONS

- Drug can decrease the frequency and force of uterine contractions. Has been used as a tocolytic agent (suppresses uterine contractions) to inhibit premature labor.
- If used to treat seizures, institute appropriate seizure precautions.
- **I.V. use:** If necessary, dilute to a maximum concentration of 20%. Infuse no faster than 150 mg/minute (1.5 ml/minute of a 10% solution or 0.75 ml/minute of a 20% solution). Drug is compatible with D_5W.
- Monitor vital signs every 15 minutes when giving drug I.V.
- Watch for respiratory depression and signs of heart block. Respirations should be approximately 16 breaths/minute before each dose.
- Monitor fluid intake and output. Urine output should be 100 ml or more in 4-hour period before each dose.
- Keep I.V. calcium gluconate available to reverse magnesium intoxication; however, use cautiously in patients undergoing digitalization because of danger of arrhythmias.
- Check blood magnesium levels after repeated doses. Disappearance of knee-jerk and patellar reflexes is a sign of pending magnesium toxicity.
- Signs of hypermagnesemia begin to appear at blood levels of 4 mEq/liter.
- Maximum infusion rate is 150 mg/minute. Rapid drip will induce uncomfortable feeling of heat.
- Observe neonates for signs of magnesium toxicity, including neuromuscular or respiratory depression, when giving drug I.V. to toxemic mothers within 24 hours before delivery.

mephenytoin

Mesantoin

Pregnancy Risk Category: C

HOW SUPPLIED

Tablets: 100 mg

ACTION

Mechanism: Stabilizes neuronal membranes and limits seizure activity

*Liquid form contains alcohol.
**May contain tartrazine.

by either increasing efflux or decreasing influx of sodium ions across cell membranes in the motor cortex during generation of nerve impulses. Hydantoin derivative.
Duration: half-life of drug and active metabolite nirvanol, 95 to 144 hours.

INDICATIONS & DOSAGE
Generalized tonic-clonic or complex-partial seizures –
Adults: 50 to 100 mg P.O. daily. May increase by 50 to 100 mg at weekly intervals up to 200 mg P.O. t.i.d.
Children: initially, 50 to 100 mg P.O. daily or 100 to 450 mg/m² P.O. daily in three divided doses. May increase slowly by 50 to 100 mg at weekly intervals up to 200 mg P.O. t.i.d., divided q 8 hours. Dosage must be adjusted individually.

ADVERSE REACTIONS
CNS: ataxia, *drowsiness,* fatigue, irritability, choreiform movements, depression, tremor, sleeplessness, dizziness (usually transient).
EENT: conjunctivitis, diplopia, nystagmus, gingival hyperplasia (with prolonged use).
GI: nausea and vomiting (with prolonged use).
Hematologic: ***leukopenia, neutropenia, agranulocytosis, thrombocytopenia, pancytopenia,*** eosinophilia.
Skin: *rashes,* ***exfoliative dermatitis,*** hypertrichosis, photosensitivity.
Other: edema, dysarthria, lymphadenopathy, polyarthropathy, ***pulmonary fibrosis.***

INTERACTIONS
Antihistamines, chloramphenicol, cimetidine, diazepam, disulfiram, isoniazid, phenylbutazone, salicylates, sulfamethizole, valproate: ethotoin activity and toxicity; monitor closely.
Diazoxide: decreased mephenytoin activity. Monitor closely.
Ethanol (chronic use), folic acid: decreased ethotoin activity; monitor closely.

CONTRAINDICATIONS
- Contraindicated in patients with hydantoin hypersensitivity.
- Use cautiously in patients receiving other hydantoin derivatives.

NURSING CONSIDERATIONS
- Periodically monitor liver function studies with long-term use. Check CBC and platelet count before therapy and periodically thereafter. Discontinue drug if neutrophil count becomes less than 1,600/mm³.
- Never withdraw drug suddenly because seizures may worsen. Call the doctor if adverse reactions develop.
- Therapeutic blood level of mephenytoin and its active metabolite is 25 to 40 mcg/ml.
- Caution patients that heavy alchol use may diminish drug's benefits.
- Potentially life-threatening blood dyscrasias limit this drug's usefulness.
- Tell patients to notify the doctor if fever, sore throat, bleeding, or rash occurs.
- Advise patients to avoid driving or other hazardous activities that require mental alertness until CNS effects are known.
- This drug has been associated with photosensitivity reactions. Advise patients to use a sunblock, wear protective clothing, and avoid prolonged exposure to sunlight.

mephobarbital
Mebaral
Controlled Substance Schedule IV
Pregnancy Risk Category: D

HOW SUPPLIED
Tablets: 32 mg, 50 mg, 100 mg

ACTION
Mechanism: Depresses monosynaptic and polysynaptic transmission in

the CNS and increases the threshold for seizure activity in the motor cortex. Some activity comes from phenobarbital, an active metabolite. A barbiturate.
Onset: about 60 minutes. **Duration:** half-life of phenobarbital, 75 to 126 hours; effects persist 10 to 12 hours.

INDICATIONS & DOSAGE
Generalized tonic-clonic or absence seizures –
Adults: 400 to 600 mg P.O. daily or in divided doses.
Children: 6 to 8 mg/kg P.O. daily, divided q 6 to 8 hours (smaller doses are given initially and increased over 4 to 5 days as needed).

ADVERSE REACTIONS
CNS: *dizziness,* headache, *hangover,* confusion, paradoxical excitation, exacerbation of existing pain, drowsiness.
CV: hypotension, bradycardia.
GI: nausea, vomiting, epigastric pain.
Hematologic: megaloblastic anemia, ***agranulocytosis,*** thrombocytopenia, enhanced porphyria.
Respiratory: ***respiratory depression.***
Skin: urticaria, morbilliform rash, blisters, purpura, ***erythema multiforme.***
Other: allergic reactions (facial edema).

INTERACTIONS
Chloramphenicol, MAO inhibitors, valproic acid: potentiated barbiturate effect. Monitor patient for increased CNS and respiratory depression.
Corticosteroids, digitoxin, doxycycline, estrogens and oral contraceptives, oral anticoagulants, tricyclic antidepressants: mephobarbital may enhance the metabolism of these drugs. Monitor for decreased effect.
Ethanol or other CNS depressants, including narcotic analgesics: excessive CNS depression. Use cautiously.
Griseofulvin: decreased absorption of griseofulvin.
Rifampin: may decrease barbiturate levels. Monitor for decreased effect.

CONTRAINDICATIONS
- Contraindicated in patients with barbiturate hypersensitivity, porphyria, or respiratory disease with dyspnea or obstruction.
- Use cautiously in patients with hepatic, renal, cardiac, or respiratory function impairment; myasthenia gravis; or myxedema.

NURSING CONSIDERATIONS
- Never withdraw suddenly because seizures may worsen. Call the doctor at once if adverse reactions develop.
- Advise patients to avoid driving or other potentially hazardous activities that require mental alertness until CNS effects are known.
- Advise adults with nighttime seizures to take total or largest dose at night.
- Three-quarters of drug is metabolized to phenobarbital within 24 hours; therapeutic blood levels as phenobarbital are 15 to 40 mcg/ml.
- Periodically monitor CBC, and BUN and creatinine levels.
- Patients who use oral contraceptives should consider alternate birth control methods because drug may enhance contraceptive hormone metabolism and decrease its effectiveness.
- Suppresses REM sleep. When drug is discontinued, patient may experience increased dreaming.
- Store in light-resistant container.

methsuximide (mesuximide)
Celontin

Pregnancy Risk Category: C

HOW SUPPLIED
Capsules: 150 mg, 300 mg

*Liquid form contains alcohol. *Common* reactions are in italics; ***life-threatening,*** in bold italics.
**May contain tartrazine.

ACTION
Mechanism: Increases seizure threshold. Reduces the paroxysmal spike-and-wave pattern of absence seizures by depressing nerve transmission in the motor cortex. A succinimide derivative.
Duration: half-life of parent drug, 1 to 3 hours; of active metabolites, 36 to 45 hours.

INDICATIONS & DOSAGE
Refractory absence seizures –
Adults and children: initially, 300 mg P.O. daily. May increase by 300 mg daily at weekly intervals. Maximum daily dosage is 1.2 g in divided doses.

ADVERSE REACTIONS
CNS: *drowsiness, ataxia, dizziness,* irritability, nervousness, headache, insomnia, confusion, depression, aggressiveness.
EENT: blurred vision, photophobia, periorbital edema.
GI: *nausea, vomiting, anorexia,* diarrhea, weight loss, abdominal or epigastric pain.
Hematologic: eosinophilia, ***aplastic anemia, leukopenia,*** monocytosis, ***pancytopenia.***
Skin: urticaria, pruritic and erythematous rashes.

INTERACTIONS
None significant.

CONTRAINDICATIONS
• Contraindicated in patients with hypersensitivity to succinimide derivatives.
• Use cautiously in patients with hepatic or renal dysfunction.

NURSING CONSIDERATIONS
• Therapeutic serum level is 10 to 40 mcg/ml.
• Never change or withdraw drug suddenly. Abrupt withdrawal may precipitate absence seizures. Call the doctor immediately if adverse reactions develop.
• Advise patients to avoid driving or other hazardous activities that require mental alertness until CNS effects are known.
• Check CBC, urinalysis, and liver function tests periodically.
• Tell patients to call the doctor promptly if lupuslike syndrome develops.
• Caution patients that this drug may color urine pink or brown.

paramethadione
Paradione* **

Pregnancy Risk Category: D

HOW SUPPLIED
Capsules: 150 mg, 300 mg
Oral solution: 300 mg/ml (65% alcohol) with dropper

ACTION
Mechanism: Raises the threshold for cortical seizures but does not modify seizure pattern. Decreases projection of focal activity and reduces both repetitive spinal-cord transmission and spike-and-wave patterns of absence (petit mal) seizures.
Peak: Serum levels peak 30 minutes to 1 hour after a dose. **Duration:** half-life, 12 to 24 hours.

INDICATIONS & DOSAGE
Refractory absence seizures –
Adults: initially, 300 mg P.O. t.i.d. May increase by 300 mg weekly, up to 600 mg q.i.d., if needed.
Children over 6 years: 0.9 g P.O. daily in divided doses t.i.d. or q.i.d.
Children 2 to 6 years: 0.6 g P.O. daily in divided doses t.i.d. or q.i.d.
Children under 2 years: 0.3 g P.O. daily in divided doses b.i.d.

ADVERSE REACTIONS
CNS: *drowsiness,* fatigue, vertigo, headache, paresthesia, irritability, myasthenic syndrome.
CV: hypertension, hypotension.
EENT: day-blindness (hemeralopia), photophobia, diplopia, epistaxis, retinal hemorrhage, bleeding gums.
GI: nausea, vomiting, abdominal pain, weight loss.
GU: albuminuria, vaginal bleeding.
Hematologic: ***neutropenia, leukopenia,*** eosinophilia, ***thrombocytopenia, pancytopenia, agranulocytosis, hypoplastic and aplastic anemia.***
Hepatic: abnormal liver function tests.
Skin: acneiform or morbilliform rash, ***exfoliative dermatitis, erythema multiforme,*** petechiae, alopecia, photosensitivity.
Other: lymphadenopathy, lupuslike syndrome.

INTERACTIONS
None significant.

CONTRAINDICATIONS
- Contraindicated in patients with renal and hepatic dysfunction or severe blood dyscrasia.
- Use cautiously in patients with retinal or optic nerve diseases.

NURSING CONSIDERATIONS
- Advise patients to call the doctor at once if nausea, dizziness, and visual disturbances occur because they may be signs of overdosage.
- Never withdraw drug suddenly because seizures may worsen. Call the doctor at once if adverse reactions develop.
- Discontinue drug if scotomata or signs of hepatitis, systemic lupus erythematosus, lymphadenopathy, skin rash, nephrosis, hair loss, or generalized tonic-clonic seizures appear.
- Tell patients to report sore throat, fever, malaise, bruises, petechiae, or epistaxis to the doctor immediately.
- Drug has been associated with photosensitivity reactions. Advise patients to use a sunblock, wear protective clothing, and avoid prolonged exposure to sunlight.
- Suggest that patients wear dark glasses if bright light blurs vision. Tell patients to notify the doctor if this occurs.
- Advise patients to avoid driving or other potentially hazardous activities that require mental alertness until the CNS effects of the drug are known.
- Monitor liver function studies and urinalysis before therapy; then monthly.
- Before administering oral solution, dilute it with water because it contains 65% alcohol.
- Give drug with food or milk to minimize GI upset.
- Monitor CBC. Discontinue drug if neutrophil count falls below 2,500/mm^3.

phenacemide (phenacetylcarbamide)
Phenurone

Pregnancy Risk Category: D

HOW SUPPLIED
Tablets: 500 mg

ACTION
Mechanism: Stabilizes neuronal membranes and limits seizure activity by either increasing efflux or decreasing influx of sodium ions across cell membranes in the motor cortex during generation of nerve impulses. Hydantoin derivative.
Peak: Serum levels peak 1 to 2 hours after a dose. **Duration:** half-life, 22 to 25 hours.

INDICATIONS & DOSAGE
Refractory, complex-partial, generalized tonic-clonic, absence, and atypical absence seizures –
Adults: 500 mg P.O. t.i.d. May in-

crease by 500 mg P.O. daily at weekly intervals up to a maximum of 5 g daily.
Children 5 to 10 years: 250 mg P.O. t.i.d. May increase by 250 mg daily at weekly intervals, up to a maximum of 1.5 g daily.

ADVERSE REACTIONS
CNS: drowsiness, dizziness, insomnia, headache, paresthesia, ***depression, suicidal tendencies,*** aggressiveness.
GI: anorexia, weight loss.
GU: nephritis with marked albuminuria.
Hematologic: *aplastic anemia, agranulocytosis,* leukopenia.
Hepatic: hepatitis, jaundice.
Skin: rashes.

INTERACTIONS
Ethotoin: paranoia. Use together cautiously.
Other anticonvulsants: enhanced risk of toxicity.

CONTRAINDICATIONS
- Contraindicated in patients with preexisting personality disturbances or in patients achieving satisfactory seizure control with other anticonvulsants.
- Use cautiously in patients with hepatic dysfunction or history of allergy, and when a hydantoin derivative is used concomitantly.
- Extremely toxic. Use drug only when other anticonvulsants are ineffective.

NURSING CONSIDERATIONS
- Check liver function tests, CBCs, and urinalyses before and at monthly intervals during therapy.
- Tell patients to report sore throat or fever to the doctor immediately.
- Warn patients to avoid activities that require alertness or good psychomotor coordination until CNS effects are known.
- Never withdraw suddenly. Call the doctor at once if adverse reactions develop.
- Tell the patient's family to watch for personality or psychological changes and report them to the doctor at once.
- When phenacemide replaces another anticonvulsant, increase phenacemide dosage slowly while slowly decreasing the dosage of the drug being discontinued to maintain adequate seizure control.
- Notify the doctor if the patient develops jaundice or other signs of hepatitis, abnormal urinary findings, or WBC count below 4,000/mm³.

phenobarbital (phenobarbitone)
Ancalixir†, Barbita, Solfoton

phenobarbital sodium (phenobarbitone sodium)
Luminal Sodium†

Controlled Substance Schedule IV
Pregnancy Risk Category: D

HOW SUPPLIED
Tablets: 8 mg, 15 mg, 16 mg, 30 mg, 32 mg, 60 mg, 65 mg, 100 mg
Capsules: 16 mg
Elixir:* 15 mg/5 ml, 20 mg/5 ml
Injection: 30 mg/ml, 60 mg/ml, 65 mg/ml, 130 mg/ml
Powder for injection: 120 mg/ampule

ACTION
Mechanism: Depresses monosynaptic and polysynaptic transmission in the CNS and increases the threshold for seizure activity in the motor cortex. As a sedative, probably interferes with transmission of impulses from the thalamus to the cortex of the brain. A barbiturate.
Onset: within 15 minutes of I.V. injection, 20 to 60 minutes after I.M. injection, within 60 minutes of oral administration. **Peak:** Peak effects occur 15 to 30 minutes after I.V. in-

jection, 1 to 6 hours after I.M. injection, 8 to 10 hours after oral administration. **Duration:** effects persist 10 to 12 hours.

INDICATIONS & DOSAGE

All forms of epilepsy, febrile seizures in children –
Adults: 100 to 200 mg P.O. daily, divided t.i.d. or given as single dose h.s.
Children: 4 to 6 mg/kg P.O. daily, usually divided q 12 hours. It can, however, be administered once daily, usually h.s.
Status epilepticus –
Adults: 10 mg/kg as I.V. infusion no faster than 50 mg/minute. May give up to 20 mg/kg total. Administer in acute care or emergency area only.
Children: 5 to 10 mg/kg I.V. May repeat q 10 to 15 minutes up to total of 20 mg/kg. I.V. injection rate should not exceed 50 mg/minute.
Sedation –
Adults: 30 to 120 mg P.O. daily in two or three divided doses.
Children: 3 to 5 mg/kg P.O. daily divided t.i.d.
Insomnia –
Adults: 100 to 320 mg P.O. or I.M.
Children: 3 to 5 mg/kg.
Preoperative sedation –
Adults: 100 to 200 mg I.M. 60 to 90 minutes before surgery.
Children: 16 to 100 mg I.M. 60 to 90 minutes before surgery.
Hyperbilirubinemia –
Neonates: 7 mg/kg/day P.O. from first to fifth day of life; or 5 mg/kg/day I.M. on first day, repeated P.O. on second to seventh days.
Chronic cholestasis –
Adults and children ages 12 and older: 90 to 180 mg P.O. daily in two or three divided doses.
Children under age 12: 3 to 12 mg/kg/day P.O. in two or three divided doses.

ADVERSE REACTIONS

CNS: *drowsiness, lethargy, hangover,* paradoxical excitement in elderly patients.
CV: bradycardia, hypotension.
GI: nausea, vomiting.
Hematologic: exacerbation of porphyria.
Respiratory: ***respiratory depression.***
Skin: rash, ***erythema multiforme, Stevens-Johnson syndrome,*** urticaria; pain, swelling, thrombophlebitis, necrosis, nerve injury at injection site.
Other: ***angioedema.***

INTERACTIONS

Chloramphenicol, MAO inhibitors, valproic acid: potentiated barbiturate effect. Monitor patient for increased CNS and respiratory depression.
Corticosteroids, digitoxin, doxycycline, estrogens and oral contraceptives, oral anticoagulants, tricyclic antidepressants: mephobarbital may enhance the metabolism of these drugs. Monitor for decreased effect.
Diazepam: increased effects of both drugs. Use together cautiously.
Ethanol or other CNS depressants, including narcotic analgesics: excessive CNS depression. Use cautiously.
Griseofulvin: decreased absorption of griseofulvin.
Mephobarbital, primidone: excessive phenobarbital blood levels; monitor closely.
Rifampin: may decrease barbiturate levels. Monitor for decreased effect.
Valproic acid: increased phenobarbital levels. Monitor for toxicity.

CONTRAINDICATIONS

- Contraindicated in patients with barbiturate hypersensitivity, porphyria, hepatic dysfunction, respiratory disease with dyspnea or obstruction, and nephritis; and in breast-feeding patients.
- Use cautiously in patients with hyperthyroidism, diabetes mellitus, and

anemia, and in elderly or debilitated patients.

NURSING CONSIDERATIONS

- Elderly patients are more sensitive to the drug's effects.
- Watch for signs of barbiturate toxicity: coma, asthmatic breathing, cyanosis, clammy skin, and hypotension. Overdose can be fatal.
- Advise patients to avoid driving or other potentially hazardous activities that require mental alertness until CNS effects are known.
- Don't stop drug abruptly because seizures may worsen. Call the doctor immediately if adverse reactions develop.
- Full therapeutic effects not seen for 2 to 3 weeks, except when loading dose is used.
- Therapeutic blood levels are 15 to 40 mcg/ml.
- Make sure patients are aware that phenobarbital is available in different milligram strengths and sizes.
- Patients using oral contraceptives should consider alternate birth control methods because drug may enhance contraceptive hormone metabolism and decrease its effect.
- **I.V. use:** Reserve I.V. injection for emergency treatment and give slowly under close supervision. Monitor respirations closely. When administering I.V., do not give more than 60 mg/minute. Have resuscitation equipment available.
- Give I.M. injection deeply. Superficial injection may cause pain, sterile abscess, and tissue sloughing.
- Do not use injectable solution if it contains a precipitate.
- Do not mix parenteral form with acidic solutions; precipitation may result.

phensuximide

Milontin

Pregnancy Risk Category: D

HOW SUPPLIED

Capsules: 500 mg

ACTION

Mechanism: Increases seizure threshold. Reduces the paroxysmal spike-and-wave pattern of absence seizures by depressing nerve transmission in the motor cortex. A succinimide derivative.

Peak: Serum levels peak in 1 to 4 hours. **Duration:** half-life, 5 to 12 hours.

INDICATIONS & DOSAGE

Absence seizures –

Adults and children: 500 mg to 1 g P.O. b.i.d. to t.i.d.

ADVERSE REACTIONS

CNS: muscular weakness, *drowsiness,* dizziness, ataxia, headache.

GI: nausea, vomiting, anorexia.

GU: urinary frequency, renal damage, hematuria.

Hematologic: transient leukopenia, ***aplastic anemia, pancytopenia, agranulocytosis.***

Skin: pruritus, eruptions, erythema.

Other: lupuslike syndrome.

INTERACTIONS

None significant.

CONTRAINDICATIONS

- Contraindicated in patients with hypersensitivity to succinimide derivatives.
- Use cautiously in patients with hepatic or renal disease.

NURSING CONSIDERATIONS

- Therapeutic blood level is 40 to 80 mcg/ml.
- May increase incidence of generalized tonic-clonic seizures if used

alone to treat patients with mixed seizure types.

- Never withdraw drug suddenly. Abrupt withdrawal may precipitate absence seizures. Call the doctor immediately if adverse reactions develop.
- Advise patients to avoid driving or other potentially hazardous activities that require mental alertness until the CNS effects of the drug are known.
- Check CBC every 3 to 4 months; urinalysis and liver function tests every 6 months.
- Tell patients to report lupuslike symptoms immediately.
- Caution patients that this drug may color urine pink or red to reddish brown.

phenytoin (diphenylhydantoin)

Dilantin, Dilantin Infatabs, Dilantin-30 Pediatric, Dilantin-125

phenytoin sodium

Dilantin, Phenytex

phenytoin sodium (extended)

Dilantin Kapseals

Pregnancy Risk Category: D

HOW SUPPLIED

phenytoin
Tablets (chewable): 50 mg
Oral suspension: 30 mg/5 ml, 125 mg/5 ml
phenytoin sodium
Capsules: 30 mg (27.6-mg base), 100 mg (92-mg base)
Injection: 50 mg/ml (46-mg base)
phenytoin sodium (extended)
Capsules: 30 mg (27.6-mg base), 100 mg (92-mg base)

ACTION

Mechanism: Stabilizes neuronal membranes and limits seizure activity by either increasing efflux or decreasing influx of sodium ions across cell membranes in the motor cortex during generation of nerve impulses. When used to treat digitalis glycoside-induced arrhythmias, produces antiarrhythmic effect by normalizing sodium influx to Purkinje's fibers. Hydantoin derivative.
Peak: Peak levels occur immediately after I.V. injection, 1½ to 3 hours after tablets or oral solution, 4 to 12 hours after extended capsules. **Duration:** elimination half-life averages 22 hours (dose-dependent).

INDICATIONS & DOSAGE

Generalized tonic-clonic seizures, status epilepticus, nonepileptic seizures (post-head trauma, Reye's syndrome) –
Adults: loading dose is 900 mg to 1.5 g I.V. no faster than 50 mg/minute or P.O. divided t.i.d.; then start maintenance dosage of 300 mg P.O. daily (extended only) or divided t.i.d.
Children: loading dose is 15 mg/kg I.V. no faster than 50 mg/minute or P.O. divided q 8 to 12 hours; then start maintenance dosage of 5 to 7 mg/kg P.O. or I.V. daily, divided q 12 hours.
For patient who has not received phenytoin previously or has no detectable drug level, use loading dose –
Adults: 900 mg to 1.5 g I.V. divided into t.i.d. no faster than 50 mg/minute. Do not exceed 500 mg each dose.
Children: 15 mg/kg I.V. no faster than 50 mg/minute.
For patient who has been receiving phenytoin but has missed one or more doses and has subtherapeutic levels of the drug –
Adults: 100 to 300 mg I.V. no faster than 50 mg/minute.
Children: 5 to 7 mg/kg I.V. no faster than 50 mg/minute. May repeat lower dose in 30 minutes p.r.n.
Neuritic pain (migraine, trigeminal neuralgia, Bell's palsy) –
Adults: 200 to 400 mg P.O. daily.

Ventricular arrhythmias unresponsive to lidocaine or procainamide; supraventricular and ventricular arrhythmias induced by digitalis glycosides – **Adults:** loading dose is 1 g P.O. divided over first 24 hours, followed by 500 mg daily for 2 days, then maintenance dose of 100 mg P.O. b.i.d. or q.i.d., or 100 mg I.V. q 5 minutes until arrhythmias subside, adverse reactions develop, or 1 g has been given. Infusion rate should never exceed 50 mg/minute (slow I.V. push).

Or administer entire loading dose of 1 g I.V. slowly at 25 mg/minute, or dilute in 0.9% sodium chloride solution. I.M. dose not recommended because of pain and erratic absorption. **Children:** 3 to 8 mg/kg/day P.O. or slow I.V. or 250 mg/m²/day given as single dose or in two divided doses.

ADVERSE REACTIONS

CNS: *ataxia, slurred speech, confusion,* dizziness, insomnia, nervousness, twitching, headache.
CV: hypotension, ***ventricular fibrillation.***
EENT: *nystagmus, diplopia,* blurred vision, *gingival hyperplasia (especially in children).*
GI: *nausea, vomiting.*
Hematologic: ***thrombocytopenia, leukopenia, agranulocytosis, pancytopenia,*** macrocytosis, megaloblastic anemia.
Hepatic: ***toxic hepatitis.***
Skin: scarlatiniform or morbilliform rash; bullous, *exfoliative,* or purpuric dermatitis; ***Stevens-Johnson syndrome;*** lupus erythematosus; *hirsutism;* ***toxic epidermal necrolysis;*** photosensitivity; pain, necrosis, and inflammation at injection site; discoloration of skin ("purple glove syndrome") if given by I.V. push in back of hand.
Other: periarteritis nodosa, lymphadenopathy, hyperglycemia, osteomalacia, hypertrichosis.

INTERACTIONS

Amiodarone, antihistamines, chloramphenicol, cimetidine, cycloserine, diazepam, disulfiram, influenza vaccine, isoniazid, phenylbutazone, salicylates, sulfamethizole, valproate: monitor for increased phenytoin activity and toxicity.
Dexamethasone, diazoxide, ethanol (chronic use), folic acid: decreased phenytoin activity; monitor closely.
Oral tube feedings with Osmolite or Isocal: may interfere with absorption of oral phenytoin. Schedule feedings as far as possible from drug administration.

CONTRAINDICATIONS

- Contraindicated in patients with phenacemide or hydantoin hypersensitivity, bradycardia, SA or AV block, or Stokes-Adams syndrome.
- Use cautiously in patients with hepatic or renal dysfunction, hypotension, myocardial insufficiency, and respiratory depression; in elderly or debilitated patients; and in patients receiving other hydantoin derivatives.

NURSING CONSIDERATIONS

- Elderly patients tend to metabolize phenytoin slowly and may require lower dosages.
- If using to treat seizures, take appropriate precautions.
- Phenytoin requirements usually increase during pregnancy. Monitor serum levels closely.
- Don't withdraw drug suddenly because seizures may worsen. Call the doctor at once if adverse reactions develop.
- Advise patients to avoid driving or other potentially hazardous activities that require mental alertness until CNS effects are known.
- Monitor CBC and serum calcium levels every 6 months, and periodically monitor hepatic function. If megaloblastic anemia is evident, the

doctor may order folic acid and vitamin B_{12}.

• Caution patients that this drug may color urine pink, red, or reddish-brown.

• Stress importance of good oral hygiene and regular dental examinations. Gingivectomy may be necessary periodically if dental hygiene is poor.

• Drug should be discontinued if rash appears. If rash is scarlet or measles-like, drug may be resumed after rash clears. If rash reappears, therapy should be discontinued. If rash is exfoliative, purpuric, or bullous, don't resume drug.

• Divided doses given with or after meals may decrease GI adverse reactions.

• Shake suspension well before each dose. Use tablets or capsules, if possible.

• Therapeutic phenytoin blood level is 10 to 20 mcg/ml.

• Heavy alcohol use may diminish drug's benefits.

• Mononucleosis may decrease phenytoin levels. Monitor for increased seizure activity.

• Dilantin brand and Bolar generic capsules are the only oral forms that can be given once daily. Toxic levels may result if any other brand is given once daily. Dilantin brand tablets and oral suspension should not be taken once daily.

• Advise patient not to change brands or dosage forms once stabilized on therapy.

• Suspension available as 30 mg/5 ml or 125 mg/5 ml. Read label carefully.

• Therapy with phenytoin may cause laboratory test interferences, including reduced serum protein-bound iodine and free thyroxine levels without clinical signs of hypothyroidism; a slight decrease in urinary 17-hydroxysteroid and 17-ketosteroid levels; increased urinary 6-ß hydroxycortisol excretion and serum levels of alkaline phosphatase or γ-glutamyltransferase; and decreased values for dexamethasone suppression or metyrapone tests.

• **I.V. use:** Administer slowly (50 mg/minute) as I.V. bolus. If giving as an infusion, don't mix drug with D_5W because it will precipitate. Clear I.V. tubing first with 0.9% sodium chloride solution. Never use cloudy solution. May mix with this solution if necessary and give as an infusion over 30 to 60 minutes when possible. Infusion must begin within 1 hour after preparation and should run through an in-line filter. Discard 4 hours after preparation.

• Check patency of I.V. catheter before administering. Extravasation has caused severe local tissue damage.

• Check vital signs, blood pressure, and ECG during I.V. administration.

• Avoid administering phenytoin by I.V. push into veins on the back of the hand to avoid discoloration known as purple glove syndrome. Inject into larger veins or central venous catheter if available.

• Do not give I.M. unless dosage adjustments are made. Drug may precipitate at injection site, cause pain, and be erratically absorbed.

• Use only clear solution for injection. A slight yellow color is acceptable. Don't refrigerate.

primidone

Apo-Primidone†, Myidone, Mysoline, PMS-Primidone†, Sertan†

Pregnancy Risk Category: D

HOW SUPPLIED

Tablets: 50 mg, 250 mg

Oral suspension: 250 mg/5 ml

ACTION

Mechanism: Unknown, but some activity may be caused by phenylethyl-

*Liquid form contains alcohol. *Common* reactions are in italics; ***life-threatening,*** in bold italics.

**May contain tartrazine.

malonamide (PEMA) and phenobarbital, which are active metabolites.
Peak: Serum levels peak in 3 to 4 hours. **Duration:** half-life of primidone, 3 to 23 hours; of PEMA, 10 to 25 hours; of phenobarbital, 75 to 126 hours.

INDICATIONS & DOSAGE
Generalized tonic-clonic seizures, complex-partial seizures –
Adults and children over 8 years: 250 mg P.O. daily. Increase by 250 mg weekly, up to maximum of 2 g daily, divided q.i.d.
Children under 8 years: 125 mg P.O. daily. Increase by 125 mg weekly, up to maximum of 25 mg/kg daily, divided q.i.d.

ADVERSE REACTIONS
CNS: *drowsiness, ataxia,* emotional disturbances, vertigo, hyperirritability, fatigue.
EENT: *diplopia,* nystagmus, edema of the eyelids.
GI: anorexia, *nausea, vomiting,* thirst.
GU: impotence, polyuria.
Hematologic: leukopenia, eosinophilia.
Respiratory: ***respiratory depression.***
Skin: morbilliform rash, alopecia.
Other: edema.

INTERACTIONS
Carbamazepine: increased primidone levels. Observe for toxicity.
Phenytoin: stimulated conversion of primidone to phenobarbital. Observe for increased phenobarbital effect.

CONTRAINDICATIONS
- Contraindicated in patients with phenobarbital hypersensitivity or porphyria.

NURSING CONSIDERATIONS
- Don't withdraw drug suddenly because seizures may worsen. Call the doctor if adverse reactions develop.
- Advise patients to avoid driving or other potentially hazardous activities that require mental alertness until CNS effects are known.
- Full therapeutic response may take 2 weeks or more.
- Therapeutic blood level of primidone is 5 to 12 mcg/ml. Therapeutic blood level of phenobarbital is 15 to 40 mcg/ml.
- Monitor CBC and routine blood chemistry every 6 months.
- Shake liquid suspension well.

trimethadione
Tridione, Tridone Dulcets
Pregnancy Risk Category: D

HOW SUPPLIED
Capsules: 300 mg
Tablets (chewable): 150 mg
Oral solution: 200 mg/5 ml

ACTION
Mechanism: Raises the threshold for cortical seizure but does not modify seizure pattern. Decreases projection of focal activity and reduces both repetitive spinal-cord transmission and spike-and-wave patterns of absence (petit mal) seizures. An oxazolidinedione derivative.
Duration: half-life of trimethadione, 11 to 16 hours; of dimethadione, an active metabolite, 10 days.

INDICATIONS & DOSAGE
Refractory absence seizures –
Adults and children over 13 years: initially, 300 mg P.O. t.i.d. May increase by 300 mg P.O. daily at weekly intervals to a maximum of 600 mg P.O. q.i.d.
Children: 13 mg/kg P.O. t.i.d. or 335 mg/m^2 P.O. t.i.d.; alternatively, give according to age.
Children under 2 years: 100 mg P.O. t.i.d.
Children 2 to 6 years: 200 mg P.O. t.i.d.

Children 6 to 13 years: 300 mg P.O. t.i.d.

ADVERSE REACTIONS
CNS: *drowsiness,* fatigue, *malaise,* insomnia, dizziness, headache, paresthesia, irritability.
CV: hypertension, hypotension.
EENT: *day-blindness (hemeralopia),* diplopia, photophobia, epistaxis, retinal hemorrhage.
GI: nausea, vomiting, anorexia, abdominal pain, bleeding gums.
GU: nephrosis, albuminuria, vaginal bleeding.
Hematologic: ***neutropenia, leukopenia,*** eosinophilia, ***thrombocytopenia, pancytopenia, agranulocytosis, hypoplastic and aplastic anemia.***
Hepatic: abnormal liver function tests.
Skin: acneiform and morbilliform rash, ***exfoliative dermatitis, erythema multiforme,*** petechiae, alopecia, photosensitivity.
Other: lymphadenopathy, lupuslike syndrome, myasthenia-like syndrome.

INTERACTIONS
None significant.

CONTRAINDICATIONS
- Contraindicated in patients with paramethadione and trimethadione hypersensitivity, severe blood dyscrasia, or hepatic dysfunction.
- Use with extreme caution in patients with retinal and optic nerve diseases.

NURSING CONSIDERATIONS
- Don't withdraw drug suddenly. Abrupt withdrawal may precipitate absence seizures. Call doctor immediately if adverse reactions develop.
- Check CBC, hepatic function, and urinalysis before starting therapy and monthly thereafter. Drug should be stopped if neutrophil count falls below 2,500/mm³.
- Watch for impending toxicity; may precipitate tonic-clonic seizure.
- Warn patients to report skin rash, alopecia, sore throat, fever, bruises, or epistaxis to the doctor immediately.
- Advise patients to avoid driving or other potentially hazardous activities that require mental alertness until the CNS effects of the drug are known.
- Advise patients to use a sunblock, wear protective clothing, and avoid prolonged exposure to sunlight.
- Suggest sunglasses if bright light blurs the patients' vision. Tell patients to notify the doctor if this occurs.
- If scotomata or rash develops, drug should be discontinued.
- May increase risk of tonic-clonic seizures if used alone to treat patients who have mixed types of seizures.

---

valproate sodium
Depakene Syrup, Epilim‡, Myproic Acid Syrup

valproic acid
Depakene, Myproic Acid

divalproex sodium
Depakote, Depakote Sprinkle, Epival†, Valcote‡

Pregnancy Risk Category: D

HOW SUPPLIED
valproate sodium
Syrup: 250 mg/ml‡
valproic acid
Tablets (enteric-coated): 200 mg‡, 500 mg‡
Crushable tablets: 100 mg‡
Capsules: 250 mg
Syrup: 200 mg/5 ml‡
divalproex sodium
Capsules (delayed-release): 125 mg
Tablets (enteric-coated): 125 mg, 250 mg, 500 mg

ACTION
Mechanism: Increases brain levels of gamma-aminobutyric acid, which transmits inhibitory nerve impulses in the CNS.
Peak: Serum levels peak within 1 to 4

hours after capsules or syrup; 3 to 4 hours after tablets and delayed-release capsules. **Duration:** half-life, variable from 6 to 16 hours.

INDICATIONS & DOSAGE

Simple and complex absence seizures, mixed seizure types (including absence seizures), investigationally in generalized, tonic-clonic seizures – **Adults and children:** initially, 15 mg/kg P.O. daily divided b.i.d. or t.i.d.; then may increase by 5 to 10 mg/kg daily at weekly intervals up to maximum of 60 mg/kg daily, divided b.i.d. or t.i.d.

ADVERSE REACTIONS

Because drug is usually used in combination with other anticonvulsants, adverse reactions reported may not be caused by valproic acid alone.

CNS: *sedation,* emotional upset, depression, psychosis, aggression, hyperactivity, behavioral deterioration, muscle weakness, tremor.

EENT: stomatitis.

GI: *nausea, vomiting,* indigestion, diarrhea, abdominal cramps, constipation, increased appetite and weight gain, *anorexia,* ***pancreatitis.*** *(Note:* lower incidence of GI effects with divalproex.)

Hematologic: inhibited platelet aggregation, thrombocytopenia, increased bleeding time.

Hepatic: *elevated enzymes,* ***toxic hepatitis.***

Other: alopecia, elevated serum ammonia.

INTERACTIONS

Antacids, aspirin: May cause valproic acid toxicity. Use together cautiously and monitor blood levels.

Ethanol: excessive CNS depression. Avoid concomitant use.

Phenobarbital: increased phenobarbital levels.

Phenytoin: increased or decreased phenytoin levels.

CONTRAINDICATIONS

- Contraindicated in patients with hepatic dysfunction.
- Use cautiously in children under 2 years, in children with congenital metabolic disorders or mental retardation, in patients with organic brain disease, and in those taking multiple anticonvulsants.

NURSING CONSIDERATIONS

- Tell patients not to discontinue the drug suddenly because sudden withdrawal may worsen seizures. Call the doctor at once if adverse reactions develop.
- Monitor liver function studies, platelet counts, and PT before starting drug and periodically thereafter.
- Serious or fatal hepatotoxicity may follow nonspecific symptoms, such as malaise, fever, and lethargy.
- Advise patients to avoid driving or other potentially hazardous activities that require mental alertness until the CNS effects of the drug are known.
- To reduce adverse GI effects, this drug may be taken with food or milk.
- Advise patients against chewing capsules; irritation of mouth and throat may result.
- May need to reduce dosage if tremors occur.
- May produce false-positive test results for ketones in urine.
- Keep out of children's reach.
- Syrup shouldn't be mixed with carbonated beverages; may be irritating to mouth and throat.
- Don't administer syrup to patients who need sodium restriction. Check with the doctor.
- Valproic acid has been used investigationally to prevent recurrent febrile seizures in children.

30

Antidepressants

amitriptyline hydrochloride
amoxapine
bupropion hydrochloride
clomipramine hydrochloride
desipramine hydrochloride
doxepin hydrochloride
fluoxetine hydrochloride
imipramine hydrochloride
imipramine pamoate
isocarboxazid
maprotiline hydrochloride
nortriptyline hydrochloride
paroxetine hydrochloride
phenelzine sulfate
protriptyline hydrochloride
sertraline hydrochloride
tranylcypromine sulfate
trazodone hydrochloride
trimipramine maleate
venlafaxine hydrochloride

COMBINATION PRODUCTS

ETRAFON: perphenazine 2 mg and amitriptyline hydrochloride 25 mg.
ETRAFON 2-10: perphenazine 2 mg and amitriptyline hydrochloride 10 mg.
ETRAFON-A: perphenazine 4 mg and amitriptyline hydrochloride 10 mg.
ETRAFON-FORTE: perphenazine 4 mg and amitriptyline hydrochloride 25 mg.
LIMBITROL 5-12.5: chlordiazepoxide 5 mg and amitriptyline hydrochloride 12.5 mg.
LIMBITROL 10-25: chlordiazepoxide 10 mg and amitriptyline hydrochloride 25 mg.
TRIAVIL 2-10, TRIAVIL 4-10, TRIAVIL 2-25, TRIAVIL 4-25 are products identical to the Etrafon products listed above. Triavil is also available as TRIAVIL 4-50 (perphenazine 4 mg and amitriptyline hydrochloride 50 mg).

amitriptyline hydrochloride

Apo-Amitriptyline†, Elavil, Emitrip, Endep, Enovil, Levate†, Novo-Triptyn†, PMS-Amitriptyline, Tryptanol‡

amitriptyline pamoate

Elavil†

Pregnancy Risk Category: D

HOW SUPPLIED

hydrochloride
Tablets: 10 mg, 25 mg, 50 mg, 75 mg, 100 mg, 150 mg
Injection: 10 mg/ml
pamoate
Syrup: 10 mg/5 ml

ACTION

Mechanism: A tricyclic antidepressant (TCA) that increases the amount of norepinephrine or serotonin, or both, in the CNS by blocking their reuptake by the presynaptic neurons.
Onset: therapeutic effect, several weeks. **Peak:** Serum levels peak in 2 to 12 hours. **Duration:** elimination half-life, 10 to 50 hours.

INDICATIONS & DOSAGE

Depression –
Adults: 50 to 100 mg P.O. h.s., increasing to 200 mg daily; maximum dosage is 300 mg daily, if needed. Or 20 to 30 mg I.M. q.i.d.; alternatively, entire I.M. dose can be given h.s.
Elderly patients and adolescents: 30 mg P.O. daily in divided doses. May be increased to 150 mg.

ADVERSE REACTIONS

CNS: *drowsiness, dizziness,* excitation, tremors, weakness, confusion, headache, nervousness, EEG alter-

*Liquid form contains alcohol.
**May contain tartrazine.

Common reactions are in italics; ***life-threatening,*** in bold italics.

ations, ***seizures,*** extrapyramidal reactions.
CV: *orthostatic hypotension, tachycardia, ECG changes,* hypertension.
EENT: *blurred vision,* tinnitus, mydriasis.
GI: *dry mouth, constipation,* nausea, vomiting, anorexia, paralytic ileus.
GU: *urine retention.*
Skin: rash, urticaria, photosensitivity.
Other: *diaphoresis,* hypersensitivity reaction.
After abrupt withdrawal of long-term therapy: nausea, headache, malaise (does not indicate addiction).

INTERACTIONS
Barbiturates, CNS depressants, ethanol: enhanced CNS depression. Avoid concomitant use.
Cimetidine, methylphenidate: increased TCA blood levels. Monitor for enhanced antidepressant effect.
Epinephrine, norepinephrine: increased hypertensive effect. Use with caution.
MAO inhibitors: may cause severe excitation, hyperpyrexia, or seizures, usually with high dosage. Use with caution.

CONTRAINDICATIONS
- Contraindicated during acute recovery phase of MI, in patients with history of seizure disorders, and in those with prostatic hyperplasia.
- Use cautiously in patients at risk for suicide; in patients with urine retention, acute angle-closure glaucoma, increased intraocular pressure, cardiovascular disease, impaired hepatic function, or thyroid disease; and in patients receiving thyroid medications, electroconvulsive therapy, or elective surgery.

NURSING CONSIDERATIONS
- Do not withdraw drug abruptly.
- Because of hypertensive episodes during surgery in patients receiving TCAs, gradually discontinue drug several days before surgery.
- If signs of psychosis occur or increase, expect doctor to reduce dosage. Record mood changes. Monitor patients for suicidal tendencies, and allow a minimum supply of the drug.
- Warn patients to avoid activities that require alertness and good psychomotor coordination until CNS effects of drug are known. Drowsiness and dizziness usually subside after a few weeks.
- Advise patients to take full dose h.s., but warn them of possible morning orthostatic hypotension.
- Amitriptyline has strong anticholinergic effects and is one of the most sedating TCAs.
- Tell patients to avoid alcohol while taking this drug.
- Dry mouth may be relieved with sugarless hard candy or gum. Saliva substitutes may be necessary.
- Check for urine retention and constipation. Increase fluids and suggest stool softener or high-fiber diet as needed.
- Advise patients to consult their doctors before taking any other prescription or OTC medications.
- To prevent photosensitivity reactions, advise patients to use a sunblock, wear protective clothing, and avoid prolonged exposure to strong sunlight.
- Has been used to treat patients with intractable hiccups, chronic severe pain, and eating disorders (bulimia or anorexia nervosa).

amoxapine
Asendin
Pregnancy Risk Category: C

HOW SUPPLIED
Tablets: 25 mg, 50 mg, 100 mg, 150 mg

ACTION

Mechanism: A tricyclic antidepressant (TCA) that increases the amount of norepinephrine or serotonin, or both, in the CNS by blocking their reuptake by the presynaptic neurons.
Onset: antidepressant effect, 2 to 4 weeks. **Duration:** plasma half-life, 8 to 30 hours.

INDICATIONS & DOSAGE

Depression –
Adults: initial dose, 50 mg P.O. t.i.d. May increase to 100 mg t.i.d. on third day of treatment. Increases above 300 mg daily should be made only if 300 mg daily has been ineffective during a trial period of at least 2 weeks. When effective dosage is established, entire dosage (not to exceed 300 mg) may be given h.s. Maximum dosage is 600 mg in hospitalized patients.

ADVERSE REACTIONS

CNS: *drowsiness, dizziness,* excitation, tremors, weakness, confusion, headache, nervousness, *tardive dyskinesia* (especially in elderly women); EEG changes, ***seizures,*** extrapyramidal reactions (rarely), ***neuroleptic malignant syndrome*** (high fever, tachycardia, tachypnea, profuse diaphoresis).
CV: *orthostatic hypotension, tachycardia, ECG changes,* hypertension.
EENT: *blurred vision,* tinnitus, mydriasis.
GI: *dry mouth, constipation,* nausea, vomiting, anorexia, paralytic ileus.
GU: *urine retention, acute renal failure (with overdose).*
Skin: rash, urticaria, photosensitivity.
Other: *diaphoresis,* weight gain and craving for sweets, hypersensitivity reaction.
After abrupt withdrawal of long-term therapy: nausea, headache, malaise (does not indicate addiction).

INTERACTIONS

Barbiturates: decreased TCA blood levels. Monitor for decreased antidepressant effect.
Cimetidine, methylphenidate, oral contraceptives: may increase amoxapine serum levels. Monitor for increased adverse effects.
Clonidine, epinephrine, norepinephrine: increased hypertensive effect. Use with caution.
CNS depressants, ethanol: enhanced CNS depression. Avoid concomitant use.
MAO inhibitors: may cause severe excitation, hyperpyrexia, or seizures, usually with high dosage. Use with caution.

CONTRAINDICATIONS

- Contraindicated in acute recovery phase of MI, in patients with history of seizure disorders, and in patients with prostatic hyperplasia.
- Use cautiously in patients at risk for suicide; in patients with urine retention, acute angle-closure glaucoma, increased intraocular pressure, cardiovascular disease, impaired hepatic function, or thyroid disease; and in patients receiving thyroid medications, electroconvulsive therapy, or elective surgery.

NURSING CONSIDERATIONS

- Reduce dosage in elderly or debilitated persons and adolescents.
- Do not withdraw drug abruptly.
- Because hypertensive episodes have occurred during surgery in patients receiving TCAs, gradually discontinue drug several days before surgery.
- Expect delay of 2 weeks or more before noticeable effect. Full effect may take 4 weeks or more.
- If signs of psychosis occur or increase, reduce dosage. Record mood changes. Monitor patients for suicidal tendencies, and allow them only a minimum supply of the drug.

- Monitor for signs and symptoms of tardive dyskinesia, especially in elderly women.
- Warn patient to avoid activities that require alertness and good psychomotor coordination until CNS effects of the drug are known. Drowsiness and dizziness usually subside after first few weeks.
- Whenever possible, patient should take full dose h.s.
- Amoxapine therapy has been associated with neuroleptic malignant syndrome, a rare but life-threatening syndrome usually seen with phenothiazines. Discontinue drug immediately and institute appropriate therapy if symptoms occur.
- Relieve dry mouth with sugarless hard candy or gum. Saliva substitutes may be necessary.
- Check for urine retention and constipation. Increase fluids to lessen constipation. Suggest stool softener or high-fiber diet, if needed.
- Some patients may experience photosensitivity reactions. Advise the patient to use a sunblock, wear protective clothing, and avoid prolonged exposure to strong sunlight.

bupropion hydrochloride

Wellbutrin

Pregnancy Risk Category: B

HOW SUPPLIED

Tablets: 75 mg, 100 mg

ACTION

Mechanism: Bupropion is not a tricyclic antidepressant, does not inhibit MAO, and is a weak inhibitor of norepinephrine, dopamine, and serotonin reuptake. Exact mechanism unknown. **Onset:** antidepressant effect, 2 weeks or longer. **Peak:** Serum levels peak within 1 to 3 hours. **Duration:** elimination half-life, about 14 hours.

INDICATIONS & DOSAGE

Depression –

Adults: initially, 100 mg P.O. b.i.d. Dosage may be increased after 3 days to 100 mg P.O. t.i.d. If no response occurs after several weeks of therapy, dosage may be increased to 150 mg t.i.d.

ADVERSE REACTIONS

CNS: *headache,* akathisia, ***seizures,*** *agitation,* anxiety, *confusion,* delusions, euphoria, hostility, impaired sleep quality, insomnia, sedation, sensory disturbance, tremor.
CV: ***arrhythmias,*** hypertension, hypotension, palpitations, syncope, tachycardia.
EENT: auditory disturbance, blurred vision.
GI: dry mouth, gustatory disturbance, appetite increase, constipation, dyspepsia, nausea, vomiting.
GU: impotence, menstrual complaints, urinary frequency.
Skin: pruritus, rash, cutaneous temperature disturbance.
Other: arthritis, fever and chills, diaphoresis, decreased libido.

INTERACTIONS

Ethanol, levodopa, phenothiazines, MAO inhibitors, or tricyclic antidepressants, or recent and rapid withdrawal of benzodiazepines: increased risk of adverse reactions, including seizures.

CONTRAINDICATIONS

- Contraindicated in patients who are allergic to the drug, who have taken MAO inhibitors within the previous 14 days, and in patients with seizure disorders. Also contraindicated in patients with a history of bulimia or anorexia nervosa because of a higher incidence of seizures. Patients who experience seizures often have predisposing factors, including history of head trauma or prior seizures, or CNS tumors, or they may be taking a drug that lowers the seizure threshold.

NURSING CONSIDERATIONS

- From 28% to 30% of patients taking this drug may experience a 5-lb or greater weight loss. Consider this if weight loss is a major factor in the patient's depressive illness.
- Antidepressants can cause manic episodes during the depressed phase of bipolar disorder.
- Many patients experience a period of increased restlessness, especially at initiation of therapy. This may include agitation, insomnia, and anxiety.
- About one half of patients treated at dosages up to 450 mg/day may experience seizures. At dosages of 600 mg/day, the incidence of seizures increases about tenfold. Risk of seizure may be minimized by not exceeding 450 mg/day and by administering daily dosage in three to four equally divided doses.
- Advise patients to take the drug as scheduled, and to take each day's dosage in three divided doses to minimize the risk of seizures.
- Tell patients to avoid alcohol while taking this drug, because it may contribute to the development of seizures.
- Animal data suggest that bupropion may induce drug metabolizing enzymes, decreasing the effectiveness of other drugs taken concomitantly.
- Advise patients to consult their doctor before taking any other prescription or OTC medications.
- Advise patients to avoid hazardous activities that require alertness, and good psychomotor coordination until CNS effects of the drug are known.

clomipramine hydrochloride

Anafranil

Pregnancy Risk Category: C

HOW SUPPLIED

Capsules: 25 mg, 50 mg, 75 mg

ACTION

Mechanism: A tricyclic antidepressant (TCA) that selectively inhibits reuptake of serotonin.
Onset: 2 weeks or longer. **Duration:** elimination half-life, 21 to 31 hours.

INDICATIONS & DOSAGE

Obsessive-compulsive disorder–
Adults: initially, 25 mg P.O. daily in divided doses with meals, gradually increasing to 100 mg daily during first 2 weeks. Maximum dosage is 250 mg/day in divided doses with meals. After titration, total daily dosage may be given h.s.
Children and adolescents: initially, 25 mg P.O. daily, gradually increasing to daily maximum of 3 mg/kg or 100 mg P.O., whichever is smaller; given in divided doses with meals during first 2 weeks. Maximum daily dosage is 3 mg/kg or 200 mg, whichever is smaller; may be given h.s. after titration.

Maintenance dosage in children, adolescents, and adults is the lowest effective dose h.s. Periodic reassessment and adjustment necessary.

ADVERSE REACTIONS

CNS: *somnolence, tremor, dizziness,* headache, insomnia, *nervousness, myoclonus, fatigue, EEG changes,* ***seizures,*** extrapyramidal reactions, asthenia, aggressiveness.
CV: postural hypotension, palpitations, tachycardia.
EENT: otitis media (children), *abnormal vision,* laryngitis, pharyngitis, rhinitis.
GI: *dry mouth, constipation, nausea, dyspepsia, increased appetite,* diarrhea, *anorexia,* abdominal pain, eructation, *nausea.*
GU: *micturition disorder,* urinary tract infection, dysmenorrhea, *ejaculation failure,* impotence.

*Liquid form contains alcohol. *Common* reactions are in italics; ***life-threatening,*** in bold italics.
**May contain tartrazine.

Hematologic: anemia, bone marrow suppression.
Skin: *diaphoresis,* rash, pruritus, photosensitivity, dry skin.
Other: myalgia, weight gain, *altered libido.*

INTERACTIONS
Barbiturates: decreased TCA blood levels. Monitor for decreased antidepressant effect.
Cimetidine, methylphenidate: increased TCA blood levels. Monitor for enhanced antidepressant effect.
Clonidine, epinephrine, norepinephrine: increased hypertensive effect. Use with caution.
CNS depressants, ethanol: enhanced CNS depression. Avoid concomitant use.
MAO inhibitors: may cause hyperpyretic crisis, seizures, coma, or death. Don't use together.

CONTRAINDICATIONS
- Contraindicated during acute recovery period after MI.
- Use cautiously in patients with history of seizure disorders or with brain damage of varying etiology; in patients receiving other seizure threshold-lowering drugs; in patients at risk for suicide; in patients with urine retention, acute angle-closure glaucoma, increased intraocular pressure, cardiovascular disease, impaired hepatic function, or thyroid disease; in patients with tumors of the adrenal medulla; and in patients receiving thyroid medication, electroconvulsive therapy, or elective surgery.

NURSING CONSIDERATIONS
- Do not withdraw drug abruptly.
- Because of hypertensive episodes during surgery in patients receiving TCAs, gradually discontinue drug several days before surgery.
- Warn patients to avoid hazardous activities requiring alertness and good psychomotor coordination, especially during titration. Daytime sedation and dizziness may occur.
- Total daily dose may be taken at bedtime after titration. During titration, dosage may be divided and given.
- Tell patients to avoid alcohol while taking this drug.
- Relieve dry mouth with sugarless candy or gum. Saliva substitutes may be necessary.
- Monitor for urine retention and constipation. Increase fluids, and suggest stool softener or high-fiber diet as needed.
- To prevent photosensitivity reactions, advise patients to use sunblock, wear protective clothing, and avoid prolonged exposure to strong sunlight.

desipramine hydrochloride
Norpramin**, Pertofran‡, Pertofrane

Pregnancy Risk Category: C

HOW SUPPLIED
Tablets: 10 mg, 25 mg, 50 mg, 75 mg, 100 mg, 150 mg
Capsules: 25 mg, 50 mg

ACTION
Mechanism: A tricyclic antidepressant (TCA) that increases the amount of norepinephrine or serotonin, or both, in the CNS by blocking their reuptake by the presynaptic neurons.
Onset: antidepressant effect, 2 to 4 weeks or longer. **Duration:** elimination half-life, 12 to 27 hours.

INDICATIONS & DOSAGE
Depression –
Adults: 75 to 150 mg P.O. daily in divided doses, increasing to maximum of 300 mg daily. Or entire dosage can be given at h.s.
Elderly patients and adolescents: 25 to 50 mg P.O. daily, increasing gradually to maximum of 100 mg daily.

ADVERSE REACTIONS

CNS: *drowsiness, dizziness,* excitation, tremors, weakness, confusion, headache, nervousness, EEG changes, ***seizures,*** extrapyramidal reactions.
CV: orthostatic hypotension, *tachycardia, ECG changes,* hypertension (especially during surgery).
EENT: *blurred vision,* tinnitus, mydriasis.
GI: *dry mouth, constipation,* nausea, vomiting, anorexia, paralytic ileus.
GU: *urine retention.*
Skin: rash, urticaria, photosensitivity.
Other: *diaphoresis,* hypersensitivity reaction.
After abrupt withdrawal of long-term therapy: nausea, headache, malaise (does not indicate addiction).

INTERACTIONS

Barbiturates, CNS depressants, ethanol: enhanced CNS depression. Avoid concomitant use.
Cimetidine, methylphenidate: may increase desipramine serum levels. Monitor for adverse reactions.
Clonidine, epinephrine, norepinephrine: increased hypertensive effect. Use with caution.
MAO inhibitors: may cause severe excitation, hyperpyrexia, or seizures, usually with high dose. Use with caution.

CONTRAINDICATIONS

- Contraindicated during acute recovery phase of MI, in patients with history of seizure disorders, and in patients with prostatic hyperplasia.
- Use cautiously in patients at risk for suicide; in patients with cardiovascular disease, urine retention, acute angle-closure glaucoma, blood dyscrasia, impaired hepatic function, or thyroid disease; and in patients receiving thyroid medications, electroconvulsive therapy, or elective surgery.

NURSING CONSIDERATIONS

- Do not withdraw drug abruptly.
- Because of hypertensive episodes during surgery in patients receiving TCAs, gradually discontinue drug several days before surgery.
- If signs of psychosis occur or increase, expect the doctor to reduce dosage. Record mood changes. Monitor patients for suicidal tendencies, and allow a minimum supply of the drug.
- Warn patients to avoid hazardous activities that require alertness and good psychomotor coordination until CNS effects of the drug are known. Drowsiness and dizziness usually subside after a few weeks.
- Advise patients to take full dose h.s.
- Because desipramine produces less anticholinergic effects than other TCAs, it is often prescribed for cardiac patients.
- Produces less sedation than amitriptyline or doxepin and does not usually cause orthostatic hypotension.
- Tell patients to avoid alcohol while taking this drug because it may antagonize effects of desipramine.
- Relieve dry mouth with sugarless hard candy or gum. Saliva substitutes may be necessary.
- Check for urine retention and constipation. Increase fluids, and suggest stool softener or high-fiber diet, as needed.
- Advise patients to consult their doctors before taking any other prescription or OTC medications.
- To prevent photosensitivity reactions, advise patients to use sunblock, wear protective clothing, and avoid prolonged exposure to strong sunlight.

doxepin hydrochloride

Deptran‡, Novo-Doxepin†, Sinequan, Triadapin†

Pregnancy Risk Category: C

HOW SUPPLIED
Capsules: 10 mg, 25 mg, 50 mg, 75 mg, 100 mg, 150 mg
Oral concentrate: 10 mg/ml

ACTION
Mechanism: A tricyclic antidepressant (TCA) that increases the amount of norepinephrine or serotonin, or both, in the CNS by blocking their reuptake by the presynaptic neurons.
Onset: antidepressant effect, 2 to 4 weeks or longer. **Duration:** elimination half-life, 11 to 23 hours.

INDICATIONS & DOSAGE
Depression –
Adults: initially, 50 to 75 mg P.O. daily in divided doses, to maximum of 300 mg daily. Or, entire dosage may be given h.s.

ADVERSE REACTIONS
CNS: *drowsiness, dizziness,* excitation, tremors, weakness, confusion, headache, nervousness, EEG changes, ***seizures,*** extrapyramidal reactions.
CV: *orthostatic hypotension, tachycardia, ECG changes,* hypertension.
EENT: *blurred vision,* tinnitus, mydriasis.
GI: *dry mouth, glossitis, constipation,* nausea, vomiting, anorexia, paralytic ileus.
GU: *urine retention.*
Skin: rash, urticaria, photosensitivity.
Other: *diaphoresis,* hypersensitivity reaction.
After abrupt withdrawal of long-term therapy: nausea, headache, malaise (does not indicate addiction).

INTERACTIONS
Barbiturates, CNS depressants, ethanol: enhanced CNS depression. Avoid concomitant use.
Cimetidine, methylphenidate: may increase doxepin serum levels. Monitor for increased adverse reactions.
Clonidine, epinephrine, norepinephrine: increased hypertensive effect. Use with caution.
MAO inhibitors: may cause severe excitation, hyperpyrexia, or seizures, usually with high dose. Use with caution.

CONTRAINDICATIONS
- Contraindicated during the acute recovery phase of MI or in patients with acute angle-closure glaucoma, prostatic hyperplasia, or history of seizures.
- Use cautiously in patients with urine retention, cardiovascular disease, impaired hepatic function, or thyroid disease; and in patients at risk for suicide.

NURSING CONSIDERATIONS
- Reduce dosage in elderly or debilitated patients, adolescents, and those receiving other medications (especially anticholinergics).
- Well tolerated by elderly patients.
- May be useful for chronic, severe neurogenic pain.
- Dilute oral concentrate with 120 ml of water, milk, or juice (orange, grapefruit, tomato, prune, or pineapple). Incompatible with carbonated beverages.
- Do not withdraw drug abruptly.
- Because of hypertensive episodes during surgery in patients receiving TCAs, gradually discontinue drug several days before surgery.
- If signs of psychosis occur or increase, expect doctor to reduce dosage. Record mood changes. Monitor patients for suicidal tendencies, and allow a minimum supply of the drug.
- Warn patients to avoid hazardous activities that require alertness and good psychomotor coordination until CNS effects of the drug are known. Drowsiness and dizziness usually subside after a few weeks.
- Advise patients to take full dose h.s. but warn them of possible morning orthostatic hypotension.

• Doxepin has strong anticholinergic effects; one of the most sedating TCAs.
• Tell patients to avoid alcohol while taking this drug.
• Relieve dry mouth with sugarless hard candy or gum. Saliva substitutes may be necessary.
• Check for urine retention and constipation. Increase fluids, and suggest stool softener or high-fiber diet, as needed.
• Advise patients to consult their doctors before taking any other prescription or OTC medications.
• To prevent photosensitivity reactions, advise patients to use sunblock, wear protective clothing, and avoid prolonged exposure to strong sunlight.

fluoxetine hydrochloride

Prozac, Prozac-20‡

Pregnancy Risk Category: B

HOW SUPPLIED

Pulvules: 10 mg, 20 mg
Oral solution: 20 mg/5 ml

ACTION

Mechanism: Inhibits the CNS neuronal uptake of serotonin. Not a tricyclic derivative; considered an atypical antidepressant.
Onset: antidepressant effect, 2 to 4 weeks or longer. **Peak:** Serum levels peak in 6 to 8 hours. **Duration:** elimination half-life of fluoxetine, 2 to 3 days; of active metabolite norfluoxetine, 7 to 9 days.

INDICATIONS & DOSAGE

Short-term management of depressive illness –
Adults: initially, 20 mg P.O. in the morning; dosage increased according to patient response. May be given b.i.d. in the morning and at noon. Maximum dosage is 80 mg/day.

ADVERSE REACTIONS

CNS: *nervousness, anxiety, insomnia, headache, drowsiness, tremor, dizziness, asthenia,* abnormal dreams.
CV: palpitations, flushing, bradycardia, ***arrhythmias***.
EENT: nasal congestion, pharyngitis, cough, sinusitis, visual disturbances, tinnitus.
GI: *nausea, diarrhea, dry mouth, anorexia, dyspepsia,* constipation, abdominal pain, vomiting, taste change, flatulence, increased appetite.
GU: sexual dysfunction, urine retention.
Respiratory: upper respiratory infection, respiratory distress.
Skin: *rash, pruritus, urticaria.*
Other: flulike syndrome, muscle pain, *weight loss,* edema, lymphadenopathy, diaphoresis.

INTERACTIONS

Flecainide, carbamazepine, vinblastine: increased serum levels of these drugs. Monitor serum levels and the patient for adverse effects.
Insulin, oral antidiabetic agents: altered blood glucose levels and possible altered requirements for antidiabetic medication. Adjust dosage as ordered.
Lithium, tricyclic antidepressants: risk of increased adverse CNS effects. Avoid concomitant use.
Phenytoin: increased plasma phenytoin levels and risk of toxicity. Monitor serum phenytoin levels and adjust dosage as ordered.
Tryptophan: increased toxic reaction exhibited by agitation, GI distress, and restlessness. Do not use together.

CONTRAINDICATIONS

• Contraindicated in patients hypersensitive to the drug and in patients taking MAO inhibitors within 14 days of starting therapy.
• Use cautiously in patients at high risk for suicide and in patients with history of hepatic, renal, or cardio-

vascular disease; diabetes mellitus; or history of seizures.

NURSING CONSIDERATIONS

- Elderly or debilitated patients and patients with renal or hepatic dysfunction may require lower dosages or less frequent dosing.
- Less sedating than other antidepressants, but may cause dizziness or drowsiness in some patients. Warn patients to avoid driving or other hazardous activities that require alertness and good psychomotor coordination until CNS effects of the drug are known.
- Tell patients to avoid taking drug in the afternoon because fluoxetine commonly causes nervousness and insomnia.
- Use antihistamines or topical corticosteroids to treat rashes or pruritus.
- Advise patients to consult their doctors before taking any other prescription or OTC medications.
- Warn patients to avoid food high in tryptophan, including meats, poultry, fish, liver, kidney, eggs, nuts, peanut butter, broad beans, and wheat germ.

---

imipramine hydrochloride

Apo-Imipramine†, Imiprin‡, Impril†, Janimine**, Melipramine‡, Norfranil, Novo-Pramine†, Tipramine, Tofranil**

imipramine pamoate

Tofranil-PM**

Pregnancy Risk Category: D

HOW SUPPLIED

hydrochloride

Tablets: 10 mg, 25 mg, 50 mg

Injection: 12.5 mg/ml

pamoate

Capsules: 75 mg, 100 mg, 125 mg, 150 mg

ACTION

Mechanism: A tricyclic antidepressant (TCA) that increases the amount of norepinephrine or serotonin, or both, in the CNS by blocking their reuptake by the presynaptic neurons.

Onset: antidepressant effect, 2 to 4 weeks or longer. **Duration:** elimination half-life, 11 to 25 hours.

INDICATIONS & DOSAGE

Depression –

Adults: 75 to 100 mg P.O. or I.M. daily in divided doses, increased 25- to 50-mg increments up to maximum dosage of 300 mg daily. Or, entire dosage may be given h.s. (using pamoate salt).

Childhood enuresis –

Children 6 years and over: 25 mg P.O. 1 hour before bedtime. If no response within 1 week, increase to 50 mg if child is under 12 years; increase to 75 mg for children 12 years and over. In either case, do not exceed 2.5 mg/kg/day.

ADVERSE REACTIONS

CNS: *drowsiness, dizziness,* excitation, tremors, weakness, confusion, headache, nervousness, EEG changes, *seizures,* extrapyramidal reactions.

CV: *orthostatic hypotension, tachycardia, ECG changes,* hypertension.

EENT: *blurred vision,* tinnitus, mydriasis.

GI: *dry mouth, constipation,* nausea, vomiting, anorexia, paralytic ileus.

GU: *urine retention.*

Skin: rash, urticaria, photosensitivity.

Other: *diaphoresis,* hypersensitivity reaction.

After abrupt withdrawal of long-term therapy: nausea, headache, malaise (does not indicate addiction).

INTERACTIONS

Barbiturates, CNS depressants, ethanol: enhanced CNS depression. Avoid concomitant use.

Cimetidine, methylphenidate: may increase imipramine serum levels. Monitor for adverse reactions.
Clonidine, epinephrine, norepinephrine: increased hypertensive effect. Use with caution.
MAO inhibitors: may cause severe excitation, hyperpyrexia, or seizures, usually with high dose. Use with caution.

CONTRAINDICATIONS
- Contraindicated during acute recovery phase of MI, in patients with history of seizure disorders, and in those with prostatic hyperplasia.
- Use with extreme caution in patients at risk for suicide; in patients with urine retention, acute angle-closure glaucoma, increased intraocular pressure, cardiovascular disease, blood dyscrasia, impaired hepatic function, or thyroid disease; and in patients receiving thyroid medications, electroconvulsive therapy, or elective surgery. Injectable form contains sulfites, which may cause allergic reactions in hypersensitive individuals.

NURSING CONSIDERATIONS
- Reduce dosage in elderly or debilitated persons, adolescents, and patients with aggravated psychotic symptoms.
- Dosages greater than 200 mg daily are not recommended for outpatients.
- Do not withdraw drug abruptly.
- Because of hypertensive episodes during surgery in patients receiving TCAs, gradually discontinue drug several days before surgery.
- If signs of psychosis occur or increase, expect doctor to reduce dosage. Record mood changes. Monitor patients for suicidal tendencies, and only a minimum supply of the drug.
- Warn patients to avoid hazardous activities that require alertness and good psychomotor coordination until CNS effects of the drug are known. Drowsiness and dizziness usually subside after a few weeks.
- Advise patients to take full dose at bedtime but warn them of possible morning orthostatic hypotension.
- Tell patients to avoid alcohol while taking this drug.
- May be useful for chronic, severe neurogenic pain.
- If the child is an "early night" bedwetter, it may be more effective to divide dosage and administer the first dose earlier in the day.
- To prevent relapse in children receiving the drug for enuresis, withdraw dosage gradually.
- Check for urine retention and constipation. Increase fluids, and suggest stool softener, or a high-fiber diet as needed.
- Relieve dry mouth with sugarless hard candy or gum. Saliva substitutes may be necessary.
- Advise patients to consult their doctors before taking any other prescription or OTC medications.
- To prevent photosensitivity reactions, advise patient to use sunblock, wear protective clothing, and avoid prolonged exposure to strong sunlight.

isocarboxazid
Marplan

Pregnancy Risk Category: C

HOW SUPPLIED
Tablets: 10 mg

ACTION
Mechanism: An MAO inhibitor that promotes accumulation of neurotransmitters by inhibiting their metabolism.
Onset: antidepressant effects, 2 to 4 weeks or longer. **Peak:** Plasma levels peak within 3 to 5 hours. **Duration:** recovery of MAO activity, about 10 days after therapy is stopped.

INDICATIONS & DOSAGE
Depression –
Adults: 30 mg P.O. daily in divided doses. Reduce to 10 to 20 mg daily when condition improves. Not recommended for children under 16 years.

ADVERSE REACTIONS
CNS: *dizziness,* vertigo, weakness, headache, hyperactivity, hyperreflexia, tremors, muscle twitching, mania, *insomnia,* confusion, memory impairment, fatigue.
CV: *orthostatic hypotension,* ***arrhythmias,*** paradoxical hypertension.
EENT: blurred vision.
GI: dry mouth, *anorexia,* nausea, diarrhea, constipation.
Skin: rash.
Other: peripheral edema, diaphoresis, weight changes, altered libido.
After abrupt withdrawal from drug therapy: restlessness, anxiety, hallucinations, headache, weakness.

INTERACTIONS
Amphetamines, antihistamines, ephedrine, levodopa, meperidine, metaraminol, methylphenidate, phenylephrine, phenylpropanolamine, sympathomimetics: enhanced pressor effects of these drugs. Avoid concomitant use.
Barbiturates, dextromethorphan, ethanol, methotrimeprazine, narcotics, other sedatives, tricyclic antidepressants: unpredictable interactions. Use these agents with caution and in reduced dosages.
Insulin, oral antidiabetic agents: increased risk of hypoglycemia. Use with caution in reduced dosages.
Foods high in tyramine, tryptophan: risk of hypertensive crisis. Avoid concomitant use.

CONTRAINDICATIONS
- Contraindicated in elderly or debilitated patients; in patients with severe hepatic or renal impairment, CHF, pheochromocytoma, hypertension, or cardiovascular or cerebrovascular disease; and in patients with severe or frequent headaches.
- Contraindicated with foods containing tryptophan or tyramine; during therapy with other MAO inhibitors (including phenelzine, tranylcypromine) or within 10 days of such therapy; and within 10 days of elective surgery requiring general anesthetic, cocaine, or local anesthetic containing sympathomimetic vasoconstrictors.
- Use cautiously with other psychotropic drugs or with spinal anesthetics; in hyperactive, agitated, or schizophrenic patients; in patients at risk for suicide; and in patients with Parkinson's disease, diabetes, or seizure disorders.

NURSING CONSIDERATIONS
- Obtain baseline blood pressure and heart rate readings, CBC, and liver function tests before beginning therapy, and continue to monitor throughout treatment.
- Dosage is usually reduced to maintenance level as soon as possible.
- Do not withdraw drug abruptly.
- In most patients, MAO inhibitors should be discontinued 14 days before elective surgery to avoid drug interactions that may occur during anesthetic procedure.
- Because MAO inhibitors may alleviate chest pain in patients with angina, warn such patients to moderate activities and avoid overexertion.
- To prevent dizziness from orthostatic hypotension, tell patient to get out of bed slowly, sitting up first for 1 minute. Supervise walking.
- Monitor patients closely for suicidal tendencies, and allow a minimum supply of the drug.
- If the patient develops symptoms of overdosage (palpitations, frequent headaches, or severe orthostatic hypotension), withhold dose and notify the doctor.

- Have phentolamine available to counteract severe hypertension.
- Weigh patients biweekly. Teach patients how to check for edema and urine retention.
- Warn patients to avoid foods high in tryptophan (broad beans) or tyramine (aged cheese, Chianti wine, beer, avocados, chicken livers, chocolate, bananas, soy sauce, meat tenderizers, salami, bologna) and large amounts of caffeine.
- Tell patients to avoid alcohol while taking this drug.
- Advise patients to consult their doctor before taking any other prescription or OTC medications. Severe adverse effects can occur if MAO inhibitors are taken with OTC cold, hay fever, or diet preparations.
- Continue precautions 10 days after discontinuation of the drug because it has long-lasting effects.

maprotiline hydrochloride

Ludiomil

Pregnancy Risk Category: B

HOW SUPPLIED

Tablets: 25 mg, 50 mg, 75 mg

ACTION

Mechanism: A tetracyclic antidepressant similar to tricyclic derivatives. Increases the amount of norepinephrine or serotonin, or both, in the CNS by blocking their reuptake by the presynaptic neurons.

Onset: 3 to 7 days. **Peak:** Serum levels peak 12 hours after dose, antidepressant effect, 2 to 4 weeks or longer. **Duration:** elimination half-life, 43 hours; active metabolite half-life, 60 to 90 hours.

INDICATIONS & DOSAGE

Depression –

Adults: initial dose, 75 mg P.O. daily for patients with mild to moderate depression, increased to 150 mg daily, if needed. Maximum dosage is 225 mg daily in patients who are not hospitalized. Severely depressed, hospitalized patients may receive up to 300 mg daily.

ADVERSE REACTIONS

CNS: *drowsiness, dizziness,* excitation, ***seizures,*** tremor, weakness, confusion, headache, nervousness, extrapyramidal reactions.

CV: *orthostatic hypotension, tachycardia, ECG changes.*

EENT: *blurred vision,* tinnitus, mydriasis.

GI: dry mouth, *constipation,* nausea, vomiting, anorexia, paralytic ileus.

GU: *urine retention.*

Skin: rash, urticaria, photosensitivity.

Other: *diaphoresis,* hypersensitivity reaction.

After abrupt withdrawal of long-term therapy: nausea, headache, malaise (does not indicate addiction).

INTERACTIONS

Barbiturates: decreased maprotiline blood levels. Monitor for decreased antidepressant effect.

Cimetidine, methylphenidate: may increase maprotiline serum levels. Monitor for adverse reactions.

Clonidine, epinephrine, norepinephrine: increased hypertensive effect. Use with caution.

CNS depressants, ethanol: enhanced CNS depression. Avoid concomitant use.

MAO inhibitors: may cause severe excitation, hyperpyrexia, or seizures, usually with high dose. Use with caution.

CONTRAINDICATIONS

- Contraindicated during acute recovery phase of MI and in prostatic hyperplasia.
- Use cautiously in patients at risk for suicide; in patients with a history of seizures; in patients with urine reten-

tion, acute angle-closure glaucoma, cardiovascular disease, blood dyscrasia, impaired hepatic function, or thyroid disease; and in patients receiving thyroid medications, electroconvulsive therapy, or elective surgery.

NURSING CONSIDERATIONS

- Reduce dosage in elderly or debilitated patients and adolescents.
- Do not withdraw drug abruptly.
- Because maprotiline shares toxic potentials with tricyclic antidepressants and may cause hypertensive episodes during surgery, gradually discontinue drug several days before surgery.
- If signs of psychosis occur or increase, expect doctor to reduce dosage. Record mood changes. Monitor patients for suicidal tendencies, and allow a minimum supply of the drug.
- Warn patients to avoid activities that require alertness and good psychomotor coordination until CNS effects of the drug are known. Drowsiness and dizziness usually subside after a few weeks.
- Tell patients to avoid alcohol while taking this drug.
- Advise patients to take full dose h.s., but warn them of possible morning orthostatic hypotension.
- Relieve dry mouth with sugarless hard candy or gum. Saliva substitutes may be necessary.
- Check for urine retention and constipation. Increase fluids, and suggest stool softener or high-fiber diet, as needed.
- Advise patients to consult their doctors before taking any other prescription or OTC medications.
- To prevent photosensitivity reactions, advise patients to use sunblock, wear protective clothing, and avoid prolonged exposure to strong sunlight.

nortriptyline hydrochloride

Allegron‡, Aventyl*, Nortab‡, Pamelor*

Pregnancy Risk Category: D

HOW SUPPLIED

Tablets: 10 mg‡, 25 mg‡
Capsules: 10 mg, 25 mg, 50 mg, 75 mg
Oral solution: 10 mg/5 ml (4% alcohol)

ACTION

Mechanism: A tricyclic antidepressant (TCA) that increases the amount of norepinephrine or serotonin, or both, in the CNS by blocking their reuptake by the presynaptic neurons.
Onset: therapeutic effect, 2 to 4 weeks or longer. **Duration:** elimination half-life, 18 to 44 hours.

INDICATIONS & DOSAGE

Depression—
Adults: 25 mg P.O. t.i.d. or q.i.d., gradually increasing to maximum of 150 mg daily. Or, entire dosage may be given h.s.

ADVERSE REACTIONS

CNS: *drowsiness, dizziness,* excitation, ***seizures,*** tremor, weakness, confusion, headache, nervousness, EEG changes, extrapyramidal reactions.
CV: *tachycardia, ECG changes,* hypertension.
EENT: *blurred vision,* tinnitus, mydriasis.
GI: dry mouth, *constipation,* nausea, vomiting, anorexia, paralytic ileus.
GU: *urine retention.*
Skin: rash, urticaria, photosensitivity.
Other: *diaphoresis,* hypersensitivity reaction.
After abrupt withdrawal of long-term therapy: nausea, headache, malaise (does not indicate addiction).

INTERACTIONS

Barbiturates, CNS depressants, ethanol: enhanced CNS depression. Avoid concomitant use.
Cimetidine, methylphenidate: may increase nortriptyline serum levels. Monitor for adverse reactions.
Clonidine, epinephrine, norepinephrine: increased hypertensive effect. Use with caution.
MAO inhibitors: may cause severe excitation, hyperpyrexia, or seizures, usually with high dosage. Use with caution.

CONTRAINDICATIONS

- Contraindicated during acute recovery phase of MI, in patients with history of seizure disorders, or in those with prostatic hyperplasia.
- Use cautiously in patients at risk for suicide; in patients with urine retention, glaucoma, cardiovascular disease, blood dyscrasia, impaired hepatic function, or thyroid disease; and in patients receiving thyroid medications, electroconvulsive therapy, or elective surgery.

NURSING CONSIDERATIONS

- Reduce dosage in elderly or debilitated patients and adolescents.
- Do not withdraw drug abruptly.
- Because hypertensive episodes have occurred during surgery in patients receiving TCAs, gradually discontinue drug several days before surgery.
- If signs of psychosis occur or increase, expect doctor to reduce dosage. Record mood changes. Monitor patients for suicidal tendencies, and allow a minimum supply of the drug.
- Warn patients to avoid activities that require alertness and good psychomotor coordination until CNS effects of the drug are known. Drowsiness and dizziness usually subside after a few weeks.
- Whenever possible, advise patients to take full dose h.s. to reduce the risk of orthostatic hypotension.
- Has anticholinergic effects similar to other TCAs.
- Tell patients to avoid alcohol while taking this drug.
- Relieve dry mouth with sugarless hard candy or gum. Saliva substitutes may be necessary.
- Check for urine retention and constipation. Increase fluids, and suggest stool softener or high-fiber diet, as needed.
- Advise patients to consult their doctors before taking any other prescription or OTC medications.
- To prevent photosensitivity reactions, advise patients to use sunblock, wear protective clothing, and avoid prolonged exposure to strong sunlight.

paroxetine hydrochloride

Paxil

Pregnancy Risk Category: B

HOW SUPPLIED

Tablets: 20 mg, 30 mg

ACTION

Mechanism: Blocks reuptake of serotonin (5-hydroxytryptamine; 5-HT) into nerve terminals within the CNS.
Onset: therapeutic effect, 2 to 4 weeks or longer. **Peak:** Steady-state levels are reached after about 10 days.

INDICATIONS & DOSAGE

Depression –
Adults: initially, 20 mg P.O. daily, preferably in the morning as indicated, increase dosage in 10-mg/day increments, at 1-week intervals, to a maximum of 50 mg daily.
Elderly or debilitated patients; patients with severe hepatic or renal disease: initially, 10 mg P.O. daily, preferably in the morning as indicated, increase dosage in 10-mg/day increments, at 1-week intervals, to a maximum of 40 mg daily.

ADVERSE REACTIONS

CNS: blurred vision, *somnolence, dizziness, insomnia, tremor, nervousness,* anxiety, paresthesia.
CV: palpitations, vasodilation, postural hypotension.
EENT: lump or tightness in throat, dysgeusia.
GI: *dry mouth, nausea, constipation, diarrhea, decreased appetite,* flatulence, vomiting, dyspepsia, increased appetite.
GU: *ejaculatory disturbances, male genital disorders* (including anorgasmy, erectile difficulties, delayed ejaculation or orgasm, impotence, and sexual dysfunction), urinary frequency, other urinary disorder, female genital disorder (including anorgasmy, difficulty with orgasm).
Skin: rash.
Other: *asthenia, diaphoresis,* hyponatremia, myopathy, myalgia, myasthenia, decreased libido.

INTERACTIONS

Cimetidine: decreased hepatic metabolism of paroxetine, leading to risk of toxicity. Dosage adjustments may be necessary.
Digoxin: may decrease digoxin levels. Monitor closely.
MAO inhibitors: may increase risk of serious, sometimes fatal, adverse reactions. Avoid concomitant use.
Phenobarbital, phenytoin: may alter pharmacokinetics of both drugs. Dosage adjustments may be necessary.
Procyclidine: may increase procyclidine levels. Monitor for excessive anticholinergic effects.
Tryptophan: may increase incidence of adverse reactions, such as diaphoresis, headache, nausea, and dizziness. Avoid concomitant use.
Warfarin: increased risk of bleeding. Avoid concomitant use.

CONTRAINDICATIONS

- Contraindicated in patients taking MAO inhibitors.
- Use cautiously in patients with a history of seizure disorders or mania; in patients with hepatic or renal impairment; or in those with severe, concomitant systemic illness.
- Use cautiously in breast-feeding patients, because drug is excreted in breast milk.

NURSING CONSIDERATIONS

- Don't administer paroxetine with, or within 14 days of discontinuing, MAO inhibitor therapy. Allow at least 2 weeks after discontinuing paroxetine before starting treatment with an MAO inhibitor.
- If signs of psychosis occur or increase, expect doctor to reduce dosage. Record mood changes. Monitor patients for suicidal tendencies, and allow them only a minimum supply of the drug.
- Use cautiously in patients at risk for volume depletion, and monitor appropriately.
- Overdosage is usually associated with nausea, vomiting, drowsiness, sinus tachycardia, and dilated pupils. No specific antidote exists for the drug, and forced diuresis, dialysis, hemoperfusion, or exchange transfusion is believed to be of little benefit. Establish and maintain an airway, and perform gastric evacuation. Activated charcoal (20 to 30 g) may be administered every 4 to 6 hours for the first 24 to 48 hours after ingestion. Provide supportive care with frequent monitoring of vital signs.
- Warn patients to avoid foods high in tryptophan, including meats, poultry, fish, liver, kidney, eggs, nuts, peanut butter, broad beans, and wheat germ.
- Warn patients to avoid activities that require alertness and good psychomotor coordination until CNS effects of drug are known.

phenelzine sulfate

Nardil

Pregnancy Risk Category: C

HOW SUPPLIED

Tablets: 15 mg

ACTION

Mechanism: An MAO inhibitor that promotes accumulation of neurotransmitters by inhibiting their metabolism.

Onset: therapeutic effect, 2 to 4 weeks or longer. **Peak:** Plasma levels peak in 2 to 4 hours. **Duration:** recovery of MAO activity, about 10 days after therapy is stopped.

INDICATIONS & DOSAGE

Depression –

Adults: 45 mg P.O. daily in divided doses, increasing rapidly to 60 mg daily. Then dosage can usually be reduced to 15 mg daily. Maximum dosage is 90 mg daily.

ADVERSE REACTIONS

CNS: *dizziness,* vertigo, headache, hyperactivity, hyperreflexia, tremors, muscle twitching, mania, jitters, *insomnia,* confusion, memory impairment, drowsiness, weakness, fatigue.

CV: paradoxical hypertension, palpitations, *orthostatic hypotension,* ***arrhythmias.***

GI: dry mouth, *anorexia,* nausea, constipation.

Other: peripheral edema, diaphoresis, weight changes.

INTERACTIONS

Amphetamines, antihistamines, ephedrine, levodopa, meperidine, metaraminol, methylphenidate, phenylephrine, phenylpropanolamine, sympathomimetics: enhanced pressor effects. Avoid concomitant use.

Barbiturates, dextromethorphan, ethanol, methotrimeprazine, narcotics, other sedatives, tricyclic antidepressants: unpredictable interaction. Use these agents with caution and in reduced dosage.

Insulin, oral antidiabetic agents: increased risk of hypoglycemia. Use with caution and in reduced dosages.

Foods high in tryptophan, tyramine: may precipitate hypertensive crisis. Avoid concomitant use.

CONTRAINDICATIONS

- Contraindicated in elderly or debilitated patients; in patients with hepatic impairment, CHF, pheochromocytoma, hypertension, cardiovascular or cerebrovascular disease; or in patients with severe or frequent headaches.
- Contraindicated during therapy with other MAO inhibitors (isocarboxazid, tranylcypromine) or within 10 days of such therapy; within 10 days of elective surgery requiring general anesthetic, cocaine, or local anesthetic containing sympathomimetic vasoconstrictors; and in hyperactive, agitated, or schizophrenic patients.
- Use cautiously with antihypertensive agents containing thiazide diuretics, with spinal anesthetics, and in patients at risk for suicide or with diabetes, seizure disorders, or Parkinson's disease.

NURSING CONSIDERATIONS

- Obtain baseline blood pressure and heart rate readings, CBC, and liver function tests before therapy, and continue to monitor throughout treatment.
- Dosage is usually reduced to maintenance level as soon as possible.
- In most patients, discontinue MAO inhibitors 14 days before elective surgery to avoid drug interactions that may occur during the anesthetic procedure.
- Because MAO inhibitors may alleviate chest pain in patients with angina, warn such patients to moderate activities to prevent overexertion.
- Warn patients about the probability

*Liquid form contains alcohol.
**May contain tartrazine.

Common reactions are in italics; ***life-threatening,*** in bold italics.

of orthostatic hypotension. Supervise walking. Tell patients to get out of bed slowly, sitting up first for 1 minute.
- Monitor patients closely for suicidal tendencies, and allow a minimum supply of the drug.
- If patients develop symptoms of overdose (severe hypotension, palpitations, or frequent headaches), withhold dose and notify the doctor.
- Have phentolamine available to combat severe hypertension.
- Warn patients to avoid foods high in tryptophan (broad beans) or tyramine (aged cheese, Chianti wine, beer, avocados, chicken livers, chocolate, bananas, soy sauce, meat tenderizers, salami, bologna) and large amounts of caffeine.
- Tell patients to avoid alcohol while taking drug.
- Advise patients to consult their doctor before taking any other prescription or OTC medications. Severe adverse effects can occur if MAO inhibitors are taken with OTC cold, hay fever, or diet preparations.
- Continue precautions 10 days after stopping drug because it has long-lasting effects.
- Store drug in tight container, away from heat and light.

protriptyline hydrochloride

Triptil†, Vivactil

Pregnancy Risk Category: C

HOW SUPPLIED

Tablets: 5 mg, 10 mg

ACTION

Mechanism: A tricyclic antidepressant (TCA) that increases the amount of norepinephrine or serotonin, or both, in the CNS by blocking their reuptake by the presynaptic neurons.
Onset: therapeutic effect, 2 to 4 weeks or longer. **Duration:** elimination half-life, 67 to 89 hours.

INDICATIONS & DOSAGE

Depression –
Adults: 15 to 40 mg P.O. daily in divided doses, increasing gradually to maximum of 60 mg daily.

ADVERSE REACTIONS

CNS: excitation, ***seizures,*** tremor, weakness, confusion, headache, nervousness, EEG changes, extrapyramidal reactions.
CV: *tachycardia, ECG changes,* orthostatic hypotension, hypertension.
EENT: *blurred vision,* tinnitus, mydriasis.
GI: *dry mouth, constipation,* nausea, vomiting, anorexia, paralytic ileus.
GU: *urine retention.*
Skin: rash, urticaria, photosensitivity.
Other: *diaphoresis,* hypersensitivity reaction.
After abrupt withdrawal of long-term therapy: nausea, headache, malaise (does not indicate addiction).

INTERACTIONS

Barbiturates: decreased TCA blood levels. Monitor for decreased antidepressant effect.
Cimetidine, methylphenidate: may increase protriptyline serum levels. Monitor for adverse reactions.
Clonidine, epinephrine, norepinephrine: increased hypertensive effect. Use with caution.
CNS depressants, ethanol: enhanced CNS depression. Avoid concomitant use.
MAO inhibitors: may cause severe excitation, hyperpyrexia, seizures, or death, usually with high dose. Use with caution.

CONTRAINDICATIONS

- Contraindicated during acute recovery phase of MI, in patients with prostatic hyperplasia, and in those with seizure disorders.
- Use cautiously in elderly patients; in patients at risk for suicide; in pa-

tients with urine retention, increased intraocular pressure, cardiovascular disease, blood dyscrasia, impaired hepatic function, or thyroid disease; and in patients receiving thyroid medications, electroconvulsive therapy, or elective surgery.

NURSING CONSIDERATIONS

- Reduce dosage in elderly or debilitated patients and adolescents.
- Do not withdraw drug abruptly.
- Because of hypertensive episodes during surgery in patients receiving TCAs, gradually discontinue drug several days before surgery.
- If signs of psychosis occur or increase, expect doctor to reduce dosage. Record mood changes. Monitor patients for suicidal tendencies, and allow a minimum supply of the drug.
- Protriptyline has low potential for producing orthostatic hypotension and is the least sedating of the TCAs. It may even have amphetamine-like effects. To prevent insomnia, avoid late-day dosing.
- Protriptyline has high anticholinergic effects.
- Relieve dry mouth with sugarless hard candy or gum. Saliva substitutes may be necessary.
- Check for urine retention and constipation. Increase fluids, and suggest stool softener or high-fiber diet, as needed.
- Tell patients to avoid alcohol while taking this drug.
- Advise patients to consult their doctor before taking any other prescription or OTC medications.
- To prevent photosensitivity reactions, advise patients to use sunblock, wear protective clothing, and avoid prolonged exposure to strong sunlight.
- Used investigationally to treat patients with obstructive sleep apnea.

sertraline hydrochloride

Zoloft

Pregnancy Risk Category: B

HOW SUPPLIED

Tablets: 50 mg, 100 mg

ACTION

Mechanism: An antidepressant chemically unrelated to tricyclic, tetracyclic, or any other currently available agents. Probably acts by blocking the reuptake of serotonin (5-hydroxytryptamine; 5-HT) into presynaptic neurons in the CNS, prolonging the action of 5-HT.
Onset: 2 to 4 weeks. **Peak:** Serum levels peak 4½ to 8½ hours after dose. **Duration:** elimination half-life of sertraline, about 24 hours; of active metabolite N-desmethylsertraline, 62 to 104 hours.

INDICATIONS & DOSAGE

Depression, obsessive-compulsive disorder –
Adults: 50 mg P.O. daily. Adjust dosage as tolerated and p.r.n.; clinical trials involved dosage of 50 to 200 mg daily. Dosage adjustments should be made at intervals of no less than 1 week.

ADVERSE REACTIONS

CNS: *headache, tremor, dizziness, insomnia, somnolence,* syncope, paresthesia, hypoesthesia, hyperesthesia, twitching, hypertonia, confusion, ataxia, abnormal coordination or gait, vertigo, hyperkinesia, hypokinesia, mania.
CV: palpitations, chest pain, postural hypotension, hypertension, hypotension, edema, peripheral ischemia, tachycardia.
EENT: nystagmus.
GI: *dry mouth, nausea, diarrhea, loose stools, dyspepsia,* vomiting, flatulence, anorexia, abdominal pain, increased appetite, dysphagia.

GU: male sexual dysfunction.
Skin: rash, acne, alopecia, pruritus, erythematous or maculopapular rash, cold or clammy skin, dry skin.
Other: *diaphoresis,* flushing, myalgia.

INTERACTIONS

Diazepam, tolbutamide: decreased clearance of these drugs. Clinical significance unknown; however, monitor patients for increased drug effects.
MAO inhibitors: may cause serious mental status changes, hyperthermia, autonomic instability, rapid fluctuations of vital signs, delirium, coma, and death. Avoid concomitant use.
Warfarin, other highly protein-bound drugs: may increase plasma levels of sertraline or other highly bound drug. Small (8%) increases in PT have been seen with concomitant use of warfarin. Monitor closely.

CONTRAINDICATIONS

- Contraindicated in patients hypersensitive to the drug, and in patients taking an MAO inhibitor within 14 days of starting therapy.
- Use cautiously in patients with hepatic impairment or seizure disorders, in patients with history of drug abuse, or in patients at risk for suicide.
- Use cautiously with other highly protein-bound drugs, such as warfarin; sertraline is 98% bound to plasma proteins.

NURSING CONSIDERATIONS

- Administer sertraline once daily, either in the morning or evening. May be given with or without food.
- Do not administer sertraline with, or within 14 days of discontinuing, MAO inhibitor therapy. Allow 14 days after discontinuing sertraline before starting treatment with an MAO inhibitor.
- Record mood changes. Monitor patients for suicidal tendencies, and allow a minimum supply of the drug.
- May change several laboratory values – increases in serum cholesterol and triglyceride levels, decreases in uric acid concentrations, and elevations in AST, and ALT (usually within the first 9 weeks of therapy). AST and ALT values return to normal after discontinuing drug; clinical significance is unknown.
- Patients who improve during the first 8 weeks of therapy will probably continue to respond to the drug; however, information is limited about use for longer than 16 weeks. Periodically monitor effectiveness during prolonged use. It is unknown if periodic dosage adjustments are necessary to maintain effectiveness.
- Advise patients to use caution when performing hazardous tasks that require alertness and to avoid alcohol while taking this drug. Drugs that influence the CNS may impair judgment.
- Caution patients to check with their doctors or pharmacists before taking any OTC medications.

tranylcypromine sulfate

Parnate

Pregnancy Risk Category: C

HOW SUPPLIED

Tablets: 10 mg

ACTION

Mechanism: An MAO inhibitor that promotes accumulation of neurotransmitters by inhibiting MAO.
Onset: therapeutic effect, 2 to 4 weeks or longer. **Peak:** Plasma levels peak in 1 to 3½ hours. **Duration:** recover of MAO activity, about 10 days after therapy ends.

INDICATIONS & DOSAGE

Depression –
Adults: 10 mg P.O. b.i.d. Increase to maximum of 30 mg daily, if neces-

sary, after 2 weeks. Not recommended for children under 16 years.

ADVERSE REACTIONS

CNS: *dizziness,* vertigo, headache, hyperactivity, hyperreflexia, tremors, muscle twitching, mania, jitters, confusion, memory impairment, fatigue.
CV: *orthostatic hypotension,* ***arrhythmias,*** paradoxical hypertension, palpitations.
EENT: blurred vision.
GI: dry mouth, *anorexia,* nausea, diarrhea, constipation, abdominal pain.
GU: impotence.
Skin: rash.
Other: peripheral edema, diaphoresis, weight changes, chills, altered libido.

INTERACTIONS

Amphetamines, antihistamines, ephedrine, levodopa, meperidine, metaraminol, methylphenidate, phenylephrine, phenylpropanolamine, sympathomimetics: enhanced pressor effects of these drugs. Avoid concomitant use.
Barbiturates, dextromethorphan, ethanol, methotrimeprazine, narcotics, other sedatives, tricyclic antidepressants: enhanced adverse CNS effects. Use with caution and in reduced dosage.
Insulin, oral antidiabetic agents: increased risk of hypoglycemia. Use with caution and in reduced dosages.
Foods high in tryptophan, tyramine: may cause hypertensive crisis. Avoid concomitant use.

CONTRAINDICATIONS

- Contraindicated in patients with severe hepatic or renal impairment, CHF, pheochromocytoma, hypertension, or cardiovascular or cerebrovascular disease; in patients with severe or frequent headaches; and in patients taking antihypertensives or diuretics.
- Contraindicated in elderly or debilitated patients; in patients for whom close supervision is not possible; and in hyperactive, agitated, or schizophrenic patients.
- Also contraindicated with foods containing tryptophan or tyramine; during therapy with other MAO inhibitors (phenelzine, isocarboxazid) or within 7 days of such therapy; and within 7 days of elective surgery requiring general anesthetic, cocaine, or local anesthetic containing sympathomimetic vasoconstrictors.
- Use cautiously with antiparkinsonian drugs or spinal anesthetics; in patients with renal disease, diabetes, seizure disorder, Parkinson's disease, and hyperthyroidism; and in patients at risk for suicide.

NURSING CONSIDERATIONS

- Obtain baseline blood pressure and heart rate readings, CBC, and liver function tests before beginning therapy, and continue to monitor throughout treatment.
- Dosage is usually reduced to maintenance level as soon as possible.
- Do not withdraw drug abruptly.
- In most patients, discontinue MAO inhibitors 14 days before elective surgery to avoid drug interactions that may occur during the anesthetic procedure.
- Because MAO inhibitors may alleviate chest pain in patients with angina, warn such patients to moderate activities to avoid overexertion.
- To prevent dizziness resulting from orthostatic hypotension, tell patients to get out of bed slowly, sitting up for 1 minute first.
- Monitor patients for suicidal tendencies, and allow them only a minimum supply of the drug.
- If patients develop symptoms of overdose (palpitations, severe hypotension, or frequent headaches), withhold dose and notify the doctor.
- Have phentolamine available to combat severe hypertension.

• MAO inhibitor most often reported to cause hypertensive crisis with ingestion of foods high in tyramine, including aged cheese, Chianti wine, beer, avocados, chicken livers, chocolate, bananas, soy sauce, meat tenderizers, salami, bologna. Warn patients to avoid foods high in tyramine or tryptophan and large amounts of caffeine.
• Tell patients to avoid alcohol while taking this drug.
• Advise patients to consult their doctors before taking any other prescription or OTC medications. Severe adverse effects can occur if MAO inhibitors are taken with OTC cold, hay fever, or diet preparations.
• Continue precautions for 7 days after stopping drug; effects are long lasting.

trazodone hydrochloride

Desyrel, Trazon, Trialodine

Pregnancy Risk Category: C

HOW SUPPLIED
Tablets: 50 mg, 100 mg, 150 mg, 300 mg

ACTION
Mechanism: Inhibits serotonin uptake in the brain. Not a tricyclic derivative; considered an atypical antidepressant.
Onset: antidepressant effects, 2 to 4 weeks or longer. **Peak:** Plasma levels peak after 1 hour if taken on an empty stomach, 2 hours if taken with food.
Duration: terminal elimination half-life, about 5 to 9 hours.

INDICATIONS & DOSAGE
Depression –
Adults: initial dosage, 150 mg P.O. daily in divided doses; can be increased by 50 mg daily q 3 to 4 days. Average dosage ranges from 150 mg to 400 mg daily. Maximum dosage is 600 mg.

ADVERSE REACTIONS
CNS: *drowsiness, dizziness,* nervousness, fatigue, confusion, tremors, weakness, hostility, anger, nightmares, vivid dreams.
CV: orthostatic hypotension, tachycardia, bradycardia.
EENT: blurred vision, tinnitus.
GI: dry mouth, dysgeusia, constipation, nausea, vomiting, anorexia.
GU: urine retention, priapism possibly leading to impotence, hematuria.
Hematologic: anemia.
Skin: rash, urticaria.
Other: diaphoresis.

INTERACTIONS
Antihypertensives: increased hypotensive effect of trazodone. Antihypertensive dosage may have to be decreased.
Clonidine, CNS depressants, ethanol: enhanced CNS depression.
Digoxin, phenytoin: may increase serum levels of these drugs. Monitor for toxicity.
MAO inhibitors: no clinical experience. Use together very cautiously.

CONTRAINDICATIONS
• Contraindicated during initial recovery phase of MI.
• Avoid concurrent administration with electroconvulsive therapy.
• Use cautiously in patients with cardiac disease, in patients at risk for suicide, and in patients receiving CNS depressants.

NURSING CONSIDERATIONS
• Priapism is a potential problem in men taking trazodone; may require surgical intervention.
• Record mood changes. Monitor patients for suicidal tendencies, and allow minimum supply of the drug.
• Teach patients' families how to recognize signs of suicidal tendency or ideation.
• Warn patients to avoid activities that require alertness and good psy-

chomotor coordination until CNS effects of the drug are known. Drowsiness and dizziness usually subside after the first few weeks.
• Administer after meals or a light snack for optimal absorption and to decrease incidence of dizziness.
• Anticholinergic and adverse cardiac effects are minimal.

trimipramine maleate

Apo-Trimip†, Novo-Triptamine†, Rhotrimine†, Surmontil
Pregnancy Risk Category: C

HOW SUPPLIED

Tablets: 25 mg‡
Capsules: 25 mg, 50 mg, 100 mg

ACTION

Mechanism: A tricyclic antidepressant (TCA) that increases the amount of norepinephrine or serotonin, or both, in the CNS by blocking their reuptake by the presynaptic neurons.
Onset: antidepressant effects, 2 to 4 weeks or longer. **Peak:** Plasma concentration peak in 2 hours. **Duration:** plasma half-life, 9 hours.

INDICATIONS & DOSAGE

Depression –
Adults: 75 mg P.O. daily in divided doses, increased to 200 mg daily. Dosages over 300 mg daily not recommended.

ADVERSE REACTIONS

CNS: *drowsiness, dizziness,* excitation, tremors, weakness, confusion, headache, nervousness, EEG changes, ***seizures,*** extrapyramidal reactions.
CV: *orthostatic hypotension, tachycardia, ECG changes,* hypertension.
EENT: *blurred vision,* tinnitus, mydriasis.
GI: *dry mouth, constipation,* nausea, vomiting, anorexia, paralytic ileus.
GU: *urine retention.*
Skin: rash, urticaria, photosensitivity.
Other: *diaphoresis,* hypersensitivity reaction.
After abrupt withdrawal of long-term therapy: nausea, headache, malaise (does not indicate addiction).

INTERACTIONS

Barbiturates: decreased TCA blood levels. Monitor for decreased antidepressant effect.
Cimetidine, methylphenidate: may increase trimipramine serum levels. Monitor for increased adverse reactions.
Clonidine, epinephrine, norepinephrine: increased hypertensive effect. Use with caution.
CNS depressants, ethanol: enhanced CNS depression. Avoid concomitant use.
MAO inhibitors: may cause severe excitation, hyperpyrexia, or seizures, usually with high dose. Use with caution.

CONTRAINDICATIONS

• Contraindicated during acute recovery phase of MI; in patients with prostatic hyperplasia or seizure disorders; in patients at risk for suicide; and in patients receiving electroconvulsive therapy, thyroid drugs, or elective surgery.
• Use with extreme caution in patients with CV disease, urine retention, acute angle-closure glaucoma, increased intraocular pressure, thyroid disease, blood dyscrasia, or impaired hepatic function.

NURSING CONSIDERATIONS

• Reduce dosage in elderly or debilitated persons and adolescents.
• Do not withdraw drug abruptly.
• Because of hypertensive episodes during surgery in patients receiving TCAs, gradually discontinue drug several days before surgery.
• If signs of psychosis occur or in-

crease, expect doctor to reduce dosage. Record mood changes. Monitor patients for suicidal tendencies, and allow a minimum supply of the drug.
• Warn patients to avoid hazardous activities that require alertness and good psychomotor coordination until CNS effects of the drug are known. Drowsiness and dizziness usually subside after a few weeks.
• To avoid daytime sedation, tell patients to take full dose h.s. Warn them about possible morning orthostatic hypotension.
• Tell patients to avoid alcohol while taking this drug.
• Relieve dry mouth with sugarless hard candy or gum. Saliva substitutes may be necessary.
• Effectiveness in enuresis may decrease with long-term use.
• Check for urine retention and constipation. Increase fluids, and suggest stool softener or high-fiber diet, as needed.
• Advise patients to consult their doctors before taking any other prescription or OTC medications.
• To prevent photosensitivity reactions, advise patients to use sunblock, wear protective clothing, and avoid prolonged exposure to strong sunlight.

venlafaxine hydrochloride

Effexor

Pregnancy Risk Category: C

HOW SUPPLIED

Tablets: 25 mg, 37.5 mg, 50 mg, 75 mg, 100 mg

ACTION

Mechanism: Blocks reuptake of norepinephrine and serotonin into neurons in CNS.
Onset: days to weeks. **Peak:** Steady-state plasma levels are reached after 3 days of therapy. **Duration:** elimination half life of venlafaxine, about 5 hours; of its major active metabolite, about 11 hours.

INDICATIONS & DOSAGE

Depression –
Adults: initially 75 mg P.O. daily, in two or three divided doses with food. Increase dosage as tolerated p.r.n. in increments of 75 mg/day at intervals of no less than 4 days. For moderately depressed outpatients, usual maximum dosage is 225 mg/day; in certain severely depressed patients, dosage may be as high as 375 mg/day.

ADVERSE REACTIONS

CNS: *headache, somnolence, dizziness, nervousness,* insomnia, anxiety.
CV: *hypertension.*
EENT: *blurred vision.*
GI: *nausea, constipation, vomiting, dry mouth.*
GU: *abnormal ejaculation, impotence.*
Other: *tremor, diaphoresis,* asthenia, weight loss.

INTERACTIONS

MAO inhibitors: may precipitate a syndrome similar to neuroleptic malignant syndrome (myoclonus, hyperthermia, seizures, and death). Do not start venlafaxine within 14 days of discontinuing therapy with an MAO inhibitor, and don't start MAO inhibitor therapy within 7 days of stopping venlafaxine.

CONTRAINDICATIONS

• Contraindicated in patients hypersensitive to the drug. Also contraindicated for use within 14 days of an MAO inhibitor.
• Use cautiously in patients with renal or hepatic impairment, and in those with history of mania or seizures.

NURSING CONSIDERATIONS

• Total daily dosage should be reduced by 50% in patients with hepatic impairment. In patients with moderate renal impairment (glomerular filtration rate of 10 to 70 ml/minute), total daily dosage should be reduced by 25%. In patients undergoing hemodialysis, withold dose until dialysis session is completed and reduce daily dosage by 50%.

- Patients who have received drug for 6 weeks or more should gradually taper dosage over a 2-week period.
- Carefully monitor blood pressure. Venlafaxine therapy is associated with sustained, dose-dependent increases in blood pressure. Greatest increases (averaging about 7 mm Hg above baseline) occur in patients taking 375 mg/day.

*Liquid form contains alcohol.
**May contain tartrazine.

31

Antianxiety agents

alprazolam
buspirone hydrochloride
chlordiazepoxide
chlordiazepoxide hydrochloride
clorazepate dipotassium
diazepam
halazepam
hydroxyzine embonate
hydroxyzine hydrochloride
hydroxyzine pamoate
lorazepam
meprobamate
oxazepam
prazepam

COMBINATION PRODUCTS

EQUAGESIC: meprobamate 200 mg and aspirin 325 mg.
LIBRAX CAPSULES: chlordiazepoxide hydrochloride 5 mg and clidinium bromide 2.5 mg.
LIMBITROL 5-12.5: chlordiazepoxide 5 mg and amitriptyline hydrochloride 12.5 mg.
LIMBITROL 10-25: chlordiazepoxide 10 mg and amitriptyline hydrochloride 25 mg.
MENRIUM 5-2: chlordiazepoxide 5 mg and esterified estrogens 0.2 mg.
MENRIUM 5-4: chlordiazepoxide 5 mg and esterified estrogens 0.4 mg.
MENRIUM 10-4: chlordiazepoxide 10 mg and esterified estrogens 0.4 mg.
MILPREM-200: meprobamate 200 mg and conjugated estrogens 0.45 mg.
MILPREM-400: meprobamate 400 mg and conjugated estrogens 0.45 mg.
PMB 200: meprobamate 200 mg and conjugated estrogens 0.45 mg.
PMB 400: meprobamate 400 mg and conjugated estrogens 0.45 mg.

alprazolam

Apo-Alpraz†, Novo-Alprazol†, Nu-Alpraz†, Xanax
Controlled Substance Schedule IV
Pregnancy Risk Category: D

HOW SUPPLIED

Tablets: 0.25 mg, 0.5 mg, 1 mg, 2 mg
Oral solution: 0.5 mg/5 ml, 1 mg/ml (concentrate)

ACTION

Mechanism: A benzodiazepine that potentiates the effects of gamma-aminobutyric acid, an inhibitory neurotransmitter, and depresses the CNS at the limbic and subcortical levels of the brain.
Peak: Serum levels peak within 1 to 2 hours of oral dose. **Duration:** elimination half-life, 11 to 16 hours.

INDICATIONS & DOSAGE

Anxiety and tension –
Adults: usual initial dose, 0.25 to 0.5 mg P.O. t.i.d. Maximum dosage is 4 mg daily in divided doses.
Elderly or debilitated patients: usual initial dose, 0.25 mg P.O. b.i.d. or t.i.d. Maximum dosage is 4 mg daily in divided doses.

ADVERSE REACTIONS

CNS: *drowsiness, light-headedness,* headache, confusion, hostility, anterograde amnesia, restlessness, psychosis, ***suicidal tendencies.***
CV: transient hypotension, tachycardia.
EENT: visual disturbances.
GI: dry mouth, nausea, vomiting, constipation, discomfort.
GU: incontinence, urine retention, menstrual irregularities.

INTERACTIONS
Cimetidine: increased sedation. Monitor carefully.
Digoxin: may increase serum levels of digoxin, increasing toxicity. Monitor closely.
Ethanol, other CNS depressants: increased CNS depression. Avoid concomitant use.
Smoking: increased clearance of benzodiazepines. Monitor for lack of effect.
Tricyclic antidepressants: increased plasma levels of tricyclic antidepressants. Monitor for toxicity.

CONTRAINDICATIONS
• Contraindicated in patients with acute angle-closure glaucoma, psychoses, or anxiety-free psychiatric disorders.
• Use cautiously in patients with hepatic or renal disease and in elderly or debilitated patients.

NURSING CONSIDERATIONS
• Do not withdraw drug abruptly after long-term use; withdrawal symptoms may occur. Abuse or addiction is possible.
• Drug should not be prescribed for everyday stress or for long-term use (more than 4 months).
• Monitor liver, renal, and hematopoietic function studies periodically in patients receiving repeated or prolonged therapy.
• Alprazolam is more rapidly metabolized and excreted than most other benzodiazepines, with a lower incidence of lethargy than other drugs of this class.
• Warn patients to avoid hazardous activities that require alertness and good psychomotor coordination until CNS effects of the drug are known.
• Tell patients to avoid alcohol while taking this drug.
• If alprazolam overdose occurs, flumazenil (a specific benzodiazepine antagonist) may be useful. Alprazolam's duration of action is longer than flumazenil's; resedation possible.
• May be effective for depression.

buspirone hydrochloride
BuSpar

Pregnancy Risk Category: B

HOW SUPPLIED
Tablets: 5 mg, 10 mg

ACTION
Mechanism: May inhibit neuronal firing and reduce 5-HT turnover in cortical, amygdaloid, and septohippocampal tissue.
Onset: therapeutic effect, 1 to 2 weeks; optimal results, 3 to 4 weeks.
Peak: Serum levels peak within 40 to 90. **Duration:** half-life, 2 to 3 hours.

INDICATIONS & DOSAGE
Anxiety disorders; short-term relief of anxiety–
Adults: initially, 5 mg P.O. t.i.d. Dosage may be increased at 3-day intervals. Usual maintenance dosage is 20 to 30 mg daily in divided doses. Do not exceed 60 mg/day.

ADVERSE REACTIONS
CNS: *dizziness, drowsiness,* nervousness, excitement, insomnia, headache.
GI: dry mouth, nausea, diarrhea.
Other: fatigue.

INTERACTIONS
Ethanol, other CNS depressants: increased CNS depression. Avoid concomitant use.
MAO inhibitors: may elevate blood pressure. Avoid concomitant use.

CONTRAINDICATIONS
• Contraindicated in patients hypersensitive to the drug.
• Use cautiously in patients with hepatic or renal failure.

NURSING CONSIDERATIONS

- Unlike the benzodiazepines, buspirone is not an effective anticonvulsant or skeletal muscle relaxant.
- Buspirone is less sedating than other anxiolytics and does not produce any serious functional impairment. However, CNS effects in individual patients may be unpredictable.
- Warn patients to avoid hazardous activities that require alertness and good psychomotor coordination until CNS effects of the drug are known.
- Tell patients to take drug with food.
- Before initiating buspirone therapy in patients already being treated with benzodiazepines, warn them against stopping the benzodiazepine abruptly; withdrawal reaction may occur.
- Has shown no potential for abuse and has not been classified as a controlled substance. However, it is not recommended to relieve everyday stress.

chlordiazepoxide

Librium, Libritabs

chlordiazepoxide hydrochloride

Apo-Chlordiazepoxide†, Librium, Lipoxide, Novopoxide†, Solium†
Controlled Substance Schedule IV

Pregnancy Risk Category: D

HOW SUPPLIED

chlordiazepoxide
Tablets: 5 mg, 10 mg, 25 mg
chlordiazepoxide hydrochloride
Capsules: 5 mg, 10 mg, 25 mg
Powder for injection: 100 mg/ampule

ACTION

Mechanism: Depresses the CNS at the limbic and subcortical levels of the brain.
Peak: Plasma levels peak in 30 minutes to 4 hours. **Duration:** elimination half-life, 5 to 30 hours; for some active metabolites, up to 100 hours.

INDICATIONS & DOSAGE

Mild to moderate anxiety and tension –
Adults: 5 to 10 mg P.O. t.i.d. or q.i.d.
Children over 6 years: 5 mg P.O. b.i.d. to q.i.d. Maximum dosage is 10 mg P.O. b.i.d. to t.i.d.
Severe anxiety and tension –
Adults: 20 to 25 mg P.O. t.i.d. or q.i.d.
Withdrawal symptoms of acute alcoholism –
Adults: 50 to 100 mg P.O., I.M., or I.V. Maximum dosage is 300 mg daily.
Preoperative apprehension and anxiety –
Adults: 5 to 10 mg P.O. t.i.d. or q.i.d. on day preceding surgery; or 50 to 100 mg I.M. 1 hour before surgery.

Note: Parenteral form not recommended in children under 12 years.

ADVERSE REACTIONS

CNS: *drowsiness, lethargy, hangover,* fainting, restlessness, psychosis, ***suicidal tendencies.***
CV: *thrombophlebitis,* transient hypotension.
EENT: visual disturbances.
GI: nausea, vomiting, abdominal discomfort.
GU: incontinence, urine retention, menstrual irregularities.
Skin: *swelling, pain at injection site.*

INTERACTIONS

Cimetidine: increased sedation. Monitor carefully.
Digoxin: increased serum digoxin levels and risk of toxicity. Monitor closely.
Ethanol, other CNS depressants: increased CNS depression. Avoid concomitant use.
Smoking: increased clearance of benzodiazepines. Monitor for lack of effect.

CONTRAINDICATIONS
• Contraindicated in patients hypersensitive to the drug and in those with acute angle-closure glaucoma, psychoses, or anxiety-free psychiatric disorders.
• Use cautiously in patients with mental depression, psychiatric disturbances, blood dyscrasia, porphyria, hepatic or renal disease, or in patients undergoing anticoagulant therapy.

NURSING CONSIDERATIONS
• Reduce dosage in elderly or debilitated patients.
• Drug should not be prescribed regularly for everyday stress.
• Monitor liver, renal, and hematopoietic function studies periodically in patients receiving repeated or prolonged therapy.
• Possibility of abuse and addiction exists. Do not withdraw drug abruptly after long-term administration; withdrawal symptoms may occur.
• Warn patients to avoid hazardous activities that require alertness and good psychomotor coordination until CNS effects of the drug are known.
• Tell patients to avoid alcohol while taking this drug.
• Injectable form (as hydrochloride) comes as two ampules – diluent and powdered drug. Read directions carefully.
• Recommended for I.M. use only, but may be given I.V.
• **I.V. use:** Use 5 ml of 0.9% sodium chloride solution or sterile water for injection as diluent; do not give packaged diluent I.V. Administer over 1 minute.
• When giving drug I.V., be sure equipment and personnel needed for emergency airway management are available. Monitor respirations every 5 to 15 minutes and before each repeated I.V. dose.
• For I.M. use, add 2 ml of diluent to powder and agitate gently until clear. Use immediately. I.M. form may be erratically absorbed.
• Keep powder away from light and refrigerate; mix just before use and discard remainder.
• Do not mix injectable form with any other parenteral drug.
• If chlordiazepoxide overdose occurs, flumazenil (a specific benzodiazepine antagonist) may be useful. Chlordiazepoxide's duration of action is longer than flumazenil's; resedation possible.
• May cause false-positive reaction in the Gravindex pregnancy test. May also interfere with certain tests for urine 17-ketosteroids.

clorazepate dipotassium

Apo-Clorazepate†, Gen-Xene, Novoclopate†, Tranxene, Tranxene-SD, Tranxene-T-Tab
Controlled Substance Schedule IV

Pregnancy Risk Category: D

HOW SUPPLIED
Tablets: 3.75 mg, 7.5 mg, 11.25 mg, 15 mg, 22.5 mg
Capsules: 3.75 mg, 7.5 mg, 15 mg

ACTION
Mechanism: A benzodiazepine that facilitates the action of the inhibitory neurotransmitter gamma-aminobutyric acid. Depresses the CNS at the limbic and subcortical levels of the brain and suppresses the spread of seizure activity produced by epileptogenic foci in the cortex, thalamus, and limbic structures.
Onset: within 2½ hours. **Peak:** Plasma levels peak within 1 to 2 hours. **Duration:** half-lives for some active metabolites, up to 100 hours.

INDICATIONS & DOSAGE
Acute alcohol withdrawal –
Adults: day 1 – 30 mg P.O. initially, followed by 30 to 60 mg P.O. in divided doses; day 2 – 45 to 90 mg P.O.

in divided doses; day 3 – 22.5 to 45 mg P.O. in divided doses; day 4 – 15 to 30 mg P.O. in divided doses; gradually reduce dosage to 7.5 to 15 mg daily.
Anxiety –
Adults: 15 to 60 mg P.O. daily.
Adjunct in seizure disorder –
Adults and children over 12 years: Maximum recommended initial dosage is 7.5 mg P.O. t.i.d. Dosage increases should be no greater than 7.5 mg/week. Maximum dosage should not exceed 90 mg daily.
Children between 9 and 12 years: Maximum recommended initial dosage is 7.5 mg P.O. b.i.d. Dosage increases should be no greater than 7.5 mg/week. Maximum dosage should not exceed 60 mg daily.

ADVERSE REACTIONS
CNS: *drowsiness, lethargy, hangover,* fainting, restlessness, psychosis.
CV: transient hypotension.
EENT: visual disturbances.
GI: nausea, vomiting, abdominal discomfort.
GU: urine retention, incontinence.

INTERACTIONS
Cimetidine: increased sedation. Monitor carefully.
Digoxin: may increase serum levels of digoxin, increasing toxicity. Monitor closely.
Ethanol, other CNS depressants: increased CNS depression. Avoid concomitant use.
Smoking: increased clearance of benzodiazepines. Monitor for lack of effect.

CONTRAINDICATIONS
- Contraindicated in patients with acute angle-closure glaucoma, depressive neuroses, and psychotic reactions.
- Use cautiously in patients with renal or hepatic impairment.

NURSING CONSIDERATIONS
- Reduce dosage in elderly or debilitated patients.
- Drug should not be prescribed regularly for everyday stress.
- Monitor liver, renal, and hematopoietic function studies periodically in patients receiving repeated or prolonged therapy.
- Possibility of abuse and addiction exists. Do not withdraw drug abruptly after prolonged use; withdrawal symptoms may occur.
- Warn patients to avoid activities that require alertness and good psychomotor coordination until CNS effects of the drug are known.
- Tell patients to avoid alcohol while taking this drug.
- Sugarless chewing gum or hard candy can relieve dry mouth.
- If clorazepate overdose occurs, flumazenil (a specific benzodiazepine antagonist) may be useful. Clorazepate's duration of action is longer than flumazenil's; resedation possible.

diazepam
Apo-Diazepam†, Atenex‡, Diazemuls†‡, Diazepam Intensol, Ducene‡, Novodipam†, PMS Diazepam†, T-Quil, Valium, Valrelease, Vazepam, Vivol†, Zetran
Controlled Substance Schedule IV
Pregnancy Risk Category: D

HOW SUPPLIED
Tablets: 2 mg, 5 mg, 10 mg
Capsules (extended-release): 15 mg
Oral solution: 5 mg/5 ml, 5 mg/ml
Injection: 5 mg/ml
Sterile emulsion for injection: 5 mg/ml†

ACTION
Mechanism: A benzodiazepine that depresses the CNS at the limbic and subcortical levels of the brain. Suppresses spread of seizure activity pro-

duced by epileptogenic foci in the cortex, thalamus, and limbic structures.
Onset: 30 minutes after oral dose, 1 to 5 minutes after I.V. injection.
Peak: Plasma levels peak 30 minutes to 2 hours after oral dose, immediately after I.V. injection; peak levels after administration of injectable emulsion occur 15 minutes after I.V. injection, 2 hours after I.M. injection.
Duration: effects persist 3 to 8 hours after oral dose, 15 minutes to 1 hour after I.V. injection.

INDICATIONS & DOSAGE

Tension, anxiety, adjunct in seizure disorders or skeletal muscle spasm –
Adults: 2 to 10 mg P.O. t.i.d. or q.i.d. Or 15 to 30 mg of extended-release capsule once daily.
Elderly or debilitated patients: 2.5 mg P.O. b.i.d.
Children over 6 months: 1 to 2.5 mg P.O. t.i.d. or q.i.d. Alternatively, 0.12 to 0.8 mg/kg or 3.5 to 24 mg/m² P.O. daily in 3 or 4 divided doses.
Tension, anxiety, muscle spasm, endoscopic procedures, seizures –
Adults: 5 to 10 mg I.V. initially, up to 30 mg in 1 hour or possibly more for cardioversion or status epilepticus, depending on response.
Children 30 days to 5 years: 0.2 to 0.5 mg I.V. or I.M. slowly q 2 to 5 minutes to maximum of 5 mg. Repeat q 2 to 4 hours.
Children 5 years and older: 1 mg I.V. or I.M. slowly q 2 to 5 minutes to maximum of 10 mg. Repeat q 2 to 4 hours.
Tetanic muscle spasms –
Infants over 30 days: 1 to 2 mg I.M. or I.V. q 3 to 4 hours, p.r.n.
Children over 5 years: 5 to 10 mg I.M. or I.V. q 3 to 4 hours, p.r.n.
Status epilepticus –
Adults: 5 to 20 mg slow I.V. push at 2 to 5 mg/minute; may repeat q 5 to 10 minutes up to maximum total dose of 60 mg. Use 2 to 5 mg in elderly or debilitated patients. May repeat therapy in 20 to 30 minutes with caution if seizures recur.
Children: 0.1 to 0.3 mg/kg slow I.V. push at 1 mg/minute over 3 minutes; may repeat q 15 minutes for 2 doses. Maximum single dose in children under 5 years is 5 mg; in children over 5 years, 10 mg.

ADVERSE REACTIONS

CNS: *drowsiness, lethargy, hangover, ataxia,* fainting, depression, restlessness, anterograde amnesia, psychosis, slurred speech, tremor.
CV: transient hypotension, bradycardia, ***cardiovascular collapse.***
EENT: diplopia, blurred vision, nystagmus.
GI: nausea, vomiting, abdominal discomfort.
GU: incontinence, urine retention.
Respiratory: respiratory depression.
Skin: rash, urticaria, desquamation.
Other: physical or psychological dependence, ***acute abstinence syndrome*** after sudden withdrawal in physically dependent persons, *pain, phlebitis at injection site.*

INTERACTIONS

Cimetidine: increased sedation. Monitor carefully.
Digoxin: may increase serum levels of digoxin, increasing toxicity. Monitor closely.
Ethanol, other CNS depressants: increased CNS depression. Avoid concomitant use.
Phenobarbital: increased effects of both drugs. Use together cautiously.
Smoking: increased clearance of benzodiazepines. Monitor for lack of effect.

CONTRAINDICATIONS

• Contraindicated in patients in experiencing shock, coma, or acute alcohol intoxication; in patients with acute angle-closure glaucoma, psychoses, or myasthenia gravis; and in oral form for children under 6 months.

• Use cautiously in patients with blood dyscrasia, liver or kidney damage, depression, or chronic open-angle glaucoma; in elderly and debilitated patients; and in those with limited pulmonary reserve.

NURSING CONSIDERATIONS

• Reduce dosage in elderly or debilitated patients because they may be more susceptible to the adverse CNS effects of the drug.
• Drug should not be prescribed regularly for everyday stress.
• Drug of choice (I.V. form) for status epilepticus. Seizures may recur within 20 to 30 minutes of initial control because of redistribution of drug.
• Monitor periodic liver, renal, and hematopoietic function studies in patients receiving repeated or prolonged therapy.
• Possibility of abuse and addiction exists. Do not withdraw drug abruptly after long-term use; withdrawal symptoms may occur.
• Warn patients to avoid activities that require alertness and good psychomotor coordination until CNS effects of the drug are known.
• Tell patients to avoid alcohol while taking this drug.
• If diazepam overdose occurs, flumazenil (a specific benzodiazepine antagonist) may be useful. Diazepam's duration of action is longer than flumazenil's; resedation possible.
• **I.V. use:** Give at rate not to exceed 5 mg/minute. When injecting I.V., administer directly into the vein. If this is impossible, inject slowly through the infusion tubing as near to the vein insertion site as possible. Watch daily for phlebitis at injection site.
• Parenteral emulsion – a stabilized oil-in-water emulsion – should appear milky white and uniform. Avoid mixing with any other drugs or solutions, and avoid infusion sets or containers made from polyvinyl chloride. If dilution is necessary, drug may be mixed with I.V. fat emulsion. Use, the admixture within 6 hours.
• Do not store in plastic syringes.
• Do not mix injectable form with other drugs because diazepam is incompatible with most drugs.
• Avoid extravasation. Do not inject into small veins.
• Continuous infusions of 1 to 10 mg/hr have been used to prevent seizure recurrence. However, controversy exists about the use of diluted diazepam solutions for continuous I.V. infusion because of its low aqueous solubility. Under certain conditions, it may be compatible with 0.9% sodium chloride or lactated Ringer's injection, but the solution may not be stable. Consult hospital pharmacy about reconstitution and stability.
• Monitor respirations every 5 to 15 minutes and before each repeated I.V. dose. Have emergency resuscitation equipment and oxygen at bedside.
• I.V. route is the most reliable parenteral route; I.M. administration is not recommended because absorption is variable and injection is painful.
• When oral concentrate solution is used, dilute the dose just before administering. Use water, juice, or carbonated beverages, or mix with semisolid food such as applesauce or pudding.

halazepam

Paxipam
Controlled Substance Schedule IV
Pregnancy Risk Category: D

HOW SUPPLIED

Tablets: 20 mg, 40 mg

ACTION

Mechanism: Potentiates the effects of gamma-aminobutyric acid, an inhibitory neurotransmitter and depresses the CNS at the limbic and subcortical levels of the brain.
Onset: within 2 to 3 hours. **Peak:**

Serum levels peak within 1 to 3 hours.
Duration: elimination half-life, 14 hours; half-lives for some active metabolites, up to 100 hours.

INDICATIONS & DOSAGE
Anxiety and tension –
Adults: Usual dose, 20 to 40 mg P.O. t.i.d. or q.i.d. Optimal dosage is 80 to 160 mg daily.
Elderly or debilitated patients: initially, 20 mg once or twice daily.

ADVERSE REACTIONS
CNS: *drowsiness, lethargy, hangover,* fainting.
CV: transient hypotension.
GI: dry mouth, nausea and vomiting, discomfort.
Other: ***acute abstinence syndrome*** following sudden withdrawal in physically dependent persons.

INTERACTIONS
Cimetidine: increase sedation. Monitor carefully.
Digoxin: may increase serum levels of digoxin, increasing toxicity. Monitor closely.
Ethanol, other CNS depressants: increased CNS depression. Avoid concomitant use.
Smoking: increased clearance of benzodiazepines. Monitor for lack of effect.

CONTRAINDICATIONS
- Contraindicated in patients hypersensitive to the drug and in patients with acute angle-closure glaucoma, psychoses, or anxiety-free psychiatric disorders.
- Use cautiously in patients with hepatic or renal impairment.

NURSING CONSIDERATIONS
- Drug should not be prescribed for everyday stress or for long-term use (more than 4 months).
- Monitor liver, renal, and hematopoietic function studies periodically in patients receiving repeated or prolonged therapy.
- Possibility of abuse and addiction exists. Do not withdraw drug abruptly after long-term use; withdrawal symptoms may occur.
- Warn patients to avoid hazardous activities that require alertness and good psychomotor coordination until CNS effects of the drug are known.
- Tell patients to avoid alcohol while taking this drug.
- If halazepam overdose occurs, flumazenil (a specific benzodiazepine antagonist) may be useful. Halazepam's duration of action is longer than flumazenil's; resedation possible.

hydroxyzine embonate‡
Atarax

hydroxyzine hydrochloride
Anxanil, Apo-Hydroxyzine†, Atarax*, Atozine, Durrax, E-Vista, Hydroxacen, Hyzine-50, Multipax†, Novohydroxyzin†, Quiess, Vistacon, Vistaject, Vistaquel, Vistaril, Vistazine

hydroxyzine pamoate
Hy-Pam, Vamate, Vistaril

Pregnancy Risk Category: C

HOW SUPPLIED
embonate‡
Capsules: 25 mg, 50 mg
hydrochloride
Tablets: 10 mg, 25 mg, 50 mg, 100 mg
Capsules: 10 mg†‡, 25 mg†‡, 50 mg†‡
Syrup: 10 mg/5 ml
Injection: 25 mg/ml, 50 mg/ml
pamoate
Capsules: 25 mg, 50 mg, 100 mg
Oral suspension: 25 mg/5 ml

ACTION
Mechanism: A piperazine antihistamine that depresses the CNS at the

limbic and subcortical levels of the brain.
Peak: Serum levels peak about 2 hours after oral dose. **Duration:** half-life, 20 to 25 hours; effects persist 4 to 6 hours.

INDICATIONS & DOSAGE
Anxiety and tension –
Adults: 25 to 100 mg P.O. t.i.d. or q.i.d.
Anxiety, tension, hyperkinesia –
Children under 6 years: 50 mg P.O. daily in divided doses.
Children 6 years and over: 50 to 100 mg P.O. daily in divided doses.
Preoperative and postoperative adjunctive therapy –
Adults: 25 to 100 mg I.M. q 4 to 6 hours.
Children: 1.1 mg/kg I.M. q 4 to 6 hours.
Rashes, pruritus –
Adults: 25 mg P.O. t.i.d. or q.i.d.
Children under 6 years: 50 mg P.O. daily in divided doses.
Children 6 years and over: 50 to 100 mg P.O. daily in divided doses.

ADVERSE REACTIONS
CNS: *drowsiness,* involuntary motor activity.
GI: *dry mouth.*
Other: marked discomfort at site of I.M. injection.

INTERACTIONS
Ethanol, other CNS depressants: increased CNS depression. Avoid concomitant use.

CONTRAINDICATIONS
- Contraindicated in patients hypersensitive to the drug and in patients experiencing shock, comatose states, or acute asthmatic attacks.
- Use cautiously in patients with acute angle-closure glaucoma, prostatic hyperplasia, COPD, asthma, hyperthyroidism, or cardiovascular disease.

NURSING CONSIDERATIONS
- Reduce dosage in elderly or debilitated patients.
- Warn patients to avoid hazardous activities that require alertness and good psychomotor coordination until CNS effects of the drug are known.
- Tell patients to avoid alcohol while taking this drug.
- If the patient is taking other CNS drugs, observe for excessive sedation.
- Use perioperatively as an antiemetic and anxiolytic and in psychogenically induced allergic conditions, such as chronic urticaria and pruritus. Especially useful for pruritus that prevents sleep.
- Parenteral form (hydroxyzine hydrochloride) for I.M. use only. Never administer I.V. (Z-track injection is preferred.)
- Aspirate injection carefully to prevent inadvertent intravascular injection. Inject deeply into a large muscle mass.
- To relieve dry mouth, suggest sugarless hard candy or gum.
- May cause false elevations of urine 17-hydroxycorticosteroids, depending on test method used.

lorazepam
Alzapam, Apo-Lorazepam†, Ativan, Lorazepam Intensol, Novolorazem†, Nu-Loraz†
Controlled Substance Schedule IV

Pregnancy Risk Category: D

HOW SUPPLIED
Tablets: 0.5 mg, 1 mg, 2 mg
Tablets (sublingual): 0.5 mg†, 1 mg†, 2 mg†
Oral solution (concentrated): 2 mg/ml
Injection: 2 mg/ml, 4 mg/ml

ACTION
Mechanism: Depresses the CNS at the limbic and subcortical levels of the brain.
Onset: within 1 to 1½ hours after

I.M. injection, 1 to 6 hours after oral administration. **Peak:** Plasma levels peak within 1 to 1½ hours. **Duration:** half-life, 10 to 20 hours.

INDICATIONS & DOSAGE

Anxiety, tension, agitation, irritability, particularly in anxiety neuroses or organic (especially GI or CV) disorders –

Adults: 2 to 6 mg P.O. daily in divided doses. Maximum dosage is 10 mg daily.

Insomnia –

Adults: 2 to 4 mg P.O. h.s.

Premedication before operative procedure –

Adults: 0.05 mg/kg I.M. or slow I.V. injection (< 2 mg/minute). Total dosage should not exceed 4 mg.

ADVERSE REACTIONS

CNS: *drowsiness, lethargy, hangover,* fainting, anterograde amnesia, restlessness, psychosis.
CV: transient hypotension.
EENT: visual disturbances.
GI: dry mouth, abdominal discomfort.
GU: incontinence, urine retention.
Other: ***acute abstinence syndrome*** following sudden withdrawal in physically dependent persons.

INTERACTIONS

Digoxin: may increase serum levels of digoxin, increasing toxicity. Monitor closely.
Ethanol, other CNS depressants: increased CNS depression. Avoid concomitant use.
Smoking: increased clearance of benzodiazepines. Monitor for lack of effect.

CONTRAINDICATIONS

- Contraindicated in patients with acute angle-closure glaucoma, psychoses, or mental depression.
- Use cautiously in patients with organic brain syndrome, myasthenia gravis, and pulmonary, renal, or hepatic impairment.

NURSING CONSIDERATIONS

- Reduce dosage in elderly or debilitated patients. Preoperative I.V. dose not to exceed 2 mg in patients over 50.
- Do not use drug regularly for everyday stress.
- Monitor liver, renal, and hematopoietic function studies periodically in patients receiving repeated or prolonged therapy.
- Possibility of abuse and addiction exists. Do not withdraw drug abruptly after long-term use; withdrawal symptoms may occur.
- Has fewer cumulative effects than other benzodiazepines because of its short half-life.
- As a premedication before surgery, lorazepam provides substantial preoperative amnesia. Patient teaching requires extra care to ensure adequate recall. Provide written materials or inform a family member, if possible.
- Warn patients to avoid hazardous activities that require alertness or good psychomotor coordination until CNS effects of the drug are known.
- Tell patients to avoid alcohol while taking this drug.
- If lorazepam overdose occurs, flumazenil (a specific benzodiazepine antagonist) may be useful. Lorazepam's duration of action is longer than flumazenil's; resedation possible.
- **I.V. use:** Give I.V. slowly, at rate not exceeding 2 mg/minute. Dilute with an equal volume of sterile water for injection, 0.9% sodium chloride injection, or dextrose 5% injection.
- Monitor respirations every 5 to 15 minutes and before each repeated I.V. dose. Have emergency resuscitation equipment and oxygen at bedside.
- For I.M. administration, inject deeply into a muscle mass. Don't dilute.
- Refrigerate to prolong shelf life.

meprobamate

Apo-Meprobamate†, Equanil**, Meprospan-200, Meprospan-400, Miltown-200, Miltown-400, Miltown-600, Probate, Trancot
Controlled Substance Schedule IV
Pregnancy Risk Category: D

HOW SUPPLIED

Tablets: 200 mg, 400 mg, 600 mg
Capsules (sustained-release): 200 mg, 400 mg

ACTION

Mechanism: Depresses the CNS at the limbic and subcortical levels of the brain.
Duration: plasma half-life, about 10 hours.

INDICATIONS & DOSAGE

Anxiety and tension –
Adults: 1.2 to 1.6 g P.O. in three or four equally divided doses. Maximum dosage is 2.4 g daily. Alternatively, 400 to 800 mg P.O. b.i.d. as a sustained-release capsule.
Children 6 to 12 years: 100 to 200 mg P.O. b.i.d. or t.i.d. Or, 200 mg P.O. b.i.d. as a sustained-release capsule. Not recommended for children under 6 years.

ADVERSE REACTIONS

CNS: *drowsiness,* ataxia, dizziness, slurred speech, headache, vertigo, ***seizures***.
CV: palpitation, tachycardia, hypotension.
GI: anorexia, nausea, vomiting, diarrhea, stomatitis.
Hematologic: ***aplastic anemia, thrombocytopenia, leukopenia,*** eosinophilia.
Skin: pruritus, urticaria, erythematous maculopapular rash.
After abrupt withdrawal of long-term therapy: severe generalized tonic-clonic seizures.

INTERACTIONS

Ethanol, other CNS depressants: increased CNS depression. Avoid concomitant use.

CONTRAINDICATIONS

- Contraindicated in patients hypersensitive to meprobamate, carisoprodol, mebutamate, tybamate, and carbromal and in patients with renal insufficiency or porphyria.
- Use cautiously in patients with impaired hepatic or renal function, seizure disorders, or suicidal tendencies; and in patients with a history of aspirin hypersensitivity.

NURSING CONSIDERATIONS

- Reduce dosage in elderly or debilitated patients.
- Drug should not be prescribed for everyday stress.
- Possibility of abuse and addiction exists with long-term use. Withdraw drug gradually over 2 weeks to avoid withdrawal symptoms.
- Warn patients to avoid hazardous activities that require alertness and good psychomotor coordination until CNS effects of the drug are known.
- Tell patients to avoid alcohol while taking this drug.
- Give drug with meals to reduce GI distress.
- Therapeutic blood levels, 0.5 to 2 mg/100 ml; levels above 20 mg/100 ml may cause coma and death.
- Periodically monitor CBC and renal and liver function tests in patients receiving high doses.
- Tell patients to report any unusual bruising or bleeding, fever, or sore throat. These symptoms may indicate serious hematologic toxicity.
- May interfere with certain laboratory tests for urinary 17-ketogenic steroids and 17-hydroxycorticosteroids.

oxazepam

Alepam‡, Apo-Oxazepam†, Murelax‡, Novoxapam†, Ox-Pam†, Serax**, Serepax‡, Zapex†

Controlled Substance Schedule IV

Pregnancy Risk Category: C

HOW SUPPLIED

Tablets: 10 mg, 15 mg, 30 mg
Capsules: 10 mg, 15 mg, 30 mg

ACTION

Mechanism: Depresses the CNS at the limbic and subcortical levels of the brain.

Peak: Serum levels peak within 1 to 4 hours. **Duration:** elimination half-life, 5 to 15 hours.

INDICATIONS & DOSAGE

Alcohol withdrawal –
Adults: 15 to 30 mg P.O. t.i.d. or q.i.d.

Severe anxiety –
Adults: 15 to 30 mg P.O. t.i.d. or q.i.d.

Tension, mild to moderate anxiety –
Adults: 10 to 15 mg P.O. t.i.d. or q.i.d.

ADVERSE REACTIONS

CNS: *drowsiness, lethargy, hangover,* fainting.
CV: transient hypotension.
GI: nausea, vomiting, abdominal discomfort.
Hematologic: ***leukopenia (rare).***
Hepatic: ***hepatic dysfunction.***

INTERACTIONS

Digoxin: may increase serum levels of digoxin, increasing toxicity. Monitor closely.
Ethanol, cimetidine, other CNS depressants: increased CNS depression. Avoid concomitant use.
Smoking: increased clearance of benzodiazepines. Monitor for lack of effect.

CONTRAINDICATIONS

- Contraindicated in patients hypersensitive to the drug and in those with acute angle-closure glaucoma, depression, or psychoses.
- Use cautiously in patients with history of seizure disorders, drug allergies, blood dyscrasia, and renal disease.

NURSING CONSIDERATIONS

- Reduce dosage in elderly or debilitated patients.
- Possibility of abuse and addiction exists. Do not stop drug abruptly; withdrawal symptoms may occur.
- Monitor liver, renal, and hematopoietic function studies periodically in patients receiving repeated or prolonged therapy.
- Warn patients to avoid hazardous activities that require alertness or good psychomotor coordination until CNS effects of the drug are known.
- Tell patients to avoid alcohol while taking this drug.
- Has fewer cumulative effects than many other benzodiazepines because of short half-life.
- If oxazepam overdose occurs, flumazenil (a specific benzodiazepine antagonist) may be useful. Oxazepam's duration of action is longer than flumazenil's; resedation possible.

prazepam

Centrax

Controlled Substance Schedule IV

Pregnancy Risk Category: D

HOW SUPPLIED

Tablets: 5 mg, 10 mg
Capsules: 5 mg, 10 mg, 20 mg

ACTION

Mechanism: Potentiates the effects of gamma-aminobutyric acid, an inhibitory neurotransmitter. Depresses the CNS at the limbic and subcortical levels of the brain.

*Liquid form contains alcohol.
**May contain tartrazine.

Common reactions are in italics; ***life-threatening,*** in bold italics.

Peak: Serum levels peak in 2½ to 6 hours. **Duration:** elimination half-life of active metabolites, 100 hours or more.

INDICATIONS & DOSAGE
Anxiety –
Adults: 20 to 60 mg P.O. daily in divided doses, or 20 mg h.s.

ADVERSE REACTIONS
CNS: *drowsiness, lethargy, hangover,* dizziness, ataxia, fainting.
CV: transient hypotension.
GI: dry mouth, nausea, vomiting, abdominal discomfort.
Skin: rash.

INTERACTIONS
Cimetidine: increased sedation. Monitor carefully.
Digoxin: may increase serum levels of digoxin, increasing toxicity. Monitor closely.
Ethanol, other CNS depressants: increased CNS depression. Avoid concomitant use.
Smoking: increased clearance of benzodiazepines. Monitor for lack of effect.

CONTRAINDICATIONS
- Contraindicated in patients with acute angle-closure glaucoma, psychoses, or anxiety-free psychiatric disorders.
- Use cautiously in patients with renal or hepatic impairment.

NURSING CONSIDERATIONS
- Reduce dosage in elderly or debilitated patients.
- Possibility of abuse and addiction exists. Do not stop drug abruptly; withdrawal symptoms may occur.
- Prazepam should not be prescribed for everyday stress.
- Monitor liver, renal, and hematopoietic function studies periodically in patients receiving repeated or prolonged therapy.
- Warn patients to avoid activities that require alertness or good psychomotor coordination until CNS effects of the drug are known.
- Tell patients to avoid alcohol while taking this drug.
- If prazepam overdose occurs, flumazenil (a specific benzodiazepine antagonist) may be useful. Prazepam's duration of action is longer than flumazenil's; resedation possible.

32
Antipsychotics

acetophenazine maleate
chlorpromazine hydrochloride
chlorprothixene
clozapine
fluphenazine decanoate
fluphenazine enanthate
fluphenazine hydrochloride
haloperidol
haloperidol decanoate
haloperidol lactate
loxapine hydrochloride
loxapine succinate
mesoridazine besylate
molindone hydrochloride
perphenazine
pimozide
prochlorperazine
(See Chapter 50, ANTIEMETICS.)
promazine hydrochloride
risperidone
thioridazine hydrochloride
thiothixene
thiothixene hydrochloride
trifluoperazine hydrochloride

COMBINATION PRODUCTS
ETRAFON 2-10: perphenazine 2 mg and amitriptyline hydrochloride 10 mg.
ETRAFON-A: perphenazine 2 mg and amitriptyline hydrochloride 25 mg.
ETRAFON-FORTE: perphenazine 4 mg and amitriptyline hydrochloride 25 mg.
TRIAVIL 2-10, TRIAVIL 4-10, TRIAVIL 2-25 are identical to Etrafon products above; TRIAVIL 4-50: perphenazine 4 mg and amitriptyline hydrochloride 50 mg.

acetophenazine maleate
Tindal

Pregnancy Risk Category: C

HOW SUPPLIED
Tablets: 20 mg

ACTION
Mechanism: A piperazine phenothiazine that blocks postsynaptic dopamine receptors in the brain.
Onset: several weeks; varies considerably among patients. **Peak:** Plasma levels peak after about 7 days of therapy; peak therapeutic effect may not occur for 6 weeks to 6 months. **Duration:** elimination half-life, 10 to 20 hours.

INDICATIONS & DOSAGE
Psychotic disorders –
Adults: initially, 20 mg P.O. t.i.d. or q.i.d. Daily dosage ranges from 40 to 80 mg in outpatients, or 80 to 120 mg in hospitalized patients. In severe psychotic states, up to 600 mg daily has been safely administered. Use smallest effective dosage at all times.

ADVERSE REACTIONS
CNS: *extrapyramidal reactions* (high incidence), *tardive dyskinesia,* sedation (low incidence), pseudoparkinsonism, EEG changes, dizziness.
CV: *orthostatic hypotension,* tachycardia, ECG changes.
EENT: ocular changes, *blurred vision.*
GI: *dry mouth, constipation.*
GU: *urine retention,* dark urine, menstrual irregularities, gynecomastia, inhibited ejaculation.
Hepatic: cholestatic jaundice, abnormal liver function tests.
Skin: *mild photosensitivity,* allergic reactions.
Other: weight gain; increased appetite, hyperprolactinemia; rarely, ***neuroleptic malignant syndrome*** (fever,

*Liquid form contains alcohol.
**May contain tartrazine.

Common reactions are in italics; ***life-threatening,*** in bold italics.

tachycardia, tachypnea, profuse diaphoresis).
After abrupt withdrawal of long-term therapy: gastritis, nausea, vomiting, dizziness, tremors, feeling of warmth or cold, diaphoresis, tachycardia, headache, insomnia.

INTERACTIONS

Antacids: inhibited absorption of oral phenothiazines. Separate antacid and phenothiazine doses by at least 2 hours.
Barbiturates: may decrease phenothiazine effect. Observe patient.
Ethanol: increased CNS depression. Avoid concomitant use.
Other CNS depressants: increased CNS depression. Use with caution.

CONTRAINDICATIONS

- Contraindicated in patients with CNS depression, bone marrow suppression, subcortical damage, and coma, and with use of spinal or epidural anesthetic or adrenergic blockers.
- Use cautiously in elderly or debilitated patients; and in patients with hepatic disease, arteriosclerosis or cardiovascular disease (may cause sudden drop in blood pressure), exposure to extreme heat or cold (including antipyretic therapy), respiratory disorders, hypocalcemia, seizure disorders (may lower seizure threshold), severe reactions to insulin or electroconvulsive therapy, suspected brain tumor or intestinal obstruction, glaucoma, or prostatic hyperplasia.

NURSING CONSIDERATIONS

- Tardive dyskinesia may occur after prolonged use. It may not appear until months or years later and may disappear spontaneously or persist for life despite discontinuation of drug.
- Acute dystonic reactions may be treated with I.V. diphenhydramine.
- Neuroleptic malignant syndrome is rare, but frequently fatal. It is not necessarily related to length of drug use or type of neuroleptic, but over 60% of affected patients are men. Watch for symptoms.
- Withhold dose and notify doctor if patient develops symptoms of blood dyscrasia (fever, sore throat, infection, cellulitis, weakness), persistent (longer than a few hours) extrapyramidal reactions, or any such reaction during pregnancy.
- Dose of 20 mg is therapeutic equivalent of 100 mg chlorpromazine.
- Monitor therapy with weekly bilirubin tests during first month; periodic blood tests (CBC and liver function); and ophthalmic tests (long-term use).
- Have patients report urine retention or constipation.
- Tell patients to use sunblock and to wear protective clothing to avoid photosensitivity reactions.
- Tell patients that the drug may discolor the urine.
- Warn patients to avoid activities requiring alertness or good psychomotor coordination until CNS effects of the drug are known.
- Tell patients to avoid alcohol while taking this drug.
- Obtain baseline measures of blood pressure before starting therapy and monitor routinely. Watch for orthostatic hypotension; advise patient to get up slowly.
- Relieve dry mouth with sugarless gum, sour hard candy, or mouthwash.
- Do not withdraw drug abruptly unless required by severe adverse reactions.
- Patient on maintenance therapy may take medication h.s. to facilitate sleep and decrease daytime sedation.

chlorpromazine hydrochloride

Chlorpromanyl-5†, Chlorpromanyl-20†, Chlorpromanyl-40†, Largactil†‡, Novo-Chlorpromazine†, Ormazine, Thorazine, Thor-Prom

Pregnancy Risk Category: C

HOW SUPPLIED

Tablets: 10 mg, 25 mg, 50 mg, 100 mg, 200 mg
Capsules (controlled-release): 30 mg, 75 mg, 150 mg, 200 mg, 300 mg
Oral concentrate: 30 mg/ml, 100 mg/ml
Syrup: 10 mg/5ml
Injection: 25 mg/ml
Suppositories: 25 mg, 100 mg

ACTION

Mechanism: An aliphatic phenothiazine that blocks postsynaptic dopamine receptors in the brain and inhibits the medullary chemoreceptor trigger zone.
Onset: full antipsychotic effects, 6 weeks or longer. **Peak:** Plasma levels peak within 2 to 4 hours after oral dose. **Duration:** variable; elimination half-life, 10 to 20 hours; metabolites may be found in urine 6 months after last dose.

INDICATIONS & DOSAGE

Psychosis –
Adults: initially, 30 to 75 mg P.O. daily in two to four divided doses. Increase dosage by 20 to 50 mg twice weekly until symptoms are controlled. Up to 800 mg daily may be required in some patients. Or, 25 to 50 mg I.M. q 1 to 4 hours p.r.n. Switch to oral therapy as soon as possible.
Children 6 months and older: 0.55 mg/kg P.O. or I.M. q 4 to 6 hours; or 1.1 mg/kg P.R. q 6 to 8 hours. Maximum I.M. dose in children under 5 years or weighing less than 22.7 kg is 40 mg. Maximum I.M. dose in children 5 to 12 years or weighing 22.7 to 45.5 kg is 75 mg.
Nausea and vomiting –
Adults: 10 to 25 mg P.O. or I.M. q 4 to 6 hours, p.r.n.; or 50 to 100 mg P.R. q 6 to 8 hours, p.r.n.
Children 6 months and older: 0.55 mg/kg P.O. or I.M. q 4 to 6 hours; or 1.1 mg/kg P.R. q 6 to 8 hours. Maximum I.M. dose in children under 5 years or weighing less than 22.7 kg is 40 mg. Maximum I.M. dose in children 5 to 12 years or weighing 22.7 to 45.5 kg is 75 mg.
Intractable hiccups –
Adults: 25 to 50 mg P.O. or I.M. t.i.d. or q.i.d.
Mild alcohol withdrawal, acute intermittent porphyria, tetanus –
Adults: 25 to 50 mg I.M. t.i.d. or q.i.d.

ADVERSE REACTIONS

CNS: *extrapyramidal reactions* (moderate incidence), *sedation* (high incidence), *tardive dyskinesia,* pseudoparkinsonism, EEG changes, dizziness.
CV: *orthostatic hypotension,* tachycardia, ECG changes.
EENT: ocular changes, blurred vision.
GI: *dry mouth, constipation.*
GU: *urine retention,* dark urine, menstrual irregularities, gynecomastia, inhibited ejaculation.
Hematologic: transient leukopenia, ***agranulocytosis,*** hyperprolactinemia.
Hepatic: cholestatic jaundice, abnormal liver function tests.
Skin: *mild photosensitivity,* allergic reactions, *I.M. injection pain,* sterile abscess.
Other: weight gain; increased appetite; rarely, ***neuroleptic malignant syndrome*** (fever, tachycardia, tachypnea, profuse diaphoresis).
After abrupt withdrawal of long-term therapy: gastritis, nausea, vomiting, dizziness, tremors, feeling of

*Liquid form contains alcohol.
**May contain tartrazine.

Common reactions are in italics; ***life-threatening,*** in bold italics.

warmth or cold, diaphoresis, tachycardia, headache, insomnia.

INTERACTIONS

Antacids: inhibited absorption of oral phenothiazines. Separate antacid and phenothiazine doses by at least 2 hours.
Anticholinergics (including antidepressant and antiparkinsonian agents): increased anticholinergic activity, aggravated parkinsonian symptoms. Use with caution.
Barbiturates, lithium: may decrease phenothiazine effect. Observe patient.
Centrally acting antihypertensive agents: decreased antihypertensive effect.
Ethanol, other CNS depressants: increased CNS depression. Avoid concomitant use.
Propranolol: increased levels of both propranolol and chlorpromazine.

CONTRAINDICATIONS

- Contraindicated in patients experiencing CNS depression, bone marrow suppression, subcortical damage, Reye's syndrome, and coma; also contraindicated with use of spinal or epidural anesthetic or with adrenergic blocking agents.
- Use cautiously in elderly or debilitated patients; in patients with hepatic disease, arteriosclerosis or CV disease (may cause sudden drop in blood pressure), exposure to extreme heat or cold (including antipyretic therapy), respiratory disorders, hypocalcemia, seizure disorders (may lower seizure threshold), severe reactions to insulin or electroconvulsive therapy, suspected brain tumor or intestinal obstruction, glaucoma, or prostatic hyperplasia; and in acutely ill or dehydrated children.
- Use parenteral form cautiously in asthmatics and in patients allergic to sulfites.

NURSING CONSIDERATIONS

- Tardive dyskinesia may occur after prolonged use. It may not appear until months or years later and may disappear spontaneously or persist for life despite discontinuation of drug.
- Neuroleptic malignant syndrome is rare, but frequently fatal. It is not necessarily related to length of drug use or type of neuroleptic, but over 60% of affected patients are men. Watch for symptoms.
- Acute dystonic reactions may be treated with I.V. diphenhydramine.
- Withhold dose and notify doctor if patient develops jaundice, symptoms of blood dyscrasia (fever, sore throat, infection, cellulitis, weakness), persistent (longer than a few hours) extrapyramidal reactions, or any such reaction in pregnancy or in children.
- Monitor therapy with weekly bilirubin tests during first month; periodic blood tests (CBC and liver function); and ophthalmic tests (long-term use).
- Obtain baseline measures of blood pressure before starting therapy and monitor regularly. Watch for orthostatic hypotension, especially with parenteral administration. Monitor blood pressure before and after I.M. administration. Keep patient supine for 1 hour afterward and advise him to get up slowly.
- **I.V. use:** For direct injection, drug may be diluted with 0.9% sodium chloride injection and administered into a large vein or through the tubing of a free-flowing I.V. solution. Do not exceed 1 mg/minute for adults or 0.5 mg/minute for children. Drug may also be given as an intermittent I.V. infusion; dilute with 50 or 100 ml of a compatible solution and infuse over 30 minutes. Chlorpromazine is compatible with most common I.V. solutions, including D_5W, Ringer's injection, lactated Ringer's injection, and 0.9% sodium chloride injection.
- Slight yellowing of injection or concentrate is common; does not affect

potency. Discard markedly discolored solutions.
• Give deep I.M. only in upper outer quadrant of buttocks. Massage slowly afterward to prevent sterile abscess. Injection stings.
• Oral liquid and parenteral forms can cause contact dermatitis. Wear gloves when preparing solutions, and prevent any contact with skin and clothing.
• Protect liquid concentrate from light. Dilute with fruit juice, milk, or semisolid food just before administration.
• Do not withdraw drug abruptly unless required by severe adverse reactions.
• Have patients report urine retention or constipation.
• Tell patients that the drug may discolor the urine.
• Tell patients to use sunblock and to wear protective clothing to avoid photosensitivity reactions. Chlorpromazine causes higher incidence of photosensitivity than any other drug in its class.
• Warn patients to avoid activities that require alertness or good psychomotor coordination until CNS effects of the drug are known. Drowsiness and dizziness usually subside after first few weeks.
• Tell patients to avoid alcohol while taking this drug.
• Relieve dry mouth with sugarless gum, sour hard candy, or mouthwash.

chlorprothixene

Taractan**, Tarasan†

Pregnancy Risk Category: C

HOW SUPPLIED

Tablets: 10 mg, 25 mg, 50 mg, 100 mg
Oral concentrate: 100 mg/5 ml (fruit)
Injection: 12.5 mg/ml

ACTION

Mechanism: A thioxanthene that blocks postsynaptic dopamine receptors in the brain.
Onset: several weeks; varies considerably among patients. **Peak:** Plasma levels peak after about 7 days; peak therapeutic effect may not occur for 6 weeks to 6 months. **Duration:** elimination half-life, 10 to 20 hours.

INDICATIONS & DOSAGE

Psychotic disorders –
Adults: initially, 25 to 50 mg P.O. t.i.d. or q.i.d. Increase gradually to maximum of 600 mg daily.
Children over 6 years: 10 to 25 mg P.O. t.i.d. or q.i.d.
Agitation of severe neurosis, depression, schizophrenia –
Adults: 25 to 50 mg P.O. or I.M. t.i.d. or q.i.d. Increase as needed up to maximum of 600 mg.

ADVERSE REACTIONS

CNS: extrapyramidal reactions (low incidence), tardive dyskinesia, *sedation,* pseudoparkinsonism, EEG changes, dizziness.
CV: *orthostatic hypotension,* tachycardia, ECG changes.
EENT: ocular changes, *blurred vision.*
GI: *dry mouth, constipation.*
GU: *urine retention,* dark urine, menstrual irregularities, gynecomastia, inhibited ejaculation.
Hematologic: transient leukopenia, ***agranulocytosis,*** hyperprolactinemia.
Hepatic: cholestatic jaundice, abnormal liver function tests.
Skin: *mild photosensitivity,* allergic reactions, pain on I.M. injection, sterile abscess.
Other: weight gain; increased appetite; rarely, ***neuroleptic malignant syndrome*** (fever, tachycardia, tachypnea, profuse diaphoresis).
After abrupt withdrawal of long-term therapy: gastritis, nausea, vomiting, dizziness, tremors, feeling of

*Liquid form contains alcohol.
**May contain tartrazine.

warmth or cold, diaphoresis, tachycardia, headache, insomnia.

INTERACTIONS

Anticholinergics: potentiated central anticholinergic effects. Use together cautiously.
Centrally acting antihypertensives: decreased antihypertensive effect. Monitor blood pressure.
Ethanol: increased CNS depression. Avoid concomitant use.
Other CNS depressants: increased CNS depression. Use together cautiously.

CONTRAINDICATIONS

- Contraindicated in patients experiencing CNS depression, bone marrow suppression, circulatory collapse, CHF, cardiac decompensation, coronary artery or cerebrovascular disorders, subcortical damage, and coma; also contraindicated with use of spinal or epidural anesthetic or with adrenergic blocking agents.
- Use cautiously in elderly or debilitated patients; in patients with hepatic or renal disease, arteriosclerosis or CV disease (may cause sudden drop in blood pressure), exposure to extreme heat or cold (including antipyretic therapy), respiratory disorders, hypocalcemia, seizure disorders (may lower seizure threshold), severe reactions to insulin or electroconvulsive therapy, suspected brain tumor or intestinal obstruction, glaucoma, or prostatic hyperplasia; and in acutely ill or dehydrated children.

NURSING CONSIDERATIONS

- Tardive dyskinesia may occur after prolonged use. It may not appear until months or years later and may disappear spontaneously or persist for life despite discontinuation of drug.
- Neuroleptic malignant syndrome is rare, but frequently fatal. It is not necessarily related to length of drug use or type of neuroleptic, but over 60% of affected patients are men. Watch for symptoms.
- Acute dystonic reactions may be treated with I.V. diphenhydramine.
- Withhold dose and notify doctor if patient develops symptoms of blood dyscrasia (fever, sore throat, infection, cellulitis, weakness), jaundice, persistent (longer than a few hours) extrapyramidal reactions, or any such reactions in children.
- Monitor therapy with weekly bilirubin tests during first month; periodic blood tests (CBC and liver function) before and during therapy; and ophthalmic tests (long-term therapy).
- Have patients report urine retention or constipation.
- Dose of 100 mg is the therapeutic equivalent of 100 mg chlorpromazine.
- Obtain baseline measures of blood pressure before starting therapy and monitor regularly. Watch for orthostatic hypotension, especially with parenteral administration, because adrenergic blockage is high. Keep patients in a supine position for 1 hour afterward and advise them to change positions slowly.
- Give deep I.M. only in upper outer quadrant of buttocks or midlateral thigh. Massage slowly afterward to prevent sterile abscess. Injection stings.
- Dilute liquid concentrate with fruit juice, milk, or semisolid food just before administration.
- Protect medication from light. Slight yellowing of injection or concentrate is common; does not affect potency. Discard markedly discolored solutions.
- Do not withdraw drug abruptly unless required by severe adverse reactions.
- Prevent contact dermatitis by keeping drug off patients' skin and clothes. Wear gloves when preparing liquid forms of the drug.
- Tell patients to use sunblock and to

wear protective clothing to avoid photosensitivity reactions.
- Warn patients to avoid activities that require alertness or good psychomotor coordination until CNS effects of the drug are known. Drowsiness and dizziness usually subside after first few weeks.
- Tell patients to avoid alcohol while taking this drug.
- Relieve dry mouth with sugarless gum, sour hard candy, or mouthwash.

clozapine

Clozaril

Pregnancy Risk Category: B

HOW SUPPLIED

Tablets: 25 mg, 100 mg

ACTION

Mechanism: Binds to dopamine receptors (both D-1 and D-2) within the limbic system of the CNS and may interfere with adrenergic, cholinergic, histaminergic, and serotonergic receptors.
Peak: Serum levels peak in about 2½ hours. **Duration:** elimination half-life, about 8 hours; effects persist 4 to 12 hours.

INDICATIONS & DOSAGE

Schizophrenia in severely ill patients unresponsive to other therapies –
Adults: initially, 25 mg P.O. once daily or b.i.d., titrated upward at 25 to 50 mg daily (if tolerated) to 300 to 450 mg daily by the end of 2 weeks. Individual dosage is based on clinical response, patient tolerance, and adverse reactions. Subsequent dosage should not be increased more than once or twice weekly, and should not exceed 100 mg. Many patients respond to dosages of 300 to 600 mg daily, but some may require as much as 900 mg daily. Do not exceed 900 mg/day.

ADVERSE REACTIONS

CNS: *drowsiness, sedation,* ***seizures,*** *dizziness,* syncope, vertigo, headache, tremor, disturbed sleep or nightmares, restlessness, hypokinesia or akinesia, agitation, rigidity, akathisia, confusion, fatigue, insomnia, hyperkinesia, weakness, lethargy, ataxia, slurred speech, depression, myoclonia, anxiety.
CV: *tachycardia, hypotension,* hypertension, chest pain, ECG changes, orthostatic hypotension.
GI: *dry mouth, constipation,* nausea, vomiting, *salivation,* heartburn, constipation.
GU: urinary abnormalities (urinary frequency or urgency, urine retention), incontinence, abnormal ejaculation.
Hematologic: ***leukopenia, agranulocytosis.***
Skin: rash.
Other: fever, muscle pain or spasm, muscle weakness, weight gain.
After abrupt withdrawal of long-term therapy: possible abrupt recurrence of psychotic symptoms. Monitor closely.

INTERACTIONS

Anticholinergics: may potentiate anticholinergic effects of clozapine. Avoid concomitant use. Monitor blood pressure.
Antihypertensives: may potentiate hypotensive effects.
Bone marrow suppressants: may increase bone marrow toxicity. Don't use together.
Psychoactive drugs: may produce additive effects. Use together cautiously.
Warfarin, digoxin, and other highly protein-bound drugs: may increase serum levels of these drugs. Monitor closely for adverse reactions.

CONTRAINDICATIONS

- Contraindicated in patients with a history of clozapine-induced agranulocytosis; in patients with a WBC count below 3,500/mm^3; in patients with severe CNS depression or coma; in patients taking other drugs that suppress bone marrow function; and in those with myelosuppressive disorders.

• Use cautiously in patients with prostatic hyperplasia or glaucoma because clozapine has potent anticholinergic effects.

NURSING CONSIDERATIONS

• Seizures may occur, especially in patients receiving high doses.

• Warn patients to avoid hazardous activities that require alertness and good psychomotor coordination while taking this drug.

• Clozapine carries significant risk of agranulocytosis. If possible, patients should receive at least two trials of a standard antipsychotic drug therapy before clozapine therapy is initiated. Baseline WBC and differential counts are required before therapy. Monitor WBC counts weekly for at least 4 weeks after clozapine therapy is discontinued.

• When administering clozapine, ensure that WBC counts and blood tests are performed weekly. Also ensure that no more than 1-week supply of drug is distributed.

• If WBC count drops below 3,500/mm^3 after therapy is initiated or it exhibits a substantial drop from baseline, monitor patient closely for signs of infection. If WBC count is 3,000 to 3,500/mm^3 and granulocyte count is above 1,500/mm^3, perform WBC and differential count twice weekly. If WBC count drops below 3,000/mm^3 and granulocyte count drops below 1,500/mm^3, interrupt therapy and monitor the patient for signs of infection. Therapy may be cautiously restarted if WBC count returns above 3,000/mm^3 and granulocyte count returns above 1,500/mm^3. Continue monitoring of WBC and differential counts twice weekly until WBC count exceeds 3,500/mm^3.

• If the WBC count drops below 2,000/mm^3 and granulocyte count drops below 1,000/mm^3, the patient may require protective isolation. If the patient develops infection, prepare cultures according to policy and administer antibiotics as ordered. Some clinicians may perform bone marrow aspiration to assess bone marrow function. Future clozapine therapy is contraindicated in such patients.

• If clozapine therapy must be discontinued, the drug is usually withdrawn gradually (over a 1- to 2-week period). However, changes in the patient's medical condition (including the development of leukopenia) may require abrupt discontinuation of the drug. Monitor closely for the recurrence of psychotic symptoms.

• If therapy is reinstated in patients withdrawn from the drug, follow usual guidelines for dosage build-up. However, reexposure of the patient to this drug may increase the severity and risk of adverse reactions. If therapy was terminated for WBC counts below 2,000/mm^3 or granulocyte counts below 1,000/mm^3, do not continue the drug.

• Warn patients about the risk of agranulocytosis. Tell patients the drug is available only through a special monitoring program that requires weekly blood tests to monitor for agranulocytosis. Advise patients to report flulike symptoms, fever, sore throat, lethargy, malaise, or other signs of infection.

• Some patients experience transient fevers (temperature > 100.4° F, or 38° C), especially in the first 3 weeks of therapy. Monitor patients closely.

• Advise patients to check with their doctor before taking any OTC drugs or alcohol.

• Recommend ice chips or sugarless

candy or gum to help relieve dry mouth.

- Tell patients to rise slowly to avoid orthostatic hypotension.

fluphenazine decanoate

Modecate†‡, Modecate Concentrate†, Prolixin Decanoate

fluphenazine enanthate

Moditen Enanthate†, Prolixin Enanthate

fluphenazine hydrochloride

Anatensol‡*, Apo-Fluphenazine†, Moditen HCl†, Moditen HCl-HP†, Permitil* **, Permitil Concentrate, Prolixin* **, Prolixin Concentrate

Pregnancy Risk Category: C

HOW SUPPLIED

decanoate
Depot injection: 25 mg/ml
enanthate
Depot injection: 25 mg/ml
hydrochloride
Tablets: 1 mg, 2.5 mg, 5 mg, 10 mg
Oral concentrate: 5 mg/ml (contains 1% alcohol)
Elixir: 2.5 mg/5 ml (with 14% alcohol)
I.M. injection: 2.5 mg/ml

ACTION

Mechanism: A piperazine phenothiazine that blocks postsynaptic dopamine receptors in the brain.
Onset: several weeks; varies considerably among patients. **Peak:** Plasma levels peak 2 to 3 days after injection of enanthate preparation, 1 to 2 days after decanoate preparation. Peak therapeutic effect may not occur for 6 weeks to 6 months. **Duration:** elimination half-life 10 to 20 hours.

INDICATIONS & DOSAGE

Psychotic disorders –
Adults: initially, 0.5 to 10 mg (hydrochloride) P.O. daily in divided doses q 6 to 8 hours; may increase cautiously to 20 mg. Higher doses (50 to 100 mg) have been given. Maintenance dosage is 1 to 5 mg P.O. daily. I.M. doses are one-third to one-half of oral doses. Use lower dosages for elderly patients (1 to 2.5 mg daily).
Children: 0.25 to 0.75 mg (hydrochloride) P.O. daily in divided doses q 4 to 6 hours; or one-third to one-half of an oral dose I.M.; maximum dosage is 10 mg daily.
Adults and children over 12 years: 12.5 to 25 mg of long-acting esters (decanoate or enanthate) I.M. or S.C. q 1 to 6 weeks. Maintenance dosage is 25 to 100 mg, p.r.n.

ADVERSE REACTIONS

CNS: *extrapyramidal reactions* (high incidence), *tardive dyskinesia,* sedation (low incidence), pseudoparkinsonism, EEG changes, dizziness.
CV: *orthostatic hypotension,* tachycardia, ECG changes.
EENT: ocular changes, *blurred vision.*
GI: *dry mouth, constipation.*
GU: *urine retention,* dark urine, menstrual irregularities, gynecomastia, inhibited ejaculation.
Hematologic: transient leukopenia, ***agranulocytosis,*** hyperprolactinemia.
Hepatic: cholestatic jaundice, abnormal liver function tests.
Skin: *mild photosensitivity,* allergic reactions.
Other: weight gain; increased appetite; rarely, ***neuroleptic malignant syndrome*** (fever, tachycardia, tachypnea, profuse diaphoresis).
After abrupt withdrawal of long-term therapy: gastritis, nausea, vomiting, dizziness, tremors, feeling of warmth or cold, diaphoresis, tachycardia, headache, insomnia.

INTERACTIONS

Antacids: inhibited absorption of oral phenothiazines. Separate antacid and

*Liquid form contains alcohol.
**May contain tartrazine.

Common reactions are in italics; ***life-threatening,*** in bold italics.

phenothiazine doses by at least 2 hours.
Anticholinergics: increased anticholinergic effects. Avoid concomitant use.
Barbiturates, lithium: may decrease phenothiazine effect. Observe patient.
Centrally acting antihypertensives: decrease antihypertensive effect. Monitor blood pressure.
Ethanol, other CNS depressants: increased CNS depression. Avoid concomitant use.

CONTRAINDICATIONS

- Contraindicated in patients experiencing coma, CNS depression, bone marrow suppression or other blood dyscrasia, subcortical damage, liver damage, or renal insufficiency.
- Contraindicated with use of spinal or epidural anesthetic or with adrenergic blocking agents.
- Use cautiously in elderly or debilitated patients; in acutely ill or dehydrated children; in patients with hepatic disease, pheochromocytoma, arteriosclerotic, cerebrovascular or CV disease (may cause sudden drop in blood pressure); in patients with peptic ulceration, exposure to extreme heat or cold (including antipyretic therapy), respiratory disorders, hypocalcemia, seizure disorders (may lower seizure threshold), or severe reactions to insulin or electroconvulsive therapy; and in patients with suspected brain tumor or intestinal obstruction, glaucoma, or prostatic hyperplasia. Use parenteral form cautiously in asthmatic patients and patients allergic to sulfites.

NURSING CONSIDERATIONS

- Tardive dyskinesia may occur after prolonged use. It may not appear until months or years later and may disappear spontaneously or persist for life despite discontinuation of drug.
- Neuroleptic malignant syndrome is rare, but frequently fatal. It is not necessarily related to length of drug use or type of neuroleptic, but over 60% of affected patients are men. Watch for symptoms.
- Acute dystonic reactions may be treated with I.V. diphenhydramine.
- Withhold dose and notify doctor if patient develops symptoms of blood dyscrasia (fever, sore throat, infection, cellulitis, weakness), persistent (longer than a few hours) extrapyramidal reactions, or any such reactions during pregnancy or in children.
- Monitor therapy with weekly bilirubin tests during first month; periodic blood tests (CBC and liver function); and periodic renal function and ophthalmic tests (long-term use).
- Have patient report urine retention or constipation.
- Tell patients that the drug may discolor urine.
- Dose of 2 mg is therapeutic equivalent of 100 mg chlorpromazine.
- For long-acting forms (decanoate and enanthate), which are oil preparations, use a dry needle of at least 21 G. Allow 24 to 96 hours for onset of action. Note and report adverse reactions in patients taking these drug forms.
- Decanoate and enanthate forms may be given subcutaneously.
- Prolixin Concentrate and Permitil Concentrate are 10 times more concentrated than Prolixin Elixir (5 mg/ml vs. 0.5 mg/ml).
- Dilute liquid concentrate with water, fruit juice, milk, or semisolid food just before administration.
- Do not withdraw drug abruptly unless severe adverse reactions occur.
- Oral liquid and parenteral forms can cause contact dermatitis. Wear gloves when preparing solutions, and prevent contact with skin and clothing.
- Protect medication from light. Slight yellowing of injection or concentrate is common; does not affect

potency. Discard markedly discolored solutions.

- Tell patients to use sunblock and to wear protective clothing to avoid photosensitivity reactions.
- Warn patients to avoid activities that require alertness and good psychomotor coordination until CNS effects of the drug are known. Drowsiness and dizziness usually subside after first few weeks.
- Tell patients to avoid alcohol while taking this drug.
- Relieve dry mouth with sugarless gum, sour hard candy, or mouthwash.

haloperidol

Apo-Haloperidol†, Haldol**, Halperon, Novoperidol†, Peridol†, Serenace‡

haloperidol decanoate

Haldol Decanoate, Haldol LA†

haloperidol lactate

Haldol

Pregnancy Risk Category: C

HOW SUPPLIED

haloperidol
Tablets: 0.5 mg, 1 mg, 2 mg, 5 mg, 10 mg, 20 mg
haloperidol decanoate
Injection: 50 mg/ml
haloperidol lactate
Oral concentrate: 2 mg/ml
Injection: 5 mg/ml

ACTION

Mechanism: A butyrophenone that blocks postsynaptic dopamine receptors in the brain.
Onset: several weeks. **Peak:** Serum concentrations peak immediately after I.V. injection, within 20 minutes of I.M. injection (lactate), 3 to 5 hours after oral dose, about 6 days after long-acting depot injection (decanoate).

INDICATIONS & DOSAGE

Psychotic disorders –
Adults: dosage varies for each patient. Initial range, 0.5 to 5 mg P.O. b.i.d. or t.i.d.; or 2 to 5 mg I.M. q 4 to 8 hours, increasing rapidly if necessary for prompt control. Maximum dosage is 100 mg P.O. daily. Doses over 100 mg have been used for patients with severely resistant conditions.
Chronic psychotic patients who require prolonged therapy –
Adults: 50 to 100 mg I.M. haloperidol decanoate q 4 weeks.
Control of tics, vocal utterances in Tourette syndrome –
Adults: 0.5 to 5 mg P.O. b.i.d. or t.i.d., increasing to p.r.n.

ADVERSE REACTIONS

CNS: *severe extrapyramidal reactions* (high incidence), *tardive dyskinesia,* sedation (low incidence).
CV: cardiovascular effects (low incidence with therapeutic dosages).
EENT: *blurred vision.*
GU: urine retention, menstrual irregularities, gynecomastia.
Hematologic: transient leukopenia and leukocytosis.
Skin: rash.
Other: rarely, ***neuroleptic malignant syndrome*** (fever, tachycardia, tachypnea, profuse diaphoresis), dry mouth.

INTERACTIONS

Ethanol, other CNS depressants: increased CNS depression. Avoid concomitant use.
Lithium: lethargy and confusion with high doses. Monitor the patient.
Methyldopa: may cause symptoms of dementia or psychosis. Monitor the patient.

CONTRAINDICATIONS

- Contraindicated in patients experiencing parkinsonism, coma, or CNS depression.

*Liquid form contains alcohol.
**May contain tartrazine.

Common reactions are in italics; ***life-threatening,*** in bold italics.

• Use cautiously in elderly and debilitated patients; in patients with severe CV disorders, allergies, glaucoma, or urine retention; and in conjunction with anticonvulsant, anticoagulant, antiparkinsonian, or lithium medications.

NURSING CONSIDERATIONS

• Tardive dyskinesia may occur after prolonged use. It may not appear until months or years later and may disappear spontaneously or persist for life despite discontinuation of drug.
• Neuroleptic malignant syndrome is rare, but frequently fatal. It is not necessarily related to length of drug use or type of neuroleptic, but over 60% of affected patients are men. Watch for symptoms.
• Acute dystonic reactions may be treated with I.V. diphenhydramine.
• Elderly patients usually require lower initial doses and a more gradual dosage titration.
• Least sedating of the antipsychotic agents. However, warn patients to avoid activities that require alertness and good psychomotor coordination until CNS effects of the drug are known. Drowsiness and dizziness usually subside after a few weeks.
• Dose of 2 mg is therapeutic equivalent of 100 mg chlorpromazine.
• Especially useful for agitation associated with senile dementia.
• Do not administer the decanoate form I.V.
• When changing from tablets to decanoate injection, give patient 10 to 15 times the oral dose once a month (maximum 100 mg).
• Protect medication from light. Slight yellowing of injection or concentrate is common; does not affect potency. Discard markedly discolored solutions.
• Do not withdraw drug abruptly unless required by severe adverse reactions.
• Relieve dry mouth with sugarless gum, sour hard candy, or mouthwash.
• Tell the patient to avoid alcohol while taking this drug.

loxapine hydrochloride

Loxapac†, Loxitane C, Loxitane I.M.

loxapine succinate

Loxapac†, Loxitane

Pregnancy Risk Category: C

HOW SUPPLIED

hydrochloride

Oral concentrate: 25 mg/ml
Injection: 50 mg/ml

succinate

Capsules: 5 mg, 10 mg, 25 mg, 50 mg
Tablets: 5 mg†, 10 mg†, 25 mg†, 50 mg†

ACTION

Mechanism: A dibenzoxazepine that blocks postsynaptic dopamine receptors in the brain.
Onset: therapeutic effect, several weeks. **Peak:** Plasma levels peak within 1½ to 3 hours of oral dose.

INDICATIONS & DOSAGE

Psychotic disorders –
Adults: 10 mg P.O. or I.M. b.i.d. to q.i.d., rapidly increasing to 60 to 100 mg P.O. daily for most patients; dosage varies from patient to patient.

ADVERSE REACTIONS

CNS: *extrapyramidal reactions* (moderate incidence), *sedation* (moderate incidence), *tardive dyskinesia,* pseudoparkinsonism, EEG changes, dizziness.
CV: *orthostatic hypotension,* tachycardia, ECG changes.
EENT: *blurred vision.*
GI: *dry mouth, constipation.*
GU: *urine retention,* dark urine, menstrual irregularities, gynecomastia.

Hematologic: transient leukopenia.
Skin: *mild photosensitivity,* allergic reactions.
Other: weight gain; increased appetite; rarely, ***neuroleptic malignant syndrome*** (fever, tachycardia, tachypnea, profuse diaphoresis).

INTERACTIONS
Ethanol, other CNS depressants: increased CNS depression. Avoid concomitant use.

CONTRAINDICATIONS
- Contraindicated in patients experiencing coma, severe CNS depression, or drug-induced depressed states.
- Use cautiously in patients with seizure disorder, CV disorders, glaucoma, urine retention, suspected intestinal obstruction or brain tumor, and renal damage.

NURSING CONSIDERATIONS
- Tardive dyskinesia may occur after prolonged use. It may not appear until months or years later and may disappear spontaneously or persist for life despite discontinuation of drug.
- Neuroleptic malignant syndrome is rare, but frequently fatal. It is not necessarily related to length of drug use or type of neuroleptic, but over 60% of affected patients are men. Watch for symptoms.
- Acute dystonic reactions may be treated with I.V. diphenhydramine.
- Obtain baseline measures of blood pressure before starting therapy and monitor regularly. Advise patients to get up slowly to avoid orthostatic hypotension.
- Warn patients to avoid activities that require alertness and good psychomotor coordination until CNS effects of the drug are known. Drowsiness and dizziness usually subside after first few weeks.
- Tell patients to avoid alcohol while taking this drug.
- Periodic eye examinations are recommended.
- Dose of 10 mg is therapeutic equivalent of 100 mg chlorpromazine.
- Dilute liquid concentrate with orange or grapefruit juice just before giving.
- Relieve dry mouth with sugarless gum, sour hard candy, or mouthwash.

mesoridazine besylate
Serentil* **, Serentil Concentrate
Pregnancy Risk Category: C

HOW SUPPLIED
Tablets: 10 mg, 25 mg, 50 mg, 100 mg
Oral concentrate: 25 mg/ml (0.6% alcohol)
Injection: 25 mg/ml

ACTION
Mechanism: A piperidine phenothiazine and the major sulfoxide metabolite of thioridazine that blocks postsynaptic dopamine receptors in the brain.
Onset: therapeutic effect, several weeks. **Peak:** Plasma levels peak within 4 hours of I.M. or P.O. dose.

INDICATIONS & DOSAGE
Alcoholism –
Adults and children over 12 years: 25 mg P.O. b.i.d. up to maximum of 200 mg daily.
Behavioral problems associated with chronic brain syndrome –
Adults and children over 12 years: 25 mg P.O. t.i.d. up to maximum of 300 mg daily.
Psychoneurotic manifestations (anxiety) –
Adults and children over 12 years: 10 mg P.O. t.i.d. up to maximum of 150 mg daily.
Schizophrenia –
Adults and children over 12 years: initially, 50 mg P.O. t.i.d. or 25 mg I.M. repeated in 30 to 60 minutes,

*Liquid form contains alcohol.
**May contain tartrazine.

p.r.n. Maximum dosage is 400 mg daily.

ADVERSE REACTIONS

CNS: extrapyramidal reactions (low incidence), *tardive dyskinesia, sedation* (high incidence), EEG changes, dizziness.
CV: *orthostatic hypotension,* tachycardia, ECG changes.
EENT: *ocular changes, blurred vision,* pigmentary retinopathy.
GI: *dry mouth, constipation.*
GU: *urine retention,* dark urine, menstrual irregularities, gynecomastia, inhibited ejaculation.
Hematologic: transient leukopenia, ***agranulocytosis,*** hyperprolactinemia.
Hepatic: cholestatic jaundice, abnormal liver function tests.
Skin: *mild photosensitivity,* allergic reactions, pain at I.M. injection site, sterile abscess.
Other: weight gain; increased appetite; rarely, ***neuroleptic malignant syndrome*** (fever, tachycardia, tachypnea, profuse diaphoresis).
After abrupt withdrawal of long-term therapy: gastritis, nausea, vomiting, dizziness, tremors, feeling of warmth or cold, diaphoresis, tachycardia, headache, insomnia.

INTERACTIONS

Antacids: inhibited absorption of oral phenothiazines. Separate antacid and phenothiazine doses by at least 2 hours.
Anticholinergics: may increase anticholinergic effects. Use together cautiously.
Barbiturates: may decrease phenothiazine effect. Observe patient.
Ethanol: increased CNS depression. Avoid concomitant use.
Other CNS depressants: increased CNS depression. Use together cautiously.

CONTRAINDICATIONS

• Contraindicated in patients experiencing coma, CNS depression, bone marrow suppression, or subcortical damage; and with use of spinal or epidural anesthetic or adrenergic blocking agents.
• Use cautiously in elderly or debilitated patients; in acutely ill or dehydrated children; and in patients with hepatic disease, arteriosclerosis or CV disease (may cause sudden drop in blood pressure), exposure to extreme heat or cold (including antipyretic therapy), respiratory disorders, hypocalcemia, seizure disorders, severe reactions to insulin or electroconvulsive therapy, suspected brain tumor or intestinal obstruction, glaucoma, and prostatic hyperplasia.

NURSING CONSIDERATIONS

• Tardive dyskinesia may occur after prolonged use. It may not appear until months or years later and may disappear spontaneously or persist for life despite discontinuation of drug.
• Neuroleptic malignant syndrome is rare, but frequently fatal. It is not necessarily related to length of drug use or type of neuroleptic, but over 60% of affected patients are men. Watch for symptoms.
• Acute dystonic reactions may be treated with I.V. diphenhydramine.
• Withhold dose and notify the doctor if patient develops jaundice, symptoms of blood dyscrasia (fever, sore throat, infection, cellulitis, weakness), persistent (longer than a few hours) extrapyramidal reactions, or any such reactions in pregnancy or in children.
• Monitor therapy with weekly bilirubin tests during first month; periodic blood tests (CBC and liver function); and ophthalmic tests (long-term use).
• Have patients report urine retention or constipation.
• Tell patients that the drug may discolor the urine.

• Obtain baseline measures of blood pressure before starting therapy and monitor regularly. Watch for orthostatic hypotension, especially with parenteral administration; advise patients to change positions slowly.
• Dose of 50 mg is therapeutic equivalent of 100 mg chlorpromazine.
• Give deep I.M. only in upper outer quadrant of buttocks. Massage slowly afterward to prevent sterile abscess. Injection may sting.
• Oral liquid and parenteral forms may cause contact dermatitis. Wear gloves when preparing solutions,and prevent contact with skin and clothing.
• Protect medication from light. Slight yellowing of injection or concentrate is common; does not affect potency. Discard markedly discolored solutions.
• Do not withdraw drug abruptly unless required by severe adverse reactions.
• Tell patients to use sunblock and to wear protective clothing to avoid photosensitivity reactions.
• Warn patients to avoid activities that require alertness and good psychomotor coordination until CNS effects of the drug are known. Drowsiness and dizziness usually subside after a few weeks.
• Tell patients to avoid alcohol while taking this drug.
• Relieve dry mouth with sugarless gum, sour hard candy, or mouthwash.

molindone hydrochloride
Moban

Pregnancy Risk Category: C

HOW SUPPLIED
Tablets: 5 mg, 10 mg, 25 mg, 50 mg, 100 mg
Oral solution: 20 mg/ml

ACTION
Mechanism: A dihydroindolone that blocks postsynaptic dopamine receptors in the brain.
Onset: therapeutic effect, several weeks. **Peak:** Plasma levels peak in about 1½ hours. **Duration:** effects persist for about 34 to 36 hours.

INDICATIONS & DOSAGE
Psychotic disorders –
Adults: 50 to 75 mg P.O. daily, increasing to 225 mg daily initially. Doses up to 400 mg may be required.

ADVERSE REACTIONS
CNS: *extrapyramidal reactions* (moderate incidence), *tardive dyskinesia, sedation* (moderate incidence), pseudoparkinsonism, EEG changes, dizziness.
CV: *orthostatic hypotension,* tachycardia, ECG changes.
EENT: *blurred vision.*
GI: *dry mouth, constipation.*
GU: *urine retention,* dark urine, menstrual irregularities, gynecomastia, inhibited ejaculation.
Hematologic: transient leukopenia, hyperprolactinemia.
Hepatic: cholestatic jaundice, abnormal liver function tests.
Skin: *mild photosensitivity,* allergic reactions.
Other: rarely, ***neuroleptic malignant syndrome*** (fever, tachycardia, tachypnea, profuse diaphoresis).

INTERACTIONS
Ethanol, other CNS depressants: increased CNS depression. Avoid concomitant use.

CONTRAINDICATIONS
• Contraindicated in patients experiencing coma or severe CNS depression.
• Use cautiously when increased physical activity would be harmful because this agent increases activity; in patients subject to seizures (may

lower seizure threshold), at risk for suicide, and with suspected brain tumor or intestinal obstruction.

NURSING CONSIDERATIONS

- Tardive dyskinesia may occur after prolonged use. It may not appear until months or years later and may disappear spontaneously or persist for life despite discontinuation of drug.
- Neuroleptic malignant syndrome is rare, but frequently fatal. It is not necessarily related to length of drug use or type of neuroleptic, but over 60% of affected patients are men. Watch for symptoms.
- Acute dystonic reactions may be treated with I.V. diphenhydramine.
- Warn patients to avoid activities that require alertness or good psychomotor coordination until CNS effects of the drug are known. Drowsiness and dizziness usually subside after first few weeks.
- Tell patients to avoid alcohol while taking this drug.
- Relieve dry mouth with sugarless gum, sour hard candy, or mouthwash.
- Dose of 10 mg is therapeutic equivalent of 100 mg chlorpromazine.
- May be administered in a single daily dose.

perphenazine

Apo-Perphenazine†, PMS-Perphenazine†, Trilafon, Trilafon Concentrate

Pregnancy Risk Category: C

HOW SUPPLIED

Tablets: 2 mg, 4 mg, 8 mg, 16 mg
Oral concentrate: 16 mg/5ml
Syrup: 2 mg/5 ml†
Injection: 5 mg/ml

ACTION

Mechanism: Blocks postsynaptic dopamine receptors in the brain and inhibits the medullary chemoreceptor trigger zone.

Onset: antipsychotic effect, 2 weeks or longer. **Peak:** Steady-state levels are reached after several days of therapy. Peak therapeutic effects may not occur for 6 weeks to 6 months.

INDICATIONS & DOSAGE

Psychosis in hospitalized patients—
Adults: initially, 8 to 16 mg P.O. b.i.d., t.i.d., or q.i.d., increasing to 64 mg daily.
Children over 12 years: 6 to 12 mg P.O. daily in divided doses.
Mental disturbances, acute alcoholism, nausea, vomiting, hiccups—
Adults and children over 12 years: 5 to 10 mg I.M. p.r.n. Maximum dosage is 15 mg daily in ambulatory patients, 30 mg daily in hospitalized patients.

ADVERSE REACTIONS

CNS: *extrapyramidal reactions* (high incidence), *tardive dyskinesia,* sedation (low incidence), pseudoparkinsonism, EEG changes, dizziness.
CV: *orthostatic hypotension,* tachycardia, ECG changes.
EENT: ocular changes, *blurred vision.*
GI: *dry mouth, constipation.*
GU: *urine retention,* dark urine, menstrual irregularities, gynecomastia, inhibited ejaculation.
Hematologic: transient leukopenia, hyperprolactinemia, ***agranulocytosis.***
Hepatic: cholestatic jaundice, abnormal liver function tests.
Skin: *mild photosensitivity,* allergic reactions, pain at I.M. injection site, sterile abscess.
Other: weight gain; increased appetite; rarely, ***neuroleptic malignant syndrome*** (fever, tachycardia, tachypnea, profuse diaphoresis).
After abrupt withdrawal of long-term therapy: gastritis, nausea, vomiting, dizziness, tremors, feeling of warmth or cold, diaphoresis, tachycardia, headache, insomnia.

INTERACTIONS

Antacids: inhibited absorption of oral phenothiazines. Separate antacid and phenothiazine doses by at least 2 hours.

Barbiturates: may decrease phenothiazine effect. Observe patient.

Ethanol, other CNS depressants: increased CNS depression. Avoid concomitant use.

CONTRAINDICATIONS

- Contraindicated in patients experiencing coma or CNS depression, bone marrow suppression, or subcortical damage.
- Contraindicated with use of spinal or epidural anesthetic or adrenergic blocking agents.
- Use cautiously with other CNS depressants or anticholinergics; in elderly or debilitated patients; in acutely ill or dehydrated children; and in patients with hepatic disease, arteriosclerosis or CV disease (may cause sudden drop in blood pressure), exposure to extreme heat or cold (including antipyretic therapy), respiratory disorders, hypocalcemia, seizure disorders (may lower seizure threshold), severe reactions to insulin or electroconvulsive therapy, suspected brain tumor or intestinal obstruction, glaucoma, or prostatic hyperplasia.

NURSING CONSIDERATIONS

- Tardive dyskinesia may occur after prolonged use. It may not appear until months or years later and may disappear spontaneously or persist for life despite discontinuation of drug.
- Acute dystonic reactions may be treated with I.V. diphenhydramine.
- Neuroleptic malignant syndrome is rare, but frequently fatal. It is not necessarily related to length of drug use or type of neuroleptic, but over 60% of affected patients are men. Watch for symptoms.
- Withhold dose and notify doctor if patient develops jaundice, symptoms of blood dyscrasia (fever, sore throat, infection, cellulitis, weakness), or persistent (longer than a few hours) extrapyramidal reactions.
- Monitor therapy with weekly bilirubin tests during first month; periodic blood tests (CBC and liver function); and ophthalmic tests (long-term use).
- Dose of 8 mg is therapeutic equivalent of 100 mg chlorpromazine.
- Obtain baseline measures of blood pressure before starting therapy and monitor regularly. Watch for orthostatic hypotension, especially with parenteral administration. Keep patient supine for 1 hour afterward; advise him to change positions slowly.
- Give deep I.M. only in upper outer quadrant of buttocks. Massage slowly afterward to prevent sterile abscess. Injection may sting.
- Do not withdraw drug abruptly unless required by severe adverse reactions.
- Protect drug from light. Slight yellowing of injection or concentrate is common; does not affect potency. Discard markedly discolored solutions.
- Prevent contact dermatitis by keeping drug off skin and clothes. Wear gloves when preparing liquid forms.
- Dilute liquid concentrate with fruit juice, milk, carbonated beverage, or semisolid food just before giving. Exceptions: Oral concentrate causes turbidity or precipitation in colas, black coffee, grape or apple juice, or tea. Do not mix with these liquids.
- Advise patients to report urine retention or constipation.
- Tell patients to use sunblock and to wear protective clothing to avoid photosensitivity reactions.
- Warn patients to avoid activities that require alertness or good psychomotor coordination until CNS effects of the drug are known. Drowsiness and dizziness usually subside after a few weeks.

• Tell patients to avoid alcohol while taking this drug.
• Relieve dry mouth with sugarless gum, sour hard candy, or mouthwash.

pimozide
Orap

Pregnancy Risk Category: C

HOW SUPPLIED
Tablets: 2 mg

ACTION
Mechanism: Blocks dopamine receptors.
Onset: antipsychotic effect, 2 weeks or longer. **Peak:** Serum levels peak 6 to 8 hours after dose. Peak therapeutic effects may not occur for 6 weeks to 6 months. **Duration:** elimination half-life, about 29 hours.

INDICATIONS & DOSAGE
Suppression of severe motor and phonic tics in patients with Tourette syndrome –
Adults and children over 12 years: initially, 1 to 2 mg P.O. daily in divided doses. Then, increase dosage every other day. Maintenance dosage ranges from 7 to 16 mg daily.

ADVERSE REACTIONS
CNS: *parkinsonian-like symptoms,* other extrapyramidal symptoms (dystonia, akathisia, hyperreflexia, opisthotonus, oculogyric crisis), *tardive dyskinesia, sedation.*
CV: *ECG changes (prolonged QT interval),* hypotension.
EENT: visual disturbances.
GI: *dry mouth, constipation.*
GU: impotence.
Other: rarely, ***neuroleptic malignant syndrome*** (fever, tachycardia, tachypnea, profuse diaphoresis); muscle tightness.

INTERACTIONS
Ethanol, other CNS depressants: increased CNS depression. Avoid concomitant use.
Phenothiazines, tricyclic antidepressants, antiarrhythmics: increased incidence of ECG abnormalities. Monitor patient closely.

CONTRAINDICATIONS
• Contraindicated in patients with congenital long QT syndrome or history of arrhythmias, patients with severe toxic CNS depression, and patients experiencing coma.
• Use cautiously in patients with hepatic or renal dysfunction, glaucoma, and prostatic hyperplasia.

NURSING CONSIDERATIONS
• Tardive dyskinesia may occur after prolonged use. It may not appear until months or years later and may disappear spontaneously or persist for life despite discontinuation of drug.
• Neuroleptic malignant syndrome is rare, but frequently fatal. It is not necessarily related to length of drug use or type of neuroleptic, but over 60% of affected patients are men. Watch for symptoms.
• Acute dystonic reactions may be treated with I.V. diphenhydramine.
• Pimozide is not recommended for treatment of simple tics, except those associated with Tourette syndrome. Don't use in drug-induced motor and phonic tics.
• Avoid concurrent administration of other drugs that prolong the QT interval, such as antiarrhythmics.
• Perform an ECG before treatment begins and periodically thereafter. Monitor for prolonged QT interval.
• Monitor patients who are also taking anticonvulsants for increased seizure activity. Pimozide may lower the seizure threshold.
• Because pimozide may cause serious adverse effects, inform patients and their family about the drug. Pi-

mozide therapy is indicated only for patients who failed to respond to standard treatment.
- Tell patients to avoid alcohol while taking this drug.
- Warn patients not to stop taking drug abruptly and not to exceed prescribed dose.
- Tell patients to use sugarless hard candy, gum, and liquids to relieve dry mouth.

promazine hydrochloride

Primazine, Prozine-50, Sparine**

Pregnancy Risk Category: C

HOW SUPPLIED

Tablets: 25 mg, 50 mg, 100 mg
Injection: 25 mg/ml, 50 mg/ml

ACTION

Mechanism: An aliphatic phenothiazine that blocks postsynaptic dopamine receptors in the brain.
Onset: antipsychotic effect, 2 weeks or longer. **Peak:** Steady-state levels are reached after several days of therapy. Peak therapeutic effects may not occur for 6 weeks to 6 months.

INDICATIONS & DOSAGE

Psychosis –
Adults: 10 to 200 mg P.O. or I.M. q 4 to 6 hours, up to 1 g daily. For acutely agitated patients, initial dose is 50 to 150 mg I.M.; repeat within 5 to 10 minutes if necessary.
Children over 12 years: 10 to 25 mg P.O. or I.M. q 4 to 6 hours.

ADVERSE REACTIONS

CNS: *extrapyramidal reactions* (moderate incidence), *tardive dyskinesia, sedation* (high incidence), pseudoparkinsonism, EEG changes, dizziness.
CV: *orthostatic hypotension,* tachycardia, ECG changes.
EENT: ocular changes, blurred vision.
GI: *dry mouth, constipation.*
GU: *urine retention,* dark urine, menstrual irregularities, gynecomastia, inhibited ejaculation.
Hematologic: transient leukopenia, ***agranulocytosis,*** hyperprolactinemia.
Hepatic: cholestatic jaundice, abnormal liver function tests.
Skin: *mild photosensitivity,* allergic reactions, pain at I.M. injection site, sterile abscess.
Other: weight gain; increased appetite; rarely, ***neuroleptic malignant syndrome*** (fever, tachycardia, tachypnea, profuse diaphoresis).
After abrupt withdrawal of long-term therapy: gastritis, nausea, vomiting, dizziness, tremors, feeling of warmth or cold, diaphoresis, tachycardia, headache, insomnia.

INTERACTIONS

Antacids: inhibited absorption of oral phenothiazines. Use together cautiously. Separate antacid and phenothiazine doses by at least 2 hours.
Anticholinergics (including antidepressant and antiparkinsonian agents): increased anticholinergic activity, aggravated parkinsonian symptoms. Use together cautiously.
Barbiturates, lithium: may decrease phenothiazine effect. Observe patient.
Centrally acting antihypertensives: decreased antihypertensive effect. Monitor blood pressure.
Ethanol: increased CNS depression. Avoid concomitant use.
Other CNS depressants: increased CNS depression. Use together cautiously.

CONTRAINDICATIONS

- Contraindicated in patients experiencing coma or CNS depression, bone marrow suppression, or subcortical damage.
- Contraindicated with use of spinal or epidural anesthetic or with adrenergic blocking agents.
- Use cautiously in elderly or debili-

tated patients; in patients with hepatic disease, arteriosclerosis or CV disease (may cause sudden drop in blood pressure), exposure to extreme heat or cold (including antipyretic therapy), respiratory disorders, hypocalcemia, seizure disorders (may lower seizure threshold), severe reactions to insulin or electroconvulsive therapy, suspected brain tumor or intestinal obstruction, glaucoma, or prostatic hyperplasia; and in acutely ill or dehydrated children.

NURSING CONSIDERATIONS

- Tardive dyskinesia may occur after prolonged use. It may not appear until months or years later and may disappear spontaneously or persist for life despite discontinuation of drug.
- Neuroleptic malignant syndrome is rare, but frequently fatal. It is not necessarily related to length of drug use or type of neuroleptic, but over 60% of affected patients are men. Watch for symptoms.
- Acute dystonic reactions may be treated with I.V. diphenhydramine.
- Withhold dose and notify doctor if patient develops jaundice, symptoms of blood dyscrasia (fever, sore throat, infection, cellulitis, weakness), persistent (longer than a few hours) extrapyramidal reactions, or such reactions during pregnancy or in children.
- Monitor therapy with weekly bilirubin tests during first month; periodic blood tests (CBC and liver function); and ophthalmic tests (long-term use).
- Have patients report urine retention or constipation.
- Tell patients to use sunblock and to wear protective clothing to avoid photosensitivity reactions.
- Warn patients to avoid activities that require alertness or good psychomotor coordination until CNS effects of the drug are known. Drowsiness and dizziness usually subside after a few weeks.
- Tell patients to avoid alcohol while taking this drug.
- Monitor blood pressure with patient lying and standing before starting therapy, and routinely throughout course of treatment.
- Watch for orthostatic hypotension, especially with parenteral administration. Keep the patient supine for 1 hour afterward and advise patient to change positions slowly.
- Prevent contact dermatitis by keeping drug off the patient's skin and clothes. Wear gloves when preparing liquid forms.
- Give deeply I.M. only in upper outer quadrant of buttocks. Massage slowly afterward to prevent sterile abscess. Injection may sting.
- Dilute liquid concentrate with fruit juice, milk, semisolid food, or chocolate-flavored drinks just before giving. For best taste, use at least 10 ml diluent per 25 mg drug.
- Protect drug from light. Slight yellowing of injection or concentrate is common; does not affect potency. Discard markedly discolored solutions.
- Do not withdraw drug abruptly unless required by severe adverse reactions.
- Relieve dry mouth with sugarless gum, sour hard candy, or mouthwash.

risperidone

Risperdal

Pregnancy Risk Category: C

HOW SUPPLIED

Tablets: 1 mg, 2 mg, 3 mg, 4 mg

ACTION

Mechanism: Blocks dopamine and serotonin (5-HT) receptors; also blocks alpha-1, alpha-2, and histamine-1 receptors in the CNS.
Peak: Plasma levels peak in about 1 hour. **Duration:** elimination half-life, about 20 hours.

INDICATIONS & DOSAGE

Psychosis –

Adults: initially, 1 mg P.O. b.i.d. Increase in increments of 1 mg b.i.d. on the second and third day of treatment to a target dose of 3 mg b.i.d. Wait at least 1 week before adjusting dosage further.

Elderly or debilitated patients, hypotensive patients, or patients with severe renal or hepatic impairment: initially 0.5 mg P.O. b.i.d. Increase dosage in increments of 0.5 mg b.i.d. on the second and third day of treatment to a target dosage of 1.5 mg P.O. b.i.d. Wait at least 1 week before increasing dosage further.

ADVERSE REACTIONS

CNS: *somnolence, extrapyramidal symptoms, headache, insomnia, agitation, anxiety,* tardive dyskinesia, aggressive reaction.

CV: tachycardia, chest pain, orthostatic hypotension, prolonged QT interval.

EENT: rhinitis, coughing, upper respiratory infection, sinusitis, pharyngitis, abnormal vision.

GI: *constipation, nausea, vomiting, dyspepsia.*

Skin: rash, dry skin, photosensitivity.

Other: arthralgia, back pain, fever, ***neuroleptic malignant syndrome.***

INTERACTIONS

Carbamazepine: increased clearance of risperidone, leading to decreased effectiveness. Monitor closely.

Clozapine: decreased clearance of risperidone, increasing toxicity. Monitor closely.

Ethanol, CNS depressants: additive CNS depression. Avoid concomitant use.

Levodopa: antagonized effects. Don't use together.

CONTRAINDICATIONS

- Contraindicated in patients hypersensitive to the drug. Also contraindicated in breast-feeding patients.
- Use cautiously in patients with prolonged QT interval, a condition associated with torsades de pointes, a life-threatening arrhythmia. Patients at risk include those with congenital heart abnormalities, bradycardia, or electrolyte imbalances and those using other drugs that also prolong QT interval. Also use cautiously in patients with a history of breast cancer. Many breast cancers are prolactin-dependent; risperidone raises serum prolactin levels.

NURSING CONSIDERATIONS

- Tardive dyskinesia may occur after prolonged use. It may not appear until months or years later and may disappear spontaneously or persist for life despite discontinuation of drug.
- Neuroleptic malignant syndrome is rare, but frequently fatal. It is not necessarily related to length of drug use or type of neuroleptic, but over 60% of affected patients are men. Watch for symptoms.
- Tell patients to use sunblock and to wear protective clothing to avoid photosensitivity reactions.
- Advise patients to use caution in hot weather to prevent heat stroke because the drug may interfere with thermoregulation.
- Warn patients to avoid activities that require alertness or good psychomotor coordination until CNS effects of the drug are known. Drowsiness and dizziness usually subside after a few days.
- Tell patients to avoid alcohol while taking this drug.
- Obtain baseline measures of blood pressure before starting therapy and monitor regularly. Watch for orthostatic hypotension, especially during initial dosage titration. Warn patient to rise slowly, avoid hot showers, and

use extra caution during the first few days of therapy to avoid fainting.

• Tell patients to notify their doctors if they are or plan to become pregnant during therapy.

thioridazine hydrochloride

Aldazine‡, Apo-Thioridazine†, Mellaril*, Mellaril Concenrate, Novoridazine†, PMS Thioridazine†

Pregnancy Risk Category: C

HOW SUPPLIED

Tablets: 10 mg, 15 mg, 25 mg, 50 mg, 100 mg, 150 mg, 200 mg
Oral suspension: 10 mg/5 ml, 25 mg/5 ml, 100 mg/5 ml
Oral concentrate: 30 mg/ml, 100 mg/ml (3% to 4.2% alcohol)

ACTION

Mechanism: A piperidine phenothiazine that blocks postsynaptic dopamine receptors in the brain.
Onset: antipsychotic effect, 2 weeks or longer. **Peak:** Steady-state levels are reached after several days of therapy. Peak therapeutic effects may not occur for 6 weeks to 6 months.

INDICATIONS & DOSAGE

Psychosis –
Adults: initially, 25 to 100 mg P.O. t.i.d., with gradual increments up to 800 mg daily in divided doses, if needed. Dosage varies.
Depressive neurosis, alcohol withdrawal, dementia in elderly patients, behavioral problems in children –
Adults: initially, 25 mg P.O. t.i.d. Maintenance dosage is 20 to 200 mg daily.
Children over 2 years: 0.5 to 3 mg/kg P.O. daily in divided doses.

ADVERSE REACTIONS

CNS: extrapyramidal reactions (low incidence), *tardive dyskinesia, sedation* (high incidence), EEG changes, dizziness.
CV: *orthostatic hypotension,* tachycardia, ECG changes.
EENT: *ocular changes, blurred vision,* pigmentary retinopathy.
GI: *dry mouth, constipation.*
GU: *urine retention,* dark urine, menstrual irregularities, gynecomastia, inhibited ejaculation.
Hematologic: transient leukopenia, ***agranulocytosis,*** hyperprolactinemia.
Hepatic: cholestatic jaundice.
Skin: *mild photosensitivity,* allergic reactions.
Other: weight gain; increased appetite; rarely, ***neuroleptic malignant syndrome*** (fever, tachycardia, tachypnea, profuse diaphoresis).
After abrupt withdrawal of long-term therapy: gastritis, nausea, vomiting, dizziness, tremors, feeling of warmth or cold, diaphoresis, tachycardia, headache, insomnia.

INTERACTIONS

Antacids: inhibited absorption of oral phenothiazines. Separate antacid and phenothiazine doses by at least 2 hours.
Barbiturates, lithium: may decrease phenothiazine effect. Observe patient.
Centrally acting antihypertensives: decreased antihypertensive effect. Monitor blood pressure.
Ethanol: increased CNS depression. Avoid concomitant use.
Other CNS depressants: increased CNS depression. Use together cautiously.

CONTRAINDICATIONS

• Contraindicated in patients experiencing coma or CNS depression, bone marrow suppression, hypertensive or hypotensive cardiac disease, or subcortical damage.
• Contraindicated with use of spinal or epidural anesthetic or with adrenergic blocking agents.
• Use cautiously in elderly or debilitated patients; in patients with hepatic

disease, arteriosclerosis or CV disease (may cause sudden drop in blood pressure), exposure to extreme heat or cold (including antipyretic therapy), respiratory disorders, hypocalcemia, seizure disorders, severe reactions to insulin or electroconvulsive therapy, suspected brain tumor or intestinal obstruction, glaucoma, or prostatic hypertrophy; and in acutely ill or dehydrated children.

NURSING CONSIDERATIONS

• Tardive dyskinesia may occur after prolonged use. It may not appear until months or years later and may disappear spontaneously or persist for life despite discontinuation of drug.
• Neuroleptic malignant syndrome is rare, but frequently fatal. It is not necessarily related to length of drug use or type of neuroleptic, but over 60% of affected patients are men. Watch for symptoms.
• Acute dystonic reactions may be treated with I.V. diphenhydramine.
• Withhold dose and notify the doctor if patient develops jaundice, symptoms of blood dyscrasia (fever, sore throat, infection, cellulitis, weakness), or persistent (longer than a few hours) extrapyramidal reactions, or such reactions during pregnancy or in children.
• Monitor therapy with weekly bilirubin tests during first month; periodic blood tests (CBC and liver function); and ophthalmic tests (long-term therapy).
• Remember that different liquid formulations have different concentrations.
• Dilute liquid concentrate with water or fruit juice just before giving.
• Be sure to shake suspension well before using.
• Prevent contact dermatitis by keeping drug off skin and clothes. Wear gloves when preparing liquid forms.
• Do not withdraw abruptly unless required by severe adverse reactions.
• Dose of 100 mg is therapeutic equivalent of 100 mg chlorpromazine.
• Dosage above 800 mg may be associated with ocular toxicity (pigmentary retinopathy).
• Have patients report urine retention or constipation.
• Tell patients that drug may discolor the urine.
• Tell patients to watch for and notify doctor of blurred vision.
• Tell patients to use sunblock and to wear protective clothing to avoid photosensitivity reactions.
• Warn patients to avoid activities that require alertness or good psychomotor coordination until CNS effects of the drug are known. Drowsiness and dizziness usually subside after a few weeks.
• Tell patients to avoid alcohol while taking this drug.
• Watch for orthostatic hypotension, especially with parenteral administration. Advise patient to change positions slowly.
• Relieve dry mouth with sugarless gum, sour hard candy, or mouthwash.

thiothixene
Navane

thiothixene hydrochloride
Navane*

Pregnancy Risk Category: C

HOW SUPPLIED

thiothixene
Capsules: 1 mg, 2 mg, 5 mg, 10 mg, 20 mg
thiothixene hydrochloride
Oral concentrate: 5 mg/ml (7% alcohol)
Injection: 2 mg/ml, 5 mg/ml

ACTION

Mechanism: A thioxanthene that blocks postsynaptic dopamine receptors in the brain.
Onset: antipsychotic effect, 2 weeks

or longer. **Peak:** Steady-state levels occur after several days of therapy. Peak therapeutic effects may not occur for 6 weeks to 6 months.

INDICATIONS & DOSAGE

Acute agitation –
Adults: 4 mg I.M. b.i.d. to q.i.d. Maximum dosage is 30 mg daily I.M. Change to P.O. as soon as possible.
Mild to moderate psychosis –
Adults: initially, 2 mg P.O. t.i.d. May increase gradually to 15 mg daily.
Severe psychosis –
Adults: initially, 5 mg P.O. b.i.d. May increase gradually to 15 to 30 mg daily. Maximum recommended dosage is 60 mg daily. Not recommended in children under 12 years.

ADVERSE REACTIONS

CNS: *extrapyramidal reactions* (high incidence), *tardive dyskinesia,* sedation (low incidence), pseudoparkinsonism, EEG changes, dizziness.
CV: *orthostatic hypotension,* tachycardia, ECG changes.
EENT: ocular changes, *blurred vision.*
GI: *dry mouth, constipation.*
GU: *urine retention,* dark urine, menstrual irregularities, gynecomastia, inhibited ejaculation.
Hematologic: transient leukopenia, ***agranulocytosis,*** hyperprolactinemia.
Hepatic: cholestatic jaundice.
Skin: *mild photosensitivity,* allergic reactions, pain at I.M. injection site, sterile abscess.
Other: weight gain; increased appetite; rarely, ***neuroleptic malignant syndrome*** (fever, tachycardia, tachypnea, profuse diaphoresis).
After abrupt withdrawal of long-term therapy: gastritis, nausea, vomiting, dizziness, tremors, feeling of warmth or cold, diaphoresis, tachycardia, headache, insomnia.

INTERACTIONS

Ethanol, other CNS depressants: increased CNS depression. Avoid concomitant use.

CONTRAINDICATIONS

- Contraindicated in patients experiencing convulsive seizures, circulatory collapse, coma, CNS depression, blood dyscrasia, bone marrow suppression, alcohol withdrawal, akathisia or restlessness, or subcortical damage.
- Contraindicated with use of spinal or epidural anesthetic or with adrenergic blocking agents.
- Use cautiously with other CNS depressants and anticholinergics; in elderly or debilitated patients; and in patients with hepatic disease, arteriosclerosis or CV disease (may cause sudden drop in blood pressure), exposure to extreme heat or cold (including antipyretic therapy) or excessive sunlight, respiratory disorders, hypocalcemia, severe reactions to insulin or electroconvulsive therapy, suspected brain tumor or intestinal obstruction, glaucoma, and prostatic hyperplasia.

NURSING CONSIDERATIONS

- Tardive dyskinesia may occur after prolonged use; may not appear until months or years later and may disappear spontaneously or persist for life, despite discontinuation of drug.
- Neuroleptic malignant syndrome rare, but frequently fatal. Not necessarily related to length of drug use or type of neuroleptic, but over 60% of affected patients are men. Watch for symptoms.
- Acute dystonic reactions may be treated with I.V. diphenhydramine.
- Withhold dose and notify doctor if patient develops jaundice, symptoms of blood dyscrasia (fever, sore throat, infection, cellulitis, weakness), persistent (longer than a few hours) ex-

trapyramidal reactions, or any such reactions during pregnancy.

- Monitor therapy with weekly bilirubin tests during first month; periodic blood tests (CBC and liver function); and ophthalmic tests (long-term use).
- Have patient report urine retention or constipation.
- Watch for orthostatic hypotension, especially with parenteral administration. Keep the patient in supine position for 1 hour afterward and advise him to change positions slowly.
- Dose of 4 mg is therapeutic equivalent of 100 mg chlorpromazine.
- Give I.M. only in upper outer quadrant of buttocks or midlateral thigh. Massage slowly afterward to prevent sterile abscess. Injection may sting.
- Slight yellowing of injection or concentrate is common; does not affect potency. Discard markedly discolored solutions.
- Refrigerate I.M. form.
- Dilute liquid concentrate with fruit juice, milk, or semisolid food just before administering.
- Prevent contact dermatitis by keeping drug off skin and clothes. Wear gloves when preparing liquid forms.
- Do not withdraw abruptly unless required by severe adverse reactions.
- Relieve dry mouth with sugarless gum, sour hard candy, or mouthwash.
- Tell patients to use sunblock and to wear protective clothing to avoid photosensitivity reactions.
- Warn patients to avoid activities that require alertness or good psychomotor coordination until CNS effects of the drug are known. Drowsiness and dizziness usually subside after a few weeks.
- Tell patients to avoid alcohol while taking this drug.

trifluoperazine hydrochloride

Apo-Trifluoperazine†, Calmazine‡, Novo-Flurazine†, PMS-Trifluoperazine†, Solazine†, Stelazine, Stelazine Concentrate, Terfluzine†, Terfluzine Concentrate†

Pregnancy Risk Category: C

HOW SUPPLIED

Tablets (regular and film-coated): 1 mg, 2 mg, 5 mg, 10 mg
Oral concentrate: 10 mg/ml
Injection: 2 mg/ml

ACTION

Mechanism: A piperazine phenothiazine that blocks postsynaptic dopamine receptors in the brain.
Onset: antipsychotic effect may not be apparent for 2 weeks or longer.
Peak: Steady-state levels occur after several days of therapy. Peak therapeutic effects may not occur for 6 weeks to 6 months.

INDICATIONS & DOSAGE

Anxiety states –
Adults: 1 to 2 mg P.O. b.i.d.
Schizophrenia and other psychotic disorders –
Adults: *outpatients* – 1 to 2 mg P.O. b.i.d., up to 4 mg daily; *hospitalized patients* – 2 to 5 mg P.O. b.i.d., gradually increased to 40 mg daily. Or 1 to 2 mg I.M. q 4 to 6 hours, p.r.n.
Children 6 to 12 years (hospitalized or under close supervision): 1 mg P.O. daily or b.i.d.; may increase gradually to 15 mg daily.

ADVERSE REACTIONS

CNS: *extrapyramidal reactions* (high incidence), *tardive dyskinesia,* sedation (low incidence), pseudoparkinsonism, EEG changes, dizziness.
CV: *orthostatic hypotension,* tachycardia, ECG changes.

EENT: ocular changes, *blurred vision.*
GI: *dry mouth, constipation.*
GU: *urine retention,* dark urine, menstrual irregularities, gynecomastia, inhibited ejaculation.
Hematologic: transient leukopenia, ***agranulocytosis,*** hyperprolactinemia.
Hepatic: cholestatic jaundice.
Skin: *mild photosensitivity,* allergic reactions, pain at I.M. injection site, sterile abscess.
Other: weight gain; increased appetite; rarely, ***neuroleptic malignant syndrome*** (fever, tachycardia, tachypnea, profuse diaphoresis).
After abrupt withdrawal of long-term therapy: gastritis, nausea, vomiting, dizziness, tremors, feeling of warmth or cold, diaphoresis, tachycardia, headache, insomnia.

INTERACTIONS
Antacids: inhibited absorption of oral phenothiazines. Separate antacid and phenothiazine doses by at least 2 hours.
Barbiturates, lithium: may decrease phenothiazine effect. Monitor the patient.
Centrally acting antihypertensives: decreased antihypertensive effect. Monitor blood pressure.
Ethanol: increased CNS depression. Avoid concomitant use.
Other CNS depressants: increased CNS depression. Use together cautiously.

CONTRAINDICATIONS
• Contraindicated in patients experiencing coma, CNS depression, bone marrow suppression, or subcortical damage.
• Contraindicated with use of spinal or epidural anesthetic or with adrenergic blocking agents.
• Use cautiously in elderly or debilitated patients; in patients with hepatic disease, arteriosclerosis or CV disease (may cause drop in blood pressure), exposure to extreme heat or cold (including antipyretic therapy), respiratory disorders, hypocalcemia, seizure disorders, severe reactions to insulin or electroconvulsive therapy, suspected brain tumor or intestinal obstruction, glaucoma, or prostatic hyperplasia; and in acutely ill or dehydrated children.

NURSING CONSIDERATIONS
• Dose of 5 mg is therapeutic equivalent of 100 mg chlorpromazine.
• Tardive dyskinesia may occur after prolonged use. It may not appear until months or years later, and may disappear spontaneously or persist for life despite discontinuation of drug.
• Neuroleptic malignant syndrome is rare, but frequently fatal. It is not necessarily related to length of drug use or type of neuroleptic, but over 60% of affected patients are men. Watch for symptoms.
• Treat acute dystonic reactions with I.V. diphenhydramine.
• Withhold dose and notify doctor if patient develops jaundice, symptoms of blood dyscrasia (fever, sore throat, infection, cellulitis, weakness), persistent (longer than a few hours) extrapyramidal reactions, or any such reactions during pregnancy or in children.
• Monitor therapy with weekly bilirubin tests during first month; periodic blood tests (CBC and liver function); and ophthalmic tests (long-term use).
• Have patients report urine retention or constipation.
• Watch for orthostatic hypotension, especially with parenteral administration. Keep the patient supine for 1 hour afterward, and advise him to change positions slowly.
• Give deeply I.M. only in upper outer quadrant of buttocks. Massage slowly afterward to prevent sterile abscess. Injection may sting.
• Dilute liquid concentrate with 60 ml of tomato or fruit juice, carbonated

beverages, coffee, tea, milk, water, or semisolid food just before giving.

- Prevent contact dermatitis by keeping drug off skin and clothes. Wear gloves when preparing liquid forms.
- Do not withdraw drug abruptly unless severe adverse reactions occur.
- Protect drug from light. Slight yellowing of injection or concentrate is common; does not affect potency. Discard markedly discolored solutions.
- Tell patients to use sunblock and to wear protective clothing to avoid photosensitivity reactions.
- Warn patients to avoid activities that require alertness or good psychomotor coordination until CNS effects of the drug are known. Drowsiness and dizziness usually subside after a few weeks.
- Tell patients to avoid alcohol while taking this drug.
- Relieve dry mouth with sugarless gum, sour hard candy, or mouthwash.

*Liquid form contains alcohol.
**May contain tartrazine.

Common reactions are in italics; ***life-threatening,*** in bold italics.

33
Cerebral stimulants

amphetamine sulfate
benzphetamine hydrochloride
caffeine
dextroamphetamine sulfate
diethylpropion hydrochloride
fenfluramine hydrochloride
mazindol
methamphetamine hydrochloride
methylphenidate hydrochloride
pemoline
phendimetrazine tartrate
phentermine hydrochloride

COMBINATION PRODUCTS
None.

amphetamine sulfate
Controlled Substance Schedule II

Pregnancy Risk Category: C

HOW SUPPLIED
Tablets: 5 mg, 10 mg

ACTION
Mechanism: Promotes nerve impulse transmission by releasing stored norepinephrine from nerve terminals in the brain. Main sites of activity appears to be the cerebral cortex and the reticular activating system.
Onset: within 3 hours. **Duration:** about 10 hours.

INDICATIONS & DOSAGE
Attention deficit disorder with hyperactivity –
Children 3 to 5 years: 2.5 mg P.O. daily, with 2.5-mg increments weekly, p.r.n.
Children 6 years and older: 5 mg P.O. daily, with 5-mg increments weekly, p.r.n.
Narcolepsy –
Adults: 5 to 60 mg P.O. daily in divided doses.
Children 6 to 12 years: 5 mg P.O. daily, with 5-mg increments weekly, p.r.n.
Children over 12 years: 10 mg P.O. daily, with 10-mg increments weekly, p.r.n.
Short-term adjunct in exogenous obesity –
Adults: 5 to 30 mg daily in divided doses 30 to 60 minutes before meals. Not recommended for children under 12 years.

ADVERSE REACTIONS
CNS: *restlessness,* tremor, *hyperactivity, talkativeness, insomnia,* irritability, dizziness, headache, chills, dysphoria.
CV: *tachycardia, palpitations,* hypertension, hypotension.
GI: dry mouth, metallic taste, nausea, vomiting, cramps, diarrhea, constipation, anorexia, weight loss.
GU: impotence.
Skin: urticaria.
Other: altered libido.

INTERACTIONS
Ammonium chloride, ascorbic acid: decreased serum levels and increased renal excretion of amphetamine. Monitor for decreased amphetamine effect.
Antacids, sodium bicarbonate, acetazolamide: increased renal reabsorption. Monitor for enhanced effect.
Antihypertensives: reversal of antihypertensive action. Monitor blood pressure.
Caffeine: may increase amphetamine and related amine effects. Avoid concomitant use.
Haloperidol, phenothiazines, tricyclic antidepressants: increased CNS effect. Avoid concomitant use.
Insulin, oral antidiabetic agents: may

decrease antidiabetic agent requirements. Monitor blood glucose level. *MAO inhibitors:* severe hypertension; possible hypertensive crisis. Don't use together or within 14 days after an MAO inhibitor has been discontinued.

CONTRAINDICATIONS

• Contraindicated in patients with symptomatic CV disease, hyperthyroidism, nephritis, angina pectoris, moderate to severe hypertension, parkinsonism due to arteriosclerosis, certain types of glaucoma, advanced arteriosclerosis, or in patients in agitated states or with history of drug abuse. Not recommended for children under 3 years.
• Use cautiously in patients with diabetes mellitus; in elderly, debilitated, or hyperexcitable patients; and in children with Tourette syndrome.

NURSING CONSIDERATIONS

• Habituation or psychic dependence may occur, especially in patients with history of drug addiction. Avoid prolonged administration. When used long-term, lower dosage gradually to prevent acute rebound depression.
• Not recommended for first-line treatment of obesity or for treatment of obesity in children under 12 years. Use as an anorexigenic agent is prohibited in some states.
• Make sure obese patient is on a weight-reduction program. Give drug 30 to 60 minutes before meals. Monitor dietary intake and count calories, if necessary.
• Fatigue may result as drug effects wear off. The patient will need more rest.
• Tell the patient to avoid drinks containing caffeine, which increase the effects of amphetamines and related amines.
• Tell the patient to report signs of excessive stimulation.
• Urine acidification enhances renal excretion of the drug; urine alkalinization enhances renal reabsorption and recycling.
• If tolerance to anorexigenic effect develops, discontinue drug.
• Should not be used to combat fatigue.
• Warn the patient to avoid activities that require alertness or good psychomotor coordination until CNS effects of the drug are known.
• Use as analeptic is usually discouraged because CNS stimulation superimposed on CNS depression can lead to neuronal instability and seizures.
• To avoid sleep interference, give at least 6 hours before bedtime.

benzphetamine hydrochloride

Didrex**

Controlled Substance Schedule III

Pregnancy Risk Category: X

HOW SUPPLIED

Tablets: 25 mg, 50 mg

ACTION

Mechanism: Promotes nerve impulse transmission by releasing stored norepinephrine from nerve terminals in the brain. Main sites of activity appears to be the cerebral cortex and the reticular activating system.
Onset: within 1 hour. **Peak:** Peak effects occur in 4 to 6 hours. **Duration:** elimination half-life, about 5 hours.

INDICATIONS & DOSAGE

Short-term adjunct in exogenous obesity –
Adults: 25 to 50 mg P.O. daily, b.i.d. or t.i.d.

ADVERSE REACTIONS

CNS: *restlessness,* tremor, *hyperactivity, talkativeness, insomnia,* irritability, dizziness, headache, chills, dysphoria.

CV: *tachycardia, palpitations,* hypertension, hypotension.
GI: dry mouth, metallic taste, nausea, vomiting, cramps, diarrhea, constipation, anorexia, weight loss.
GU: impotence.
Skin: urticaria.
Other: altered libido.

INTERACTIONS

Ammonium chloride, ascorbic acid: decreased serum levels and increased renal excretion of benzphetamine.
Antacids, sodium bicarbonate, acetazolamide: increased renal reabsorption. Monitor for enhanced effects.
Caffeine: may increase amphetamine and related amine effects. Avoid concomitant use.
Insulin, oral antidiabetic agents: may decrease antidiabetic agent requirement. Monitor blood glucose levels.
MAO inhibitors: severe hypertension; possible hypertensive crisis. Don't use together or within 14 days after MAO inhibitor has been discontinued.
Phenothiazines, haloperidol, tricyclic antidepressants: increased CNS effects. Avoid concomitant use.

CONTRAINDICATIONS

- Contraindicated in patients with symptomatic CV disease, hyperthyroidism, nephritis, angina pectoris, moderate to severe hypertension, parkinsonism due to arteriosclerosis, certain types of glaucoma, advanced arteriosclerosis, agitated states, or in patients with history of drug abuse.
- Use cautiously in patients with diabetes mellitus and in elderly, debilitated, or hyperexcitable patients.

NURSING CONSIDERATIONS

- Habituation or psychic dependence may occur, especially in patients with history of drug addiction. Avoid prolonged administration. When used long-term, lower dosage gradually to prevent acute rebound depression.
- Use in conjunction with a weight-reduction program. Monitor dietary intake and count calories, if necessary. Give 30 to 60 minutes before meals.
- Fatigue may result as drug effects wear off. The patient will need more rest.
- Tell patients to avoid drinks containing caffeine, which increase the effects of amphetamines and related amines.
- Tell the patient to report signs of excessive stimulation.
- Urine acidification enhances renal excretion of the drug; urine alkalinization enhances renal reabsorption and recycling.
- If tolerance to anorexigenic effect develops, discontinue drug.
- Warn the patient to avoid activities that require alertness or good psychomotor coordination until CNS effects of the drug are known.
- To avoid sleep interference, give drug at least 6 hours before bedtime.

caffeine

Caffedrine Caplets◇, Dexitac◇, No Doz◇, Quick Pep◇, Vivarin◇

Pregnancy Risk Category: B

HOW SUPPLIED

Tablets: 100 mg◇, 150 mg◇, 200 mg◇
Capsules (timed-release): 200 mg◇, 250 mg◇
Injection: caffeine (125 mg/ml) with sodium benzoate (125 mg/ml)

ACTION

Mechanism: Inhibits phosphodiesterase, the enzyme that degrades cAMP.
Peak: Serum levels peak within 50 to 75 minutes after oral administration.
Duration: elimination half-life, 3 to 7 hours.

INDICATIONS & DOSAGE
CNS stimulant –
Adults: 100 to 200 mg anhydrous caffeine P.O.
Neonatal apnea –
Neonates: 20 mg/kg P.O., or I.V. as a loading dose. Follow in 2 or 3 days with a maintenance dose of 5 to 10 mg/kg P.O. or I.V. daily or b.i.d.

ADVERSE REACTIONS
CNS: *stimulation, insomnia,* restlessness, nervousness, mild delirium, headache, excitement, agitation, muscle tremors, twitches.
CV: *tachycardia, palpitations.*
GI: nausea, vomiting.
GU: *diuresis.*
Skin: hyperesthesia.
Other: dehydration, fever, hyperglycemia, abrupt withdrawal symptoms (headache, irritability).

INTERACTIONS
Cimetidine, fluoroquinolones, oral contraceptives, phenylpropanolamine, theophylline, beta-adrenergic agonists: excessive CNS stimulation. Avoid concomitant use.

CONTRAINDICATIONS
- Contraindicated in patients with gastric or duodenal ulceration, arrhythmias, or just after MI.

NURSING CONSIDERATIONS
- Tolerance or psychological dependence may develop.
- Be alert for signs of overdose: GI pain, mild delirium, insomnia, diuresis, dehydration, and fever. Treat with short-acting barbiturates, gastric emesis, or lavage.
- Single dose should not exceed 1 g.
- Caffeine-containing beverages should be restricted in patients who experience palpitations. Caffeine content: cola beverages, 17 to 55 mg/180 ml; tea, 40 to 100 mg/180 ml; instant coffee, 60 to 180 mg/180 ml; brewed coffee, 100 to 150 mg/180 ml; decaffeinated coffee, 1 to 6 mg/180 ml.
- Caffeine is included in many OTC analgesic preparations. Evidence conflicts regarding whether it increases pain relief.
- Caffeine does not reverse alcohol intoxication or CNS depressant effects of alcohol. Overvigorous therapy with caffeine may aggravate depression in an already depressed patient.
- Sudden discontinuation of caffeine may cause headache and irritability.
- **I.V. use:** Treatment of neonatal apnea is an off-label indication. Caffeine and sodium benzoate injection is not recommended for use in neonatal apnea because of benzoate's association with fatal gasping syndrome in neonates. Solution must be made by pharmacist, using caffeine citrate powder.
- For neonatal apnea, therapeutic serum caffeine levels are 5 to 20 mcg/ml.
- Used experimentally to treat certain types of vascular headaches.

dextroamphetamine sulfate
Dexedrine***, Dexedrine Spansule, Oxydess II, Robese, Spancap #1
Controlled Substance Schedule II
Pregnancy Risk Category: C

HOW SUPPLIED
Tablets: 5 mg, 10 mg
Capsules (sustained-release): 5 mg, 10 mg, 15 mg

ACTION
Mechanism: Promotes nerve impulse transmission by releasing stored norepinephrine from nerve terminals in the brain. Main sites of activity appears to be the cerebral cortex and the reticular activating system. In children with hyperkinesia, amphetamines have a paradoxical calming effect.
Onset: within 1 hour. **Peak:** Peak ef-

*Liquid form contains alcohol. *Common* reactions are in italics; ***life-threatening,*** in bold italics.
**May contain tartrazine.

fects occur in about 4 to 6 hours.
Duration: elimination half-life, about 5 hours.

INDICATIONS & DOSAGE

Narcolepsy –
Adults: 5 to 60 mg P.O. daily in divided doses.
Children 6 to 12 years: 5 mg P.O. daily, with 5-mg increments weekly, p.r.n.
Children over 12 years: 10 mg P.O. daily, with 10-mg increments weekly, p.r.n.
Short-term adjunct in exogenous obesity –
Adults: single 10- to 15-mg long-acting capsule, up to 30 mg daily; or in divided doses, 5 to 10 mg ½ hour before meals.
Attention deficit disorder with hyperactivity –
Children 3 to 5 years: 2.5 mg P.O. daily, with 2.5-mg increments weekly, p.r.n.
Children 6 years and older: 5 mg P.O. once daily or b.i.d., with 5-mg increments weekly, p.r.n.

ADVERSE REACTIONS

CNS: *restlessness,* tremor, *hyperactivity, talkativeness, insomnia,* irritability, dizziness, headache, chills, overstimulation, dysphoria.
CV: *tachycardia, palpitations,* hypertension, hypotension.
GI: dry mouth, metallic taste, nausea, vomiting, cramps, diarrhea, constipation, anorexia, weight loss.
GU: impotence.
Skin: urticaria.
Other: altered libido.

INTERACTIONS

Ammonium chloride, ascorbic acid: decreased blood levels and increased renal clearance of dextroamphetamine. Monitor for decreased amphetamine effects.
Antacids, sodium bicarbonate, acetazolamide: increased renal reabsorption. Monitor for enhanced amphetamine effects.
Caffeine: may increase amphetamine and related amine effects.
Insulin, oral antidiabetic agents: may decrease antidiabetic agent requirements. Monitor blood glucose levels.
MAO inhibitors: severe hypertension; possible hypertensive crisis. Don't use together or within 14 days after MAO inhibitor has been discontinued.
Phenothiazines, haloperidol, tricyclic antidepressants: increased CNS effects. Avoid concomitant use.

CONTRAINDICATIONS

- Contraindicated in patients with hyperthyroidism, nephritis, severe hypertension, angina pectoris or other severe CV disease, some types of glaucoma, and in patients with history of drug abuse.
- Use cautiously in patients with diabetes mellitus or seizure disorder; in elderly, debilitated, or hyperexcitable patients; and in children with Tourette syndrome.

NURSING CONSIDERATIONS

- Habituation or psychic dependence may occur, especially in patients with history of drug addiction. Avoid prolonged administration. When used long-term, lower dosage gradually to prevent acute rebound depression.
- Not recommended for first-line treatment of obesity. Use as an anorexigenic agent is prohibited in some states.
- Make sure the obese patient is on a weight-reduction program. Give 30 to 60 minutes before meals.
- Give at least 6 hours before bedtime to avoid sleep interference.
- Fatigue may result as drug effects wear off. Patients will need more rest.
- Tell the patient to avoid drinks containing caffeine, which increase the effects of amphetamines and related amines.

- Have patients report signs of excessive stimulation.
- Urine acidification enhances renal excretion of the drug ; urine alkalinization enhances renal reabsorption and recycling.
- If tolerance to anorexigenic effect develops, discontinue drug.
- Don't use to prevent fatigue.
- Warn patients to avoid activities that require alertness or good psychomotor coordination until CNS effects of the drug are known.
- Use as analeptic is usually discouraged because CNS stimulation superimposed on CNS depression can lead to neuronal instability and seizures.

diethylpropion hydrochloride

Nobesine†, M-Orexic, Nobesine-75†, Propion†, Tenuate, Tenuate Dospan, Tepanil, Tepanil Ten-Tab
Controlled Substance Schedule IV

Pregnancy Risk Category: B

HOW SUPPLIED

Tablets: 25 mg
Tablets (extended-release): 75 mg
Capsules (extended-release): 75 mg†

ACTION

Mechanism: Promotes nerve impulse transmission by releasing stored norepinephrine from nerve terminals in the brain. Main sites of activity appears to be the cerebral cortex and the reticular activating system.
Duration: half-life, 4 to 6 hours; effects of regular-release tablets persist for 4 hours; effects of extended-release tablets and capsules, 12 hours.

INDICATIONS & DOSAGE

Short-term adjunct in exogenous obesity–
Adults: 25 mg P.O. before meals, t.i.d.; or 75 mg extended-release tablet or capsule P.O. in midmorning.

ADVERSE REACTIONS

CNS: headache, *nervousness,* dizziness.
CV: *tachycardia, palpitations,* elevated blood pressure, ***pulmonary hypertension.***
EENT: blurred vision.
GI: dry mouth, nausea, abdominal cramps, diarrhea, constipation.
GU: impotence, menstrual changes.
Hematologic: decreased blood glucose levels.
Skin: urticaria.
Other: altered libido.

INTERACTIONS

Caffeine: may increase amphetamine and related amine effects. Avoid concomitant use.
Guanethidine: decrease antihypertensive effect. Monitor blood pressure.
Insulin, oral antidiabetic agents: may decrease antidiabetic agent requirements. Monitor blood glucose levels.
MAO inhibitors: hypertension; possible hypertensive crisis. Don't use together or within 14 days after MAO inhibitor has been discontinued.

CONTRAINDICATIONS

- Contraindicated in patients with hyperthyroidism, hypertension, angina pectoris, severe CV disease, glaucoma, or history of drug abuse.
- Use cautiously in patients with seizure disorder or diabetes mellitus, or in hyperexcitable patients.

NURSING CONSIDERATIONS

- Habituation or psychic dependence may occur.
- May alter insulin requirements. Monitor blood and urine sugars.
- If tolerance to anorexigenic effect develops, discontinue drug.
- Be sure the patient is also on a weight-reduction program.
- Can be used to stop nighttime eating.
- Give drug at least 6 hours before

bedtime to avoid sleep interference although it rarely causes insomnia.
• Fatigue may result as drug effects wear off. The patient will need more rest.
• Tell the patient to avoid drinks containing caffeine, which increase the effects of amphetamines and related amines.
• Tell the patient to report signs of excessive stimulation.
• Urine acidification enhances renal excretion of the drug; urine alkalinization enhances renal reabsorption and recycling.
• Use as analeptic is usually discouraged, because CNS stimulation superimposed on CNS depression can lead to neuronal instability and seizures.

fenfluramine hydrochloride

Ponderal†, Ponderal Pacaps†, Ponderax‡, Ponderax Pacaps‡, Pondimin, Pondimin Extentabs
Controlled Substance Schedule IV

Pregnancy Risk Category: C

HOW SUPPLIED

Tablets: 20 mg, 40 mg
Capsules (sustained-release): 60 mg†‡

ACTION

Mechanism: Stimulates ventromedial nucleus of the hypothalamus. May also affect serotonin metabolism.
Duration: half-life, 11 to 30 hours; effects persist for 4 to 6 hours.

INDICATIONS & DOSAGE

Short-term adjunct in exogenous obesity –
Adults: initially, 20 mg P.O. t.i.d., before meals. Maximum dosage is 40 mg t.i.d. Adjust dosage according to patient response.

ADVERSE REACTIONS

CNS: *drowsiness,* dizziness, incoordination, headache, euphoria or depression, anxiety, *insomnia,* weakness, fatigue, agitation.
CV: *palpitations,* hypotension, hypertension, chest pain.
EENT: eye irritation, blurred vision.
GI: dry mouth, *diarrhea,* nausea, vomiting, abdominal pain, constipation.
GU: dysuria, increased urinary frequency, impotence.
Skin: rash, urticaria, burning sensation.
Other: diaphoresis, chills, fever, increased libido.

INTERACTIONS

Centrally acting antihypertensives: decreased antihypertensive effect. Monitor blood pressure.
Ethanol, CNS depressants: enhanced CNS depression. Don't use togehter.
Insulin, oral antidiabetic agents: may decrease antidiabetic agent requirements. Monitor blood glucose levels.
MAO inhibitors: severe hypertension; possible hypertensive crisis. Don't use together or within 14 days after an MAO inhibitor has been discontinued.

CONTRAINDICATIONS

• Contraindicated in patients with glaucoma, hypersensitivity to sympathomimetic amines, symptomatic CV disease, alcoholism, or history of drug abuse.
• Use cautiously in patients with hypertension, history of mental depression, and diabetes mellitus.

NURSING CONSIDERATIONS

• Differs pharmacologically from amphetamines; it produces CNS depression more often than stimulation.
• Have patients report signs of excessive sedation, depression, or excessive stimulation. Monitor blood pressure.
• Make sure patient is on a weight-reduction program.
• Tolerance or physical or psychic de-

pendence may occur. Avoid prolonged administration.
• Tell patient to avoid alcohol while taking this drug.
• Do not discontinue abruptly; may precipitate an acute depressive reaction.
• Effective for treating autistic children.

mazindol

Mazanor, Sanorex
Controlled Substance Schedule IV
Pregnancy Risk Category: C

HOW SUPPLIED

Tablets: 1 mg, 2 mg

ACTION

Mechanism: Inhibits neuronal uptake of norepinephrine and dopamine.
Duration: half-life, 10 hours; effects persist 10 to 15 hours.

INDICATIONS & DOSAGE

Short-term adjunct in exogenous obesity –
Adults: 1 mg P.O. t.i.d. 1 hour before meals, or 2 mg daily 1 hour before lunch. Use lowest effective dosage.

ADVERSE REACTIONS

CNS: *nervousness,* restlessness, dizziness, *insomnia,* dysphoria, headache, depression, drowsiness, weakness, tremor.
CV: *palpitations, tachycardia.*
GI: dry mouth, dysgeusia, nausea, constipation, diarrhea.
GU: urinary hestitancy, impotence.
Hematologic: decreased blood glucose levels.
Skin: rash, clamminess, pallor.
Other: shivering, diaphoresis, altered libido.

INTERACTIONS

Caffeine: may increase amphetamine and related amine effects. Avoid concomitant use.
Centrally acting antihypertensives: decreased antihypertensive effect. Monitor blood pressure.
Insulin, oral antidiabetic agents: may decrease antidiabetic agent requirements. Monitor blood glucose levels.
MAO inhibitors: severe hypertension; possible hypertensive crisis. Don't use together or within 14 days after an MAO inhibitor has been discontinued.

CONTRAINDICATIONS

• Contraindicated in patients with glaucoma, CV disease (including arrhythmias), and in patients in agitated states or with history of drug abuse.
• Use cautiously in patients with diabetes mellitus, hypertension, and hyperexcitability states.

NURSING CONSIDERATIONS

• Tolerance or physical or psychic dependence may develop. Avoid prolonged use.
• Make sure the patient is also on a weight-reduction program.
• Warn the patient to avoid activities that require alertness or good psychomotor coordination until CNS effects of the drug are known.
• Fatigue may result as drug effects wear off. The patient will need more rest.
• Give at least 6 hours before bedtime to avoid sleep interference.
• Tell the patient to avoid drinks containing caffeine, which increase the effects of amphetamines and related amines.
• Tell the patient to report signs of excessive stimulation.

methamphetamine hydrochloride

Desoxyn, Desoxyn Gradumet
Controlled Substance Schedule II
Pregnancy Risk Category: C

HOW SUPPLIED
Tablets: 5 mg, 10 mg
Tablets (long-acting): 5 mg, 10 mg, 15 mg**

ACTION
Mechanism: Promotes nerve impulse transmission by releasing stored norepinephrine from nerve terminals in the brain. Main sites of activity appears to be the cerebral cortex and the reticular activating system. In children with hyperkinesia, amphetamines have a paradoxical calming effect.
Onset: within 1 hour. **Peak:** Peak effects occur in about 4 to 6 hours.
Duration: elimination half-life, about 5 hours.

INDICATIONS & DOSAGE
Attention deficit disorder with hyperactivity –
Children 6 years and older: 2.5 to 5 mg P.O. once daily or b.i.d., with 5-mg increments weekly, p.r.n. Usual effective dosage is 20 to 25 mg daily.
Short-term adjunct in exogenous obesity –
Adults: 2.5 to 5 mg P.O. once daily to t.i.d., 30 minutes before meals; or 1 long-acting 5- to 15-mg tablet daily before breakfast.

ADVERSE REACTIONS
CNS: *nervousness, insomnia,* irritability, *talkativeness,* dizziness, headache, hyperexcitability, tremor.
CV: hypertension, hypotension, *tachycardia, palpitations,* arrhythmias.
EENT: blurred vision, mydriasis.
GI: dry mouth, metallic taste, nausea, vomiting, abdominal cramps, diarrhea, constipation, anorexia.
GU: impotence.
Skin: urticaria.
Other: altered libido.

INTERACTIONS
Ammonium chloride, ascorbic acid: decreased serum levels and increased renal excretion of methamphetamine. Monitor for decreased amphetamine effects.
Antacids, sodium bicarbonate, acetazolamide: increased renal reabsorption. Monitor for enhanced effects.
Caffeine: may increase amphetamine and related amine effects. Avoid concomitant use.
Insulin, oral antidiabetic agents: may decrease antidiabetic agent requirements. Monitor blood glucose levels.
MAO inhibitors: severe hypertension; possible hypertensive crisis. Don't use together or within 14 days after MAO inhibitor has been discontinued.
Phenothiazines, haloperidol, tricyclic antidepressants: increased CNS effects. Avoid concomitant use.

CONTRAINDICATIONS
- Contraindicated in patients with hypertension, hyperthyroidism, nephritis, angina pectoris or other severe CV disease, glaucoma, parkinsonism due to arteriosclerosis, or history of drug abuse, or in agitated patients.
- Use cautiously in patients with diabetes mellitus; in patients who are elderly, debilitated, asthenic, psychopathic, or who have a history of suicidal or homicidal tendencies; and in children with Tourette syndrome.

NURSING CONSIDERATIONS
- Habituation and psychic and physical dependence may occur, especially in patients with history of drug addiction. Avoid prolonged administration. When used long-term, lower dosage gradually to prevent rebound hypertension.
- Warn the patient of high potential for abuse. Do not use to prevent fatigue.
- If tolerance to anorexigenic effect develops, discontinue drug.

• Not recommended for first-line treatment of obesity. Use as an anorexigenic agent is prohibited in some states.
• When used for obesity, be sure patient is on a weight-reduction program.
• May alter insulin needs in patients with diabetes. Monitor blood and urine sugars.
• Urine acidification enhances renal excretion of the drug; urine alkalinization enhances renal reabsorption and recycling.
• Tell the patient to avoid drinks containing caffeine, which increase the effects of amphetamines and related amines.
• Have the patient report signs of excessive stimulation.
• Warn the patient to avoid activities that require alertness or good psychomotor coordination until CNS effects of the drug are known.
• Give at least 6 hours before bedtime to avoid sleep interference.
• Never crush sustained-release tablets.

methylphenidate hydrochloride

PMS-Methylphenidate‡, Ritalin, Ritalin-SR

Controlled Substance Schedule II

Pregnancy Risk Category: C

HOW SUPPLIED

Tablets: 5 mg, 10 mg, 20 mg
Tablets (sustained-release): 20 mg

ACTION

Mechanism: Promotes nerve impulse transmission by releasing stored norepinephrine from nerve terminals in the brain. Main sites of activity appears to be the cerebral cortex and the reticular activating system. In children with hyperkinesia, amphetamines have a paradoxical calming effect.

Peak: Peak levels occur about 2 hours after regular-release tablets, 4 or 5 hours after sustained-release tablets.
Duration: effects persist 6 to 8 hours after sustained-release tablets.

INDICATIONS & DOSAGE

Attention deficit disorder with hyperactivity (ADDH) –
Children 6 years and older: initial dose, 5 to 10 mg P.O. daily before breakfast and lunch, with 5- to 10-mg increments weekly p.r.n., up to 60 mg daily.
Narcolepsy –
Adults: 10 mg P.O. b.i.d. or t.i.d. ½ hour before meals. Dosage varies with patient needs, ranging from 5 to 50 mg daily.

ADVERSE REACTIONS

CNS: *nervousness, insomnia,* Tourette syndrome, dizziness, headache, akathisia, dyskinesia, ***seizures.***
CV: *palpitations,* angina, *tachycardia,* changes in blood pressure and pulse rate.
EENT: dry throat.
GI: nausea, abdominal pain, anorexia, weight loss.
Hematologic: thrombocytopenia, thrombocytopenic purpura.
Skin: rash, urticaria, ***exfoliative dermatitis, erythema multiforme.***
Other: growth suppression.

INTERACTIONS

Caffeine: may increase amphetamine and related amine effects. Avoid concomitant use.
Centrally acting antihypertensives: decreased antihypertensive effect. Monitor blood pressure.
MAO inhibitors: severe hypertension; possible hypertensive crisis. Don't use together or within 14 days after an MAO inhibitor has been discontinued.
Tricyclic antidepressants: increased plasma levels of these drugs. Avoid concomitant use.

CONTRAINDICATIONS

- Contraindicated in patients with symptomatic cardiac disease, hyperthyroidism, moderate to severe hypertension, angina pectoris, advanced arteriosclerosis, severe endogenous or exogenous depression, glaucoma, parkinsonism, history of drug abuse or dependency, or history of marked anxiety, tension, or agitation.
- Use cautiously in elderly, debilitated, or hyperexcitable patients, and those with history of CV disease, diabetes, or seizures.

NURSING CONSIDERATIONS

- May precipitate Tourette syndrome in children. Monitor especially at start of therapy.
- Observe for signs of excessive stimulation. Monitor blood pressure.
- Periodic CBC, differential, and platelet counts advised with long-term use.
- Monitor height and weight in children on prolonged therapy. May delay "growth spurt," but children will attain normal height when drug is discontinued.
- Monitor blood and urine sugars.
- May decrease seizure threshold in patients with seizure disorders. Advise patients to notify doctor if seizure occurs.
- Drug of choice for ADDH. Usually discontinued after puberty.
- Tolerance or psychic dependence may develop, especially in patients with history of drug addiction. Avoid long-term use because of high abuse potential. After long-term use, lower dosage gradually to prevent acute rebound depression.
- Do not be use to prevent fatigue.
- Fatigue may result as drug effects wear off. The patient will need more rest.
- Tell the patient to avoid drinks containing caffeine, which increase the effects of amphetamines and related amines.
- Warn the patient to avoid activities that require alertness or good psychomotor coordination until CNS effects of the drug are known.
- Warn the patient against chewing sustained-release tablets.
- Give at least 6 hours before bedtime to prevent insomnia. Administer after meals to reduce appetite-suppressive effects.

pemoline

Cylert, Cylert Chewable
Controlled Substance Schedule IV

Pregnancy Risk Category: B

HOW SUPPLIED

Tablets: 18.75 mg, 37.5 mg, 75 mg
Tablets (chewable): 37.5 mg

ACTION

Mechanism: Promotes nerve impulse transmission by releasing stored norepinephrine from nerve terminals in the brain. Main sites of activity appears to be the cerebral cortex and the reticular activating system.
Peak: Serum levels peak 2 to 4 hours after dose. Steady-state levels occur within 2 to 3 days. Peak therapeutic effect occurs after 3 to 4 weeks.
Duration: elimination half-life, 12 hours.

INDICATIONS & DOSAGE

Attention deficit disorder with hyperactivity –
Children 6 years and older: initially, 37.5 mg P.O. in the morning. Daily dosage can be raised by 18.75 mg weekly. Effective dosage range is 56.25 to 75 mg daily; maximum dosage is 112.5 mg daily.

ADVERSE REACTIONS

CNS: *insomnia,* malaise, dyskinetic movements, irritability, fatigue, mild depression, dizziness, headache, drowsiness, hallucinations, nervous-

ness (large doses), ***seizures,*** *Tourette syndrome,* psychosis.
CV: *tachycardia* (large doses).
GI: anorexia, abdominal pain, nausea, diarrhea.
Hepatic: elevated liver enzymes.
Skin: rash.

INTERACTIONS
Insulin, oral antidiabetic agents: may decrease antidiabetic agent requirements. Monitor blood glucose levels.

CONTRAINDICATIONS
- Contraindicated in patients with hepatic dysfunction and in children under 6 years.
- Use cautiously in patients with impaired renal function or history of Tourette syndrome. Drug may accumulate.

NURSING CONSIDERATIONS
- May precipitate Tourette syndrome in children. Monitor especially at start of therapy.
- Closely monitor patients on long-term therapy for possible blood or hepatic function abnormalities and for growth suppression.
- Structurally dissimilar to amphetamines or methylphenidate. However, may produce similar adverse reactions, including lowered seizure threshold. Has greater potential for abuse and dependence than previously thought.
- To avoid sleep interference, give at least 6 hours before bedtime.

phendimetrazine tartrate

Adipost, Anorex, Appecon, Bontril PDM, Bontril Slow Release, Dyrexan OD, Malibar A, Melfiat 105 Unicelles, Metra, Neocurb, Obalan, Obe-Del, Obezine, Panrexin M, Panrexin MTP, Parzine, Phendiet, Phendiet-105, Phendimet, Phentra, Phenzine, Prelu-2, PT-105, Rexigen, Rexigen Forte, Tega-Nil, Trimcaps, Trimstat, Wehless, Weightrol, Wescoid, X-Trozine, X-Trozine LA

Controlled Substance Schedule IV
Pregnancy Risk Category: C

HOW SUPPLIED
Tablets: 35 mg
Capsules: 35 mg
Capsules (sustained-release): 105 mg

ACTION
Mechanism: Promotes nerve impulse transmission by releasing stored norepinephrine from nerve terminals in the brain. Main sites of activity appears to be the cerebral cortex and the reticular activating system.
Duration: elimination half-life, 5 to 12½ hours; effects persist about 4 hours.

INDICATIONS & DOSAGE
Short-term adjunct in exogenous obesity –
Adults: 35 mg P.O. b.i.d. to t.i.d., 1 hour before meals. Maximum dosage is 70 mg t.i.d. Use lowest effective dosage and adjust to individual response.

ADVERSE REACTIONS
CNS: *nervousness,* dizziness, *insomnia,* tremor, headache.
CV: *tachycardia, palpitations,* elevated blood pressure.
EENT: blurred vision.
GI: dry mouth, nausea, abdominal cramps, diarrhea, constipation.
GU: dysuria.

INTERACTIONS
Ammonium chloride, ascorbic acid: decreased serum levels and increased renal excretion of phendimetrazine. Monitor for decreased phendimetrazine effects.
Antacids, sodium bicarbonate, acetazolamide: increased renal reabsorption. Monitor for enhanced effects.
Caffeine: may increase CNS stimulation. Avoid concomitant use.
MAO inhibitors: severe hypertension; possible hypertensive crisis. Don't use together or within 14 days after MAO inhibitor has been discontinued.
Phenothiazines, haloperidol, tricyclic antidepressants: increased CNS effect. Avoid concomitant use.

CONTRAINDICATIONS
- Contraindicated in patients with hyperthyroidism, hypertension, angina pectoris or other severe CV disease, or glaucoma.
- Use cautiously in patients with diabetes mellitus and in patients in hyperexcitability states or with history of drug addiction.

NURSING CONSIDERATIONS
- Warn the patient to avoid activities that require alertness or good psychomotor coordination until CNS effects of the drug are known.
- Make sure the patient is also on a weight-reduction program.
- Habituation and tolerance can develop. Not advised for prolonged use.
- Fatigue may result as drug effects wear off. The patient will need more rest.
- Tell the patient to avoid drinks containing caffeine, which increase the effects of amphetamines and related amines.
- Tell the patient to report signs of excessive stimulation.
- Urine acidification enhances renal excretion of the drug; urine alkalinization enhances renal reabsorption and recycling.
- Give at least 6 hours before bedtime to avoid sleep interference.

phentermine hydrochloride
Adipex-P, Duromine‡, Fastin, Obe-Mar, Obe-Nix, Obephen, Oby-Trim, Panshape, Phentercot, Phentride, Phentride Caplets, Phentrol, Phentrol-2, Phentrol-4, Phentrol-5, T-Diet
Teramin, Wilpowr, Zantryl
Controlled Substance Schedule IV
Pregnancy Risk Category: C

HOW SUPPLIED
Tablets: 8 mg, 15 mg, 18.75 mg, 30 mg, 37.5 mg
Capsules: 8 mg, 15 mg, 18.75 mg, 30 mg, 37.5 mg
Capsules (resin complex, sustained-release): 15 mg, 30 mg

ACTION
Mechanism: Promotes nerve impulse transmission by releasing stored norepinephrine from nerve terminals in the brain. Main sites of activity appears to be the cerebral cortex and the reticular activating system.
Duration: effects persist 4 hours for capsules and tablets; 12 to 14 hours for sustained-release resin complex.

INDICATIONS & DOSAGE
Short-term adjunct in exogenous obesity –
Adults: 8 mg P.O. t.i.d. ½ hour before meals; or 15 to 30 mg daily before breakfast (resin complex).

ADVERSE REACTIONS
CNS: *nervousness,* dizziness, *insomnia.*
CV: *palpitations, tachycardia,* increased blood pressure.
GI: dry mouth, dysgeusia, nausea, constipation, diarrhea.
GU: impotence.

Skin: urticaria.
Other: altered libido.

INTERACTIONS

Ammonium chloride, ascorbic acid: decreased plasma levels and increased renal excretion of phentermine. Monitor for decreased phentermine effects.
Antacids, sodium bicarbonate, acetazolamide: increased renal reabsorption. Monitor for enhanced effects.
Caffeine: may increase CNS stimulation.
Insulin, oral antidiabetic agents: may decrease antidiabetic agent requirements. Monitor blood glucose levels.
MAO inhibitors: severe hypertension; possible hypertensive crisis. Don't use together or within 14 days aftern MAO inhibitor has been discontinued.
Phenothiazines, haloperidol, tricyclic antidepressants: increased CNS effects. Avoid concomitant use.

CONTRAINDICATIONS

- Contraindicated in patients with hyperthyroidism, hypertension, angina pectoris or other severe CV disease, or glaucoma.
- Use cautiously in patients in hyperexcitability states or with history of drug addiction.

NURSING CONSIDERATIONS

- Tolerance or dependence may develop. Avoid prolonged administration.
- Use in conjunction with a weight-reduction program. Give 30 minutes before meals.
- Fatigue may result as drug effects wear off. The patient will need more rest.
- Tell the patient to avoid drinks containing caffeine, which increase the effects of amphetamines and related amines.
- Tell the patient to report signs of excessive stimulation.
- Urine acidification enhances renal excretion of the drug; urine alkalinization enhances renal reabsorption and recycling.
- Give at least 6 hours before bedtime to avoid sleep interference.

*Liquid form contains alcohol.
**May contain tartrazine.

Common reactions are in italics; ***life-threatening,*** in bold italics.

34
Antiparkinsonian agents

amantadine hydrochloride
(See Chapter 17, ANTIVIRALS.)
benztropine mesylate
biperiden hydrochloride
biperiden lactate
bromocriptine mesylate
carbidopa-levodopa
levodopa
pergolide mesylate
procyclidine hydrochloride
selegiline hydrochloride
trihexyphenidyl hydrochloride

COMBINATION PRODUCTS
MADOPAR‡: levodopa 200 mg and benserazine 50 mg.
MADOPAR HBS‡: levodopa 100 mg and benserazine 25 mg.
MADOPAR Q‡: levodopa 50 mg and benserazine 12.5 mg.
SINEMET 10/100: carbidopa 10 mg and levodopa 100 mg.
SINEMET 25/100: carbidopa 25 mg and levodopa 100 mg.
SINEMET 25/250: carbidopa 25 mg and levodopa 250 mg.
SINEMET CR: carbidopa 50 mg and levodopa 200 mg, in extended-release tablets.

benztropine mesylate
Apo-Benztropine†, Bensylate†, Cogentin, PMS Benztropine†

Pregnancy Risk Category: C

HOW SUPPLIED
Tablets: 0.5 mg, 1 mg, 2 mg
Injection: 1 mg/ml in 2-ml ampules

ACTION
Mechanism: Blocks central cholinergic receptors, helping to balance cholinergic activity in the basal ganglia.
Onset: within 15 minutes of parenteral use, or within 1 to 2 hours of oral use. **Peak:** full effect, 2 to 3 days.
Duration: effects persist 24 hours.

INDICATIONS & DOSAGE
Acute dystonic reaction –
Adults: 1 to 2 mg I.V. or I.M. followed by 1 to 2 mg P.O. b.i.d. to prevent recurrence.
Parkinsonism –
Adults: 0.5 to 6 mg P.O. daily. Initial dose is 0.5 mg to 1 mg. Increase by 0.5 mg q 5 to 6 days. Adjust dosage to meet individual requirements. Usual dosage is 1 to 2 mg/day.

ADVERSE REACTIONS
CNS: disorientation, restlessness, irritability, incoherence, hallucinations, headache, sedation, depression, muscular weakness.
CV: palpitations, tachycardia, paradoxical bradycardia, flushing.
EENT: dilated pupils, blurred vision, photophobia, difficulty swallowing.
GI: dry mouth, *constipation,* nausea, vomiting, epigastric distress.
GU: urinary hesitancy, urine retention.

Some adverse reactions may be due to pending atropine-like toxicity and are dose related.

INTERACTIONS
Amantadine, phenothiazines, tricyclic antidepressants: additive anticholinergic adverse reactions, such as confusion and hallucinations. Reduce dosage before administering.

CONTRAINDICATIONS
- Contraindicated in patients with acute angle-closure glaucoma.
- Use cautiously in patients with prostatic hyperplasia, tardive dyskinesia, or tendency to tachycardia; and in elderly or debilitated patients.

NURSING CONSIDERATIONS
- Monitor vital signs carefully. Watch closely for adverse reactions, especially in elderly or debilitated patients. Call the doctor promptly.
- Produces atropine-like adverse reactions and may aggravate tardive dyskinesia.
- Never discontinue this drug abruptly. Dosage must be reduced gradually.
- **I.V. use:** Rarely used because of small difference in onset as compared to I.M. route.
- To help prevent GI distress, administer after meals.
- Warn patient to avoid activities that require alertness until CNS effects of the drug are known. If the patient is to receive single daily dose, give h.s.
- Advise patient to report signs of urinary hesitancy or urine retention.
- Watch for intermittent constipation, distention, and abdominal pain; may be onset of paralytic ileus.
- Relieve dry mouth with cool drinks, ice chips, sugarless gum, or hard candy.
- Advise patient to limit activities during hot weather because drug-induced anhydrosis may result in hyperthermia.

biperiden hydrochloride
Akineton

biperiden lactate
Akineton Lactate

Pregnancy Risk Category: C

HOW SUPPLIED
hydrochloride
Tablets: 2 mg
lactate
Injection: 5 mg/ml in 1-ml ampules

ACTION
Mechanism: Blocks central cholinergic receptors, helping to balance cholinergic activity in the basal ganglia.
Onset: within 15 minutes of parenteral use, within 1 hour of oral use.
Duration: effects persist 1 to 8 hours after I.V. use, 6 to 12 hours after oral use.

INDICATIONS & DOSAGE
Extrapyramidal disorders –
Adults: 2 to 6 mg P.O. daily, b.i.d., or t.i.d., depending on severity. Usual dose is 2 mg daily, or 2 mg I.M. or I.V. q ½ hour, not to exceed four doses or 8 mg total daily.
Parkinsonism –
Adults: 2 mg P.O. t.i.d. to q.i.d. Some patients may require as much as 16 mg per day.

ADVERSE REACTIONS
CNS: disorientation, euphoria, restlessness, irritability, incoherence, dizziness, increased tremor.
CV: transient postural hypotension (with parenteral use).
EENT: blurred vision.
GI: dry mouth, *constipation,* nausea, vomiting, epigastric distress.
GU: urinary hesitancy, urine retention.
Skin: rash, urticaria.

Adverse reactions are dose-related and may resemble atropine toxicity.

INTERACTIONS
Amantadine, phenothiazines, tricyclic antidepressants: excessive CNS anticholinergic effects. Avoid concomitant use.
Antacids: decreased biperiden absorption. Administer antacids at least 1 hour after biperiden.

CONTRAINDICATIONS
- Contraindicated in patients hypersensitive to the drug.
- Use cautiously in patients with prostatism, arrhythmias, acute angle-closure glaucoma, and seizure disorder.

NURSING CONSIDERATIONS

- Monitor vital signs carefully. Watch closely for adverse reactions, especially in elderly or debilitated patients. Call the doctor promptly.
- Tolerance may develop, requiring increased dosage.
- In severe parkinsonism, tremors may increase as spasticity is relieved.
- **I.V. use:** Administer very slowly.
- When giving parenterally, keep patient in a supine position. Parenteral administration may cause transient postural hypotension and coordination disturbances.
- To decrease GI adverse effects, give oral doses with or after meals.
- Because of possible dizziness, help patient when he gets out of bed.
- Warn the patient to avoid activities that require alertness until CNS effects of the drug are known.
- Advise the patient to report signs of urinary hesitancy or urine retention.
- Relieve dry mouth with cool drinks, ice chips, sugarless gum, or hard candy.

bromocriptine mesylate

Parlodel

Pregnancy Risk Category: C

HOW SUPPLIED

Tablets: 2.5 mg
Capsules: 5 mg

ACTION

Mechanism: Inhibits secretion of prolactin and acts as a dopamine-receptor agonist by activating postsynaptic dopamine receptors.
Onset: antiparkinsonian effects, 30 to 90 minutes; effects on serum prolactin, within 2 hours. **Peak:** Antiparkinsonian effects peak in 2 hours. Peak effects on serum prolactin occur within 8 hours. **Duration:** antiparkinsonian effects, 12 to 18 hours; effects on serum prolactin, about 24 hours

INDICATIONS & DOSAGE

Amenorrhea and galactorrhea associated with hyperprolactinemia; female infertility –
Adults: 1.25 to 2.5 mg P.O. daily. Increase dosage by 2.5 mg daily at 3- to 7-day intervals until desired effect is achieved. Safety and efficacy of doses greater than 100 mg daily have not been established.
Prevention of postpartum lactation –
Adults: 2.5 mg P.O. b.i.d. with meals for 14 days. Treatment may be extended for up to 21 days, if necessary.
Parkinson's disease –
Adults: 1.25 mg P.O. b.i.d. with meals. Dosage may be increased q 14 to 28 days, up to 100 mg daily.
Acromegaly –
Adults: 1.25 to 2.5 mg P.O. for 3 days. An additional 1.25 to 2.5 mg may be added q 3 to 7 days until patient receives therapeutic benefit.

ADVERSE REACTIONS

CNS: confusion, hallucinations, uncontrolled body movements, *dizziness, headache,* fatigue, mania, delusions, nervousness, insomnia, depression, ***seizures.***
CV: *hypotension,* orthostatic hypotension, hypertension, stroke, syncope.
EENT: nasal congestion, tinnitus, blurred vision.
GI: *nausea,* vomiting, *abdominal cramps,* constipation, diarrhea.
GU: urine retention, urinary frequency.
Respiratory: ***pulmonary infiltration and pleural effusion.***
Skin: coolness and pallor of fingers and toes.

INTERACTIONS

Antihypertensives: increased hypotensive effects. Adjust dosage of the antihypertensive.
Haloperidol, loxapine, phenothiazines, methyldopa, metoclopramide,

MAO inhibitors, reserpine: interferes with bromocriptine's effects. Dosage increase of bromocriptine may be required.
Levodopa: additive effects. Adjust dosage of levodopa.
Oral contraceptives, estrogens, progestins: interfere with effects of bromocriptine. Concurrent use not recommended.

CONTRAINDICATIONS
- Contraindicated in patients with hypersensitivity to ergot derivatives.
- Use cautiously in patients with preexisting psychiatric disorders and impaired renal function.

NURSING CONSIDERATIONS
- Examine patients carefully for pituitary tumor (Forbes-Albright syndrome). Use of bromocriptine will not affect tumor size although it may alleviate amenorrhea or galactorrhea.
- Baseline and periodic evaluations of cardiac, liver, renal, and hematopoietic function are recommended during prolonged therapy.
- Patients with impaired renal function may require dosage adjustments.
- May lead to early postpartum conception. Test for pregnancy every 4 weeks or whenever period is missed after menses resumes.
- Advise patients to use contraceptive methods other than oral contraceptives or subdermal implants during treatment.
- Monitor blood pressure closely in patients who receive bromocriptine for suppression of postpartum lactation. In such patients, transient hypotension is common; however, hypertension, seizures, and stroke have also been reported.
- Incidence of adverse reactions is high (about 68%), particularly at beginning of therapy; however, most are mild to moderate, with nausea as the most common. Minimize adverse reactions by gradually titrating doses to effective levels. Adverse reactions are more frequent when drug is used for Parkinson's disease.
- Orthostatic hypotension is common. Advise patients to avoid dizziness and fainting by rising slowly to an upright position and avoiding sudden position changes.
- Recurrence rates when used to treat amenorrhea or galactorrhea associated with hyperprolactinemia range from 70% to 80%.
- Advise patients that it may take 6 to 8 weeks or longer for menses to resume and galactorrhea to be suppressed.
- When therapy is discontinued, patients may experience mild to moderate rebound breast secretion, congestion, or engorgement.
- Give drug with meals.
- For Parkinson's disease, bromocriptine is usually given in addition to either levodopa or carbidopa-levodopa.

carbidopa-levodopa
Sinemet, Sinemet CR

Pregnancy Risk Category: C

HOW SUPPLIED
Tablets: carbidopa 10 mg with levodopa 100 mg (Sinemet 10-100), carbidopa 25 mg with levodopa 100 mg (Sinemet 25-100), carbidopa 25 mg with levodopa 250 mg (Sinemet 25-250)
Tablets (extended-release): carbidopa 50 mg with levodopa 200 mg (Sinemet CR)

ACTION
Mechanism: Levodopa is decarboxylated to dopamine, countering the depletion of striatal dopamine in extrapyramidal centers. Carbidopa inhibits the peripheral decarboxylation of levodopa without affecting levodopa's metabolism within the CNS. Therefore, more levodopa is available

to be decarboxylated to dopamine in the brain.
Peak: Peak serum levels occur in about 40 minutes for regular-release tablets, or 2½ hours for extended-release tablets. **Duration:** half-life of carbidopa, about 2 hours; of levodopa (when taken with carbidopa), 2 to 15 hours.

INDICATIONS & DOSAGE
Idiopathic Parkinson's disease, postencephalitic parkinsonism, and symptomatic parkinsonism resulting from carbon monoxide or manganese intoxication –
Adults: 3 to 6 tablets of 25 mg carbidopa/100 mg levodopa daily in divided doses. Increase dosage by 1 tablet every day or every other day as necessary. Substitute 25 mg carbidopa/250 mg levodopa or 10 mg carbidopa/100 mg levodopa tablets as required to obtain maximum response. Do not exceed 8 tablets of 25 mg carbidopa/250 mg levodopa daily. Optimum daily dosage must be determined by careful titration for each patient.

Patients treated with conventional tablets may receive extended-release tablets; dosage is calculated on current levodopa intake. Initially, give extended-release tablets equal to 10% more levodopa per day; increase as needed and tolerated to 30% more levodopa per day. Administer in divided doses at intervals of 4 to 8 hours.

ADVERSE REACTIONS
CNS: *choreiform, dystonic, dyskinetic movements; involuntary grimacing, head movements, myoclonic body jerks, ataxia,* tremors, muscle twitching; bradykinetic episodes; psychiatric disturbances, memory loss, nervousness, anxiety, disturbing dreams, euphoria, malaise, fatigue; severe depression, suicidal tendencies, dementia, delirium, hallucinations (may necessitate reduction or withdrawal of drug).
CV: *orthostatic hypotension,* ***cardiac irregularities,*** flushing, hypertension, phlebitis.
EENT: blepharospasm, blurred vision, diplopia, mydriasis or miosis, widening of palpebral fissures, activation of latent Horner's syndrome, oculogyric crises, nasal discharge, sialorrhea.
GI: *dry mouth,* bitter taste, *nausea, vomiting, anorexia,* weight loss may occur at start of therapy; constipation; flatulence; diarrhea; *epigastric pain. bleeding* (rare).
GU: urinary frequency, urine retention, urinary incontinence, darkened urine, excessive and inappropriate sexual behavior, priapism.
Hematologic: ***hemolytic anemia.***
Hepatic: hepatotoxicity.
Other: dark perspiration, hyperventilation, hiccups.

INTERACTIONS
Antihypertensives: additive hypotensive effects. Use together cautiously.
MAO inhibitors: risk of severe hypertension. Avoid concomitant use.
Papaverine, phenytoin: antagonism of antiparkinsonian actions. Don't use together.
Phenothiazines and other antipsychotics: may antagonize antiparkinsonian actions. Use together cautiously.

CONTRAINDICATIONS
- Contraindicated in patients with acute angle-closure glaucoma, melanoma, or undiagnosed skin lesions.
- Use cautiously in patients with cardiovascular, renal, hepatic, and pulmonary disorders; in patients with history of peptic ulceration, psychiatric illness, MI with residual arrhythmias, bronchial asthma, emphysema, and endocrine disease.

NURSING CONSIDERATIONS

• If the patient is being treated with levodopa, discontinue at least 8 hours before starting carbidopa-levodopa.

• Carefully monitor patients also receiving antihypertensives. Discontinue MAO inhibitors at least 2 weeks before therapy is begun.

• Adjust dosage according to patient's response and tolerance to drug. Therapeutic and adverse reactions occur more rapidly with carbidopa-levodopa than with levodopa alone. Observe and monitor vital signs, especially while adjusting dosage. Report significant changes.

• At least 70 mg of the carbidopa component should be given daily to effectively block peripheral dopa decarboxylase.

• Carbidopa (Lodosyn) as a single agent is available from Merck Sharp & Dohme at the doctor's request.

• Assess the patient for signs and symptoms of GI intolerance. To minimize GI upset, tell patient to take the drug with food.

• Pyridoxine (vitamin B_6) does not reverse the beneficial effects of carbidopa-levodopa. Multivitamins can be taken without losing control of symptoms.

• Warn the patient of possible dizziness and orthostatic hypotension, especially at start of therapy. Tell the patient to change position slowly and dangle legs before getting out of bed. Elastic stockings may control this adverse reaction in some patients.

• Muscle twitching and blepharospasm (twitching of eyelids) may be early signs of drug overdosage; report immediately.

• Patients receiving long-term therapy should be tested regularly for diabetes and acromegaly and should have periodic tests of liver, renal, and hematopoietic function.

• If therapy is interrupted temporarily, give the usual daily dosage as soon as patient resumes oral medication.

• Carbidopa-levodopa typically decreases amount of levodopa needed by 75%, reducing the incidence of adverse reactions.

• Instruct the patient to report adverse reactions and therapeutic effects.

• Warn the patient and his family not to increase dosage without doctor's orders.

• Depending on reagent and test method used, expect possible false-positive increases in levels of uric acid, urine ketones, catecholamines, and vanillylmandelic acid.

• False-positive tests for urine glucose can occur if reagents using copper sulfate are used; false-negative results can occur with tests that use glucose enzymatic methods. An accurate measure can be obtained if the paper strip is only partially immersed in the urine sample. Urine will migrate up the strip, as with an ascending chromatographic system. Read only the top of the strip.

levodopa

Dopar, Larodopa

Pregnancy Risk Category: C

HOW SUPPLIED

Tablets: 100 mg, 250 mg, 500 mg
Capsules: 100 mg, 250 mg, 500 mg

ACTION

Mechanism: Levodopa is decarboxylated to dopamine, countering the depletion of striatal dopamine in extrapyramidal centers, which is thought to produce parkinsonism.
Onset: maximal effects, 3 weeks to 6 months. **Peak:** Plasma levels peak in ½ to 2 hours. **Duration:** varies, usually 5 hours.

INDICATIONS & DOSAGE
Idiopathic parkinsonism, postencephalitic parkinsonism, and symptomatic parkinsonism after carbon monoxide or manganese intoxication or in association with cerebral arteriosclerosis –
Adults and children over 12 years: initially, 0.5 to 1 g P.O. daily, b.i.d., t.i.d., or q.i.d. with food; increase by no more than 0.75 g daily q 3 to 7 days, until usual maximum of 8 g is reached. Carefully adjust dosage to individual requirements, tolerance, and response. Higher dosage requires close supervision.

ADVERSE REACTIONS
CNS: *aggressive behavior; choreiform, dystonic, and dyskinetic movements; involuntary grimacing, head movements, myoclonic body jerks, ataxia, tremors, muscle twitching, bradykinetic episode, psychiatric disturbances, memory loss, mood changes, nervousness, anxiety, disturbing dreams, euphoria, malaise, fatigue, severe depression, suicidal tendencies, dementia, delirium, hallucinations* (may necessitate reduction or withdrawal of drug).
CV: *orthostatic hypotension,* cardiac irregularities, flushing, hypertension, phlebitis.
EENT: blepharospasm, blurred vision, diplopia, mydriasis or miosis, widening of palpebral fissures, activation of latent Horner's syndrome, oculogyric crises, nasal discharge, sialorrhea.
GI: dry mouth, bitter taste, *nausea, vomiting, anorexia,* weight loss may occur at start of therapy, constipation, flatulence, diarrhea, epigastric pain.
GU: urinary frequency, urine retention, incontinence, darkened urine, excessive and inappropriate sexual behavior, priapism.
Hematologic: ***hemolytic anemia,*** leukopenia.
Hepatic: hepatotoxicity.
Other: dark perspiration, hyperventilation, hiccups.

INTERACTIONS
Antacids: increased absorption of levodopa. Administer antacids 1 hour after levodopa.
Cocaine, sympathomimetics, inhalational halogenated anesthetics: increased risk of arrhythmias. Monitor the patient closely.
MAO inhibitors, furazolidone, procarbazine: risk of severe hypertension. Avoid concomitant use.
Metoclopramide: accelerated gastric emptying of levodopa. Give metoclopramide 1 hour after levodopa.
Papaverine, phenothiazines and other antipsychotics, phenytoin, rauwolfia alkaloids: decreased levodopa effect.
Pyridoxine: reversal of antiparkinsonian effects. Check vitamin preparations and nutritional supplements for pyridoxine (vitamin B_6) content. Don't give together.
Foods high in protein: decreased absorption of levodopa. Don't give levodopa with high-protein foods.

CONTRAINDICATIONS
- Contraindicated in patients with acute angle-closure glaucoma, melanoma, or undiagnosed skin lesions.
- Use cautiously in patients with cardiovascular, renal, liver, and pulmonary disorders; peptic ulceration; psychiatric illness; MI with residual arrhythmias; bronchial asthma; emphysema; and endocrine disease.

NURSING CONSIDERATIONS
- Observe and monitor vital signs, especially while adjusting dosage. Report significant changes.
- Assess the patient for signs and symptoms of GI intolerance. To minimize GI upset, tell the patient to take the drug with food. However, taking the drug with high-protein meals can impair absorption and reduce effectiveness.

- For patients who have difficult swallowing pills, crush tablets and mix with applesauce or baby food fruits.
- Advise the patient and his family that multivitamin preparations, fortified cereals, and certain OTC medications may contain pyridoxine (vitamin B_6), which can block the effects of levodopa by enhancing its peripheral metabolism.
- Warn the patient of possible dizziness and orthostatic hypotension, especially at start of therapy. Tell the patient to change position slowly and dangle legs before getting out of bed. Elastic stockings may control this adverse reaction in some patients.
- Muscle twitching and blepharospasm (twitching of eyelids) may be early signs of drug overdosage; report immediately.
- Patients receiving long-term therapy should be tested regularly for diabetes and acromegaly; periodically monitor renal, liver, and hematopoietic function.
- If therapy is interrupted for a long time, adjust drug gradually to previous level.
- Patients who must undergo surgery should continue levodopa as long as oral intake is permitted, generally 6 to 24 hours before surgery. Drug should be resumed as soon as patient is able to take oral medication.
- Protect from heat, light, and moisture. If preparation darkens, it has lost potency and should be discarded.
- A doctor-supervised period of drug discontinuance (called a drug holiday) may reestablish the effectiveness of a lower dosage regimen.
- Carbidopa-levodopa typically decreases amount of levodopa needed by 75%, reducing the incidence of adverse reactions.
- Warn the patient and his family not to increase dosage without the doctor's orders. Daily dosage should not exceed 8 g.
- Coombs' test occasionally becomes positive during extended use. Expect uric acid elevations with colorimetric method but not with uricase method.
- Alkaline phosphatase, AST, ALT, lactate dehydrogenase, bilirubin, BUN, and protein-bound iodine show transient elevations in patients receiving levodopa; WBC, hemoglobin, and hematocrit show occasional reduction.
- Depending on reagent and test method used, expect possible false-positive increases in levels of uric acid, urine ketones, catecholamines, and vanillylmandelic acid, depending on reagent and test method used.
- False-positive tests for urine glucose can occur if reagents using copper sulfate are used; false-negative results can occur with tests that use glucose enzymatic methods. An accurate measure can be obtained if the paper strip is only partially immersed in the urine sample. Urine will migrate up the strip, as with an ascending chromatographic system. Read only the top of the strip.

pergolide mesylate

Permax

Pregnancy Risk Category: B

HOW SUPPLIED

Tablets: 0.05 mg, 0.25 mg, 1 mg

ACTION

Mechanism: A dopamine agonist that directly stimulates dopamine receptors in the nigrostriatal system.

INDICATIONS & DOSAGE

Adjunctive treatment to carbidopa-levodopa in the management of the symptoms associated with Parkinson's disease –

Adults: initially, 0.05 mg P.O. daily for the first 2 days. Gradually increase dosage by 0.1 to 0.15 mg every third day over the next 12 days of therapy.

Subsequent dosage can be increased by 0.25 mg every third day until optimum response is seen. The drug is usually administered in divided doses t.i.d. Gradual reductions in carbidopa-levodopa dosage may be made during dosage titration.

ADVERSE REACTIONS

CNS: headache, asthenia, *dyskinesia, dizziness, hallucinations,* dystonia, confusion, *somnolence,* insomnia, anxiety, depression, tremor, abnormal dreams, personality disorder, psychosis, abnormal gait, akathisia, extrapyramidal syndrome, incoordination, akinesia, hypertonia, neuralgia, speech disorder, twitching.
CV: *orthostatic hypotension,* vasodilation, palpitations, hypotension, syncope, hypertension, ***arrhythmias, MI.***
EENT: *rhinitis,* epistaxis, abnormal vision, diplopia, eye disorder.
GI: dry mouth, dysgeusia, abdominal pain, *nausea, constipation,* diarrhea, dyspepsia, anorexia, vomiting.
GU: urinary frequency, urinary tract infection, hematuria.
Skin: rash, diaphoresis, paresthesia.
Other: flulike syndrome, accident or injury; chest, neck, and back pain; chills; infection; facial, peripheral, or generalized edema; weight gain; arthralgia; bursitis; myalgia.

Note: The above adverse reactions, although not always attributable to the drug, occurred in > 1% of the study population.

INTERACTIONS

Phenothiazines, butyrophenones, thioxanthenes, metoclopramide, other dopamine antagonists: may antagonize the effects of pergolide. Avoid concomitant use.

CONTRAINDICATIONS

- Contraindicated in patients hypersensitive to the drug or to ergot alkaloids.

NURSING CONSIDERATIONS

- Inform patients of potential adverse reactions, especially hallucinations and confusion (27% incidence).
- Symptomatic orthostatic or sustained hypotension may occur in some patients, especially at the start of therapy.
- Warn patients to avoid activities that could result in injury from orthostatic hypotension and syncope.

procyclidine hydrochloride

Kemadrin, PMS Procyclidine†, Procyclid†

Pregnancy Risk Category: C

HOW SUPPLIED

Tablets: 5 mg

ACTION

Mechanism: Blocks central cholinergic receptors, helping to balance cholinergic activity in the basal ganglia.
Onset: within 1 hour. **Peak:** Peak effects occur in 1 to 3 hours. **Duration:** effects persist about 4 hours.

INDICATIONS & DOSAGE

Parkinsonism, muscle rigidity –
Adults: initially, 2 to 2.5 mg P.O. t.i.d., after meals. Increase gradually as needed. Usual dosage range is 20 to 30 mg/day, but some patients may require up to 60 mg daily.

Also used to relieve extrapyramidal dysfunction that accompanies treatment with phenothiazines and rauwolfia derivatives. Also controls excessive salivation from neuroleptic medications.

ADVERSE REACTIONS

CNS: light-headedness, giddiness.
EENT: blurred vision, mydriasis.
GI: *dry mouth, constipation,* nausea, vomiting, epigastric distress.
Skin: rash.
Other: muscle weakness.

INTERACTIONS
None significant.

CONTRAINDICATIONS
- Contraindicated in patients with acute angle-closure glaucoma.
- Use cautiously in patients with tachycardia, hypotension, urine retention, and prostatic hyperplasia.

NURSING CONSIDERATIONS
- Watch closely for mental confusion, disorientation, agitation, hallucinations, and psychotic symptoms, especially in elderly patients. Call the doctor promptly if these occur.
- In severe parkinsonism, tremors may increase as spasticity is relieved.
- To minimize GI distress, give after meals.
- Warn the patient to avoid activities that require alertness until CNS effects of the drug are known.
- Relieve dry mouth with cool drinks, ice chips, sugarless gum, or hard candy.

selegiline hydrochloride (L-deprenyl hydrochloride)
Eldepryl

Pregnancy Risk Category: C

HOW SUPPLIED
Tablets: 5 mg

ACTION
Mechanism: Probably acts by selectively inhibiting MAO type B (found mostly in the brain). At higher-than-recommended doses, it is a nonselective inhibitor of MAO, including MAO type A (found in the GI tract). It also may directly increase dopaminergic activity by decreasing the reuptake of dopamine into nerve cells. Its active metabolites, amphetamine and methamphetamine, may contribute to this effect.
Peak: Plasma levels peak in about 2 hours. **Duration:** elimination half-life, about 39 hours.

INDICATIONS & DOSAGE
Adjunctive treatment to carbidopa-levodopa in the management of the symptoms associated with Parkinson's disease –
Adults: 10 mg P.O. daily, taken as 5 mg at breakfast and 5 mg at lunch. After 2 or 3 days of therapy, begin gradual decrease of carbidopa-levodopa dosage.

ADVERSE REACTIONS
CNS: *dizziness,* increased tremor, chorea, loss of balance, restlessness, increased bradykinesia, facial grimace, stiff neck, dyskinesia, involuntary movements, twitching, increased apraxia, behavioral changes, tiredness, headache.
CV: orthostatic hypotension, hypertension, hypotension, ***arrhythmias,*** palpitations, new or increased anginal pain, tachycardia, peripheral edema, syncope.
EENT: blepharospasm.
GI: dry mouth, dysgeusia, *nausea,* vomiting, constipation, weight loss, anorexia or poor appetite, dysphagia, diarrhea, heartburn.
GU: slow urination, transient nocturia, prostatic hyperplasia, urinary hesitancy, urinary frequency, urine retention, sexual dysfunction.
Skin: rash, hair loss.
Other: malaise, diaphoresis.

INTERACTIONS
Adrenergic agents: possible increased pressor response, particularly in patients who have taken an overdose of selegiline. Use together cautiously.
Foods high in tyramine: possible hypertensive crisis. Monitor blood pressure.

CONTRAINDICATIONS
- Contraindicated in patients with hypersensitivity to the drug.

NURSING CONSIDERATIONS

- Warn patients to move cautiously at the start of therapy because they may experience dizziness.
- Some patients experience increased adverse reactions associated with levodopa and require a 10% to 30% reduction of carbidopa-levodopa dosage.
- Inform patients about possibile interaction with tyramine-containing foods. They should immediately report any symptoms of hypertension, including severe headache. However, at the recommended dosage, the drug does not interact with tyramine. No dietary restrictions are necessary.
- Advise patients not to take more than 10 mg daily, because a greater amount will not improve efficacy and it may increase adverse reactions.

trihexyphenidyl hydrochloride

Aparkane†, Apo-Trihex†, Artane*, Artane Sequels, Novohexidyl†, Trihexane, Trihexy-2, Trihexy-5

Pregnancy Risk Category: C

HOW SUPPLIED

Tablets: 2 mg, 5 mg
Capsules (sustained-release): 5 mg
Elixir: 2 mg/5 ml

ACTION

Mechanism: Blocks central cholinergic receptors, helping to balance cholinergic activity in the basal ganglia.
Onset: within 1 hour. **Duration:** effects persist 6 to 12 hours.

INDICATIONS & DOSAGE

Drug-induced parkinsonism –
Adults: 1 mg P.O. first day, 2 mg second day; then increase by 2 mg q 3 to 5 days until total of 6 to 10 mg is given daily. Usually given t.i.d. with meals and p.r.n., q.i.d. (last dose before bedtime) or switch to extended-release form b.i.d. Postencephalitic parkinsonism may require total daily dosage of 12 to 15 mg.

ADVERSE REACTIONS

CNS: nervousness, dizziness, headache, restlessness, hallucinations, euphoria, amnesia.
CV: tachycardia.
EENT: blurred vision, mydriasis, increased intraocular pressure (IOP).
GI: *dry mouth,* constipation, *nausea.*
GU: urinary hesitancy, urine retention.

INTERACTIONS

Amantadine: additive anticholinergic adverse reactions, such as confusion and hallucinations. Reduce dosage of trihexyphenidyl before administering.

CONTRAINDICATIONS

- Contraindicated in patients hypersensitive to the drug.
- Use cautiously in patients with acute angle-closure glaucoma; cardiac, hepatic, or renal disorders; hypertension; obstructive disease of the GI and GU tracts; possible prostatic hyperplasia; those with arteriosclerosis or history of drug hypersensitivities; and patients over 60 years.

NURSING CONSIDERATIONS

- Dosage may need to be gradually increased in patients who develop a tolerance to the drug.
- Gonioscopic evaluation and monitoring of IOP are needed, especially in patients over 40 years.
- Adverse reactions are dose-related and usually transient.
- Advise the patient to report signs of urinary hesitancy or urine retention.
- May cause nausea if given before meals.
- Tell patient to avoid activities that require alertness until CNS effects of the drug are known.
- Relieve dry mouth with cool drinks, ice chips, sugarless gum, or hard candy.

35

Miscellaneous CNS agents

disulfiram
lithium carbonate
lithium citrate
nicotine polacrilex
nicotine transdermal system
sumatriptan succinate
tacrine hydrochloride

COMBINATION PRODUCTS
None.

disulfiram

Antabuse, Cronetal, Ro-Sulfiram-500

Pregnancy Risk Category: X

HOW SUPPLIED
Tablets: 250 mg, 500 mg

ACTION
Mechanism: Blocks oxidation of ethanol at the acetaldehyde stage. Excess acetaldehyde produces a highly unpleasant reaction in the presence of even small amounts of ethanol.
Onset: 1 to 2 hours. **Duration:** effects persist 14 days after drug discontinuation.

INDICATIONS & DOSAGE
Adjunct in management of chronic alcoholism –
Adults: 500 mg P.O. as a single dose in the morning for 1 to 2 weeks. Can be taken in evening if drowsiness occurs. Maintenance: 125 to 500 mg P.O. daily (average dosage 250 mg) until permanent self-control is established. Treatment may continue for months or years.

ADVERSE REACTIONS
CNS: drowsiness, headache, fatigue, delirium, depression, neuritis, peripheral neuritis, polyneuritis.
EENT: optic neuritis.
GI: metallic or garlic aftertaste.
GU: impotence.
Skin: acneiform or allergic dermatitis.
Other: disulfiram reaction (precipitated by ethanol use), which may include flushing, throbbing headache, dyspnea, nausea, copious vomiting, diaphoresis, thirst, chest pain, palpitations, hyperventilation, hypotension, syncope, anxiety, weakness, blurred vision, confusion. ***In severe reactions – respiratory depression, cardiovascular collapse, arrhythmias, MI, acute CHF, seizures, unconsciousness, or death.***

INTERACTIONS
Alfentanil: prolonged duration of effect. Closely monitor patient.
Anticoagulants: increased anticoagulant effect. Adjust dosage of anticoagulant.
Bacampicillin: lowered concentrations of ethanol and acetaldehyde.
CNS depressants: increased CNS depression. Use together cautiously.
Ethanol: precipitated disulfiram reaction. Do not use concomitantly.
Isoniazid: ataxia or marked change in behavior. Do not use concomitantly.
Metronidazole: psychotic reaction. Do not use concomitantly.
Midazolam: increased plasma levels of midazolam. Use together cautiously.
Paraldehyde: toxic levels of acetaldehyde. Do not use concomitantly.
Phenytoin: increase blood levels of phenytoin. Monitor phenytoin blood levels and expect the doctor to adjust phenytoin dosages.
Tricyclic antidepressants, especially amitriptyline: transient delirium. Closely monitor the patient.

CONTRAINDICATIONS
• Contraindicated during alcohol intoxication and within 12 hours of alcohol ingestion; in patients with psychoses, myocardial disease, or coronary occlusion; in patients receiving metronidazole, paraldehyde, alcohol, or alcohol-containing preparations; and in pregnancy.
• Use cautiously in patients with diabetes mellitus, hypothyroidism, seizure disorder, cerebral damage, nephritis, hepatic cirrhosis or insufficiency, abnormal EEG, and multiple drug dependence.

NURSING CONSIDERATIONS
• Use only under close medical and nursing supervision. Never administer until the patient has abstained from alcohol for at least 12 hours. Patients should clearly understand consequences of disulfiram therapy and give permission for its use. Use drug only in patients who are cooperative, well motivated, and receiving supportive psychiatric therapy.
• Complete physical examination and laboratory studies, including CBC, SMA-12, and transaminase, should precede therapy and be repeated regularly.
• Warn patients to avoid all sources of alcohol (for example, sauces and cough syrups). Even external application of liniments, shaving lotion, and back-rub preparations may precipitate disulfiram reaction. Tell patients that alcohol reaction may occur as long as 2 weeks after single dose of disulfiram; the longer patients remain on drug, the more sensitive they will become to alcohol.
• Patients should wear a bracelet or carry a card supplied by drug manufacturer identifying them as disulfiram user. *Note:* Mild reactions may occur in sensitive patients with blood alcohol levels of 5 to 10 mg/100 ml; symptoms are fully developed at 50 mg/100 ml; unconsciousness typically occurs at 125 to 150 mg/100 ml level. Reaction may last from ½ hour to several hours, or as long as alcohol remains in blood.
• Caution patient's family that disulfiram should never be given to the patient without his knowledge; severe reaction or death could result if the patient ingested alcohol.
• Reassure patients that disulfiram-induced adverse reactions (unrelated to concomitant alcohol use), such as drowsiness, fatigue, impotence, headache, peripheral neuritis, and metallic or garlic taste, subside after about 2 weeks of therapy.

lithium carbonate
Carbolith†, Duralith†, Eskalith, Eskalith CR, Lithane**, Lithicarb‡, Lithizine†, Lithonate, Lithotabs, Priadel‡

lithium citrate
Cibalith-S*

Pregnancy Risk Category: D

HOW SUPPLIED
carbonate
Tablets: 250 mg‡, 300 mg (300 mg = 8.12 mEq lithium)
Tablets (controlled-release): 400 mg‡, 450 mg
Capsules: 150 mg, 300 mg, 600 mg
citrate
Syrup (sugarless): 300 mg/5 ml (0.3% alcohol)

ACTION
Mechanism: Alters chemical transmitters in the CNS, possibly by interfering with ionic pump mechanisms in brain cells and may compete with or replace sodium ions.
Onset: clinical effects, within 1 to 3 weeks of initiating therapy. **Peak:** Serum levels peak within 1 to 4 hours.

INDICATIONS & DOSAGE
Prevention or control of mania—
Adults: 300 to 600 mg P.O. up to q.i.d., increasing on the basis of blood levels to achieve optimal dosage. Recommended therapeutic lithium blood levels: 1 to 1.5 mEq/L for acute mania; 0.6 to 1.2 mEq/L for maintenance therapy; and 2 mEq/L as maximum.

Note: 5 ml lithium citrate (liquid) contains 8 mEq lithium, equal to 300 mg lithium carbonate.

ADVERSE REACTIONS
CNS: tremors, drowsiness, headache, confusion, restlessness, dizziness, psychomotor retardation, stupor, lethargy, ***coma,*** blackouts, epileptiform seizures, EEG changes, worsened organic brain syndrome, impaired speech, ataxia, muscle weakness, incoordination, hyperexcitability.
CV: *reversible ECG changes,* ***arrhythmias,*** hypotension, ***peripheral vascular collapse,*** allergic vasculitis.
EENT: tinnitus, impaired vision.
GI: dry mouth, metallic taste, nausea, vomiting, anorexia, diarrhea, *thirst.*
GU: *polyuria,* glycosuria, incontinence, renal toxicity with long-term use.
Hematologic: *leukocytosis of 14,000 to 18,000/mm³* (reversible).
Skin: pruritus, rash, diminished or lost sensation, drying and thinning of hair.
Other: transient hyperglycemia, goiter, hypothyroidism (lowered T_3, T_4, and protein-bound iodine, but elevated ^{131}I uptake), hyponatremia, ankle and wrist edema.

INTERACTIONS
Aminophylline, sodium bicarbonate, sodium chloride: increased lithium excretion. Avoid salt loads and monitor lithium levels.
Carbamazepine, probenecid, indomethacin, methyldopa, piroxicam: increased effect of lithium. Monitor for lithium toxicity.
Diuretics: increased reabsorption of lithium by kidneys, with possible toxic effect. Use with extreme caution, and monitor lithium and electrolyte levels (especially sodium).
Haloperidol, thioridazine: encephalopathic syndrome (lethargy, tremors, extrapyramidal symptoms). Watch for syndrome, and stop drug if it occurs.
Neuromuscular blockers: may cause prolonged paralysis or weakness. Monitor patient closely.
Thyroid hormones: may induce hypothyroidism. Don't use together.

CONTRAINDICATIONS
• Contraindicated if therapy cannot be closely monitored.
• Use cautiously with haloperidol, other antipsychotics, neuromuscular blockers, and diuretics; in elderly or debilitated patients; and in patients with thyroid disease, seizure disorder, renal or cardiovascular disease, brain damage, severe debilitation or dehydration, and sodium depletion.

NURSING CONSIDERATIONS
• Monitor baseline ECG, thyroid and renal studies, as well as electrolyte levels. Monitor lithium blood levels 8 to 12 hours after first dose, usually before morning dose, two or three times weekly first month, then weekly to monthly on maintenance.
• Determination of lithium blood concentration is crucial to the safe use of the drug. Do not use in patients who can't have regular lithium blood level checks.
• Explain to patients that lithium has a narrow therapeutic margin of safety. A blood level that is even slightly too high can be dangerous.
• With blood levels of lithium below 1.5 mEq/L, adverse reactions usually remain mild.
• Administer with plenty of water and after meals to minimize GI upset.

• Check fluid intake and output, especially when surgery is scheduled.
• Check urine for specific gravity and report level below 1.005, which may indicate diabetes insipidus.
• May alter glucose tolerance in diabetics. Monitor blood glucose closely.
• Warn patients and their families to watch for signs of toxicity (diarrhea, vomiting, drowsiness, muscular weakness, ataxia) and to expect transient nausea, polyuria, thirst, and discomfort during first few days. Patients should withhold one dose and call the doctor if toxic symptoms appear, but not stop drug abruptly.
• Weigh the patient daily; check for signs of edema or sudden weight gain.
• Adjust fluid and salt ingestion to compensate if excessive loss occurs through protracted diaphoresis or diarrhea. Under normal conditions, patients should have fluid intake of 2,500 to 3,000 ml daily and a balanced diet with adequate salt intake.
• Perform outpatient follow-up of thyroid and renal functions every 6 to 12 months. Palpate thyroid to check for enlargement.
• Warn ambulatory patients to avoid hazardous activities that require alertness and good psychomotor coordination until CNS effects of the drug are known.
• Tell patients not to switch brands of lithium or to take other prescription or OTC drugs without their doctor's guidance.
• Patients should carry medical identification card.
• Used investigationally to increase WBC count cells in patients undergoing cancer chemotherapy and to treat cluster headaches, aggression, organic brain syndrome, tardive dyskinesia, and SIADH.

nicotine polacrilex (nicotine resin complex)

Nicorette, Nicorette DS

Pregnancy Risk Category: X

HOW SUPPLIED

Chewing gum: 2 mg/square, 4 mg/square

ACTION

Mechanism: Provides nicotine, which stimulates nicotinic acetylcholine receptors in the CNS, neuromuscular junction, autonomic ganglia, and adrenal medulla.
Peak: Serum levels peak within 15 to 30 minutes after the patient begins to chew the gum. **Duration:** variable; nicotine half-life, 1 to 2 hours; cotinine (major metabolite) half-life, 15 to 20 hours.

INDICATIONS & DOSAGE

Relief of nicotine withdrawal symptoms in patients undergoing smoking cessation –
Adults: initiate therapy with 2-mg squares; highly dependant patients should start treatment with 4-mg squares. Patients should chew one piece of gum slowly and intermittently for 30 minutes whenever the urge to smoke occurs. Most patients require 9 to 12 pieces of gum daily during the first month. For patients using 4 mg squares, don't exceed 20 pieces daily. For patients using 2 mg squares, don't exceed 30 pieces daily.

ADVERSE REACTIONS

CNS: dizziness, light-headedness.
CV: atrial fibrillation.
EENT: throat soreness, jaw muscle ache (from chewing).
GI: nausea, vomiting, indigestion.
Other: hiccups.

INTERACTIONS

Beta blockers, propoxyphene, propranolol, xanthine bronchodilators:

decreased metabolism of these agents, increasing therapeutic effects. Dosage adjustments of these agents may be necessary.

CONTRAINDICATIONS

- Contraindicated in nonsmokers; in patients with recent MI, life-threatening arrhythmias, severe or worsening angina pectoris, active temporomandibular joint disease; and during pregnancy.
- Use cautiously in patients with hyperthyroidism, pheochromocytoma, or insulin-dependent diabetes.

NURSING CONSIDERATIONS

- Smokers most likely to benefit from nicotine gum are those with high "physical" nicotine dependence – those who smoke more than 15 cigarettes daily, prefer brands of cigarettes with high nicotine levels, usually inhale the smoke, smoke the first cigarette within 30 minutes of arising, find the first morning cigarette the hardest to give up, smoke most frequently during the morning, find it difficult to refrain from smoking in places where it's forbidden, or smoke even when ill and confined to bed during the day.
- Instruct patients to chew gum slowly and intermittently (chew several times, then place between cheek and gums) for about 30 minutes to promote slow and even buccal absorption of nicotine. Fast chewing tends to produce more adverse reactions.
- Successful abstainers will begin gradually withdrawing gum usage after 3 months. Use of the gum for longer than 6 months is not recommended. For gradual withdrawal, cut gum in halves or quarters and mix with other sugar-free gum.
- Emphasize the importance of withdrawing the gum gradually.
- Gum is sugar-free and usually doesn't stick to dentures.
- Be sure the patient reads and understands the patient instruction sheet included in the package.

nicotine transdermal system

Habitrol, Nicoderm, Prostep

Pregnancy Risk Category: D

HOW SUPPLIED

Transdermal system: designed to release nicotine at a fixed rate.
Habitrol – 21 mg/day, 14 mg/day, 11 mg/day
Nicoderm – 21 mg/day, 14 mg/day, 11 mg/day
Prostep – 22 mg/day, 11 mg/day

ACTION

Mechanism: Provides nicotine, which stimulates nicotinic acetylcholine receptors in the CNS, neuromuscular junction, autonomic ganglia, and adrenal medulla.
Peak: Users of Habitrol exhibit peak serum levels 5 to 6 hours after application; Nicoderm, 4 hours after application; ProStep, 9 hours after application. **Duration:** variable; nicotine half-life, 1 to 2 hours; of cotinine (the major metabolite) 15 to 20 hours.

INDICATIONS & DOSAGE

Relief of nicotine withdrawal symptoms in patients undergoing smoking cessation –
Adults: apply one transdermal patch to a nonhairy part of the upper trunk or upper outer arm. After 24 hours, removethe patch and apply a new one to a different site. Dosage varies slightly with echa produc.
Nicoderm, Habitrol – initially, apply one 21-mg/day patch daily for 6 weeks. Then, taper dosage to 14 mg/day for 2 to 4 weeks. Finally, taper dosage to 7 mg/day if necessary. Nicotine substitution and gradual withdrawal should take 8 to 12 weeks. Patients who weigh under 100 lb (45.5 kg), who have cardiovascular disease,

or who smoke less than one-half pack of cigarettes per day should start therapy with the 14-mg/day system.
Prostep – initially, apply one 22-mg/day patch daily for 4 to 8 weeks. Patients who weigh under 100 lb should start therapy with the 11-mg/day system. Those who have successfully stopped smoking during this period may discontinue the drug. If therapy was initiated with the 22-mg/day system, patient may be treated for an additional 2 to 4 weeks at the lower dosage (11 mg/day). Nicotine substitution and gradual withdrawal should take 6 to 12 weeks.

ADVERSE REACTIONS

CNS: somnolence, dizziness, *headache, insomnia.*
EENT: pharyngitis, sinusitis.
GI: abdominal pain, constipation, dyspepsia, nausea.
GU: dysmenorrhea.
Skin: *local or systemic erythema, pruritus, burning at application site,* cutaneous hypersensitivity, rash.
Other: back pain, myalgia, diaphoresis.

INTERACTIONS

Acetaminophen, caffeine, imipramine, oxazepam, pentazocine, propranolol, theophylline: may decrease induction of hepatic enzymes that help metabolize certain drugs. Dosage reductions may be necessary.
Adrenergic agonists, such as isoproterenol or phenylephrine: may decrease circulating catecholamines. Dosage increases may be necessary.
Adrenergic antagonists, such as prazosin or labetalol: may decrease circulating catecholamines. Dosage reductions may be necessary.
Insulin: may increase amount of subcutaneous insulin absorbed. Dosage reduction of insulin may be necessary.

CONTRAINDICATIONS

- Contraindicated in patients with hypersensitivity to nicotine or any component of the transdermal system.
- Use with extreme caution, and only after educational and behavioral interventions have failed, in patients with recent MI, serious arrhythmias, or worsening angina pectoris, or during pregnancy.
- Use cautiously in elderly patients and in those with renal or hepatic insufficiency, endocrine disease, peptic ulcer disease, or hypertension.

NURSING CONSIDERATIONS

- Drug therapy alone is usually not sufficient to wean patients from use of tobacco. Behavior modification therapy may provide better results.
- Because nicotine can be addictive and toxic, use cautiously in all patients. Risks of nicotine administration must be weighed against the hazards associated with patient's likelihood of continued smoking while using the transdermal system. Patients should be warned not to smoke. If they continue to smoke while using the system, they may experience serious adverse effects because peak serum nicotine levels will be substantially higher than those achieved by smoking alone.
- Patients who cannot stop cigarette smoking during the initial 4 weeks of therapy will probably not benefit from the continued use of the drug. Patients who were unsuccessful may benefit from counseling to identify factors that led to treatment failure. Encourage patient to minimize or eliminate factors contributing to treatment failure and to try again, possibly after some interval before the next attempt.
- Use of the transdermal system for more than 3 months should be discouraged. Chronic nicotine consumption by any route can be dangerous and habit-forming.
- Tell patients who experience persis-

tent or severe local skin reactions or generalized rash to immediately discontinue use of the patch and contact the doctor.

- Advise patients to apply the patch promptly because the nicotine can evaporate from the transdermal system once it is removed from its protective packaging. Patch should not be altered in any way (folded or cut) before application. Do not store in temperatures above 86° F (30° C).
- Teach patients proper disposal of the transdermal system. After removal, fold the patch in half, bringing the adhesive sides together. If the system comes in a protective pouch, place the used patch in the pouch that contained the new system. Careful disposal is necessary to prevent accidental poisoning of children or pets.
- Health care workers' exposure to nicotine within transdermal systems is probably minimal; however, avoid unnecessary contact with the system. Wash hands with water alone because soap can enhance absorption.
- Be sure the patient reads and understands the patient information that is dispensed with the drug.

sumatriptan succinate

Imitrex

Pregnancy Risk Category: C

HOW SUPPLIED

Tablets: 100 mg (base)†

Injection: 6 mg/0.5 ml (12 mg/ml) in 0.5-ml prefilled syringes and vials

ACTION

Mechanism: Selectively activates vascular serotonin (5-hydroxytryptamine, 5-HT) receptors. Stimulation of the specific receptor subtype 5-HT_1, present on cranial arteries and the dura mater, causes vasoconstriction of cerebral vessels but has minimal effects on systemic vessels, tissue perfusion, and blood pressure.

Onset: within 10 to 20 minutes after S.C. injection, or 30 minutes after oral administration. **Peak:** Serum levels peak about 12 minutes after S.C. injection, within 1½ hours after oral administration. Peak effect occurs within 1 to 2 hours after S.C. administration, within 2 to 4 hours after oral administration. **Duration:** half-life, about 2 hours.

INDICATIONS & DOSAGE

Acute migraine attacks (with or without aura) –

Adults: 6 mg S.C. May be repeated after a minimum of 1 hour. Maximum recommended dosage is two 6-mg injections daily.

Where available, give 100 mg P.O. If a beneficial response occurs, repeat dosage in 4 hours. Do not give more than 300 mg P.O. within 24 hours.

ADVERSE REACTIONS

CNS: *dizziness, vertigo,* drowsiness, headache, anxiety, malaise, fatigue, weakness, dysphagia.

CV: ***atrial fibrillation, ventricular fibrillation, ventricular tachycardia, MI, ECG changes such as ischemic ST-segment elevation*** (rare).

EENT: discomfort of throat, nasal cavity or sinus, mouth, jaw, or tongue; visual alterations.

GI: abdominal discomfort.

Skin: local reactions, flushing.

Other: *tingling; warm or hot sensation; burning sensation; heaviness, pressure or tightness;* feeling strange; tight feeling in head; cold sensation; pressure or tightness in chest; neck pain; myalgia; muscle cramps; diaphoresis.

INTERACTIONS

Ergot and ergot derivatives: prolonged vasospastic effects. Don't use these drugs and sumatriptan within 24 hours of sumatriptan.

CONTRAINDICATIONS
- Contraindicated in patients with hypersensitivity to the drug; in patients with hypertension or with ischemic heart disease, such as angina pectoris, Prinzmetal's angina, history of MI, or documented silent ischemia; in patients with hemiplegic or basilar migraine; and in patients taking ergotamine.
- Use cautiously in patients who are pregnant or intend to become pregnant.
- Use cautiously in patients who may have unrecognized coronary artery disease (CAD), such as postmenopausal women; male patients over age 40; or patients with risk factors such as hypertension, hypercholesterolemia, obesity, diabetes, smoking, or family history of CAD.

NURSING CONSIDERATIONS
- Serious adverse cardiac effects can follow S.C. administration of this drug, but such events are rare. When giving the drug to patients at risk for unrecognized CAD, consider administering the first dose in the doctor's office.
- After S.C. injection, most patients experience relief within 1 to 2 hours.
- Redness or pain at the injection site should subside within 1 hour after the injection.
- Studies haven't confirmed benefit from second S.C. dose received after minimum of 1 hour.
- Be sure patients understand that drug is intended only to treat a migraine attack, not to prevent or reduce the number of attacks.
- Tell patients drug may be given at any time during a migraine attack, but preferable as soon as symptoms appear.
- Drug is available in a spring-loaded injector system that facilitates self-administration. Review detailed information with patient. Be sure the patient understands how to load the injector, administer the injection, and dispose of the used syringes.
- Tell patients who are pregnant or intend to become pregnant not to use this drug. Advise them to discuss with the doctor the risks and benefits of using the drug during pregnancy.
- Tell patients who feel persistent or severe chest pain to call the doctor immediately. Patients who feel pain or tightness in the throat or experience wheezing, heart throbbing, rash, lumps, hives, or swollen eyelids, face, or lips should stop using the drug and call the doctor.

tacrine hydrochloride
Cognex

Pregnancy Risk Category: C

HOW SUPPLIED
Tablets: 10 mg, 20 mg, 30 mg, 40 mg

ACTION
Mechanism: Reversibly inhibits the enzyme cholinesterase in the CNS, allowing the buildup of acetylcholine and thereby temporarily improving cognitive function in patients with Alzheimer's disease.
Peak: Plasma concentrations peak within 1 to 2 hours. Steady-state plasma levels are reached within 24 to 36 hours. **Duration:** elimination half-life, 2 to 4 hours.

INDICATIONS & DOSAGE
Mild to moderate dementia of the Alzheimer's type –
Adults: initially, 10 mg P.O. q.i.d. If the patient tolerates treatment and there are no transaminase elevations, increase to 20 mg P.O. q.i.d. After 6 weeks, titrate dosage upward to 30 mg P.O. q.i.d. If still tolerated, increase to 40 mg P.O. q.i.d. after another 6 weeks.

ADVERSE REACTIONS

CNS: anorexia, agitation, ataxia.
GI: nausea, vomiting, diarrhea, dyspepsia, loose stools, changes in stool color.
Skin: rash, jaundice.
Other: *elevations in transaminases* (especially ALT), myalgia.

INTERACTIONS

Anticholinergics: may decrease the effectiveness of anticholinergics. Monitor closely.
Cholinesterase inhibitors, cholinergics (such as bethanechol): additive effects. Monitor for toxicity.
Succinylcholine: enhanced neuromuscular blockade and prolonged duration of action. Monitor closely.
Theophylline: increased theophylline serum levels and prolonged theophylline half-life. Carefully monitor theophylline plasma levels, and adjust dosage as ordered.
Food: decreased absorption of tacrine if taken concomitantly. Take drug 1 hour before a meal.

CONTRAINDICATIONS

• Contraindicated in patients hypersensitive to the drug or acridine derivatives. Also contraindicated in patients who have previously developed tacrine-related jaundice, which has been confirmed with an elevated total bilirubin level of more than 3 mg/dl.
• Use cautiously in patients with sick sinus syndrome or bradycardia; in patients at risk for peptic ulceration (including patients taking NSAIDs, or patients with history of peptic ulceration); and in patients with history of hepatic disease. Also use cautiously in patients with renal disease, asthma, prostatic hyperplasia, or other urinary outflow impairment.

NURSING CONSIDERATIONS

• Have the patient take the drug between meals whenever possible. If GI upset becomes a problem, the drug may be taken with meals, although doing so may reduce plasma levels by 30% to 40%.
• Monitor serum ALT levels weekly for the first 18 weeks of therapy. If ALT is modestly elevated after the first 18 weeks of monitoring (twice the upper limit of normal), continue weekly monitoring. If no problems are detected, decrease frequency to once every 3 months. On each occasion that dosage is increased, resume weekly monitoring for at least 6 weeks.
• If the drug is discontinued for 4 weeks or more, the full dose titration and monitoring schedule must be restarted.
• Patient and family members should understand that this drug does not alter the underlying degenerative disease, but can alleviate symptoms. Effect of therapy depends upon drug administration at regular intervals.
• Remind caregivers that dosage titration is an integral part of the safe use of this drug. Abrupt discontinuation or a large reduction in daily dosage (80 mg/day or more) may precipitate behavioral disturbances and a decline in cognitive function.
• Advise the patient and caregivers to immediately report any significant adverse effects or changes in status.

36

Cholinergics (parasympathomimetics)

ambenonium chloride
bethanechol chloride
edrophonium chloride
neostigmine bromide
neostigmine methylsulfate
physostigmine salicylate
pyridostigmine bromide

COMBINATION PRODUCTS
None.

ambenonium chloride
Mytelase
Pregnancy Risk Category: C

HOW SUPPLIED
Tablets: 10 mg

ACTION
Mechanism: Inhibits the destruction of acetylcholine released from the parasympathetic and somatic efferent nerves. Acetylcholine accumulates, promoting increased stimulation of the receptor.
Onset: 20 to 30 minutes. **Duration:** 3 to 8 hours.

INDICATIONS & DOSAGE
Symptomatic treatment of myasthenia gravis in patients who cannot take neostigmine bromide or pyridostigmine bromide –
Adults: dosage individualized for each patient, but usually ranges from 5 to 25 mg P.O. t.i.d. to q.i.d. Starting dose usually is 5 mg P.O. t.i.d. to q.i.d. Increase gradually and adjust at 1- to 2-day intervals to avoid drug accumulation and overdosage. Usual dosage range is 15 to 100 mg daily, but some patients may require as much as 75 mg b.i.d. to q.i.d.

ADVERSE REACTIONS
CNS: headache, dizziness, muscle weakness, incoordination, ***seizures,*** mental confusion, jitters, sweating.
CV: bradycardia, hypotension.
EENT: miosis, blurred vision.
GI: *nausea, vomiting, diarrhea, abdominal cramps,* increased salivation.
GU: urinary frequency, incontinence.
Respiratory: bronchospasm, ***bronchoconstriction,*** increased bronchial secretions, ***respiratory paralysis.***
Other: muscle cramps.

INTERACTIONS
Aminoglycosides, anesthetics, atropine, corticosteroids, magnesium, procainamide, quinidine: decreased cholinergic effects. Dosage adjustment may be necessary.
Mecamylamine, other ganglionic blockers: increased toxicity. Avoid concomitant use.

CONTRAINDICATIONS
- Contraindicated in patients with mechanical obstruction of intestine or urinary tract, bradycardia, or hypotension.
- Use with extreme caution in patients with bronchial asthma. Use cautiously in patients with epilepsy, recent coronary occlusion, vagotonia, hyperthyroidism, arrhythmias, postoperative atelectasis, and pneumonia.

NURSING CONSIDERATIONS
- Avoid large dose in patients with decreased GI motility or megacolon.
- Discontinue all other cholinergics before administering this drug.
- Give with milk or food to produce fewer muscarinic adverse reactions.
- Administer each dose exactly as ordered, on time. Amount and frequency of dosage should vary with

the patient's activity level. The doctor will probably order larger doses when the patient is fatigued, for example, in the afternoon and at mealtime.

- Seek approval when indicated for hospitalized patients to have bedside supply of tablets. Patients with long-standing disease often insist on taking pills themselves.
- Monitor vital signs frequently, especially respirations, and document. Always have atropine injection available and be prepared to give 0.5 mg S.C. or slow I.V. push as ordered. Provide respiratory support as needed.
- Watch the patient very closely for adverse reactions, particularly if total dosage is greater than 200 mg daily. When adverse reactions indicate drug toxicity, notify the doctor immediately.
- If muscle weakness is severe, the doctor must determine if caused by drug toxicity or exacerbation of myasthenia gravis. A test dose of edrophonium I.V. will aggravate drug-induced weakness but will temporarily relieve weakness resulting from the disease.
- Weakness occurring 30 to 60 minutes after taking dose is a warning sign of drug toxicity. Notify the doctor immediately.
- Record the patient's variations in muscle strength. Show the patient how to monitor himself.
- When given for myasthenia gravis, explain that this drug will relieve symptoms of ptosis, double vision, difficulty in chewing and swallowing, and trunk and limb weakness. Stress the importance of taking this drug exactly as ordered.
- Explain to the patient and his family that ambenonium chloride is a chronic drug. Teach them about the disease and the drug's effect on symptoms.
- Patients may develop resistance to drug.
- Advise patients to wear medical identification bracelets indicating myasthenia gravis.

bethanechol chloride

Duvoid, Urabeth, Urecholine, Urocarb Liquid‡, Urocarb Tablets‡

Pregnancy Risk Category: C

HOW SUPPLIED

Tablets: 5 mg, 10 mg, 25 mg, 50 mg
Injection: 5 mg/ml

ACTION

Mechanism: Binds to cholinergic (muscarinic) receptors, mimicking the action of acetylcholine.
Onset: within 5 to 15 minutes of S.C. dose, within 30 to 90 minutes of oral dose. **Peak:** Effects occur 15 to 30 minutes after S.C. administration, about 1 hour after oral dose. **Duration:** persists for about 2 hours after S.C. administration, up to 6 hours after oral administration, depending upon dose.

INDICATIONS & DOSAGE

Acute postoperative and postpartum nonobstructive (functional) urine retention, neurogenic atony of urinary bladder with retention, abdominal distention, megacolon, or reflux esophagitis caused by low esophageal sphincter pressure –
Adults: 10 to 30 mg P.O. b.i.d. to q.i.d. Or, 2.5 to 10 mg S.C. Never give I.M. or I.V. When used for urine retention, some patients may require 50 to 100 mg P.O. per dose. Use such doses with extreme caution.

Test dose is 2.5 mg S.C. repeated at 15- to 30-minute intervals to total of 4 doses to determine the minimal effective dose; then use minimal effective dose q 6 to 8 hours. All doses must be adjusted individually.
Children: 0.6 mg/kg/day P.O. in 3 or 4 divided doses, or 0.15 to 0.2 mg/kg/day S.C. in 3 or 4 divided doses.

ADVERSE REACTIONS
CNS: headache, malaise.
CV: bradycardia, hypotension, ***cardiac arrest,*** reflex tachycardia.
EENT: lacrimation, miosis.
GI: *abdominal cramps, diarrhea,* salivation, nausea, vomiting, belching, borborygmus, esophageal spasms.
GU: urinary urgency.
Respiratory: ***bronchoconstriction,*** increased bronchial secretions.
Skin: flushing, sweating.

INTERACTIONS
Atropine, anticholinergic agents, procainamide, quinidine: may reverse cholinergic effects. Observe for lack of drug effect.
Cholinergic agonists, anticholinergic agents: may cause additive effects, or increase toxicity. Avoid concomitant use.
Ganglionic blockers: may cause hypotension. Avoid concomitant use.

CONTRAINDICATIONS
• Contraindicated in patients with uncertain strength or integrity of bladder wall; when increased muscular activity of GI or urinary tract is harmful; in patients with mechanical obstructions of GI or urinary tract; in patients with hyperthyroidism, peptic ulceration, latent or active bronchial asthma, cardiac or coronary artery disease, vagotonia, epilepsy, Parkinson's disease, bradycardia, chronic obstructive pulmonary disease, and hypotension.
• Bethanechol increases pancreatic secretion, raising serum levels of amylase and lipase. Because drug causes a spasm in the sphincter of Oddi, it may raise serum bilirubin and AST levels and increase sulfobromophthalein retention.
• Use cautiously in patients with hypertension, vasomotor instability, peritonitis, and other acute inflammatory conditions of GI tract.

NURSING CONSIDERATIONS
• Give on empty stomach; otherwise, may cause nausea and vomiting.
• Poor and variable oral absorption requires larger oral doses. Oral and S.C. doses are *not* interchangeable.
• Monitor vital signs frequently, especially respirations. Always have atropine injection available and be prepared to give 0.5 mg S.C. or slow I.V. push as ordered. Provide respiratory support if needed.
• *Never* give I.M. or I.V.; could cause circulatory collapse, hypotension, severe abdominal cramping, bloody diarrhea, shock, or cardiac arrest.
• Edrophonium not effective against muscle relaxation. Watch for toxicity, especially with S.C. administration.
• Watch closely for adverse reactions that may indicate drug toxicity.
• If used to treat urine retention, ensure that bedpan is available. Monitor fluid intake and output.
• When used to prevent abdominal distention and GI distress, the doctor may order a rectal tube inserted to help gas passage.

edrophonium chloride
Enlon, Reversol, Tensilon

Pregnancy Risk Category: C

HOW SUPPLIED
Injection: 10 mg/ml in 1-ml ampules or 10-ml vials

ACTION
Mechanism: Inhibits the destruction of acetylcholine released from the parasympathetic and somatic efferent nerves. Acetylcholine accumulates, promoting increased stimulation of the receptor. Edrophonium has a very short duration of action.
Onset: occurs within 30 to 60 seconds of I.V. administration, within 2 to 10 minutes of I.M. injection. **Duration:** 5 to 10 minutes after I.V. in-

jection, 5 to 30 minutes after I.M. injection.

INDICATIONS & DOSAGE

As a curare antagonist (to reverse nondepolarizing neuromuscular blocking action) –

Adults: 10 mg I.V. given over 30 to 45 seconds. Dose may be repeated as necessary to 40 mg maximum dosage. Larger dosages may potentiate effect of curare.

Diagnostic aid in myasthenia gravis (Tensilon test) –

Adults: 1 to 2 mg I.V. within 15 to 30 seconds, then 8 mg if no response (increase in muscular strength). Alternatively, give 10 mg I.M. If cholinergic reaction occurs, give 2 mg I.M. 30 minutes later to rule out false-negative response.

Children over 34 kg: 2 mg I.V. If no response within 45 seconds, give 1 mg q 45 seconds to maximum of 10 mg. Alternatively, give 5 mg I.M.

Children up to 34 kg: 1 mg I.V. If no response within 45 seconds, give 1 mg q 45 seconds to maximum of 5 mg. Alternatively, give 2 mg I.M.

I.M. route may be used in children because of difficulty with I.V. route: for children under 34 kg, inject 2 mg I.M.; children over 34 kg, 5 mg I.M. Expect same reactions as with I.V. test, but these appear after 2- to 10-minute delay.

Infants: 0.5 mg to 1 mg I.M. or S.C.

To differentiate myasthenic crisis from cholinergic crisis –

Adults: 1 mg I.V. If no response in 1 minute, repeat dose once. Increased muscular strength confirms myasthenic crisis; no increase or exaggerated weakness confirms cholinergic crisis.

Paroxysmal supraventricular tachycardia –

Adults: 5 to 10 mg I.V. given over 1 minute or less. Alternatively, give a test dose of 2 mg I.V., followed by 2 mg every minute for a total of 10 mg I.V. If heart rate decreases, infuse at 0.25 mg/minute; increase as needed to a maximum of 2 mg/minute.

Children: 2 mg slow I.V.

ADVERSE REACTIONS

CNS: ***seizures,*** weakness, dysarthria, dysphagia, sweating.

CV: hypotension, bradycardia, AV block.

EENT: excessive lacrimation, diplopia, miosis, conjunctival hyperemia.

GI: nausea, vomiting, *diarrhea, abdominal cramps,* excessive salivation.

GU: urinary frequency, incontinence.

Respiratory: ***paralysis, bronchospasm, laryngospasm,*** increased bronchial secretions.

Other: muscle cramps, muscle fasciculation.

INTERACTIONS

Aminoglycosides, anesthetics: prolonged or enhanced muscle weakness. Monitor closely.

Corticosteroids, magnesium, procainamide, quinidine: may antagonize cholinergic effects. Observe for lack of drug effect.

Digitalis glycosides: may increase the heart's sensitivity to edrophonium. Use together cautiously.

CONTRAINDICATIONS

- Contraindicated in patients with mechanical obstruction of intestine or urinary tract, bradycardia, or hypotension.
- Use with extreme caution in patients with bronchial asthma. Use cautiously in patients with hyperthyroidism, cardiac disease, peptic ulceration, and arrhythmias (especially AV block and bradycardia).

NURSING CONSIDERATIONS

- Effective against muscle relaxation induced by decamethonium bromide and succinylcholine chloride.
- This cholinergic has the most rapid

onset but shortest duration; therefore, do not use to treat myasthenia gravis.
- Stop all other cholinergics before giving this drug.
- Monitor vital signs frequently, especially respirations. Always have atropine injection available and be prepared to give 0.5 mg S.C. or slow I.V. push as ordered. Provide respiratory support as needed.
- **I.V. use:** For easier parenteral administration, use tuberculin syringe with an I.V. needle. When giving drug to differentiate myasthenic crisis from cholinergic crisis, observe patient's muscle strength closely.
- Continuous I.V. infusions have been used to control atrial tachycardia or supraventricular tachycardia associated with Wolff-Parkinson-White syndrome, which is unresponsive to digitalis glycosides.
- Watch closely for adverse reactions; may indicate toxicity.

neostigmine bromide
Prostigmin Bromide

neostigmine methylsulfate
Prostigmin

Pregnancy Risk Category: C

HOW SUPPLIED
bromide
Tablets: 15 mg
methylsulfate
Injection: 0.25 mg/ml, 0.5 mg/ml, 1 mg/ml

ACTION
Mechanism: An anticholinesterase agent that inhibits the destruction of acetylcholine released from the parasympathetic and somatic efferent nerves. Acetylcholine accumulates, promoting increased stimulation of the receptor.
Onset: 10 to 30 minutes after I.M. or I.V. injection, 2 to 4 hours after oral use. **Peak:** Effects occur 20 to 30 minutes after I.M. or I.V. administration. **Duration:** 2½ to 4 hours after I.M. injection.

INDICATIONS & DOSAGE
Treatment of myasthenia gravis –
Adults: 15 to 30 mg P.O. t.i.d. (range is 15 to 375 mg daily); or 0.5 to 2 mg S.C., I.M., or I.V. q 1 to 3 hours.
Children: 7.5 to 15 mg P.O. t.i.d. to q.i.d.

Dosage must be individualized, depending on response and tolerance of adverse effects. Therapy may be required day and night.

Diagnosis of myasthenia gravis –
Adults: 0.022 mg/kg I.M. 30 minutes after 0.4 to 0.6 mg of atropine sulfate.
Children: 0.025 to 0.04 mg/kg. I.M. after 0.11 mg/kg atropine sulfate S.C.

Postoperative abdominal distention and bladder atony –
Adults: 0.5 to 1 mg I.M. or S.C. q 4 to 6 hours.

Postoperative ileus –
Adults: 0.25 to 1 mg I.M. or S.C. q 4 to 6 hours.
Neonates and infants: 0.04 mg/kg I.M. q 6 hours.

Antidote for nondepolarizing neuromuscular blocking agents –
Adults: 0.5 to 2.5 mg I.V. slowly. Repeat p.r.n. to a total of 5 mg. Give 0.6 to 1.2 mg atropine sulfate I.V. before antidote dose.

Note: 1:1,000 solution of injectable solution contains 1 mg/ml; 1:2,000 solution contains 0.5 mg/ml.

ADVERSE REACTIONS
CNS: dizziness, headache, muscle weakness, mental confusion, jitters, sweating.
CV: bradycardia, hypotension.
EENT: blurred vision, lacrimation, miosis.
GI: *nausea, vomiting, diarrhea, abdominal cramps,* excessive salivation.
GU: urinary frequency.
Respiratory: ***depression, bronchospasm, bronchoconstriction.***

Skin: rash (bromide).
Other: *muscle cramps,* muscle fasciculations.

INTERACTIONS

Atropine, anticholinergic agents, corticosteroids, magnesium sulfate, procainamide, aminoglycosides, quinidine: may antagonize neostigmine-induced enhancements in muscle strength. Observe for lack of drug effect.

CONTRAINDICATIONS

- Contraindicated in patients with hypersensitivity to cholinergics or to bromide, mechanical obstruction of the intestine or urinary tract, bradycardia, or hypotension.
- Use with extreme caution in patients with bronchial asthma. Use cautiously in patients with seizure disorders, recent coronary occlusion, peritonitis, vagotonia, hyperthyroidism, cardiac arrhythmias, and peptic ulceration.

NURSING CONSIDERATIONS

- Reduce GI adverse reactions by taking drug with milk or food.
- Although frequently used to reverse the effects of nondepolarizing neuromuscular blockers in postsurgical patients, neostigmine may actually worsen the blockade produced by succinylcholine.
- Stop all other cholinergics before giving this drug.
- Monitor vital signs frequently, especially respirations. Have atropine injection available and be prepared to give as ordered; provide respiratory support as needed.
- When using for myasthenia gravis, explain that this drug will relieve ptosis, double vision, difficulty in chewing and swallowing, and trunk and limb weakness. Stress importance of taking drug exactly as ordered. Explain that drug may have to be taken for life.
- In myasthenia gravis, schedule dose before periods of fatigue. For example, if the patient has dysphagia, schedule dose 30 minutes before each meal.
- Optimum dosage is difficult to judge. Monitor and document the patient's response after each dose. Observe closely for improvement in strength, vision, and ptosis 45 to 60 minutes after each dose. Show the patient how to observe and record variations in muscle strength.
- **I.V. use:** Give at a slow, controlled rate not to exceed 1 mg/minute in adults and 0.5 mg/minute in children.
- If muscle weakness is severe, the doctor determines if it is caused by drug-induced toxicity or exacerbation of myasthenia gravis. Test dose of edrophonium I.V. will aggravate drug-induced weakness but will temporarily relieve weakness caused by disease.
- I.M. neostigmine may be used instead of edrophonium to diagnose myasthenia gravis. May be preferable to edrophonium when limb weakness is the only symptom.
- Hospitalized patients with long-standing myasthenia gravis may request bedside supply of tablets. Caution patients to take each dose precisely as ordered.
- Seek approval for self-medication program according to hospital policy, but continue to oversee medication regimen.
- When used to prevent abdominal distention and GI distress, the doctor may order a rectal tube inserted to help gas passage.
- Advise patients to wear medical identification bracelets indicating myasthenia gravis.
- Patients sometimes develop a resistance to neostigmine.

physostigmine salicylate (eserine salicylate)

Antilirium

Pregnancy Risk Category: C

HOW SUPPLIED

Injection: 1 mg/ml

ACTION

Mechanism: Inhibits the destruction of acetylcholine released from the parasympathetic and somatic efferent nerves. Acetylcholine accumulates, promoting increased stimulation of the receptor.

Onset: occurs within 3 to 5 minutes of injection. **Peak:** Effects occur within 5 minutes of I.V. injection, or 20 to 30 minutes after I.M. injection. **Duration:** 30 to 60 minutes after parenteral use.

INDICATIONS & DOSAGE

To reverse the CNS toxicity associated with tricyclic antidepressant (TCA) and anticholinergic poisoning–

Adults: 0.5 to 2 mg I.M. or I.V. (1 mg/minute I.V.) repeated every 20 minutes as necessary if life-threatening signs recur (coma, seizures, arrhythmias). Additional doses of 1 to 4 mg I.M. or I.V. every 30 to 60 minutes may be given.

Children: 0.02 mg/kg I.M. or I.V. Repeat every 5 to 10 minutes until response is obtained. Maximum dosage is 2 mg.

Used investigationally to improve cognitive function in patients with Alzheimer's disease. Investigators have used 0.5 mg P.O. q 2 hours, increasing to 2 to 2.5 mg P.O. q 2 hours, 6 or 7 times a day. Maximum dosage is 16 mg/day.

ADVERSE REACTIONS

CNS: ***seizures,*** hallucinations, muscular twitching, muscle weakness, ataxia, *restlessness, excitability, sweating.*

CV: irregular pulse, palpitations, bradycardia, hypotension.

EENT: miosis.

GI: nausea, vomiting, epigastric pain, *diarrhea, excessive salivation.*

GU: urinary urgency.

Respiratory: ***bronchospasm,*** bronchial constriction, dyspnea.

INTERACTIONS

Atropine, anticholinergic agents, procainamide, quinidine: may reverse cholinergic effects. Observe for lack of drug effect.

Ganglionic blockers: may decrease blood pressure. Avoid concomitant use.

CONTRAINDICATIONS

- Contraindicated in patients with mechanical obstruction of intestine or urogenital tract, bronchial asthma, gangrene, diabetes, CV disease, acute angle-closure glaucoma, or vagotonia.
- Use cautiously in patients with bradycardia, hypotension, seizure disorder, Parkinson's disease, hyperthyroidism, and peptic ulceration.

NURSING CONSIDERATIONS

- Only cholinergic that crosses blood-brain barrier; therefore only one useful for treating CNS effects of anticholinergic or TCA toxicity.
- Monitor vital signs frequently, especially respirations. Position the patient to ease breathing. Have atropine injection available and be prepared to give 0.5 mg S.C. or slow I.V. push as ordered. Provide respiratory support as needed. Best administered in presence of a doctor.
- **I.V. use:** Give I.V. at controlled rate; use direct injection at no more than 1 mg/minute.
- Use only clear solution. Darkening may indicate loss of potency.
- Effectiveness often immediate and dramatic but may be transient and may require repeat doses.

• Watch closely for adverse reactions, particularly CNS disturbances. Use side rails if the patient becomes restless or hallucinates. Adverse reactions may indicate drug toxicity.

pyridostigmine bromide

Mestinon*, Mestinon Supraspan†, Mestinon Timespan, Regonol

Pregnancy Risk Category: C

HOW SUPPLIED

Tablets: 60 mg
Tablets (extended-release): 180 mg
Syrup: 60 mg/5 ml
Injection: 5 mg/ml in 2-ml ampules or 5-ml vials

ACTION

Mechanism: Inhibits the destruction of acetylcholine released from the parasympathetic and somatic efferent nerves. Acetylcholine accumulates, promoting increased stimulation of the receptor.
Onset: within 2 to 5 minutes of I.V. injection, 15 minutes following I.M. injection, 30 to 45 minutes after oral ingestion of regular-release tablets or syrup, 30 to 60 minutes following ingestion of extended-release tablets.
Peak: Effects occur within 1 to 2 hours of oral administration. **Duration:** 2 to 3 hours after parenteral use, 3 to 6 hours after regular-release tablets or syrup, 6 to 12 hours after extended-release tablets.

INDICATIONS & DOSAGE

Antidote for nondepolarizing neuromuscular blocking agents –
Adults: 10 to 20 mg I.V. preceded by atropine sulfate 0.6 to 1.2 mg I.V.
Myasthenia gravis –
Adults: 60 to 120 mg P.O. q 3 or 4 hours. Usual dosage is 600 mg daily but higher dosage may be needed (up to 1,500 mg daily). Give 1/30 of oral dosage I.M. or I.V. Dosage must be adjusted for each patient, depending on response and tolerance of adverse effects. Alternatively, may give 180 to 540 mg timed-release tablets (1 to 3 tablets) b.i.d., with at least 6 hours between doses.
Children: 7 mg/kg or 200 mg/m^2 daily in 5 or 6 divided doses.
Supportive treatment of neonates born to myasthenic mothers –
Neonates: 0.05 to 0.15 mg/kg I.M. q 4 to 6 hours. Gradually decrease daily dosage until drug can be withdrawn.

ADVERSE REACTIONS

CNS: headache (with high doses), weakness, sweating, ***seizures.***
CV: bradycardia, hypotension, thrombophlebitis.
EENT: miosis.
GI: abdominal cramps, nausea, vomiting, diarrhea, excessive salivation.
Respiratory: ***bronchospasm, bronchoconstriction,*** increased bronchial secretions.
Skin: rash.
Other: muscle cramps, muscle fasciculations.

INTERACTIONS

Aminoglycosides, anesthetics: may decrease response to pyridostigmine. Use together cautiously.
Atropine, anticholinergic agents, corticosteroids, magnesium, procainamide, quinidine: may antagonize cholinergic effects. Observe for lack of drug effect.
Ganglionic blockers: increased risk of hypotension. Monitor closely.

CONTRAINDICATIONS

• Contraindicated in patients with mechanical obstruction of intestine or urinary tract, bradycardia, or hypotension. Use with extreme caution in patients with bronchial asthma.
• Use cautiously in patients who have epilepsy, recent coronary occlusion, vagotonia, hyperthyroidism, arrhythmias, and peptic ulceration. Avoid

large doses in patients with decreased GI motility.

NURSING CONSIDERATIONS

- Optimum dosage is difficult to judge. Monitor and document patient's response after each dose.
- Stop all other cholinergics before giving this drug.
- **I.V. use:** Administer I.V. injection no faster than 1 mg/minute. If I.V. administration is too rapid, bradycardia and seizures may result. Monitor vital signs frequently, especially respirations. Position patient to ease breathing. Have atropine injection available and be prepared to give as ordered; provide respiratory support as needed.
- If muscle weakness is severe, the doctor determines if it is caused by drug-induced toxicity or exacerbation of myasthenia gravis. Test dose of edrophonium. I.V. will aggravate drug-induced weakness but will temporarily relieve weakness caused by disease.
- When using for myasthenia gravis, stress importance of taking drug exactly as ordered, on time, in evenly spaced doses. If the doctor has ordered extended-release tablets, explain that patients must take tablets at the same time each day, at least 6 hours apart. Explain that patients may have to take drug for life.
- Drug has longest duration of the cholinergics used for myasthenia gravis.
- Advise patients to wear medical identification bracelets indicating myasthenia gravis.
- Use by oral route to treat senility associated with Alzheimer's disease.
- Don't crush the timed-release (Timespan or Supraspan) tablets.
- Available as sweet syrup for patients who have difficulty swallowing. Give over ice chips if the patient can't tolerate flavor.
- Obtain a doctor's order for a hospitalized patient to have bedside supply of tablets to take himself. Patients with long-standing disease often insist on self-administration.
- In the United States, Regonol contains benzyl ethanol preservative that may cause toxicity in neonates if administered in high doses. The Canadian formulation of this drug does not contain benzyl ethanol.

37

Anticholinergics

atropine sulfate
(See Chapter 20, ANTIARRHYTHMICS.)
belladonna leaf
clidinium bromide
dicyclomine hydrochloride
glycopyrrolate
hyoscyamine
hyoscyamine sulfate
isopropamide iodide
levorotatory alkaloids of belladonna
mepenzolate bromide
methantheline bromide
methscopolamine bromide
oxyphencyclimine hydrochloride
propantheline bromide
scopolamine
scopolamine butylbromide
scopolamine hydrobromide

COMBINATION PRODUCTS

BARBIDONNA ELIXIR*: atropine sulfate 0.034 mg/5 ml, phenobarbital 21.6 mg/5 ml, hyoscyamine hydrobromide or sulfate 0.174 mg/5 ml, scopolamine hydrobromide 0.01 mg/5 ml, and ethanol 15%.
BARBIDONNA NO. 2 TABLETS: atropine sulfate 0.025 mg, scopolamine hydrobromide 0.0074 mg, hyoscyamine hydrobromide or sulfate 0.1286 mg, and phenobarbital 32 mg.
BARBIDONNA TABLETS: atropine sulfate 0.025 mg, scopolamine hydrobromide 0.0074 mg, hyoscyamine hydrobromide or sulfate 0.1286 mg, and phenobarbital 16 mg.
CHARDONNA-2: belladonna extract 15 mg and phenobarbital 15 mg.
DONNATAL ELIXIR*: atropine sulfate 0.0194 mg/5 ml, scopolamine hydrobromide 0.0065 mg/5 ml, ethanol 23%, hyoscyamine hydrobromide or sulfate 0.1037 mg/5 ml, and phenobarbital 16 mg/5 ml.
DONNATAL EXTENTABS: atropine sulfate 0.0582 mg, scopolamine hydrobromide 0.0195 mg, hyoscyamine sulfate 0.3111 mg, and phenobarbital 48.6 mg.
DONNATAL NO. 2 TABLETS: atropine sulfate 0.0194 mg, scopolamine hydrobromide 0.0065 mg, hyoscyamine hydrobromide or sulfate 0.1037 mg, and phenobarbital 32.4 mg.
DONNATAL TABLETS AND CAPSULES: atropine sulfate 0.0194 mg, scopolamine hydrobromide 0.0065 mg, hyoscyamine hydrobromide or sulfate 0.1037 mg, and phenobarbital 16 mg.
KINESED TABLETS: atropine sulfate 0.02 mg, scopolamine hydrobromide 0.007 mg, hyoscyamine hydrobromide or sulfate 0.1 mg, and phenobarbital 16 mg.
LIBRAX CAPSULES: clidinium bromide 2.5 mg and chlordiazepoxide hydrochloride 5 mg.
ROBINUL FORTE TABLETS: glycopyrrolate 2 mg and phenobarbital 16.2 mg.
ROBINUL TABLETS: glycopyrrolate 1 mg and phenobarbital 16.2 mg.

belladonna leaf

(used to prepare extract and tincture)
Belladonna Tincture USP*
Pregnancy Risk Category: C

HOW SUPPLIED

Tablets: 15 mg
Oral solution: 27 to 33 mg belladonna alkaloids/100 ml in 67% alcohol solution

ACTION

Mechanism: Blocks acetylcholine, which decreases GI motility and inhibits gastric acid secretion.

*Liquid form contains alcohol.
**May contain tartrazine.

Onset: within 1 to 2 hours of administration. **Duration:** about 4 hours.

INDICATIONS & DOSAGE

Adjunctive therapy for peptic ulceration, irritable bowel syndrome, functional G.I. disorders, and neurogenic bowel disturbances –
Adults: 15 mg P.O. t.i.d. or q.i.d. of extract; 0.3 to 1 ml t.i.d. or q.i.d. of tincture.
Children: 0.1 ml/kg or 2.5 ml/m^2 tincture P.O. t.i.d. to q.i.d. Total dosage should not exceed 3.5 ml/day.

ADVERSE REACTIONS

CNS: headache, insomnia, drowsiness, dizziness, *confusion or excitement in elderly patients,* nervousness, weakness.
CV: *palpitations,* tachycardia.
EENT: *blurred vision,* mydriasis, increased ocular tension, cycloplegia, photophobia.
GI: *dry mouth,* dysphagia, heartburn, loss of taste, *constipation,* nausea, vomiting.
GU: *urinary hesitancy, urine retention,* impotence.
Skin: urticaria, decreased sweating or possible anhidrosis, other dermal manifestations.
Other: fever, allergic reactions.

Overdosage may cause curare-like effects, such as respiratory paralysis.

INTERACTIONS

Amantadine, antihistamines, antiparkinsonian agents, disopyramide, glutethimide, meperidine, phenothiazines, procainamide, quinidine: additive adverse effects. Avoid concomitant use.
Antacids: decreased absorption of orally administered anticholinergics. Separate administration times by 2 to 3 hours.
Ketoconazole: anticholinergics may interfere with ketoconazole absorption. Avoid concomitant use.
Methotrimeprazine: anticholinergics may enhance risk of extrapyramidal reactions. Avoid concomitant use.

CONTRAINDICATIONS

- Contraindicated in patients with acute angle-closure glaucoma, obstructive uropathy, obstructive disease of GI tract, severe ulcerative colitis, myasthenia gravis, hypersensitivity to anticholinergics, paralytic ileus, intestinal atony, unstable cardiovascular status in acute hemorrhage, or toxic megacolon.
- Use cautiously in patients with autonomic neuropathy, hyperthyroidism, coronary artery disease, arrhythmias, CHF, hypertension, hiatal hernia associated with reflux esophagitis, hepatic or renal disease, and ulcerative colitis; or in patients over 40 years because of increased incidence of glaucoma. Also use cautiously in patients in hot or humid environments. Drug-induced heatstroke can develop.

NURSING CONSIDERATIONS

- Give 30 minutes to 1 hour before meals and h.s. Bedtime dose can be larger; give at least 2 hours after last meal of the day.
- Administer smaller doses to elderly patients.
- Monitor the patient's vital signs and urine output carefully.
- Instruct the patient to avoid driving and other hazardous activities if he is drowsy, dizzy, or has blurred vision; to drink plenty of fluids to help prevent constipation; and to report any skin rash or local eruption.
- Sugarless gum or hard candy may relieve dry mouth.

clidinium bromide

Quarzan

Pregnancy Risk Category: C

HOW SUPPLIED

Capsules: 2.5 mg, 5 mg

ACTION

Mechanism: Blocks acetylcholine, which decreases GI motility and inhibits gastric acid secretion.
Onset: within 1 hour of administration. **Duration:** up to 3 hours.

INDICATIONS & DOSAGE

Adjunctive therapy for peptic ulcerations –
Adults: 2.5 to 5 mg P.O. t.i.d. or q.i.d. before meals and h.s.
Elderly or debilitated patients: 2.5 mg P.O. t.i.d.

ADVERSE REACTIONS

CNS: headache, insomnia, drowsiness, dizziness, *confusion or excitement in elderly patients,* nervousness, weakness.
CV: *palpitations,* tachycardia.
EENT: *blurred vision,* mydriasis, increased ocular tension, cycloplegia, photophobia.
GI: *dry mouth,* dysphagia, heartburn, loss of taste, nausea, vomiting, *paralytic ileus, constipation.*
GU: *urinary hesitancy, urine retention,* impotence.
Skin: urticaria, decreased sweating or possible anhidrosis, other dermal manifestations.
Other: fever, allergic reactions.

Overdosage may cause curare-like effects, such as respiratory paralysis.

INTERACTIONS

Amantadine, antihistamines, antiparkinsonian agents, disopyramide, glutethimide, meperidine, phenothiazines, procainamide, quinidine: additive adverse effects. Avoid concomitant use.
Antacids: decreased absorption of orally administered anticholinergics. Separate administration times by 2 to 3 hours.
Ketoconazole: anticholinergics may interfere with ketoconazole absorption. Avoid concomitant use.
Methotrimeprazine: anticholinergics may enhance risk of extrapyramidal reactions. Avoid concomitant use.

CONTRAINDICATIONS

- Contraindicated in patients with acute angle-closure glaucoma, obstructive uropathy, obstructive disease of GI tract, severe ulcerative colitis, myasthenia gravis, hypersensitivity to anticholinergics, paralytic ileus, intestinal atony, unstable cardiovascular status in acute hemorrhage, or toxic megacolon.
- Use cautiously in patients with autonomic neuropathy, hyperthyroidism, coronary artery disease, arrhythmias, CHF, hypertension, hiatal hernia associated with reflux esophagitis, hepatic or renal disease, and ulcerative colitis; or in patients over 40 years because of increased incidence of glaucoma. Also use cautiously in patients in hot or humid environments. Drug-induced heatstroke may develop.

NURSING CONSIDERATIONS

- No conclusive evidence exists that clidinium aids in healing, decreasing recurrence of, or preventing complications of peptic ulcerations.
- Give 30 minutes to 1 hour before meals and h.s. Bedtime dose can be larger; give at least 2 hours after last meal of the day.
- Dosage should be individualized according to severity of symptoms and occurrence of adverse reactions.
- Dysphagia may cause aspiration.
- Monitor the patient's vital signs and urine output carefully.
- Instruct the patient to avoid driving and other hazardous activities if he is drowsy, dizzy, or has blurred vision; to drink plenty of fluids to help prevent constipation; and to report any rash or skin eruption.
- Sugarless gum or hard candy may relieve dry mouth.

dicyclomine hydrochloride

Antispas, A-Spas, Bentyl, Bentylol†, Di-Spaz, Formulex†, Lomine†, Merbentyl‡, Neoquess Injection, Or-Tyl, Spasmoban†, Spasmoject

Pregnancy Risk Category: B

HOW SUPPLIED

Tablets: 10 mg‡, 20 mg
Capsules: 10 mg, 20 mg
Syrup: 5 mg/5 ml‡, 10 mg/5 ml
Injection: 10 mg/ml

ACTION

Mechanism: Exerts a nonspecific, direct spasmolytic action on smooth muscle. Also possesses local anesthetic properties that may be partly responsible for spasmolysis.
Peak: Peak effects occur 1 to 1½ hours after administration. **Duration:** terminal elimination half-life, 9 to 10 hours.

INDICATIONS & DOSAGE

Adjunctive therapy for peptic ulcerations, irritable bowel syndrome, and other functional GI disorders –
Adults: 10 to 20 mg P.O. t.i.d. or q.i.d.; 20 mg I.M. q 4 to 6 hours.
Children 2 years and older: 10 mg P.O. t.i.d. or q.i.d.
Children 6 months to 2 years: 5 to 10 mg P.O. t.i.d. to q.i.d.

ADVERSE REACTIONS

CNS: *headache; dizziness;* insomnia; drowsiness; nervousness, confusion, excitement (in elderly patients).
CV: *palpitations,* tachycardia.
EENT: blurred vision, increased intraocular pressure, mydriasis.
GI: nausea, vomiting, *constipation, dry mouth,* abdominal distention, heartburn, paralytic ileus.
GU: *urinary hesitancy, urine retention,* impotence.
Skin: urticaria, decreased sweating or possible anhidrosis, other dermal manifestations.
Other: fever, allergic reactions. Dicyclomine is a synthetic tertiary derivative that may have atropine-like adverse reactions.

Overdosage may cause curare-like effects, such as respiratory paralysis.

INTERACTIONS

Amantadine, antihistamines, antiparkinsonian agents, disopyramide, glutethimide, meperidine, phenothiazines, procainamide, quinidine: additive adverse effects. Avoid concomitant use.
Antacids: decreased absorption of orally administered anticholinergics. Separate administration times by 2 to 3 hours.
Ketoconazole: anticholinergics may interfere with ketoconazole absorption. Avoid concomitant use.
Methotrimeprazine: anticholinergics may enhance risk of extrapyramidal reactions. Avoid concomitant use.

CONTRAINDICATIONS

- Contraindicated in patients with obstructive uropathy, obstructive disease of GI tract, severe ulcerative colitis, myasthenia gravis, hypersensitivity to anticholinergics, paralytic ileus, intestinal atony, unstable cardiovascular status in acute hemorrhage, or toxic megacolon. Also contraindicated in children under 6 months. Seizures, asphyxia, hypotonia, and coma have been reported.
- Use cautiously in patients with autonomic neuropathy, acute angle-closure glaucoma, hyperthyroidism, coronary artery disease, arrhythmias, CHF, hypertension, hiatal hernia associated with reflux esophagitis, hepatic or renal disease, and ulcerative colitis; or in patients over 40 years because of increased incidence of glaucoma. Also use cautiously in patients in hot or humid environments. Drug-induced heatstroke can develop.

NURSING CONSIDERATIONS

- Always adjust dosage according to patient's needs and response. Doses up to 40 mg P.O. q.i.d. have been used in adults, but safety and efficacy for more than 2 weeks has not been established.
- Give 30 minutes to 1 hour before meals and h.s.. Bedtime dose can be larger; give at least 2 hours after last meal of the day.
- Monitor patient's vital signs and urine output carefully.
- Not for S.C. or I.V. use.
- Instruct the patient to avoid driving and other hazardous activities if he is drowsy, dizzy, or has blurred vision; to drink plenty of fluids to help prevent constipation; and to report any rash or skin eruption.
- Gum or sugarless hard candy may relieve dry mouth.

glycopyrrolate

Robinul, Robinul Forte

Pregnancy Risk Category: B

HOW SUPPLIED

Tablets: 1 mg, 2 mg
Injection: 0.2 mg/ml

ACTION

Mechanism: Inhibits cholinergic (muscarinic) actions of acetylcholine on autonomic effectors innervated by postganglionic cholinergic nerves.
Onset: 1 minute after I.V. injection, 15 to 30 minutes after S.C. or I.M. injection. **Peak:** Effects occur 30 to 45 minutes after I.M. injection. **Duration:** vagal blocking effects, about 3 hours; effect on secretions, up to 7 hours.

INDICATIONS & DOSAGE

Blockade of cholinergic adverse effects caused by anticholinesterase agents used to reverse neuromuscular blockade –
Adults and children: 0.2 mg I.V. for each 1 mg neostigmine or 5 mg of pyridostigmine. May be given I.V. without dilution or may be added to dextrose injection and given by infusion.

Preoperatively to diminish secretions and block cardiac vagal reflexes –
Adults: 0.0044 mg/lb of body weight I.M. 30 to 60 minutes before anesthesia.
Children 2 years and older: 0.0044 mg/kg I.M. 30 to 60 minutes before anesthesia.
Children under 2 years: 0.0088 mg/kg I.M. 30 minutes before anesthesia.

Adjunctive therapy in peptic ulcerations and other GI disorders –
Adults: 1 to 2 mg P.O. t.i.d. or 0.1 mg I.M. t.i.d. or q.i.d. Dosage must be individualized. Maximum P.O. dosage is 8 mg/day.

ADVERSE REACTIONS

CNS: disorientation, irritability, incoherence, weakness, nervousness, drowsiness, dizziness, headache, confusion or excitement (in elderly patients).
CV: palpitations, tachycardia, paradoxical bradycardia.
EENT: *dilated pupils, blurred vision,* photophobia, increased intraocular pressure, difficulty swallowing.
GI: *constipation, dry mouth,* nausea, vomiting, epigastric distress.
GU: *urinary hesitancy, urine retention,* impotence.
Respiratory: *bronchial plugging.*
Skin: urticaria, decreased sweating or anhidrosis, other dermal manifestations.
Other: burning at injection site, fever, loss of taste, abdominal distention.

INTERACTIONS

Amantadine, antihistamines, antiparkinsonian agents, disopyramide, glutethimide, meperidine, phenothiazines, procainamide, quinidine: ad-

ditive adverse effects. Avoid concomitant use.
Antacids: decreased absorption of orally administered anticholinergics. Separate administration times by 2 to 3 hours.
Ketoconazole: anticholinergics may interfere with ketoconazole absorption. Avoid concomitant use.
Methotrimeprazine: anticholinergics may enhance risk of extrapyramidal reactions. Avoid concomitant use.

CONTRAINDICATIONS
- Contraindicated in patients with acute angle-closure glaucoma, obstructive uropathy, obstructive disease of the GI tract, myasthenia gravis, paralytic ileus, intestinal atony, unstable cardiovascular status in acute hemorrhage, or toxic megacolon.
- Use cautiously in patients with autonomic neuropathy, hyperthyroidism, coronary artery disease, arrhythmias, CHF, hypertension, hiatal hernia associated with reflux esophagitis, hepatic or renal disease, and ulcerative colitis; and in patients over 40 years because of increased incidence of glaucoma. Use with caution in patients in hot or humid environments. Drug-induced heatstroke is possible.

NURSING CONSIDERATIONS
- Monitor vital signs carefully. Watch closely for adverse reactions, especially in elderly or debilitated patients. Call the doctor promptly if they occur.
- Advise patients to report signs of urinary hesitancy or urine retention.
- Administer 30 minutes to 1 hour before meals.
- Elderly patients typically receive smaller dosages.
- Check all dosages carefully; slight overdose lead to toxicity.
- Warn patients to avoid activities that require alertness until CNS effects are known.
- **I.V. use:** Administer by direct injection without dilution. Alternatively, inject into the tubing of a free-flowing I.V. solution.
- Don't mix with I.V. solution containing sodium bicarbonate or alkaline solutions with a pH > 6. Alkaline drugs, such as barbiturates (thiopental, methohexital, secobarbital, pentobarbital), chloramphenicol, dexamethasone, dimenhydrinate, diazepam, methylprednisolone, and pentazocine are incompatible with glycopyrrolate.

hyoscyamine
Cystospaz

hyoscyamine sulfate
Anaspaz, Bellaspaz, Cystospaz, Cystospaz-M, Gastrosed, Levsin*, Levsin S/L, Levsinex Timecaps, Neoquess

Pregnancy Risk Category: C

HOW SUPPLIED
hyoscyamine
Tablets: 0.15 mg
hyoscyamine sulfate
Tablets: 0.125 mg, 0.13 mg, 0.15 mg
Capsules (extended-release): 0.375 mg
Elixir: 125 mcg/5 ml
Oral solution: 0.125 mg/ml
Injection: 0.5 mg/ml

ACTION
Mechanism: Competitively blocks acetylcholine, which decreases GI motility and inhibits gastric acid secretion.
Onset: within 2 minutes after I.V. injection, 5 to 20 minutes after oral elixer, 20 to 30 minutes after oral tablets. **Peak:** Effects occur 15 to 30 minutes after parenteral use, or 30 to 60 minutes after oral use. **Duration:** 4 to 12 hours.

INDICATIONS & DOSAGE

GI tract disorders caused by spasm; adjunctive therapy for peptic ulcerations –

Adults: 0.125 to 0.25 mg P.O. or sublingually t.i.d. or q.i.d. before meals and h.s.; extended-release form 0.375 mg P.O. q 8 to 12 hours; or 0.25 to 0.5 mg (1 or 2 ml) I.M., I.V., or S.C. b.i.d. to q.i.d. (Substitute oral medication when symptoms are controlled.)

Children 2 to 10 years: half of adult dose P.O., not to exceed 1.5 mg daily.

Children under 2 years: one-quarter of adult dose P.O.

ADVERSE REACTIONS

CNS: headache, insomnia, drowsiness, dizziness, *confusion or excitement in elderly patients,* nervousness, weakness.

CV: *palpitations,* tachycardia.

EENT: *blurred vision,* mydriasis, increased ocular tension, cycloplegia, photophobia.

GI: *dry mouth,* dysphagia, *constipation,* heartburn, loss of taste, nausea, vomiting, *paralytic ileus.*

GU: *urinary hesitancy, urine retention,* impotence.

Skin: urticaria, decreased sweating or possible anhidrosis, other dermal manifestations.

Other: fever, allergic reactions.

Overdosage may cause curare-like effects, such as respiratory paralysis.

INTERACTIONS

Amantadine, antihistamines, antiparkinsonian agents, disopyramide, glutethimide, meperidine, phenothiazines, procainamide, quinidine: additive adverse effects. Avoid concomitant use.

Antacids: decreased absorption of orally administered anticholinergics. Separate administration times by 2 to 3 hours.

Ketoconazole: anticholinergics may interfere with ketoconazole absorption. Avoid concomitant use.

Methotrimeprazine: anticholinergics may enhance risk of extrapyramidal reactions. Avoid concomitant use.

CONTRAINDICATIONS

- Contraindicated in patients with acute angle-closure glaucoma, obstructive uropathy, obstructive disease of GI tract, severe ulcerative colitis, myasthenia gravis, hypersensitivity to anticholinergics, paralytic ileus, intestinal atony, unstable cardiovascular status in acute hemorrhage, or toxic megacolon.
- Use cautiously in patients with autonomic neuropathy, hyperthyroidism, coronary artery disease, arrhythmias, CHF, hypertension, hiatal hernia associated with reflux esophagitis, hepatic or renal disease, and ulcerative colitis; or in patients over 40 years because of the increased incidence of glaucoma. Also use cautiously in patients in hot or humid environments. Drug-induced heatstroke can develop.
- Injection contains sodium metabisulfite, which may cause allergic reaction in certain individuals.

NURSING CONSIDERATIONS

- Give 30 minutes to 1 hour before meals and h.s. Bedtime dose can be larger; give at least 2 hours after the last meal of the day.
- Monitor the patient's vital signs and urine output carefully.
- Instruct the patient to avoid driving and other hazardous activities if he is drowsy, dizzy, or has blurred vision; to drink plenty of fluids to help prevent constipation; and to report any rash or skin eruption.
- Gum or sugarless hard candy may relieve dry mouth.

isopropamide iodide

Darbid, Tyrimide‡

Pregnancy Risk Category: C

HOW SUPPLIED

Tablets: 5 mg

ACTION

Mechanism: Blocks acetylcholine, resulting in decreased GI motility and reduced gastric acid secretion.

Duration: 10 to 12 hours.

INDICATIONS & DOSAGE

Adjunctive therapy for peptic ulceration, irritable bowel syndrome –

Adults and children over 12 years: 5 mg P.O. q 12 hours. Some patients may require 10 mg or more b.i.d.

Adjust dosage to individual patient's needs.

ADVERSE REACTIONS

CNS: headache, insomnia, drowsiness, dizziness, *confusion or excitement in elderly patients,* nervousness, weakness.

CV: *palpitations,* tachycardia.

EENT: *blurred vision,* mydriasis, increased ocular tension, cycloplegia, photophobia.

GI: *dry mouth,* dysphagia, heartburn, loss of taste, nausea, vomiting, *constipation, paralytic ileus.*

GU: *urinary hesitancy, urine retention,* impotence.

Skin: urticaria, decreased sweating or possible anhidrosis, other dermal manifestations, iodine skin rash.

Other: fever, allergic reactions.

Overdosage may cause curare-like effects, such as respiratory paralysis.

INTERACTIONS

Amantadine, antihistamines, antiparkinsonian agents, disopyramide, glutethimide, meperidine, phenothiazines, procainamide, quinidine: additive adverse effects. Avoid concomitant use.

Antacids: decreased absorption of orally administered anticholinergics. Separate administration times by 2 to 3 hours.

Ketoconazole: anticholinergics may interfere with ketoconazole absorption. Avoid concomitant use.

Methotrimeprazine: anticholinergics may enhance risk of extrapyramidal reactions. Avoid concomitant use.

CONTRAINDICATIONS

- Contraindicated in patients with hypersensitivity to iodine or anticholinergics, acute angle-closure glaucoma, obstructive uropathy, obstructive disease of GI tract, severe ulcerative colitis, myasthenia gravis, paralytic ileus, intestinal atony, unstable cardiovascular status in acute hemorrhage, or toxic megacolon.
- Use cautiously in patients with autonomic neuropathy, hyperthyroidism, coronary artery disease, cardiac arrhythmias, CHF, hypertension, hiatal hernia associated with reflux esophagitis, hepatic or renal disease, and ulcerative colitis; or in patients over 40 years because of increased incidence of glaucoma. Also use cautiously in patients in hot or humid environments. Drug-induced heatstroke can develop.

NURSING CONSIDERATIONS

- Give 30 minutes to 1 hour before meals and h.s. Bedtime dose can be larger; give at least 2 hours after the last meal of the day.
- Single dose produces 10- to 12-hour antisecretory effect and GI antispasmodic effect.
- Because isopropamide interferes with the 24-hour ^{131}I uptake test and may interfere with determinations of protein-bound iodine, discontinue drug 1 week before thyroid function tests.
- Monitor the patient's vital signs and urine output carefully.
- Instruct the patient to avoid driving

and other hazardous activities if he is drowsy, dizzy, or has blurred vision; to drink plenty of fluids to help prevent constipation; and to report any rash or skin eruption.
- Gum or sugarless hard candy may relieve dry mouth.

levorotatory alkaloids of belladonna

Bellafoline

Pregnancy Risk Category: C

HOW SUPPLIED

Tablets: 0.25 mg

ACTION

Mechanism: Blocks acetylcholine, which decreases GI motility and inhibits gastric acid secretion.
Duration: 4 to 6 hours.

INDICATIONS & DOSAGE

Adjunctive therapy for peptic ulceration, irritable bowel syndrome, and functional GI disorders –
Adults: 0.25 to 0.5 mg P.O. t.i.d.
Children over 6 years: 0.125 to 0.25 mg P.O. t.i.d.

ADVERSE REACTIONS

CNS: headache, insomnia, drowsiness, dizziness, *confusion or excitement in elderly patients,* nervousness, weakness.
CV: *palpitations,* tachycardia.
EENT: *blurred vision,* mydriasis, increased ocular tension, cycloplegia, photophobia.
GI: *dry mouth,* dysphagia, heartburn, loss of taste, *constipation, paralytic ileus.*
GU: *urinary hesitancy, urine retention,* impotence.
Skin: urticaria, decreased sweating or possible anhidrosis, other dermal manifestations.
Other: fever, allergic reactions.

Overdosage may cause curare-like effects, such as repiratory paralysis.

INTERACTIONS

Amantadine, antihistamines, antiparkinsonian agents, disopyramide, glutethimide, meperidine, phenothiazines, procainamide, quinidine: additive adverse effects. Avoid concomitant use.
Antacids: decreased absorption of orally administered anticholinergics. Separate administration times by 2 to 3 hours.
Ketoconazole: anticholinergics may interfere with ketoconazole absorption. Avoid concomitant use.
Methotrimeprazine: anticholinergics may enhance risk of extrapyramidal reactions. Avoid concomitant use.

CONTRAINDICATIONS

- Contraindicated in patients with acute angle-closure glaucoma, obstructive uropathy, obstructive disease of GI tract, severe ulcerative colitis, myasthenia gravis, hypersensitivity to anticholinergics, paralytic ileus, intestinal atony, unstable cardiovascular status in acute hemorrhage, or toxic megacolon.
- Use cautiously in patients with autonomic neuropathy, hyperthyroidism, coronary artery disease, arrhythmias, CHF, hypertension, hiatal hernia associated with reflux esophagitis, hepatic or renal disease, and ulcerative colitis; or in patients over 40 years because of increased incidence of glaucoma. Also use cautiously in patients in hot or humid environments. Drug-induced heatstroke can develop.

NURSING CONSIDERATIONS

- Administer 30 minutes to 1 hour before meals.
- Monitor the patient's vital signs and urine output carefully.
- Instruct the patient to avoid driving and other hazardous activities if he is drowsy, dizzy, or has blurred vision; to drink plenty of fluids to help pre-

vent constipation; and to report any rash or skin eruption.
• Sugarless gum or hard candy may relieve dry mouth.

mepenzolate bromide
Cantil**

Pregnancy Risk Category: C

HOW SUPPLIED
Tablets: 25 mg

ACTION
Mechanism: Blocks acetylcholine, which decreases GI motility and inhibits gastric acid secretion.
Duration: 4 to 6 hours.

INDICATIONS & DOSAGE
Adjunctive therapy in treating peptic ulceration, irritable bowel syndrome, and neurologic bowel disturbances–
Adults: 25 to 50 mg P.O. t.i.d. to q.i.d. with meals and h.s. Adjust dosage to individual patient's needs.

ADVERSE REACTIONS
CNS: headache, insomnia, drowsiness, dizziness, *confusion or excitement in elderly patients,* nervousness, weakness.
CV: *palpitations,* tachycardia.
EENT: *blurred vision,* mydriasis, increased ocular tension, cycloplegia, photophobia.
GI: *dry mouth,* dysphagia, heartburn, loss of taste, nausea, *constipation,* vomiting, *paralytic ileus.*
GU: *urinary hesitancy, urine retention,* impotence.
Skin: urticaria, decreased sweating or possible anhidrosis, other dermal manifestations.
Other: fever, allergic reactions.

Overdosage may cause curare-like effects, such as respiratory paralysis.

INTERACTIONS
Amantadine, antihistamines, antiparkinsonian agents, disopyramide, glutethimide, meperidine, phenothiazines, procainamide, quinidine: additive adverse effects. Avoid concomitant use.
Antacids: decreased absorption of orally administered anticholinergics. Separate administration times by 2 to 3 hours.
Ketoconazole: anticholinergics may interfere with ketoconazole absorption. Avoid concomitant use.
Methotrimeprazine: anticholinergics may enhance risk of extrapyramidal reactions. Avoid concomitant use.

CONTRAINDICATIONS
• Contraindicated in patients with acute angle-closure glaucoma, obstructive uropathy, obstructive disease of GI tract, severe ulcerative colitis, myasthenia gravis, hypersensitivity to anticholinergics, paralytic ileus, intestinal atony, unstable cardiovascular status in acute hemorrhage, or toxic megacolon. Contains tartrazine, which may precipitate an allergic reaction in certain individuals, especially those hypersensitive to aspirin.
• Use cautiously in patients with autonomic neuropathy, hyperthyroidism, coronary artery disease, arrhythmias, CHF, hypertension, hiatal hernia associated with reflux esophagitis, hepatic or renal disease, and ulcerative colitis; or in patients over 40 years because of increased incidence of glaucoma. Also use cautiously in patients in hot or humid environments. Drug-induced heatstroke can develop.

NURSING CONSIDERATIONS
• Give with meals and h.s.
• Monitor the patient's vital signs and urine output carefully.
• Instruct the patient to avoid driving and other hazardous activities if he is drowsy, dizzy, or has blurred vision; to drink plenty of fluids to help pre-

vent constipation; and to report any rash or skin eruption.

• Sugarless gum or hard candy may relieve dry mouth.

methantheline bromide

Banthine

Pregnancy Risk Category: C

HOW SUPPLIED

Tablets: 50 mg

ACTION

Mechanism: Blocks acetylcholine, which decreases GI motility and inhibits gastric acid secretion.

Onset: within 30 to 45 minutes.

Duration: 4 to 6 hours.

INDICATIONS & DOSAGE

Adjunctive therapy in peptic ulceration, pylorospasm, spastic colon, biliary dyskinesia, pancreatitis, neurogenic bladder, and certain forms of gastritis –

Adults: 50 to 100 mg P.O. q 6 hours.

Children over 1 year: 12.5 to 50 mg P.O. q.i.d.

Children under 1 year: 12.5 to 25 mg P.O. q.i.d.

Neonates: 12.5 mg P.O. b.i.d. to t.i.d.

ADVERSE REACTIONS

CNS: headache, insomnia, drowsiness, dizziness, *confusion or excitement in elderly patients,* nervousness, weakness.

CV: *palpitations,* tachycardia.

EENT: *blurred vision,* mydriasis, increased ocular tension, cycloplegia, photophobia.

GI: *dry mouth,* dysphagia, *constipation,* heartburn, loss of taste, nausea, vomiting, *paralytic ileus.*

GU: *urinary hesitancy, urine retention,* impotence.

Skin: urticaria, decreased sweating or possible anhidrosis, other dermal manifestations.

Other: fever, allergic reactions.

Overdosage may cause curare-like effects, such as respiratory paralysis.

INTERACTIONS

Amantadine, antihistamines, antiparkinsonian agents, disopyramide, glutethimide, meperidine, phenothiazines, procainamide, quinidine: additive adverse effects. Avoid concomitant use.

Antacids: decreased absorption of orally administered anticholinergics. Separate administration times by 2 to 3 hours.

Ketoconazole: anticholinergics may interfere with ketoconazole absorption. Avoid concomitant use.

Methotrimeprazine: anticholinergics may enhance risk of extrapyramidal reactions. Avoid concomitant use.

CONTRAINDICATIONS

• Contraindicated in patients with acute angle-closure glaucoma, obstructive uropathy, obstructive disease of GI tract, severe ulcerative colitis, myasthenia gravis, hypersensitivity to anticholinergics, paralytic ileus, intestinal atony, unstable cardiovascular status in acute hemorrhage, or toxic megacolon.

• Use cautiously in patients with autonomic neuropathy, hyperthyroidism, coronary artery disease, arrhythmias, CHF, hypertension, hiatal hernia associated with reflux esophagitis, hepatic or renal disease, and ulcerative colitis; or in patients over 40 years because of the increased incidence of glaucoma. Also use cautiously in patients in hot or humid environments. Drug-induced heatstroke can develop.

NURSING CONSIDERATIONS

• Give 30 minutes to 1 hour before meals and h.s. Bedtime dose can be larger; give at least 2 hours after the last meal of the day.

• If taking antihistamines, the patient

may experience increased dryness of mouth.

- Monitor the patient's vital signs and urine output carefully.
- Instruct the patient to avoid driving and other hazardous activities if he is drowsy, dizzy, or has blurred vision; to drink plenty of fluids to help prevent constipation; and to report any rash or skin eruption.
- Sugarless gum or hard candy may relieve dry mouth.

methscopolamine bromide

Pamine

Pregnancy Risk Category: C

HOW SUPPLIED

Tablets: 2.5 mg

ACTION

Mechanism: Blocks acetylcholine, which decreases GI motility and inhibits gastric acid secretion.

Duration: 4 to 6 hours.

INDICATIONS & DOSAGE

Adjunctive therapy in peptic ulceration disease and irritable bowel syndrome –

Adults: 2.5 to 5 mg P.O. one-half hour before meals and h.s.

Children: 0.2 mg/kg or 6 mg/m^2 P.O. daily in four divided doses with meals and h.s.

ADVERSE REACTIONS

CNS: headache, insomnia, dizziness, *confusion or excitement in elderly patients,* nervousness, weakness.

CV: *palpitations,* tachycardia.

EENT: *blurred vision,* mydriasis, increased ocular tension, cycloplegia, photophobia.

GI: *dry mouth,* dysphagia, *constipation,* heartburn, loss of taste, nausea, vomiting, *paralytic ileus.*

GU: *urinary hesitancy, urine retention,* impotence.

Skin: urticaria, decreased sweating or possible anhidrosis, other dermal manifestations.

Other: fever, allergic reactions.

Overdosage may cause curare-like effects, such as respiratory paralysis.

INTERACTIONS

Amantadine, antihistamines, antiparkinsonian agents, disopyramide, glutethimide, meperidine, phenothiazines, procainamide, quinidine: additive adverse effects. Avoid concomitant use.

Antacids: decreased absorption of orally administered anticholinergics. Separate administration times by 2 to 3 hours.

Ketoconazole: anticholinergics may interfere with ketoconazole absorption. Avoid concomitant use.

Methotrimeprazine: anticholinergics may enhance risk of extrapyramidal reactions. Avoid concomitant use.

CONTRAINDICATIONS

- Contraindicated in patients with acute angle-closure glaucoma, obstructive uropathy, obstructive disease of GI tract, severe ulcerative colitis, myasthenia gravis, hypersensitivity to anticholinergics, paralytic ileus, intestinal atony, unstable cardiovascular status in acute hemorrhage, or toxic megacolon.
- Use cautiously in patients with autonomic neuropathy, hyperthyroidism, coronary artery disease, arrhythmias, CHF, hypertension, hiatal hernia associated with reflux esophagitis, hepatic or renal disease, and ulcerative colitis; or in patients over 40 years because of increased incidence of glaucoma. Also use cautiously in patients in hot or humid environments. Drug-induced heatstroke can develop.

NURSING CONSIDERATIONS

- Give 30 minutes to 1 hour before meals and h.s. Bedtime dose can be

larger; give at least 2 hours after last meal of the day.
• Monitor the patient's vital signs and urine output carefully.
• Instruct the patient to avoid driving and other hazardous activities if he is drowsy, dizzy, or has blurred vision; to drink plenty of fluids to help prevent constipation; and to report any rash or skin eruption.
• Sugarless gum or hard candy may relieve dry mouth.

oxyphencyclimine hydrochloride

Daricon

Pregnancy Risk Category: C

HOW SUPPLIED

Tablets: 10 mg

ACTION

Mechanism: Exerts a nonspecific, direct spasmolytic action on smooth muscle. Also competitively blocks acetylcholine at muscarinic cholinergic receptors, and possesses local anesthetic properties that may be partly responsible for spasmolysis.
Onset: within 1 to 2 hours. **Duration:** more than 12 hours.

INDICATIONS & DOSAGE

Adjunctive treatment of peptic ulceration disease and irritable bowel syndrome –
Adults: 10 mg P.O. b.i.d. in the morning and h.s., or 5 mg b.i.d. or t.i.d.

ADVERSE REACTIONS

CNS: *headache,* insomnia, drowsiness, *dizziness.*
CV: *palpitations,* tachycardia.
EENT: *blurred vision,* mydriasis, increased intraocular pressure, cycloplegia, photophobia.
GI: *constipation,* nausea, vomiting, *paralytic ileus, dry mouth.*
GU: *urinary hesitancy, urine retention,* impotence.
Skin: urticaria, decreased sweating or possible anhidrosis, other dermal manifestations.
Other: fever, allergic reactions.

Overdosage may cause curare-like effects, such as respiratory paralysis.

INTERACTIONS

Amantadine, antihistamines, antiparkinsonian agents, disopyramide, glutethimide, meperidine, phenothiazines, procainamide, quinidine: additive adverse effects. Avoid concomitant use.
Antacids: decreased absorption of orally administered anticholinergics. Separate administration times by 2 to 3 hours.
Ketoconazole: anticholinergics may interfere with ketoconazole absorption. Avoid concomitant use.
Methotrimeprazine: anticholinergics may enhance risk of extrapyramidal reactions. Avoid concomitant use.

CONTRAINDICATIONS

• Contraindicated in patients with acute angle-closure glaucoma, obstructive uropathy, obstructive disease of GI tract, severe ulcerative colitis, myasthenia gravis, hypersensitivity to anticholinergics, paralytic ileus, intestinal atony, unstable cardiovascular status in acute hemorrhage, or toxic megacolon.
• Use cautiously in patients with autonomic neuropathy, hyperthyroidism, coronary artery disease, arrhythmias, CHF, hypertension, hiatal hernia associated with reflux esophagitis, hepatic or renal disease, and ulcerative colitis; or in patients over 40 years because of increased incidence of glaucoma. Also use cautiously in patients in hot or humid environments. Drug-induced heatstroke can develop.

NURSING CONSIDERATIONS
- Give 30 minutes to 1 hour before breakfast and h.s.
- Monitor the patient's vital signs and urine output carefully.
- Instruct the patient to avoid driving and other hazardous activities if he is drowsy, dizzy, or has blurred vision; to drink plenty of fluids to help prevent constipation; and to report any rash or skin eruption.
- Sugarless gum or hard candy may relieve dry mouth.

propantheline bromide

Norpanth, Pantheline‡, Pro-Banthine, Propanthel†

Pregnancy Risk Category: C

HOW SUPPLIED
Tablets: 7.5 mg, 15 mg

ACTION
Mechanism: Blocks acetylcholine, which decreases GI motility and inhibits gastric acid secretion.
Duration: about 6 hours.

INDICATIONS & DOSAGE
Adjunctive treatment of peptic ulceration, irritable bowel syndrome, and other GI disorders; to reduce duodenal motility during diagnostic radiologic procedures –
Adults: 15 mg P.O. t.i.d. before meals, and 30 mg h.s. q.i.d.
Elderly patients: 7.5 mg P.O. t.i.d. before meals.
Children: 375 mcg/kg or 10 mg/m² P.O. q.i.d.

Drug may be used in conjunction with a histamine-2 receptor antagonist to treat Zollinger-Ellison syndrome.

ADVERSE REACTIONS
CNS: headache, insomnia, drowsiness, dizziness, *confusion or excitement in elderly patients,* nervousness, weakness.
CV: *palpitations,* tachycardia.
EENT: *blurred vision,* mydriasis, increased ocular tension, cycloplegia, photophobia.
GI: *dry mouth,* dysphagia, constipation, heartburn, loss of taste, nausea, vomiting, paralytic ileus.
GU: *urinary hesitancy, urine retention,* impotence.
Skin: urticaria, decreased sweating or possible anhidrosis, other dermal manifestations.
Other: fever, allergic reactions.

Overdosage may cause curare-like effects, such as respiratory paralysis.

INTERACTIONS
Amantadine, antihistamines, antiparkinsonian agents, disopyramide, glutethimide, meperidine, phenothiazines, procainamide, quinidine: additive adverse effects. Avoid concomitant use.
Antacids: decreased absorption of orally administered anticholinergics. Separate administration times by 2 to 3 hours.
Ketoconazole: anticholinergics may interfere with ketoconazole absorption. Avoid concomitant use.
Methotrimeprazine: anticholinergics may enhance risk of extrapyramidal reactions. Avoid concomitant use.

CONTRAINDICATIONS
- Contraindicated in patients with acute angle-closure glaucoma, obstructive uropathy, obstructive disease of GI tract, severe ulcerative colitis, myasthenia gravis, hypersensitivity to anticholinergics, paralytic ileus, intestinal atony, unstable cardiovascular status in acute hemorrhage, or toxic megacolon.
- Use cautiously in patients with autonomic neuropathy, hyperthyroidism, coronary artery disease, arrhythmias, CHF, hypertension, hiatal hernia associated with reflux esophagitis, hepatic or renal disease, and ulcerative colitis; or in patients over 40

years because of the increased incidence of glaucoma. Also use cautiously in patients in hot or humid environments. Drug-induced heatstroke can develop.

NURSING CONSIDERATIONS
- Give 30 minutes to 1 hour before meals and h.s. Bedtime doses can be larger; give at least 2 hours after last meal of the day.
- Monitor the patient's vital signs and urine output carefully.
- Instruct the patient to avoid driving and other hazardous activities if he is drowsy, dizzy, or has blurred vision; to drink plenty of fluids to help prevent constipation; and to report any rash or skin eruption.
- Sugarless gum or hard candy may relieve dry mouth.

---

scopolamine (hyoscine)
Scop‡, Transderm-Scōp, Transderm-V†

scopolamine butylbromide (hyoscine butylbromide)
Buscopan†‡

scopolamine hydrobromide (hyoscine hydrobromide)

Pregnancy Risk Category: C

HOW SUPPLIED
scopolamine
Transdermal patch: 1.5 mg
scopolamine butylbromide
Capsules: 0.25 mg
Suppositories: 10 mg†
Tablets: 10 mg†
scopolamine hydrobromide
Injection: 0.3, 0.4, 0.5, 0.6, and 1 mg/ml in 1-ml vials and ampules; 0.86 mg/ml in 0.5-ml ampules

ACTION
Mechanism: Inhibits muscarinic actions of acetylcholine on autonomic effectors innervated by postganglionic cholinergic neurons. May also affect neural pathways originating in the labyrinth to inhibit nausea and vomiting.
Onset: 15 to 30 minutes after I.M. or S.C. administration, 10 minutes after I.V. injection, within 4 hours of application of transdermal patch. **Peak:** Effects occur within 1 hour of oral administration, 50 to 80 minutes after I.V. injection, 1 to 2 hours after I.M. use. **Duration:** about 2 hours after I.V. use, 4 to 8 hours after I.M. injection, 72 hours after applying transdermal system.

INDICATIONS & DOSAGE
Postencephalitic parkinsonism and other spastic states –
Adults: 0.5 to 1 mg P.O. t.i.d. to q.i.d.; 0.3 to 0.6 mg S.C., I.M., or I.V. (with suitable dilution) t.i.d. to q.i.d.
Children: 0.006 mg/kg or 0.2 mg/m^2 P.O. or S.C. t.i.d. to q.i.d.
Infants 4 to 7 months: 100 mcg I.M. or S.C.
Preoperatively to reduce secretions and block cardiac vagal reflexes –
Adults: 0.4 to 0.6 mg S.C. 30 to 60 minutes before induction of anesthesia.
Children 8 to 12 years: 300 mcg I.M. or I.V.
Children 3 to 8 years: 200 mcg I.M. or I.V.
Children 7 months to 3 years: 150 mcg I.M. or I.V.
Infants 4 to 7 months: 100 mcg I.M. or I.V.
Prevention of nausea and vomiting associated with motion sickness –
Adults: one Transderm-Scōp or Transderm-V patch (a circular flat unit) programmed to deliver 0.5 mg scopolamine daily over 3 days (72 hours), applied to the skin behind the ear several hours before the antiemetic is required.

Not recommended for children.

Dysmenorrhea† –
Adults: 10 to 20 mg P.O. t.i.d. to q.i.d., or 10 mg rectally t.i.d. or q.i.d.

ADVERSE REACTIONS
CNS: disorientation, restlessness, irritability, dizziness, drowsiness, headache.
CV: palpitations, tachycardia, paradoxical bradycardia.
EENT: dilated pupils, blurred vision, photophobia, increased intraocular pressure, difficulty swallowing.
GI: *constipation, dry mouth, nausea, vomiting, epigastric distress.*
GU: urinary hesitancy, urine retention.
Respiratory: bronchial plugging, depressed respirations.
Skin: rash, flushing, dryness.
Other: fever.

Adverse reactions may be caused by pending atropine-like toxicity and are dose related. Individual tolerance varies greatly.

Many adverse reactions (such as dry mouth, constipation) are an expected extension of the drug's pharmacologic activity.

INTERACTIONS
Centrally acting anticholinergics (tricyclic antidepressants, phenothiazines): increased CNS adverse reactions.
Digoxin: increased digoxin levels.
Ethnol, CNS depressants: increased CNS depression.

CONTRAINDICATIONS
• Contraindicated in patients with acute angle-closure glaucoma, obstructive uropathy, obstructive disease of the GI tract, asthma, chronic pulmonary disease, myasthenia gravis, paralytic ileus, intestinal atony, unstable cardiovascular status in acute hemorrhage, or toxic megacolon.
• Use cautiously in patients with autonomic neuropathy, hyperthyroidism, coronary artery disease, arrhythmias, CHF, hypertension, hiatal hernia associated with reflux esophagitis, hepatic or renal disease, and ulcerative colitis; in patients over 40 years because of the increased incidence of glaucoma; and in children under 6 years. Also use cautiously in patients in hot or humid environments. Drug-induced heatstroke possible.

NURSING CONSIDERATIONS
• Wash and dry hands thoroughly before and after applying the transdermal patch on dry skin behind the ear and before touching the eye, as pupil may dilate. After removing the system, discard it. Wash hands and application site thoroughly.
• Transdermal method releases a controlled therapeutic amount of scopolamine. Transderm-Scōp is effective if applied 2 to 3 hours before experiencing motion, but more effective if used 12 hours before. Therefore, advise the patient to apply patch the night before a planned trip.
• In therapeutic doses, scopolamine may produce amnesia, drowsiness, and euphoria; may need to reorient the patient.
• If patch becomes displaced, remove and replace it with another patch on a fresh skin site behind the ear.
• Withdrawal symptoms (nausea, vomiting, headache, dizziness) can occur if the transdermal system is used longer than 72 hours.
• Advise patients to report signs of urinary hesitancy or urine retention.
• Some patients become temporarily excited or disoriented. Symptoms disappear when sedative effect is complete. Raise the bed's side rails as a precaution.
• Tolerance may develop when given over a long time.
• **I.V. use:** Intermittent and continuous infusions are not recommended. For direct injection, dilute with sterile

water and inject diluted drug at ordered rate through patent I.V. line.
- Protect I.V. solutions from freezing and light, and store at room temperature.
- Have the patient ask the pharmacist for the brochure that comes with the transdermal product.
- Warn patients against driving and other activities that require alertness until CNS effects are known.
- Sugarless gum or hard candy may help minimize dry mouth.

*Liquid form contains alcohol.
**May contain tartrazine.

Common reactions are in italics; ***life-threatening,*** in bold italics.

38

Adrenergics (sympathomimetics)

dobutamine hydrochloride
dopamine hydrochloride
mephentermine sulfate
metaraminol bitartrate
norepinephrine bitartrate
phenylephrine hydrochloride
pseudoephedrine hydrochloride
pseudoephedrine sulfate

COMBINATION PRODUCTS
ENTEX: phenylephrine hydrochloride 5 mg, phenylpropanolamine hydrochloride 45 mg, guaifenesin 400 mg.
ENTEX LIQUID: phenylephrine hydrochloride 5 mg/5 ml, phenylpropanolamine hydrochloride 20 mg/5 ml, guaifenesin 100 mg/5 ml (alcohol 5%).

dobutamine hydrochloride

Dobutrex

Pregnancy Risk Category: C

HOW SUPPLIED
Injection: 12.5 mg/ml in 20-ml vials (parenteral)

ACTION
Mechanism: Directly stimulates $beta_1$ receptors of the heart to increase myocardial contractility and stroke volume. At therapeutic doses, decreases peripheral vascular resistance (afterload), reduces ventricular filling pressure (preload), and may facilitate AV nodal conduction. Net result is increased cardiac output.
Onset: 1 to 2 minutes, up to 10 minutes if infusion rate is slow. **Peak:** Effects usually occur within 10 minutes of starting infusion. **Duration:** plasma half-life, 2 minutes.

INDICATIONS & DOSAGE
To increase cardiac output in the short-term treatment of cardiac decompensation caused by depressed contractility, such as during refractory heart failure, and as adjunct in cardiac surgery –
Adults: 2.5 to 10 mcg/kg/minute I.V. infusion. Infusion rates up to 40 mcg/kg/minute may be needed (rare).

ADVERSE REACTIONS
CNS: headache.
CV: *increased heart rate,* ***hypertension, PVCs,*** angina, nonspecific chest pain.
GI: nausea, vomiting.
Respiratory: shortness of breath.
Other: mild leg cramps or tingling sensation.

INTERACTIONS
Beta blockers: may antagonize dobutamine effects. Do not use together.
General anesthetics: greater incidence of ventricular arrhythmias.

CONTRAINDICATIONS
- Contraindicated in idiopathic hypertrophic subaortic stenosis and in patients hypersensitive to the drug or any component of the formulation. Contains sulfites, which may cause an allergic response in sensitive patients.
- Do not administer through the same I.V. line with other drugs. Drug is incompatible with heparin, hydrocortisone sodium succinate, cefazolin, cefamandole, neutral cephalothin, penicillin, and sodium ethacrynate.
- Incompatible with alkaline solutions. Do not mix with sodium bicarbonate injection. Infusions for up to 72 hours produce no more adverse effects than shorter infusions.
- Use cautiously in patients with a history of hypertension. Drug may precipitate an exaggerated pressor response.

NURSING CONSIDERATIONS

- A unique agent that increases contractility of failing heart without inducing marked tachycardia, except at high doses.
- Use with nitroprusside for additive effects.
- Because drug increases AV conduction, patients with atrial fibrillation may develop a rapid ventricular rate. Administer a digitalis glycoside before dobutamine as ordered.
- Before initiating therapy with dobutamine, correct hypovolemia with plasma volume expanders.
- **I.V. use:** Administer using a central venous catheter or large peripheral vein. Titrate infusion according to the doctor's orders and the patient's condition. Use an infusion pump.
- Dilute concentrate for injection before administration. Compatible solutions include D_5W, 0.45% sodium chloride injection, 0.9% sodium chloride injection, and lactated Ringer's injection. The contents of one vial (250 mg) diluted with 1,000 ml of solution yields a concentration of 250 mcg/ml; diluted with 500 ml, a concentration of 500 mcg/ml; diluted with 250 ml, a concentration of 1,000 mcg/ml. Maximum concentration should not exceed 5 mg/ml.
- Avoid extravasation; may cause an inflammatory response. Change I.V. sites regularly to avoid phlebitis.
- Continuously monitor ECG, blood pressure, pulmonary capillary wedge pressure, cardiac condition, and urine output.
- Monitor serum electrolytes. Drug may lower serum potassium levels.
- Oxidation of drug may slightly discolor admixtures containing dobutamine. This does not indicate a significant loss of potency provided drug is used within 24 hours of reconstitution.
- I.V. solutions remain stable for 24 hours.

dopamine hydrochloride

Dopastat, Intropin, Revimine†‡

Pregnancy Risk Category: C

HOW SUPPLIED

Injection: 40 mg/ml, 80 mg/ml, 160 mg/ml parenteral concentrate for injection for I.V. infusion; 0.8 mg/ml (200 or 400 mg) in dextrose 5%; 1.6 mg/ml (400 or 800 mg) in dextrose 5%, 3.2 mg/ml (800 mg) in dextrose 5% parenteral injection for I.V. infusion.

ACTION

Mechanism: Stimulates dopaminergic, beta-adrenergic, and alpha-adrenergic receptors of the sympathetic nervous system.

Onset: occurs within 5 minutes of starting I.V. infusion. **Duration:** subsides within 10 minutes of discontinuing infusion.

INDICATIONS & DOSAGE

To treat shock and correct hemodynamic imbalances; to improve perfusion to vital organs; to increase cardiac output; to correct hypotension; to treat acute renal failure –

Adults: initially, 2 to 5 mcg/kg/minute by I.V. infusion. Titrate dosage to desired hemodynamic or renal response; infusion may be increased by 1 to 4 mcg/kg/minute at 10 to 30 minute intervals.

ADVERSE REACTIONS

CNS: headache.

CV: ***arrhythmias,*** ectopic beats, tachycardia, anginal pain, palpitations, *hypotension.* Less frequently, bradycardia, widening of QRS complex, conduction disturbances, vasoconstriction.

GI: nausea, vomiting.

Other: necrosis and tissue sloughing with extravasation, piloerection, dyspnea.

INTERACTIONS

Beta blockers: may antagonize dopamine's effects.
Ergot alkaloids: extreme elevations in blood pressure. Don't use together.
Inhalation anesthetics: increased risk of arrhythmias or hypertension. Monitor closely.
MAO inhibitors: may cause hypertensive crisis. Avoid if possible.
Phenytoin: may lower blood pressure of dopamine-stabilized patients. Monitor carefully.

CONTRAINDICATIONS

- Contraindicated in patients with uncorrected tachyarrhythmias, pheochromocytoma, or ventricular fibrillation.
- Use cautiously in patients with occlusive vascular disease, cold injuries, diabetic endarteritis, and arterial embolism; in pregnant patients; and in those taking MAO inhibitors.

NURSING CONSIDERATIONS

- Not a substitute for blood or fluid volume deficit. If deficit exists, replace fluid before administering vasopressors.
- Acidosis decreases effectiveness of dopamine.
- During infusion, frequently monitor ECG, blood pressure, cardiac output, central venous pressure, pulmonary capillary wedge pressure, pulse rate, urine output, and color and temperature of extremities.
- Observe patients closely for adverse effects. If they develop, the doctor will adjust or discontinue dosage.
- After drug is stopped, watch closely for sudden drop in blood pressure. Taper dosages slowly to evaluate stability of blood pressure.
- Patient response depends upon dosage and pharmacologic effect. Dosages of 0.5 to 2 mcg/kg/minute predominantly stimulate dopamine receptors and produce vasodilation of the renal vasculature. Dosages of 2 to 10 mcg/kg/minute stimulate beta-adrenergic receptors. Higher doses also stimulate alpha-adrenergic receptors.
- Most patients satisfactorily maintained on less than 20 mcg/kg/minute.
- If a disproportionate rise in diastolic pressure (a marked decrease in pulse pressure) is observed in patients receiving dopamine, decrease infusion rate and observe carefully for further evidence of predominant vasoconstrictor activity, unless such an effect is desired.
- If dosages exceed 50 mcg/kg/minute, check urine output often. If urine flow decreases without hypotension, consider reducing dose.
- **I.V. use:** Use a central line or large vein, such as in the antecubital fossa, to minimize risk of extravasation. Watch infusion site carefully for signs of extravasation; if it occurs, stop infusion immediately and call doctor. Extravasation may require treatment by infiltration of the area with 5 to 10 mg phentolamine and 10 to 15 ml 0.9% sodium chloride solution. Don't mix with alkaline solutions. Use D_5W, 0.9% sodium chloride solution, or a combination of D_5W and 0.9% sodium chloride solution. Mix just before use.
- Use a continuous infusion pump to regulate flow rate.
- Do not mix other drugs in I.V. container with dopamine. Do not give alkaline drugs (for example, sodium bicarbonate, phenytoin sodium) through I.V. line containing dopamine.
- Dopamine solutions deteriorate after 24 hours. Discard at that time or earlier if solution is discolored.

mephentermine sulfate

Wyamine

Pregnancy Risk Category: C

HOW SUPPLIED

Injection: 15 mg/ml, 30 mg/ml

ACTION

Mechanism: Indirectly stimulates beta- and alpha-adrenergic receptors by releasing norepinephrine.

Onset: immediately after I.V. injection, within 5 to 15 minutes after I.M. injection. **Duration:** lasts 15 to 30 minutes after I.V. injection, 1 to 2 hours after I.M. injection.

INDICATIONS & DOSAGE

Hypotension following spinal anesthesia –

Adults: 30 to 45 mg I.V. in a single injection, then 30 mg I.V. repeated p.r.n. Maintenance of blood pressure: continuous I.V. infusion of 0.1% solution of mephentermine in D_5W.

Children: 0.4 mg/kg I.M. or I.V.

Hypotension following spinal anesthesia during obstetric procedures –

Adults: initially 15 mg I.V. p.r.n.

Prevention of hypotension during spinal anesthesia –

Adults: 30 to 45 mg I.M. 10 to 20 minutes before anesthesia.

ADVERSE REACTIONS

CNS: euphoria, nervousness, anxiety, tremor, incoherence, drowsiness, ***seizures,*** visual hallucinations (with large doses).

CV: ***arrhythmias, marked elevation of blood pressure (with large doses),*** AV block, tachycardia.

INTERACTIONS

Antihypertensives, guanethidine, phenothiazines, reserpine, nitrates: decreased effects of these adrenergic blocking agents.

Beta-adrenergic blocking agents, rauwolfia alkaloids: mutual inhibition of therapeutic effects.

CNS stimulants, mazindol, methylphenidate, sympathomimetics: increased CNS stimulation.

Digitalis glycosides, levodopa, inhalation anesthetics: increased risk of arrhythmias.

Ergot alkaloids, oxytocin: enhanced vasoconstriction.

Inhalation anesthetics: increased risk of hypertension. Monitor closely.

MAO inhibitors: may cause severe hypertension (hypertensive crisis) or arrhythmias. Don't use together.

Thyroid hormones: enhanced risk of coronary insufficiency.

Tricyclic antidepressants, maprotiline: decreased pressure of mephentermine.

CONTRAINDICATIONS

- Contraindicated in patients with concealed hemorrhage or hypotension from hemorrhage, except in emergencies; and in patients receiving phenothiazines, or who have received MAO inhibitors within 2 weeks.
- Use cautiously in patients with arteriosclerosis, cardiovascular disease, hyperthyroidism, hypertension, and chronic illness.
- May increase uterine contractions during third trimester of pregnancy.

NURSING CONSIDERATIONS

- Not a substitute for blood or fluid volume deficit. If deficit exists, replace fluid before administering vasopressors.
- Hypercapnia, hypoxia or acidosis may reduce effectiveness or increase adverse effects. Identify and correct before and during administration.
- **I.V. use:** Administer at 1 to 5 mg/minute. Can be given undiluted; I.V. drug is not irritating to tissue, and extravasation is not dangerous. To prepare 0.1% I.V. solution, add 16.6 ml of mephentermine (30 mg/ml) to 500 ml of D_5W.
- I.M. route may be used because drug is not irritating to tissue.
- Don't mix with I.V. hydralazine or epinephrine, which are physically incompatible with mephentermine.
- During infusion, frequently monitor ECG, blood pressure, cardiac output, central venous pressure, pulmonary

capillary wedge pressure, pulse rate, urine output, and color and temperature of extremities. Titrate infusion rate according to findings and the doctor's guidelines. Use a continuous infusion pump to regulate flow rate.
• During infusion, check blood pressure every 2 minutes until stabilized; then every 10 to 15 minutes.
• Monitor blood pressure until stable, even after discontinuing drug.
• Observe patients closely for adverse effects. If they develop, the doctor will adjust or discontinue dosage.

metaraminol bitartrate

Aramine

Pregnancy Risk Category: D

HOW SUPPLIED

Injection: 10 mg/ml

ACTION

Mechanism: Stimulates alpha-adrenergic receptors within the sympathetic nervous system.
Onset: 10 minutes after I.V. injection, 10 minutes after I.M. injection, 5 to 20 minutes after S.C injection.
Duration: lasts 20 minutes after I.V. injection, up to 90 minutes after S.C. or I.M. injection.

INDICATIONS & DOSAGE

Prevention of hypotension –
Adults: 2 to 10 mg I.M. or S.C.
Treatment of hypotension caused by severe shock –
Adults: 0.5 to 5 mg by direct I.V. injection, followed by I.V. infusion titrated to maintain blood pressure.
Children: 0.01 mg/kg as single I.V. injection; 1 mg/25 ml of D_5W as I.V. infusion. Adjust rate to maintain blood pressure in normal range. 0.1 mg/kg I.M. as single dose, p.r.n. Allow at least 10 minutes to elapse before increasing dose because maximum effect is not immediately apparent.

ADVERSE REACTIONS

CNS: apprehension, restlessness, dizziness, headache, tremor, weakness; with excessive use, ***seizures.***
CV: hypertension; hypotension; precordial pain; palpitations; ***arrhythmias,*** including sinus or ***ventricular tachycardia;*** bradycardia; premature supraventricular contractions; AV dissociation.
GI: nausea, vomiting.
GU: decreased urine output.
Respiratory: respiratory distress.
Skin: flushing, pallor, sweating.
Other: abscess, hyperglycemia, necrosis, sloughing upon extravasation, ***metabolic acidosis in hypovolemia,*** *increased body temperature.*

INTERACTIONS

Beta adrenergic blocking agents: mutual inhibition of drug effects, with possible hypertension, bradycardia, and heart block. Avoid concomitant use.
Cocaine, digitalis glycosides, doxapram, ergot alkaloids, general anesthetics, levodopa, maprotiline, other sympathomimetics, thyroid hormones, or tricyclic antidepressants: increased risk of adverse cardiac effects. Monitor closely.
Guanadrel, guanethidine: metaraminol may decrease the hypotensive effect of these drugs; guanadrel and guanethidine may enhance the pressor effect of metaraminol. Avoid concomitant use.
MAO inhibitors, furazolidone, procarbazine: may cause severe hypertension (hypertensive crisis). Don't use within 14 days of MAO inhibitor therapy.

CONTRAINDICATIONS

• Contraindicated in patients with peripheral or mesenteric thrombosis, pulmonary edema, hypercarbia, or acidosis; also in patients during anesthesia with cyclopropane and halogenated hydrocarbon anesthetics.

- Use cautiously in patients with heart disease, hypertension, peripheral vascular disease, thyroid disease, diabetes, cirrhosis, malaria, or sulfite sensitivity, and in patients receiving digitalis glycosides.

NURSING CONSIDERATIONS

- Do not mix metaraminol with other drugs.
- Not a substitute for blood or fluid volume deficit. If deficit exists, replace fluid before administering vasopressors.
- Blood pressure should be raised to slightly less than the patient's normal level. Be careful to avoid excessive blood pressure response. Headache may be a symptom of hypertension. Rapidly induced hypertensive response can cause acute pulmonary edema, arrhythmias, and cardiac arrest.
- Observe patients closely for adverse effects. If they develop, the doctor will adjust or discontinue dosage.
- Keep emergency drugs on hand to reverse effects of metaraminol: atropine for reflex bradycardia; phentolamine to decrease vasopressor effects; and propranolol for arrhythmias.
- When discontinuing drug, gradually slow infusion rate. Continue monitoring vital signs, watching for possible severe drop in blood pressure. Keep equipment nearby to resume drug, if necessary. Do not reinstate pressor therapy until the systolic blood pressure falls below 70 to 80 mm Hg.
- Allow at least 10 minutes between doses. Drug effects are not always immediately apparent.
- Because of prolonged action, a cumulative effect is possible. With an excessive vasopressor response, elevated blood pressure may persist after drug is stopped.
- Urine output may decrease initially, then increase as blood pressure reaches normal level. Report persistent decreased urine output.
- Closely monitor patients with diabetes; insulin dose may need to be adjusted.
- **I.V. use:** To prepare an I.V. infusion, mix 15 to 100 mg in 500 ml of 0.9% sodium chloride solution or D_5W. Adjust rate to maintain blood pressure.
- During infusion, check blood pressure every 5 minutes until stabilized; then every 15 minutes. Monitor ECG, blood pressure, cardiac output, central venous pressure, pulmonary capillary wedge pressure, pulse rate, urine output, and extremity color and temperature often. Titrate infusion rate according to findings, using the doctor's guidelines. Use a continuous infusion pump to regulate flow rate.
- Use a central venous catheter or large veins, such as in the antecubital fossa, to minimize risk of extravasation. Use a continuous infusion pump to regulate infusion flow rate and a piggyback setup so I.V. can continue if drug is stopped. Watch infusion site carefully for signs of extravasation. If it occurs, stop infusion immediately and call the doctor.
- To treat extravasation, infiltrate site promptly with 10 to 15 ml of 0.9% sodium chloride injection containing 5 to 10 mg phentolamine. Use a fine needle.
- Keep solution in light-resistant container, away from heat.

norepinephrine bitartrate (levarterenol bitartrate, noradrenaline acid tartrate)

Levophed

Pregnancy Risk Category: D

HOW SUPPLIED

Injection: 1 mg/ml

ACTION

Mechanism: Stimulates alpha- and $beta_1$-adrenergic receptors within the sympathetic nervous system.

*Liquid form contains alcohol.
**May contain tartrazine.

Common reactions are in italics; ***life-threatening,*** in bold italics.

Onset: immediately after infusion begins. **Duration:** 1 to 2 minutes after infusion ends.

INDICATIONS & DOSAGE

To restore blood pressure in acute hypotensive states –

Adults: initially, 8 to 12 mcg/minute I.V. infusion, then adjust to maintain normal blood pressure. Average maintenance dosage is 2 to 4 mcg/minute.

Children: 2 mcg/m^2/minute I.V. infusion; adjust dosage based upon patient response.

Severe hypotension during cardiac arrest –

Children: initial infusion rate is 0.1 mcg/kg/minute. Adjust rate according to patient response.

ADVERSE REACTIONS

CNS: *headache,* anxiety, weakness, dizziness, tremor, restlessness, insomnia.

CV: bradycardia, ***severe hypertension,*** marked increase in peripheral resistance, decreased cardiac output, ***arrhythmias, ventricular tachycardia, fibrillation,*** bigeminal rhythm, AV dissociation, precordial pain.

GU: decreased urine output.

Respiratory: respiratory difficulties.

Other: fever, metabolic acidosis, hyperglycemia, increased glycogenolysis, irritation with extravasation, swelling and enlargement of thyroid.

INTERACTIONS

Alpha-adrenergic blocking agents: may antagonize drug effects.

Antihistamine, ergot alkaloids, guanethidine, methyldopa: when given with sympathomimetics, may cause severe hypertension (hypertensive crisis). Don't give together.

Inhalation anesthetics: increased risk of arrhythmias. Monitor closely.

MAO inhibitors: increased risk of hypertensive crisis.

CONTRAINDICATIONS

- Contraindicated in patients with mesenteric or peripheral vascular thrombosis, profound hypoxia, hypercarbia, hypotension from blood volume deficits; and during cyclopropane and halothane anesthesia or in pregnant patients.
- *Use with extreme caution* in patients receiving MAO inhibitors or tricyclic antidepressants. Use cautiously in patients with hypertension, hyperthyroidism, severe cardiac disease, and sulfite sensitivity.

NURSING CONSIDERATIONS

- Not a substitute for blood or fluid volume deficit. If deficit exists, replace fluid before administering vasopressors.
- When discontinuing drug, gradually slow infusion rate. Continue monitoring vital signs, watching for possible severe drop in blood pressure.
- Report decreased urine output to the doctor immediately.
- Keep emergency drugs on hand to reverse effects of norepinephrine: atropine for reflex bradycardia; phentolamine for increased vasopressor effects; and propranolol for arrhythmias.
- **I.V. use:** Use a central venous catheter or a large vein, as in the antecubital fossa, to minimize risk of extravasation. Administer in dextrose 5% in 0.9% sodium chloride injection; 0.9% sodium chloride injection alone is not recommended. Use continuous infusion pump to regulate infusion flow rate and a piggyback setup so I.V. can continue if norepinephrine is stopped.
- During infusion, frequently monitor ECG, blood pressure, cardiac output, central venous pressure, pulmonary capillary wedge pressure, pulse rate, urine output, and color and temperature of extremities. Titrate infusion rate according to findings and the doctor's guidelines. Use continuous infusion pump to regulate flow rate.

In previously hypertensive patients, blood pressure should be raised no higher than 40 mm Hg below preexisting systolic pressure.

• Check site frequently for signs of extravasation. If it occurs, stop infusion immediately and call the doctor. He may counteract effect by infiltrating area with 5 to 10 mg phentolamine and 10 to 15 ml of 0.9% sodium chloride solution. Also check for blanching along course of infused vein; may progress to superficial sloughing.
• If prolonged I.V. therapy is necessary, change injection site frequently.
• Never leave patients unattended during infusion. Also, check blood pressure every 2 minutes until stabilized; then every 5 minutes.
• Norepinephrine solutions deteriorate after 24 hours.
• Store drug protected from light. Discard discolored solutions or solutions that contain a precipitate.

phenylephrine hydrochloride

Neo-Synephrine

Pregnancy Risk Category: C

HOW SUPPLIED

Injection: 10 mg/ml

ACTION

Mechanism: Predominantly stimulates alpha-adrenergic receptors in the sympathetic nervous system.
Onset: immediately after I.V. injection, within 10 to 15 minutes after S.C. or I.M. injection. **Duration:** 15 to 20 minutes after I.V injection, ½ to 2 hours after I.M. injection, 50 minutes to 1 hour after S.C. injection.

INDICATIONS & DOSAGE

Hypotensive emergencies during spinal anesthesia –
Adults: initially, 0.1 to 0.2 mg I.V., then subsequent doses of 0.1 to 0.2 mg.
Maintenance of blood pressure during spinal or inhalation anesthesia –
Adults: 2 to 3 mg S.C. or I.M. 3 or 4 minutes before anesthesia.
Children: 0.04 mg to 0.088 mg/kg S.C. or I.M.
Mild to moderate hypotension –
Adults: 2 to 5 mg S.C. or I.M.; repeat in 1 to 2 hours as needed and tolerated. Initial dose should not exceed 5 mg. Alternatively, give 0.1 to 0.5 mg I.V., not to be repeated more often than 10 to 15 minutes.
Children: 0.1 mg/kg I.M. or S.C.; repeat in 1 to 2 hours as needed and tolerated.
Paroxysmal supraventricular tachycardia –
Adults: initially, 0.5 mg rapid I.V.; subsequent doses should not exceed the preceding dose by more than 0.1 to 0.2 mg and should not exceed 1 mg.
Prolongation of spinal anesthesia –
Adults: 2 to 5 mg added to anesthetic solution.
Severe hypotension and shock (including drug-induced) –
Adults: 10 mg in 250 ml to 500 ml of D_5W or 0.9% sodium chloride injection. Start 100 to 180 mcg/minute I.V. infusion, then decrease to a maintenance infusion of 40 to 60 mcg/minute when blood pressure stabilizes.
Vasoconstrictor for regional anesthesia –
Adults: 1 mg phenylephrine added to 20 ml local anesthetic.

ADVERSE REACTIONS

CNS: *headache, restlessness, lightheadedness, weakness,* ***seizures.***
CV: palpitations, bradycardia, ***arrhythmias,*** hypertension, anginal pain, decreased cardiac output.
EENT: blurred vision.
GI: vomiting.
Skin: goose bumps, feeling of coolness.

*Liquid form contains alcohol. *Common* reactions are in italics; ***life-threatening,*** in bold italics.
**May contain tartrazine.

Other: tachyphylaxis (may occur with continued use), tissue sloughing with extravasation.

INTERACTIONS

MAO inhibitors: may cause severe hypertension (hypertensive crisis). Don't use together.

Oxytocics, tricyclic antidepressants (TCAs): increased pressor response. Observe patient.

CONTRAINDICATIONS

- Contraindicated in patients with acute angle-closure glaucoma, hypotension, ventricular tachycardia, severe coronary disease, or cardiovascular disease (including myocardial infarction), and in patients who are taking MAO inhibitors or TCAs.
- Use with extreme caution in patients with heart disease, hyperthyroidism, diabetes, severe atherosclerosis, bradycardia, partial heart block, myocardial disease, or sulfite sensitivity, and in elderly patients.

NURSING CONSIDERATIONS

- Longer acting than ephedrine and epinephrine.
- Causes little or no CNS stimulation.
- Monitor blood pressure frequently; avoid severe increase. Maintain blood pressure at slightly below the patient's normal level. In previously normotensive patients, maintain systolic blood pressure at 80 to 100 mm Hg; in previously hypertensive patients, maintain systolic blood pressure at 30 to 40 mm Hg below their usual level.
- Drug is incompatible with butacaine sulfate, alkalies, ferric salts, and oxidizing agents.
- May reverse severe increase in blood pressure with phentolamine.
- **I.V. use:** For direct injection, dilute 10 mg (1 ml) with 9 ml sterile water for injection to provide a solution containing 1 mg/ml. I.V. infusions are usually prepared by adding 10 mg of drug to 500 ml of D_5W or 0.9% sodium chloride injection. The initial infusion rate is usually 100 to 180 mcg/minute; the maintenance infusion rate is usually 40 to 60 mcg/minute.
- With prolonged I.V. infusions, avoid abrupt withdrawal. During infusion, frequently monitor ECG, blood pressure, cardiac output, central venous pressure, pulmonary capillary wedge pressure, pulse rate, urine output, and color and temperature of extremities. Titrate infusion rate according to findings and the doctor's guidelines. Use a continuous infusion pump to regulate flow rate.
- Use a central venous catheter or a large vein, as in the antecubital fossa, to minimize risk of extravasation. Use a continuous infusion pump to regulate infusion flow rate.
- To treat extravasation, infiltrate site promptly with 10 to 15 ml of 0.9% sodium chloride injection containing 5 to 10 mg phentolamine. Use a fine needle.

pseudoephedrine hydrochloride

Afrinol Repetabs◊, Allerid◊, Cenafed◊, Children's Sudafed Liquid◊, Chlor-Trimeton Non-Drowsy Formula◊, Congestac N.D. caplets†◊, Decofed◊, De Fed-60◊, Dorcol Children's Decongestant◊, Drixoral Non-Drowsy Formula◊, Efidac/24◊, Eltor 120†◊, Genaphed◊, Halofed◊, Halofed Adult Strength◊, Maxenal†◊, Myfredine◊, NeoFed◊, Novafed◊, Ornex Cold†◊, Otrivin◊, Pediacare Infant's Oral Decongestant Drops◊, Pseudo◊, Pseudofrin†◊, Pseudogest◊, Robidrine◊, Sinufed◊, Sinustat◊, Sudafed◊, Sudafed 12-Hour◊, Sudafed-60◊, Sudrin◊, Sufedrin◊

pseudoephedrine sulfate

Afrinol Repetabs, Drixoral‡

Pregnancy Risk Category: B

HOW SUPPLIED

hydrochloride

Tablets: 30 mg◊, 60 mg◊
Tablets (extended-release): 120 mg◊, 240 mg◊
Capsules: 60 mg
Capsules (extended-release): 120 mg
Oral solution: 15 mg/5 ml◊, 30 mg/5 ml◊, 7.5 mg/0.8 ml◊
Syrup: 30 mg/5 ml

sulfate

Tablets (extended-release): 120 mg (60 mg immediate release, 60 mg delayed release)◊

ACTION

Mechanism: Stimulates alpha-adrenergic receptors in the respiratory tract, producing vasoconstriction.
Onset: within 30 minutes of regular-release preparations. **Duration:** 4 to 8 hours after regular-release preparations, 12 to 24 hours after extended-release preparations.

INDICATIONS & DOSAGE

Nasal and eustachian tube decongestant –
Adults: 60 mg P.O. q 4 hours. Maximum dosage is 240 mg daily.
Children age 6 to 12: 30 mg P.O. q 4 to 6 hours. Maximum dosage is 120 mg daily.
Children age 2 to 6: 15 mg P.O. q 4 to 6 hours. Maximum dosage is 60 mg/day.
Extended-release tablets:
Adults and children over age 12: 120 mg P.O. q 12 hours, or 240 mg P.O. (Efidac/24) once daily.
Relief of nasal congestion –
Adults: 120 mg q 12 hours.

ADVERSE REACTIONS

CNS: *anxiety,* transient stimulation, tremors, dizziness, headache, insomnia, *nervousness.*
CV: arrhythmias, *palpitations,* tachycardia.
EENT: dry mouth.
GI: anorexia, nausea, vomiting.
GU: difficulty urinating.
Respiratory: respiratory difficulty.
Skin: pallor.

INTERACTIONS

Antihypertensives: may attenuate hypotensive effect.
MAO inhibitors: may cause severe hypertension (hypertensive crisis). Don't use together.

CONTRAINDICATIONS

- Contraindicated in patients with severe hypertension or severe coronary artery disease, in patients receiving MAO inhibitors, and in breast-feeding patients. Extended-release preparations are contraindicated for children under age 12.
- Use cautiously in patients with hypertension, cardiac disease, diabetes, glaucoma, hyperthyroidism, and prostatic hyperplasia.

NURSING CONSIDERATIONS

- Do not crush or break extended-release forms.
- Elderly patients are more sensitive to the drug's effects.
- Warn against using OTC products containing other sympathomimetics.
- Tell the patient to stop drug if he becomes unusually restless and to notify the doctor promptly.
- Tell the patient not to take drug within 2 hours of bedtime because it can cause insomnia.
- Tell patients to relieve dry mouth with sugarless gum or hard candy.

39

Adrenergic blockers (sympatholytics)

dihydroergotamine mesylate
ergotamine tartrate
methysergide maleate
phenoxybenzamine hydrochloride
(See Chapter 22, ANTIHYPERTENSIVES.)
propranolol hydrochloride
(See Chapter 21, ANTIANGINALS.)

COMBINATION PRODUCTS
BELLERGAL-S**, BEL-PHEN-ERGOT S, PHENERBEL-S: ergotamine tartrate 0.6 mg, levorotatory belladonna alkaloids 0.2 mg, and phenobarbital 40 mg.
CAFERGOT, ERCAF, LANATRATE, WIGRAINE: ergotamine tartrate 1 mg and caffeine 100 mg.
CAFERGOT-PB SUPPOSITORIES: ergotamine tartrate 2 mg, caffeine 100 mg, levorotatory belladonna alkaloids 0.25 mg and pentobarbital 60 mg.
CAFERGOT SUPPOSITORIES: ergotamine tartrate 2 mg and caffeine 100 mg.
ERGO-CAFF PB: ergotamine tartrate 1 mg, belladonna alkaloids 0.125 mg, caffeine 100 mg, and pentobarbital sodium 30 mg.
HYDERGINE: dihydroergocornine mesylate 0.167 mg, dihydroergocristine mesylate 0.167 mg, and dihydroergocryptine mesylate 0.167 mg.
MIGRAL: ergotamine tartrate 1 mg, caffeine 50 mg, and cyclizine hydrochloride 25 mg.
WIGRAINE SUPPOSITORIES: ergotamine tartrate 2 mg and caffeine 100 mg.

dihydroergotamine mesylate

D.H.E. 45, Dihydergot‡, Dihydroergotamine-Sandoz†

Pregnancy Risk Category: X

HOW SUPPLIED
Injection: 1 mg/ml

ACTION
Mechanism: Inhibits effects of epinephrine, norepinephrine, and other sympathomimetic amines. Also has antiserotonin effects.
Onset: within 5 minutes of I.V. injection, within 15 to 30 minutes of I.M. injection. **Peak:** Effects occur within 15 minutes of I.V. injection, 30 minutes after I.M. injection, or 15 to 45 minutes after S.C. injection. **Duration:** about 8 hours after parenteral use.

INDICATIONS & DOSAGE
To prevent or abort vascular or migraine headache –
Adults: 1 mg I.M. or I.V. May repeat q 1 to 2 hours, p.r.n., up to total of 2 mg I.V. or 3 mg I.M. per attack. Maximum weekly dosage is 6 mg.

ADVERSE REACTIONS
CNS: dizziness.
CV: numbness and tingling in fingers and toes, transient tachycardia or bradycardia, precordial distress and pain, increased arterial pressure.
GI: nausea, vomiting.
Skin: itching.
Other: weakness in legs, muscle pains in extremities, localized edema.

INTERACTIONS
Erythromycin, troleandomycin, other macrolides: may cause symptoms of

ergot toxicity. Vasopressors (nitroprusside, nifedipine, or prazosin) may be ordered to treat such an attack. Monitor closely.
Propranolol and other beta blockers: blocked natural pathway for vasodilation in patients receiving ergot alkaloids; may result in excessive vasoconstriction. Watch closely if drugs are used together.

CONTRAINDICATIONS
- Contraindicated in patients hypersensitive to the drug, during pregnancy, and in patients with peripheral and occlusive vascular disease, coronary artery disease, hypertension, hepatic or renal dysfunction, and sepsis.

NURSING CONSIDERATIONS
- Most effective when used at first sign of migraine or soon after onset.
- Avoid prolonged administration; don't exceed recommended dosage. Adjust to most effective minimal dose for best results.
- Ergotamine rebound, or an increase in frequency and duration of headache, may occur when drug is stopped.
- **I.V. use:** Continuous and intermittent infusion are not recommended. Directly inject solution into the vein over 3 minutes.
- Protect ampules from heat and light. Discard if solution is discolored.
- Instruct patients to lie down and relax in a quiet, low-light environment after administration.
- Tell patients to report any feeling of coldness in extremities or tingling of fingers and toes. Severe vasoconstriction may result in tissue damage. Keep extremities warm and administer vasodilators as ordered.
- Help patients evaluate underlying causes of stress, which may precipitate attacks.

ergotamine tartrate

Ergodryl Mono‡, Ergomar, Ergostat, Gynergen†

Pregnancy Risk Category: X

HOW SUPPLIED
Capsules: 1 mg‡
Tablets: 1 mg†
Tablets (sublingual): 2 mg
Aerosol inhaler: 360 mcg/metered spray†
Suppositories: 2 mg

ACTION
Mechanism: Inhibits effects of epinephrine, norepinephrine, and other sympathomimetic amines. Also has antiserotonin effects.
Onset: variable; partly dependent on how soon drug is taken following onset of headache symptoms. **Peak:** Plasma levels peak 2 to 3 hours after oral dose. **Duration:** variable; terminal elimination half-life, 21 hours.

INDICATIONS & DOSAGE
Vascular or migraine headache –
Adults: initially, 2 mg P.O. or S.L., then 1 to 2 mg P.O. q hour or S.L. q ½ hour, to maximum of 6 mg daily and 10 mg weekly. Alternatively, use aerosol inhaler: 1 spray (360 mcg) initially, repeated every 5 minutes p.r.n. to a maximum of 6 sprays (2.16 mg) per 24 hours or 15 sprays (5.4 mg) per week.

Patient may also use rectal suppositories. Initially, 2 mg rectally at onset of the attack, repeated in 1 hour p.r.n. Maximum dosage is 2 suppositories per attack or 5 suppositories per week.

ADVERSE REACTIONS
CV: numbness and tingling in fingers and toes, transient tachycardia or bradycardia, precordial distress and pain, increased arterial pressure, angina pectoris, peripheral vasoconstriction.

GI: nausea, vomiting, diarrhea, abdominal cramps, ischemic colitis.
Skin: itching.
Other: weakness in legs, muscle pains in extremities, localized edema, pruritus.

INTERACTIONS

Erythromycin, troleandomycin, other macrolides: may cause symptoms of ergot toxicity. Vasopressors (nitroprusside, nifedipine, or prazosin) may be ordered to treat such an attack. Monitor closely.
Propranolol and other beta blockers: blocked natural pathway for vasodilation in patients receiving ergot alkaloids; may result in excessive vasoconstriction. Watch closely if drugs are used together.

CONTRAINDICATIONS

- Contraindicated in patients with hypersensitivity to ergot alkaloids, during pregnancy, and in patients with peripheral and occlusive vascular diseases, coronary artery disease, hypertension, hepatic or renal dysfunction, or sepsis.

NURSING CONSIDERATIONS

- Most effective when used during prodromal stage of headache or as soon as possible after onset.
- Sublingual tablet is preferred during early stage of attack because of its rapid absorption. Tell patients not to eat, drink, or smoke while the tablet is dissolving.
- Avoid prolonged administration; don't exceed recommended dosage.
- Warn patients not to increase dosage without first consulting the doctor.
- Ergotamine rebound, or an increase in frequency and duration of headache, may occur if drug is suddenly discontinued.
- Provide a quiet, low-light environment to help patients relax.
- Help patient evaluate underlying causes of stress, which may precipitate attacks.
- Prolonged exposure to cold weather should be avoided whenever possible. Cold may increase many of the adverse reactions to the drug.
- Obtain an accurate dietary history from the patient to determine if a relationship exists between certain foods and onset of headache.
- Instruct patients on long-term therapy to check for and report feeling of coldness in extremities or tingling of fingers and toes. Severe vasoconstriction may result in tissue damage. Keep extremities warm and administer vasodilators as ordered.
- Instruct patients how to use inhaler correctly.

methysergide maleate

Deseril‡, Sansert**

Pregnancy Risk Category: C

HOW SUPPLIED

Tablets: 1 mg‡, 2 mg

ACTION

Mechanism: Specifically blocks serotonin (a neurotransmitter) in the peripheral nervous system. In CNS, drug acts as a serotonin agonist.
Onset: within 1 to 2 days. **Duration:** 1 to 2 days.

INDICATIONS & DOSAGE

Prevention of frequent, severe, uncontrollable, or disabling migraine or vascular headaches –
Adults: 4 to 8 mg P.O. daily with meals.
To control diarrhea caused by carcinoid disease –
Adults: initially, 2 mg P.O. t.i.d., increased p.r.n. to 4 to 16 mg t.i.d.

ADVERSE REACTIONS

CNS: insomnia, drowsiness, *euphoria, vertigo,* ataxia, *light-headedness,* hyperesthesia, weakness, hallu-

cinations or feelings of disassociation, rapid speech, lethargy.
CV: ***fibrotic thickening of cardiac valves and aorta, inferior vena cava, and common iliac branches (retroperitoneal fibrosis);*** vasoconstriction, causing chest pain, abdominal pain, vascular insufficiency of lower limbs; cold, numb, painful extremities with or without paresthesia and diminished or absent pulses; postural hypotension; tachycardia; peripheral edema; murmurs; bruits.
EENT: nasal stuffiness, visual disturbances.
GI: nausea, vomiting, diarrhea, constipation, epigastric pain.
Hematologic: neutropenia, eosinophilia.
Respiratory: ***pulmonary fibrosis,*** causing dyspnea, tightness and pain in chest, pleural friction rubs, and effusion.
Skin: hair loss, dermatitis, sweating, flushing, rash.
Other: arthralgia, myalgia.

INTERACTIONS

None significant.

CONTRAINDICATIONS

- Contraindicated in patients with severe hypertension, arteriosclerosis, peripheral vascular insufficiency, renal or hepatic disease, severe coronary artery disease (CAD), thromboembolic disorders, phlebitis or cellulitis of lower limbs, fibrotic processes, or valvular heart disease; and in debilitated patients.
- Use cautiously in patients with peptic ulcerations or suspected CAD. ECG and cardiac status evaluation advisable before giving to patients over 40 years. Use cautiously in patients sensitive to aspirin or tartrazine.

NURSING CONSIDERATIONS

- Indicated only for patients who are unresponsive to other drugs and who can be kept under close medical supervision.
- Because of its slow onset of action, do not use drug for *treatment* of migraine or vascular headache.
- Do not use to treat tension (muscle contraction) headaches.
- Monitor laboratory studies of cardiac and renal function, blood count, and sedimentation rate before and during therapy.
- Give drug for 3 weeks before evaluating effectiveness.
- GI effects may be prevented by gradual introduction of medication and by administering with meals.
- Drug may be gradually withdrawn every 6 months; then restarted after at least 3 weeks.
- Tell patients not to stop drug abruptly; may cause rebound headaches. Stop gradually over 2 to 3 weeks.
- Patients should keep daily weight record and report unusually rapid weight gain. Teach patients to check for peripheral edema. Explain and suggest low-salt diet if necessary.
- Tell patients to promptly report any of the following symptoms the doctor: cold, numb, or painful hands and feet; leg cramps when walking; and pelvic, chest, or flank pain.

40

Skeletal muscle relaxants

baclofen
carisoprodol
chlorphenesin carbamate
chlorzoxazone
cyclobenzaprine
dantrolene sodium
methocarbamol
orphenadrine citrate

COMBINATION PRODUCTS
NORGESIC: orphenadrine citrate 25 mg, aspirin 385 mg, and caffeine 30 mg.
NORGESIC FORTE: orphenadrine citrate 50 mg, aspirin 770 mg, and caffeine 60 mg.
ROBAXISAL: methocarbamol 400 mg and aspirin 325 mg.
SOMA COMPOUND: carisoprodol 200 mg and aspirin 325 mg.
SOMA COMPOUND WITH CODEINE: carisoprodol 200 mg, aspirin 325 mg, caffeine 32 mg, and codeine phosphate 16 mg.

baclofen

Clofen‡, Lioresal, Lioresal Intrathecal

Pregnancy Risk Category: C

HOW SUPPLIED
Tablets: 10 mg, 20 mg, 25 mg‡
Intrathecal injection: 500 mcg/ml, 2,000 mcg/ml

ACTION
Mechanism: Reduces transmission of impulses from the spinal cord to skeletal muscle.
Onset: hours to weeks after oral administration, ½ to 1 hour after intrathecal administration. **Peak:** Serum levels peak 2 to 3 hours after an oral dose; peak effects occur about 4 hours after intrathecal administration. **Duration:** effects of intrathecal injection, about 8 hours.

INDICATIONS & DOSAGE
Spasticity in multiple sclerosis, spinal cord injury –
Adults: initially, 5 mg P.O. t.i.d. for 3 days, 10 mg t.i.d. for 3 days, 15 mg t.i.d. for 3 days, 20 mg t.i.d. for 3 days. Increase according to response up to maximum of 80 mg daily.
Management of severe spasticity in patients who do not respond to or cannot tolerate oral baclofen therapy –
Screening phase –
Adults: After a test dose to check responsiveness, drug will be administered by an implantable infusion pump. The test dose is 1 ml of a 50-mcg/ml dilution administered into the intrathecal space by barbotage over 1 minute or more. Significantly decreased severity or frequency of muscle spasm or reduced muscle tone should be evident within 4 to 8 hours. If the response is inadequate, a second screening dose of 75 mcg/1.5 ml should be give 24 hours after the first. If response is still inadequate, a final test dose of 100 mcg/2 ml may be given 24 hours later. Patients unresponsive to the 100-mcg dose shouldn't be considered candidates for the implantable pump.
Maintenance therapy –
Adults: titrate initial dose based on the screening dose that elicited an adequate response. Double this effective dose and administer over 24 hours. However, if the screening dose efficacy was maintained for 12 hours or more, don't double the dose. After the first 24 hours, increase the dose slowly as needed and tolerated by 10% to 30% daily. During prolonged maintenance therapy, daily dose may

be increased by 10% to 40% if needed; if the patient experiences adverse effects, dosage may be decreased by 10% to 20%. Maintenance dosages have ranged from 12 mcg to 1,500 mcg daily; however, experience with dosages over 1,000 mcg daily is limited. Most patients need 300 to 800 mcg daily.

ADVERSE REACTIONS

CNS: *drowsiness, dizziness,* headache, *weakness, fatigue,* confusion, insomnia, dysarthria, ***seizures.***
CV: hypotension.
EENT: nasal congestion, blurred vision.
GI: *nausea,* constipation.
GU: urinary frequency.
Hepatic: increased AST and alkaline phosphatase.
Skin: rash, pruritus.
Other: ankle edema, excessive perspiration, hyperglycemia, weight gain.

INTERACTIONS

Ethanol, CNS depressants: increased CNS depression. Avoid concomitant use.

CONTRAINDICATIONS

- Contraindicated in patients with hypersensitivity to the drug. Do not use orally administered drug to treat muscle spasm caused by rheumatic disorders, cerebral palsy, Parkinson's disease, or CVA because efficacy hasn't been established. Do not administer intrathecal injection by I.V., I.M., S.C., or epidural route.
- Use cautiously in patients with impaired renal function or seizure disorder or when spasticity is used to maintain motor function.

NURSING CONSIDERATIONS

- Give oral form with meals or with milk to prevent GI distress.
- Oral overdosage treatment is supportive only; don't induce emesis or use a respiratory stimulant in obtunded patients.
- Amount of relief determines if dosage (and drowsiness) can be reduced.
- Used investigationally for treatment of unstable bladder.
- Watch for sensitivity reactions, such as fever, skin eruptions, and respiratory distress.
- Do not withdraw drug abruptly after long-term use unless required by severe adverse reactions; may precipitate hallucinations or rebound spasticity.
- Watch for increased incidence of seizures in epileptics.
- Advise the patient to follow the doctor's orders regarding rest and physical therapy.
- Experience with long-term intrathecal use suggests that about 10% of patients may develop tolerance to the drug. In some cases, this may be treated by hospitalizing the patient and slowly withdrawing the drug over a 2-week period.
- Tell patients to avoid activities that require alertness until CNS effects are known. Drowsiness is usually transient.
- Tell patients to avoid alcohol while taking this drug.

carisoprodol

Rela, Sodol, Soma, Soprodol, Soridol

Pregnancy Risk Category: C

HOW SUPPLIED

Tablets: 350 mg

ACTION

Mechanism: Precise mechanism unknown; drug modifies central perception of pain without modifying pain reflexes. Blocks interneuronal activity in descending reticular activating system and in spinal cord.
Onset: within 30 minutes. **Peak:** Ef-

*Liquid form contains alcohol.
**May contain tartrazine.

Common reactions are in italics; ***life-threatening,*** in bold italics.

fects occur within 4 hours. **Duration:** 4 to 6 hours.

INDICATIONS & DOSAGE
As an adjunct in acute, painful musculoskeletal conditions –
Adults and children over 12 years: 350 mg P.O. t.i.d. and h.s.

Not recommended for children under 12 years.

ADVERSE REACTIONS
CNS: *drowsiness, dizziness,* vertigo, ataxia, tremor, agitation, irritability, headache, depressive reactions, insomnia.
CV: orthostatic hypotension, tachycardia, facial flushing.
GI: nausea, vomiting, hiccups, increased bowel activity, epigastric distress.
Hematologic: eosinophilia.
Respiratory: asthmatic episodes.
Skin: rash, ***erythema multiforme,*** pruritus.
Other: fever, angioedema, ***anaphylaxis.***

INTERACTIONS
Ethanol, CNS depressants: increased CNS depression. Avoid concomitant use.

CONTRAINDICATIONS
- Contraindicated in patients with hypersensitivity to related compounds (for example, meprobamate or tybamate) or with intermittent porphyria.
- Use cautiously in patients with impaired hepatic or renal function.

NURSING CONSIDERATIONS
- Watch for idiosyncratic reactions after first to fourth dose (weakness, ataxia, visual and speech difficulties, fever, skin eruptions, and mental changes) or severe reactions, including bronchospasm, hypotension, and anaphylactic shock. Withhold dose and notify the doctor immediately of any unusual reactions.
- Record amount of relief to help the doctor determine whether dosage can be reduced.
- Do not stop drug abruptly; mild withdrawal effects, such as insomnia, headache, nausea, and abdominal cramps, may result.
- Warn patients to avoid activities that require alertness until CNS effects are known. Drowsiness is transient.
- Advise patients to avoid combining drug with alcohol or other CNS depressants.
- Advise patients to follow doctor's orders regarding rest and physical therapy.

chlorphenesin carbamate
Maolate**

Pregnancy Risk Category: C

HOW SUPPLIED
Tablets: 400 mg

ACTION
Mechanism: Precise mechanism unknown; drug modifies central perception of pain without modifying pain reflexes. Blocks interneuronal activity in descending reticular activating system and in spinal cord.
Peak: Effects occur within 1 to 3 hours. **Duration:** elimination half-life, 2½ to 5 hours.

INDICATIONS & DOSAGE
As an adjunct in short-term, acute, painful musculoskeletal conditions –
Adults: initial dose is 800 mg P.O. t.i.d. Maintenance dosage is 400 mg P.O. q.i.d. for maximum of 8 weeks.
Trigeminal neuralgia –
Adults: 400 mg P.O. upon awakening, 400 mg P.O. at noon, and 800 mg P.O. at h.s.

ADVERSE REACTIONS
CNS: *drowsiness, dizziness,* confusion, headache, weakness. Dose-re-

lated adverse reactions include paradoxical stimulation, agitation, insomnia, nervousness, headache.
GI: *nausea, GI distress.*
Hematologic: thrombocytopenia, leukopenia, ***agranulocytosis.***
Other: ***anaphylaxis.***

INTERACTIONS
Ethanol, CNS depressants: increased CNS depression. Avoid concomitant use.

CONTRAINDICATIONS
- Contraindicated in patients hypersensitive to the drug.
- Use cautiously in patients with hepatic disease or impaired renal function, and in patients hypersensitive to aspirin because tablets contain tartrazine.

NURSING CONSIDERATIONS
- Safe use for periods over 8 weeks not established.
- Take with meals or milk to prevent GI distress.
- Amount of relief determines if dosage (and drowsiness) can be reduced.
- Watch for sensitivity reactions, such as fever, skin eruptions, and respiratory distress. Withhold dose and notify doctor of unusual reactions.
- Monitor CBC and platelet studies in patients on long-term therapy. Watch for unusual bleeding and infections that may indicate hematologic dyscrasia.
- Tell patients to avoid activities that require mental alertness until adverse CNS effects are known.
- Advise patients to avoid combining drug with alcohol or other CNS depressants.

chlorzoxazone
Paraflex, Parafon Forte DSC, Strifon Forte DSC
Pregnancy Risk Category: C

HOW SUPPLIED
Tablets: 250 mg
Caplets: 500 mg

ACTION
Mechanism: Precise mechanism unknown; drug modifies central perception of pain without modifying pain reflexes. Blocks interneuronal activity in descending reticular activating system and in spinal cord.
Onset: within 1 hour. **Peak:** Effects occur within 1 to 2 hours. **Duration:** 3 to 4 hours.

INDICATIONS & DOSAGE
As an adjunct in acute, painful musculoskeletal conditions –
Adults: 250 to 750 mg P.O. t.i.d. or q.i.d.
Children: 20 mg/kg P.O. daily in divided doses t.i.d. or q.i.d.

ADVERSE REACTIONS
CNS: *drowsiness, dizziness, lightheadedness,* malaise, headache, overstimulation, tremor.
GI: anorexia, nausea, vomiting, heartburn, abdominal distress, constipation, diarrhea.
GU: urine discoloration (orange or purple-red).
Hematologic: anemia, granulocytopenia.
Hepatic: hepatic dysfunction.
Skin: urticaria, redness, itching, petechiae, bruising.

INTERACTIONS
Ethanol, CNS depressants: increased CNS depression. Avoid concomitant use.

CONTRAINDICATIONS
- Contraindicated in patients hypersensitive to the drug and in patients with impaired hepatic function.
- Use cautiously in patients with history of drug allergies.

*Liquid form contains alcohol.
**May contain tartrazine.

Common reactions are in italics; ***life-threatening,*** in bold italics.

NURSING CONSIDERATIONS

- Give with meals or milk to prevent GI distress.
- Amount of relief determines if dosage (and drowsiness) can be reduced.
- Watch for signs of hepatic dysfunction. If they occur, withhold dose and notify the doctor.
- Warn patients to avoid activities that require alertness until CNS effects are known.
- Warn patients to avoid combining with alcohol or other CNS depressants.
- Tell patients that the drug may discolor urine orange or purple-red.
- Advise patients to follow the doctor's orders regarding physical activity.

cyclobenzaprine

Flexeril

Pregnancy Risk Category: B

HOW SUPPLIED

Tablets: 10 mg

ACTION

Mechanism: Precise mechanism unknown; drug modifies central perception of pain without modifying pain reflexes. Blocks interneuronal activity in the descending reticular activating system and in the spinal cord. Drug is related to tricyclic antidepressants (TCAs) and may have similar actions.
Onset: within 1 hour. **Peak:** Effects occur in 3 to 8 hours. **Duration:** 12 to 24 hours.

INDICATIONS & DOSAGE

Short-term treatment of muscle spasm –
Adults: 10 mg P.O. t.i.d. for 7 days. Maximum dosage is 60 mg daily; maximum duration of treatment is 2 to 3 weeks.
Fibromyalgia syndrome –
Adults: 5 to 40 mg P.O. h.s. Drug has been used effectively for periods beyond 12 weeks.

ADVERSE REACTIONS

CNS: *drowsiness,* euphoria, weakness, headache, insomnia, nightmares, paresthesia, dizziness, depression, visual disturbances, ***seizures.***
CV: tachycardia.
EENT: blurred vision, dry mouth.
GI: abdominal pain, dyspepsia, peculiar taste, constipation.
GU: urine retention.
Skin: rash, urticaria, pruritus.
Other: in high doses, watch for adverse reactions like those of other tricyclic drugs.

INTERACTIONS

Anticholinergic agents: additive anticholinergic effects. Avoid concomitant use.
Ethanol, CNS depressants: may cause additive CNS depression. Avoid concomitant use.
MAO inhibitors: may exacerbate CNS depression or anticholinergic effects. Don't give within 14 days after discontinuing MAO inhibitors.

CONTRAINDICATIONS

- Contraindicated in patients who have received MAO inhibitors within 14 days; during acute recovery phase of MI; in patients with hyperthyroidism, hypersensitivity to the drug or TCAs, heart block, arrhythmias, conduction disturbances, or CHF.
- Use cautiously in patients suffering from urine retention, acute angle-closure glaucoma, increased intraocular pressure, CV disease, impaired hepatic function, and seizures; and in elderly or debilitated patients.

NURSING CONSIDERATIONS

- Nausea, headache, and malaise may occur if drug is stopped abruptly after long-term use.
- Watch for symptoms of overdose, including possible cardiotoxicity. No-

tify the doctor immediately and have physostigmine available.
• Advise patients to report urinary hesitancy or urine retention. If constipation is a problem, increase fluid intake and suggest a stool softener.
• Warn patients to avoid activities that require alertness until CNS effects are known.
• Warn patients to avoid combining with alcohol or other CNS depressants.
• Tell patients that dry mouth may be relieved with sugarless candy or gum.

dantrolene sodium

Dantrium, Dantrium I.V.

Pregnancy Risk Category: C

HOW SUPPLIED

Capsules: 25 mg, 50 mg, 100 mg
Injection: 20 mg/vial

ACTION

Mechanism: Acts directly on skeletal muscle to interfere with intracellular calcium movement.
Peak: Peak levels occur 5 hours after oral administration.

INDICATIONS & DOSAGE

Spasticity and sequelae secondary to severe chronic disorders (multiple sclerosis, cerebral palsy, spinal cord injury, stroke) –
Adults: 25 mg P.O. daily. Increase gradually in increments of 25 mg at 4- to 7-day intervals, up to 100 mg b.i.d. to q.i.d., to maximum of 400 mg daily.
Children: initially, 0.5 mg/kg P.O. b.i.d.; increase to t.i.d. then q.i.d. Gradually increase dosage as needed by 0.5 mg/kg daily to 3 mg/kg b.i.d. to q.i.d. Maximum dosage is 100 mg q.i.d.
Management of malignant hyperthermia –
Adults and children: 1 mg/kg I.V. initially; may repeat dose up to cumulative dose of 10 mg/kg.
Prevention or attenuation of malignant hyperthermia in susceptible patients who require surgery –
Adults: 4 to 8 mg/kg P.O. daily given in three to four divided doses for 1 to 2 days before procedure. Administer final dose 3 to 4 hours before procedure.
Prevention of recurrence of malignant hyperthermia –
Adults: 4 to 8 mg/kg/day P.O. given in four divided doses for up to 3 days following hyperthermic crisis.

Dantrolene has also been used to treat neuroleptic malignant syndrome.

ADVERSE REACTIONS

CNS: *muscle weakness, drowsiness,* dizziness, light-headedness, malaise, headache, confusion, nervousness, insomnia, hallucinations, ***seizures.***
CV: tachycardia, blood pressure changes.
EENT: excessive tearing, auditory or visual disturbances.
GI: anorexia, constipation, cramping, dysphagia, metallic taste, severe diarrhea, bleeding.
GU: urinary frequency, hematuria, incontinence, nocturia, dysuria, crystalluria, difficulty achieving erection.
Hepatic: hepatitis.
Respiratory: pleural effusion.
Skin: eczematous eruption, pruritus, urticaria, photosensitivity.
Other: abnormal hair growth, drooling, diaphoresis, myalgia, chills, fever.

INTERACTIONS

Ethanol, CNS depressants: increased CNS depression. Avoid concomitant use.
Verapamil (I.V.): may result in cardiovascular collapse. Stop verapamil before administering I.V. dantrolene.

CONTRAINDICATIONS

- Contraindicated in patients when spasticity is used to maintain motor function; for spasms in rheumatic disorders; in patients with active hepatic disease; and in breast-feeding patients.
- Use cautiously in patients with severely impaired cardiac or pulmonary function or preexisting hepatic disease; in women; and in patients over 35 years.

NURSING CONSIDERATIONS

- Safety and efficacy in long-term use has not been established. Do not give more than 45 days if no benefits are obtained.
- Liver function tests should be performed at the beginning of therapy.
- For optimum drug effect, give daily dosage in 4 divided doses.
- Give with meals or milk to prevent GI distress.
- Prepare oral suspension for single dose by dissolving capsule contents in juice or other suitable liquid. For multiple doses, use acid vehicle, such as citric acid in USP syrup; refrigerate. Use within several days.
- Some patients may experience difficulty swallowing during therapy. Tell patients to use caution when eating to avoid choking.
- Amount of relief in patient determines if dosage (and drowsiness) can be reduced.
- Watch for hepatitis (fever and jaundice), severe diarrhea, severe weakness, or sensitivity reactions (fever and skin eruptions). Withhold dose and notify the doctor.
- **I.V. use:** Administer as soon as malignant hyperthermia reaction is recognized. Reconstitute each vial by adding 60 ml of sterile water for injection and shaking vial until clear. Don't use a diluent that contains a bacteriostatic agent. Protect contents from light and use within 6 hours. Be careful to avoid extravasation.
- Warn patients to avoid driving and other hazardous activities until CNS effects are known.
- Advise patients to avoid combining with alcohol and other CNS depressants.
- Tell patients to avoid photosensitivity reactions by using sunblock and protective clothing; to report abdominal discomfort or GI problems immediately; and to follow the doctor's orders regarding rest and physical therapy.

methocarbamol

Delaxin, Marbaxin-750, Robaxin, Robomol-500, Robomol-750

Pregnancy Risk Category: C

HOW SUPPLIED

Tablets: 500 mg, 750 mg
Injection: 100 mg/ml

ACTION

Mechanism: Precise mechanism unknown; drug modifies central perception of pain without modifying pain reflexes. Blocks interneuronal activity in the descending reticular activating system and in the spinal cord.
Onset: immediate after I.V. use; within ½ hour after oral administration. **Peak:** Peak levels occur immediately after an I.V. injection, or within 2 hours of an oral dose. **Duration:** elimination half-life, 1 to 2 hours.

INDICATIONS & DOSAGE

As an adjunct in acute, painful musculoskeletal conditions –
Adults: 1.5 g P.O. q.i.d. for 2 to 3 days, then 1 g P.O. q.i.d., or not more than 500 mg (5 ml) I.M. into each gluteal region. May repeat q 8 hours. Or 1 to 3 g daily (10 to 30 ml) I.V. directly into vein at 3 ml/minute, or 10 ml may be added to no more than 250 ml of D_5W or 0.9% sodium chloride solution. Maximum dosage is 3 g daily.

Supportive therapy in tetanus management–
Adults: 1 to 2 g into tubing of running I.V. or 1 to 3 g in infusion bottle q 6 hours.
Children: 15 mg/kg I.V. q 6 hours.

ADVERSE REACTIONS

CNS: drowsiness, dizziness, lightheadedness, headache, syncope, mild muscular incoordination (I.M. or I.V. only), ***seizures*** (I.V. only).
CV: hypotension, bradycardia (I.M. or I.V. only).
GI: nausea, anorexia, GI upset, metallic taste.
GU: hematuria (I.V. only), discoloration of urine.
Hematologic: hemolysis, decreased hemoglobin (I.V. only).
Skin: urticaria, pruritus, rash.
Respiratory: thrombophlebitis.
Other: extravasation (I.V. only), fever, flushing, ***anaphylactic reactions*** (I.M. or I.V. only).

INTERACTIONS

Ethanol, CNS depressants: increased CNS depression. Avoid concomitant use.

CONTRAINDICATIONS

- Contraindicated in patients with hypersensitivity to the drug, impaired renal function (injectable form), myasthenia gravis, or epilepsy (injectable form); in children under 12 years (except in tetanus); and in patients receiving anticholinesterase agents.

NURSING CONSIDERATIONS

- Watch for orthostatic hypotension, especially with parenteral administration. Keep the patient supine for 15 minutes afterward, and supervise ambulation. Advise the patient to get up slowly.
- Watch for sensitivity reactions, such as fever and skin eruptions.
- Have epinephrine, antihistamines, and corticosteroids available.
- Give tablets with meals or milk to prevent GI distress.
- Prepare liquid by crushing tablets into water or sodium chloride solution. Give through nasogastric tube.
- In tetanus management, use methocarbamol with tetanus antitoxin, penicillin, tracheotomy, and aggressive supportive care. Long course of I.V. methocarbamol required.
- **I.V. use:** Dilute 10 ml of drug in not more than 250 ml of solution. Use D_5W or 0.9% sodium chloride injection. Infuse slowly; maximum rate is 300 mg (3 ml)/minute.
- Give I.M. deeply, only into upper outer quadrant of buttocks, with maximum of 5 ml in each buttock.
- Do not give S.C.
- Drug irritates veins; may cause phlebitis, aggravate seizures, and cause fainting if injected rapidly. Make sure the patient remains in a supine position during infusion. Drug is an irritant; avoid extravasation.
- Monitor CBC periodically during prolonged therapy.
- May interfere with urine tests for 5-hydroxyindoleacetic acid and vanillylmandelic acid.
- Tell patients urine may turn green, black, or brown.
- Advise patients to follow the doctor's orders regarding physical activity.
- Warn patients to avoid activities that require alertness until CNS effects are known.
- Advise patients to avoid combining with alcohol or other CNS depressants.

---

orphenadrine citrate

Banflex, Flexoject, Flexon, K-Flex, Marflex, Myolin, Neocyten, Noradex, Norflex, O-Flex, Orflagen, Orphenate

Pregnancy Risk Category: C

HOW SUPPLIED
Tablets: 100 mg
Tablets (extended-release): 100 mg
Injection: 30 mg/ml

ACTION
Mechanism: Precise mechanism unknown; drug modifies central perception of pain without modifying pain reflexes. Blocks interneuronal activity in descending reticular activating system and in spinal cord.
Onset: immediately with I.V. use, within 5 minutes of I.M. injection, or within 1 hour of oral administration.
Peak: Peak levels occur immediately after I.V. infusion, within 30 minutes of I.M. injection, within 2 hours of tablet ingestion, or within 6 to 8 hours of extended-release tablet ingestion.
Duration: half-life, about 14 hours.

INDICATIONS & DOSAGE
Adjunctive treatment in painful, acute musculoskeletal conditions –
Adults: 100 mg P.O. b.i.d., or 60 mg I.V. or I.M. q 12 hours, p.r.n. For maintenance, switch to oral therapy beginning 12 hours after last parenteral dose.

ADVERSE REACTIONS
CNS: disorientation, restlessness, irritability, weakness, *drowsiness,* headache, dizziness, hallucinations, insomnia.
CV: palpitations, tachycardia.
EENT: dilated pupils, blurred vision, difficulty swallowing, increased intraocular pressure.
GI: constipation, *dry mouth,* nausea, vomiting, paralytic ileus, epigastric distress.
GU: urinary hesitancy or urine retention.
Hematologic: ***aplastic anemia.***
Other: ***anaphylaxis.***

INTERACTIONS
Ethanol, CNS depressants: increased CNS depression. Avoid concomitant use.

CONTRAINDICATIONS
- Contraindicated in patients with acute angle-closure glaucoma; prostatic hyperplasia; pyloric, duodenal, or bladder-neck obstruction; myasthenia gravis; tachycardia; severe hepatic or renal disease; peptic ulceration; ulcerative colitis; or hypersensitivity to the drug.
- Use cautiously in elderly or debilitated patients with cardiac disease, arrhythmias or sulfite sensitivity, and in patients exposed to high temperatures.

NURSING CONSIDERATIONS
- Check all dosages carefully; a slight overdose can lead to toxicity. Early signs are excessive dry mouth, dilated pupils, blurred vision, skin flushing, and fever.
- Relieve dry mouth with cool drinks, sugarless gum, or hard candy.
- Have patients report urinary hesitancy and urine retention. Have patients void before taking the drug.
- Monitor CBC, hepatic function, and urinalysis in patients receiving long-term therapy.
- Monitor vital signs carefully.
- **I.V. use:** Inject drug over approximately 5 minutes while the patient is supine. Wait 5 to 10 minutes and then help the patient to sit up.
- When given I.V., may cause paradoxical initial bradycardia; usually disappears in 2 minutes.
- Warn patients to avoid tasks that require alertness until CNS effects are known.
- Advise patients to avoid combining with alcohol or other CNS depressants.

41

Neuromuscular blockers

atracurium besylate
doxacurium chloride
gallamine triethiodide
metocurine iodide
mivacurium chloride
pancuronium bromide
pipecuronium bromide
rocuronium bromide
succinylcholine chloride
tubocurarine chloride
vecuronium bromide

COMBINATION PRODUCTS
None.

atracurium besylate

Tracrium
Pregnancy Risk Category: C

HOW SUPPLIED
Injection: 10 mg/ml

ACTION
Mechanism: A nondepolarizing agent that prevents acetylcholine from binding to receptors on the muscle end plate, thus blocking depolarization.
Onset: within 2 minutes. **Peak:** Peak effects occur in 3 to 5 minutes. **Duration:** 25% of muscle twitch strength returns in 35 to 45 minutes; 95% recovery evident in 60 to 70 minutes.

INDICATIONS & DOSAGE
Adjunct to general anesthesia, to facilitate endotracheal intubation and to provide skeletal muscle relaxation during surgery or mechanical ventilation –
Dosage depends on anesthetic used, individual needs, and response. Dosages given here are representative and must be adjusted.
Adults and children over 2 years: 0.4 to 0.5 mg/kg by I.V. bolus. Maintenance dosage of 0.08 to 0.10 mg/kg within 20 to 45 minutes of initial dose should be administered during prolonged surgical procedures. Maintenance dosages may be administered q 12 to 25 minutes in patients receiving balanced anesthesia. For prolonged procedures, a constant infusion of 5 to 9 mcg/kg/minute may be used.
Children 1 month to 2 years: initial dose, 0.3 to 0.4 mg/kg. Frequent maintenance dosages may be needed.

ADVERSE REACTIONS
CV: bradycardia, hypotension.
Skin: skin flush, erythema, pruritus, urticaria.
Respiratory: ***prolonged dose-related apnea,*** wheezing, increased bronchial secretions.

INTERACTIONS
Aminoglycoside antibiotics (including amikacin, gentamicin, kanamycin, neomycin, streptomycin); polymyxin antibiotics (polymyxin B sulfate, colistin); clindamycin; quinidine; general anesthetics such as halothane, enflurane, and isoflurane: potentiated neuromuscular blockade, leading to increased skeletal muscle relaxation and possible respiratory paralysis. Use cautiously during surgical and postoperative periods.
Lithium, opioid analgesics: potentiated neuromuscular blockade, leading to increased skeletal muscle relaxation and possible respiratory paralysis. Use with extreme caution and reduce dose of atracurium.

CONTRAINDICATIONS
- Contraindicated in patients with hypersensitivity to the drug.

• Use cautiously in patients with CV disease, severe electrolyte disorders, bronchogenic carcinoma, hepatic or pulmonary impairment, and neuromuscular diseases and in elderly or debilitated patients.

NURSING CONSIDERATIONS

• Neuromuscular blockers don't obtund consciousness or alter the pain threshold. Sedatives or general anesthetics should be given before neuromuscular blockers are administered.
• Use this drug only under direct medical supervision by personnel skilled in the use of neuromuscular blockers and techniques for maintaining a patent airway. Don't use unless facilities and equipment for mechanical ventilation, oxygen therapy, and intubation and an antagonist are within reach.
• A nerve stimulator and train-of-four monitoring are recommended to confirm antagonism of neuromuscular blockade and recovery of muscle strength. Before attempting pharmacologic reversal with neostigmine, some evidence of spontaneous recovery (T_4:T_1 ratio > 0 or T_1 > 10% of control) should be seen.
• Prior administration of succinylcholine doesn't prolong duration of action, but quickens onset and may deepen neuromuscular blockade.
• Atracurium has a longer duration of action than succinylcholine and a shorter duration of action than *d*-tubocurarine or pancuronium.
• Keep airway clear. Have emergency respiratory support equipment (endotracheal equipment, ventilator, oxygen, atropine, edrophonium, neostigmine, and epinephrine) on hand.
• Once spontaneous recovery starts, atracurium-induced neuromuscular blockade may be reversed with an anticholinesterase agent (such as neostigmine or edrophonium). Usually administered together with an anticholinergic (such as atropine).
• Monitor respirations closely until the patient is fully recovered from neuromuscular blockade, as evidenced by tests of muscle strength (hand grip, head lift, and ability to cough).
• **I.V. use:** Drug is usually administered by rapid I.V. bolus injection but may be given by intermittent infusion or continuous infusion. At concentrations of 0.2 mg/ml to 0.5 mg/ml, atracurium is compatible for 24 hours in D_5W, 0.9% sodium chloride injection, and dextrose 5% in 0.9% sodium chloride injection.
• In lactated Ringer's injection, atracurium is stable for 8 hours at a concentration of 0.5 mg/ml. However, because of an increased rate of drug degradation in this solution, it is not recommended.
• Do not administer by I.M. injection.
• Do not mix with acidic or alkaline solutions (precipitate may form).

doxacurium chloride

Nuromax

Pregnancy Risk Category: C

HOW SUPPLIED

Injection: 1 mg/ml

ACTION

Mechanism: A nondepolarizing agent that competes with acetylcholine for receptor sites at the motor end plate; because this action may be antagonized by cholinesterase inhibitors, doxacurium is considered a competitive antagonist.
Onset: within 5 minutes. **Peak:** Peak effects are dose dependent and occur within 3 to 9 minutes. **Duration:** 1 to 4 hours.

INDICATIONS & DOSAGE

To provide skeletal muscle relaxation during surgery as an adjunct to general anesthesia –

Dosage is highly individualized. Note that all times of onset and duration of neuromuscular blockade are averages and considerable individual variation is normal.

Adults: 0.05 mg/kg rapid I.V. produces adequate conditions for endotracheal intubation in 5 minutes in about 90% of patients when used as part of a thiopental-narcotic induction technique. Lower doses may require longer delay before intubation is possible. Neuromuscular blockade at this dose will last for an average of 100 minutes.

Children over 2 years: an initial dose of 0.03 mg/kg I.V. administered during halothane anesthesia produces effective blockade in 7 minutes with duration of 30 minutes. Under the same conditions, 0.05 mg/kg produces a blockade in 4 minutes with duration of 45 minutes.

Maintenance of neuromuscular blockade during long procedures –

Adults and children: after initial dose of 0.5 mg/kg I.V., maintenance dosages of 0.005 and 0.01 mg/kg will prolong neuromuscular blockade for an average of 30 minutes. Children usually require more frequent administration of maintenance dosages.

ADVERSE REACTIONS

Respiratory: dyspnea, respiratory depression, ***respiratory insufficiency or apnea.***

Other: prolonged muscle weakness.

INTERACTIONS

Alkaline solutions (such as barbiturate solutions): physically incompatible; may form precipitate. Do not administer through same I.V. line.

Aminoglycosides (kanamycin, neomycin, streptomycin, dihydrostreptomycin, and gentamicin), bacitracin, colistin, polymyxin B, colistimethate, and tetracyclines: increased muscle weakness. Use together cautiously.

Magnesium salts: may enhance neuromuscular blockade. Monitor for excessive weakness.

Phenytoin, carbamazepine: may prolong the time to maximal block or shorten the duration of block with neuromuscular blocking agents.

Quinidine, inhalation anesthetics: may enhance the activity (or prolonged action) of nondepolarizing neuromuscular blocking agents.

CONTRAINDICATIONS

• Contraindicated in patients hypersensitive to the drug. Do not use in neonates. The drug contains benzyl ethanol, which has been associated with fatalities in newborns.

• Because of the lack of data supporting safety, this drug is not recommended for use in patients requiring prolonged mechanical ventilation in the intensive care unit, before or after nondepolarizing neuromuscular blocking agents, or during cesarean section.

• Use cautiously, possibly at reduced dosage, in debilitated patients; in patients with metastatic cancer, severe electrolyte disturbances, or neuromuscular diseases; and in patients in whom potentiation or difficulty in reversal of neuromuscular blockade is anticipated. Patients with myasthenia gravis or myasthenic syndrome (Eaton-Lambert syndrome) are particularly sensitive to the effects of nondepolarizing relaxants. Shorter-acting agents are recommended for use in such patients.

NURSING CONSIDERATIONS

• Doxacurium has no effect on consciousness or pain threshold. To avoid distress to the patient, drug should not be administered until the patient's consciousness is obtunded by general anesthetic.

• Higher initial doses may be required in patients with severe burns and in some patients with severe liver disease. Higher doses (0.8 mg/kg) will produce intubating conditions more rapidly (4 minutes), with neuromuscular blockade for 160 minutes or more. Consequently, these higher doses should be reserved for long procedures. Administration during steady-state anesthesia with enflurane, halothane, or isoflurane may allow 33% reduction of dose.

• The drug is not metabolized; it is excreted in urine and bile. Therefore, patients with renal or hepatic insufficiency may require dosage adjustment.

• Dosage should be adjusted to ideal body weight in obese patients (patients 30% or more above their ideal weight) to avoid prolonged neuromuscular blockade.

• Use drug only under direct medical supervision by personnel familiar with the use of neuromuscular blocking agents and techniques involved in maintaining a patent airway. Do not use unless facilities and equipment for mechanical ventilation, oxygen therapy, and intubation and an antagonist are within reach.

• A nerve stimulator and train-of-four monitoring are recommended to document antagonism of neuromuscular blockade and recovery of muscle strength. Before attempting pharmacologic reversal with neostigmine, some evidence of spontaneous recovery (T_4:T_1 ratio > 0 or T_1 > 10% of control) should be evident.

• Experimental evidence suggests that acid-base and electrolyte balance may influence the actions of nondepolarizing neuromuscular blockers. Alkalosis may counteract the paralysis and acidosis may enhance it.

• Because the drug has minimal vagolytic action, bradycardia during anesthesia may be common.

• Monitor respirations closely until the patient is fully recovered from neuromuscular blockade as evidenced by tests of muscle strength (hand grip, head lift, and ability to cough).

• **I.V. use:** Drug is compatible with D_5W, 0.9% sodium chloride injection, dextrose 5% in 0.9% sodium chloride injection, lactated Ringer's injection, and dextrose 5% in lactated Ringer's injection.

• When diluted as directed, doxacurium is compatible with alfentanil, fentanyl, and sufentanil.

• Diluted solutions are stable for 24 hours at room temperature; however, because reconstitution dilutes the preservative, risk of contamination increases. Recommend that the product be administered immediately after reconstitution. Unused solutions should be discarded after 8 hours.

gallamine triethiodide

Flaxedil

Pregnancy Risk Category: C

HOW SUPPLIED

Injection: 20 mg/ml

ACTION

Mechanism: A nondepolarizing agent that prevents acetylcholine from binding to the receptors on the muscle end plate, thus blocking depolarization.

Onset: 1 to 2 minutes. **Peak:** Peak effects occur in 3 to 5 minutes. **Duration:** 15 to 30 minutes.

INDICATIONS & DOSAGE

Adjunct to anesthesia to induce skeletal muscle relaxation; facilitate intubation, reduction of fractures and dislocations; lessen muscle contractions in pharmacologically or electrically induced seizures; assist with mechanical ventilation–

Dosage depends on anesthetic used, individual needs, and response. Dosages are representative and must be adjusted.

Adults and children over 1 month: initially, 1 mg/kg I.V. to maximum of 100 mg, regardless of patient's

weight; then 0.5 mg to 1 mg/kg q 30 to 40 minutes.
Children under 1 month but over 5 kg (11 lb): initially, 0.25 to 0.75 mg/kg I.V., then may give additional doses of 0.1 to 0.5 mg/kg q 30 to 40 minutes.

ADVERSE REACTIONS

CV: tachycardia.
Respiratory: ***respiratory paralysis, dose-related prolonged apnea,*** increased oropharyngeal secretions.
Other: residual muscle weakness, allergic or idiosyncratic hypersensitivity reactions.

INTERACTIONS

Aminoglycoside antibiotics (amikacin, gentamicin, kanamycin, neomycin, streptomycin); polymyxin antibiotics (polymyxin B sulfate, colistin); clindamycin; quinidine; general anesthetics (such as halothane, enflurane, isoflurane: potentiated neuromuscular blockade, leading to increased skeletal muscle relaxation and possible respiratory paralysis. Monitor closely.
Narcotic analgesics, I.V. diazepam: potentiated neuromuscular blockade, leading to increased skeletal muscle relaxation and possible respiratory paralysis. Use with extreme caution, and reduce dose of gallamine.

CONTRAINDICATIONS

- Contraindicated in patients with hypersensitivity to iodides, impaired renal function, and myasthenia gravis; in patients in shock; and in patients in whom tachycardia may be hazardous.
- Use cautiously in elderly or debilitated patients; in patients with cardiac, hepatic, or pulmonary impairment; respiratory depression, myasthenic syndrome of lung cancer or bronchogenic carcinoma, dehydration, thyroid disorders, collagen diseases, porphyria, and electrolyte disturbances; in patients sensitive to sulfites; and in patients undergoing cesarean section.

NURSING CONSIDERATIONS

- Neuromuscular blockers do not obtund consciousness or alter pain threshold. Patients should receive sedatives or general anesthetics before neuromuscular blockers are administered.
- May be preferred for patients with bradycardia.
- Use drug only under direct medical supervision by personnel skilled in the use of neuromuscular blockers and techniques for maintaining a patent airway. Do not use unless facilities and equipment for artificial respiration, mechanical ventilation, oxygen therapy, and intubation and an antagonist are within reach.
- Keep airway clear. Have emergency respiratory support equipment (endotracheal equipment, ventilator, oxygen, atropine, edrophonium, neostigmine, and epinephrine) on hand.
- A nerve stimulator and train-of-four monitoring are recommended to confirm antagonism of neuromuscular blockade and recovery of muscle strength. Before attempting pharmacologic reversal, some evidence of spontaneous recovery (T_4:T_1 ratio > 0 or T_1 > 10% of control) should exist. Reversal agents, such as neostigmine, are usually administered with an anticholinergic (such as atropine or glycopyrrolate).
- Monitor baseline electrolyte determinations (electrolyte imbalance can potentiate neuromuscular effects).
- Take vital signs every 15 minutes, especially for developing tachycardia. Notify doctor immediately of significant changes.
- Monitor respirations closely until patient is fully recovered from neuromuscular blockade, as evidenced by tests of muscle strength (hand grip, head lift, and ability to cough).

• **I.V. use:** Give by direct I.V. injection over 30 to 90 seconds.
• Protect drug from light or excessive heat; use only fresh solutions.
• Do not mix solution with meperidine or barbiturate solutions.

metocurine iodide

Metubine

Pregnancy Risk Category: C

HOW SUPPLIED

Injection: 2 mg/ml

ACTION

Mechanism: A nondepolarizing agent that prevents acetylcholine from binding to receptors on the muscle end plate, thus blocking depolarization.

Onset: 1 to 4 minutes. **Peak:** Peak effects occur in 3 to 5 minutes. **Duration:** 35 to 60 minutes; may take more than 6 hours for more than 50% of muscle twitch strength to return.

INDICATIONS & DOSAGE

Adjunct to anesthesia to induce skeletal muscle relaxation; facilitate intubation, reduction of fractures and dislocations –

Adults: 1.75 to 5.5 mg I.V.

Children 1 month to 2 years: initial dose, 0.3 to 0.4 mg.

Lessen muscle contractions in pharmacologically or electrically induced seizures –

Adults: 1.75 to 5.5 mg I.V.

Children 1 month to 2 years: initial dose, 0.3 to 0.4 mg.

ADVERSE REACTIONS

CV: hypotension secondary to histamine release, ganglionic blockade in rapid dose or overdose.

GI: reduced motility and tone.

Respiratory: ***dose-related prolonged apnea, bronchospasm.***

Other: residual muscle weakness, increased oropharyngeal secretions, allergic or idiosyncratic hypersensitivity reactions.

INTERACTIONS

Aminoglycoside antibiotics (including amikacin, gentamicin, kanamycin, neomycin, streptomycin); polymyxin antibiotics (polymyxin B sulfate, colistin); clindamycin; quinidine; general anesthetics (such as halothane, enflurane, isoflurane), furosemide, thiazide diuretics, and beta-adrenergic blocking agents: potentiated neuromuscular blockade, leading to increased skeletal muscle relaxation and possible respiratory paralysis. Use cautiously during surgical and postoperative periods.

Opioid analgesics: potentiated neuromuscular blockade, leading to increased skeletal muscle relaxation and possible respiratory paralysis. Use with extreme caution, and reduce dose of metocurine iodide.

CONTRAINDICATIONS

• Contraindicated in patients with hypersensitivity to iodides or in whom histamine release is a hazard (asthmatic or atopic patients).
• Use cautiously in elderly or debilitated patients; in patients with cardiac, renal, hepatic, or pulmonary impairment, respiratory depression, myasthenia gravis, myasthenic syndrome of lung cancer or bronchogenic cancer, dehydration, thyroid disorders, collagen diseases, porphyria, electrolyte disturbances, hyperthermia, hypotension, and shock; and (in large doses) in patients undergoing cesarean section.

NURSING CONSIDERATIONS

• Metocurine should only be used by personnel skilled in airway management.
• Keep airway clear. Have emergency respiratory support equipment (endotracheal equipment, ventilator, oxy-

gen, atropine, edrophonium, epinephrine, and neostigmine) on hand.

- Neuromuscular blockers do not obtund consciousness or alter pain threshold. Patients should receive sedatives or general anesthetics before neuromuscular blockers are administered.
- A nerve stimulator and train-of-four monitoring are recommended to document antagonism of neuromuscular blockade and recovery of muscle strength. Before attempting pharmacologic reversal with neostigmine, some evidence of spontaneous recovery (T_4:T_1 ratio > 0 or T_1 > 10% of control) should be seen. Once spontaneous recovery starts, metocurine-induced neuromuscular blockade may be reversed with an anticholinesterase agent (such as neostigmine or edrophonium). Usually administered with an anticholinergic (such as atropine).
- Dose of 1 mg is the therapeutic equivalent of 3 mg tubocurarine chloride.
- Monitor baseline electrolyte determinations (electrolyte imbalance, especially potassium, calcium, and magnesium, can potentiate neuromuscular effects) and vital signs, especially respiration.
- Monitor respirations closely until patient is fully recovered from neuromuscular blockade, as evidenced by tests of muscle strength (hand grip, head lift, and ability to cough).
- Measure fluid intake and output (renal dysfunction prolongs duration of action, because drug is mainly unchanged before excretion).
- **I.V. use:** Give by direct I.V. injection over 30 to 90 seconds. Dosage depends on anesthetic used, individual needs, and response. Dosages given are representative and must be adjusted. Administer as sustained injection over 30 to 60 seconds. Adults given cyclopropane, 2 to 4 mg I.V. (2.68 mg average); given ether, 1.5 to 3 mg I.V. (2.1 mg average); given nitrous oxide, 4 to 7 mg I.V. (4.79 mg average) with supplemental injections of 0.5 to 1 mg in 25 to 90 minutes, repeated p.r.n.
- I.M. administration is not recommended.
- Store solution away from heat and sunlight. Do not mix with barbiturates (precipitate will form). Use fresh solutions only.

mivacurium chloride

Mivacron

Pregnancy Risk Category: C

HOW SUPPLIED

Injection: 2 mg/ml in 5-ml and 10-ml vials

Infusion: 0.5 mg/ml in 50 ml of D_5W

ACTION

Mechanism: A nondepolarizing agent that competes with acetylcholine for receptor sites at the motor end plate. Because this action may be antagonized by cholinesterase inhibitors, mivacurium is considered a competitive antagonist. The drug is a mixture of three stereoisomers, each possessing neuromuscular blocking activity.

Onset: 1 to 2 minutes. **Peak:** Peak effects occur in 2 to 5 minutes. **Duration:** 95% muscle twitch strength recovery within 20 to 35 minutes.

INDICATIONS & DOSAGE

As an adjunct to general anesthesia, to facilitate endotracheal intubation, and to relax skeletal muscles during surgery or mechanical ventilation –

Adults: dosage is highly individualized. Usually, 0.15 mg/kg I.V. push over 5 to 15 seconds provides adequate muscle relaxation within 2½ minutes for endotracheal intubation. Supplemental doses of 0.1 mg/kg I.V. q 15 minutes usually sufficient to maintain muscle relaxation.

Alternatively, maintain neuromuscular blockade with a continuous infusion of 4 mcg/kg/minute begun simultaneously with the initial dose, or 9 to 10 mcg/kg/minute started after evidence of spontaneous recovery from the initial dose. When used with isoflurane or enflurane anesthesia, dosage is usually reduced about 25%. **Children 2 to 12 years:** 0.20 mg/kg I.V. push administered over 5 to 15 seconds. Neuromuscular blockade is usually evident in less than 2 minutes. Maintenance dosages are generally required more frequently in children.

Alternatively, maintain neuromuscular blockade with a continuous infusion titrated to effect. Most children respond to 5 to 31 mcg/kg/minute (average 14 mcg/kg/minute).

ADVERSE REACTIONS

CNS: dizziness.
CV: *flushing,* hypotension, tachycardia, bradycardia, arrhythmias.
Respiratory: ***bronchospasm,*** wheezing, ***respiratory insufficiency or apnea.***
Skin: rash, urticaria, erythema.
Other: prolonged muscle weakness, phlebitis, muscle spasms.

INTERACTIONS

Alkaline solutions (such as barbiturate solutions): physically incompatible; may form precipitate. Do not administer through the same I.V. line.
Aminoglycosides (kanamycin, neomycin, streptomycin, and gentamicin), bacitracin, colistin, polymyxin B, colistimethate, and tetracyclines: increased muscle weakness. Use together cautiously.
Magnesium salts: may enhance neuromuscular blockade. Monitor for excessive weakness.
Phenytoin, carbamazepine: may prolong the time to maximal blockade or shorten the duration of blockade with neuromuscular blockers.
Quinidine, inhalation anesthetics (especially isoflurane or enflurane): may enhance the activity (or prolonged action) of nondepolarizing neuromuscular blockers. Monitor for excessive weakness.

CONTRAINDICATIONS

- Contraindicated in patients hypersensitive to the drug.
- Use cautiously in patients with significant CV disease and in patients who may be adversely affected by release of histamine (such as asthmatics). To avoid hypotension, initial dose of the drug should be lower or drug should be given over longer periods of time (60 seconds).
- Also use cautiously, possibly at reduced dosage, in debilitated patients; in patients with metastatic cancer, severe electrolyte disturbances, or neuromuscular diseases; and in those in whom potentiation or difficulty in reversal of neuromuscular blockade is anticipated. Patients with myasthenia gravis or myasthenic syndrome (Eaton-Lambert syndrome) are particularly sensitive to effects of nondepolarizing relaxants. Test doses of 0.015 to 0.020 mg/kg may be used to assess the patient's sensitivity to the drug.
- Drug is metabolized to inactive compounds by plasma pseudocholinesterase. Use very cautiously, if at all, in patients who are homozygous for the atypical plasma pseudocholinesterase gene.

NURSING CONSIDERATIONS

- Use only under direct medical supervision by personnel familiar with the use of neuromuscular blockers and techniques involved in maintaining a patent airway. Do not use unless facilities and equipment for artificial respiration, mechanical ventilation, oxygen therapy, intubation, and an antagonist are within reach.
- Mivacurium, like other neuromuscular blockers, has no effect on consciousness or pain threshold. To avoid patient distress, do not administer un-

til the patient's consciousness is obtunded by the general anesthetic.

• Like other neuromuscular blockers, dosage requirements for children are higher on a mg/kg basis than those for adults. Onset and recovery of neuromuscular blockade occur more rapidly in children.

• Duration of the drug effect is increased about 150% in patients with end-stage renal disease and 300% in patients with hepatic dysfunction.

• Patients with severe burns are known to develop resistance to nondepolarizing neuromuscular blockers; however, they may also have reduced plasma pseudocholinesterase activity. Administer a test dose to assess the patient's sensitivity to the drug.

• Dosage should be adjusted to ideal body weight in obese patients (patients 30% or more above their ideal weight) because they may experience prolonged neuromuscular blockade.

• A nerve stimulator and train-of-four monitoring are recommended to document antagonism of neuromuscular blockade and recovery of muscle strength. Before attempting pharmacologic reversal with neostigmine or edrophonium, some signs of spontaneous recovery should be evident.

• Experimental evidence suggests that acid-base and electrolyte balances may influence the actions of nondepolarizing neuromuscular blockers. Alkalosis may counteract the paralysis; acidosis may enhance it.

• Monitor respirations closely until patient is fully recovered from neuromuscular blockade as evidenced by tests of muscle strength (hand grip, head lift, and ability to cough).

• **I.V. use:** Drug is compatible with D_5W, 0.9% sodium chloride injection, dextrose 5% in 0.9% sodium chloride injection, lactated Ringer's injection, and dextrose 5% in lactated Ringer's injection. Diluted solutions are stable for 24 hours at room temperature.

• When diluted as directed, mivacurium is compatible with alfentanil, fentanyl, sufentanil, droperidol, and midazolam.

• Drug is also available as premixed infusion in D_5W. After removing the protective outer wrap, check container for minor leaks by squeezing the bag before administering. Do not add any other drugs to the container, and do not use the container in series connections.

pancuronium bromide

Pavulon

Pregnancy Risk Category: C

HOW SUPPLIED

Injection: 1 mg/ml, 2 mg/ml

ACTION

Mechanism: A nondepolarizing agent that prevents acetylcholine from binding to receptors on the muscle end plate, thus blocking depolarization.

Onset: 30 to 45 seconds. **Peak:** Peak effects occur in 3 to 4½ minutes.

Duration: 35 to 45 minutes; 90% of muscle twitch strength returns within 1 hour.

INDICATIONS & DOSAGE

Adjunct to anesthesia to induce skeletal muscle relaxation; facilitate intubation; lessen muscle contractions in pharmacologically or electrically induced seizures; assist with mechanical ventilation –

Dosage depends on anesthetic used, individual needs, and response. Dosages are representative and must be adjusted.

Adults: initially, 0.04 to 0.1 mg/kg I.V.; then 0.01 mg/kg q 30 to 60 minutes.

Children over age 10: initially, 0.04 to 0.1 mg/kg I.V., then ⅕ initial dose q 30 to 60 minutes.

Dosage of 1 mg is the approximate

therapeutic equivalent of 5 mg tubocurarine chloride.

ADVERSE REACTIONS

CV: tachycardia, increased blood pressure.
Respiratory: ***prolonged dose-related apnea,*** wheezing.
Skin: transient rashes.
Other: burning sensation, excessive sweating and salivation, residual muscle weakness, allergic or idiosyncratic hypersensitivity reactions.

INTERACTIONS

Aminoglycoside antibiotics (including amikacin, gentamicin, kanamycin, neomycin, streptomycin); polymyxin antibiotics (polymyxin B sulfate, colistin); clindamycin; quinidine; general anesthetics (such as halothane, enflurane, isoflurane): potentiated neuromuscular blockade, leading to increased skeletal muscle relaxation and possible respiratory paralysis. Use cautiously during surgical and postoperative periods.
Lithium, opioid analgesics: potentiated neuromuscular blockade, leading to increased skeletal muscle relaxation and possible respiratory paralysis. Use with extreme caution, and reduce dose of pancuronium.

CONTRAINDICATIONS

- Contraindicated in patients with hypersensitivity to bromides; preexisting tachycardia; and in patients for whom even a minor increase in heart rate is undesirable.
- Use cautiously in elderly or debilitated patients; in patients with renal, hepatic, or pulmonary impairment; in patients with respiratory depression, myasthenia gravis, myasthenic syndrome of lung cancer or bronchogenic carcinoma, dehydration, thyroid disorders, collagen diseases, porphyria, electrolyte disturbances, hyperthermia, and toxemic states; and (in large doses) in patients undergoing cesarean section.

NURSING CONSIDERATIONS

- Drug does not cause histamine release or hypotension, but may raise heart rate and blood pressure.
- Pancuronium should be used only by personnel experienced in airway management.
- Have emergency respiratory support equipment (endotracheal equipment, ventilator, oxygen, atropine, edrophonium, epinephrine, and neostigmine) on hand.
- Neuromuscular blockers do not obtund consciousness or alter the pain threshold. Patients should receive sedatives or general anesthetics before neuromuscular blockers are administered.
- Monitor baseline electrolyte determinations (electrolyte imbalance can potentiate neuromuscular effects) and vital signs (watch respiration and heart rate closely).
- Measure fluid intake and output (renal dysfunction may prolong duration of action, since 25% of the drug is unchanged before excretion).
- A nerve stimulator and train-of-four monitoring are recommended to confirm antagonism of neuromuscular blockade and recovery of muscle strength. Before attempting pharmacologic reversal with neostigmine, some evidence of spontaneous recovery (T_4:T_1 ratio > 0 or T_1 > 10% of control) should be seen.
- Once spontaneous recovery starts, pancuronium-induced neuromuscular blockade may be reversed with an anticholinesterase agent (such as neostigmine or edrophonium). Usually administered with an anticholinergic (such as atropine).
- Monitor respirations closely until patient is fully recovered from neuromuscular blockade, as evidenced by tests of muscle strength (hand grip, head lift, and ability to cough).

• Allow succinylcholine effects to subside before giving pancuronium.
• **I.V. use:** Do not mix with alkaline solutions such as barbiturate solutions (precipitate will form); use only fresh solutions.
• Store in refrigerator. Do not store in plastic containers or syringes, although plastic syringes may be used for administration.

pipecuronium bromide

Arduan

Pregnancy Risk Category: C

HOW SUPPLIED

Powder for injection: 10 mg/vial

ACTION

Mechanism: A nondepolarizing muscle relaxant that competes with acetylcholine for receptor sites at the motor end-plate. Because this action may be antagonized by cholinesterase inhibitors, pipecuronium is considered a competitive antagonist.
Onset: 1 to 2 minutes. **Peak:** Peak effects occur within 5 minutes. **Duration:** 25% to 50% of muscle twitch strength returns within 24 minutes.

INDICATIONS & DOSAGE

To provide skeletal muscle relaxation during surgery as adjunct to general anesthesia –
Dosage is highly individualized. The following doses may serve as a guide for use in nonobese patients with normal renal function.
Adults and children: initially, 70 to 85 mcg/kg I.V. provides conditions considered ideal for endotracheal intubation and maintains paralysis for 1 to 2 hours. If succinylcholine is used for endotracheal intubation, initial dosages of 50 mcg/kg I.V. provide good relaxation for 45 minutes or more. Maintenance dosages of 10 to 15 mcg/kg provide relaxation for about 50 minutes.

Note: Dosage adjustments are necessary for patients with impaired renal function.

ADVERSE REACTIONS

CV: hypotension, bradycardia, hypertension, myocardial ischemia, *CVA,* thrombosis, atrial fibrillation, ***ventricular extrasystole.***
GU: anuria.
Respiratory: dyspnea, respiratory depression, ***respiratory insufficiency or apnea.***
Other: prolonged muscle weakness, increased creatinine levels.

INTERACTIONS

Aminoglycosides (kanamycin, neomycin, streptomycin, dihydrostreptomycin, and gentamicin), bacitracin, colistin, polymyxin B, colistimethate, and tetracyclines: increased muscle weakness. Use together cautiously.
Magnesium salts: may enhance neuromuscular blockade. Monitor for excessive weakness.
Quinidine, inhalation anesthetics: enhanced activity (or prolonged action) of nondepolarizing neuromuscular blocking agents.

CONTRAINDICATIONS

• Contraindicated in patients hypersensitive to the drug.
• Use with caution and with dosage adjustments in patients with renal failure because the drug is excreted by the kidneys. No information is available regarding use of the drug in patients with hepatic disease.

NURSING CONSIDERATIONS

• Use drug under direct medical supervision by persons familiar with use of neuromuscular blockers and techniques involved in maintaining a patent airway. Do not use drug unless facilities and equipment for artificial respiration, mechanical ventilation, oxygen therapy, intubation, and an antagonist are within reach.

• Because of the lack of data supporting safety, this drug is not recommended for use in patients requiring prolonged mechanical ventilation in the intensive care unit, before or after other nondepolarizing neuromuscular blockers, or during cesarean section.
• Neuromuscular blockers do not obtund consciousness or alter pain threshold. Give patients sedatives or general anesthetics before neuromuscular blockers are administered.
• Pipecuronium may be administered after succinylcholine when the latter is used to facilitate intubation. However, no evidence exists to support safe use of pipecuronium before succinylcholine to decrease adverse effects of the latter drug.
• Patients with myasthenia gravis or myasthenic syndrome (Eaton-Lambert syndrome) are particularly sensitive to the effects of nondepolarizing relaxants. Shorter-acting agents are recommended for use in such patients.
• Not recommended for use in neonates and infants younger than 3 months. Limited evidence suggests that infants and children (age 1 to 14) under balanced anesthesia or halothane anesthesia may be less sensitive than adults.
• Dosage should be adjusted to ideal body weight in obese patients (30% or more over their ideal weight) because prolonged neuromuscular blockade has been reported in such patients.
• Because the drug has minimal vagolytic action, bradycardia during anesthesia may be common.
• A nerve stimulator and train-of-four monitoring are recommended to document antagonism of neuromuscular blockade and recovery of muscle strength. Before attempting pharmacologic reversal with neostigmine, some evidence of spontaneous recovery (T_4:T_1 ratio > 0 or T_1 > 10% of control) should be evident.
• Experimental evidence suggests that acid-base and electrolyte balances may influence the actions of nondepolarizing neuromuscular blocking agents. Alkalosis may counteract the paralysis and acidosis may enhance it.
• Because of its prolonged duration of action, pipecuronium is recommended only for procedures that take 90 minutes or longer.
• Monitor respirations closely until patient is fully recovered from neuromuscular blockade, as evidenced by tests of muscle strength (hand grip, head lift, and ability to cough).
• **I.V. use:** Reconstitute with 10 ml solution before use to yield a solution of 1 mg/ml. Large volumes of diluent or addition of the drug to a hanging I.V. solution is not recommended.
• After reconstitution with sterile water for injection or other compatible I.V. solutions (such as 0.9% sodium chloride injection, D_5W, lactated Ringer's injection, dextrose 5% in saline), the drug is stable for 24 hours if refrigerated.
• After reconstitution with any solution other than bacteriostatic water for injection, discard unused drug.
• After reconstitution with bacteriostatic water for injection, the drug is stable for 5 days at room temperature or in the refrigerator. Note that bacteriostatic water contains benzyl alcohol and is not intended for use in neonates.
• Store the powder at room temperature or in the refrigerator (36° to 86° F [2° to 30° C]).

rocuronium bromide

Zemuron

Pregnancy Risk Category: B

HOW SUPPLIED

Injection: 10 mg/ml

ACTION

Mechanism: A nondepolarizing agent that prevents acetylcholine from binding to receptors on the muscle end plate, thus blocking depolarization.

Onset: within 1 minute. **Peak:** Peak effects occur within 2 minutes in most patients. **Duration:** dose dependent; 25% recovery of muscle twitch strength within 22 to 67 minutes.

INDICATIONS & DOSAGE

Adjunct to general anesthesia, to facilitate endotracheal intubation and to provide skeletal muscle relaxation during surgery or mechanical ventilation –

Dosage depends on anesthetic used, individual needs, and response. Dosages are representative and must be adjusted.

Adults and children: Initially, 0.6 mg/kg I.V. bolus. In most patients, tracheal intubation may be performed within 2 minutes; muscle paralysis should last about 22 minutes. A maintenance dosage of 0.1 mg/kg should provide an additional 12 minutes of muscle relaxation; 0.15 mg/kg will add 17 minutes; or 0.2 mg/kg will add 24 minutes to the duration of effect.

ADVERSE REACTIONS

CV: tachycardia, abnormal ECG, arrhythmias (rare).
GI: nausea, vomiting.
Respiratory: asthma.
Local: rash, edema, pruritus.
Other: hiccup.

INTERACTIONS

Aminoglycoside antibiotics (including amikacin, gentamicin, kanamycin, neomycin, streptomycin); polymyxin antibiotics (polymyxin B sulfate, colistin); anticonvulsants; clindamycin; quinidine; general anesthetics (such as halothane, enflurane, isoflurane), opiate analgesics: potentiated neuromuscular blockade, leading to increased skeletal muscle relaxation and possible respiratory paralysis. Use cautiously during surgical and postoperative periods.

CONTRAINDICATIONS

- Contraindicated in patients hypersensitive to bromides.
- Because of lack of clinical experience with the drug, it is not recommended for use during rapid sequence induction for cesarean section.
- Use cautiously in altered circulation time from cardiovascular disease, old age, and edematous states; in hepatic disease; in severe obesity; in bronchogenic carcinoma; in patients with electrolyte disturbances; and in neuromuscular disease.

NURSING CONSIDERATIONS

- Rocuronium should be used only by personnel experienced in airway management.
- Keep airway clear. Have emergency respiratory support equipment (endotracheal equipment, ventilator, oxygen, atropine, edrophonium, epinephrine, and neostigmine) on hand.
- Neuromuscular blockers do not obtund consciousness or alter the pain threshold. Patients should receive sedatives or general anesthetics before neuromuscular blockers are administered.
- Unlike many other nondepolarizing neuromuscular blockers, rocuronium has no effect on cardiovascular system. Also, the drug causes no histamine release and therefore no histamine-related hypersensitivity reactions, such as bronchospasm, hypotension, or tachycardia.
- Rocuronium is well tolerated in patients with renal failure.
- Patients with liver disease may require higher doses of the drug to achieve adequate muscle relaxation. However, such patients exhibit prolonged effects from the drug. Monitor closely.
- Prior administration of succinylcholine may enhance neuromuscular blocking effect and duration of action.
- Rocuronium provides conditions for

intubation within 3 minutes. Effect lasts 25 to 40 minutes.
• A nerve stimulator and train-of-four monitoring are recommended to confirm antagonism of neuromuscular blockade and recovery of muscle strength. Before attempting pharmacologic reversal with neostigmine, some evidence of spontaneous recovery (T_4:T_1 ratio > 0 or T_1 > 10% of control) should be seen. Once spontaneous recovery starts, rocuronium-induced neuromuscular blockade may be reversed with an anticholinesterase agent (such as neostigmine or edrophonium). Usually administered with an anticholinergic (such as atropine).
• Monitor respirations closely until patient is fully recovered from neuromuscular blockade, as evidenced by tests of muscle strength (hand grip, head lift, and ability to cough).
• **I.V. use:** usually administered by rapid I.V. injection. Alternatively, drug may be given by continuous I.V. infusion. Infusion rates are highly individualized but have ranged from 0.004 to 0.16 mg/kg/minute. Compatible solutions include D_5W, 0.9% sodium chloride injection, dextrose 5% in 0.9% sodium chloride injection, sterile water for injection, and lactated Ringer's injection.
• Store reconstituted solution in refrigerator. Discard after 24 hours.

succinylcholine chloride (suxamethonium chloride)

Anectine, Anectine Flo-Pack, Quelicin, Scoline‡, Sucostrin

Pregnancy Risk Category: C

HOW SUPPLIED
Injection: 20 mg/ml, 50 mg/ml, 100 mg/ml; 100 mg/vial, 500 mg/vial, 1 g/vial

ACTION
Mechanism: A depolarizing agent that prolongs depolarization of the muscle end plate.
Onset: 30 seconds to 1 minute after I.V. use; 2 to 3 minutes after I.M. use.
Peak: Peak effects occur in 1 to 2 minutes after I.V. use. **Duration:** 4 to 10 minutes after I.V. use, 10 to 30 minutes after I.M. use.

INDICATIONS & DOSAGE
Adjunct to anesthesia to induce skeletal muscle relaxation; facilitate intubation and assist with mechanical ventilation or orthopedic manipulations (drug of choice); lessen muscle contractions in pharmacologically or electrically induced seizures – Dosage depends on anesthetic used, individual needs, and response. Dosages are representative and must be adjusted.
Adults: 25 to 75 mg I.V., then 2.5 mg/minute, p.r.n., or 2.5 mg/kg I.M. up to maximum of 150 mg I.M. in deltoid muscle.
Children: 1 to 2 mg/kg I.M. or I.V. Maximum I.M. dosage is 150 mg. (Children may be less sensitive to succinylcholine than adults.)

ADVERSE REACTIONS
CV: bradycardia, tachycardia, hypertension, hypotension, ***arrhythmias.***
EENT: increased intraocular pressure.
Respiratory: ***prolonged respiratory depression, apnea.***
Other: malignant hyperthermia, muscle fasciculation, *postoperative muscle pain,* myoglobinemia, excessive salivation, allergic or idiosyncratic hypersensitivity reactions.

INTERACTIONS
Aminoglycoside antibiotics (including amikacin, gentamicin, kanamycin, neomycin, streptomycin); polymyxin antibiotics (polymyxin B sulfate, colistin); cholinesterase inhibitors (such as

neostigmine, pyridostigmine, edrophonium, physostigmine, or echothiophate); general anesthetics (such as halothane, enflurane, isoflurane): potentiated neuromuscular blockade, leading to increased skeletal muscle relaxation and possible respiratory paralysis. Use cautiously during surgical and postoperative periods.
Digitalis glycosides: possible cardiac arrhythmias. Use together cautiously.
Magnesium sulfate (parenterally): potentiated neuromuscular blockade, increased skeletal muscle relaxation, and possible respiratory paralysis. Use with caution, preferably with reduced doses.
MAO inhibitors, lithium, cyclophosphamide: prolonged apnea. Use with caution.
Opioid analgesics, methotrimeprazine: potentiated neuromuscular blockade, leading to increased skeletal muscle relaxation and possible respiratory paralysis. Use with extreme caution.

CONTRAINDICATIONS

- Contraindicated in patients hypersensitive to the drug, and in patients with abnormally low plasma pseudocholinesterase, acute angle-closure glaucoma, or penetrating eye injuries.
- Use cautiously in elderly or debilitated patients; in patients with personal or family history of malignant hypertension or hyperthermia; in patients with hepatic, renal, or pulmonary impairment, respiratory depression, severe burns or trauma, electrolyte imbalances, quinidine or digitalis therapy, hyperkalemia, paraplegia, spinal neuraxis injury, stroke, degenerative or dystrophic neuromuscular disease, myasthenia gravis, myasthenic syndrome of lung cancer or bronchogenic carcinoma, dehydration, thyroid disorders, collagen diseases, porphyria, fractures, muscle spasms, eye surgery, pheochromocytoma; and (in large doses) patients undergoing cesarean section.

NURSING CONSIDERATIONS

- Drug of choice for short procedures (less than 3 minutes) and for orthopedic manipulations; use caution in fractures or dislocations.
- Neuromuscular blockers do not obtund consciousness or alter the pain threshold. Patients should receive sedatives or general anesthetics before neuromuscular blockers are administered.
- Succinylcholine should be used only by personnel experienced in airway management.
- Keep airway clear. Have emergency respiratory support equipment (endotracheal equipment, ventilator, oxygen, atropine, and epinephrine) on hand.
- Unlike nondepolarizing agents, neostigmine or edrophonium may worsen neuromuscular blockade. Don't use reversing agents.
- Repeated or continuous infusions of succinylcholine alone not advised; may cause reduced response or prolonged muscle relaxation and apnea.
- Monitor baseline electrolyte determinations and vital signs (check respiration every 5 to 10 minutes during infusion).
- Monitor respirations closely until patient is fully recovered from neuromuscular blockade, as evidenced by tests of muscle strength (hand grip, head lift, and ability to cough).
- **I.V. use:** Give test dose (10 mg I.M. or I.V.) after patient has been anesthetized. Normal response (no respiratory depression or transient depression for up to 5 minutes) indicates drug may be given. Do not give if patient develops respiratory paralysis sufficient to permit endotracheal intubation. (Recovery within 30 to 60 minutes.)
- Store injectable form in refrigerator. Store powder form at room tem-

perature, tightly closed. Use immediately after reconstitution. Do not mix with alkaline solutions (thiopental sodium, sodium bicarbonate, barbiturates).

• **I.M. use:** give deep I.M., preferably high into deltoid muscle.

• Reassure patients that postoperative stiffness is normal and will soon subside.

tubocurarine chloride

Tubarine†

Pregnancy Risk Category: C

HOW SUPPLIED

Injection: 3 mg (20 units)/ml; 10 mg/ml‡

ACTION

Mechanism: A nondepolarizing agent that prevents acetylcholine from binding to receptors on the muscle end plate, thus blocking depolarization.

Onset: within 1 minute. **Peak:** Peak effects occur in 2 to 5 minutes. **Duration:** 20 to 40 minutes; 50% recovery of muscle twitch strength within 50 minutes, 90% recovery within 75 to 90 minutes.

INDICATIONS & DOSAGE

Adjunct to anesthesia to induce skeletal muscle relaxation; facilitate intubation, orthopedic manipulations – Dosage depends on anesthetic used, individual needs, and response. Dosages listed are representative and must be adjusted.

Adults: 1 unit/kg or 0.15 mg/kg I.V. slowly over 60 to 90 seconds. Average, initially, 40 to 60 units I.V. May give 20 to 30 units in 3 to 5 minutes. For longer procedures, give 20 units, p.r.n.

Children: 1 unit/kg or 0.15 mg/kg.

Assist with mechanical ventilation –

Adults and children: initially, 0.0165 mg/kg I.V. (average 1 mg or 7 units), then adjust subsequent doses to patient's response.

Lessen muscle contractions in pharmacologically or electrically induced seizures –

Adults and children: 1 unit/kg or 0.15 mg/kg over 60 to 90 seconds. Initial dosage is 20 units (3 mg) less than calculated dose.

Diagnosis of myasthenia gravis –

Adults: 4 to 33 mcg/kg as a single I.V. dose.

ADVERSE REACTIONS

CV: hypotension, circulatory depression.

Respiratory: ***respiratory depression or apnea, bronchospasm.***

Other: profound and prolonged muscle relaxation, hypersensitivity reactions, idiosyncrasy, residual muscle weakness, increased salivation.

INTERACTIONS

Aminoglycoside antibiotics (including amikacin, gentamicin, kanamycin, neomycin, streptomycin); polymyxin antibiotics (polymyxin B sulfate, colistin); general anesthetics (such as halothane, enflurane, isoflurane): potentiated neuromuscular blockade, leading to increased skeletal muscle relaxation and possible respiratory paralysis. Use cautiously during surgical and postoperative periods.

Quinidine: prolonged neuromuscular blockade. Use together with caution. Monitor closely.

Thiazide diuretics, furosemide, ethacrynic acid, amphotericin B, propranolol, methotrimeprazine, opioid analgesics: potentiated neuromuscular blockade, leading to increased respiratory paralysis. Use with extreme caution during surgical and postoperative periods.

CONTRAINDICATIONS

• Contraindicated in patients for whom histamine release is a hazard (asthmatics).

• Use cautiously in elderly or debilitated patients; in patients with hepatic or pulmonary impairment, hypothermia, respiratory depression, myasthenia gravis, myasthenic syndrome of lung cancer or bronchogenic carcinoma, dehydration, thyroid disorders, collagen diseases, porphyria, electrolyte disturbances, fractures, muscle spasms; and (in large doses) and patients undergoing cesarean section.

NURSING CONSIDERATIONS

• Only personnel experienced in airway management should use tubocurarine.
• Keep airway clear. Have emergency respiratory support equipment (endotracheal equipment, ventilator, oxygen, atropine, edrophonium, epinephrine, and neostigmine) on hand.
• Neuromuscular blockers do not obtund consciousness or alter the pain threshold. Give patients sedatives or general anesthetics before neuromuscular blockers are administered.
• Allow succinylcholine effects to subside before giving tubocurarine.
• Monitor baseline electrolyte determinations (electrolyte imbalance can potentiate neuromuscular blocking effects).
• A nerve stimulator and train-of-four monitoring are recommended to confirm antagonism of neuromuscular blockade and recovery of muscle strength. Before attempting pharmacologic reversal with neostigmine, some evidence of spontaneous recovery (T_4:T_1 ratio > 0 or T_1 > 10% of control) should be seen. Once spontaneous recovery starts, tubocurarine-induced neuromuscular blockade may be reversed with an anticholinesterase agent (such as neostigmine or edrophonium). Usually administered with an anticholinergic (such as atropine).
• Monitor respirations closely until patient is fully recovered from neuromuscular blockade, as evidenced by tests of muscle strength (hand grip, head lift, and ability to cough).
• Check vital signs every 15 minutes. Notify the doctor at once of changes.
• Measure fluid intake and output (renal dysfunction prolongs duration of action, because much of drug is unchanged before excretion).
• **I.V. use:** Give I.V. over 60 to 90 seconds.
• Do not mix with barbiturates (precipitate will form). Use only fresh solutions and discard if discolored.

vecuronium bromide

Norcuron

Pregnancy Risk Category: C

HOW SUPPLIED

Injection: 10 mg/vial

ACTION

Mechanism: A nondepolarizing agent that prevents acetylcholine from binding to receptors on the muscle end plate, thus blocking depolarization.
Onset: within 1 minute. **Peak:** Peak effects occur in 3 to 5 minutes. **Duration:** 25 to 30 minutes; 25% recovery of muscle twitch strength within 24 to 40 minutes, 95% recovery in 45 to 65 minutes.

INDICATIONS & DOSAGE

Adjunct to general anesthesia, to facilitate endotracheal intubation and to provide skeletal muscle relaxation during surgery or mechanical ventilation – Dosage depends on anesthetic used, individual needs, and response. Dosages are representative and must be adjusted.
Adults and children over age 9: initially, 0.08 to 0.10 mg/kg I.V. bolus. Maintenance dosages of 0.010 to 0.015 mg/kg within 25 to 40 minutes of initial dose should be administered during prolonged surgical procedures. Maintenance dosages may be given

q 12 to 15 minutes in patients receiving balanced anesthesia.
Children under age 9: may require a slightly higher initial dose and may also require supplementation slightly more often than adults. Alternatively, drug may be given by continuous I.V. infusion of 1 mcg/kg/minute initially, then 0.8 to 1.2 mcg/kg/minute.

ADVERSE REACTIONS
CV: transient increases in heart rate.
Respiratory: ***prolonged dose-related apnea.***
Other: redness, itching, induration.

INTERACTIONS
Aminoglycoside antibiotics (including amikacin, gentamicin, kanamycin, neomycin, streptomycin); polymyxin antibiotics (polymyxin B sulfate, colistin); clindamycin; quinidine; general anesthetics (such as halothane, enflurane, isoflurane): potentiated neuromuscular blockade, leading to increased skeletal muscle relaxation and possible respiratory paralysis. Use cautiously during surgical and postoperative periods.
Opioid analgesics: potentiated neuromuscular blockade, leading to increased skeletal muscle relaxation and possible respiratory paralysis. Use with extreme caution, and reduce dose of vecuronium.

CONTRAINDICATIONS
• Contraindicated in patients hypersensitive to bromides.
• Use cautiously in elderly patients, in patients with altered circulation time from cardiovascular disease, and edematous states; in patients with hepatic disease, severe obesity, and bronchogenic carcinoma; and in patients with electrolyte disturbances and neuromuscular disease.

NURSING CONSIDERATIONS
• Should be used only by personnel experienced in airway management.
• Keep airway clear. Have emergency respiratory support equipment (endotracheal equipment, ventilator, oxygen, atropine, edrophonium, epinephrine, and neostigmine) on hand.
• Unlike other nondepolarizing neuromuscular blockers, vecuronium has no effect on cardiovascular system. Also, the drug causes no histamine release and therefore no histamine-related hypersensitivity reactions, such as bronchospasm, hypotension, or tachycardia.
• Neuromuscular blockers do not obtund consciousness or alter the pain threshold. Give patients sedatives or general anesthetics before neuromuscular blockers are administered.
• Vecuronium is well tolerated in patients with renal failure.
• Prior administration of succinylcholine may enhance the neuromuscular blocking effect and duration of action.
• A nerve stimulator and train-of-four monitoring are recommended to confirm antagonism of neuromuscular blockade and recovery of muscle strength. Before attempting pharmacologic reversal with neostigmine, some evidence of spontaneous recovery (T_4:T_1 ratio > 0 or T_1 > 10% of control) should be seen. Once spontaneous recovery starts, vecuronium-induced neuromuscular blockade may be reversed with an anticholinesterase agent (such as neostigmine or edrophonium). Usually administered with an anticholinergic (such as atropine).
• Monitor respirations closely until patient is fully recovered from neuromuscular blockade.
• **I.V. use:** Usually administered by rapid I.V. injection. Alternatively, 10 to 20 mg may be added to 100 ml of a compatible solution and given by I.V. infusion. Compatible solutions include D_5W, 0.9% sodium chloride injection, dextrose 5% in 0.9% sodium chloride injection, and lactated Ringer's injection.
• Store reconstituted solution in refrigerator. Discard after 24 hours.
• Do not mix with alkaline solutions.

42

Antihistamines

astemizole
azatadine maleate
brompheniramine maleate
chlorpheniramine maleate
clemastine fumarate
cyproheptadine hydrochloride
dexchlorpheniramine maleate
diphenhydramine hydrochloride
loratadine
methdilazine hydrochloride
promethazine hydrochloride
promethazine theoclate
terfenadine
trimeprazine tartrate
tripelennamine citrate
tripelennamine hydrochloride
triprolidine hydrochloride

COMBINATION PRODUCTS

ALLEREST TABLETS◇: phenylpropanolamine hydrochloride 18.7 mg and chlorpheniramine maleate 2 mg.
ALLERGESIC: phenylpropanolamine hydrochloride 18.7 mg and chlorpheniramine maleate 2 mg.
BROMFED-AT: brompheniramine maleate 2 mg, dextromethorphan hydrobromide 10 mg, and pseudoephedrine hydrochloride 30 mg/5 ml.
CHLOR-TRIMETON DECONGESTANT◇: chlorpheniramine maleate 4 mg and pseudoephedrine sulfate 60 mg.
CHLOR-TRIMETON DECONGESTANT REPETABS◇: chlorpheniramine maleate 8 mg and pseudoephedrine sulfate 120 mg.
CODIMAL DH*: hydrocodone bitartrate 1.66 mg, phenylephrine hydrochloride 5 mg, pyrilamine maleate 8.33 mg, potassium guaiacolsulfonate 83.3 mg, sodium citrate 216 mg, and citric acid 50 mg.
CONDRIN-LA: phenylpropanolamine hydrochloride 75 mg and chlorpheniramine maleate 12 mg.
CONTAC CAPSULES◇: phenylpropanolamine 75 mg and chlorpheniramine maleate 8 mg.
CONTAC 12-HOUR CAPLETS◇: phenylpropanolamine 75 mg and chlorpheniramine maleate 12 mg.
CORICIDIN TABLETS◇: chlorpheniramine maleate 2 mg and acetaminophen 325 mg.
DECONADE: phenylpropanolamine hydrochloride 75 mg and chlorpheniramine maleate 12 mg.
DECONAMINE: pseudoephedrine hydrochloride 60 mg and chlorpheniramine maleate 4 mg.
DIMETAPP EXTENTABS: brompheniramine maleate 12 mg, and phenylpropanolamine hydrochloride 75 mg.
DISOPHROL CHRONOTABS◇: dexbrompheniramine maleate 6 mg and pseudoephedrine sulfate 120 mg.
DRIXORAL◇: dexbrompheniramine maleate 6 mg and pseudoephedrine sulfate 120 mg.
DRIZE: phenylpropanolamine hydrochloride 75 mg and chlorpheniramine maleate 12 mg.
FEDAHIST: pseudoephedrine hydrochloride 60 mg and chlorpheniramine maleate 4 mg.
HISTABID DURACAPS: phenylpropanolamine 75 mg and chlorpheniramine maleate 8 mg.
HISTASPAN-D: chlorpheniramine maleate 8 mg, phenylephrine hydrochloride 20 mg, and methscopolamine nitrate 2.5 mg.
NALDECON: phenylephrine hydrochloride 10 mg, phenylpropanolamine hydrochloride 40 mg, phenyltoloxamine citrate 15 mg, and chlorpheniramine maleate 5 mg.
NOLAMINE: chlorpheniramine maleate 4 mg, phenindamine tartrate 24 mg, and phenylpropanolamine hydrochloride 50 mg.

NOVAFED A: pseudoephedrine hydrochloride 120 mg and chlorpheniramine maleate 8 mg.
NOVAHISTINE ELIXIR◇*: phenylephrine 5 mg, chlorpheniramine maleate 2 mg, and alcohol 5%/5 ml.
ORAHIST: phenylpropanolamine hydrochloride 75 mg and chlorpheniramine maleate 12 mg.
ORNADE SPANSULES: phenylpropanolamine hydrochloride 75 mg and chlorpheniramine maleate 12 mg.
P-V TUSSIN: hydrocodone bitartrate 2.5 mg, pseudoephedrine hydrochloride 30 mg, and chlorpheniramine maleate 2 mg per 5 ml.
RHINEX D-LAY: acetaminophen 300 mg, salicylamide 300 mg, phenylpropanolamine hydrochloride 60 mg, and chlorpheniramine maleate 4 mg.
RONDEC: carbinoxamine maleate 4 mg and pseudoephedrine hydrochloride 60 mg.
SELDANE-D: terfenadine 60 mg and pseudoephedrine hydrochloride 120 mg.
SEMPREX-D:acrivastine 8 mg and pseudoephedrine hydrochloride 60 mg.
SUDAFED PLUS◇: pseudoephedrine hydrochloride 60 mg and chlorpheniramine maleate 4 mg.
TAVIST-D◇: clemastine fumarate 1.34 mg and phenylpropanolamine 75 mg.
TRIAMINIC-12: phenylpropanolamine hydrochloride 75 mg and chlorpheniramine maleate 12 mg.
TRIAMINIC EXTENDED-RELEASE TABLETS†: phenylpropanolamine hydrochloride 50 mg, pheniramine maleate 25 mg, and pyrilamine maleate 25 mg.
TRINALIN REPETABS: azatadine maleate 1 mg and pseudoephedrine sulfate 120 mg.

astemizole

Hismanal

Pregnancy Risk Category: C

HOW SUPPLIED

Tablets: 10 mg
Oral suspension: 2 mg/ml*‡

ACTION

Mechanism: Blocks effects of histamine at H_1 receptors. Astemizole is a nonsedating antihistamine; its chemical structure prevents entry into the CNS.
Onset: 2 to 3 days. **Peak:** Plasma levels peak 1 to 4 hours after a dose.
Duration: depends upon the duration of therapy; after long-term use, effects may last several weeks after discontinuing therapy.

INDICATIONS AND DOSAGE

Relief of symptoms associated with chronic idiopathic urticaria and seasonal allergic rhinitis –
Adults and children over 12 years: 10 mg P.O. daily. A loading dose may be given in order to achieve steady-state plasma levels quickly. Begin therapy at 30 mg on the first day, followed by 20 mg on the second day, and 10 mg daily thereafter.
Children 6 to 12 years: 5 mg P.O. daily.

ADVERSE REACTIONS

CNS: headache, nervousness, dizziness, drowsiness.
CV: arrhythmias (with high plasma levels).
EENT: dry mouth, pharyngitis, conjunctivitis.
GI: nausea, diarrhea, abdominal pain, increased appetite.
Other: arthralgia, weight gain, cholestatic jaundice.

INTERACTIONS

Itraconazole, ketoconazole, or macrolide antibiotics such as erythromycin:

†Available in Canada only. ‡Available in Australia only. ◇Available OTC.

risk of serious adverse cardiac reactions. Don't use together.

CONTRAINDICATIONS

- Contraindicated in patients hypersensitive to astemizole and in patients taking the antifungal agents itraconazole or ketoconazole or the macrolide antibiotics azithromycin, clarithromycin, erythromycin, or troleandomycin.
- Use cautiously in patients with hepatic or renal disease. Astemizole is not believed to be dialyzable.
- Also use cautiously in patients with lower respiratory diseases (including asthma); drying effects can increase the risk of bronchial mucus plug formation.

NURSING CONSIDERATIONS

- Ensure that patients know to take astemizole only once a day. If symptoms persist or worsen, warn patients not to increase dosage without consulting doctor. High doses may increase risk of arrhythmias.
- Instruct patient to take drug on an empty stomach at least 2 hours after a meal and to avoid eating for at least 1 hour after dosing.
- Warn patients to stop drug 4 days before allergy skin tests to preserve accuracy of tests.

azatadine maleate

Optimine, Zadine‡

Pregnancy Risk Category: B

HOW SUPPLIED

Tablets: 1 mg
Syrup: 0.5 mg/5 ml‡

ACTION

Mechanism: Competes with histamine for H_1-receptor sites on effector cells. Prevents, but does not reverse, histamine-mediated responses.
Onset: 15 to 60 minutes. **Peak:** Plasma levels peak within 4 hours.
Duration: 12 hours.

INDICATIONS & DOSAGE

Rhinitis, allergy symptoms, chronic urticaria –
Adults: 1 to 2 mg P.O. b.i.d. Maximum dosage is 4 mg daily.
Children over 12 years: 0.5 to 1 mg P.O. b.i.d.

Children under 12 years should use only as directed by a doctor.

ADVERSE REACTIONS

CNS: (especially in elderly patients) *drowsiness, dizziness,* vertigo, disturbed coordination.
CV: hypotension, palpitations.
GI: anorexia, nausea, vomiting, *dry mouth and throat,* epigastric distress.
GU: urine retention.
Hematologic: thrombocytopenia.
Respiratory: thick bronchial secretions.
Skin: urticaria, rash.

INTERACTIONS

CNS depressants: increased sedation. Use together cautiously.
MAO inhibitors: increased anticholinergic effects. Don't use together.

CONTRAINDICATIONS

- Contraindicated in patients with acute asthmatic attacks.
- Use cautiously in elderly patients and in patients with increased intraocular pressure, hyperthyroidism, cardiovascular or renal disease, hypertension, bronchial asthma, urine retention, prostatic hyperplasia, bladder-neck obstruction, and stenosing peptic ulcerations.
- Not recommended for breast-feeding patients because small amounts are excreted in breast milk.

NURSING CONSIDERATIONS

- Reduce GI distress by giving drug with food or milk.
- Monitor blood counts during long-term therapy; watch for signs of blood dyscrasia.

• If tolerance develops, substitute with another antihistamine.
• Warn patients to stop drug 4 days before allergy skin tests to preserve accuracy of tests.
• Warn patients to avoid alcohol and activities that require alertness until CNS response to drug is determined.
• Coffee or tea may reduce drowsiness. Sugarless gum, sour hard candy, or ice chips may relieve dry mouth.

brompheniramine maleate

Bromphen*◊, Chlorphed◊, Codimal-A, Conjec-B◊, Cophene-B, Dehist, Diamine TD, Dimetane*◊, Dimetane Extentabs◊, Dimetane-Ten◊, Histaject Modified, Nasahist B, ND-Stat Revised, Oraminic II, Veltane

Pregnancy Risk Category: C

HOW SUPPLIED
Tablets: 4 mg◊
Tablets (extended-release): 8 mg◊, 12 mg◊
Elixir: 2 mg/5 ml*◊
Injection: 10 mg/ml

ACTION
Mechanism: Competes with histamine for H_1-receptor sites on effector cells. Prevents, but does not reverse, histamine-mediated responses.
Onset: 15 to 60 minutes. **Peak:** Peak levels occur within 2 to 5 hours. Peak effects occur in 3 to 9 hours. **Duration:** 4 to 6 hours for regular-release preparations, up to 25 hours for extended-release preparations.

INDICATIONS & DOSAGE
Rhinitis, allergy symptoms –
Adults: 4 to 8 mg P.O. t.i.d. or q.i.d.; or (extended-release) 8 to 12 mg P.O. b.i.d. or t.i.d.; or 5 to 20 mg q 6 to 12 hours I.M., I.V., or S.C. Maximum dosage is 40 mg daily.
Children 6 years and over: 2 to 4 mg P.O. t.i.d. or q.i.d.; or (extended-release) 8 to 12 mg q 12 hours; or 0.5 mg/kg I.M., I.V., or S.C. daily divided t.i.d. or q.i.d.
Children under 6 years: 0.5 mg/kg P.O., I.M., I.V., or S.C. daily divided t.i.d. or q.i.d.

Note: Children under 12 years should use only as directed by a doctor.

ADVERSE REACTIONS
CNS: (especially in elderly patients) dizziness, tremors, irritability, insomnia, *drowsiness, stimulation.*
CV: hypotension, palpitations.
GI: anorexia, nausea, vomiting, *dry mouth and throat.*
GU: urine retention.
Hematologic: thrombocytopenia, ***agranulocytosis.***
Skin: urticaria, rash.
Other: (after parenteral administration) local stinging, diaphoresis, syncope.

INTERACTIONS
CNS depressants: increased sedation. Use together cautiously.
MAO inhibitors: increased anticholinergic effects. Don't use together.

CONTRAINDICATIONS
• Contraindicated in patients with acute asthmatic attacks.
• Use cautiously in elderly patients, breast-feeding patients, and in those with increased intraocular pressure, hyperthyroidism, cardiovascular or renal disease, hypertension, bronchial asthma, urine retention, prostatic hyperplasia, bladder-neck obstruction, and stenosing peptic ulcerations.
• Antihistamines are not recommended for use by breast-feeding patients because small amounts of drug are excreted in breast milk.

NURSING CONSIDERATIONS
• Reduce GI distress by giving drug with food or milk.

• Monitor blood count during long-term therapy; observe for signs of blood dyscrasia.
• **I.V. use:** Injectable form containing 10 mg/ml can be given diluted or undiluted very slowly I.V. Do not give the 100 mg/ml injection I.V.
• Warn patients to stop drug 4 days before allergy skin tests to preserve accuracy of tests.
• If tolerance develops, another antihistamine may be substituted.
• Warn patients to avoid alcohol and and to avoid activities that require alertness until adverse CNS effects of drug are known.
• Coffee or tea may reduce drowsiness. Causes less drowsiness than some other antihistamines.
• Sugarless gum, sour hard candy, or ice chips may relieve dry mouth.

chlorpheniramine maleate

Aller-Chlor*◇, Allergex‡, Chlo-Amine◇, Chlor-100◇, Chlorate◇, Chlor-Niramine◇, Chlor-Pro, Chlor-Pro 10, Chlorspan-12, Chlortab-4, Chlortab-8, Chlor-Trimeton*◇, Chlor-Trimeton 12-Hour Allergy◇, Chlor-Tripolon†◇, Genallerate◇, Novopheniram‡◇, Pfeiffer's Allergy◇, Phenetron*, Piriton‡, Pyranistan◇, Telachlor, Teldrin◇, Trymegen◇

Pregnancy Risk Category: B

HOW SUPPLIED

Tablets: 4 mg◇
Tablets (chewable): 2 mg◇
Tablets (timed-release): 8 mg◇, 12 mg◇
Capsules (timed-release): 8 mg◇, 12 mg◇
Syrup: 2 mg/5 ml*◇
Injection: 10 mg/ml, 100 mg/ml

ACTION

Mechanism: Competes with histamine for H_1-receptor sites on effector cells. Prevents, but does not reverse, histamine-mediated responses.
Onset: 15 to 60 minutes. **Peak:** Peak concentrations occur 2 to 6 hours after oral dose, or immediately after I.V. injection. Peak effect occurs in 6 hours after oral dose. **Duration:** 4 to 8 hours.

INDICATIONS & DOSAGE

Rhinitis, allergy symptoms –
Adults: 4 mg P.O. q 4 to 6 hours, not to exceed 24 mg/day; or (timed-release) 8 to 12 mg P.O. every 8 to 12 hours; or 5 to 40 mg I.M., I.V., or S.C. as a single dose.
Children 6 to 12 years: 2 mg P.O. q 4 to 6 hours, not to exceed 12 mg/day. Alternatively, may give 8 mg (timed-release) h.s.
Children 2 to 6 years: 1 mg P.O. q 4 to 6 hours.

Note: Children under 12 years should use only as directed by a doctor.

ADVERSE REACTIONS

CNS: *stimulation,* sedation, *drowsiness* (especially in elderly patients), excitability (in children).
CV: hypotension, palpitations.
GI: epigastric distress, *dry mouth.*
GU: urine retention.
Respiratory: thick bronchial secretions.
Skin: rash, urticaria.
Other: (after parenteral administration) local stinging, burning sensation, pallor, weak pulse, transient hypotension.

INTERACTIONS

CNS depressants: increased sedation. Use together cautiously.
MAO inhibitors: increased anticholinergic effects. Don't use together.

CONTRAINDICATIONS

• Contraindicated in patients with acute asthmatic attacks.
• Use cautiously in elderly patients

*Liquid form contains alcohol. *Common* reactions are in italics; ***life-threatening,*** in bold italics.
**May contain tartrazine.

and in those with increased intraocular pressure, hyperthyroidism, cardiovascular or renal disease, hypertension, bronchial asthma, urine retention, prostatic hyperplasia, bladder-neck obstruction, and stenosing peptic ulcerations.
• Antihistamines are not recommended for breast-feeding patients because small amounts of drug are excreted in breast milk.

NURSING CONSIDERATIONS
• If symptoms occur during or after parenteral dose, discontinue drug. Notify the doctor.
• If tolerance develops, substitute with another antihistamine.
• **I.V. use:** Drug is available in 10 mg/ml ampules for I.V. use; do not give the 100 mg/ml strength I.V. Chlorpheniramine is compatible with most I.V. solutions. Give injection over 1 minute.
• Warn patients to stop drug 4 days before allergy skin tests to preserve accuracy of tests.
• Warn patients to avoid alcohol and other CNS depressants and to avoid driving or other activities that require alertness until CNS response to drug is determined.
• Coffee or tea may reduce drowsiness. Sugarless gum, sour hard candy, or ice chips may relieve dry mouth.

clemastine fumarate
Tavist-1 ◊, Tavist

Pregnancy Risk Category: C

HOW SUPPLIED
Tablets: 1.34 mg ◊, 2.68 mg
Syrup: 0.67 mg per 5 ml

ACTION
Mechanism: Competes with histamine for H_1-receptor sites on effector cells. Prevents, but does not reverse, histamine-mediated responses.
Onset: 15 to 60 minutes. **Peak:** Peak levels occur in 2 to 4 hours; peak effects occur in 5 to 7 hours. **Duration:** 12 hours.

INDICATIONS & DOSAGE
Rhinitis, allergy symptoms –
Adults and children 12 years and over: 1.34 mg P.O. q 12 hours, or 2.68 mg P.O. 1 to 3 times a day as needed.
Children 6 to 12 years: 0.67 to 1.34 mg P.O. b.i.d.
Children under 6 years: Use only as directed by a physician.
Note: Children under 12 years should use only as directed by a doctor.

ADVERSE REACTIONS
CNS: (especially in elderly patients) *sedation, drowsiness.*
CV: hypotension, palpitations, tachycardia.
GI: epigastric distress, anorexia, nausea, vomiting, constipation, *dry mouth.*
GU: urine retention.
Hematologic: hemolytic anemia, thrombocytopenia, ***agranulocytosis.***
Respiratory: thick bronchial secretions.
Skin: rash, urticaria.

INTERACTIONS
CNS depressants: increased sedation. Use together cautiously.
MAO inhibitors: increased anticholinergic effects. Don't use together.

CONTRAINDICATIONS
• Contraindicated in patients with acute asthmatic attacks.
• Use cautiously in elderly patients and in those with increased intraocular pressure, hyperthyroidism, cardiovascular or renal disease, hypertension, bronchial asthma, urine retention, prostatic hyperplasia, bladder-neck obstruction, and stenosing peptic ulcerations.
• Antihistamines are not recom-

mended for breast-feeding patients because small amounts of drug are excreted in breast milk.

NURSING CONSIDERATIONS
- If tolerance develops, substitute with another antihistamine.
- Monitor blood counts during long-term therapy; observe for signs of blood dyscrasia.
- Warn patients to stop drug 4 days before allergy skin tests to preserve accuracy of tests.
- Warn patients to avoid alcohol during therapy and to avoid driving or other activities that require alertness until CNS response to drug is determined.
- Coffee or tea may reduce drowsiness. Sugarless gum, sour hard candy, or ice chips may relieve dry mouth.

cyproheptadine hydrochloride
Periactin

Pregnancy Risk Category: B

HOW SUPPLIED
Tablets: 4 mg
Syrup: 2 mg/5 ml

ACTION
Mechanism: Competes with histamine for H_1-receptor sites on effector cells. Prevents, but does not reverse, histamine-mediated responses.
Onset: 15 to 60 minutes. **Duration:** 8 hours.

INDICATIONS & DOSAGE
Allergy symptoms, pruritus –
Adults: 4 mg P.O. t.i.d. or q.i.d. Maximum dosage is 0.5 mg/kg daily.
Children 7 to 14 years: 4 mg P.O. b.i.d. or t.i.d. Maximum dosage is 16 mg daily.
Children 2 to 6 years: 2 mg P.O. b.i.d. or t.i.d. Maximum dosage is 12 mg daily.
Note: Children under 14 years should use only as directed by a doctor.

ADVERSE REACTIONS
CNS: (especially in elderly patients) *drowsiness,* dizziness, headache, fatigue.
GI: nausea, vomiting, epigastric distress, *dry mouth.*
GU: urine retention.
Skin: rash.
Other: weight gain.

INTERACTIONS
CNS depressants: increased sedation. Use together cautiously.
MAO inhibitors: increased anticholinergic effects. Don't use together.

CONTRAINDICATIONS
- Contraindicated in patients with acute asthmatic attacks.
- Use cautiously in elderly patients and in patients with increased intraocular pressure, hyperthyroidism, cardiovascular or renal disease, hypertension, bronchial asthma, urine retention, prostatic hyperplasia, bladder-neck obstruction, and stenosing peptic ulcerations.
- Antihistamines are not recommended for breast-feeding patients because small amounts of drug are excreted in breast milk.

NURSING CONSIDERATIONS
- Reduce GI distress by giving drug with food or milk.
- Warn patients to avoid alcohol and to avoid driving or other activities that require alertness until CNS response to drug is determined.
- Coffee or tea may reduce drowsiness. Sugarless gum, sour hard candy, or ice chips may relieve dry mouth.
- If tolerance develops, substitute with another antihistamine.
- Warn patients to stop drug 4 days before allergy skin tests to preserve accuracy of tests.

dexchlorpheniramine maleate

Dexchlor, Poladex TD, Polaramine*, Polaramine Repetabs

Pregnancy Risk Category: B

HOW SUPPLIED

Tablets: 2 mg
Tablets (timed-release): 4 mg, 6 mg
Syrup: 2 mg/5 ml*

ACTION

Mechanism: Competes with histamine for H_1-receptor sites on effector cells. Prevents, but does not reverse, histamine-mediated responses.
Onset: 15 to 60 minutes. **Duration:** 4 to 8 hours.

INDICATIONS & DOSAGE

Rhinitis, allergy symptoms, contact dermatitis, pruritus –
Adults: 2 mg P.O. q 4 to 6 hours, not to exceed 12 mg/day; or (timed-release) 4 to 6 mg b.i.d. or t.i.d.
Children age 6 to 12: 1 mg P.O. q 4 to 6 hours, not to exceed 6 mg/day; or 4 mg (timed-release tablet) h.s.
Children age 2 to 6: 0.5 mg P.O. q 4 to 6 hours, not to exceed 3 mg/day.

Note: Children under age 6 should use only as directed by a doctor. Do not use timed-release tablets for children younger than age 6.

ADVERSE REACTIONS

CNS: (especially in elderly patients) *drowsiness,* dizziness, *stimulation.*
GI: nausea, *dry mouth.*
GU: polyuria, dysuria, urine retention.

INTERACTIONS

CNS depressants: increased sedation. Use together cautiously.
MAO inhibitors: increased anticholinergic effects. Don't use together.

CONTRAINDICATIONS

- Contraindicated in patients with acute asthmatic attacks.
- Use cautiously in elderly patients and in patients with increased intraocular pressure, hyperthyroidism, cardiovascular or renal disease, hypertension, bronchial asthma, urine retention, prostatic hyperplasia, bladder-neck obstruction, and stenosing peptic ulcerations.
- Antihistamines are not recommended for use by breast-feeding patients because small amounts of drug are excreted in breast milk.

NURSING CONSIDERATIONS

- Warn patients to avoid alcohol and to avoid driving or other activities that require alertness until CNS response to drug is determined.
- Coffee or tea may reduce drowsiness. Sugarless gum, sour hard candy, or ice chips may relieve dry mouth.
- If tolerance develops, substitute another antihistamine.
- Warn patients to stop drug 4 days before allergy skin tests to preserve accuracy of tests.

diphenhydramine hydrochloride

Allerdryl†◊, AllerMax Caplets◊, Aller-med◊, Banophen◊, Banophen Caplets◊, Beldin◊, Belix◊, Bena-D 10, Bena-D 50, Benadryl◊, Benadryl 25◊, Benadryl Kapseals◊, Benahist 10, Benahist 50, Ben-Allergin-50, Benoject-10, Benoject-50, Benylin Cough◊, Bydramine Cough◊, Compoz◊, Diphenacen-50, Diphenadryl◊, Diphen Cough◊, Diphenhist◊, Diphenhist Captabs◊, Dormarex 2◊, Fynex◊, Genahist◊, Gen-D-phen◊, Hydramine◊, Hydramine Cough◊, Hydramyn◊, Hydril◊, Hyrexin-50, Insomnal†◊, Nervine Nighttime Sleep Aid◊, Nidryl◊, Noradryl◊, Nordryl◊

Hydril◊, Hyrexin-50, Insomnal†◊, Nervine Nighttime Sleep Aid◊, Nidryl◊, Noradryl◊, Nordryl◊, Nordryl Cough◊, Nytol Maximum Strength◊, Nytol with DPH◊, Phendry◊, Phendry Children's Allergy Medicine◊, Sleep-Eze 3◊, Sominex Formula 2◊, Tusstat◊, Twilite Caplets◊, Uni-Bent Cough◊, Wehdryl-10, Wehdryl-50

Pregnancy Risk Category: B

HOW SUPPLIED

Tablets: 25 mg◊, 50 mg◊
Capsules: 25 mg◊, 50 mg◊
Elixir: 12.5 mg/5 ml (14% alcohol)*◊
Syrup: 12.5 mg/5 ml◊, 13.3 mg/5 ml (5% alcohol)◊
Injection: 10 mg/ml, 50 mg/ml

ACTION

Mechanism: Competes with histamine for H_1-receptor sites on effector cells. Prevents, but does not reverse, histamine-mediated responses, particularly histamine's effects on the smooth muscle of the bronchial tubes, GI tract, uterus, and blood vessels. Structurally related to local anesthetics, diphenhydramine provides local anesthesia by preventing initiation and transmission of nerve impulses. Also suppresses cough reflex by a direct effect in the medulla of the brain.
Onset: within 15 minutes of oral administration, immediately after I.V. injection. **Peak:** Serum levels peak and drug effects occur 1 to 4 hours after administration. **Duration:** 6 to 8 hours.

INDICATIONS & DOSAGE

Rhinitis, allergy symptoms, motion sickness, Parkinson's disease –
Adults: 25 to 50 mg P.O. t.i.d. or q.i.d.; or 10 to 50 mg deep I.M. or I.V. Maximum I.M. or I.V. dosage is 400 mg daily.
Children under 12 years: 5 mg/kg daily P.O., deep I.M., or I.V. divided q.i.d. Maximum dosage is 300 mg daily.
Sedation –
Adults: 25 to 50 mg P.O., or deep I.M., p.r.n.
Nighttime sleep aid –
Adults: 50 mg P.O. h.s.
Nonproductive cough –
Adults: 25 mg P.O. q 4 hours (not to exceed 150 mg daily).
Children 6 to 12 years: 12.5 mg P.O. q 4 hours (not to exceed 75 mg daily).
Children 2 to 6 years: 6.25 mg P.O. q 4 hours (not to exceed 37.5 mg daily).

Note: Children under 12 years should use only as directed by a doctor.

ADVERSE REACTIONS

CNS: (especially in elderly patients) *drowsiness,* confusion, insomnia, headache, vertigo.
CV: palpitations.
EENT: diplopia.
GI: *nausea,* vomiting, diarrhea, *dry mouth,* constipation.
GU: dysuria, urine retention.
Respiratory: nasal stuffiness.
Skin: urticaria, photosensitivity.

INTERACTIONS

CNS depressants: increased sedation. Use together cautiously.
MAO inhibitors: increased anticholinergic effects. Don't use together.

CONTRAINDICATIONS

- Contraindicated in patients hypersensitive to the drug, and during acute asthmatic attacks.
- Use cautiously in patients with acute angle-closure glaucoma, prostatic hyperplasia, pyloroduodenal and bladder-neck obstruction, and stenosing peptic ulcerations; in newborns; and in asthmatic, hypertensive, or cardiac patients.
- Antihistamines are not recommended for breast-feeding patients

because small amounts of drug are excreted in breast milk.

NURSING CONSIDERATIONS
- Reduce GI distress by giving drug with food or milk.
- One of most sedating antihistamines; often used as a hypnotic.
- Use with epinephrine in anaphylaxis.
- Alternate injection sites to prevent irritation. Administer deep I.M. into large muscle.
- Warn patients to avoid alcohol and to avoid driving or other hazardous activities that require alertness until CNS response to drug is determined.
- Coffee or tea may reduce drowsiness. Sugarless gum, sour hard candy, or ice chips may relieve dry mouth.
- If tolerance develops, substitute another antihistamine.
- For use to prevent motion sickness, instruct patients to take 30 minutes before travel.
- Warn patients to stop drug 4 days before allergy skin tests to preserve accuracy of tests.
- Warn patients of possible photosensitivity. Advise use of a sunblock.

loratadine

Claratyne‡, Claritin

Pregnancy Risk Category: B

HOW SUPPLIED
Tablets: 10 mg

ACTION
Mechanism: Blocks effects of histamine at H_1 receptors. Loratadine is a nonsedating antihistamine; its chemical structure prevents entry into the CNS.
Onset: 30 minutes. **Peak:** Peak effects occur in 4 to 6 hours. **Duration:** at least 24 hours.

INDICATIONS & DOSAGE
Symptomatic treatment of seasonal allergic rhinitis –
Adults and children 12 years and over: 10 mg P.O. daily. Patients with hepatic failure should start therapy with 10 mg every other day.

ADVERSE REACTIONS
CNS: headache, somnolence, fatigue.
GI: dry mouth.

INTERACTIONS
None significant.

CONTRAINDICATIONS
- Contraindicated in patients hypersensitive to the drug.
- Use cautiously and in lower dosages in patients with liver failure to prevent accumulation of drug and its active metabolites. Also use cautiously with drugs that are known to impair hepatic drug metabolism. Studies to rule out drug interactions have not been performed.
- Use cautiously in breast-feeding patients because trace amounts of drug are found in human breast milk.

NURSING CONSIDERATIONS
- Although administration with food causes only small changes in drug absorption, give loratadine on an empty stomach. Instruct patients to take drug at least 2 hours after a meal and to avoid eating for at least 1 hour after taking drug.
- Ensure that patients know to take drug only once daily. If symptoms persist or worsen, patients should contact the doctor.
- Warn patients to stop taking drug 4 days before allergy skin tests to preserve accuracy of tests.

methdilazine hydrochloride

Dilosyn †‡ Tacaryl*

Pregnancy Risk Category: C

HOW SUPPLIED
Tablets: 8 mg
Tablets (chewable): 3.6 mg methdilazine (equal to 4 mg methdilazine hydrochloride)
Syrup: 4 mg/5 ml*

ACTION
Mechanism: Competes with histamine for H_1-receptor sites on effector cells. Prevents, but does not reverse, histamine-mediated responses. A phenothiazine derivative.
Onset: 15 to 60 minutes. **Duration:** 6 to 12 hours.

INDICATIONS & DOSAGE
Allergic rhinitis, pruritus –
Adults: 8 mg P.O. b.i.d. to q.i.d. or (chewable tablets) 7.2 mg P.O. b.i.d. to q.i.d.
Children over 3 years: 4 mg P.O. b.i.d. to q.i.d. or (chewable tablets) 3.6 mg P.O. b.i.d. to q.i.d.

ADVERSE REACTIONS
CNS: (especially in elderly patients) *drowsiness,* dizziness, headache.
GI: nausea, *dry mouth and throat.*
GU: urine retention.
Hepatic: cholestatic jaundice.
Skin: rash.

INTERACTIONS
CNS depressants: increased sedation. Use together cautiously.
MAO inhibitors: increased anticholinergic effects. Don't use together.
Phenothiazines: increased effects. Don't use together.

CONTRAINDICATIONS
- Contraindicated in patients experiencing acute asthmatic attacks.
- Use cautiously in elderly or debilitated patients; acutely ill or dehydrated children; in patients with a history of seizures; in those with pulmonary, hepatic, or cardiovascular disease; and in patients with asthma, hypertension, prostatic hyperplasia, bladder-neck obstruction, CNS depression, and stenosing peptic ulcerationations.
- Antihistamines are not recommended for breast-feeding patients because small amounts of drug are excreted in breast milk.

NURSING CONSIDERATIONS
- If tolerance develops, substitute another antihistamine.
- Reduce GI distress by giving drug with food or milk.
- Available as chewable tablet for children. Instruct child to chew completely and swallow promptly; may cause local anesthetic effect in mouth, which increases the risk of choking.
- Warn patients to avoid alcohol and to avoid driving or other activities that require alertness until CNS response to drug is determined.
- Coffee or tea may reduce drowsiness. Sugarless gum, sour hard candy, or ice chips may relieve dry mouth.
- Warn patients to stop drug 4 days before allergy skin to preserve accuracy of tests.

promethazine hydrochloride
Anergan 25, Anergan 50, Histanil†, Pentazine, Phenameth, Phenazine 25, Phenazine 50, Phencen-50, Phenergan*, Phenergan-Fortis*, Phenergan-Plain*, Phenoject-50, PMS-Promethazine†, Pro-50, Prometh-25, Prometh-50, Promethegan, Prothazine†*, Prorex-25, Prorex-50, Prothazine Plain, V-Gan-25, V-Gan-50

promethazine theoclate
Avomine‡

Pregnancy Risk Category: C

*Liquid form contains alcohol.
**May contain tartrazine.

HOW SUPPLIED
hydrochloride
Tablets: 12.5 mg, 25 mg, 50 mg
Syrup: 5 mg/5 ml‡*, 6.25 mg/5 ml*, 10 mg/5 ml*, 25 mg/5 ml*
Injection: 25 mg/ml, 50 mg/ml
Suppositories: 12.5 mg, 25 mg, 50 mg
theoclate
Tablets: 25 mg‡

ACTION
Mechanism: Competes with histamine for H_1-receptor sites on effector cells. Prevents, but does not reverse, histamine-mediated responses. A phenothiazine derivative.
Onset: 15 to 60 minutes after oral administration, 20 minutes after rectal use. **Duration:** 6 to 12 hours.

INDICATIONS & DOSAGE
Motion sickness –
Adults: 25 mg P.O. b.i.d.
Children: 1 mg/kg P.O., I.M., or P.R. b.i.d.
Nausea –
Adults: 12.5 to 25 mg P.O., I.M., or P.R. q 4 to 6 hours, p.r.n.
Children: 1 mg/kg I.M. or P.R. q 4 to 6 hours, p.r.n.
Rhinitis, allergy symptoms –
Adults: 12.5 mg P.O. q.i.d.; or 25 mg P.O. h.s.
Children: 6.25 to 12.5 mg P.O. t.i.d. or 25 mg P.O. or P.R. h.s.
Sedation –
Adults: 25 to 50 mg P.O. or I.M. h.s. or p.r.n.
Children: 12.5 to 25 mg P.O., I.M., or P.R. h.s.
Routine preoperative or postoperative sedation or adjunct to analgesics –
Adults: 25 to 50 mg I.M., I.V., or P.O.
Children: 12.5 to 25 mg I.M., I.V., or P.O.

ADVERSE REACTIONS
CNS: (especially in elderly patients) *sedation,* confusion, restlessness, tremors, *drowsiness.*
CV: hypotension.
EENT: transient myopia, nasal congestion.
GI: anorexia, nausea, vomiting, constipation, *dry mouth.*
GU: urine retention.
Hematologic: leukopenia, ***agranulocytosis.***
Other: photosensitivity.

INTERACTIONS
Anticholinergics, tricyclic antidepressants, phenothiazines: increased effects. Don't give together.
Ethanol, CNS depressants: increased sedation. Use together cautiously.
MAO inhibitors: increased anticholinergic effects. Don't use together.
Levodopa: promethazine may decrease levodopa's antiparkinsonian action. Avoid concomitant use.
Lithium: promethazine may reduce GI absorption or enhance renal elimination of lithium. Avoid concomitant use.

CONTRAINDICATIONS
- Contraindicated in patients with increased intraocular pressure, intestinal obstruction, prostatic hyperplasia, bladder-neck obstruction, seizure disorders, bone-marrow depression, coma, CNS depression, stenosing peptic ulcerations, and in newborns and acutely ill or dehydrated children.
- Use cautiously in patients with pulmonary, hepatic, or cardiovascular disease; asthma; hypertension; bone-marrow depression; in elderly or debilitated patients; and in patients with a history of seizures.
- Antihistamines are not recommended for breast-feeding patients because small amounts of drug are excreted in breast milk.

NURSING CONSIDERATIONS
- Reduce GI distress by giving drug with food or milk.
- Pronounced sedative effect limits use in many ambulatory patients.

• When treating motion sickness, tell patients to take first dose 30 to 60 minutes before travel. On succeeding days of travel, he should take dose upon rising and with evening meal.
• In patients scheduled for a myelogram, discontinue drug 48 hours before procedure and do not resume drug until 24 hours after procedure because of the risk of seizures.
• Warn patient to stop drug 4 days before allergy skin tests to preserve accuracy of tests.
• May cause false-positive immunologic urine pregnancy test (Gravindex). Also may interfere with blood grouping in ABO system.
• Inject deep I.M. into large muscle mass. Don't administer S.C. Rotate injection sites.
• **I.V. use:** Don't give in a concentration greater than 25 mg/ml or at a rate exceeding 25 mg/minute. Shield I.V. infusion from direct light.
• Used as an adjunct to analgesics (usually to increase sedation); promethazine has no analgesic activity.
• May be safely mixed with meperidine (Demerol) in the same syringe.
• Warn patients about possible photosensitivity and precautions to avoid it.
• Warn patients to avoid alcohol and to avoid driving or other activities that require alertness until CNS response to drug is determined.
• Coffee or tea may reduce drowsiness. Sugarless gum, sour hard candy, or ice chips may relieve dry mouth.

terfenadine

Seldane, Seldane Caplets†, Teldane‡

Pregnancy Risk Category: C

HOW SUPPLIED

Tablets: 60 mg, 120 mg†
Oral suspension†: 6 mg/ml

ACTION

Mechanism: Competes with histamine for H_1-receptor sites on effector cells. Prevents, but does not reverse, histamine-mediated responses.
Onset: about 1 hour. **Peak:** Peak effects occur in 3 to 4 hours. Peak levels occur about 2 hours after an oral dose. **Duration:** over 12 hours.

INDICATIONS & DOSAGE

Rhinitis, allergy symptoms –
Adults and children over 12 years: 60 mg P.O. b.i.d. to t.i.d., or 120 mg once a day.
Children 6 to 12 years: 30 to 60 mg P.O. b.i.d.
Children 3 to 5 years: 15 mg P.O. b.i.d.

ADVERSE REACTIONS

CNS: fatigue, dizziness, *headache,* sedation.
CV: ***arrhythmias*** (with high blood levels).
EENT: dry throat and mouth.
GI: abdominal distress, nausea.
Respiratory: nasal stuffiness.
Other: alopecia, cholestatic jaundice.

INTERACTIONS

Cimetidine, ciprofloxacin, itraconazole, ketoconazole, macrolide antibiotics (erythromycin, troleandomycin): decreased hepatic metabolism of terfenadine, leading to increased serum levels and risk of serious arrhythmias. Avoid concomitant use.

CONTRAINDICATIONS

• Contraindicated in patients hypersensitive to terfenadine and in those taking the antifungal agents itraconazole or ketoconazole or the macrolide antibiotics.

NURSING CONSIDERATIONS

• Tablets must be broken for children's dosages.
• Terfenadine does not cause the degree of drowsiness and sedation asso-

ciated with other antihistamines because it does not cross blood-brain barrier; its anticholinergic and antiserotonin effects are mild.

- Keep patients well hydrated. Drug may cause a mild anticholinergic drying effect in patients with lower airway disease, such as asthma.
- Instruct patients not to exceed prescribed dose. If overdose occurs, monitor patient for arrhythmias.

trimeprazine tartrate

Panectyl†, Temaril*, Vallergan‡

Pregnancy Risk Category: C

HOW SUPPLIED

Tablets: 2.5 mg, 10 mg‡
Spansule capsules (sustained-release): 5 mg
Syrup: 2.5 mg/5 ml*, 7.5 mg/5 ml*‡, 30 mg/5 ml*‡

ACTION

Mechanism: Competes with histamine for H_1-receptor sites on effector cells. Prevents, but does not reverse, histamine-mediated responses. A phenothiazine derivative.
Onset: 15 to 60 minutes. **Duration:** 3 to 6 hours.

INDICATIONS & DOSAGE

Pruritus –
Adults: 2.5 mg P.O. q.i.d.; or (timed-release) 5 mg P.O. b.i.d.
Children 3 to 12 years: 2.5 mg P.O. h.s. or t.i.d., p.r.n.
Children 6 months to 3 years: 1.25 mg P.O. h.s. or t.i.d., p.r.n.
Note: Children under 12 years should use only as directed by a doctor.

ADVERSE REACTIONS

CNS: (especially in elderly patients) drowsiness, dizziness, confusion, headache, restlessness, tremors, irritability, insomnia; (in children) paradoxical excitation.
CV: hypotension, palpitations, tachycardia.
GI: anorexia, nausea, vomiting, *dry mouth and throat.*
GU: urinary frequency, urine retention.
Hematologic: ***agranulocytosis,*** leukopenia.
Skin: urticaria, rash, *photosensitivity.*

INTERACTIONS

Anticholinergics, MAO inhibitors, phenothiazines, tricyclic antidepressants: increased anticholinergic effect. Don't use together.
Ethanol, CNS depressants: increased sedation. Use together cautiously.
Levodopa: trimeprazine may block levodopa's antiparkinsonian effects. Don't use together.
Lithium: trimeprazine may decrease GI absorption and enhance renal excretion of lithium. Don't use together.

CONTRAINDICATIONS

- Contraindicated in patients with acute asthmatic attacks.
- Use cautiously in patients with pulmonary, hepatic, or cardiovascular disease; asthma; hypertension; acute angle-closure glaucoma; intestinal obstruction; prostatic hyperplasia; bladder-neck obstruction; seizure disorder; bone-marrow depression; coma; CNS depression; stenosing peptic ulcerations; in elderly or debilitated patients; and in acutely ill or dehydrated children.
- Antihistamines are not recommended for use by breast-feeding patients because small amounts of drug are excreted in breast milk.

NURSING CONSIDERATIONS

- Reduce GI distress by giving drug with food or milk.
- Monitor blood counts during long-term therapy.
- In patients scheduled for a myelogram, discontinue drug 48 hours be-

fore procedure; do not continue drug until 24 hours after the procedure because of the risk of seizures.
- Warn patients to avoid alcohol and to avoid driving or other activities that require alertness until CNS response to drug is determined.
- Coffee or tea may reduce drowsiness. Sugarless gum, sour hard candy, or ice chips may relieve dry mouth.
- Warn patients about risk of photosensitivity. Recommend use of a sunblock. If photosensitivity occurs, tell the patient to discontinue drug and call the doctor.
- Warn patients to stop drug 4 days before allergy skin tests to preserve accuracy of tests.

tripelennamine citrate

PBZ*

tripelennamine hydrochloride

PBZ, PBZ-SR, Pelamine, Pyribenzamine

Pregnancy Risk Category: B

HOW SUPPLIED

citrate

Elixir: 37.5 mg/5 ml (equivalent to 25 mg/5 ml tripelennamine hydrochloride)*

hydrochloride

Tablets: 25 mg, 50 mg

Tablets (extended-release): 100 mg

ACTION

Mechanism: Competes with histamine for H_1-receptor sites on effector cells. Prevents, but does not reverse, histamine-mediated responses.

Onset: 15 to 60 minutes. **Duration:** 4 to 6 hours.

INDICATIONS & DOSAGE

Rhinitis, allergy symptoms –

Adults: 25 to 50 mg P.O. q 4 to 6 hours; or (extended-release) 100 mg b.i.d. or t.i.d. Maximum dosage is 600 mg daily.

Children: 5 mg/kg P.O. daily in four to six divided doses. Maximum dosage is 300 mg daily.

ADVERSE REACTIONS

CNS: (especially in elderly patients) *drowsiness,* dizziness, confusion, restlessness, tremors, irritability, insomnia.

CV: palpitations.

GI: anorexia, diarrhea or constipation, *nausea, vomiting, dry mouth.*

GU: urinary frequency, urine retention.

Skin: urticaria, rash.

Other: thick bronchial secretions.

INTERACTIONS

CNS depressants: increased sedation. Use together cautiously.

MAO inhibitors: increased anticholinergic effects. Don't use together.

CONTRAINDICATIONS

- Contraindicated in patients experiencing acute asthmatic attacks.
- Use cautiously in elderly patients, and in patients with increased intraocular pressure, hyperthyroidism, CV or renal disease, hypertension, bronchial asthma, urine retention, prostatic hyperplasia, bladder-neck obstruction, and stenosing peptic ulcerations. Do not use extended-release preparations children.
- Anthistamines are not recommended for breast-feeding patients because small amounts of drug are excreted in breast milk.

NURSING CONSIDERATIONS

- Warn patients to avoid alcohol and to avoid driving or other activities that require alertness until CNS response to drug is determined.
- Reduce GI distress by giving drug with food or milk.
- Coffee or tea may reduce drowsi-

*Liquid form contains alcohol.
**May contain tartrazine.

Common reactions are in italics; ***life-threatening,*** in bold italics.

ness. Sugarless gum, sour hard candy, or ice chips may relieve dry mouth.
- If tolerance develops, substitute another antihistamine.
- Warn patients to stop drug 4 days before allergy skin tests to preserve accuracy of tests.

triprolidine hydrochloride
Alleract◊, Myidyl
Pregnancy Risk Category: C

HOW SUPPLIED
Tablets: 2.5 mg◊
Syrup:* 1.25 mg/5 ml◊

ACTION
Mechanism: Competes with histamine for H_1-receptor sites on effector cells. Prevents, but does not reverse, histamine-mediated responses.
Onset: 15 to 60 minutes. **Peak:** Peak levels occur in about 2 hours. Peak effects occur in 2 to 3 hours. **Duration:** 4 to 8 hours.

INDICATIONS & DOSAGE
Colds and allergy symptoms –
Adults: 2.5 mg P.O. q 4 to 6 hours. Maximum dosage is 10 mg/day.
Children 6 years and over: 1.25 mg P.O. q 4 to 6 hours. Maximum dosage is 5 mg/day.
Children 4 to 6 years: 0.9 mg P.O. q 4 to 6 hours. Maximum dosage is 3.75 mg/day.
Children 2 to 4 years: 0.6 mg P.O. q 4 to 6 hours. Maximum dosage is 2.5 mg/day.
Children 4 months to 2 years: 0.3 mg P.O. q 4 to 6 hours. Maximum dosage is 1.25 mg/day.
Note: Children under 12 years should use only as directed by a doctor.

ADVERSE REACTIONS
CNS: (especially in elderly patients) *drowsiness,* dizziness, confusion, restlessness, insomnia, *stimulation.*
GI: anorexia, diarrhea or constipation, nausea, vomiting, *dry mouth.*
GU: urinary frequency, urine retention.
Skin: urticaria, rash.

INTERACTIONS
CNS depressants: increased sedation.
MAO inhibitors: increased anticholinergic effects. Don't use together.

CONTRAINDICATIONS
- Contraindicated in patients experiencing acute asthma attacks.
- Use cautiously in elderly patients and in those with increased intraocular pressure, hyperthyroidism, cardiovascular or renal disease, hypertension, diabetes mellitus, bronchial asthma, urine retention, prostatic hyperplasia, bladder-neck obstruction, and stenosing peptic ulcerations.
- Antihistamines are not recommended for breast-feeding patients because small amounts of drug are excreted in breast milk.

NURSING CONSIDERATIONS
- Reduce GI distress by giving drug with food or milk.
- Warn patients to avoid alcohol and to avoid driving or other activities that require alertness until CNS response to drug is determined.
- Coffee or tea may reduce drowsiness. Sugarless gum, sour hard candy, or ice chips may relieve dry mouth.
- Warn patients to stop drug 4 days before allergy skin tests to preserve accuracy of tests.

43

Bronchodilators

albuterol
albulterol sulfate
aminophylline
atropine sulfate
(See Chapter 20, ANTIARRHYTHMICS.)
bitolterol mesylate
dyphylline
ephedrine sulfate
epinephrine
epinephrine bitartrate
epinephrine hydrochloride
ethylnorepinephrine hydrochloride
ipratropium bromide
isoetharine hydrochloride
isoetharine mesylate
isoproterenol
isoproterenol hydrochloride
isoproterenol sulfate
metaproterenol sulfate
oxtriphylline
pirbuterol
salmeterol xinafoate
terbutaline sulfate
theophylline
theophylline sodium glycinate

COMBINATION PRODUCTS

Inhalants

DUO-MEDIHALER: isoproterenol hydrochloride 0.16 mg and phenylephrine bitartrate 0.24 mg per dose.

Oral bronchodilators

BRONCHIAL CAPSULES: 150 mg theophylline and 90 mg guaifenesin.
BRONCHOBID DURACAPS: theophylline 260 mg and ephedrine hydrochloride 35 mg.
BRONDECON TABLETS: 200 mg oxtriphylline and 100 mg guaifenesin.
DILOR-G TABLETS: 200 mg dyphylline and 200 mg guaifenesin.
DYFLEX-G TABLETS: 200 mg dyphylline and 200 mg guaifenesin.
DYLINE-GG TABLETS: 200 mg dyphylline and 200 mg guaifenesin.
ENTEX LA: phenylpropanolamine hydrochloride 75 mg and guaifenesin 400 mg.
GLYCERYL-T CAPSULES: 150 mg theophylline and 90 mg guaifenesin.
LANOPHYLLIN-GG CAPSULES: 150 mg theophylline and 90 mg guaifenesin.
MARAX*: theophylline 130 mg, ephedrine sulfate 25 mg, and hydroxyzine hydrochloride 10 mg.
NEOTHYLLINE-GG TABLETS: 200 mg dyphylline and 200 mg guaifenesin.
QUADRINAL: theophylline calcium salicylate 65 mg, ephedrine hydrochloride 24 mg, potassium iodide 320 mg, and phenobarbital 24 mg.
QUIBRON CAPSULES: 150 mg theophylline and 90 mg guaifenesin.
QUIBRON PLUS*: theophylline 150 mg, ephedrine hydrochloride 25 mg, guaifenesin 100 mg, and butabarbital 20 mg.
TEDRAL◇: theophylline 130 mg, ephedrine hydrochloride 24 mg, and phenobarbital 8 mg.
TEDRAL SA: theophylline 180 mg, ephedrine hydrochloride 48 mg, and phenobarbital 25 mg.
THALFED◇: theophylline 120 mg, ephedrine hydrochloride 25 mg, and phenobarbital 8 mg.

Decongestants

ACTIFED◇: pseudoephedrine hydrochloride 60 mg and triprolidine hydrochloride 2.5 mg.
CONGESPIRIN◇: phenylephrine hydrochloride 1.25 mg and acetaminophen 81 mg.
DRISTAN◇: phenylephrine hydrochloride 5 mg, chlorpheniramine maleate 2 mg, and acetaminophen 325 mg.
HISTASPAN-PLUS: phenylephrine hy-

*Liquid form contains alcohol.
**May contain tartrazine.

drochloride 20 mg and chlorpheniramine maleate 8 mg.
NALDECON: phenylpropanolamine hydrochloride 40 mg, phenylephrine hydrochloride 10 mg, chlorpheniramine maleate 5 mg, and phenyltoloxamine citrate 15 mg.
ORNEX◇: phenylpropanolamine hydrochloride 18 mg and acetaminophen 325 mg.
PHENERGAN-D: pseudoephedrine hydrochloride 60 mg and promethazine hydrochloride 6.25 mg.

albuterol (salbutamol)

Asmol‡, Proventil, Respolin‡, Ventolin

albuterol sulfate (salbutamol sulphate)

Proventil, Proventil Repetabs, Respolin Autohaler Inhalation Device‡, Respolin Inhaler‡, Respolin Respirator Solution‡, Ventolin, Ventolin Obstetric Injection‡, Ventolin Rotacaps, Volmax

Pregnancy Risk Category: C

HOW SUPPLIED

albuterol
Aerosol inhaler: 90 mcg/metered spray, 100 mcg/metered spray‡
albuterol sulfate
Capsules for inhalation: 200 mcg
Tablets: 2 mg, 4 mg
Tablets (extended-release): 4 mg, 8 mg
Syrup: 2 mg/5 ml
Solution for inhalation: 0.083%, 0.5%
Injection: 1 mg/ml‡

ACTION

Mechanism: Relaxes bronchial and uterine smooth muscle by acting on beta$_2$-adrenergic receptors.
Onset: within 5 to 15 minutes after inhalation; within 15 to 30 minutes after oral administration. **Peak:** Peak effect occurs 1 to 1½ hours after inhalation, or 2 to 3 hours after oral administration. **Duration:** 3 to 6 hours after inhalation; about 8 hours after oral administration; about 12 hours for extended release preparations.

INDICATIONS & DOSAGE

To prevent or treat bronchospasm in patients with reversible obstructive airway disease –
Adults and children 12 years and older: dosage and frequency vary with dosage form.
Aerosol inhalation: – 1 to 2 inhalations q 4 to 6 hours. More frequent administration or a greater number of inhalations is not recommended.
Solution for inhalation: – 2.5 mg 3 or 4 times a day by nebulizer. To prepare solution, use 0.5 ml of the 0.5% solution diluted with 2.5 ml of 0.9% sodium chloride. Alternatively, use 3 ml of the 0.083% solution.
Capsules for inhalation: – 200 mcg inhaled every 4 to 6 hours using a Rotahaler inhalation device. Some patients may need 400 mcg q 4 to 6 hours.
Oral tablets – 2 to 4 mg t.i.d. or q.i.d. Maximum dosage is 8 mg q.i.d.
Extended-release tablets – 4 to 8 mg q 12 hours. Maximum dosage is 16 mg b.i.d.
Children 6 to 13 years: 2 mg (1 teaspoonful) P.O. t.i.d. or q.i.d.
Children 2 to 5 years: 0.1 mg/kg P.O. t.i.d., not to exceed 2 mg (1 teaspoonful) t.i.d.
Adults over 65 years: 2 mg P.O. t.i.d. or q.i.d.
To prevent exercise-induced asthma –
Adults: 2 inhalations 15 minutes before exercise.
Prevention of premature labor‡ –
Adults: initially, 10 mcg/minute by continuous I.V. infusion (use an infusion pump). Dosage should be increased in 10-minute intervals until the desired response is achieved.

ADVERSE REACTIONS

CNS: *tremor, nervousness,* dizziness, insomnia, headache.
CV: tachycardia, palpitations, hypertension.
EENT: drying and irritation of nose and throat (with inhaled form).
GI: heartburn, nausea, vomiting.
Respiratory: ***bronchospasm.***
Other: muscle cramps, hypokalemia (with high doses).

INTERACTIONS

CNS stimulants: increased CNS stimulation. Avoid concomitant use.
Levodopa: risk of arrhythmias. Monitor closely.
MAO inhibitors, tricyclic antidepressants: increased adverse cardiovascular effects.
Propranolol and other beta blockers: mutual antagonism. Monitor patient carefully.

CONTRAINDICATIONS

- Contraindicated in patients hypersensitive to the drug or any component of the formulation.
- Use cautiously in patients with cardiovascular disorders, including coronary insufficiency and hypertension; in patients with hyperthyroidism or diabetes mellitus; and in patients who are unusually responsive to adrenergics.
- Albuterol reportedly produces less cardiac stimulation than other sympathomimetics, especially isoproterenol.

NURSING CONSIDERATIONS

- Patients may use tablets and aerosol concomitantly. Monitor closely for toxicity.
- Teach patients to perform oral inhalation correctly. Give the following instructions for using metered-dose inhaler:
  - Clear nasal passages and throat.
  - Breathe out, expelling as much air from lungs as possible.
  - Place mouthpiece well into mouth as dose from inhaler is released, and inhale deeply.
  - Hold breath for several seconds, remove mouthpiece, and exhale slowly.
- If more than one inhalation is ordered, advise patient to wait at least 2 minutes before repeating procedure.
- Tell patients who are also using a steroid inhaler to use the bronchodilator first, then wait about 5 minutes before using the steroid. This allows bronchodilator to open air passages for maximum effectiveness.
- When used to prevent premature labor, monitor maternal heart rate closely. It should not exceed 140 beats/minute.
- After uterine contractions have ceased, drip rate of drug should be maintained for 1 hour, then gradually tapered at 50% increments in six hourly intervals. Do not continue infusions for more than 48 hours. If therapy needs to continue over 48 hours, doctor may prescribe 4 to 8 mg P.O. q.i.d.
- **I.V. use:** I.V. form (where available) may be used to prepare infusion using sodium chloride injection, glucose injection, or sodium chloride and glucose injection. Do not administer drug without dilution. Do not mix with any other medication. Discard unused dilution after 24 hours.
- Aerosol form may be prescribed for use 15 minutes before exercise to prevent exercise-induced bronchospasm.
- Warn patients about possibility of paradoxical bronchospasm. If this occurs, discontinue drug immediately.
- Pleasant-tasting syrup may be taken by children as young as 2 years. Contains no alcohol or sugar.

aminophylline (theophylline ethylenediamine)

Aminophyllin, Cardophyllin‡, Corophyllin†, Phyllocontin, Phyllocontin-350, Somophyllin, Somophyllin-DF

Pregnancy Risk Category: C

HOW SUPPLIED

Tablets: 100 mg, 200 mg
Tablets (extended-release): 225 mg, 350 mg†
Oral liquid: 105 mg/5 ml
Injection: 250 mg/10 ml, 500 mg/20 ml, 500 mg/2 ml, 100 mg/100 ml in 0.45% sodium chloride, 200 mg/100 ml in 0.45% sodium chloride
Rectal solution: 300 mg/5 ml
Rectal suppositories: 250 mg, 500 mg

ACTION

Mechanism: Inhibits phosphodiesterase, the enzyme that degrades cAMP. Results in relaxation of smooth muscle of the bronchial airways and pulmonary blood vessels.
Onset: 15 minutes after I.V. injection, 15 to 60 minutes after oral solution or tablets, 15 to 30 minutes after rectal solution. **Peak:** Peak serum levels occur immediately after I.V. infusion; within 1 hour of oral solution; 2 hours after oral, uncoated tablets; 4 to 7 hours after extended-release capsules or tablets; 1 to 2 hours after a retention enema. **Duration:** variable – in healthy adults with asthma, half-life about 9 hours; more than 24 hours in adults with cor pulmonale, heart failure, COPD, or liver disease; about 5 hours in patients who smoke or have smoked in the last 2 to 3 years; 24 hours or more in neonates and infants to age 6 months; about 4 hours in children over age 6 months.

INDICATIONS & DOSAGE

Symptomatic relief of bronchospasm –
Patients not currently receiving theophylline who require rapid relief of symptoms: loading dose is 6 mg/kg (equivalent to 4.7 mg/kg anhydrous theophylline) I.V. (less than or equal to 25 mg/minute), then maintenance infusion.
Adults (nonsmokers): 0.7 mg/kg/hour for 12 hours; then 0.5 mg/kg/hour.
Otherwise healthy adult smokers: 1 mg/kg/hour for 12 hours; then 0.8 mg/kg/hour.
Older patients and adults with cor pulmonale: 0.6 mg/kg/hour for 12 hours; then 0.3 mg/kg/hour.
Adults with CHF or liver disease: 0.5 mg/kg/hour for 12 hours; then 0.1 to 0.2 mg/kg/hour.
Children 9 to 16 years: 1 mg/kg/hour for 12 hours; then 0.8 mg/kg/hour.
Children 6 months to 9 years: 1.2 mg/kg/hour for 12 hours; then 1 mg/kg/hour.
Patients currently receiving theophylline: aminophylline infusions of 0.63 mg/kg (0.5 mg/kg anhydrous theophylline) will increase plasma levels of theophylline by 1 mcg/ml. Some clinicians recommend a dose of 3.1 mg/kg (2.5 mg/kg anhydrous theophylline) if no obvious signs of theophylline toxicity are present.
Chronic bronchial asthma –
Adults: 600 to 1,600 mg P.O. daily divided t.i.d. or q.i.d.
Children: 12 mg/kg P.O. daily divided t.i.d. or q.i.d.
Adjunctive treatment of neonatal apnea –
Neonates: 5.7 mg/kg I.V. as a loading dose, followed by 2.3 mg/kg/day I.V. in 2 or 3 divided doses.

ADVERSE REACTIONS

CNS: *nervousness, restlessness, dizziness,* headache, *insomnia,* light-headedness, ***seizures,*** muscle twitching.
CV: *palpitations, sinus tachycardia,* extrasystoles, flushing, marked hypotension, increase in respiratory rate.
GI: *nausea, vomiting, anorexia,* bitter

aftertaste, dyspepsia, heavy feeling in stomach, diarrhea.
Skin: urticaria.
Other: rectal suppositories may cause irritation.

INTERACTIONS

Adenosine: decreased antiarrhythmic effectiveness. Higher doses of adenosine may be necessary.
Alkali-sensitive drugs: reduced activity. Do not add to I.V. fluids containing aminophylline.
Barbiturates, carbamazepine, nicotine, phenytoin, rifampin: enhanced metabolism and decreased theophylline blood levels. Monitor for decreased aminophylline effect.
Beta-adrenergic blockers: antagonism. Propranolol and nadolol, especially, may cause bronchospasm in sensitive patients. Use together cautiously.
Cimetidine, influenza virus vaccine, macrolide antibiotics (such as erythromycin), oral contraceptives, quinolone antibiotics (such as ciprofloxacin): decreased hepatic clearance of theophylline; elevated theophylline levels. Monitor for signs of toxicity.

CONTRAINDICATIONS

- Contraindicated in patients hypersensitive to xanthine compounds (caffeine, theobromine) and in patients with preexisting arrhythmias, especially tachyarrhythmias.
- Use cautiously in young children; in elderly patients with CHF or other cardiac or circulatory impairment, cor pulmonale, or hepatic disease; in patients with active peptic ulceration because drug may increase volume and acidity of gastric secretions; and in patients with hyperthyroidism or diabetes mellitus.

NURSING CONSIDERATIONS

- Relieve GI symptoms by giving oral drug with full glass of water at meals, although food in stomach delays absorption. No evidence exists that antacids reduce GI adverse reactions. Enteric-coated tablets may also delay and impair absorption.
- Monitor vital signs; measure and record fluid intake and output. Expected clinical effects include improvement in quality of pulse and respiration.
- Aminophylline is a soluble salt of theophylline. Adjust dosage by monitoring response, tolerance, pulmonary function, and serum theophylline levels. Theophylline concentrations should range from 10 to 20 mcg/ml; toxicity has been reported with levels above 20 mcg/ml.
- Patients who experience urticaria may still tolerate other theophylline preparations. Urticaria may be caused by the ethylene diamine salt.
- Warn patients to check with the doctor or pharmacist before combining aminophylline with other drugs. OTC remedies may contain ephedrine in combination with theophylline salts; excessive CNS stimulation may result.
- Before giving loading dose, ensure that patient has not had recent theophylline therapy.
- **I.V. use:** I.V. drug administration can cause burning; dilute with compatible I.V. solution and inject at a rate no faster than 25 mg/minute. Drug is compatible with most I.V. solutions except invert sugar, fructose, and fat emulsion.
- Suppositories are slowly and erratically absorbed; retention enemas may be absorbed more rapidly. Administer rectal preparations if patients cannot take drug orally. Schedule after evacuation, if possible; may be retained better if given before meal. Advise patients to remain recumbent 15 to 20 minutes after insertion.
- Advise patients to avoid switching brand without first checking with the doctor.
- Supply instructions for home care

and dosage schedule. Some patients may require an around-the-clock dosage schedule.
• Warn patients with allergies that exposure to allergens may exacerbate bronchospasm.
• Warn elderly patients of dizziness, a common adverse reaction at start of therapy.

bitolterol mesylate

Tornalate

Pregnancy Risk Category: C

HOW SUPPLIED

Aerosol inhaler: 370 mcg/metered spray

ACTION

Mechanism: Relaxes bronchial smooth muscle by acting on $beta_2$-adrenergic receptors.
Onset: 3 to 4 minutes. **Peak:** Peak effects occur within ½ to 1 hour. **Duration:** 5 to 8 hours.

INDICATIONS & DOSAGE

To prevent or treat bronchial asthma and bronchospasm –
Adults and children over 12 years: to treat bronchospasm, two inhalations at an interval of at least 1 to 3 minutes followed by a third inhalation, if needed. To prevent bronchospasm, the usual dose is two inhalations q 8 hours. In either case, dose should never exceed three inhalations q 6 hours or two inhalations q 4 hours.

ADVERSE REACTIONS

CNS: *tremors,* nervousness, headache, dizziness, light-headedness.
CV: palpitations, chest discomfort, tachycardia.
EENT: throat irritation, cough.
GI: nausea.
Other: dyspnea, *hypersensitivity.*

INTERACTIONS

None significant.

CONTRAINDICATIONS

• Contraindicated in patients hypersensitive to the drug.
• Use cautiously in patients with ischemic heart disease or hypertension, hyperthyroidism, diabetes mellitus, cardiac arrhythmias, and seizure disorders.

NURSING CONSIDERATIONS

• Monitor blood pressure regularly.
• Advise patients not to exceed recommended dosages. Too frequent use may cause tachycardia.
• Remind patients that beneficial effects last for up to 8 hours, longer than most other similar bronchodilators.
• Has rapid onset of action (about 3 to 4 minutes). Peak effect occurs in 30 to 60 minutes.
• Teach patients to perform oral inhalation correctly. Give the following instructions for using a metered-dose inhaler:
  – Clear nasal passages and throat.
  – Breathe out, expelling as much air from lungs as possible.
  – Place mouthpiece well into mouth as dose from inhaler is released, and inhale deeply.
  – Hold breath for several seconds, remove mouthpiece, and exhale slowly.
• If more than one inhalation is ordered, tell the patient to wait at least 2 minutes before repeating procedure.
• Tell patients who are also using a steroid inhaler to use bronchodilator first, then wait about 5 minutes before using steroid. This allows the bronchodilator to open air passages for maximum effectiveness.

dyphylline

Dilor*, Dilor-400, Dyflex, Dyflex-400, Lufyllin*, Lufyllin-400, Neothylline, Protophylline†, Thylline

Pregnancy Risk Category: C

HOW SUPPLIED

Tablets: 200 mg
Elixir: 100 mg/15 ml, 160 mg/15 ml*
Injection: 250 mg/ml

ACTION

Mechanism: Inhibits phosphodiesterase, the enzyme that degrades cAMP. Results in relaxation of smooth muscle of the bronchial airways and pulmonary blood vessels.
Onset: 15 minutes to 1 hour. **Peak:** Peak levels occur within 1 hour.
Duration: 4 to 6 hours; plasma half-life, 2 to 2½ hours.

INDICATIONS & DOSAGE

Relief of acute and chronic bronchial asthma and reversible bronchospasm associated with chronic bronchitis and emphysema –
Adults: 15 mg/kg P.O. q 6 hours. I.M. route is rarely used, but patients may receive 250 to 500 mg I.M. injected slowly at 6-hour intervals. Dosage should be decreased in patients with renal insufficiency.

ADVERSE REACTIONS

CNS: *restlessness, dizziness,* headache, *insomnia,* light-headedness, ***seizures,*** muscle twitching.
CV: *palpitations, sinus tachycardia,* extrasystoles, flushing, marked hypotension, increase in respiratory rate.
GI: *nausea, vomiting, anorexia,* bitter aftertaste, dyspepsia, heavy feeling in stomach.
Skin: urticaria.

INTERACTIONS

Probenecid: increased serum dyphylline levels. Monitor for adverse effects.

CONTRAINDICATIONS

- Contraindicated in patients with hypersensitivity to xanthine compounds (caffeine, theobromine) or with preexisting arrhythmias, especially tachycardias.
- Use cautiously in young children; in elderly patients with CHF, any impaired cardiac or circulatory function, cor pulmonale, renal or hepatic disease; and in patients with peptic ulceration, hyperthyroidism, or diabetes mellitus.

NURSING CONSIDERATIONS

- Monitor vital signs; measure and record fluid intake and output. Expected clinical effects include improvement in quality of pulse and respiration.
- Relieve gastric irritation by giving oral drug after meals; no evidence exists that antacids reduce this adverse reaction. May produce less gastric discomfort than theophylline.
- Discard injectable dyphylline if precipitate is present. Protect from light.
- Dyphylline is a theophylline analog; unlike other derivatives such as aminophylline, it is not converted to theophylline in the bloodstream. No routine plasma assays exists for determining effective blood levels.
- Do not administer I.V.
- Warn patients to check with the doctor or pharmacist before taking any other drugs. OTC remedies may contain ephedrine in combination with theophylline salts; excessive CNS stimulation may result.
- Warn elderly patients of dizziness, a common adverse reaction at start of therapy.
- Supply instructions for home care and dosage schedule.

ephedrine sulfate

Ephed II

Pregnancy Risk Category: C

HOW SUPPLIED

Tablets: 30 mg‡
Capsules: 25 mg, 50 mg
Syrup: 11 mg/5 ml, 20 mg/5 ml
Injection: 25 mg/ml, 50 mg/ml

ACTION

Mechanism: Stimulates alpha- and beta-adrenergic receptors; a direct- and indirect-acting sympathomimetic.
Onset: within 5 minutes of I.V. use, 10 to 20 minutes of I.M. use, 15 to 60 minutes after oral use. **Duration:** 30 minutes to 1 hour after I.M. or S.C. use; 3 to 5 hours after oral use.

INDICATIONS & DOSAGE

To correct hypotension, to support ventricular rate in Adams-Stokes syndrome –
Adults: 25 to 50 mg I.M. or S.C., or 10 to 25 mg I.V. p.r.n. to maximum of 150 mg/24 hours.
Children: 3 mg/kg or 100 mg/m² S.C. or I.V. daily, in four to six divided doses.
Bronchodilator or nasal decongestant –
Adults and children over age 12: 12.5 to 50 mg P.O. b.i.d., t.i.d., or q.i.d. Maximum dosage is 400 mg daily in six to eight divided doses.
Children over age 2: 2 to 3 mg/kg P.O. daily in four to six divided doses.

ADVERSE REACTIONS

CNS: *insomnia, nervousness,* dizziness, headache, muscle weakness, diaphoresis, euphoria, confusion, delirium.
CV: *palpitations,* tachycardia, hypertension.
EENT: dryness of nose and throat.
GI: nausea, vomiting, anorexia.
GU: urine retention, painful urination due to visceral sphincter spasm.

INTERACTIONS

Acetazolamide: increased serum ephedrine levels. Monitor for toxicity.
Alpha-adrenergic blocking agents: unopposed beta-adrenergic effects, resulting in hypotension.
Antihypertensives: decreased effects.
Beta-adrenergic blocking agents: unopposed alpha-adrenergic effects, resulting in hypertension.
Digitalis glycosides, general anesthetics (halogenated hydrocarbons): increased risk of ventricular arrhythmias.
Ergot alkaloids: enhanced vasoconstrictor activity.
Guanadrel, guanethidine: enhanced pressor effects of ephedrine.
Levodopa: enhanced risk of ventricular arrhythmias.
MAO inhibitors and tricyclic antidepressants: when given with sympathomimetics, may cause severe hypertension (hypertensive crisis).
Methyldopa: may inhibit effects of ephedrine. Use together cautiously.

CONTRAINDICATIONS

- Contraindicated in patients with porphyria, severe coronary artery disease, arrhythmias, acute angle-closure glaucoma, or psychoneurosis; and in patients on MAO-inhibitor therapy.
- Use cautiously in elderly patients and those with hypertension, hyperthyroidism, nervous or excitable states, cardiovascular disease, and prostatic hyperplasia.

NURSING CONSIDERATIONS

- Hypoxia, hypercapnia, and acidosis, which may reduce effectiveness or increase the incidence of adverse reactions, must be identified and corrected before or during ephedrine administration.
- This drug is not a substitute for blood or fluid volume replenishment. Correct volume deficit before administering vasopressors.

• Effectiveness decreases after 2 to 3 weeks, as tolerance develops. May need to increase dosage. Drug is not addictive.
• **I.V. use:** Give 10 to 25 mg by I.V. injection slowly; repeat in 5 to 10 minutes if necessary. Compatible with most common I.V. solutions.
• To prevent insomnia, avoid giving within 2 hours before bedtime.
• Warn patients not to take OTC drugs that contain ephedrine without informing the doctor.

epinephrine (adrenaline)
Adrenalin◇, Bronkaid Mist◇, Bronkaid Mistometer†, Primatene Mist ◇

epinephrine bitartrate
AsthmaHaler◇, Broniten Mist◇, Bronkaid Mist Suspension◇, Medihaler-Epi◇, Primatene Mist Suspension◇

epinephrine hydrochloride
Adrenalin Chloride◇, Epi-Pen, Epi-Pen Jr., Sus-Phrine

Pregnancy Risk Category: C

HOW SUPPLIED
Aerosol inhaler: 160 mcg◇, 200 mcg◇, 250 mcg/metered spray◇
Nebulizer inhaler: 1% (1:100)†◇, 1.25%†◇, 2.25%†◇
Injection: 0.01 mg/ml (1:100,000), 0.1 mg/ml (1:10,000), 0.5 mg/ml (1:2,000), 1 mg/ml (1:1,000) parenteral; 5 mg/ml (1:200) parenteral suspension

ACTION
Mechanism: Stimulates alpha- and beta-adrenergic receptors within the sympathetic nervous system.
Onset: immediately after I.V. injection, 3 to 5 minutes after inhalation, 6 to 15 minutes after S.C. injection, variable after I.M. use. **Peak:** Peak effects occur within 5 minutes of I.V. administration, or within 30 minutes of S.C. injection. **Duration:** 1 to 3 hours after inhalation, less than 1 to about 4 hours after parenteral use.

INDICATIONS & DOSAGE
Bronchospasm, hypersensitivity reactions, anaphylaxis –
Adults: 0.1 to 0.5 ml of 1:1,000 S.C. or I.M. Repeat q 10 to 15 minutes, p.r.n. Or 0.1 to 0.25 ml 1:1,000 I.V.
Children: 0.01 ml (10 mcg) of 1:1,000/kg S.C. Repeat q 20 minutes to 4 hours, p.r.n.; 0.005 ml/kg of 1:200 (Sus-Phrine). Repeat q 8 to 12 hours, p.r.n.
Hemostasis –
Adults: 1:50,000 to 1:1,000, applied topically.
Acute asthmatic attacks (inhalation) –
Adults and children: 1 or 2 inhalations of 1:100 or 2.25% racemic, q 1 to 5 minutes until relief is obtained; 0.2 mg/dose usual content.
To prolong local anesthetic effect –
Adults and children: 0.2 to 0.4 ml of 1:1,000 intraspinal; 1:500,000 to 1:50,000 local mixed with local anesthetic.
To restore cardiac rhythm in cardiac arrest –
Adults: 0.5 to 1 mg I.V. or into endotracheal tube. May be given intracardiac if no I.V. route or intratracheal route available. Some clinicians advocate higher dose (up to 5 mg), especially in patients who don't respond to usual I.V dose. Following initial I.V. administration, may be infused I.V. at a rate of 1 to 4 mcg/minute.
Children: 10 mcg/kg I.V. or 5 to 10 mcg (0.05 to 0.1 ml of 1:10,000)/kg intracardiac.
Note: 1 mg = 1 ml of 1:1,000 or 10 ml of 1:10,000.

ADVERSE REACTIONS
CNS: *nervousness,* tremor, euphoria, anxiety, coldness of extremities, vertigo, *headache,* diaphoresis, disorientation, agitation. In patients with Par-

kinson's disease, the drug increases rigidity and tremor.
CV: *palpitations;* widened pulse pressure; ***hypertension; tachycardia; ventricular fibrillation; CVA;*** anginal pain; ECG changes, including a decrease in the T wave amplitude.
Other: pulmonary edema, dyspnea, pallor, hyperglycemia, glycosuria.

INTERACTIONS

Alpha-adrenergic blocking agents: hypotension due to unopposed beta-adrenergic effects.
Beta blockers, such as propranolol: vasoconstriction and reflex bradycardia. Monitor patient carefully.
Digitalis glycosides, general anesthetics (halogenated hydrocarbons): increased risk of ventricular arrhythmias.
Doxapram, mazindol, methylphenidate: enhanced CNS stimulation or pressor effects.
Ergot alkaloids: enhanced vasoconstrictor activity.
Guanadrel, guanethidine: enhanced pressor effects of epinephrine.
Levodopa: enhanced risk of cardiac arrhythmias.
MAO inhibitors: increased risk of hypertensive crisis.
Tricyclic antidepressants, antihistamines, thyroid hormones: when given with sympathomimetics, may cause severe adverse cardiac effects. Avoid giving together.

CONTRAINDICATIONS

- Contraindicated in patients with acute angle-closure glaucoma, suffering shock (other than anaphylactic shock), organic brain damage, cardiac dilation, or coronary insufficiency. Also contraindicated in patients during general anesthesia with halogenated hydrocarbons or cyclopropane and in patients in labor (may delay second stage).
- Use with extreme caution in patients with long-standing bronchial asthma and emphysema who have developed degenerative heart disease. Also use cautiously in elderly patients and those with hyperthyroidism, angina, hypertension, psychoneurosis, and diabetes.

NURSING CONSIDERATIONS

- Drug of choice in emergency treatment of acute anaphylactic reactions.
- Epinephrine is rapidly destroyed by oxidizing agents, such as iodine, chromates, nitrates, nitrites, oxygen, and salts of easily reducible metals (such as iron).
- Discard epinephrine solutions after 24 hours or if solution is discolored or contains precipitate. Keep solution in light-resistant container, and don't remove before use.
- **I.V. use:** Don't mix with alkaline solutions. Use D_5W, 0.9% sodium chloride injection, lactated Ringer's injection, or combinations of dextrose in sodium chloride. Mix just before use.
- Avoid I.M. administration of parenteral suspension into buttocks. Gas gangrene may occur because epinephrine reduces oxygen tension of the tissues, encouraging the growth of contaminating organisms.
- When administering I.V., monitor blood pressure, heart rate, and ECG when therapy is initiated and frequently thereafter.
- Massage site after I.M. injection to counteract possible vasoconstriction. Repeated local injection can cause necrosis at site from vasoconstriction.
- Observe patients closely for adverse reactions. If adverse reactions develop, the doctor will adjust dosage or discontinue drug.
- If a sharp blood pressure rise occurs, rapid-acting vasodilators, such as nitrites or alpha-adrenergic blocking agents, can be given to counteract the marked pressor effect of large doses of epinephrine.
- If patient has acute hypersensitivity

reactions, for example reaction to bee stings, it may be necessary to instruct him to self-inject epinephrine at home.

- Teach patients to perform oral inhalation correctly. Give the following instructions for using a metered-dose inhaler:
  - Clear nasal passages and throat.
  - Breathe out, expelling as much air from lungs as possible.
  - Place mouthpiece well into mouth as dose from inhaler is released, and inhale deeply.
  - Hold breath for several seconds, remove mouthpiece, and exhale slowly.
- If more than one inhalation is ordered, tell patients to wait at least 2 minutes before repeating procedure.
- Tell patients who are also using a steroid inhaler to use the bronchodilator first, to open air passages for maximum effectiveness. Then wait about 5 minutes before using steroid.

ethylnorepinephrine hydrochloride

Bronkephrine

Pregnancy Risk Category: C

HOW SUPPLIED

Injection: 2 mg/ml

ACTION

Mechanism: Relaxes bronchial smooth muscle by acting on beta-adrenergic receptors.
Onset: 6 to 12 minutes. **Duration:** 1 to 2 hours.

INDICATIONS & DOSAGE

Bronchospasm caused by asthma –
Adults: 0.6 to 2 mg S.C. or I.M.
Children: 0.2 to 1 mg S.C. or I.M.

ADVERSE REACTIONS

CNS: *headache,* dizziness.
CV: changes in blood pressure, *elevation in pulse rate,* palpitations.
GI: nausea.

INTERACTIONS

Beta blockers: mutual inhibition of clinical effects.
CNS stimulants, xanthine derivatives: enhanced CNS stimulation.
Digitalis glycosides, levodopa, halogenated inhalation anesthetics, cyclopropane: increased risk of arrhythmias. Monitor closely.
Nitrates, antihypertensives: decreased effects of these agents.
Rauwolfia alkaloids, sympathomimetics: enhanced effects.
Thyroid hormones: increased risk of coronary insufficiency.

CONTRAINDICATIONS

- Contraindicated in patients hypersensitive to the drug; in patients with tachyarrhythmias, tachycardia caused by digitalis toxicity, acute angle-closure glaucoma, or shock; and in patients receiving general anesthesia with cyclopropane or halogenated inhalation anesthetics.
- Use cautiously in patients with cardiovascular disease or a history of stroke.

NURSING CONSIDERATIONS

- Safer than epinephrine for use in hypertensive or severely ill patients in whom significant pressor effects are undesirable.
- Valuable for use in children because of low incidence of adverse reactions; may be useful in diabetic asthmatics due to low glycogenolytic activity.
- Choose anatomic injection site carefully to avoid inadvertent intraneural or intravascular injection.

ipratropium bromide

Atrovent

Pregnancy Risk Category: B

HOW SUPPLIED
Inhaler: each metered dose supplies 18 mcg
Solution (for nebulizer): 0.025% (250 mcg/ml)‡
Nasal spray: each metered dose supplies 20 mcg

ACTION
Mechanism: Inhibits vagally mediated reflexes by antagonizing acetylcholine. An anticholinergic.
Onset: 5 to 15 minutes. **Peak:** Peak effects occur in 1 to 2 hours. **Duration:** usually 3 to 4 hours; up to 6 hours in some patients.

INDICATIONS & DOSAGE
Bronchospasm associated with COPD–
Adults: 1 to 2 inhalations q.i.d. Additional inhalations may be needed. However, total inhalations should not exceed 12 in 24 hours. Alternatively, use inhalation solution where available. Give 250 to 500 mcg dissolved in 0.9% sodium chloride and administer by nebulizer every 4 to 6 hours.
Children age 5 to 12: give 125 to 250 mcg nebulizer solution dissolved in 0.9% sodium chloride and administer by nebulizer every 4 to 6 hours.
Seasonal allergic rhinitis‡–
Adults: 2 sprays in each nostril b.i.d. Increase to t.i.d. or q.i.d. if needed. Maximum dosage is 8 sprays in each nostril daily.

ADVERSE REACTIONS
CNS: nervousness, dizziness, headache.
CV: palpitations.
EENT: cough, blurred vision.
GI: nausea, GI distress, dry mouth.
Skin: rash.

INTERACTIONS
Anticholinergics: increased anticholinergic effects. Avoid concomitant use.
Cromolyn sodium: will form a precipitate if mixed in the same nebulizer. Don't use together.

CONTRAINDICATIONS
• Contraindicated in patients hypersensitive to the drug.
• Use cautiously in patients with acute angle-closure glaucoma, prostatic hyperplasia, and bladder-neck obstruction.

NURSING CONSIDERATIONS
• Ipratropium is the first anticholinergic bronchodilator available as an aerosol. Works by a different mechanism from either the adrenergics or theophylline compounds.
• Tell patients to avoid accidentally spraying into eyes. Temporary blurring of vision may result.
• Teach patients to perform oral inhalation correctly. Give the following instructions for using a metered-dose inhaler:
  – Clear nasal passages and throat.
  – Breathe out, expelling as much air from lungs as possible.
  – Place mouthpiece well into mouth as dose from inhaler is released, and inhale deeply.
  – Hold breath for several seconds, remove mouthpiece, and exhale slowly.
• If more than one inhalation is ordered, tell patients to wait at least 2 minutes before repeating procedure.
• Tell patients if a dose is missed to take as soon as remembered, unless it's almost time for the next dose. In that case, skip the missed dose. Do not double-dose.
• Tell patients who are also using a steroid inhaler to use ipratropium first, then wait about 5 minutes before using the steroid. This allows the bronchodilator to open air passages for maximum effectiveness.
• Warn patients that ipratropium bromide is not effective for treating acute episodes of bronchospasm where rapid response is required.

• Advise the patient to use sugarless hard candy, gum, or a saliva substitute.

isoetharine hydrochloride

Arm-a-Med Isoetharine, Bronkosol, Dey-Dose Isoetharine, Dey-Dose Isoetharine S/F, Dey-Lute Isoetharine, Dispos-a-Med Isoetharine

isoetharine mesylate

Bronkometer

Pregnancy Risk Category: C

HOW SUPPLIED
Aerosol inhaler: 340 mcg/metered spray
Nebulizer inhaler: 0.062%, 0.08%, 0.1%, 0.125%, 0.14%, 0.167%, 0.17%, 0.2%, 0.25%, 0.5%, 1% solution

ACTION
Mechanism: Relaxes bronchial smooth muscle by acting on beta$_2$-adrenergic receptors.
Onset: 1 to 6 minutes. **Peak:** Peak effects occur within 15 to 60 minutes.
Duration: 1 to 4 hours.

INDICATIONS & DOSAGE
Bronchial asthma and reversible bronchospasm that may occur with bronchitis and emphysema –
Adults: (hydrochloride) administered by hand nebulizer, oxygen aerosolization, or IPPB.

Method	*Dose*	*Dilutions*
Hand	3 to 7 inhalations	undiluted
Oxygen aerosolization	0.5 ml	1:3 with saline
IPPB	0.5 ml	1:3 with saline

Adults: (mesylate) 1 to 2 inhalations. Occasionally, more may be required.

ADVERSE REACTIONS
CNS: *tremor, headache,* dizziness, excitement.
CV: *palpitations,* increased heart rate.
GI: nausea, vomiting.

INTERACTIONS
Cyclopropane, digitalis glycosides, levodopa, halogenated inhalation anesthetics: increased risk of arrhythmias. Monitor closely.
Propranolol and other beta blockers: blocked bronchodilating effect of isoetharine. Monitor patient carefully if used together.

CONTRAINDICATIONS
• Contraindicated in patients hypersensitive to the drug; in patients with tachyarrhythmias, tachycardia caused by digitalis toxicity, acute angle-closure glaucoma, or shock; and in patients receiving general anesthesia with cyclopropane or halogenated inhalation anesthetics.
• Use cautiously in patients with hyperthyroidism, hypertension, or coronary disease, and in patients hypersensitive to sympathomimetics.

NURSING CONSIDERATIONS
• Excessive use can lead to decreased effectiveness.
• Monitor for severe paradoxical bronchoconstriction after excessive use. Discontinue immediately if bronchoconstriction occurs.
• Although isoetharine has minimal effects on the heart, use cautiously in patients receiving general anesthetics that sensitize the myocardium to sympathomimetic drugs.
• Teach patients to perform oral inhalation correctly. Give the following instructions for using a metered-dose inhaler:
  – Clear nasal passages and throat.
  – Breathe out, expelling as much air from lungs as possible.
  – Place mouthpiece well into

mouth as dose from inhaler is released, and inhale deeply.
– Hold breath for several seconds, remove mouthpiece, and exhale slowly.

- If more than one inhalation is ordered, tell patients to wait at least 2 minutes before repeating procedure.
- Tell patients who are also using a steroid inhaler to use the bronchodilator first, then wait about 5 minutes before using the steroid. This allows the bronchodilator to open air passages for maximum effectiveness.
- Due to oxidation of drug when diluted with water, pink sputum mimicking hemoptysis may occur after inhaling isoetharine solution. Tell patients not to be concerned.

isoproterenol (isoprenaline)

Aerolone, Dey-Dose Isoproterenol, Dispos-a-Med Isoproterenol, Isuprel, Vapo-Iso

isoproterenol hydrochloride

Isuprel, Isuprel Glossets, Isuprel Mistometer, Norisodrine Aerotrol

isoproterenol sulfate

Medihaler-Iso

Pregnancy Risk Category: C

HOW SUPPLIED

isoproterenol
Nebulizer inhaler: 0.25%, 0.5%, 1%
isoproterenol hydrochloride
Tablets (sublingual): 10 mg, 15 mg
Aerosol inhaler: 120 mcg or 131 mcg/metered spray
Injection: 200 mcg/ml
isoproterenol sulfate
Aerosol inhaler: 80 mcg/metered spray

ACTION

Mechanism: Relaxes bronchial smooth muscle by acting on $beta_2$-adrenergic receptors. As a cardiac stimulant, acts on $beta_1$-adrenergic receptors in the heart.
Onset: immediately after I.V. use, 2 to 5 minutes after inhalation, 15 to 30 minutes after S.L. use. **Duration:** ½ to 2 hours after inhalation, less than 1 hour after I.V. use, 1 to 2 hours after S.L. use.

INDICATIONS & DOSAGE

Bronchial asthma and reversible bronchospasm –
Adults: 10 to 15 mg (hydrochloride) S.L. q 6 to 8 hours.
Children: 5 to 10 mg (hydrochloride) S.L. q 6 to 8 hours. Not recommended for children under 6 years.
Bronchospasm –
Adults and children: (sulfate) acute dyspneic episodes: 1 inhalation initially. May repeat if needed after 2 to 5 minutes.

Maintenance dosage is 1 to 2 inhalations q.i.d. to 6 times daily. May repeat once more 10 minutes after second dose. Not more than 3 doses should be administered for each attack.

Heart block and ventricular arrhythmias –
Adults: (hydrochloride) initially, 0.02 to 0.06 mg I.V. Subsequent doses 0.01 to 0.2 mg I.V. or 5 mcg/minute I.V.; or 0.2 mg I.M. initially, then 0.02 to 1 mg, p.r.n.
Children: (hydrochloride) may give half of initial adult dose.
Shock –
Adults and children: (hydrochloride) 0.5 to 5 mcg/minute by continuous I.V. infusion. Usual concentration is 1 mg (5 ml) in 500 ml D_5W. Adjust rate according to heart rate, central venous pressure (CVP), blood pressure, and urine flow.

ADVERSE REACTIONS

CNS: *headache,* mild tremor, weakness, dizziness, nervousness, insomnia.
CV: *palpitations, tachycardia, an-*

ginal pain; blood pressure may rise and then fall.
GI: nausea, vomiting.
Respiratory: ***bronchial edema and inflammation.***
Other: diaphoresis, flushing of face, hyperglycemia.

INTERACTIONS

Epinephrine: increased risk of arrhythmias.
Propranolol and other beta blockers: blocked bronchodilating effect of isoproterenol. Monitor patient carefully if used together.

CONTRAINDICATIONS

- Contraindicated in patients with tachycardia caused by digitalis intoxication; in patients with preexisting arrhythmias, especially tachycardia, because chronotropic effect on the heart may aggravate such disorders; and in patients with recent MI.
- Use cautiously in patients with coronary insufficiency, diabetes, or hyperthyroidism.

NURSING CONSIDERATIONS

- Not a substitute for blood or fluid volume deficit. Replace volume deficit before administering vasopressors.
- Isoproterenol may cause a slight rise in systolic blood pressure and a slight to marked drop in diastolic blood pressure.
- **I.V. use:** Give by direct injection or I.V. infusion. For infusion, drug may be diluted with most common I.V. solutions. Do not use sodium bicarbonate injection; drug decomposes rapidly in alkaline solutions.
- If heart rate exceeds 110 beats/minute, consider decreasing infusion rate or temporarily stopping infusion. Doses sufficient to increase the heart rate to more than 130 beats/minute may induce ventricular arrhythmias.
- When administering I.V. isoproterenol for shock, closely monitor blood pressure, CVP, ECG, arterial blood gas measurements, and urine output. Carefully adjust infusion rate according to these measurements. Use a continuous infusion pump to regulate infusion flow rate.
- Teach patients to perform oral inhalation correctly. Give the following instructions for using a metered-dose inhaler:
  - Clear nasal passages and throat.
  - Breathe out, expelling as much air from lungs as possible.
  - Place mouthpiece well into mouth as dose from inhaler is released, and inhale deeply.
  - Hold breath for several seconds, remove mouthpiece, and exhale slowly.
- If more than one inhalation is ordered, tell patients to wait at least 2 minutes before repeating procedure.
- Tell patients who are also using a steroid inhaler to use the bronchodilator first, then wait about 5 minutes before using the steroid. This allows the bronchodilator to open air passages for maximum effectiveness.
- Follow same instructions for metered powder nebulizer, although deep inhalation is not necessary.
- If via inhalation with oxygen, be sure oxygen concentration will not suppress respiratory drive.
- May aggravate ventilation perfusion abnormalities; even while ease of breathing is improved, arterial oxygen tension may fall paradoxically.
- Do not use injection or inhalation solution if it is discolored or contains precipitate.
- Warn patients using oral inhalant that drug may turn sputum and saliva pink.
- Teach patients to take sublingual tablet properly. Instruct patients to hold tablet under tongue, and not to swallow saliva until tablet dissolves and is absorbed. Instruct patients to rinse mouth with water between doses to help prevent oropharynx dryness.
- Caution patients that prolonged use

of sublingual tablets can cause tooth decay.

- If possible, don't give h.s.; it interrupts sleep patterns.
- Patients may develop a tolerance to this drug; warn against overuse.
- Observe patients closely for adverse reactions. Tell patients to discontinue drug immediately if it causes precordial distress or anginal pain, or if an increase in chest tightness or dyspnea occurs.

metaproterenol sulfate

Alupent, Arm-A-Med Metaproterenol, Dey-Dose Metaproterenol, Dey-Lute Metaproterenol, Metaprel

Pregnancy Risk Category: C

HOW SUPPLIED

Tablets: 10 mg, 20 mg
Syrup: 10 mg/5 ml
Aerosol inhaler: 0.65 mg/metered spray
Nebulizer inhaler: 0.6%, 5% solution

ACTION

Mechanism: Relaxes bronchial smooth muscle by acting on beta$_2$-adrenergic receptors.
Onset: within 1 hour. **Peak:** Peak effects occur within 1 hour. **Duration:** 1.5 hours after inhalation, 1 to 4 hours after oral use.

INDICATIONS & DOSAGE

Acute episodes of bronchial asthma –
Adults and children: 2 to 3 inhalations. Do not repeat inhalations more often than q 3 to 4 hours. Do not exceed 12 inhalations daily.
Bronchial asthma and reversible bronchospasm –
Adults: 20 mg P.O. q 6 to 8 hours.
Children over 9 years or over 27 kg: 20 mg P.O. q 6 to 8 hours (0.4 mg to 0.9 mg/kg/dose t.i.d.).
Children 6 to 9 years or less than 27 kg: 10 mg P.O. q 6 to 8 hours (0.4 mg to 0.9 mg/kg/dose t.i.d.).

Not recommended for children under 6 years.

ADVERSE REACTIONS

CNS: nervousness, weakness, drowsiness, tremor.
CV: tachycardia, hypertension, palpitations; ***cardiac arrest (with excessive use).***
GI: vomiting, nausea, bad taste in mouth.
Respiratory: paradoxical bronchiolar constriction with excessive use.

INTERACTIONS

Levodopa: risk of arrhythmias. Avoid concomitant use.
Propranolol and other beta blockers: blocked bronchodilating effect of metaproterenol. Monitor patient carefully if used together.

CONTRAINDICATIONS

- Contraindicated in patients with tachycardia and arrhythmias associated with tachycardia. Use cautiously in patients with hypertension, coronary artery disease, hyperthyroidism, and diabetes.
- Safe use of inhalant in children under 12 years not established.

NURSING CONSIDERATIONS

- Teach patients to administer metered dose correctly, as follows: shake container; administer aerosol while inhaling deeply on mouthpiece of inhaler holding breath for a few seconds; exhale slowly through nose. Allow 2 minutes between inhalations. Store drug in light-resistant container.
- Metaproterenol inhalations should precede steroid inhalations (when prescribed) by 10 to 15 minutes to maximize therapy.
- Warn patients to discontinue immediately if paradoxical bronchospasm occurs.
- Metaproterenol reportedly produces

less cardiac stimulation than other sympathomimetics, especially isoproterenol.
- Patients may use tablets and aerosol concomitantly. Monitor closely for toxicity.
- Inhalant solution can be administered by IPPB diluted in saline solution or via a hand nebulizer at full strength.
- Tell patients who are also using a steroid inhaler to use the bronchodilator first, then wait about 5 minutes before using the steroid. This allows bronchodilator to open air passages for maximum effectiveness.
- If more than one inhalation is ordered, tell patients to wait at least 2 minutes before repeating procedure.
- Warn patients to notify doctor if no response is derived from dosage or to request dosage adjustments.

oxtriphylline (choline theophyllinate)

Choledyl*

Pregnancy Risk Category: C

HOW SUPPLIED

Tablets: 100 mg, 200 mg
Tablets (extended-release): 400 mg, 600 mg
Tablets (delayed-release): 100 mg, 200 mg
Elixir:* 100 mg/5 ml
Syrup: 50 mg/5 ml

ACTION

Mechanism: Inhibits phosphodiesterase, the enzyme that degrades cAMP. Results in relaxation of smooth muscle of the bronchial airways and pulmonary blood vessels. Oxtriphylline is equivalent to 64% anhydrous theophylline.
Onset: 15 to 60 minutes. **Peak:** Peak effects occur within 1 hour after oral solution, or within 2 hours of oral tablets. **Duration:** varies – half-life in healthy adults with asthma, about 9 hours; more than 24 hours in adults with cor pulmonale, heart failure, COPD, or liver disease; about 5 hours in patients who smoke or have smoked in the last 2 to 3 years; 24 hours or more in neonates and infants to age 6 months; about 4 hours in children over age 6.

INDICATIONS & DOSAGE

Acute bronchial asthma and reversible bronchospasm associated with chronic bronchitis and emphysema –
Adults and children over 12 years: 6 to 8 mg/kg (up to a maximum of 400 mg) P.O. daily, in 3 or 4 divided doses; or 400 to 600 mg extended-release form P.O. q 12 hours, then adjust dosage based upon serum theophylline levels.
Children 2 to 12 years: 4 mg/kg P.O. q 6 hours. Adjust as needed to maintain therapeutic levels of theophylline (10 to 20 mcg/ml).

ADVERSE REACTIONS

CNS: *restlessness, dizziness,* headache, *insomnia,* light-headedness, ***seizures,*** muscle twitching.
CV: *palpitations, sinus tachycardia,* extrasystoles, flushing, marked hypotension.
GI: *nausea, vomiting, anorexia,* bitter aftertaste, dyspepsia, heavy feeling in stomach.
Respiratory: increased respiratory rate.
Skin: urticaria.

INTERACTIONS

Adenosine: decreased antiarrhythmic effectiveness. Higher doses of adenosine may be necessary.
Barbiturates, carbamazepine, nicotine, phenytoin, rifampin: enhanced metabolism and decreased theophylline blood levels. Monitor for decreased effect.
Beta-adrenergic blockers: antagonism. Propranolol and nadolol, especially, may cause bronchospasm in

*Liquid form contains alcohol.
**May contain tartrazine.

sensitive patients. Use together cautiously.
Cimetidine, influenza virus vaccine, macrolide antibiotics (such as erythromycin), oral contraceptives, quinolone antibiotics (such as ciprofloxacin): decreased hepatic clearance of theophylline; elevated theophylline levels. Monitor for signs of toxicity.

CONTRAINDICATIONS
• Contraindicated in patients hypersensitive to xanthines (caffeine, theobromine); and in patients with preexisting arrhythmias, especially tachyarrhythmias.
• Use cautiously in young children; in elderly patients with CHF or other cardiac or circulatory impairment, cor pulmonale, or hepatic disease; in patients with active peptic ulceration because drug may increase volume and acidity of gastric secretions; and in patients with hyperthyroidism or diabetes mellitus.

NURSING CONSIDERATIONS
• Oxtriphylline is a soluble salt of theophylline. Adjust dosage by monitoring response, tolerance, pulmonary function, and serum theophylline levels. Ensure that theophylline concentrations range from 10 to 20 mcg/ml; toxicity has been reported with levels above 20 mcg/ml.
• Administer drug after meals and h.s.
• Store at 15° to 30° C (59° to 86° F). Protect elixir from light and tablets from moisture.
• Monitor therapy carefully. Individuals metabolize theophyllines at different rates. Dosage adjustments are necessary in the elderly, in patients with CHF, cor pulmonale, hepatic disease, and in smokers.
• Tell patients to report GI distress, palpitations, irritability, restlessness, nervousness, or insomnia; may indicate excessive CNS stimulation.
• Do not combine with products containing ephedrine; excessive CNS stimulation (nervousness, tremors, akathisia) may result.

pirbuterol
Maxair

Pregnancy Risk Category: C

HOW SUPPLIED
Inhaler: 0.2 mg/metered dose

ACTION
Mechanism: Relaxes bronchial smooth muscle by acting on beta$_2$-adrenergic receptors.
Onset: within 5 minutes. **Peak:** Peak effects occur in 30 to 60 minutes.
Duration: 5 hours.

INDICATIONS AND DOSAGE
Prevention and reversal of bronchospasm, asthma –
Adults: 1 or 2 inhalations (0.2 to 0.4 mg) repeated q 4 to 6 hours. Not to exceed 12 inhalations daily.

ADVERSE REACTIONS
CNS: tremors, nervousness, dizziness, insomnia, headache.
CV: tachycardia, palpitations, increased blood pressure.
EENT: drying or irritation of throat.

INTERACTIONS
Propranolol and other beta-adrenergic blocking agents: decreased bronchodilating effects.

CONTRAINDICATIONS
• Contraindicated in patients hypersensitive to pirbuterol or other adrenergics, and in patients with digitalis toxicity or arrhythmias associated with tachycardia.

NURSING CONSIDERATIONS
• Teach patients to perform oral inhalation correctly. Give the following instructions for using a metered-dose inhaler:

– Clear nasal passages and throat.
– Breathe out, expelling as much air from lungs as possible.
– Place mouthpiece well into mouth as dose from inhaler is released, and inhale deeply.
– Hold breath for several seconds, remove mouthpiece, and exhale slowly.

• If more than one inhalation is ordered, tell patients to wait at least 2 minutes before repeating procedure.
• Tell patients who are also using a steroid inhaler to use the bronchodilator first, then wait about 5 minutes before using the steroid. This allows the bronchodilator to open air passages for maximum effectiveness.
• Tell patients who experience increased bronchospasm after using drug to call the doctor.
• Advise patients to seek medical attention if a previously effective dosage does not control symptoms; this may signify worsening of the disease.

salmeterol xinafoate

Serevent

Pregnancy Risk Category: C

HOW SUPPLIED

Inhalation aerosol: 21 mcg per metered spray

ACTION

Mechanism: Selectively activates beta$_2$-adrenergic receptors, which results in bronchodilation. Also blocks the release of allergic mediators from mast cells lining the respiratory tract.
Onset: 10 to 20 minutes. **Peak:** Peak effects occur after about 3 hours; plasma levels peak within 45 minutes, but drug acts locally in the lung and its action is not dependent upon plasma levels. **Duration:** about 12 hours.

INDICATIONS & DOSAGE

Long-term maintenance treatment of asthma; prevention of bronchospasm in patients with nocturnal asthma or reversible obstructive airway disease who require regular treatment with short-acting beta agonists –
Adults and children over 12 years: two inhalations twice daily in the morning and evening.

ADVERSE REACTIONS

CNS: headache, sinus headache, tremor.
CV: tachycardia, palpitations.
EENT: upper respiratory infection, nasopharyngitis, nasal cavity or sinus disorder.
GI: stomach ache.
Respiratory: cough, lower respiratory infection, ***bronchospasm.***
Other: hypersensitivity reactions such as rash, urticaria.

INTERACTIONS

Beta-adrenergic agonists, theophylline or other methylxanthines: possible adverse cardiac effects with excessive use. Monitor closely.
MAO inhibitors: risk of severe adverse cardiovascular effects. Avoid use within 14 days of MAO therapy.
Tricyclic antidepressants: risk of moderate to severe adverse cardiovascular effects. Use with extreme caution.

CONTRAINDICATIONS

• Contraindicated in patients hypersensitive to the drug or any component of the formulation.
• Use cautiously in patients with coronary insufficiency, cardiac arrhythmias, hypertension, or other cardiovascular disorders; thyrotoxicosis; seizure disorders; and in patients who are unusually responsive to sympathomimetics.
• Because other beta agonists have precipitated adverse effects in diabetic patients, use cautiously in diabetic patients.

NURSING CONSIDERATIONS

- Remind patients to take drug at approximately 12-hour intervals for optimum effect and to take the drug even when feeling better.
- Tell patients to contact the doctor if the short-acting agonist no longer provides sufficient relief, or if more than four inhalations are being used per day. This may be a sign that the asthma symptoms are worsening. Do not increase the dosage of salmeterol.
- Although this drug is a beta agonist, do not use to treat acute bronchospasm. Patients must be provided with a short-acting beta agonist (such as albuterol) to treat such exacerbations. Instruct patients who are already receiving short-acting beta agonists to discontinue the regular daily-dosing regimen for the drug. They should continue to use the short-acting agent as needed if they experience asthma symptoms while taking salmeterol.
- If patients are taking an inhaled corticosteroid, they should continue to use it on a regular basis. Warn patients not to take any other medications without the doctor's consent.
- If the patient is taking the drug to prevent exercise-induced bronchospasm, he should take it 30 to 60 minutes before exercise.

terbutaline sulfate

Brethaire, Brethine, Bricanyl

Pregnancy Risk Category: B

HOW SUPPLIED

Tablets: 2.5 mg, 5 mg
Aerosol inhaler: 200 mcg/metered spray
Injection: 1 mg/ml

ACTION

Mechanism: Relaxes bronchial smooth muscle by acting on beta$_2$-adrenergic receptors. Also relaxes uterine muscle.

Onset: within 15 minutes of S.C. injection, 5 to 30 minutes after inhalation, 1 to 2 hours after oral use. **Peak:** Peak effects occur within 15 minutes to 1 hour of S.C. injection, 1 to 2 hours after inhalation, or 2 to 3 hours after oral use. **Duration:** about 1.5 to 4 hours after S.C. injection, 3 to 6 hours after inhalation, or 4 to 8 hours after oral use.

INDICATIONS & DOSAGE

Bronchospasm in patients with reversible obstructive airway disease –
Adults and children over 11 years: 2 inhalations separated by a 60-second interval, repeated q 4 to 6 hours. May also administer 2.5 to 5 mg P.O. or 0.25 mg S.C. q 8 hours.
Premature labor –
Women: 0.01 mg/minute by I.V. infusion. Increase by 0.005 mg q 10 minutes up to 0.025 mg/minute or until contractions cease. Or, give 0.25 mg S.C. hourly until contractions cease. Maintenance dosage is 5 mg P.O. q 4 hours for 48 hours, then 5 mg q 6 hours.

ADVERSE REACTIONS

CNS: *nervousness, tremors, headache,* drowsiness, sweating.
CV: palpitations, increased heart rate.
EENT: drying and irritation of nose and throat (with inhaled form).
GI: vomiting, nausea.
Respiratory: ***paradoxical bronchospasm with prolonged usage.***
Other: hypokalemia (with high doses).

INTERACTIONS

CNS stimulants: increased CNS stimulation. Avoid concomitant use.
Digitalis glycosides, levodopa, halogenated inhalation anesthetics, cyclopropane: increased risk of arrhythmias. Monitor closely.
Levodopa: increased risk of arrhythmias. Avoid concomitant use.

MAO inhibitors: when given with sympathomimetics, may cause severe hypertension (hypertensive crisis). Don't use together.
Propranolol and other beta blockers: blocked bronchodilating effects of terbutaline.

CONTRAINDICATIONS

- Contraindicated in patients hypersensitive to the drug; in patients with tachyarrhythmias, tachycardia caused by digitalis toxicity, acute angle-closure glaucoma, or shock.
- Use cautiously in patients with diabetes, hypertension, hyperthyroidism, severe cardiac disease, and arrhythmias.
- Although not approved by FDA for treatment of preterm labor, it is considered very effective and is used in many hospitals. Monitor neonates for hypoglycemia.

NURSING CONSIDERATIONS

- Protect injection from light. Do not use if discolored.
- Give S.C. injections in lateral deltoid area.
- Patients may use tablets and aerosol concomitantly. Monitor closely for toxicity.
- Teach patients to perform oral inhalation correctly. Give the following instructions for using a metered-dose inhaler:
  - Clear nasal passages and throat.
  - Breathe out, expelling as much air from lungs as possible.
  - Place mouthpiece well into mouth as dose from inhaler is released, and inhale deeply.
  - Hold breath for several seconds, remove mouthpiece, and exhale slowly.
- If more than one inhalation is ordered, tell patients to wait at least 2 minutes before repeating procedure.
- Tell patients who are also using a steroid inhaler to use bronchodilator first, then wait about 5 minutes before using steroid. This allows bronchodilator to open air passages for maximum effectiveness.
- Warn patients to discontinue the drug immediately if paradoxical bronchospasm occurs.
- Tolerance may develop with prolonged use.
- Ensure that patients and family members understand why drug is necessary.

---

theophylline

Immediate-release liquids: Accurbron*, Aquaphyllin, Asmalix*, Bronkodyl*, Elixicon, Elixomin*, Elixophyllin*, Lanophyllin*, Lixolin, Slo-Phyllin, Theolair, Theon*
Immediate-release tablets and capsules: Bronkodyl, Elixophyllin, Nuelin‡, Slo-Phyllin, Somophyllin-T
Timed-release tablets: Constant-T, Duraphyl, Quibron-T/SR, Respbid, Sustaire, Theo-Dur, Theolair-SR, Theo-Time, Uniphyl
Timed-release capsules: Aerolate, Elixophyllin SR, Nuelin-SR‡, Slo-bid Gyrocaps, Slo-Phyllin, Somophyllin-CRT, Theo-24, Theobid Duracaps, Theobid Jr. Duracaps, Theochron, Theo-Dur Sprinkle, Theospan SR, Theovent Long-acting

theophylline sodium glycinate

Acet-Am†, Synophylate

Pregnancy Risk Category: C

HOW SUPPLIED

theophylline
Tablets: 100 mg, 125 mg, 200 mg, 225 mg, 250 mg, 300 mg
Tablets (chewable): 100 mg
Tablets (extended-release): 100 mg, 200 mg, 250 mg, 300 mg, 400 mg, 500 mg
Capsules: 50 mg, 100 mg, 200 mg, 250 mg

Capsules (extended-release): 50 mg, 60 mg, 65 mg, 75 mg, 100 mg, 125 mg, 130 mg, 200 mg, 250 mg, 260 mg, 300 mg
Elixir: 27 mg/5 ml, 50 mg/5 ml*
Oral solution: 27 mg/5 ml, 53 mg/5 ml
Oral suspension: 100 mg/5 ml
Syrup: 27 mg/5 ml, 50 mg/5 ml
Dextrose 5% injection: 200 mg in 50 ml or 100 ml; 400 mg in 100 ml, 250 ml, 500 ml, or 1,000 ml; 800 mg in 500 ml or 1,000 ml
theophylline sodium glycinate
Elixir: 110 mg/5 ml (equivalent to 55 mg anhydrous theophylline/5 ml)

ACTION
Mechanism: Inhibits phosphodiesterase, the enzyme that degrades cAMP. Results in relaxation of smooth muscle of the bronchial airways and pulmonary blood vessels.
Onset: within 15 minutes of I.V. use, 15 minutes to 1 hour after oral use.
Peak: Peak effects occur 15 to 30 minutes after I.V. use, or 1 to 2 hours after oral use. **Duration:** half-life, 9 hours; may be more than 24 hours in adults with cor pulmonale, heart failure, COPD, or liver disease; 5 hours, in patients who smoke or have smoked in the last 2 to 3 years; 24 hours or more in neonates and infants to age 6 months; about 4 hours in children over age 6 months.

INDICATIONS & DOSAGE
Prophylaxis and symptomatic relief of bronchial asthma, bronchospasm of chronic bronchitis and emphysema –
Adults: 6 mg/kg P.O. followed by 2 to 3 mg/kg q 6 hours for 2 doses. Maintenance dosage is 1 to 3 mg/kg q 8 to 12 hours.
Children 9 to 16 years: 6 mg/kg P.O. followed by 3 mg/kg q 6 hours for 3 doses. Maintenance dosage is 3 mg/kg q 6 hours.
Children 6 months to 9 years: 6 mg/kg P.O. followed by 4 mg/kg q 6 hours for 3 doses. Maintenance dosage is 4 mg/kg q 6 hours.

Most oral timed-release forms are given q 8 to 12 hours. Several products, however, may be given q 24 hours.
Symptomatic relief of bronchial asthma, pulmonary emphysema, and chronic bronchitis –
Adults: 330 to 660 mg (sodium glycinate) P.O. q 6 to 8 hours, after meals.
Children over 12 years: 220 to 330 mg (sodium glycinate) P.O. q 6 to 8 hours.
Children 6 to 12 years: 330 mg (sodium glycinate) P.O. q 6 to 8 hours.
Children 3 to 6 years: 110 to 165 mg (sodium glycinate) P.O. q 6 to 8 hours.
Children 1 to 3 years: 55 to 110 mg (sodium glycinate) P.O. q 6 to 8 hours.
Parenteral theophylline for patients not currently receiving theophylline –
Loading dose: 4.7 mg/kg I.V. slowly; then maintenance infusion.
Adults (nonsmokers): 0.55 mg/kg/hour for 12 hours, then 0.39 mg/kg/hour.
Otherwise-healthy adult smokers: 0.79 mg/kg/hour for 12 hours; then 0.63 mg/kg/hour.
Older adults with cor pulmonale: 0.47 mg/kg/hour for 12 hours; then 0.24 mg/kg/hour.
Adults with CHF or liver disease: 0.38 mg/kg/hour for 12 hours; then 0.08 to 0.16 mg/kg/hour.
Children 9 to 16 years: 0.79 mg/kg/hour for 12 hours; then 0.63 mg/kg/hour.
Children 6 months to 9 years: 0.95 mg/kg/hour for 12 hours; then 0.79 mg/kg/hour.

Switch to oral theophylline as soon as patient shows adequate improvement.
Symptomatic relief of bronchospasm in patients currently receiving theophylline –

Adults and children: each 0.5 mg/kg I.V. or P.O. (loading dose) will increase plasma levels by 1 mcg/ml. Ideally, dose is based upon current theophylline level. In emergency situations, some clinicians recommend a 2.5 mg/kg P.O. dose of rapidly absorbed form if no obvious signs of theophylline toxicity are present.
Adjunctive treatment of neonatal apnea –
Neonates: 5 mg/kg I.V. as a loading dose, followed by 2 mg/kg/day in two or three divided doses.

ADVERSE REACTIONS
CNS: *restlessness, dizziness,* headache, *insomnia,* light-headedness, *seizures,* muscle twitching.
CV: *palpitations, sinus tachycardia,* extrasystoles, flushing, marked hypotension.
GI: *nausea, vomiting, anorexia,* bitter aftertaste, dyspepsia, heavy feeling in stomach, diarrhea.
Respiratory: increased respiratory rate.
Skin: urticaria.

INTERACTIONS
Adenosine: decreased antiarrhythmic effectiveness. Higher doses of adenosine may be necessary.
Barbiturates, carbamazepine, nicotine, phenytoin, rifampin: enhanced metabolism and decreased theophylline blood levels. Monitor for decreased effect.
Beta-adrenergic blockers: antagonism. Propranolol and nadolol, especially, may cause bronchospasm in sensitive patients. Use together cautiously.
Cimetidine, influenza virus vaccine, macrolide antibiotics (such as erythromycin), oral contraceptives, quinolone antibiotics (such as ciprofloxacin), caffeine: decreased hepatic clearance of theophylline; elevated theophylline levels. Monitor for signs of toxicity.

Patients taking Theo-24 should take it on an empty stomach because food accelerates the drug's absorption.

CONTRAINDICATIONS
- Contraindicated in patients hypersensitive to xanthine compounds (caffeine, theobromine) and in patients with preexisting arrhythmias, especially tachyarrhythmias.
- Use cautiously in young children; in elderly patients with CHF or other circulatory impairment, cor pulmonale, renal or hepatic disease; and in patients with peptic ulceration, hyperthyroidism, or diabetes mellitus.

NURSING CONSIDERATIONS
- Be careful not to confuse sustained-release dosage forms with standard-release dosage forms.
- Individuals metabolize xanthines at different rates; determine dosage by monitoring response, tolerance, pulmonary function, and serum theophylline levels. Serum theophylline concentrations should range from 10 to 20 mcg/ml; toxicity has been reported with levels above 20 mcg/ml.
- Monitor vital signs; measure and record fluid intake and output. Expected clinical effects include improvement in quality of pulse and respiration.
- Relieve GI symptoms by taking oral drug with full glass of water after meals, although food in stomach delays absorption.
- Warn patient not to dissolve, crush, or chew slow-release products. Small children unable to swallow these can ingest (without chewing) the contents of bead-filled capsules sprinkled over soft food.
- Daily dosage may need to be decreased in patients with CHF or hepatic disease, or in elderly patients, because metabolism and excretion may be decreased. Monitor carefully, using blood levels, observation, examination, and patient interview. Give

drug around the clock, using sustained-release product at bedtime.

- Drug dosage may need to be increased in cigarette smokers and in habitual marijuana smokers because smoking causes the drug to be metabolized faster.
- **I.V. use:** Use commercially available infusion solution, or mix drug in D_5W. Use infusion pump for continuous infusion.
- Supply instructions for home care and dosage schedule.
- Warn patients to take the drug regularly, as directed. Patients tend to want to take extra "breathing pills."
- Warn patients to check with the doctor or pharmacist about *any* other drugs used. OTC remedies may contain ephedrine in combination with theophylline salts; excessive CNS stimulation may result.
- Warn elderly patients of dizziness, a common adverse reaction at start of therapy.

44

Expectorants and antitussives

acetylcysteine
ammonium chloride
(See Chapter 63, ACIDIFIER AND ALKALINIZERS.)
benzonatate
codeine phosphate
(See Chapter 27, NARCOTIC AND OPIOID ANALGESICS.)
codeine sulfate
(See Chapter 27, NARCOTIC AND OPIOID ANALGESICS.)
dextromethorphan hydrobromide
diphenhydramine hydrochloride
(See Chapter 42, ANTIHISTAMINES.)
guaifenesin
hydromorphone hydrochloride
(See Chapter 27, NARCOTIC AND OPIOID ANALGESICS.)
terpin hydrate

COMBINATION PRODUCTS

Preparations are available in the following combinations:

- expectorants with decongestants or antihistamines, or both
- antitussives with decongestants or antihistamines, or both
- expectorants and antitussives
- expectorants and antitussives with decongestants or antihistamines, or both.

acetylcysteine

Airbron†, Mucomyst, Mucosol, Parvolex†‡

Pregnancy Risk Category: B

HOW SUPPLIED

Solution: 10%, 20%
Injection: 200 mg/ml†‡

ACTION

Mechanism: A mucolytic that increases production of respiratory tract fluids to help liquefy and reduce the viscosity of tenacious secretions. Also restores liver stores of glutathione to treat acetaminophen toxicity.
Onset: immediate. **Peak:** Peak mucolytic effects occur in 5 to 10 minutes.

INDICATIONS & DOSAGE

Pneumonia, bronchitis, tuberculosis, cystic fibrosis, emphysema, atelectasis (adjunct), complications of thoracic surgery and CV surgery –
Adults and children: 1 to 2 ml 10% to 20% solution by direct instillation into trachea as often as every hour; or 3 to 5 ml 20% solution or 6 to 10 ml 10% solution by mouthpiece t.i.d. or q.i.d. Alternatively, give 300 mg/kg by I.V. infusion.
Acetaminophen toxicity –
Adults and children: initially, 140 mg/kg P.O., followed by 70 mg/kg q 4 hours for 17 doses (a total of 1,330 mg/kg). Or give 300 mg/kg by I.V. infusion.

ADVERSE REACTIONS

EENT: *rhinorrhea, hemoptysis.*
GI: *stomatitis, nausea, vomiting.*
Respiratory: ***bronchospasm*** (especially in asthmatics).

INTERACTIONS

Activated charcoal: limits acetylcysteine's effectiveness. Avoid concomitant use in treating acetaminophen toxicity.

CONTRAINDICATIONS

- Contraindicated in patients hypersensitive to the drug.
- Use cautiously in patients with asthma or severe respiratory insufficiency and in elderly or debilitated patients.

NURSING CONSIDERATIONS

- Drug may have a foul taste or smell that some patients find distressing.
- Use plastic, glass, stainless steel, or another nonreactive metal when administering by nebulization. Hand-bulb nebulizers are not recommended because output is too small and particle size too large.
- Physically or chemically incompatible with tetracyclines, erythromycin lactobionate, amphotericin B, and ampicillin sodium. If administered by aerosol inhalation, these drugs should be nebulized separately. Iodized oil, trypsin, and hydrogen peroxide are physically incompatible with acetylcysteine; don't add to nebulizer.
- Monitor cough type and frequency. or maximum effect, instruct patient to clear his airway by coughing before aerosol administration.
- Acetylcysteine is administered to treat acetaminophen overdose within 24 hours after ingestion. Start treatment immediately; do not wait for results of acetaminophen blood levels.
- When used orally to treat acetaminophen overdose, dilute oral doses with cola, fruit juice, or water before administering. Dilute the 20% solution to a concentration of 5% (add 3 ml of diluent to each ml of acetylcysteine). If patient vomits within 1 hour of receiving loading or maintenance dose, repeat dose.
- **I.V. use:** To prepare I.V. infusion, dilute calculated dose in D_5W. Dilute initial dose (150 mg/kg) in 200 ml of D_5W and infuse over 15 minutes. Dilute second dose of 50 mg/kg in 500 ml of D_5W and give over 4 hours. Dilute final dose of 100 mg/kg in 1,000 ml of D_5W and infuse over 16 hours.
- After opening, store in refrigerator; use within 96 hours.

benzonatate

Tessalon

Pregnancy Risk Category: C

HOW SUPPLIED

Capsules: 100 mg

ACTION

Mechanism: Suppresses the cough reflex by direct action on the cough center in the medulla. Also has local anesthetic action.
Onset: 15 to 20 minutes. **Duration:** up to 8 hours.

INDICATIONS & DOSAGE

Nonproductive cough –
Adults and children over 10 years: 100 mg P.O. t.i.d.; up to 600 mg daily.
Children under 10 years: 8 mg/kg P.O. in three to six divided doses.

ADVERSE REACTIONS

CNS: dizziness, drowsiness, headache, restlessness, ***seizures.***
EENT: nasal congestion, burning sensation in eyes.
GI: nausea, constipation.
Skin: rash.
Other: chills.

INTERACTIONS

None significant.

CONTRAINDICATIONS

- Contraindicated in patients hypersensitive to the drug.
- Use cautiously in patients hypersensitive to ester-type local anesthetics because cross-sensitivity reactions may occur.

NURSING CONSIDERATIONS

- Warn patients not to chew capsules or dissolve in mouth. Produces either local anesthesia that may result in aspiration or CNS stimulation that may cause restlessness, tremor, and possibly seizures.

• Don't use benzonatate when cough is a valuable diagnostic sign or is beneficial (as after thoracic surgery).
• Monitor cough type and frequency.
• Use with percussion and chest vibration.
• Maintain fluid intake to help liquefy sputum.

dextromethorphan hydrobromide

Balminil D.M.◇, Benylin DM◇, Broncho-Grippol-DM†, Children's Hold◇, DM Syrup◇, Hold◇, Koffex†, Mediquell◇, Neo-DM†, Ornex-DM 15◇, Ornex-DM 30◇, Pertussin Cough Suppressant◇, Pertussin CS◇, Pertussin ES◇, Robidex†, Robitussin Pediatric◇, Sedatuss†, St. Joseph for Children◇, Sucrets Cough Control Formula◇, Trocal◇, Vicks Formula 44 Pediatric Formula◇. More commonly available in combination products such as Anti-Tuss DM Expectorant◇, Baytussin DM◇, Benylin Expectorant Cough Formula◇, Cheracol D Cough◇, Codistan No. 1◇, Efficol Cough Whip◇, Extra Action Cough◇, 2/G DM Cough◇, Glycotuss dM◇, Guiamid D.M. Liquid◇, Guiatuss-DM◇, Halotussin DM Expectorant◇, Kolephrin GG/DM◇, Mytussin DM◇, Naldecon Senior DX◇, Pertussin CS◇, Quektuss◇, Rhinosyn-DMX Expectorant◇, Robitussin DM◇, Silexin Cough◇, Tolu-Sed DM Cough◇, Tuss-DM◇, Unproco◇, Vicks Children's Cough◇

Pregnancy Risk Category: C

HOW SUPPLIED

Chewable pieces: 15 mg◇
Liquid (extended-release): 30 mg/5 ml◇
Lozenges: 5 mg◇
Syrup: 5 mg/5 ml*◇, 7.5 mg/5 ml*◇, 10 mg/5 ml*◇, 15 mg/5 ml*◇

ACTION

Mechanism: An antitussive that suppresses the cough reflex by direct action on the cough center in the medulla.
Onset: within 30 minutes of oral ingestion. **Duration:** 3 to 6 hours with conventional dosage forms; up to 12 hours with extended-release forms.

INDICATIONS & DOSAGE

Nonproductive cough –
Adults: 10 to 20 mg P.O. q 4 hours, or 30 mg q 6 to 8 hours. Or, give 60 mg b.i.d. (controlled-release liquid). Maximum dosage is 120 mg daily.
Children 2 to 6 years: 2.5 to 5 mg P.O. q 4 hours, or 7.5 mg q 6 to 8 hours. Maximum dosage is 30 mg daily.
Children 6 to 12 years: 5 to 10 mg P.O. q 4 hours, or 15 mg q 6 to 8 hours. Or, give 30 mg b.i.d. (controlled-release liquid). Maximum dosage is 60 mg daily.

Dosages for children under 2 years must be individualized.

ADVERSE REACTIONS

CNS: drowsiness, dizziness.
GI: nausea, vomiting, stomach pain.

INTERACTIONS

MAO inhibitors: risk of hypotension, coma, hyperpyrexia, and death. Avoid concomitant use.

CONTRAINDICATIONS

• Contraindicated in patients currently taking MAO inhibitors or within 2 weeks of discontinuing MAO inhibitors.
• Don't use dextromethorphan when cough is a valuable diagnostic sign or is beneficial (as after thoracic surgery).

NURSING CONSIDERATIONS

• Drug produces no analgesia or addiction and little or no CNS depression.

- Use drug with chest percussion and vibration.
- Monitor cough type and frequency.
- Dextromethorphan 15 to 30 mg is equivalent to 8 to 15 mg codeine as an antitussive.

guaifenesin (glyceryl guaiacolate)

Anti-Tuss*◇, Balminil Expectorant†, Baytussin◇, Breonesin◇, Cremacoat 2◇, Gee-Gee◇, GG-CEN*◇, Glyate*◇, Glycotuss◇, Glytuss◇, Guiatuss*◇, Halotussin◇, Humibid L.A.◇, Hytuss◇, Hytuss-2X◇, Naldecon Senior EX◇, Neo-Spec†, Nortussin◇, Resyl†◇, Robafen◇, Robitussin*◇, S-T Expectorant◇

Pregnancy Risk Category: C

HOW SUPPLIED

Tablets: 100 mg◇, 200 mg◇
Capsules: 200 mg◇
Capsules (extended-release): 300 mg
Syrup: 67 mg/5 ml*◇, 100 mg/5 ml*◇

ACTION

Mechanism: Increases production of respiratory tract fluids to help liquefy and reduce the viscosity of tenacious secretions.
Duration: up to 4 hours for regular-release preparations, 12 hours for extended-release preparations.

INDICATIONS & DOSAGE

Expectorant –
Adults: 100 to 400 mg P.O. q 4 hours, or 600 to 1,200 mg (extended-release capsules) q 12 hours. Maximum dosage is 2,400 mg daily.
Children 2 to 6 years: 50 to 100 mg P.O. q 4 hours. Maximum dosage is 300 mg daily.
Children 6 to 12 years: 100 to 200 mg P.O. q 4 hours. Maximum dosage is 600 mg daily.

ADVERSE REACTIONS

CNS: drowsiness.
GI: stomach pain, diarrhea, vomiting, and nausea occur with large doses.

INTERACTIONS

Heparin: increased risk of bleeding. Use together cautiously.

CONTRAINDICATIONS

- Contraindicated in patients hypersensitive to the drug.

NURSING CONSIDERATIONS

- Drug may interfere with certain laboratory tests for 5-hydroxyindoleacetic acid and vanillylmandelic acid.
- Drug is used to liquefy thick, tenacious sputum, but efficacy has not been established. Advise patients to take each dose with a glass of water; increasing fluid intake may prove beneficial.
- Monitor cough type and frequency. Ensure that patients understand that persistent cough may indicate a serious condition and that they should contact a doctor if cough lasts longer than 1 week, recurs frequently, or is associated with high fever, rash, or severe headache.
- Encourage deep-breathing exercises.

terpin hydrate*◇

Pregnancy Risk Category: C

HOW SUPPLIED

Elixir: 85 mg/5 ml (43% ethanol)*◇

ACTION

Mechanism: Increases production of respiratory tract fluids to help liquefy and reduce the viscosity of thick secretions.
Duration: 4 to 6 hours.

†Available in Canada only. ‡Available in Australia only. ◇Available OTC.

INDICATIONS & DOSAGE
Excessive bronchial secretions –
Adults: 5 to 10 ml P.O. q 4 to 6 hours. Don't exceed 70 ml/day.

ADVERSE REACTIONS
GI: nausea, vomiting.

INTERACTIONS
None significant.

CONTRAINDICATIONS
- Contraindicated in patients with peptic ulceration or severe diabetes mellitus.

NURSING CONSIDERATIONS
- Efficacy as an expectorant has not been established.
- Terpin hydrate has a high ethanol content (86 proof). Don't give in large doses during pregnancy or to children. Consider risk and benefit in breast-feeding patients.
- Monitor cough type and frequency.
- Tell patients to take each dose with a full glass of water to liquefy secretions.

45

Miscellaneous respiratory agents

alpha-1 proteinase inhibitor (human)
beclomethasone dipropionate
beractant
colfosceril palmitate
cromolyn sodium
dexamethasone sodium phosphate inhalation
dornase alfa
flunisolide
nedocromil sodium
triamcinolone acetonide

COMBINATION PRODUCTS
None.

alpha-1 proteinase inhibitor (human)

Prolastin

Pregnancy Risk Category: C

HOW SUPPLIED
Injection: 500 mg, 1,000 mg

ACTION
Mechanism: Replaces alpha$_1$-proteinase in patients with alpha$_1$-antitrypsin deficiency.
Onset: within a few weeks. **Peak:** Serum levels peak immediately after I.V. infusion. **Duration:** half-life, about 4½ days.

INDICATIONS & DOSAGE
Chronic replacement therapy in patients with congenital alpha$_1$-antitrypsin deficiency and demonstrable panacinar emphysema –
Adults: 60 mg/kg I.V. once weekly. May give at a rate of 0.08 ml/kg/minute or greater.

ADVERSE REACTIONS
Hematologic: possible viral transmission.

INTERACTIONS
Cigarette smoke: blocks drug's effects. Patients should not smoke.

CONTRAINDICATIONS
• Contraindicated in patients hypersensitive to the drug and in those with selective immunoglobulin A (IgA) deficiency caused by antibodies against IgA.

NURSING CONSIDERATIONS
• Explain to patients that product has been treated to minimize the risk of transmission of hepatitis and AIDS.
• Many commercial assays for alpha$_1$-proteinase inhibitor measure immunoreactivity of the protein and not inhibitor activity. Monitoring serum level may not accurately reflect clinical response.
• **I.V. use:** Store powder for injection in the refrigerator (36° to 46° F [2° to 8° C]). Reconstitute using the supplied diluent (sterile water for injection). After reconstitution, administer within 3 hours. Inject directly into vein; intermittent or continuous infusion is not recommended.

beclomethasone dipropionate

Aldecin Inhaler‡, Beclodisk†, Becloforte Inhaler‡, Beclovent, Beclovent Rotacaps†, Vanceril

Pregnancy Risk Category: C

HOW SUPPLIED
Oral inhalation aerosol: 42 mcg/metered spray, 50 mcg/metered spray‡
Powder for inhalation: 100 mcg, 200 mcg

ACTION

Mechanism: Decreases inflammation, mainly by stabilizing leukocyte lysosomal membranes.

Onset: 1 to 4 weeks. **Duration:** plasma half-life, average of 15 hours.

INDICATIONS & DOSAGE

Steroid-dependent asthma –

Adults: 2 to 4 inhalations t.i.d. or q.i.d. Maximum dosage is 20 inhalations daily.

Children 6 to 12 years: 1 to 2 inhalations t.i.d. or q.i.d. Maximum dosage is 10 inhalations daily.

ADVERSE REACTIONS

EENT: hoarseness, fungal infections of throat, throat irritation.

GI: dry mouth, fungal infections of mouth.

INTERACTIONS

None significant.

CONTRAINDICATIONS

• Contraindicated in patients hypersensitive to any component of the formulation (fluorocarbons, oleic acid) and in those with systemic fungal infections or status asthmaticus. Not for use in patients with asthma controlled by bronchodilators or other noncorticosteroids alone or for those with nonasthmatic bronchial diseases.

NURSING CONSIDERATIONS

• Taper oral glucocorticoid therapy slowly. Acute adrenal insufficiency and death have occurred in asthmatics who changed abruptly from oral corticosteroids to beclomethasone. Be sure patients report symptoms associated with corticosteroid withdrawal, including fatigue, weakness, arthralgia, orthostatic hypotension, and dyspnea.

• Periodic measurement of growth and development may be necessary during high-dose or prolonged therapy in children.

• During times of stress (trauma, surgery, or infection) systemic corticosteroids may be needed to prevent adrenal insufficiency in previously steroid-dependent patients.

• Instruct patients to carry a card indicating need for supplemental systemic glucocorticoids during stress.

• Tell patients requiring a bronchodilator to use it several minutes before beclomethasone.

• Advise patients to allow 1 minute to elapse before taking subsequent puffs of medication and to hold breath for a few seconds to enhance action of drug.

• Inform patients that beclomethasone doesn't provide relief for acute asthma attacks.

• Instruct patients to contact their doctor if response to therapy decreases or if symptoms don't improve within 3 weeks; dose may have to be adjusted. Tell patients not to exceed recommended dose on their own.

• Check mucous membranes frequently for signs of fungal infection.

• Tell patients to prevent oral fungal infections by gargling or rinsing mouth with water after each use, but not to swallow the water.

• Tell patients to keep inhaler clean and unobstructed. Wash with warm water and dry thoroughly.

• A spacer device may help ensure delivery of the proper dose.

• Store medication between 36° and 86° F (2° and 30° C). Advise patients to ensure delivery of the proper dose by gently warming canister to room temperature before using. Some patients carry the canister in a pocket to keep it warm.

beractant (natural lung surfactant)

Survanta

HOW SUPPLIED

Suspension for intratracheal instillation: 25 mg/ml

ACTION

Mechanism: Lowers the surface tension on alveolar surfaces during respiration and stabilizes the alveoli against collapse. An extract of bovine lung containing neutral lipids, fatty acids, surfactant-associated proteins, and phospholipids that mimics naturally occurring surfactant; palmitic acid, palmitin, and dipalmitoylphosphatidylcholine are added to standardize the solution's composition.
Onset: ½ to 2 hours. **Duration:** 2 to 3 days.

INDICATIONS & DOSAGE

Prevention of respiratory distress syndrome (RDS) or hyaline membrane disease in premature neonates weighing 1,250 g or less at birth or having symptoms consistent with surfactant deficiency –
Neonates: 4 ml/kg intratracheally; administer each dose in four quarter-doses, with a hand-held ventilation bag between quarter-doses at a rate of 60 breaths/minute and sufficient oxygen to prevent cyanosis. Give drug as soon as possible, preferably within 15 minutes of birth. Repeat in 6 hours if respiratory distress continues. Give no more than four doses in 48 hours.
Rescue treatment of RDS in premature infants –
Neonates: 4 ml/kg intratracheally; before administering, increase ventilator rate to 60 breaths/minute with an inspiratory time of 0.5 second and a fraction of inspired oxygen (FIO_2) of 1. Administer each dose in four quarter-doses, with a hand-held ventilation bag between quarter-doses at a rate of 60 breaths/minute and sufficient oxygen to prevent cyanosis. Give dose as soon as RDS is confirmed by X-ray, preferably within 8 hours of birth. Repeat in 6 hours if respiratory distress continues. Give no more than four doses in 48 hours.

ADVERSE REACTIONS

CV: transient bradycardia, vasoconstriction, hypotension.
Hematologic: decreased oxygen saturation, hypocarbia, hypercarbia.
Other: endotracheal tube reflux or blockage, pallor, ***apnea.***

INTERACTIONS

None significant.

CONTRAINDICATIONS

None reported.

NURSING CONSIDERATIONS

- Beractant should be administered only by personnel familiar with the care of clinically unstable premature neonates. Such personnel should have knowledge of neonatal intubation and airway management.
- Accurate determination of weight is essential to proper measurement of dosage.
- Continuous monitoring of ECG and transcutaneous oxygen saturation are essential; frequent arterial blood pressure monitoring and frequent arterial blood gas sampling are highly desirable.
- Continuously monitor the neonate before, during, and after beractant administration. The endotracheal tube may be suctioned before giving the drug; allow the neonate to stabilize before proceeding with administration.
- Transient bradycardia and oxygen desaturation are common after dosing.
- Know that beractant can rapidly affect oxygenation and lung compliance. Peak ventilator inspiratory pressures may need to be adjusted if chest expansion improves substantially after drug administration. Adjust immediately because lung overdistention and fatal pulmonary air leak may result.
- Refrigerate at 36° to 46° F (2° to 8° C). Warm before administration by

allowing drug to stand at room temperature for at least 20 minutes or by holding in hand for at least 8 minutes. Do not use artificial warming methods. Unopened vials that have been warmed to room temperature may be returned to the refrigerator within 8 hours; however, warm and return drug to the refrigerator only once. Vials are for single use only – discard unused drug.

- Beractant does not require sonication or reconstitution before use. Inspect contents before giving; ensure that the color is off-white to light brown and the contents uniform. If settling occurs, swirl vial gently; do not shake. Some foaming is normal.
- Use a large-bore needle (20G or larger) to draw up drug; do not use a filter. Administer the drug using a #5 French end-hole catheter. Premeasure and shorten the catheter before use. Fill the catheter with beractant and discard any excess drug so only the total dose to be given remains in the syringe. Insert catheter into the neonate's endotracheal tube; make sure the catheter tip protrudes just beyond the end of the tube above the neonate's carina. Do not instill drug into a main-stem bronchus.
- Homogeneous distribution of the drug is important. In clinical trials, each dose of the drug was given in four quarter-doses, with the patient positioned differently after each administration. Each quarter-dose was given over 2 to 3 seconds; the catheter was removed and the patient ventilated between quarter-doses. With the head and body inclined slightly downward, the first quarter-dose was given with the head turned to the right; the second quarter-dose, with the head turned to the left. Then the head and body were inclined slightly upward; the third quarter-dose was given with the head turned to the right; the fourth quarter-dose, with the head turned to the left.
- Immediately after administration, moist breath sounds and crackles can occur. *Do not* suction the neonate for 1 hour unless other signs of airway obstruction are evident.
- Audiovisual materials that describe dosage and administration procedures are available from the manufacturer.

colfosceril palmitate

Exosurf Neonatal

HOW SUPPLIED

Suspension for intratracheal instillation: 10 ml

ACTION

Mechanism: Replaces a major component of naturally occurring lung surfactant (dipalmitoylphosphatidylcholine), which is deficient in premature neonates. The mixture also contains cetyl ethanol (which acts as a spreading agent between the air-fluid interface) and tyloxapol, a long chain ethanol polymer (which acts as a dispersant).

Duration: about 1 week.

INDICATIONS & DOSAGE

Prevention of respiratory distress syndrome (RDS) in neonates weighing less than 1,350 g at risk for developing RDS; prophylactic treatment of neonates weighing 1,350 g or more with evidence of pulmonary insufficiency –

Neonates: administer 5 ml/kg intratracheally as soon as possible after delivery. If neonate is maintained on a mechanical ventilator, repeat dosage 12 and 24 hours later.

Rescue treatment of neonates with RDS –

Neonates: administer 5 ml/kg intratracheally as soon as possible after diagnosis of RDS. If the neonate is still mechanically ventilated, administer a second dose of 5 ml/kg 12 hours later.

ADVERSE REACTIONS
Respiratory: ***pulmonary hemorrhage.***

INTERACTIONS
None significant.

CONTRAINDICATIONS
• None reported.

NURSING CONSIDERATIONS
• Colfosceril should be administered only by personnel familiar with the care of clinically unstable premature neonates. Such personnel should have knowledge of neonatal intubation and airway management.
• Accurate determination of weight is essential to proper measurement of dosage.
• Know that colfosceril can rapidly affect oxygenation and lung compliance. Peak ventilator inspiratory pressures may need to be adjusted if chest expansion improves substantially after drug administration. Adjust immediately because lung overdistention and fatal pulmonary air leak may result.
• If the neonate becomes pink and the transcutaneous oxygen saturation exceeds 95%, reduce fraction of inspired oxygen (FIO_2) in a stepwise fashion until the saturation is 90% to 95%. Do so immediately because hyperoxia (an excess of systemic oxygen) may result.
• Reduce ventilator rate immediately if the transcutaneous or arterial carbon dioxide measurements are less than 30 mm Hg. Failure to reduce the rate may result in hypocarbia, which can reduce blood flow to the brain.
• Monitor neonates for pulmonary hemorrhage.
• Continuous monitoring of ECG and transcutaneous oxygen saturation are essential; frequent arterial blood pressure monitoring and frequent arterial blood gas sampling are highly desirable. Continuously monitor the neonate before, during, and after drug administration.
• Reconstitute drug immediately before use with the supplied preservative-free sterile water for injection. Do not use solutions that contain antibacterial preservatives. After reconstitution, drug is stable for up to 12 hours at 36° to 86° F (2° to 30° C). Fill a 10-ml syringe with the supplied 8 ml of diluent using an 18G or 19G needle. Then, pierce the top of the vial and allow the vacuum to draw in the sterile water. Do not use vials without a vacuum. Aspirate as much of the 8 ml as possible out of vial while maintaining vacuum. Quickly release the syringe plunger. Repeat this final step at least three or four times to ensure adequate mixing of the vial contents.
• When drawing up the dose, use liquid below the froth. Each 8-ml vial contains sufficient material to administer a 5 ml/kg dose to a neonate weighing up to 1,600 g.
• Note that the suspension should have a homogeneous, milky white appearance. Do not use vials that appear to contain large flakes. If the suspension appears to separate, the vial may be shaken gently or swirled to resuspend the material.
• Suction the neonate before administering drug. Do not suction for 2 hours after dosing unless it is necessary.
• Special endotracheal tube adapters are available with each kit of surfactant. Ensure that adapter used corresponds to the inside diameter of the neonate's endotracheal tube. Insert the adapter into the tube with a twisting motion and connect to the ventilator circuit. To administer the drug (in half-doses, 2.5 ml), remove the cap from side port of the adapter and attach syringe; do not interrupt mechanical ventilation. After dosing, remember to reattach cap.
• Instill each half-dose slowly over 1 to 2 minutes (30 to 50 mechanical

breaths) in small bursts timed with inspiration. Administer first half-dose with the neonate in the midline position; then turn the neonate's head and torso 45 degrees to the right for 30 seconds to assist distribution of drug. Return the neonate to the midline position for the second half-dose and again administer over 1 to 2 minutes. After the second half-dose, turn the neonate's head and torso 45 degrees to the left for 30 seconds.

• When administering, monitor the neonate's facial expressions, skin color, chest expansion, heart rate, and endotracheal tube patency and position. If the neonate becomes dusky or agitated, heart rate slows, drug backs up in the endotracheal tube, or oxygen saturation decreases by more than 15%, discontinue the drug and modify peak inspiratory pressure, ventilator rate, or FIO_2 as ordered. Note that rapid improvements in lung function may require rapid reductions in peak inspiratory pressure, ventilator rate, or FIO_2.

cromolyn sodium (sodium cromoglycate)

Gastrocrom, Intal, Intal Inhaler, Intal Spincaps†, Nalcrom, Nasalcrom, Opticrom, Rynacrom†

Pregnancy Risk Category: B

HOW SUPPLIED

Capsules (for oral solution): 100 mg
Aerosol: 800 mcg/metered spray
Nasal solution: 5.2 mg/metered spray (40 mg/ml)
Solution (for nebulization): 20 mg/2 ml
Ophthalmic solution: 4% (with benzalkonium chloride 0.01%, EDTA 0.01%, and phenylethyl ethanol 0.4%)

ACTION

Mechanism: Inhibits the degranulation of sensitized mast cells that occurs after a patient's exposure to specific antigens. Also inhibits release of histamine and slow-reacting substance of anaphylaxis.
Onset: after 2 to 4 weeks of regular use. **Duration:** about 4 weeks.

INDICATIONS & DOSAGE

Adjunct in severe perennial bronchial asthma –
Adults and children over 5 years: 2 metered sprays using inhaler q.i.d. at regular intervals. Also available as an aqueous solution administered through a nebulizer.
Prevention and treatment of allergic rhinitis –
Adults and children over 5 years: 1 spray in each nostril t.i.d or q.i.d. Give as ordered up to six times daily.
Prevention of exercise-induced bronchospasm –
Adults and children over 5 years: 2 metered sprays inhaled no more than 1 hour before anticipated exercise.
Allergic ocular disorders –
Adults and children 4 years and older: 1 to 2 drops in each eye four to six times daily at regular intervals.
Systemic mastocytosis –
Adults: 100 to 200 mg P.O. q.i.d.
Food allergy –
Adults: 200 mg P.O. q.i.d. 15 to 20 minutes before meals. If results are not satisfactory in 2 to 3 weeks, double dosage.
Children under 2 years: up to 20 mg/kg P.O. daily.
Children 2 to 13 years: 100 mg P.O. q.i.d. 15 to 20 minutes before meals. If results are not satisfacory in 2 to 3 weeks, double dosage. Do not exceed 40 mg/kg daily.
Inflammatory bowel disease –
Adults: 200 mg P.O. q.i.d. 15 to 20 minutes before meals.
Children 2 to 14 years: 100 mg P.O. q.i.d. 15 to 20 minutes before meals.

ADVERSE REACTIONS
CNS: dizziness, headache.
EENT: *irritation of the throat and trachea,* nasal congestion, pharyngeal irritation.
GI: nausea, esophagitis.
GU: dysuria, urinary frequency.
Respiratory: ***bronchospasm*** after inhalation of dry powder; *cough,* wheezing, *eosinophilic pneumonia.*
Skin: rash, urticaria.
Other: joint swelling and pain, lacrimation, swollen parotid gland, ***angioedema.***

INTERACTIONS
None significant.

CONTRAINDICATIONS
• Contraindicated in patients experiencing acute asthma attacks and status asthmaticus because drug will only prevent attacks.
• Also contraindicated in premature neonates.
• Use cautiously in patients with coronary artery disease or a history of arrhythmias.
• Administer with caution in children. Use of cromolyn oral inhalation solution is *not* recommended in children under 2 years; cromolyn powder or aerosol for oral inhalation, not in children under 5 years; and cromolyn nasal solution, not in children under 6 years.

NURSING CONSIDERATIONS
• Discontinue if the patient develops eosinophilic pneumonia, indicated by eosinophilia and infiltrates on chest X-ray.
• Watch for recurrence of asthmatic symptoms when dosage is decreased, especially when corticosteroids are also used.
• Use only when acute episode has been controlled, airway is cleared, and the patient can inhale independently.
• Esophagitis may be relieved by antacids or a glass of milk.
• Dissolve powder in capsules for oral dose in hot water and further dilute with cold water before ingestion. Do not mix with fruit juice, milk, or food.
• Safety and efficacy of cromlyn sodium ophthalmic solution in children under 4 years has not been established.
• Oral cromolyn sodium should be used in full-term neonates and infants *only* for a severe, incapacitating disease when benefits clearly outweigh the risks.

dexamethasone sodium phosphate inhalation

Decadron Respihaler

Pregnancy Risk Category: C

HOW SUPPLIED
Oral inhalation aerosol: 100 mcg/metered spray

ACTION
Mechanism: Decreases inflammation, mainly by stabilizing leukocyte lysosomal membranes.
Onset: 1 to 4 weeks.

INDICATIONS & DOSAGE
Steroid-dependent asthma –
Adults: initially, 3 inhalations t.i.d. or q.i.d. Decrease as needed and tolerated; most patients respond to 2 inhalations b.i.d. Maximum dosage is 12 inhalations daily.
Children 6 to 12 years: 2 inhalations t.i.d. or q.i.d. Maximum dosage is 8 inhalations daily.

ADVERSE REACTIONS
EENT: hoarseness, fungal infections of throat, throat irritation.
GI: dry mouth, fungal infections of mouth.

INTERACTIONS
None significant.

CONTRAINDICATIONS
• Contraindicated in patients hypersensitive to any component of the formulation (fluorocarbons, ethanol) and in those with status asthmaticus or systemic fungal infections. Not for use in patients with asthma controlled by bronchodilators or other noncorticosteroids alone or for those with nonasthmatic bronchial diseases.

NURSING CONSIDERATIONS
• Taper oral glucocorticoid therapy slowly. Acute adrenal insufficiency and death have occurred in asthmatics who changed abruptly from oral corticosteroids to inhaled steroids. Be sure patients report symptoms associated with corticosteroid withdrawal, including fatigue, weakness, arthralgia, orthostatic hypotension, and dyspnea.
• With prolonged use of high doses, systemic effects are likely because up to 50% of a dose is absorbed.
• Conduct periodic measurements of growth and development during high-dose or prolonged therapy in children.
• During times of stress (trauma, surgery, or infection), systemic corticosteroids may be needed to prevent adrenal insufficiency in previously steroid-dependent patients.
• Instruct patients to carry a card indicating need for supplemental systemic glucocorticoids during stress.
• Advise patients requiring bronchodilator to use it several minutes before dexamethasone.
• Tell patients to allow 1 minute to elapse before taking subsequent puffs of medication and to hold breath for a few seconds to enhance action of drug.
• Inform patients that dexamethasone doesn't provide relief for acute asthma attacks.
• Instruct patients to contact their doctor if response to therapy decreases or if symptoms don't improve within 3 weeks of initiating therapy; the doctor may adjust the dose. Tell patients not to exceed recommended dose on their own.
• Check mucous membranes frequently for signs of fungal infection.
• Advise patients to prevent oral fungal infections by gargling or rinsing mouth with water after each use, but not to swallow water.
• Teach patients to keep inhaler clean and unobstructed. Wash with warm water and dry thoroughly.
• A spacer device may help ensure delivery of the proper dose of medication.
• Store medication between 36° and 86° F (2° and 30° C). Tell patients that this medication needs to be at room temperature when used. If the canister is cold, the proper dose may not be delivered.
• Advise patients to ensure delivery of the proper dose by gently warming the canister to room temperature before using. Some patients carry the canister in a pocket to keep it warm.

dornase alfa
Pulmozyme

Pregnancy Risk Category: B

HOW SUPPLIED
Inhalation solution: 2.5 mg/ampule

ACTION
Mechanism: Hydrolyzes DNA in sputum of cystic fibrosis patients, causing decreased visosity and elasticity of pulmonary secretions.
Peak: Peak increases in baseline measurement of amount of air exhaled in first second of expiration occur after about 9 days of therapy.

INDICATIONS & DOSAGE
To improve pulmonary function and decrease the frequency of moderate to severe respiratory infections in patients with cystic fibrosis –

Adults and children 5 years and over: one ampule (2.5 mg) inhaled once daily. Treatment usually takes 10 to 15 minutes. Use drug only with an approved nebulizer.

ADVERSE REACTIONS
EENT: *pharyngitis,* voice alteration, laryngitis, conjunctivitis.
Skin: rash, urticaria.
Other: chest pain.

INTERACTIONS
None significant.

CONTRAINDICATIONS
• Contraindicated in patients hypersensitive to the drug or Chinese Hamster Ovary cell products.

NURSING CONSIDERATIONS
• Use in conjunction with other standard therapies for cystic fibrosis.
• Administer only with the following nebulizers and compressors: the Hudson T Up-draft II disposable jet nebulizer and the Marquest Acorn II disposable jet nebulizer in conjunction with the Pulmo-Aide compressor or the PARI LC Jet† reusable nebulizer in conjunction with the PARI PRONEB compressor.
• Do not mix with other drugs in the nebulizer. Doing so could lead to a physical or chemical reaction that may inactivate dornase alfa.
• Remind the patient to breathe only through his mouth when using the nebulizer. If this is difficult, suggest use of a nose clip.
• Tell the patient that if he begins coughing during treatment to turn off the nebulizer without spilling the drug. To resume treatment, the patient should turn on the nebulizer and continue breathing through the mouthpiece until the nebulizer cup is empty or mist is no longer produced.
• Discard cloudy or discolored solution.
• Refrigerate drug in its protective foil pouch.
• Safety and efficacy in children under 5 years or with forced vital capacity less than 40% have not been established.

flunisolide
AeroBid

Pregnancy Risk Category: C

HOW SUPPLIED
Oral inhalant: 250 mcg/metered spray (50 inhalations/container)

ACTION
Mechanism: Decreases inflammation, mainly by stabilizing leukocyte lysosomal membranes.
Onset: after 1 to 4 weeks of therapy.
Peak: Plasma levels peak 1 to 2 hours after a dose. **Duration:** plasma half-life, 1½ to 2 hours.

INDICATIONS & DOSAGE
Steroid-dependent asthma –
Adults and children over 6 years: 2 inhalations (500 mcg) b.i.d. Don't exceed 4 inhalations b.i.d.

ADVERSE REACTIONS
CNS: headache.
EENT: watery eyes, throat irritation, hoarseness, nasopharyngeal fungal infections.
GI: nausea, vomiting, dry mouth.

INTERACTIONS
None significant.

CONTRAINDICATIONS
• Contraindicated in patients hypersensitive to the drug and in those with status asthmaticus or respiratory infections. Not recommended for use in patients with asthma controlled by bronchodilators or other noncorticosteroids alone or for those with nonasthmatic bronchial diseases.

NURSING CONSIDERATIONS

- Advise parents of children receiving long-term therapy that the child should have periodic growth measurements and be checked for evidence of hypothalamic-pituitary-adrenal axis suppression.
- Teach patients to check mucous membranes frequently for signs of fungal infection.
- Patients can prevent oral fungal infections by gargling or rinsing mouth with water after each inhaler use. Caution patients not to swallow the water.
- Withdraw drug slowly in patients who have received long-term oral corticosteroid therapy.
- Teach patients to keep inhaler clean and unobstructed. Wash with warm water and dry thoroughly after use.
- Tell patient who is also using a bronchodilator to use it several minutes before flunisolide.
- Instruct patients to allow 1 minute to elapse before repeating inhalations and to hold breath for a few seconds to enhance drug's action.
- Warn patients that flunisolide doesn't relieve emergency asthma attacks.
- A spacer device may help to ensure proper dosage administration.
- Store medication between 36° and 86° F (2° and 30° C).
- Advise patients to ensure delivery of the proper dose by gently warming the canister to room temperature before using. Some patients carry the canister in a pocket to keep it warm.

nedocromil sodium

Tilade

Pregnancy Risk Category: C

HOW SUPPLIED

Inhalation aerosol: 1.75 mg/activation

ACTION

Mechanism: Reduces inflammatory changes in the airway by blocking the release of inflammation mediators, such as leukotrienes, histamine, and prostaglandins, from mast cells and eosinophils, monocytes, neutrophils, macrophages, and other immune cells.

Onset: about 1 week.

INDICATIONS & DOSAGE

Maintenance in mild-to-moderate reversible obstructive airway disease – **Adults:** 2 inhalations q.i.d., preferably at regular intervals.

ADVERSE REACTIONS

CNS: headache.
GI: nausea, vomiting.
Other: *unpleasant taste.*

INTERACTIONS

None significant.

CONTRAINDICATIONS

- Contraindicated in patients hypersensitive to the formulation or in patients with an acute asthmatic attack or acute bronchospasm.

NURSING CONSIDERATIONS

- Warn the patient that nedocromil has no direct bronchodilating action and cannot replace bronchodilators during an acute asthmatic attack.
- Tell the patient that drug is an adjunct to the regular bronchodilator regimen and may reduce the need for corticosteroids or bronchodilators.
- Emphasize to the patient that regular use of the drug will help him feel better. Most patients report benefits after 1 week of use; some require longer treatment before any improvement.
- Teach the patient how to use the inhaler. Instruct him to shake canister immediately before use and to invert it just before actuation.
- Advise the patient to clean inhaler at least twice a week and to remove canister before rinsing inhaler in hot

running water. Allow inhaler to air dry overnight.

• In some patients, bronchospasm may be prevented by a single dose of drug before activities that precipitate asthma, such as exercise or exposure to cold air, pollutants, or allergens.

triamcinolone acetonide

Azmacort

Pregnancy Risk Category: D

HOW SUPPLIED

Inhalation aerosol: 100 mcg/metered spray

ACTION

Mechanism: Decreases inflammation, mainly by stabilizing leukocyte lysosomal membranes.

Onset: after 1 to 2 weeks of regular use. **Peak:** Plasma levels peak 1 to 2 hours after a dose. **Duration:** plasma half-life, 1 to 2 hours.

INDICATIONS & DOSAGE

Asthma –

Adults: 2 inhalations t.i.d. to q.i.d. Maximum dosage is 16 inhalations daily.

Children 6 to 12 years: 1 to 2 inhalations t.i.d. to q.i.d. Maximum dosage is 12 inhalations daily.

ADVERSE REACTIONS

Most adverse reactions to corticosteroids are dose- or duration-dependent.

EENT: dry or irritated nose or throat, hoarseness.

Respiratory: cough.

Other: *oral candidiasis,* dry or irritated tongue or mouth.

INTERACTIONS

None significant.

CONTRAINDICATIONS

• Contraindicated in patients hypersensitive to any component of the formulation and in those with status asthmaticus. Not for use in patients with asthma controlled by bronchodilators or other noncorticosteroids alone or in those with nonasthmatic bronchial diseases.

• It is not known if drug is excreted in breast milk. Because of the risk of severe adverse effects, breast-feeding is not recommended.

NURSING CONSIDERATIONS

• Taper oral therapy slowly.

• Instruct patients to carry a card indicating their need for supplemental systemic glucocorticoids during stress.

• Patients requiring a bronchodilator should use it several minutes before triamcinolone. Tell patients to allow 1 minute to elapse before repeat inhalations and to hold breath for a few seconds to enhance drug's action.

• Inform patients that inhaled corticosteroids don't provide relief for emergency asthma attacks.

• Instruct patients to contact their doctor if response to therapy decreases; the doctor may adjust the dose. Tell patients not to exceed recommended dose on their own.

• Teach patients to check mucous membranes frequently for signs of fungal infection.

• Tell patients to prevent oral fungal infections by gargling or rinsing mouth with water after each use of the inhaler, but not to swallow the water.

• Tell patients to keep inhaler clean and unobstructed. Wash with warm water and dry thoroughly after use.

• Store medication between 36° and 86° F (2° and 30° C).

• Advise patients to ensure delivery of the proper dose of medication by gently warming the canister to room temperature before using. Some patients carry the canister in a pocket to keep it warm.

46

Antacids, adsorbents, and antiflatulents

aluminum carbonate
aluminum hydroxide
aluminum phosphate
calcium carbonate
dihydroxyaluminum sodium carbonate
magaldrate
magnesium oxide
magnesium hydroxide
(See Chapter 49, LAXATIVES.)
simethicone
sodium bicarbonate
(See Chapter 63, ACIDIFIER AND ALKALINIZERS.)

COMBINATION PRODUCTS

ALKA-SELTZER, MEDI-SELTZER◇: sodium bicarbonate 1,916 mg, aspirin 325 mg, and citric acid 1,000 mg.
ALKA-SELTZER WITHOUT ASPIRIN◇: sodium bicarbonate 958 mg, citric acid 832 mg, and potassium bicarbonate 312 mg.
ALUDROX SUSPENSION◇: aluminum hydroxide 307 mg and magnesium hydroxide 103 mg.
CAMALOX TABLETS◇: aluminum hydroxide 225 mg, magnesium hydroxide 200 mg, and calcium carbonate 250 mg.
DELCID SUSPENSION◇: aluminum hydroxide 600 mg and magnesium hydroxide 665 mg.
DI-GEL LIQUID◇: aluminum hydroxide 200 mg, magnesium hydroxide 200 mg, and simethicone 20 mg.
EXTRA STRENGTH MAALOX TABLETS◇: aluminum hydroxide 400 mg and magnesium hydroxide 400 mg.
FLATULEX: simethicone 80 mg and activated charcoal 250 mg.
GAVISCON◇: aluminum hydroxide 31.7 mg and magnesium carbonate 137 mg.
GELUSIL◇: aluminum hydroxide 200 mg, magnesium hydroxide 200 mg, and simethicone 25 mg.
GELUSIL-II◇: aluminum hydroxide 400 mg, magnesium hydroxide 400 mg, and simethicone 30 mg.
MAALOX NO. 1◇: aluminum hydroxide 200 mg and magnesium hydroxide 200 mg.
MAALOX PLUS TABLETS◇: aluminum hydroxide 200 mg, magnesium hydroxide 200 mg, and simethicone 25 mg.
MAALOX TC TABLETS◇: aluminum hydroxide 600 mg and magnesium hydroxide 300 mg.
MAGNATRIL◇: aluminum hydroxide 260 mg, magnesium hydroxide 130 mg, and magnesium trisilicate 455 mg.
MYLANTA TABLETS◇: aluminum hydroxide 200 mg, magnesium hydroxide 200 mg, and simethicone 20 mg.
MYLANTA-II TABLETS◇: aluminum hydroxide 400 mg, magnesium hydroxide 400 mg, and simethicone 40 mg.
RIOPAN PLUS CHEW TABLETS◇: magaldrate 540 mg and simethicone 20 mg.
RIOPAN PLUS SUSPENSION◇: magaldrate 540 mg and simethicone 20 mg/5 ml.
TITRALAC LIQUID◇: calcium carbonate 1,000 mg in glycine.
TITRALAC TABLETS◇: calcium carbonate 420 mg and glycine 150 mg.
UNIVOL†◇: aluminum hydroxide and magnesium carbonate co-dried gel 300 mg and magnesium hydroxide 100 mg.
WINGEL◇: aluminum hydroxide 180 mg and magnesium hydroxide 160 mg.

aluminum carbonate

Basaljel◇

Pregnancy Risk Category: C

HOW SUPPLIED

Tablets or capsules: aluminum hydroxide equivalent 500 mg◇
Oral suspension: aluminum hydroxide equivalent 400 mg/5 ml◇

ACTION

Mechanism: An antacid that reduces total acid load in the GI tract, elevates gastric pH to reduce pepsin activity, strengthens the gastric mucosal barrier, and increases esophageal sphincter tone.
Onset: about 20 minutes. **Duration:** less than 1 hour.

INDICATIONS & DOSAGE

Antacid –
Adults: 5 to 10 ml of suspension P.O., p.r.n.; or 1 to 2 tablets or capsules P.O., p.r.n. Maximum dosage is 24 capsules, tablets, or teaspoonfuls per 24 hours.
To prevent formation of urinary phosphate stones (with low-phosphate diet) –
Adults: 15 to 30 ml of suspension in water or juice P.O. 1 hour after meals and h.s.; or 2 to 6 tablets or capsules 1 hour after meals and h.s.

ADVERSE REACTIONS

GI: anorexia, *constipation,* intestinal obstruction.
Other: hypophosphatemia.

INTERACTIONS

Allopurinol, antibiotics (including quinolones and tetracyclines), diflunisal, digoxin, iron, isoniazid, penicillamine, phenothiazines, quinidine: decreased pharmacologic effect because of possible impaired absorption. Separate administration times.
Enteric-coated drugs: may release prematurely in stomach. Separate doses by at least 1 hour.

CONTRAINDICATIONS

- Use cautiously in elderly patients, especially those with decreased GI motility (those receiving antidiarrheals, antispasmodics, or anticholinergics), dehydration, fluid restriction, chronic renal disease, and suspected intestinal obstruction.

NURSING CONSIDERATIONS

- Record amount and consistency of stools. Manage constipation with laxatives or stool softeners; alternate with magnesium-containing antacids (if the patient does not have renal disease).
- Shake suspension well; give with small amount of water or fruit juice to facilitate passage. When administering through nasogastric tube, make sure tube is placed correctly and is patent; after instilling, flush tube with water to ensure passage to stomach and to clear tube.
- Watch long-term, high-dose use in patients on restricted sodium intake. Each tablet, capsule, or 5 ml of suspension contains about 3 mg of sodium.
- Warn patients not to take aluminum carbonate indiscriminately or to switch antacids without their doctor's advice.
- Because drug contains aluminum, it is used in patients with renal failure to help control hyperphosphatemia by binding phosphate in the GI tract.
- Monitor serum phosphate levels.
- Watch for symptoms of hypophosphatemia with prolonged use (anorexia, malaise, muscle weakness); can also lead to resorption of calcium and bone demineralization.
- Basaljel liquid contains no sugar.

aluminum hydroxide

ALternaGEL◊, Alu-Cap◊, Alu-Tab◊, Amphojel◊, Basaljel◊, Dialume◊, Nephrox◊

Pregnancy Risk Category: C

HOW SUPPLIED

Tablets: 300 mg◊, 600 mg◊
Capsules: 475 mg◊, 500 mg◊
Oral suspension: 320 mg/5 ml◊, 600 mg/5 ml◊

ACTION

Mechanism: An antacid that reduces total acid load in the GI tract, elevates gastric pH to reduce pepsin activity, strengthens the gastric mucosal barrier, and increases esophageal sphincter tone.

Onset: varies by dosage form; liquids are more rapid-acting than tablets or capsules. **Duration:** varies with gastric emptying time; 20 to 60 minutes in fasting patients, 3 hours when taken after meals.

INDICATIONS & DOSAGE

Antacid–
Adults: 600 mg P.O. (5 to 10 ml of most products) 1 hour after meals and h.s.; 300- or 600-mg tablet, chewed before swallowing, taken with milk or water five to six times daily after meals and h.s.

Hyperphosphatemia–
Adults: 500 mg to 2 g P.O. b.i.d. to q.i.d.

ADVERSE REACTIONS

GI: anorexia, *constipation,* intestinal obstruction.
Other: hypophosphatemia.

INTERACTIONS

Allopurinol, antibiotics (including quinolones and tetracyclines), diflunisal, digoxin, iron, isoniazid, penicillamine, phenothiazines, quinidine: decreased pharmacologic effect because of possible impaired absorption. Separate administration times.
Enteric-coated drugs: may release prematurely in stomach. Separate doses by at least 1 hour.

CONTRAINDICATIONS

- Use cautiously in elderly patients, especially those with decreased GI motility (those receiving antidiarrheals, antispasmodics, or anticholinergics), dehydration, fluid restriction, chronic renal disease, and suspected intestinal obstruction.

NURSING CONSIDERATIONS

- Record amount and consistency of stools. Manage constipation with laxatives or stool softeners; alternate with magnesium-containing antacids (if the patient does not have renal disease).
- Shake suspension well; give with small amount of milk or water to facilitate passage. When administering through nasogastric tube, make sure tube is placed correctly and is patent; after instilling, flush tube with water to ensure passage to stomach and to clear tube.
- Watch long-term, high-dose use in patient on restricted sodium intake. Each tablet, capsule, or 5 ml of suspension contains 2 to 3 mg of sodium.
- Advise patients not to take aluminum hydroxide indiscriminately or to switch antacids without their doctor's advice.
- Because drug contains aluminum, it is used in patients with renal failure to help control hyperphosphatemia by binding phosphate in the GI tract.
- Monitor serum phosphate levels.
- Watch for symptoms of hypophosphatemia with prolonged use (anorexia, malaise, and muscle weakness); can also lead to resorption of calcium and bone demineralization.

aluminum phosphate

Phosphaljel◇

Pregnancy Risk Category: C

HOW SUPPLIED

Oral suspension: 233 mg/5 ml◇

ACTION

Mechanism: Provides supplemental phosphate.

Onset: about 20 minutes. **Duration:** about 1 hour.

INDICATIONS & DOSAGE

To reduce fecal elimination of phosphorus –

Adults: 15 to 30 ml undiluted P.O. q 2 hours between meals and h.s.

ADVERSE REACTIONS

GI: *constipation,* intestinal obstruction.

INTERACTIONS

Ciprofloxacin and other quinolones, tetracyclines: decreased antibiotic effect. Separate administration times.

Enteric-coated drugs: may release prematurely in stomach. Separate doses by at least 1 hour.

CONTRAINDICATIONS

- Use cautiously in elderly patients, especially those with decreased GI motility (those receiving antidiarrheals, antispasmodics, or anticholinergics), dehydration, fluid restriction, chronic renal disease, and suspected intestinal obstruction.

NURSING CONSIDERATIONS

- Record amount and consistency of stools. Manage constipation with laxatives or stool softeners; alternate with magnesium-containing antacids (if the patient does not have renal disease).
- Shake suspension well; give alone or with small amount of milk or water. When administering through nasogastric tube, make sure tube is placed correctly and is patent; after instilling, flush tube with water to ensure passage to stomach and to clear tube.
- Watch long-term, high-dose use in patients on restricted sodium intake.
- Advise patients not to take aluminum phosphate indiscriminately or to switch antacids without their doctor's advice.
- This drug is a very weak antacid.
- Can reverse hypophosphatemia induced by aluminum hydroxide.
- Phosphaljel contains no sugar.

calcium carbonate

Alka-Mints◇, Amitone◇, Calcilac◇, Calcimax‡, Calglycine◇, Cal-Sup‡, Chooz◇, Dicarbosil◇, Effercal-600‡, Equilet◇, Genalac◇, Mallamint◇, Rolaids Calcium Rich◇, Titracid◇, Titralac◇,Titralac Extra Strength◇, Titralac Plus◇, Tums◇, Tums E-X◇, Tums Liquid Extra Strength◇

Pregnancy Risk Category: C

HOW SUPPLIED

Calcium carbonate contains 40% calcium; 20 mEq calcium/g.

Tablets: 350 mg◇, 420 mg◇, 500 mg◇, 650 mg, 750 mg, 850 mg, 1,250 mg‡

Chewing gum: 500 mg/piece

Oral suspension: 1 g/5 ml◇

ACTION

Mechanism: An antacid that reduces total acid load in the GI tract, elevates gastric pH to reduce pepsin activity, strengthens the gastric mucosal barrier, and increases esophageal sphincter tone.

Onset: immediate. **Duration:** 2 to 4 hours.

INDICATIONS & DOSAGE

Antacid, calcium supplement –

Adults: 350 mg to 1.25 g P.O. four to

†Available in Canada only. ‡Available in Australia only. ◇Available OTC.

six times daily, chewed well and taken with water; or 1 g of suspension (5 ml of most products) or 2 pieces of chewing gum 1 hour after meals and h.s.

ADVERSE REACTIONS
GI: *constipation,* gastric distention, flatulence, rebound hyperacidity, *nausea.*

INTERACTIONS
Allopurinol, antibiotics (including quinolones and tetracyclines), diflunisal, digoxin, iron, isoniazid, penicillamine, phenothiazines, quinidine: decreased pharmacologic effect because of possible impaired absorption. Separate administration times.
Enteric-coated drugs: may release prematurely in stomach. Separate doses by at least 1 hour.
Milk and other foods high in vitamin D: possible milk-alkali syndrome (headache, confusion, distaste for food, nausea, vomiting, hypercalcemia, hypercalciuria, calcinosis, and hypophosphatemia). Avoid concomitant use.

CONTRAINDICATIONS
- Contraindicated in patients with severe renal disease.
- Use cautiously in elderly patients, especially those with decreased GI motility (those receiving antidiarrheals, antispasmodics, or anticholinergics), dehydration, fluid restriction, chronic renal disease, and suspected intestinal obstruction.

NURSING CONSIDERATIONS
- Record amount and consistency of stools. Manage constipation with laxatives or stool softeners.
- Watch for symptoms of hypercalcemia (nausea, vomiting, headache, mental confusion, and anorexia).
- Monitor serum calcium levels, especially in patients with mild renal impairment.
- Advise patients not to take calcium carbonate indiscriminately or to switch antacids without their doctor's advice.

dihydroxyaluminum sodium carbonate

Rolaids◊

Pregnancy Risk Category: C

HOW SUPPLIED
Tablets: 334 mg◊

ACTION
Mechanism: An antacid that reduces total acid load in the GI tract, elevates gastric pH to reduce pepsin activity, strengthens the gastric mucosal barrier, and increases esophageal sphincter tone.
Onset: immediate. **Duration:** 1 to 2 hours.

INDICATIONS & DOSAGE
Antacid –
Adults: 1 to 2 tablets (334 to 668 mg), chewed well, p.r.n.

ADVERSE REACTIONS
GI: anorexia, *constipation,* intestinal obstruction.

INTERACTIONS
Allopurinol, antibiotics (including quinolones and tetracyclines), diflunisal, digoxin, iron, isoniazid, penicillamine, phenothiazines, quinidine: decreased pharmacologic effect because of possible impaired absorption. Separate administration times.
Enteric-coated drugs: may release prematurely in stomach. Separate doses by at least 1 hour.

CONTRAINDICATIONS
- Use cautiously in elderly patients, especially those with decreased GI motility (those receiving antidiarrheals, antispasmodics, or anticholinergics), dehydration, fluid restric-

tion, chronic renal disease, and suspected intestinal obstruction.

NURSING CONSIDERATIONS

- Has high sodium content (53 mg/tablet) and may increase sodium and water retention. Watch long-term, high-dose use in patients on restricted sodium intake.
- Record amount and consistency of stools. Manage constipation with laxatives or stool softeners; alternate with magnesium-containing antacids (if the patient does not have renal disease).
- Advise patient not to take dihydroxyaluminum sodium carbonate indiscriminately.

magaldrate (aluminum-magnesium complex)

Antiflux†, Lowsium◊, Riopan◊

Pregnancy Risk Category: C

HOW SUPPLIED

Tablets: 480 mg◊
Tablets (chewable): 480 mg◊
Oral suspension: 540 mg/5 ml◊, 1,080 mg/5 ml◊

ACTION

Mechanism: An antacid that reduces total acid load in the GI tract, elevates gastric pH to reduce pepsin activity, strengthens the gastric mucosal barrier, and increases esophageal sphincter tone.
Onset: 10 to 20 minutes. **Duration:** 2 to 4 hours.

INDICATIONS & DOSAGE

Antacid –
Adults: 540 to 1,080 mg (5 to 10 ml) of suspension P.O. with water between meals and h.s.; or 480 to 960 mg tablets(1 to 2 tablets) P.O. with water between meals and h.s.; or 480 to 960 mg chewable tablets (1 to 2 tablets) P.O., chewed before swallowing, between meals and h.s.

ADVERSE REACTIONS

GI: mild constipation or diarrhea.

INTERACTIONS

Allopurinol, antibiotics (including quinolones and tetracyclines), diflunisal, digoxin, iron, isoniazid, penicillamine, phenothiazines, quinidine: decreased pharmacologic effect because of possible impaired absorption. Separate administration times.
Enteric-coated drugs: may release prematurely in stomach. Separate doses by at least 1 hour.

CONTRAINDICATIONS

- Contraindicated in patients with severe renal disease.
- Use cautiously in elderly patients, especially those with decreased GI motility (those receiving antidiarrheals, antispasmodics, or anticholinergics), dehydration, fluid restriction, and mild kidney impairment.

NURSING CONSIDERATIONS

- Record amount and consistency of stools.
- Shake suspension well; give with water to facilitate passage. When giving through nasogastric tube, make sure tube is placed properly and is patent. After instilling, flush tube with water to ensure passage to stomach and to clear tube.
- Monitor serum magnesium in patients with mild kidney impairment. Symptomatic hypermagnesemia usually occurs only in severe renal failure.
- Not typically used in patients with renal failure (although it contains aluminum) to help control hypophosphatemia because it contains magnesium, which may accumulate.
- Very low sodium content; good for patients on restricted sodium intake.
- Advise patients not to take magaldrate indiscriminately or to switch antacids without their doctor's advice.

magnesium oxide

Mag-Ox 400◇, Maox◇, Par-Mag◇, Uro-Mag◇

Pregnancy Risk Category: C

HOW SUPPLIED

Tablets: 400 mg◇, 420 mg◇
Capsules: 140 mg◇
Oral suspension: 7.75%◇

ACTION

Mechanism: An antacid that reduces total acid load in the GI tract, elevates gastric pH to reduce pepsin activity, strengthens the gastric mucosal barrier, and increases esophageal sphincter tone.
Onset: immediate. **Duration:** less than 1 hour.

INDICATIONS & DOSAGE

Antacid –
Adults: 140 mg P.O. with water or milk after meals and h.s.
Laxative –
Adults: 4 g P.O. with water or milk, usually h.s.
Oral replacement therapy in mild hypomagnesemia –
Adults: 400 to 840 mg P.O. daily. Monitor serum magnesium response.

ADVERSE REACTIONS

GI: *diarrhea,* nausea, abdominal pain.
Other: hypermagnesemia.

INTERACTIONS

Allopurinol, antibiotics (including quinolones and tetracyclines), diflunisal, digoxin, iron, isoniazid, penicillamine, phenothiazines, quinidine: decreased pharmacologic effect because of possible impaired absorption. Separate administration times.
Enteric-coated drugs: may release prematurely in stomach. Separate doses by at least 1 hour.

CONTRAINDICATIONS

- Contraindicated in patients with severe renal disease.
- Use cautiously in elderly patients and in those with mild renal impairment.

NURSING CONSIDERATIONS

- With prolonged use and some degree of renal impairment, watch for symptoms of hypermagnesemia (hypotension, nausea, vomiting, depressed reflexes, respiratory depression, and coma). Monitor serum magnesium levels.
- When used as laxative, do not give other oral drugs 1 to 2 hours before or after treatment.
- If diarrhea occurs, suggest alternative preparation.
- Advise patients not to take magnesium oxide indiscriminately or to switch antacids without their doctor's advice.

simethicone

Extra Strength Gas-X◇, Gas-Relief◇, Gas-X◇, Maximum Strength Gas-Relief◇, Maximum Strength Phazyme◇, Mylanta Gas◇, Mylanta Gas Maximum Strength◇, Mylanta Gas Regular Strength◇, Mylicon-80◇, Mylicon-125◇, Ovol†, Ovol-40†, Ovol-80†, Phazyme◇, Phazyme 55◇, Phazyme 95◇

Pregnancy Risk Category: C

HOW SUPPLIED

Tablets: 40 mg◇, 50 mg◇, 60 mg◇, 80 mg◇, 95 mg◇, 125 mg◇
Capsules: 125 mg
Drops: 40 mg/0.6 ml◇

ACTION

Mechanism: By its defoaming action, disperses or prevents formation of mucus-surrounded gas pockets in the GI tract.
Onset: immediate.

INDICATIONS & DOSAGE
Flatulence, functional gastric bloating –
Adults and children over 12 years: 40 to 125 mg after each meal and h.s.

ADVERSE REACTIONS
GI: expulsion of excessive liberated gas as belching, rectal flatus.

INTERACTIONS
None significant.

CONTRAINDICATIONS
- Contraindicated in patients hypersensitive to the drug.

NURSING CONSIDERATIONS
- Advise patients that medication does not prevent formation of gas.
- Tell patients to chew tablet before swallowing.

47
Digestants

chenodiol
monoctanoin
pancreatin
pancrelipase
ursodiol

COMBINATION PRODUCTS
BILRON: bile salts 150 mg and iron 300 mg.
DONNAZYME TABLETS: pancreatin 300 mg, pepsin 150 mg, bile salts 150 mg, hyoscyamine sulfate 0.0518 mg, atropine sulfate 0.0097 mg, scopolamine hydrobromide 0.0033 mg, and phenobarbital 8.1 mg.
ENTOZYME TABLETS: pancreatin 300 mg, pepsin 250 mg, and bile salts 150 mg.
PANCREASE CAPSULES: lipase 4,000 units, protease 25,000 units, and amylase 20,000 units in enteric-coated microspheres.

chenodiol (chenodeoxycholic acid)
Chenix

Pregnancy Risk Category: X

HOW SUPPLIED
Tablets: 250 mg

ACTION
Mechanism: Suppresses hepatic synthesis of both cholesterol and cholic acid. These actions contribute to biliary cholesterol desaturation and gradual dissolution of gallstones.
Peak: Peak levels occur 50 minutes to 2 hours after a dose.

INDICATIONS & DOSAGE
Dissolution of radiolucent cholesterol stones (gallstones) when systemic disease or age precludes surgery –
Adults: 250 mg P.O. b.i.d. for the first 2 weeks, followed, as tolerated, by weekly increases of 250 mg/day, up to 13 to 16 mg/kg/day for up to 24 months.

ADVERSE REACTIONS
GI: *diarrhea,* cramps, heartburn, constipation, nausea, vomiting, anorexia, epigastric distress.
Hepatic: reversible elevated hepatic enzymes, possible liver toxicity.

INTERACTIONS
Aluminum-containing antacids, cholestyramine, clofibrate, colestipol, estrogens, oral contraceptives: decreased chenodiol effect. Monitor the patient carefully.

CONTRAINDICATIONS
- Contraindicated in patients with known hepatocyte dysfunction, a gallbladder confirmed as nonvisualizing after two consecutive single doses of dye, radiopaque or radiolucent bile pigment stones, or gallstone complications or compelling reasons for gallbladder surgery, including unremitting acute cholecystitis, cholangitis, biliary obstruction, gallstone pancreatitis, or biliary GI fistula.

NURSING CONSIDERATIONS
- Treatment should be reserved for carefully selected patients.
- Particularly effective in the dissolution of small, floatable gallstones.
- Monitor AST and ALT levels monthly for the first 3 months every 3 months thereafter for duration of therapy.
- Final dosage should not be less than 10 mg/kg/day; lower dosages are usually ineffective.
- Diarrhea occurs in 30% to 40% of all patients. The doctor may reduce

dosage until diarrhea subsides; he may also prescribe antidiarrheals. In some patients, however, persistent diarrhea will require discontinuation of chenodiol therapy.
• Monitor liver function tests periodically and oral cholecystogram or ultrasonogram every 6 to 9 months to observe for gallstone dissolution.
• Encourage compliance with the prescribed drug regimen and with scheduled follow-up appointments.
• Tell patients to report worsening symptoms, such as sudden right upper quadrant pain, nausea, and vomiting, immediately.

monoctanoin

Moctanin

Pregnancy Risk Category: C

HOW SUPPLIED

Infusion: 120-ml bottles

ACTION

Mechanism: Dissolves gallstones by rendering them more soluble.
Onset: 7 to 10 days.

INDICATIONS & DOSAGE

To solubilize cholesterol gallstones that are retained in the biliary tract after cholecystectomy –
Adults: administer as a continuous infusion for 7 to 21 days through a catheter inserted directly into the common bile duct via a T tube. Don't exceed a rate of 3 to 5 ml/hour at a pressure of 10 cm H_2O.

ADVERSE REACTIONS

GI: *pain and discomfort, nausea, vomiting, diarrhea,* anorexia, indigestion.
Other: metabolic acidosis, fever.

INTERACTIONS

None significant.

CONTRAINDICATIONS

• Contraindicated in patients with jaundice, biliary tract infection, or a history of recent duodenal ulceration or jejunitis.

NURSING CONSIDERATIONS

• Monoctanoin treatment should be only initiated by individuals experienced in infusion therapy.
• Not to be administered parenterally; for biliary tract infusion only.
• Because impaired liver function may lead to metabolic acidosis during monoctanoin administration, routine liver function tests should be performed before perfusion therapy begins.
• Dilute each vial with sterile water for injection. Diluting the drug will reduce solution viscosity and enhance bathing of the stone.
• Pressure must be kept below 15 cm H_2O. Keeping the pressure at 10 cm H_2O will help minimize GI and biliary tract irritation.
• Use a peristaltic infusion pump to regulate the infusion. Outpatients may use a battery-operated portable pump.
• Warm the solution to 60° to 80° F (16° to 27° C) before perfusion. Temperature of the solution should not fall below 65° F (18° C) during administration.
• Reduce GI symptoms by slowing the infusion rate or discontinuing infusion during meals.

pancreatin

Bioglan Panazyme‡, Creon, Creon 25, Dizymes Tablets◇, Donnazyme, 8X Pancreatin 900 mg◇, Entozyme, 4X Pancreatin 600 mg◇, Hi-Vegi-Lip Tablets◇, Pancrezyme 4X Tablets◇

Pregnancy Risk Category: C

HOW SUPPLIED

Bioglan Panazyme‡
Tablets: 468 mg pancreatin, 7,200

units lipase, 656 units protease, and 9,200 units amylase
Creon
Capsules (enteric-coated microspheres): 300 mg pancreatin, 8,000 units lipase, 13,000 units protease, and 30,000 units amylase
Creon 25
Capsules (enteric-coated microspheres): 300 mg pancreatin, 25,000 units lipase, 62,500 units protease, and 74,700 units amylase
Dizymes
Tablets (enteric-coated): 250 mg pancreatin, 6,750 units lipase, 41,250 units protease, and 43,750 units amylase ◇
Donnazyme
Tablets: 500 mg pancreatin, 1,000 units lipase, 12,500 units protease, and 12,500 units amylase
8X Pancreatin 900 mg
Tablets (enteric-coated): 7,200 mg pancreatin, 22,500 units lipase, 180,000 units protease, and 180,000 units amylase ◇
Entozyme
Tablets: 500 mg pancreatin, 600 units lipase, 7,500 units protease, and 7,500 units amylase
4X Pancreatin 600 mg
Tablets (enteric-coated): 2,400 mg pancreatin, 12,000 units lipase, 60,000 units protease, and 60,000 units amylase ◇
Hi-Vegi-Lip
Tablets (enteric-coated): 2,400 mg pancreatin, 12,000 units lipase, 60,000 units protease, and 60,000 units amylase ◇
Pancrezyme 4X
Tablets (enteric-coated): 2,400 mg pancreatin, 12,000 units lipase, 60,000 units protease, and 60,000 units amylase ◇

ACTION

Mechanism: Replaces endogenous exocrine pancreatic enzymes and aids digestion of starches, fats, and proteins.
Duration: 1 to 2 hours.

INDICATIONS & DOSAGE

Exocrine pancreatic secretion insufficiency; digestive aid in diseases associated with deficiency of pancreatic enzymes, such as cystic fibrosis –
Adults and children: dosage varies with condition being treated. Usual initial dosage is 8,000 to 24,000 units of lipase activity with each meal or snack.

ADVERSE REACTIONS

GI: nausea, diarrhea with high doses.
Other: hyperuricosuria (with high doses).

INTERACTIONS

Antacids: may negate pancreatin's beneficial effect. Avoid concomitant use.

CONTRAINDICATIONS

- Use cautiously in patients hypersensitive to pork. Bovine preparations are available for these patients but are less effective.

NURSING CONSIDERATIONS

- Minimal USP standards dictate that each milligram of bovine or porcine pancreatin contain lipase 2 units, protease 25 units, and amylase 25 units.
- Balance fat, protein, and starch intake properly to avoid indigestion. Dosage varies according to degree of maldigestion and malabsorption, amount of fat in diet, and enzyme activity of individual preparations.
- Decreased number of bowel movements and improved stool consistency indicate effective therapy.
- Not effective in GI disorders unrelated to pancreatic enzyme deficiency.
- Enteric coating on some products may reduce availability of enzyme in upper portion of jejunum.
- Store in airtight containers at room temperature.

• Don't crush or chew enteric-coated dosage forms. However, capsules containing enteric-coated microspheres may be opened and the contents sprinkled on a small quantity of soft food or applesauce.

pancrelipase

Cotazym Capsules, Cotazym-S Capsules, Creon 10 Capsules, Ilozyme Tablets, Ku-Zyme HP Capsules, Pancrease Capsules, Pancrease MT4, Pancrease MT10, Pancrease MT16, Pancrelipase Capsules, Protilase Capsules, Ultrase MT 12, Ultrase MT 16, Ultrase MT 24, Viokase Powder, Viokase Tablets, Zymase Capsules

Pregnancy Risk Category: C

HOW SUPPLIED

Cotazym

Capsules: 8,000 units lipase, 30,000 units protease, 30,000 units amylase, and 25 mg calcium carbonate

Cotazym-S

Capsules (enteric-coated spheres): 5,000 units lipase, 20,000 units protease, and 20,000 units amylase

Creon

Capsules (enteric-coated microspheres): 10,000 units lipase, 13,000 units protease, and 30,000 units amylase

Ilozyme

Tablets: 11,000 units lipase, 30,000 units protease, and 30,000 units amylase

Ku-Zyme HP

Capsules: 8,000 units lipase, 30,000 units protease, and 30,000 units amylase

Pancrease

Capsules (enteric-coated microspheres): 4,000 units lipase, 25,000 units protease, and 20,000 units amylase

Pancrease MT4

Capsules (enteric-coated microtablets): 4,000 units lipase, 12,000 units protease, and 30,000 units amylase

Pancrease MT10

Capsules (enteric-coated microtablets): 10,000 units lipase, 30,000 units protease, and 30,000 units amylase

Pancrease MT16

Capsules (enteric-coated microtablets): 16,000 units lipase, 48,000 units protease, and 48,000 units amylase

Pancrelipase

Capsules (enteric-coated pellets): 4,000 units lipase, 25,000 units protease, and 20,000 units amylase

Protilase

Capsules (enteric-coated spheres): 4,000 units lipase, 25,000 units protease, and 20,000 units amylase

Ultrase MT 12

Capsules (delayed-release): 12,000 units lipase, 39,000 units protease, and 39,000 units amylase

Ultrase MT 16

Capsules (delayed-release): 20,000 units lipase, 65,000 units protease, and 65,000 units amylase

Ultrase MT 24

Capsules (delayed-release): 24,000 units lipase, 78,000 units protease, and 78,000 units amylase

Viokase

Tablets: 8,000 units lipase, 30,000 units protease, and 30,000 units amylase

Powder: 16,800 units lipase, 70,000 units protease, and 70,000 units amylase per 0.7 g powder

Zymase

Capsules (enteric-coated spheres): 12,000 units lipase, 24,000 units protease, and 24,000 units amylase

ACTION

Mechanism: Replaces endogenous exocrine pancreatic enzymes and aids digestion of starches, fats, and proteins.

Onset: varies with gastric emptying time.

INDICATIONS & DOSAGE
Exocrine pancreatic secretion insufficiency, cystic fibrosis in adults and children, steatorrhea and other disorders of fat metabolism secondary to insufficient pancreatic enzymes –
Adults and children: titrate dose to patient's response. Usual initial dosage is 8,000 to 24,000 units of lipase activity with each meal or snack.

ADVERSE REACTIONS
GI: *nausea,* cramping, diarrhea (high doses).

INTERACTIONS
Antacids: may destroy enteric coating and result in enhanced degradation of pancrelipase. Avoid concomitant use.

CONTRAINDICATIONS
• Contraindicated in patients with severe hypersensitivity to pork.

NURSING CONSIDERATIONS
• Minimal USP standards dictate that each mg of pancrelipase contain 24 units lipase, 100 units protease, and 100 units amylase.
• Use only after confirmed diagnosis of exocrine pancreatic insufficiency. Not effective in GI disorders unrelated to enzyme deficiency.
• Lipase activity greater than with other pancreatic enzymes.
• For infants, mix powder with applesauce and give with meals. Avoid contact with or inhalation of powder because it may be very irritating. Older children may take capsules with food.
• Dosage varies with degree of maldigestion and malabsorption, amount of fat in diet, and enzyme activity of individual preparations.
• Adequate replacement decreases number of bowel movements and improves stool consistency.
• Enteric coating on some products may reduce availability of enzyme in upper portion of jejunum.
• Don't crush or chew enteric-coated dosage forms.

ursodiol

Actigall

Pregnancy Risk Category: B

HOW SUPPLIED
Capsules: 300 mg

ACTION
Mechanism: A naturally occurring bile acid that suppresses hepatic synthesis and secretion of cholesterol as well as intestinal cholesterol absorption. After long-term administration, ursodiol can solubilize cholesterol from gallstones.
Peak: Peak concentrations occur 1 to 3 hours after a dose.

INDICATIONS & DOSAGE
Dissolution of gallstones less than 20 mm in diameter in patients who are poor surgical candidates or refuse surgery –
Adults: 8 to 10 mg/kg P.O. daily in two or three divided doses. Most patients receive 300 mg b.i.d.

ADVERSE REACTIONS
CNS: headache, fatigue, anxiety, depression, sleep disorders.
EENT: rhinitis.
GI: nausea, vomiting, dyspepsia, metallic taste, abdominal pain, biliary pain, cholecystitis, diarrhea, constipation, stomatitis, flatulence.
Respiratory: cough.
Skin: pruritus, rash, dry skin, urticaria, itching, hair thinning.
Other: arthralgia, myalgia, back pain.

INTERACTIONS
Aluminum-containing antacids, cholestyramine, colestipol: bind ursodiol and prevent its absorption.

Clofibrate, estrogens, oral contraceptives: increased hepatic cholesterol secretion; may counteract the effects of ursodiol.

CONTRAINDICATIONS

- Contraindicated in patients hypersensitive to ursodiol or other bile acids.
- Also contraindicated in patients with chronic hepatic disease, acute cholecystitis, cholangitis, biliary obstruction, gallstone pancreatitis, or biliary-GI fistulae.

NURSING CONSIDERATIONS

- Therapy is usually long-term, with ultrasound images of the gallbladder taken at 6-month intervals. If partial stone dissolution does not occur within 12 months, eventual success is unlikely. Safety of use for longer than 24 months has not been established.
- Ursodiol will not dissolve calcified cholesterol stones, radiolucent bile pigment stones, or radiopaque stones.
- The relapse rate after bile acid therapy may be as high as 50% after 5 years. Tell patients about alternative therapies, including "watchful waiting" (no intervention) and cholecystectomy.
- Monitor liver function tests, including AST and ALT, at the beginning of therapy and after 1 month, 3 months, and every 6 months during ursodiol therapy. Abnormal tests may indicate a worsening of the disease. A theoretical risk exists that a hepatotoxic metabolite of ursodiol may be formed in some patients.

48

Antidiarrheals

bismuth subgallate
bismuth subsalicylate
calcium polycarbophil
(See Chapter 49, LAXATIVES.)
difenoxin hydrochloride and atropine sulfate
diphenoxylate hydrochloride and atropine sulfate
kaolin and pectin mixtures
loperamide
octreotide acetate
opium tincture
opium tincture, camphorated

COMBINATION PRODUCTS

DONNAGEL-PG*: powdered opium 24 mg, kaolin 6 g, pectin 142.8 mg, hyoscyamine sulfate 0.1037 mg, atropine sulfate 0.0194 mg, scopolamine hydrobromide 0.0065 mg, and alcohol 5% in 30-ml suspension.
DONNAGEL SUSPENSION*: kaolin 6 g, pectin 142.8 mg, hyoscyamine sulfate 0.1037 mg, atropine sulfate 0.0194 mg, scopolamine hydrobromide 0.0065 mg, and alcohol 3.8% in 30-ml suspension.
PAREPECTOLIN*: opium 15 mg (equivalent to paregoric 3.7 ml), kaolin 5.85 g, pectin 162 mg, and alcohol 0.69% in 30-ml suspension.

---

bismuth subgallate

Devrom◊

bismuth subsalicylate

Maximum Strength Pepto-Bismol Liquid◊, Pepto-Bismol◊

Pregnancy Risk Category: C (D in 3rd trimester)

HOW SUPPLIED

subgallate
Tablets (chewable): 200 mg◊

subsalicylate
Tablets (chewable): 262.5 mg◊
Oral suspension: 262.5 mg/15 ml◊, 525 mg/15 ml◊

ACTION

Mechanism: Has a mild water-binding capacity; also may adsorb toxins and provide protective coating for mucosa.
Onset: within 1 hour.

INDICATIONS & DOSAGE

Mild, nonspecific diarrhea –
Adults: 1 to 2 tablets (subgallate) P.O. chewed or swallowed whole t.i.d.; or 30 ml or 2 tablets (subsalicylate) q ½ to 1 hour, up to a maximum of eight doses and for no longer than 2 days.
Children 3 to 6 years: 5 ml or ⅓ tablet P.O.
Children 6 to 9 years: 10 ml or ⅔ tablet P.O.
Children 9 to 12 years: 15 ml or 1 tablet P.O.
Prevention and treatment of traveler's diarrhea (turista) –
Adults: prophylactically, 60 ml (subsalicylate) P.O. q.i.d. during the first 2 weeks of travel. During acute illness, give 30 to 60 ml q 30 minutes for a total of eight doses. Alternatively, give 2 tablets q.i.d. for up to 3 weeks.

ADVERSE REACTIONS

GI: temporary darkening of tongue and stools.
Other: salicylism (high doses).

INTERACTIONS

Aspirin, other salicylates: risk of salicylate toxicity. Monitor closely.
Oral anticoagulants, oral antidiabetic agents: theoretical risk of increased

*Liquid form contains alcohol.
**May contain tartrazine.

effects of these agents after high doses of bismuth subsalicylate. Monitor the patient closely.
Probenecid: theoretical risk of decreased uricosuric effects after high doses of bismuth subsalicylate. Monitor the patient closely.
Tetracycline: decreased tetracycline absorption. Separate administration times by at least 2 hours.

CONTRAINDICATIONS
• Contraindicated in patients hypersensitive to salicylates.
• Use cautiously in patients already taking aspirin. Discontinue if tinnitus occurs.

NURSING CONSIDERATIONS
• Advise patients that bismuth subsalicylate contains a large amount of salicylate (each tablet provides 102 mg salicylate; the regular-strength liquid provides 130 mg/15 ml, and the extra-strength liquid yields 230 mg/15 ml).
• Tell patients to call their doctor if diarrhea persists for more than 2 days or is accompanied by high fever.
• Avoid use before GI radiologic procedures because bismuth is radiopaque and may interfere with X-rays.
• Consult with the doctor before giving bismuth subsalicylate to children or teenagers during or after recovery from the flu or chicken pox.
• Instruct patients to chew tablets well or to shake liquid before measuring dose.
• Both the liquid and tablet forms of Pepto-Bismol are effective against traveler's diarrhea. Tablets may be more convenient to carry.
• Has been used investigationally to treat peptic ulceration disease, especially when ulcerations are associated with *Helicobacter pylori* infection.

difenoxin hydrochloride and atropine sulfate

Lyspafen‡, Motofen
Controlled Substance Schedule IV
Pregnancy Risk Category: C

HOW SUPPLIED
Tablets: 0.5 mg (with atropine sulphate, 0.025 mg)‡, 1 mg (with atropine sulfate, 0.025 mg)

ACTION
Mechanism: Exerts a direct effect on the intestinal wall to slow motility.
Onset: within 30 minutes. **Peak:** Peak levels occur within 40 to 60 minutes. **Duration:** elimination half-life, 12 to 24 hours.

INDICATIONS AND DOSAGE
Adjunct in acute nonspecific diarrhea and acute exacerbations of chronic functional diarrhea –
Adults: initially, 2 mg P.O., then 1 mg P.O. after each loose bowel movement. Do not exceed total dosage of 8 mg daily. Not recommended for use longer than 2 days.

ADVERSE REACTIONS
CNS: dizziness, light-headedness, drowsiness, headache, fatigue, nervousness, insomnia, confusion.
EENT: burning eyes, blurred vision.
GI: nausea, vomiting, dry mouth, epigastric distress, constipation.

INTERACTIONS
Barbiturates, CNS depressants, ethanol, narcotics, tranquilizers: enhanced CNS depression. Closely monitor patients.
MAO inhibitors: potential hypertensive crisis. Avoid concomitant use.

CONTRAINDICATIONS
• Contraindicated in patients hypersensitive to difenoxin or atropine, in children under 2 years, and in patients

with diarrhea from pseudomembranous colitis associated with antibiotics.
- Contraindicated in patients with jaundice and in those with diarrhea from organisms that may penetrate the intestinal mucosa (including toxigenic *Escherichia coli, Salmonella,* or *Shigella*).
- Use cautiously in patients with a history of drug abuse or in those currently receiving drugs with a high abuse potential. Difenoxin is the principal metabolite of diphenoxylate and is chemically related to meperidine.

NURSING CONSIDERATIONS
- Atropine has been added to difenoxin to prevent abuse. The small dosage of atropine is unlikely to cause any significant clinical problems, but patients may experience dry mouth, tachycardia, urine retention, and flushing. Monitor for these effects.
- Advise patients to avoid hazardous activities that may require mental alertness, such as driving or operating heavy machinery, until CNS effects of the drug are known.
- Monitor patients closely for fluid and electrolyte imbalance. Difenoxin-induced decreases in peristalsis may result in fluid retention in the colon, with subsequent dehydration and possibly delayed difenoxin intoxication.
- Advise patients to adhere to dosing schedule. Overdose with difenoxin may cause respiratory depression and coma. Encourage storing drug out of children's reach.
- For overdose, observe patient for at least 48 hours. Respiratory depression may occur up to 30 hours after ingestion. Use gastric lavage, establishment of a patent airway, and mechanically assisted ventilation to treat overdose and naloxone to reverse respiratory depression. Because difenoxin has a longer duration of action than naloxone, repeated injections of naloxone are necessary.

diphenoxylate hydrochloride and atropine sulfate

Diphenatol, Lofene, Logen, Lomanate, Lomotil*, Lonox, Lo-Trol, Nor-Mil

Controlled Substance Schedule V

Pregnancy Risk Category: C

HOW SUPPLIED

Tablets: 2.5 mg (with atropine sulfate, 0.025 mg)

Liquid: 2.5 mg/5 ml (with atropine sulfate, 0.025 mg/5 ml)*

ACTION

Mechanism: Increases smooth muscle tone in the GI tract, inhibits motility and propulsion, and diminishes secretions.

Onset: antidiarrheal activity, 45 to 60 minutes after ingestion. **Peak:** Plasma levels peak about 3 hours after ingestion. **Duration:** 3 to 4 hours; plasma half-life of diphenoxylate, about 2½ hours, of active metabolites, 14 hours.

INDICATIONS & DOSAGE

Acute, nonspecific diarrhea –

Adults: initially, 5 mg P.O. q.i.d., then adjust dosage.

Children 2 to 12 years: 0.3 to 0.4 mg/kg P.O. (liquid form) daily in four divided doses. For maintenance, reduce initial dose as needed up to 75%.

ADVERSE REACTIONS

CNS: *sedation, dizziness,* headache, drowsiness, lethargy, restlessness, depression, euphoria.

CV: tachycardia.

EENT: mydriasis.

GI: *dry mouth,* nausea, vomiting, abdominal discomfort or distention, ***paralytic ileus,*** anorexia, fluid retention in bowel (may mask depletion of extracellular fluid and electrolytes, especially in young children treated for acute gastroenteritis), possible

physical dependence with long-term use.
GU: urine retention.
Respiratory: respiratory depression.
Skin: pruritus, giant urticaria, rash.
Other: ***angioedema.***

INTERACTIONS
Barbiturates, CNS depressants, ethanol, narcotics, tranquilizers: enhanced CNS depression. Closely monitor patients.
MAO inhibitors: potential hypertensive crisis. Avoid concomitant use.

CONTRAINDICATIONS
• Contraindicated in patients with acute diarrhea resulting from poison until toxic material is eliminated from GI tract, acute diarrhea caused by organisms that penetrate intestinal mucosa, or diarrhea resulting from antibiotic-induced pseudomembranous enterocolitis; also contraindicated in jaundiced patients and children under 2 years.
• Use cautiously in children; in patients with hepatic disease, narcotic dependence, or acute ulcerative colitis; and in pregnant patients. Stop therapy immediately if abdominal distention or other signs of toxic megacolon develop.

NURSING CONSIDERATIONS
• Advise patients to avoid hazardous activities such as driving until CNS effects of the drug are known.
• Risk of physical dependence increases with high dosage and long-term use. Atropine sulfate is included to discourage abuse.
• Drug is unlikely to be effective if no response occurs within 48 hours.
• Warn patients not to use drug to treat acute diarrhea for longer than 2 days and to seek medical attention if diarrhea continues.
• Tell patients not to exceed recommended dosage. Use naloxone as ordered to treat respiratory depression caused by overdose.
• Dehydration, especially in young children, may increase risk of delayed toxicity. Correct fluid and electrolyte disturbances before starting drug.
• Dose of 2.5 mg is as effective as 5 ml camphorated tincture of opium.
• Not indicated for treating antibiotic-induced diarrhea.

kaolin and pectin mixtures

Donnagel-MB*†, Kao-Con†, Kaopectate◇, Kaopectate Concentrate◇, Kao-tin◇, Kapectolin◇, K-P◇, K-Pek◇

Pregnancy Risk Category: C

HOW SUPPLIED
Oral suspension: 5.2 mg kaolin and 260 mg pectin per 30 ml◇ (K-P◇); 5.85 g kaolin and 130 mg pectin per 30 ml◇ (Kaopectate◇, Kao-tin◇, Kapectolin◇, K-Pek◇); 5.91 g kaolin and 132 mg pectin per 30 ml◇ (Kaopectate◇), 6 g kaolin and 130 mg pectin per 30 ml◇ (Kaopectate†◇); 6 g kaolin and 143 mg pectin per 30 ml◇, with 3.8% ethanol (Donnagel-MB*†); 8.7 g kaolin and 195 mg pectin per 30 ml◇ (Kaopectate Concentrate◇); 8.8 g kaolin and 195 mg pectin per 30 ml◇ (Kao-Con†, Kaopectate Concentrate†◇)

ACTION
Mechanism: Decreases the stool's fluid content, although *total* water loss seems to remain the same.
Onset: 2 to 3 hours.

INDICATIONS & DOSAGE
Mild, nonspecific diarrhea –
Adults: 60 to 120 ml P.O. after each bowel movement.
Children 3 to 6 years: 15 to 30 ml P.O. after each bowel movement.
Children 6 to 12 years: 30 to 60 ml P.O. after each bowel movement.

Children over 12 years: 60 ml P.O. after each bowel movement.

ADVERSE REACTIONS
GI: drug absorbs nutrients, drugs, and enzymes; fecal impaction or ulceration in infants and elderly or debilitated patients after chronic use; constipation.

INTERACTIONS
Orally administered drugs: adsorption may occur. Separate administration times by at least 2 to 3 hours.

CONTRAINDICATIONS
• Contraindicated in patients with suspected obstructive bowel lesions and in children under 3 years.

NURSING CONSIDERATIONS
• Advise patients not to use drug for more than 2 days.
• Do not use drug to replace specific therapy for underlying cause.

loperamide
Imodium, Imodium A-D◇

Pregnancy Risk Category: B

HOW SUPPLIED
Tablets: 2 mg
Capsules: 2 mg◇
Oral liquid: 1 mg/5 ml◇

ACTION
Mechanism: Inhibits peristaltic activity, prolonging transit of intestinal contents.
Peak: Peak plasma levels occur about 2½ hours after oral liquid, 4 to 5 hours after capsules. **Duration:** about 24 hours; half-life, 9 to 14 hours.

INDICATIONS & DOSAGE
Acute, nonspecific diarrhea –
Adults: initially, 4 mg P.O., then 2 mg after each unformed stool. Maximum dosage is 16 mg daily.
Children 2 to 5 years: 5 ml P.O. t.i.d. on first day. If diarrhea persists, contact doctor.
Children 5 to 8 years: 10 ml P.O. b.i.d. on first day. If diarrhea persists, contact doctor.
Children 8 to 12 years: 10 ml t.i.d. P.O. on first day. (Subsequent doses of 5 ml/10 kg of body weight may be administered after each unformed stool.) Maximum dosage is 6 mg daily.
Chronic diarrhea –
Adults: initially, 4 mg P.O., then 2 mg after each unformed stool until diarrhea subsides. Adjust dosage to individual response.

ADVERSE REACTIONS
CNS: drowsiness, fatigue, dizziness.
GI: dry mouth; abdominal pain, distention, or discomfort; *constipation;* nausea; vomiting.
Skin: rash.

INTERACTIONS
None significant.

CONTRAINDICATIONS
• Contraindicated in patients with acute diarrhea resulting from poison until toxic material is removed from GI tract, in acute diarrhea caused by organisms that penetrate intestinal mucosa, and when constipation must be avoided. Also contraindicated in children under 2 years.
• Use cautiously in patients with severe prostatic hyperplasia, hepatic disease, and history of opioid dependence.

NURSING CONSIDERATIONS
• Stop drug immediately if abdominal distention or other symptoms develop in acute colitis.
• In acute diarrhea, discontinue drug and seek medical attention if no improvement occurs within 48 hours; in chronic diarrhea, discontinue drug if no improvement occurs after giving 16 mg daily for at least 10 days.

• Advise patients not to exceed recommended dosage.
• Produces antidiarrheal action similar to diphenoxylate but without as many adverse CNS effects.

octreotide acetate

Sandostatin
Pregnancy Risk Category: B

HOW SUPPLIED

Injection: 0.05 mg, 0.1 mg, 0.5 mg

ACTION

Mechanism: Mimics the action of naturally occurring somatostatin.
Onset: within 30 minutes. **Peak:** Peak levels occur within ½ hour.
Duration: up to 12 hours.

INDICATIONS & DOSAGE

Flushing and diarrhea associated with carcinoid tumors –
Adults: 0.1 to 0.6 mg daily S.C. in two to four divided doses for the first 2 weeks of therapy (usual daily dosage is 0.3 mg). Base subsequent dosage on individual response.
Watery diarrhea associated with vasoactive intestinal polypeptide (secreting) tumors (VIPomas) –
Adults: 0.2 to 0.3 mg daily S.C. in two to four divided doses for the first 2 weeks of therapy. Base subsequent dosage on individual response; typically, don't exceed 0.45 mg daily.
Severe, refractory diarrhea in patients with AIDS –
Adults: 0.1 to 1.8 mg S.C. daily in divided doses.

ADVERSE REACTIONS

CNS: dizziness, light-headedness, fatigue.
GI: *nausea, diarrhea, abdominal pain or discomfort,* loose stools, vomiting, fat malabsorption.
Skin: flushing, edema, wheal, erythema or pain at injection site.
Other: hyperglycemia, hypoglycemia, hypothyroidism.

INTERACTIONS

Cyclosporine: may decrease plasma levels of cyclosporine.

CONTRAINDICATIONS

• Contraindicated in patients hypersensitive to the drug or any of its components.

NURSING CONSIDERATIONS

• May be associated with development of cholelithiasis by either altering gallbladder motility or fat absorption. Monitor patients regularly for gallbladder disease, and tell them to report any signs of abdominal discomfort.
• Half-life may be altered in patients in end-stage renal failure who are receiving dialysis.
• Monitor baseline and periodic thyroid function tests.
• Monitor laboratory tests, such as urine 5-hydroxyindoleacetic acid, plasma serotonin, and plasma substance P (for carcinoid tumors), and plasma vasoactive intestinal peptide for VIPomas.
• Mild, transient hypoglycemia or hyperglycemia may occur during octreotide therapy. Monitor closely for symptoms of glucose imbalance.
• Insulin-dependent diabetic patients and patients receiving oral antidiabetic agents or oral diazoxide may require dosage adjustments during therapy.
• Octreotide therapy may alter fluid and electrolyte balance and may require adjustment of other drugs used to control symptoms of the disease, such as beta blockers.

opium tincture*

Controlled Substance Schedule II

opium tincture, camphorated* (paregoric)

Controlled Substance Schedule III

Pregnancy Risk Category: B (D for prolonged use or high doses at term)

HOW SUPPLIED

opium tincture

Oral solution: equivalent to morphine 10 mg/ml*

opium tincture, camphorated

Oral solution: Each 5 ml contains morphine, 2 mg; anise oil, 0.2 ml; benzoic acid, 20 mg; camphor, 20 mg; glycerin, 0.2 ml; and ethanol to make 5 ml*

ACTION

Mechanism: Increases smooth muscle tone in the GI tract, inhibits motility and propulsion, and diminishes secretions.

Onset: 1 to 2 hours.

INDICATIONS & DOSAGE

Acute, nonspecific diarrhea –

Adults: 0.6 ml opium tincture (range 0.3 to 1 ml) P.O. q.i.d. Maximum dosage is 6 ml daily. Or, 5 to 10 ml camphorated tincture of opium daily, b.i.d., t.i.d., or q.i.d. until diarrhea subsides.

Children: 0.25 to 0.5 ml/kg camphorated tincture of opium P.O. daily, b.i.d., t.i.d., or q.i.d. until diarrhea subsides.

ADVERSE REACTIONS

CNS: dizziness, light-headedness.

GI: nausea, vomiting, physical dependence after long-term use.

INTERACTIONS

None significant.

CONTRAINDICATIONS

- Contraindicated in patients with acute diarrhea resulting from poison until toxic material is removed from GI tract or diarrhea caused by organisms that penetrate intestinal mucosa.
- Use cautiously in patients with asthma, prostatic hyperplasia, hepatic disease, and opioid dependence.

NURSING CONSIDERATIONS

- Advise patients against using drug for more than 2 days; risk of physical dependence increases with long-term use.
- An effective and prompt-acting antidiarrheal, but unique because dosage can be adjusted precisely to patient's needs.
- Opium content of opium tincture is 25 times greater than camphorated tincture of opium. Camphorated tincture of opium is more dilute, and teaspoonful doses are easier to measure than dropper quantities of opium tincture.
- Milky fluid forms when camphorated tincture of opium is added to water.
- Camphorated tincture of opium 0.06 to 0.5 ml daily has been used to treat infants with mild narcotic physical dependence.
- Store in tightly capped, light-resistant container.
- Mix with sufficient water to ensure passage to stomach.
- For overdose, use the narcotic antagonist naloxone, as ordered, to reverse respiratory depression.

*Liquid form contains alcohol.
**May contain tartrazine.

49

Laxatives

bisacodyl
calcium polycarbophil
cascara sagrada
cascara sagrada aromatic fluidextract
cascara sagrada fluidextract
castor oil
docusate calcium
docusate potassium
docusate sodium
glycerin
lactulose
magnesium citrate
magnesium hydroxide
magnesium sulfate
methylcellulose
mineral oil
phenolphthalein, white
phenolphthalein, yellow
polyethylene glycol-electrolyte solution
psyllium
senna
sodium phosphates

COMBINATION PRODUCTS

AGORAL◊: mineral oil 28% and white phenolphthalein 1.3% in emulsion, with tragacanth, agar, egg albumin, acacia, and glycerin.
DIALOSE-PLUS◊: docusate potassium 100 mg and casanthranol 30 mg.
DIOLAX◊: docusate sodium 100 mg and casanthranol 50 mg.
DOXIDAN◊: docusate calcium 60 mg and phenolphthalein 65 mg.
D-S-S PLUS◊: docusate sodium 100 mg and casanthranol 30 mg.
HALEY'S M-O◊: mineral oil (25%) and magnesium hydroxide.
KONDREMUL WITH CASCARA◊: heavy mineral oil 55%, cascara sagrada extract 660 mg/15 ml, and Irish moss as emulsifier.
KONDREMUL WITH PHENOLPHTHALEIN◊: heavy mineral oil 55%, white phenolphthalein 150 mg/15 ml, and Irish moss as emulsifier.
MODANE PLUS◊: docusate sodium 100 mg and phenolphthalein 60 mg.
PERI-COLACE◊ (capsules): docusate sodium 100 mg and casanthranol 30 mg.
PERI-COLACE◊ (syrup): docusate sodium 60 mg and casanthranol 30 mg/15 ml.
SENOKOT-S◊: docusate sodium 50 mg and standardized senna concentrate 187 mg.
UNILAX◊: docusate sodium 230 mg and yellow phenolphthalein 130 mg.

bisacodyl

Bisac-Evac◊, Bisacolax†◊, Bisalax‡, Bisco-Lax**◊, Carter's Little Pills◊, Dacodyl◊, Deficol◊, Dulcolax◊, Durolax‡, Fleet Bisacodyl◊, Fleet Bisacodyl Prep◊, Fleet Laxative◊, Laxit†◊, Theralax◊

Pregnancy Risk Category: C

HOW SUPPLIED

Tablets (enteric-coated): 5 mg◊
Enema: 0.33 mg/dl◊, 10 mg/5 ml (microenema)‡
Powder for rectal solution (bisacodyl tannex): 1.5 mg bisacodyl and 2.5 g tannic acid
Suppositories: 5 mg◊, 10 mg◊

ACTION

Mechanism: A stimulant laxative that increases peristalsis by direct effect on the smooth muscle of the intestine. Thought to either irritate the musculature or stimulate the colonic intramural plexus. Also promotes fluid accumulation in the colon and small intestine.
Onset: 15 to 60 minutes after suppos-

†Available in Canada only. ‡Available in Australia only. ◊Available OTC.

itory, 6 to 12 hours after oral administration.

INDICATIONS & DOSAGE

Chronic constipation; preparation for delivery, surgery, or rectal or bowel examination –

Adults: 10 to 15 mg P.O. in evening or before breakfast. Give up to 30 mg as needed and ordered, or 10 mg P.R. for evacuation before examination or surgery.

Children under 2 years: 5 mg P.R.

Children 2 to 5 years: 10 mg P.R.

Children 6 years and older: 5 to 10 mg P.O. or 10 mg P.R.

ADVERSE REACTIONS

CNS: muscle weakness with excessive use.

GI: *nausea, vomiting, abdominal cramps,* diarrhea with high doses, *burning sensation in rectum* (with suppositories), laxative dependence with long-term or excessive use.

Other: alkalosis, hypokalemia, tetany, protein-losing enteropathy in excessive use, fluid and electrolyte imbalance.

INTERACTIONS

None significant.

CONTRAINDICATIONS

- Contraindicated in patients with abdominal pain, nausea, vomiting, or other symptoms of appendicitis or acute surgical abdomen and in those with rectal fissures or ulcerated hemorrhoids.

NURSING CONSIDERATIONS

- Advise the patient to swallow enteric-coated tablet whole to avoid GI irritation. Don't give within 1 hour of milk or antacid intake.
- Soft, formed stool usually produced 15 to 60 minutes after rectal administration. Time administration of drug so as not to interfere with scheduled activities or sleep.
- Use tablets and suppositories together to clean the colon before and after surgery and before barium enema.
- Insert suppository as high as possible into the rectum, and try to position the suppository against the rectal wall. Avoid embedding within fecal material because this may delay the onset of action.
- Use for short-term treatment. A stimulant laxative, this type of laxative is most abused. Discourage excessive use.
- Store tablets and suppositories at a temperature below 86° F (30° C).
- Before giving for constipation, determine if the patient has adequate fluid intake, exercise, and diet. Tell him that dietary sources of bulk include bran and other cereals, fresh fruit, and vegetables.
- Advise the patient to report adverse effects to the doctor.

calcium polycarbophil

Equalactin◇, Fiberall◇, FiberCon◇, FiberLax◇, FiberNorm◇, Mitrolan◇

Pregnancy Risk Category: C

HOW SUPPLIED

Tablets: 500 mg◇, 625 mg◇, 1,250 mg◇

Tablets (chewable): 500 mg◇

ACTION

Mechanism: A bulk-forming laxative that absorbs water and expands to increase bulk and moisture content of the stool. The increased bulk encourages peristalsis and bowel movement. As an antidiarrheal, absorbs free fecal water, thereby producing formed stools.

Onset: 12 to 24 hours. **Peak:** Peak effects may not occur for up to 3 days.

INDICATIONS & DOSAGE
Constipation (Equalactin and Mitrolan must be chewed before swallowing) –
Adults: 1 g P.O. q.i.d. as required. Maximum dosage is 6 g in 24-hour period.
Children 2 to 6 years: 500 mg P.O. b.i.d. as required. Maximum dosage is 1.5 g in 24-hour period.
Children 6 to 12 years: 500 mg P.O. t.i.d. as required. Maximum dosage is 3 g in 24-hour period.
Diarrhea associated with irritable bowel syndrome, as well as acute nonspecific diarrhea (Mitrolan must be chewed before swallowing) –
Adults: 1 g P.O. q.i.d. as required. Maximum dosage is 6 g in 24-hour period.
Children 2 to 6 years: 500 mg P.O. b.i.d. as required. Maximum dosage is 1.5 g in 24-hour period.
Children 6 to 12 years: 500 mg P.O. t.i.d. as required. Maximum dosage is 3 g in 24-hour period.

ADVERSE REACTIONS
GI: abdominal fullness and increased flatus, intestinal obstruction.
Other: laxative dependence with long-term or excessive use.

INTERACTIONS
None significant.

CONTRAINDICATIONS
- Contraindicated in patients with signs of GI obstruction, and in children under 2 years.

NURSING CONSIDERATIONS
- Rectal bleeding or failure to respond to therapy may indicate need for surgery.
- For severe diarrhea, repeat dose every half hour, but do not exceed maximum daily dosage.
- Before giving for constipation, determine if the patient has adequate fluid intake, exercise, and diet. Tell him that dietary sources of bulk include bran and other cereals, fresh fruit, and vegetables.
- Advise the patient to chew Equalactin or Mitrolan tablets thoroughly and to drink a full glass of water with each dose. When used as an antidiarrheal, tell the patient not to drink a glass of water.

cascara sagrada ◊

cascara sagrada aromatic fluidextract* ◊

cascara sagrada fluidextract* ◊

Pregnancy Risk Category: C

HOW SUPPLIED
Tablets: 325 mg ◊
Aromatic fluidextract: 1 g/ml* ◊
Fluidextract: 1 g/ml* ◊

ACTION
Mechanism: A stimulant laxative that increases peristalsis by direct effect on the smooth muscle of the intestine. Thought to either irritate the musculature or stimulate the colonic intramural plexus. Also promotes fluid accumulation in the colon and small intestine.
Onset: 6 to 10 hours.

INDICATIONS & DOSAGE
Acute constipation; preparation for bowel or rectal examination –
Adults: 325 mg cascara sagrada tablets P.O. h.s.; or 1 ml fluidextract daily; or 5 ml aromatic fluidextract daily.
Children under 2 years: ¼ adult dose.
Children 2 to 12 years: ½ adult dose.

ADVERSE REACTIONS
GI: *nausea;* vomiting; diarrhea; loss of normal bowel function with exces-

sive use; *abdominal cramps,* especially in severe constipation; malabsorption of nutrients; "cathartic colon" (syndrome resembling ulcerative colitis radiologically and pathologically) in chronic misuse; discoloration of rectal mucosa after long-term use.
Other: hypokalemia, protein enteropathy, electrolyte imbalance with excessive use, laxative dependence with long-term or excessive use.

INTERACTIONS
None significant.

CONTRAINDICATIONS
- Contraindicated in patients with abdominal pain, nausea, vomiting, or other symptoms of appendicitis or acute surgical abdomen; acute surgical delirium; fecal impaction; and intestinal obstruction or perforation.
- Use cautiously when rectal bleeding is present.

NURSING CONSIDERATIONS
- Aromatic cascara fluidextract is less active and less bitter than nonaromatic fluidextract.
- Liquid preparations are more reliable than solid dosage forms.
- Before giving for constipation, determine if the patient has adequate fluid intake, exercise, and diet. Tell him that dietary sources of bulk include bran and other cereals, fresh fruit, and vegetables.
- May turn alkaline urine red-pink and acidic urine yellow-brown.
- Monitor serum electrolytes during prolonged use.

castor oil
Alphamul◇, Emulsoil◇, Fleet Flavored Castor Oil◇, Kellogg's Castor Oil◇, Minims Castor Oil‡◇, Neoloid◇, Purge◇

Pregnancy Risk Category: X

HOW SUPPLIED
Oral liquid: 36.4% (Neoloid◇), 60% (Alphamul◇), 67% (Fleet◇), 95% (Purge◇, Emulsoil◇), 100% (Kellogg's◇, Minims◇).

ACTION
Mechanism: A stimulant laxative that increases peristalsis by direct effect on the smooth muscle of the intestine. Thought to either irritate the musculature or stimulate the colonic intramural plexus. Also promotes fluid accumulation in the colon and small intestine.
Onset: 2 to 6 hours.

INDICATIONS & DOSAGE
Preparation for rectal or bowel examination or for surgery; acute constipation (rarely) –
Adults: 15 to 60 ml P.O.
Infants: up to 4 ml P.O. Increased dose produces no greater effect.
Children under 2 years: 1.25 to 7.5 ml P.O.
Children over 2 years: 5 to 15 ml P.O.

ADVERSE REACTIONS
GI: *nausea;* vomiting; diarrhea; loss of normal bowel function with excessive use; *abdominal cramps,* especially in severe constipation; malabsorption of nutrients; "cathartic colon" (syndrome resembling ulcerative colitis radiologically and pathologically) in chronic misuse, laxative dependence with long-term or excessive use. May cause constipation after catharsis.
GU: pelvic congestion in menstruating women.
Other: hypokalemia, protein-losing enteropathy, other electrolyte imbalances with excessive use.

INTERACTIONS
None significant.

CONTRAINDICATIONS

- Contraindicated in patients with ulcerative bowel lesions; abdominal pain, nausea, vomiting, or other symptoms of appendicitis or acute surgical abdomen; and anal or rectal fissures, fecal impaction, or intestinal obstruction or perforation; and during menstruation or pregnancy.
- Use cautiously in patients with rectal bleeding.

NURSING CONSIDERATIONS

- Failure to respond to drug may indicate acute condition requiring surgery.
- Give castor oil with juice or carbonated beverage to mask oily taste. Tell the patient to stir mixture and drink it promptly. Ice held in the mouth before taking drug will help prevent tasting it.
- Time drug administration so that it doesn't interfere with scheduled activities or sleep.
- Give on empty stomach for best results.
- Emulsion is better tolerated but is more expensive. Shake emulsion well before measuring dose. Store below 40° F (4.4° C). Don't freeze.
- Tell the patient not to expect another bowel movement for 1 to 2 days after castor oil has emptied bowel.
- Monitor serum electrolytes during prolonged use.
- Typically used before diagnostic testing or therapy requiring thorough evacuation of GI tract.
- Use short-term to treat acute constipation not responsive to milder laxatives. Not recommended for routine use.
- Before giving for constipation, determine if the patient has adequate fluid intake, exercise, and diet. Tell him that dietary sources of bulk include bran and other cereals, fresh fruit, and vegetables.
- Increased intestinal motility lessens absorption of concomitantly administered oral drugs. Separate administration times.
- Castor oil affects the small intestine. Regular use may cause excessive loss of water and salt.

docusate calcium (dioctyl calcium sulfosuccinate)

Pro-Cal-Sof◇, Surfak◇

docusate potassium (dioctyl potassium sulfosuccinate)

Dialose◇, Diocto-K◇, Kasof◇

docusate sodium (dioctyl sodium sulfosuccinate)

Afko-Lube◇, Colace◇, Coloxyl‡, Coloxyl Enema Concentrate‡, D-S-S◇, Di-Sosul◇, Diocto◇, Dioeze◇, Diosuccin◇, Dio-Sul◇, Disonate◇, Di-Sosul◇, DOK-250◇, DOK Liquid◇, Doss◇, Doss 300◇, Doxinate◇, D-S-S◇, Duosol◇, Genasoft◇, Laxinate 100◇, Modane Soft◇, Molatoc◇, Pro-Sof◇, Pro-Sof Liquid Concentrate◇, Pro-Sof Liquid Plus◇, Regulax SS◇, Regulex†◇, Regutol◇, Stulex◇, Therevac Plus◇, Therevac-SB◇

Pregnancy Risk Category: C

HOW SUPPLIED

calcium

Capsules: 50 mg◇, 240 mg◇

potassium

Capsules: 100 mg◇, 240 mg◇

sodium

Tablets: 100 mg◇

Capsules: 50 mg◇, 60 mg◇, 100 mg◇, 240 mg◇, 250 mg◇

Oral liquid: 150 mg/15 ml◇

Oral solution: 50 mg/ml◇

Syrup: 50 mg/15 ml◇, 60 mg/15 ml◇

Enema concentrate: 18 g/100 ml (must be diluted)‡

†Available in Canada only. ‡Available in Australia only. ◇Available OTC.

ACTION

Mechanism: A stool softener that reduces surface tension of interfacing liquid contents of the bowel. This detergent activity promotes incorporation of additional liquid into the stool, forming a softer mass.

Onset: variable; usually within 24 to 72 hours.

INDICATIONS & DOSAGE

Stool softener–

Adults and older children: 50 to 300 mg (sodium, calcium, or potassium) P.O. daily until bowel movements are normal. Alternatively, give enema (where available). Dilute 1:24 with sterile water before administration, and give 100 to 150 ml (retention enema), 300 to 500 ml (evacuation enema), or 0.5 to 1.5 liters (flushing enema).

Children under 3 years: 10 to 40 mg (sodium) P.O. daily.

Children 3 to 6 years: 20 to 60 mg (sodium) P.O. daily.

Children 6 to 12 years: 40 to 120 mg (sodium) P.O. daily.

Use higher dosages for initial therapy. Adjust dosage to individual response. Usual dosage in children and adults with minimal needs is 50 to 150 mg (calcium) P.O. daily.

ADVERSE REACTIONS

EENT: throat irritation.

GI: bitter taste, mild abdominal cramping, diarrhea, laxative dependence with long-term or excessive use.

INTERACTIONS

Mineral oil: may increase mineral oil absorption and cause lipoid pneumonia. Separate administration times.

CONTRAINDICATIONS

- Contraindicated in patients hypersensitive to the drug and in those with intestinal obstruction, undiagnosed abdominal pain, vomiting or other signs of appendicitis, fecal impaction, or acute surgical abdomen.

NURSING CONSIDERATIONS

- Use only occasionally and don't use for more than 1 week without the doctor's knowledge.
- Give liquid in milk, fruit juice, or infant formula to mask bitter taste.
- Not for use in treating existing constipation, but prevents constipation from developing.
- Laxative of choice for patients who should not strain during defecation, including patients recovering from MI or rectal surgery; those with rectal or anal disease that makes passage of firm stool difficult; or those with postpartum constipation.
- Acts within 24 to 48 hours to produce firm, semisolid stool.
- Doesn't stimulate intestinal peristaltic movements.
- Discontinue if severe cramping occurs.
- Store at 59° to 86° F (15° to 30° C), and protect liquid from light.
- Before giving for constipation, determine if the patient has adequate fluid intake, exercise, and diet. Tell him that dietary sources of bulk include bran and other cereals, fresh fruit, and vegetables.

glycerin

Fleet Babylax◊, Sani-Supp◊

Pregnancy Risk Category: C •

HOW SUPPLIED

Enema (pediatric): 4 ml/applicator◊

Suppositories: adult, children, and infant sizes◊

ACTION

Mechanism: A hyperosmolar laxative that draws water from the tissues into the feces and thus stimulates evacuation.

Onset: 15 to 60 minutes.

*Liquid form contains alcohol.
**May contain tartrazine.

Common reactions are in italics; ***life-threatening,*** in bold italics.

INDICATIONS & DOSAGE
Constipation –
Adults and children over 6 years: 3 g as a rectal suppository or 5 to 15 ml as an enema.
Children under 6 years: 1 to 1.5 g as a rectal suppository; or 2 to 5 ml as an enema.

ADVERSE REACTIONS
GI: *cramping pain,* rectal discomfort, hyperemia of rectal mucosa.

INTERACTIONS
None significant.

CONTRAINDICATIONS
• Contraindicated in patients hypersensitive to the drug and in those with intestinal obstruction, undiagnosed abdominal pain, vomiting or other signs of appendicitis, fecal impaction, or acute surgical abdomen.

NURSING CONSIDERATIONS
• Use mainly to reestablish proper toilet habits in laxative-dependent patients.
• Must be retained for at least 15 minutes; usually acts within 1 hour. Entire suppository need not melt to be effective.

lactulose

Cephulac, Cholac, Chronulac, Constilac, Duphalac, Enulose, Generlac, Lactulax†, Portalac

Pregnancy Risk Category: B

HOW SUPPLIED
Syrup: 10 g/15 ml

ACTION
Mechanism: Produces an osmotic effect in the colon. Resulting distention promotes peristalsis. Also decreases blood ammonia, probably as a result of bacterial degradation, which decreases the pH of colon contents.
Onset: 24 to 48 hours.

INDICATIONS & DOSAGE
Constipation –
Adults: 15 to 30 ml P.O. daily.
To prevent and treat portal-systemic encephalopathy, including hepatic precoma and coma in patients with severe hepatic disease –
Adults: initially, 20 to 30 g (30 to 45 ml) P.O. t.i.d. or q.i.d., until two or three soft stools are produced daily. Usual dosage is 60 to 100 g daily in divided doses. Alternatively, give by retention enema in at least 100 ml of fluid.

ADVERSE REACTIONS
GI: abdominal cramps, belching, diarrhea, gaseous distention, flatulence.
Other: hypernatremia.

INTERACTIONS
Antibotics, orally administered neomycin, antacids: decreased effectiveness of lactulose. Avoid concomitant use.

CONTRAINDICATIONS
• Contraindicated in patients on a low-galactose diet.
• Use cautiously in patients with diabetes mellitus.

NURSING CONSIDERATIONS
• Reduce dosage if diarrhea occurs. Replace fluid loss.
• Monitor serum sodium for possible hypernatremia, especially when giving in higher doses to treat hepatic encephalopathy.
• To minimize sweet taste, dilute with water or fruit juice or give with food.
• Enema not commercially available but may be prepared by adding 200 g (300 ml) to 700 ml of water or 0.9% sodium chloride solution. The diluted solution is administered as a retention enema for 30 to 60 minutes. Use a rectal balloon catheter.
• If the enema is not retained for at least 30 minutes, repeat dose.

• Store at room temperature, preferably below 86° F (30° C). Don't freeze.

magnesium citrate (citrate of magnesia)
Citroma◇, Citro-Mag†

magnesium hydroxide (milk of magnesia)
M.O.M.◇

magnesium sulfate (epsom salts)◇

Pregnancy Risk Category: B

HOW SUPPLIED
citrate
Oral solution: approximately 168 mEq magnesium/240 ml◇
hydroxide
Oral suspension: 7% to 8.5% (approximately 80 mEq magnesium/30 ml)◇
sulfate
Granules: approximately 40 mEq magnesium/5 g◇

ACTION
Mechanism: A saline laxative that produces an osmotic effect in the small intestine by drawing water into the intestinal lumen.
Onset: ½ to 3 hours.

INDICATIONS & DOSAGE
Constipation; to evacuate bowel before surgery–
Adults and children over 6 years: 15 g magnesium sulfate P.O. in glass of water; or 10 to 20 ml concentrated milk of magnesia; or 15 to 60 ml milk of magnesia; or 5 to 10 oz magnesium citrate h.s.
Children 2 to 6 years: 5 to 15 ml milk of magnesia P.O.
Antacid–
Adults: 5 to 15 ml milk of magnesia P.O. t.i.d. or q.i.d.

ADVERSE REACTIONS
GI: *abdominal cramping, nausea, diarrhea,* laxative dependence with long-term or excessive use.
Other: fluid and electrolyte disturbances with daily use.

INTERACTIONS
Orally administered drugs: impaired absorption. Separate administration times.

CONTRAINDICATIONS
• Contraindicated in patients with abdominal pain, nausea, vomiting, or other symptoms of appendicitis or acute surgical abdomen and in those with myocardial damage, heart block, imminent delivery, fecal impaction, rectal fissures, intestinal obstruction or perforation, or renal disease.
• Use cautiously in patients with rectal bleeding.

NURSING CONSIDERATIONS
• Shake suspension well; give with large amount of water when used as laxative. When administering through nasogastric tube, make sure tube is placed properly and is patent. After instilling, flush tube with water to ensure passage to stomach and maintain tube patency.
• For short-term therapy; don't use longer than 1 week.
• Drug produces watery stool in 3 to 6 hours. Time drug administration so that it doesn't interfere with scheduled activities or sleep.
• Magnesium sulfate is more potent than other saline laxatives.
• Before giving for constipation, determine if the patient has adequate fluid intake, exercise, and diet. Tell him that dietary sources of bulk include bran and other cereals, fresh fruit, and vegetables.
• Chill magnesium citrate before use to make it more palatable.
• Monitor serum electrolytes during prolonged use. Magnesium may accu-

mulate in patients with renal insufficiency.

• Warn patients that frequent or prolonged use as a laxative may cause dependence.

methylcellulose

Citrucel◊, Cologel◊

Pregnancy Risk Category: C

HOW SUPPLIED

Powder: 2 g/heaping tablespoon◊
Tablets: 500 mg◊

ACTION

Mechanism: A bulk-forming laxative that absorbs water and expands to increase bulk and moisture content of the stool. The increased bulk encourages peristalsis and bowel movement.
Onset: 12 to 24 hours. **Peak:** Peak effects may not occur for up to 3 days.

INDICATIONS & DOSAGE

Chronic constipation –
Adults: 1 heaping tablespoon in 8 oz (240 ml) cold water daily to t.i.d.
Children 6 to 12 years: 1 level tablespoon in 4 oz (120 ml) cold water daily to t.i.d.

ADVERSE REACTIONS

GI: *nausea,* vomiting, diarrhea (all after excessive use); esophageal, gastric, small intestinal, or colonic strictures when drug is chewed or taken in dry form; *abdominal cramps,* especially in severe constipation, laxative dependence with long-term or excessive use.

INTERACTIONS

None significant.

CONTRAINDICATIONS

• Contraindicated in patients with abdominal pain, nausea, vomiting, or other symptoms of appendicitis or acute surgical abdomen and in those with intestinal obstruction or ulceration, disabling adhesions, or difficulty swallowing.

NURSING CONSIDERATIONS

• Tell the patient to take drug with at least 8 oz of pleasant-tasting liquid to mask grittiness.
• Especially useful in debilitated patients and in those with postpartum constipation, irritable bowel syndrome, diverticulitis, and colostomies. Also useful to treat laxative abuse and to empty colon before barium enema examinations.
• Before giving for constipation, determine if the patient has adequate fluid intake, exercise, and diet. Tell him that dietary sources of bulk include bran and other cereals, fresh fruit, and vegetables.
• Not absorbed systemically; nontoxic.

mineral oil (liquid petrolatum)

Agoral Plain◊, Fleet Mineral Oil◊, Kondremul◊, Kondremul Plain◊, Lansoyl†, Liqui-Doss◊, Milkinol◊, Neo-Cultol◊, Petrogalar Plain◊, Zymenol◊

Pregnancy Risk Category: C

HOW SUPPLIED

Emulsion: 50%◊
Oral liquid: in pints, quarts, gallons◊
Enema: 120 ml◊, 133 ml◊

ACTION

Mechanism: A lubricant laxative that increases water retention in the stool by creating a barrier between colon wall and feces that prevents colonic reabsorption of fecal water.
Onset: 6 to 8 hours.

INDICATIONS & DOSAGE

Constipation; preparation for bowel studies or surgery –
Adults: 5 to 45 ml P.O. h.s.; or 120 ml P.R. (enema).

Children: 5 to 20 ml P.O. h.s.; or 30 to 60 ml P.R. (enema).

ADVERSE REACTIONS
GI: *nausea;* vomiting; diarrhea with excessive use; *abdominal cramps,* especially in severe constipation; decreased absorption of nutrients and fat-soluble vitamins, resulting in deficiency; slowed healing after hemorrhoidectomy.
Other: laxative dependence with long-term or excessive use, pruritus, ***lipid pneumonitis.***

INTERACTIONS
Docusate salts: may increase mineral oil absorption and cause lipid pneumonia. Separate administration times.
Fat-soluble vitamins (A, D, E, K): possible decreased absorption after prolonged administration.

CONTRAINDICATIONS
- Contraindicated in patients with abdominal pain, nausea, vomiting, or other symptoms of appendicitis or acute surgical abdomen and in those with fecal impaction or intestinal obstruction or perforation. Enema contraindicated in children under 2 years.
- Use cautiously in young children; in elderly or debilitated patients because of susceptibility to lipid pneumonitis through aspiration, absorption, and transport from intestinal mucosa; and in patients with rectal bleeding.

NURSING CONSIDERATIONS
- Give drug on an empty stomach because it delays passage of food from stomach; drug is more active on an empty stomach.
- Advise patient to take drug only at bedtime and not to take for more than 1 week.
- Give with fruit juices or carbonated drinks to disguise taste.
- Use when the patient needs to ease the strain of evacuation.
- To avoid soiling clothing, advise the patient of possible rectal leakage from excessive dosages.
- Before giving for constipation, determine if the patient has adequate fluid intake, exercise, and diet. Tell him that dietary sources of bulk include bran and other cereals, fresh fruit, and vegetables.

phenolphthalein, white
Alophen Pills◇, Feen-A-Mint◇, Medilax◇, Modane◇, Modane Mild◇, Phenolax Wafers**◇, Prulet◇

phenolphthalein, yellow
Espotabs◇, Evac-U-Gen◇, Evac-U-Lax◇, Ex-Lax◇, Ex-Lax Maximum Relief Formula◇, Ex-Lax Pills◇, Feen-A-Mint Gum◇, Lax-Pills◇

Pregnancy Risk Category: C

HOW SUPPLIED
white
Tablets: 60 mg◇, 65 mg◇
Tablets (chewable): 60 mg◇, 64.8 mg◇
yellow
Tablets (chewable): 80 mg◇, 90 mg◇, 97.2 mg◇
Chewing gum: 97.2 mg◇

ACTION
Mechanism: A stimulant laxative that increases peristalsis by direct effect on the smooth muscle of the intestine. Thought either to irritate the musculature or stimulate the colonic intramural plexus. Also promotes fluid accumulation in the colon and small intestine.
Onset: 6 to 10 hours. **Duration:** effects persist 3 to 4 days.

INDICATIONS & DOSAGE
Constipation –
Adults and children over 12 years: 30 to 270 mg P.O., preferably h.s.
Children 6 to 11 years: 30 to 60 mg P.O. h.s.

*Liquid form contains alcohol.
**May contain tartrazine.

Common reactions are in italics; ***life-threatening,*** in bold italics.

Children 2 to 5 years: 15 to 30 mg P.O. h.s.

ADVERSE REACTIONS

GI: diarrhea; *colic in large doses;* factitious nausea; vomiting; loss of normal bowel function with excessive use; *abdominal cramps,* especially in severe constipation; malabsorption of nutrients; "cathartic colon" (syndrome resembling ulcerative colitis radiologically and pathologically) with chronic misuse; reddish discoloration in alkaline feces or urine, laxative dependence with long-term or excessive use.
Skin: dermatitis, pruritus, rash, pigmentation.
Other: hypersensitivity reactions.

INTERACTIONS

None significant.

CONTRAINDICATIONS

• Contraindicated in patients with abdominal pain, nausea, vomiting, or other symptoms of appendicitis or acute surgical abdomen; in patients with fecal impaction or intestinal obstruction or perforation; and in children under 2 years.
• Use cautiously in patients with rectal bleeding.

NURSING CONSIDERATIONS

• Time drug administration so that it doesn't interfere with scheduled activities or sleep.
• Phenolphthalein may cause drug-induced dermatoses. Warn the patient to avoid excessive sun exposure, not to use drug with any other product containing phenolphthalein, and to discontinue use if dermatoses occur.
• Before giving for constipation, determine if the patient has adequate fluid intake, exercise, and diet. Tell him that dietary sources of bulk include bran and other cereals, fresh fruit, and vegetables.
• May discolor alkaline urine red-pink and acidic urine yellow-brown.
• Children may mistake for candy. Keep out of reach.
• Yellow phenolphthalein has been reported to be two to three times as potent as white phenolphthalein, but this has not been proved in clinical studies.

polyethylene glycol-electrolyte solution

Colovage, CoLyte, Glycoprep‡, GoLYTELY, NuLYTELY, OCL

Pregnancy Risk Category: C

HOW SUPPLIED

Powder for oral solution: polyethylene glycol (PEG) 3350 (6 g), anhydrous sodium sulfate (568 mg), sodium chloride (146 mg), potassium chloride (74.5 mg) per 100 ml (Colovage); PEG 3350 (120 g), sodium sulfate (3.36 g), sodium chloride (2.92 g), potassium chloride (1.49 g) per 2 liters (CoLyte); PEG 3350 (60 g), sodium chloride (1.46 g), potassium chloride (745 mg), sodium bicarbonate (1.68 g), sodium sulfate (5.68 g) per liter (Glycoprep‡); PEG 3350 (236 g), sodium sulfate (22.74 g), sodium bicarbonate (6.74g), sodium chloride (5.86 g), potassium chloride (2.97 g) per 4.8 liter (GoLYTELY); PEG 3350 (420 g), sodium bicarbonate (5.72 g), sodium chloride (11.2 g), potassium chloride (1.48 g) per 4 liters (NuLYTELY); PEG 3350 (6 g), sodium sulfate decahydrate (1.29 g), sodium chloride (146 mg), potassium chloride (75 mg), polysorbate-80 (30 mg) per 100 ml (OCL)

ACTION

Mechanism: PEG 3350, a nonabsorbable solution, acts as an osmotic agent. Sodium sulfate greatly reduces sodium absorption. The electrolyte concentration causes virtually no net absorption or secretion of ions.

Onset: ½ to 1 hour.

INDICATIONS & DOSAGE
Bowel preparation before GI examination –
Adults: 240 ml P.O. q 10 minutes until 4 liters are consumed. Typically, administer 4 hours before examination, allowing 3 hours for drinking and 1 hour for bowel evacuation.
Children 3 weeks to 18 years: 25 to 40 ml/kg/hour for 4 to 10 hours.

ADVERSE REACTIONS
GI: *nausea, bloating, cramps, vomiting.*

INTERACTIONS
Orally administered drugs: decreased absorption if administered within 1 hour of starting therapy. Administer at least 2 to 3 hours before starting therapy.

CONTRAINDICATIONS
- Contraindicated in patients with GI obstruction or perforation, gastric retention, toxic colitis, or megacolon.

NURSING CONSIDERATIONS
- If administered to semiconscious patients or to patients with impaired gag reflex, take care to prevent aspiration.
- No major shifts in fluid or electrolyte balance have been reported.
- Orally administered solution induces diarrhea (onset 30 to 60 minutes) that rapidly cleans the bowel, usually within 4 hours. Administer solution early in the morning if the patient is scheduled for a midmorning examination.
- May be less useful as a preparation for barium enema because it may interfere with barium coating of the colonic mucosa. To avoid interference, administer solution the evening before the examination.
- Have the patient fast for 3 to 4 hours before taking the solution and thereafter ingest only clear fluids until the examination is complete.
- Use tap water to reconstitute powder. Shake vigorously to ensure that all powder is dissolved. Refigerate reconstituted solution but use within 48 hours.
- Do not add flavoring or additional ingredients to the solution or administer chilled solution. Hypothermia has been reported after ingestion of large amounts of chilled solution.

psyllium

Alramucil◇, Cillium◇, Fiberall◇, Fibrepur†◇, Hydrocil Instant◇, Karacil†◇, Konsyl◇, Metamucil◇, Metamucil Instant Mix◇, Metamucil Sugar Free◇, Modane◇, Naturacil◇, Perdiem Plain◇, Pro-Lax◇, Prodiem†◇, Reguloid◇, Serutan◇, Siblin◇, Syllact◇ Versabran◇, V-Lax◇

Pregnancy Risk Category: C

HOW SUPPLIED
Chewable pieces: 1.7 g/piece◇
Effervescent powder: 3.4 g/packet◇, 3.7 g/packet◇
Granules: 2.5 g/tsp◇, 4.03 g/tsp◇
Powder: 3.3 g/tsp◇, 3.4 g/tsp◇, 3.5 g/tsp◇, 4.94 g/tsp◇
Wafers: 3.4 g/wafer◇

ACTION
Mechanism: A bulk-forming laxative that absorbs water and expands to increase bulk and moisture content of the stool, encouraging peristalsis and bowel movement.
Onset: 12 to 24 hours. **Peak:** Peak effects may not occur for 3 days.

INDICATIONS & DOSAGE
Constipation; bowel management –
Adults: 1 to 2 rounded teaspoonfuls P.O. in full glass of liquid daily, b.i.d., or t.i.d., followed by second glass of liquid; or 1 packet dissolved in water daily, b.i.d., or t.i.d.

Children over 6 years: 1 level teaspoonful P.O. in half a glass of liquid h.s.

ADVERSE REACTIONS
GI: nausea, vomiting, diarrhea (all after excessive use); esophageal, gastric, small intestinal, or colonic strictures when drug is taken in dry form; abdominal cramps, especially in severe constipation.

INTERACTIONS
None significant.

CONTRAINDICATIONS
• Contraindicated in patients with abdominal pain, nausea, vomiting, or other symptoms of appendicitis and in those with intestinal obstruction or ulceration, disabling adhesions, or difficulty swallowing.

NURSING CONSIDERATIONS
• Teach the patient how to properly mix medication. To enhance effect and prevent intestinal obstruction, tell the patient to take drug with plenty of water. Advise the patient that inhaling powder may cause allergic reactions.
• In diabetic patients, use brand of psyllium that does not contain sugar. Check label.
• Mix with at least 8 oz (240 ml) of cold, pleasant-tasting liquid such as orange juice to mask grittiness, and stir only a few seconds. Have the patient drink mixture immediately so it does not congeal. Follow with additional glass of liquid.
• Before giving for constipation, determine if the patient has adequate fluid intake, exercise, and diet. Tell him that dietary sources of bulk include bran and other cereals, fresh fruit, and vegetables.
• May reduce appetite if taken before meals.
• Laxative effect usually occurs in 12 to 24 hours, but may be delayed 3 days.
• For dosages in children under 6 years, consult the doctor.
• Not absorbed systemically; nontoxic. Especially useful in debilitated patients and those with postpartum constipation, irritable bowel syndrome, and diverticular disease. Also useful to treat chronic laxative abuse and in combination with other laxatives to empty colon before barium enema examinations.

senna

Black-Draught◇, Fletcher's Castoria◇, Lax-Senna◇, Senexon◇, Senokot◇, Senolax◇, X-Prep Liquid*◇

Pregnancy Risk Category: C

HOW SUPPLIED
Tablets: 187 mg◇, 217 mg◇, 600 mg◇
Granules: 326 mg/tsp◇, 1.65 g/½ tsp◇
Suppositories: 652 mg◇
Syrup: 218 mg/5 ml◇

ACTION
Mechanism: A stimulant laxative that increases peristalsis by direct effect on the smooth muscle of the intestine. Thought to either irritate the musculature or stimulate the colonic intramural plexus. Also promotes fluid accumulation in the colon and small intestine.
Onset: 6 to 10 hours.

INDICATIONS & DOSAGE
Acute constipation; preparation for bowel or rectal examination –
Adults: dosage range for Senokot is 1 to 8 tablets P.O.; ½ to 4 teaspoonfuls of granules added to liquid P.O.; 1 to 2 suppositories P.R., h.s.; or 1 to 4 teaspoonfuls syrup P.O., h.s. Dosage for Black-Draught is 2 tablets or ¼ to ½ level teaspoonfuls of granules mixed with water.

X-Prep Liquid used solely as single dose for preradiographic bowel evacu-

ation. Give 20 g powder dissolved in juice or 75 ml liquid P.O. between 2 p.m. and 4 p.m. on day before X-ray procedure. Use in divided doses, if needed, for elderly or debilitated patients.
Children over 27 kg: half adult dose of tablets, granules, or syrup (except Black-Draught tablets and granules – not recommended for children).
Children 1 month to 1 year: 1.25 to 2.5 ml Senokot syrup P.O. h.s.

ADVERSE REACTIONS
GI: *nausea;* vomiting; diarrhea; loss of normal bowel function with excessive use; *abdominal cramps,* especially in severe constipation; malabsorption of nutrients; "cathartic colon" (syndrome resembling ulcerative colitis radiologically) with chronic misuse; may cause constipation after catharsis; yellow or yellow-green cast to feces; diarrhea in breast-feeding infants of mothers receiving senna; darkened pigmentation of rectal mucosa with long-term use (usually reversible within 4 to 12 months after stopping drug), with excessive use – laxative dependence.
GU: red-pink discoloration in alkaline urine; yellow-brown color to acidic urine.
Other: protein-losing enteropathy, electrolyte imbalance (such as hypokalemia).

INTERACTIONS
None significant.

CONTRAINDICATIONS
- Contraindicated in patients with ulcerative bowel lesions and in those with nausea, vomiting, abdominal pain, or other symptoms of appendicitis or acute surgical abdomen; fecal impaction; or intestinal obstruction or perforation.

NURSING CONSIDERATIONS
- Use for short-term treatment.
- Avoid exposing product to excessive heat or light.
- Before giving for constipation, determine if the patient has adequate fluid intake, exercise, and diet. Tell him that dietary sources of bulk include bran and other cereals, fresh fruit, and vegetables.
- Limit diet to clear liquids after X-Prep Liquid is taken.
- Senna is one of the most effective laxatives for counteracting constipation caused by narcotic analgesics.

sodium phosphates
Fleet Phospho-Soda◊

Pregnancy Risk Category: C

HOW SUPPLIED
Liquid: 2.4 g/5 ml sodium phosphate and 900 mg sodium biphosphate/5 ml◊
Enema: 160 mg/ml sodium phosphate and 60 mg/ml sodium biphosphate◊

ACTION
Mechanism: A saline laxative that produces an osmotic effect in the small intestine by drawing water into the intestinal lumen.
Onset: ½ to 3 hours after oral use, 5 to 10 minutes after enema.

INDICATIONS & DOSAGE
Constipation –
Adults: 20 to 30 ml solution mixed with 120 ml cold water P.O.; or 60 to 135 ml P.R. (enema).
Children: 5 to 15 ml solution mixed with 120 ml of cold water P.O.; or 67.5 ml P.R. (enema).

ADVERSE REACTIONS
GI: *abdominal cramping.*
Other: fluid and electrolyte disturbances (hypernatremia, hyperphosphatemia) with daily use; laxative de-

pendence with long-term or excessive use.

INTERACTIONS
None significant.

CONTRAINDICATIONS
- Contraindicated in patients with abdominal pain, nausea, vomiting, or other symptoms of appendicitis or acute surgical abdomen; intestinal obstruction or perforation; edema; CHF; megacolon; or impaired renal function and in patients on sodium-restricted diets.
- Use cautiously in patients with large hemorrhoids or anal excoriations.

NURSING CONSIDERATIONS
- Before giving for constipation, determine if the patient has adequate fluid intake, exercise, and diet. Tell him that dietary sources of bulk include bran and other cereals, fresh fruit, and vegetables.
- Up to 10% of sodium content of drug may be absorbed.
- Also used to prepare for barium edema or sigmoidoscopy, to treat fecal impaction or hypercalcemia, or as a phosphate replacement.

50

Antiemetics

benzquinamide hydrochloride
buclizine hydrochloride
chlorpromazine hydrochloride
(See Chapter 32, ANTIPSYCHOTICS.)
cyclizine hydrochloride
cyclizine lactate
dimenhydrinate
diphenidol hydrochloride
dronabinol
granisetron hydrochloride
meclizine hydrochloride
metoclopramide hydrochloride
ondansetron hydrochloride
perphenazine
(See Chapter 32, ANTIPSYCHOTICS.)
prochlorperazine
prochlorperazine edisylate
prochlorperazine maleate
promethazine hydrochloride
(See Chapter 42, ANTIHISTAMINES.)
scopolamine
(See Chapter 37, ANTICHOLINERGICS.)
thiethylperazine maleate
trimethobenzamide hydrochloride

COMBINATION PRODUCTS
None.

benzquinamide hydrochloride

Emete-Con

Pregnancy Risk Category: C

HOW SUPPLIED
Injection: 50 mg/vial

ACTION
Mechanism: Acts on the chemoreceptor trigger zone to inhibit nausea and vomiting.
Onset: within 15 minutes. **Peak:** Blood levels peak immediately after I.V. injection or within 30 minutes after I.M. injection. **Duration:** 3 to 4 hours.

INDICATIONS & DOSAGE
Nausea and vomiting associated with anesthesia and surgery –
Adults: 50 mg I.M. (0.5 mg/kg to 1 mg/kg). Repeat in 1 hour and thereafter q 3 to 4 hours, p.r.n.; or 25 mg (0.2 mg/kg to 0.4 mg/kg) I.V. as a single dose, administered slowly (25 mg/minute).

ADVERSE REACTIONS
CNS: *drowsiness,* fatigue, insomnia, restlessness, headache, excitation, tremor, twitching, dizziness.
CV: sudden rise in blood pressure and transient arrhythmias (premature atrial and ventricular contractions, atrial fibrillation) after I.V. administration; hypertension; hypotension.
EENT: salivation, blurred vision.
GI: anorexia, nausea, dry mouth.
Skin: urticaria, rash.
Other: muscle weakness, flushing, hiccups, sweating, chills, fever.

INTERACTIONS
CNS depressants, ethanol: enhanced CNS depression. Avoid concomitant use.

CONTRAINDICATIONS
- Contraindicated for I.V. use in patients with CV disease and within 15 minutes of administering preanesthetic or CV drugs.

NURSING CONSIDERATIONS
- Monitor blood pressure frequently.
- Like other antiemetics, drug may mask symptoms of ototoxicity, brain tumor, or intestinal obstruction.
- For I.M. use, give injections in large muscle mass. Use deltoid area only if well developed.
- **I.V. use:** Reconstitute drug with 2.2 ml of sterile water for injection or

bacteriostatic water containing benzyl ethanol or parabens. Do not dilute further. Inject directly and slowly (25 mg/minute).
• Do not reconstitute with 0.9% sodium chloride injection.
• Reconstituted solution is stable for 14 days at room temperature. Store dry powder and reconstituted solution in a light-resistant container.

buclizine hydrochloride

Bucladin-S**

Pregnancy Risk Category: C

HOW SUPPLIED
Tablets (chewable): 50 mg

ACTION
Mechanism: An antihistamine that may affect neural pathways originating in the labyrinth to inhibit nausea and vomiting, but exact mechanism of action is unknown.
Duration: 4 to 6 hours.

INDICATIONS & DOSAGE
Motion sickness (prevention) –
Adults: 50 mg P.O. at least ½ hour before beginning travel. If needed, repeat another 50 mg after 4 to 6 hours.
Vertigo –
Adults: 50 mg P.O., up to 150 mg daily in severe cases. Maintenance dosage is 50 mg b.i.d.

ADVERSE REACTIONS
CNS: *drowsiness,* headache, dizziness, jitters.
EENT: blurred vision.
GI: dry mouth.
GU: urine retention.

INTERACTIONS
CNS depressants, ethanol: additive CNS depression. Avoid concomitant use.

CONTRAINDICATIONS
• Contraindicated in patients hypersensitive to the drug. Contains tartrazine, which may precipitate allergic reactions in certain individuals, including those allergic to aspirin.
• Use cautiously in patients with glaucoma or GU or GI obstruction and in elderly males with possible prostatic hyperplasia.

NURSING CONSIDERATIONS
• Advise patients against driving and other activities that require alertness until CNS effects of the drug are known.
• Like other antiemetics, drug may mask symptoms of ototoxicity, intestinal obstruction, or brain tumor.
• Tell patients to place tablets in mouth and allow to dissolve without water, chew, or swallow them whole.

cyclizine hydrochloride

Marezine◇

cyclizine lactate

Marzine†

Pregnancy Risk Category: B

HOW SUPPLIED
hydrochloride
Tablets: 50 mg◇
lactate
Injection: 50 mg/ml†

ACTION
Mechanism: An antihistamine that may affect neural pathways originating in the labyrinth to inhibit nausea and vomiting, but the exact mechanism of action is unknown.
Onset: ½ to 1 hour. **Duration:** 4 to 6 hours.

INDICATIONS & DOSAGE
Motion sickness (prevention and treatment) –
Adults: 50 mg P.O. (hydrochloride) ½ hour before travel, then q 4 to 6

†Available in Canada only. ‡Available in Australia only. ◇Available OTC.

hours, p.r.n., to maximum of 200 mg daily; or 50 mg I.M. (lactate) q 4 to 6 hours, p.r.n.
Postoperative vomiting (prevention) –
Adults: 50 mg I.M. (lactate) preoperatively or 20 to 30 minutes before expected termination of surgery; then postoperatively 50 mg I.M. (lactate) q 4 to 6 hours, p.r.n.
Motion sickness and postoperative vomiting –
Children 6 to 12 years: 3 mg/kg (lactate) I.M. divided t.i.d.; or 25 mg (hydrochloride) P.O. q 4 to 6 hours, p.r.n., to a maximum of 75 mg daily.

ADVERSE REACTIONS
CNS: *drowsiness,* dizziness, auditory and visual hallucinations.
CV: hypotension.
EENT: blurred vision.
GI: constipation, dry mouth.
GU: urine retention.

INTERACTIONS
CNS depressants, ethanol: additive CNS depression. Avoid concomitant use.

CONTRAINDICATIONS
• Contraindicated in patients hypersensitive to the drug and in children under 6 years.
• Use cautiously in patients with glaucoma, GU or GI obstruction, or heart failure and in elderly males with possible prostatic hyperplasia.

NURSING CONSIDERATIONS
• Advise patients against driving and other activities that require alertness until CNS effects of the drug are known.
• Like other antiemetics, drug may mask symptoms of ototoxicity, brain tumor, or intestinal obstruction.
• Store in cool place. When stored at room temperature, injection may turn slightly yellow; this change does not indicate loss of potency.

dimenhydrinate

Andrumin‡, Apo-Dimenhydrinate†, Calm X◇, Children's Dramamine◇, Dimetabs, Dinate, Dommanate, Dramamine◇*, Dramamine Chewable◇**, Dramamine Liquid◇*, Dramanate, Dramocen, Dramoject, Dymenate, Gravol†, Gravol L/A†, Hydrate, Marmine◇, Nauseatol†, Nico-Vert◇, Novodimenate†, PMS-Dimenhydrinate†, Tega-Vert◇, Travamine†, Travs‡, Triptone Caplets◇, Vertab

Pregnancy Risk Category: B

HOW SUPPLIED
Tablets: 50 mg◇
Tablets (chewable): 50 mg◇
Capsules: 50 mg◇
Elixir: 15 mg/5 ml†
Syrup: 12.5 mg/4 ml*◇, 15.62 mg/5 ml
Injection: 50 mg/ml

ACTION
Mechanism: An antihistamine that may affect neural pathways originating in the labyrinth to inhibit nausea and vomiting. Exact mechanism of action is unknown.
Onset: immediately after I.V. injection, within 15 to 20 minutes of I.M. injection, within 20 to 30 minutes of oral administration. **Duration:** 3 to 6 hours.

INDICATIONS & DOSAGE
Motion sickness (treatment and prevention) –
Adults: 50 mg P.O. q 4 hours, or 100 mg q 4 hours if drowsiness is not objectionable; 50 mg I.M., p.r.n.; or 50 mg I.V. diluted in 10 ml sodium chloride injection, injected over 2 minutes. Maximum dosage is 400 mg daily.
Children: 1.25 mg/kg P.O. or I.M. in divided doses q.i.d. Maximum dos-

age is 300 mg daily. Don't use in children under 2 years.
Prophylaxis of Ménière's disease –
Adults: 25 to 50 mg P.O. t.i.d.
Acute episodes of Ménière's disease –
Adults: 50 mg I.M.

ADVERSE REACTIONS
CNS: *drowsiness,* headache, incoordination, dizziness.
CV: palpitations, hypotension.
EENT: blurred vision, tinnitus, dry respiratory passages.
GI: dry mouth.

INTERACTIONS
CNS depressants, ethanol: additive CNS depression. Avoid concomitant use.

CONTRAINDICATIONS
- Contraindicated in patients hypersensitive to the drug.
- Use cautiously in patients with seizures, acute angle-closure glaucoma, or enlarged prostate gland.

NURSING CONSIDERATIONS
- Advise patients against driving and other activities that require alertness until CNS effects of the drug are known.
- Like other antiemetics, drug may mask symptoms of ototoxicity, brain tumor, or intestinal obstruction.
- **I.V. use:** Before administration, dilute each ml of drug with 10 ml of sterile water for injection, D_5W, or 0.9% sodium chloride injection. Give by direct injection over not less than 2 minutes.
- Undiluted solution is irritating to veins and may cause sclerosis.
- Because incompatibilities are common, avoid mixing parenteral preparation with other drugs.

diphenidol hydrochloride
Vontrol**

Pregnancy Risk Category: C

HOW SUPPLIED
Tablets: 25 mg

ACTION
Mechanism: Diminishes labrynthine function and vestibular stimulation and influences the chemoreceptor trigger zone to inhibit nausea and vomiting.
Peak: Blood levels peak 1½ to 3 hours after a dose. **Duration:** elimination half-life, about 4 hours.

INDICATIONS & DOSAGE
Peripheral (labyrinthine) dizziness –
Adults: 25 to 50 mg P.O. q 4 hours, p.r.n.
Nausea and vomiting –
Adults: 25 to 50 mg P.O. q 4 hours, p.r.n.
Children over 23 kg: 0.88 mg/kg P.O. q 4 hours, not to exceed 5.5 mg/kg/24 hours. Usual dose is 25 mg.

ADVERSE REACTIONS
CNS: *drowsiness,* dizziness, sleep disturbances, *confusion,* auditory and visual hallucinations and disorientation.
CV: transient hypotension.
GI: dry mouth, nausea, indigestion, heartburn.
Skin: urticaria.

INTERACTIONS
None significant.

CONTRAINDICATIONS
- Contraindicated in patients with anuria.
- Use cautiously in patients with glaucoma, pyloric stenosis, pylorospasm, obstructive lesions of GI or GU tract, prostatic hyperplasia, or organic cardiospasm.

NURSING CONSIDERATIONS
- Stop drug if auditory or visual hallucinations, disorientation, or confusion occur.
- Like other antiemetics, drug may mask symptoms of ototoxicity, brain tumor, intestinal obstruction, or other conditions.
- Closely supervise patients. Patients are usually hospitalized when receiving drug. Monitor fluid intake and output; report any changes.

dronabinol (tetrahydrocannabinol)
Marinol
Controlled Substance Schedule II
Pregnancy Risk Category: B

HOW SUPPLIED
Capsules: 2.5 mg, 5 mg, 10 mg

ACTION
Mechanism: A derivative of marijuana. Antiemetic and appetite stimulant effects are produced through an unknown action in the CNS.
Peak: Blood levels peak 2 to 3 hours after an oral dose. **Duration:** elimination half-life, about 36 hours.

INDICATIONS & DOSAGE
Nausea and vomiting associated with cancer chemotherapy –
Adults: 5 mg/m^2 P.O. 1 to 3 hours before administration of chemotherapy. Then give same dose q 2 to 4 hours after chemotherapy for a total of four to six doses per day. If needed, increase dosage in increments of 2.5 mg/m^2 to a maximum of 15 mg/m^2 per dose.
Anorexia and weight loss in patients with AIDS –
Adults: 2.5 mg P.O. b.i.d. before lunch and dinner.

ADVERSE REACTIONS
CNS: *dizziness, drowsiness, euphoria, ataxia,* depersonalization, disorientation, hallucinations, headache, irritability, memory lapse, muddled thinking, paranoia, perceptual difficulties, weakness, paresthesia.
CV: tachycardia, orthostatic hypotension.
GI: *dry mouth.*
Other: visual distortions.

INTERACTIONS
CNS depressants, ethanol, psychotomimetic substances, sedatives: additive effects. Avoid concomitant use.

CONTRAINDICATIONS
- Contraindicated in patients hypersensitive to sesame oil or marijuana and in those with nausea and vomiting from any cause other than cancer chemotherapy or anorexia and weight loss from any cause other than AIDS.
- Use cautiously in elderly patients and those with hypertension, heart disease, and psychiatric illness.

NURSING CONSIDERATIONS
- Advise the patient against hazardous activities that require alertness until the CNS effects of the drug are known.
- Expect this drug to be prescribed only for patients who have not responded satisfactorily to other antiemetics.
- Drug's effects may persist for days after treatment ends.
- Dronabinol is the principal active substance present in *Cannabis sativa* (marijuana). This substance can produce both physical and psychic dependence and has high potential for abuse.
- CNS effects are intensified at higher drug dosages.
- To prevent panic and anxiety, tell the patient drug may induce unusual changes in mood or other adverse behavioral effects.
- Warn family members to ensure that the patient is supervised by a responsible person during and immediately after treatment.

granisetron hydrochloride
Kytril

Pregnancy Risk Category: B

HOW SUPPLIED
Injection: 1 mg/ml

ACTION
Mechanism: A selective antagonist of a specific type of serotonin receptor (5-HT_3) located in the CNS at the area postrema (chemoreceptor trigger zone) and in the peripheral nervous system on nerve terminals of the vagus nerve. Drug's blocking action may occur at both sites.
Duration: half-life, highly variable; average of about 5 hours.

INDICATIONS & DOSAGE
Prevention of nausea and vomiting associated with emetogenic cancer chemotherapy –
Adults and children ages 2 to 16: 10 mcg/kg I.V. infused over 5 minutes. Begin infusion within 30 minutes before administration of chemotherapy.

ADVERSE REACTIONS
CNS: *headache, asthenia,* somnolence.
CV: hypertension.
GI: diarrhea, constipation.
Other: taste disorder, fever.

INTERACTIONS
None significant.

CONTRAINDICATIONS
• Contraindicated in patients hypersensitive to the drug.

NURSING CONSIDERATIONS
• **I.V. use:** Dilute drug with 0.9% sodium chloride injection or D_5W to a volume of 20 to 50 ml. Infuse over 5 minutes. Diluted solutions are stable for 24 hours at room temperature.
• Do not mix with other drugs; data regarding compatibility is limited.

meclizine hydrochloride (meclozine hydrochloride)
Ancolan‡, Antivert, Antivert/25◇, Antivert/50, Bonamine†, Bonine◇, Dizmiss◇, D-Vert 15, D-Vert 30, Meni-D, Ru-Vert M

Pregnancy Risk Category: B

HOW SUPPLIED
Tablets: 12.5 mg, 25 mg◇, 50 mg
Tablets (chewable): 25 mg◇
Capsules: 15 mg, 25 mg, 30 mg

ACTION
Mechanism: An antihistamine that may affect neural pathways originating in the labyrinth to inhibit nausea and vomiting. Exact mechanism of action is unknown.
Onset: about 1 hour. **Duration:** 8 to 24 hours.

INDICATIONS & DOSAGE
Dizziness –
Adults: 25 to 100 mg P.O. daily in divided doses. Dosage varies with patient response. Maximum dosage is 200 mg daily.
Motion sickness –
Adults: 25 to 50 mg P.O. 1 hour before travel, repeated daily for duration of journey.

ADVERSE REACTIONS
CNS: *drowsiness,* fatigue.
EENT: blurred vision.
GI: dry mouth.

INTERACTIONS
CNS depressants: increased drowsiness.

CONTRAINDICATIONS
• Contraindicated in patients hypersensitive to the drug.
• Use cautiously in patients with glaucoma or GU or GI obstruction and in elderly males with possible prostatic hyperplasia.

NURSING CONSIDERATIONS
- Advise patients against driving and other hazardous activities that require alertness until CNS effects of the drug are known.
- Like other antiemetics, drug may mask symptoms of ototoxicity, brain tumor, or intestinal obstruction.

metoclopramide hydrochloride

Apo-Metoclop†, Clopra, Emex†, Maxeran†, Maxolon, Maxolon High Dose‡, Octamide, Octamide PFS, Pramin‡, Reclomide, Reglan

Pregnancy Risk Category: B

HOW SUPPLIED
Tablets: 5 mg, 10 mg
Syrup: 5 mg/5 ml
Injection: 5 mg/ml

ACTION
Mechanism: Stimulates motility of the upper GI tract by increasing lower esophageal sphincter tone and blocks dopamine receptors at the chemoreceptor trigger zone.
Onset: within 1 to 3 minutes of I.V. administration, 10 to 15 minutes after I.M. injection, 30 to 60 minutes after oral ingestion. **Duration:** 1 to 2 hours; terminal elimination half-life, 2 ½ to 6 hours.

INDICATIONS & DOSAGE
Prevention or reduction of nausea and vomiting induced by cisplatin and other chemotherapeutic agents –
Adults: 2 mg/kg I.V. q 2 hours for five doses, beginning 30 minutes before cisplatin administration.
Prevention or reduction of postoperative nausea and vomiting –
Adults: 10 to 20 mg I.M. near the end of the surgical procedure, repeated q 4 to 6 hours p.r.n.
To facilitate small-bowel intubation and to aid in radiologic examinations –
Adults: 10 mg (2 ml) I.V. as a single dose over 1 to 2 minutes.
Children under 6 years: 0.1 mg/kg I.V.
Children 6 to 14 years: 2.5 to 5 mg I.V. (0.5 to 1 ml).
Delayed gastric emptying secondary to diabetic gastroparesis –
Adults: 10 mg P.O. 30 minutes before meals and h.s. for 2 to 8 weeks, depending on response.
Gastroesophageal reflux disease –
Adults: 10 to 15 mg P.O. q.i.d., p.r.n., 30 minutes before meals.

ADVERSE REACTIONS
CNS: *restlessness, anxiety, drowsiness,* fatigue, *lassitude,* insomnia, headache, dizziness, extrapyramidal symptoms, tardive dyskinesia, dystonic reactions, sedation.
CV: transient hypertension.
GI: nausea, bowel disturbances.
Skin: rash.
Other: fever, prolactin secretion, loss of libido.

INTERACTIONS
Anticholinergics, opioid analgesics: antagonized GI motility effects of metoclopramide. Use together cautiously.
Butyrophenones, phenothiazines: increased risk of extrapyramidal effects. Monitor closely.
CNS depressants, ethanol: additive CNS depression. Avoid concomitant use.

CONTRAINDICATIONS
- Contraindicated in patients in which stimulation of GI motility might be dangerous (hemorrhage, obstruction, or perforation) and in those with pheochromocytoma or seizure disorder.
- Use cautiously in elderly patients because they are more likely to experience tardive dyskinesia. After I.V. administration, young adults and chil-

dren are more likely to suffer extrapyramidal symptoms.

NURSING CONSIDERATIONS

- Safety and effectiveness have not been established for therapy that continues longer than 12 weeks.
- **I.V. use:** Lower doses (10 mg or less) may be given by direct injection over 1 to 2 minutes. Doses larger than 10 mg should be diluted in 50 ml of a compatible diluent and infused over at least 15 minutes. Protection from light is unnecessary if the infusion mixture is administered within 24 hours.
- Compatible with D_5W, 0.9% sodium chloride injection, and dextrose 5% in sodium chloride 0.45%.
- Monitor blood pressure frequently in patients receiving I.V. dosage.
- Use diphenhydramine 25 mg I.V. to counteract the extrapyramidal adverse effects associated with high metoclopramide doses.
- Advise patients to avoid activities requiring alertness for 2 hours after taking each dose.
- Oral form is being used investigationally to treat nausea and vomiting.

ondansetron hydrochloride

Zofran

Pregnancy Risk Category: B

HOW SUPPLIED

Tablets: 4 mg, 8 mg
Injection: 2 mg/ml

ACTION

Mechanism: A selective antagonist of a specific type of serotonin receptor (5-HT_3) located in the CNS at the area postrema (chemoreceptor trigger zone) and in the peripheral nervous system on nerve terminals of the vagus nerve. Drug's blocking action may occur at both sites.
Duration: elimination half-life, about 4 hours.

INDICATIONS & DOSAGE

Prevention of nausea and vomiting associated with emetogenic chemotherapy –
Adults and children over 12 years: 8 mg P.O. 30 minutes before start of chemotherapy. Follow with 8 mg 4 and 8 hours after first dose. Then follow with 8 mg q 8 hours for 1 to 2 days. Alternatively, administer a single dose of 32 mg by I.V. infusion over 15 minutes beginning 30 minutes before chemotherapy; give three doses of 0.15 mg/kg I.V. Give first dose 30 minutes before chemotherapy; administer subsequent doses 4 and 8 hours after first dose. Infuse drug over 15 minutes.
Children 4 to 11 years: 4 mg P.O. 30 minutes before start of chemotherapy. Follow with 4 mg 4 and 8 hours after first dose. Then follow with 4 mg q 8 hours for 1 to 2 days. Alternatively, administer a single dose of 32 mg by I.V. infusion over 15 minutes beginning 30 minutes before chemotherapy; or give three doses of 0.15 mg/kg I.V. Give first dose 30 minutes before chemotherapy; administer subsequent doses 4 and 8 hours after first dose. Infuse drug over 15 minutes.
Prevention of postoperative nausea and vomiting –
Adults and children over 12 years: 4 mg I.V. (undiluted) over 2 to 5 minutes.

ADVERSE REACTIONS

CNS: headache.
GI: *diarrhea, constipation.*
Hepatic: transient elevations in AST and ALT levels.
Respiratory: ***bronchospasm (rare).***
Skin: rash.

INTERACTIONS

Drugs that alter hepatic drug metabolizing enzymes, such as phenobarbital or cimetidine: may alter pharmacokinetics of ondansetron. No dosage adjustment appears necessary.

CONTRAINDICATIONS

• Contraindicated in patients hypersensitive to the drug.
• Use cautiously in patients with liver failure. Limit daily dosage (oral or I.V.) to 8 mg.

NURSING CONSIDERATIONS

• **I.V. use:** Dilute drug in 50 ml of D_5W injection or 0.9% sodium chloride injection before administration. Drug is also stable for up to 48 hours after dilution in 5% dextrose in 0.9% sodium chloride injection, 5% dextrose in 0.45% sodium chloride injection, and 3% sodium chloride injection.

---

prochlorperazine

Compazine, PMS-Prochlorperazine†, Prorazin†, Stemetil†‡

prochlorperazine edisylate

Compa-Z, Compazine, Cotranzine, Ultrazine-10

prochlorperazine maleate

Anti-Naus‡, Chlorpazine, Compazine Spansule, PMS-Prochlorperazine†, Prorazin†, Stemetil†‡

Pregnancy Risk Category: C

HOW SUPPLIED

prochlorperazine
Injection: 5 mg/ml
Suppositories: 2.5 mg, 5 mg, 25 mg
prochlorperazine edisylate
Syrup: 1 mg/ml
prochlorperazine maleate
Tablets: 5 mg, 10 mg, 25 mg
Capsules (sustained-release): 10 mg, 15 mg, 30 mg

ACTION

Mechanism: Acts on the chemoreceptor trigger zone to inhibit nausea and vomiting; in larger doses, partially depresses the vomiting center.
Onset: 30 to 40 minutes after oral use, 60 minutes after rectal use, 10 to 20 minutes after I.M. use. **Duration:** 3 to 4 hours after regular-release preparations, 10 to 12 hours after sustained-release preparations.

INDICATIONS & DOSAGE

Preoperative nausea control –
Adults: 5 to 10 mg I.M. 1 to 2 hours before induction of anesthesia; repeat once in 30 minutes, if necessary. Or, 5 to 10 mg I.V. 15 to 30 minutes before induction of anesthesia; repeat once if necessary.
Severe nausea and vomiting –
Adults: 5 to 10 mg P.O., t.i.d. or q.i.d.; 15 mg sustained-release form P.O. on arising; 10 mg sustained-release form P.O. q 12 hours; 25 mg P.R., b.i.d.; or 5 to 10 mg I.M. repeated q 3 to 4 hours, p.r.n. Maximum I.M. dosage is 40 mg daily.
Children 9 to 13 kg: 2.5 mg P.O. or P.R. daily or b.i.d. Maximum dosage is 7.5 mg daily. Or give 0.132 mg/kg by deep I.M. injection. Control usually is obtained with one dose.
Children 14 to 17 kg: 2.5 mg P.O. or P.R., b.i.d. or t.i.d. Maximum dosage is 10 mg daily. Or give 0.132 mg/kg by deep I.M. injection. Control usually is obtained with one dose.
Children 18 to 39 kg: 2.5 mg P.O. or P.R., t.i.d.; or 5 mg P.O. or P.R., b.i.d. Maximum dosage is 15 mg daily. Or, give 0.132 mg/kg by deep I.M. injection. Control usually is obtained with one dose.
To manage symptoms of psychotic disorders –
Adults: 5 to 10 mg, P.O. t.i.d. or q.i.d.
Children 2 to 12 years: 2.5 mg P.O. or P.R., b.i.d. or t.i.d. Do not exceed 10 mg on day 1. Increase dosage gradually to recommended maximum (if necessary). In children 2 to 5 years, maximum daily dosage is 25 mg. In children 6 to 10 years, maximum daily dosage is 25 mg.

To manage symptoms of severe psychoses –
Adults: 10 to 20 mg I.M. repeated in 1 to 4 hours, if needed. Rarely, patients may receive 10 to 20 mg q 4 to 6 hours. Institute oral therapy after symptoms are controlled.
Children 2 to 12 years: 0.13 mg/kg I.M.
Excessive anxiety –
Adults: 5 to 10 mg by deep I.M. injection q 3 to 4 hours, not to exceed 40 mg daily; or 5 to 10 mg P.O., t.i.d. or q.i.d. Alternatively, give 15 mg extended-release capsule once daily or 10 mg extended-release capsule q 12 hours.

ADVERSE REACTIONS
CNS: *extrapyramidal reactions,* sedation, pseudoparkinsonism, EEG changes, dizziness.
CV: *orthostatic hypotension,* tachycardia, ECG changes.
EENT: *ocular changes, blurred vision.*
GI: *dry mouth, constipation.*
GU: *urine retention,* dark urine, menstrual irregularities, inhibited ejaculation.
Hematologic: *transient leukopenia,* ***agranulocytosis.***
Hepatic: *cholestatic jaundice.*
Skin: *mild photosensitivity,* allergic reactions, ***exfoliative dermatitis.***
Other: hyperprolactinemia, gynecomastia, weight gain, increased appetite.

INTERACTIONS
Antacids: inhibited absorption of oral phenothiazines. Separate antacid and phenothiazine doses by at least 2 hours.
Anticholinergics, including antidepressants and antiparkinsonian agents: increased anticholinergic activity and aggravated parkinsonian symptoms. Use together cautiously.
Barbiturates: may decrease phenothiazine effect. Monitor patient for decreased antiemetic effect.

CONTRAINDICATIONS
• Contraindicated in patients hypersensitive to phenothiazines and in those with CNS depression, bone marrow suppression, or subcortical damage; during pediatric surgery; when using spinal or epidural anesthetic, adrenergic blockers, or ethanol; in those experiencing coma or depression, and in children under age 2.
• Use cautiously in combination with other CNS depressants; in patients with hepatic disease, arteriosclerosis or CV disease (may cause sudden drop in blood pressure), exposure to extreme heat or cold (including antipyretic therapy), respiratory disorders, hypocalcemia, seizure disorders or severe reactions to insulin or electroshock therapy, suspected brain tumor or intestinal obstruction, glaucoma, or prostatic hyperplasia; and in acutely ill, dehydrated, or vomiting children.
• Use cautiously and in reduced dosage in elderly or debilitated patients.

NURSING CONSIDERATIONS
• Use only when vomiting can't be controlled by other measures or when only a few doses are required. If more than four doses are needed in 24 hours, notify the doctor.
• Not effective to treat motion sickness.
• To prevent contact dermatitis, avoid getting concentrate or injection solution on hands or clothing.
• Dilute oral solution with tomato or fruit juice, milk, coffee, carbonated beverage, tea, water, soup, or pudding.
• Monitor CBC and liver function studies during prolonged therapy.
• Advise patients to wear protective clothing when exposed to sunlight.
• **I.V. use:** 15 to 30 minutes before in-

duction, add 20 mg of prochlperazine per liter of D_5W and 0.9% sodium chloride solution. Flow should not exceed 5 mg/minute. Maximum parenteral dosage is 40 mg daily. Infuse slowly, never as a bolus injection.

• Watch for orthostatic hypotension, especially when giving I.V.

• For I.M. use, inject deeply into upper outer quadrant of gluteal region.

• Do not give subcutaneously or mix in syringe with another drug.

• Store in light-resistant container. Slight yellowing does not affect potency; discard extremely discolored solutions.

thiethylperazine maleate

Norzine, Torecan**

Pregnancy Risk Category: C

HOW SUPPLIED

Tablets: 10 mg
Injection: 5 mg/ml
Suppositories: 10 mg

ACTION

Mechanism: Acts on the chemoreceptor trigger zone to inhibit nausea and vomiting.
Onset: 30 minutes. **Duration:** 4 hours.

INDICATIONS & DOSAGE

Nausea and vomiting–
Adults: 10 mg P.O., I.M., or P.R. daily, b.i.d. or t.i.d.

ADVERSE REACTIONS

CNS: *extrapyramidal reactions* (high incidence), sedation (low incidence), pseudoparkinsonism, EEG changes, dizziness, confusion (especially in elderly patients).
CV: *orthostatic hypotension,* tachycardia, ECG changes.
EENT: *ocular changes, blurred vision.*
GI: *dry mouth, constipation.*
GU: *urine retention,* dark urine, menstrual irregularities, inhibited ejaculation.
Hematologic: *transient leukopenia,* ***agranulocytosis.***
Hepatic: *cholestatic jaundice.*
Skin: *mild photosensitivity,* allergic reactions.
Other: hyperprolactinemia, gynecomastia, weight gain, increased appetite.

INTERACTIONS

Antacids: inhibited absorption of oral phenothiazines. Separate antacid and phenothiazine dosage by at least 2 hours.
Anticholinergics, including antidepressants and antiparkinsonian agents: increased anticholinergic activity and increased risk of parkinsonian-like symptoms. Use together cautiously.
Barbiturates: may decrease phenothiazine effect. Monitor for decreased antiemetic effect.

CONTRAINDICATIONS

• Contraindicated in patients hypersensitive to phenothiazines, in those with severe CNS depression or hepatic disease, and in patients experiencing coma.

NURSING CONSIDERATIONS

• Don't give I.V. May cause severe hypotension.

• For nausea and vomiting associated with anesthesia and surgery, give deep I.M. injection on or shortly before terminating anesthesia.

• May effectively treat dizziness but not motion sickness.

• Use only when vomiting can't be controlled by other measures or when only a few doses are required.

• Advise patients about hypotension and suggest they stay in bed for 1 hour after receiving drug.

• Store suppositories tightly covered and at temperatures below 77° F (25° C).

• If drug gets on skin, wash off at once to prevent contact dermatitis.

trimethobenzamide hydrochloride

Arrestin, Benzacot, Bio-Gan, Stemetic, Tebamide, Tegamide, T-Gen, Ticon, Tigan, Triban, Tribenzagan

Pregnancy Risk Category: C

HOW SUPPLIED

Capsules: 100 mg, 250 mg
Injection: 100 mg/ml
Suppositories: 100 mg, 200 mg

ACTION

Mechanism: Acts on the chemoreceptor trigger zone to inhibit nausea and vomiting.
Onset: 10 to 20 minutes after oral administration, 15 to 35 minutes after I.M. administration. **Duration:** 2 to 3 hours after I.M. administration, 3 to 4 hours after oral administration.

INDICATIONS & DOSAGE

Nausea and vomiting–
Adults: 250 mg P.O., t.i.d. or q.i.d.; or 200 mg I.M. or P.R., t.i.d. or q.i.d.
Prevention of postoperative nausea and vomiting–
Adults: 200 mg I.M. or P.R. as a single dose before or during surgery; if needed, repeat 3 hours after termination of anesthesia, p.r.n. Limit use to prolonged vomiting of known etiology.
Children under 13 kg: 100 mg P.R. t.i.d. or q.i.d.
Children 13 to 40 kg: 100 to 200 mg P.O. or P.R. t.i.d. or q.i.d.

ADVERSE REACTIONS

CNS: *drowsiness,* dizziness (in large doses).
CV: hypotension.
GI: diarrhea, exaggeration of preexisting nausea (in large doses).
Hepatic: *liver toxicity.*
Skin: skin hypersensitivity reaction.
Other: pain, stinging, burning, redness, swelling at I.M. injection site.

INTERACTIONS

CNS depressants, ethanol: additive CNS depression. Avoid concomitant use.

CONTRAINDICATIONS

• Contraindicated in children with viral illness (a possible cause of vomiting in children); may contribute to development of Reye's syndrome, a potentially fatal acute childhood encephalopathy, characterized by fatty degeneration of the liver.
• Suppositories contraindicated in patients hypersensitive to benzocaine hydrochloride or similar local anesthetic.

NURSING CONSIDERATIONS

• Withhold drug if skin hypersensitivity reaction occurs.
• Like other antiemetics, may mask signs of overdosage of toxic agents or symptoms of intestinal obstruction, brain tumor, or other conditions.
• For I.M. administration, inject deeply into upper outer quadrant of gluteal region to reduce pain and local irritation.
• Advise patients of the possibility of drowsiness and dizziness, and caution against driving or other activities requiring alertness until CNS effects of the drug are known.
• Refrigerate suppositories.

51

Antiulcer agents

cimetidine
famotidine
misoprostol
nizatidine
omeprazole
ranitidine hydrochloride
sucralfate

COMBINATION PRODUCTS
None.

cimetidine

Tagamet

Pregnancy Risk Category: B

HOW SUPPLIED
Tablets: 200 mg, 300 mg, 400 mg, 800 mg
Oral liquid: 300 mg/5 ml
Effervescent tablets: 800 mg‡
Injection: 100 mg/ml‡, 150 mg/ml; 300 mg in 50 ml 0.9% sodium chloride solution injection

ACTION
Mechanism: Competitively inhibits the action of histamine (H_2) at receptor sites of the parietal cells, decreasing gastric acid secretion.
Onset: 45 to 60 minutes. **Peak:** Plasma levels peak 45 to 90 minutes after oral dose. **Duration:** plasma elimination half-life, about 2 hours; therapeutic effects last 4 to 8 hours.

INDICATIONS & DOSAGE
Duodenal ulceration (short-term treatment) –
Adults and children over 16 years: 800 mg P.O. h.s. Alternatively, give 400 mg P.O. b.i.d. or 300 mg q.i.d. (with meals and h.s.). Continue treatment for 4 to 6 weeks unless endoscopy shows healing. For maintenance therapy, give 400 mg h.s. For parenteral therapy, give 300 mg diluted to 20 ml with 0.9% sodium chloride solution or other compatible I.V. solution by I.V. push over 1 to 2 minutes q 6 hours; or 300 mg diluted in 50 ml D_5W or other compatible I.V. solution by I.V. infusion over 15 to 20 minutes q 6 hours; or 300 mg I.M. q 6 hours (no dilution necessary). To increase dosage, give 300-mg doses more frequently to maximum daily dosage of 2,400 mg. Alternatively, give 900 mg/day (37.5 mg/hour) diluted in 100 to 1,000 ml of compatible solution by continuous I.V. infusion.
Duodenal ulceration prophylaxis –
Adults and children over 16 years: 400 mg P.O. h.s.
Active benign gastric ulceration –
Adults: 300 mg P.O. q.i.d. with meals and h.s. for up to 8 weeks.
Pathologic hypersecretory conditions (such as Zollinger-Ellison syndrome, systemic mastocytosis, and multiple endocrine adenomas) –
Adults and children over 16 years: 300 mg P.O. q.i.d. with meals and h.s.; adjust to individual needs. Maximum daily dosage is 2,400 mg.
For parenteral therapy, give 300 mg diluted to 20 ml with 0.9% sodium chloride solution or other compatible I.V. solution by I.V. push over 1 to 2 minutes q 6 hours; or 300 mg diluted in 50 ml dextrose 5% solution or other compatible I.V. solution by I.V. infusion over 15 to 20 minutes q 6 hours. To increase dosage, give 300-mg doses more frequently to maximum daily dosage of 2,400 mg.
Gastroesophageal reflux disease –
Adults: 800 mg P.O. b.i.d. or 400 mg q.i.d. before meals and h.s.
Prevention of upper GI bleeding in critically ill patients –
Adults: 50 mg/hour by continuous

I.V. infusion for up to 7 days. Give 25 mg/hour to patients with creatinine clearance below 30 ml/minute/1.73 m^2.

ADVERSE REACTIONS

CNS: mental confusion, dizziness, headaches, peripheral neuropathy.
CV: bradycardia.
GI: *mild and transient diarrhea.*
GU: transient elevations in serum creatinine levels.
Hematologic: ***agranulocytosis, neutropenia, thrombocytopenia, aplastic anemia*** (rare).
Hepatic: jaundice (rare).
Skin: acnelike rash, urticaria.
Other: hypersensitivity reactions, muscle pain, mild gynecomastia after use longer than 1 month.

INTERACTIONS

Antacids: interference with cimetidine absorption. Separate administration by at least 1 hour if possible.
Lidocaine, phenytoin, propranolol, some benzodiazepines, warfarin: inhibited hepatic microsomal enzyme metabolism of these drugs. Monitor serum levels of these drugs.

CONTRAINDICATIONS

- Contraindicated in patients hypersensitive to the drug.
- Use cautiously in elderly or debilitated patients because they may be more susceptible to cimetidine-induced mental confusion.

NURSING CONSIDERATIONS

- **I.V. use:** Don't infuse I.V. too rapidly; may cause bradycardia. When administering cimetidine I.V. in 100 ml of diluent solution, do not infuse so rapidly that circulatory overload is produced. Some authorities recommend infusing drug over at least 30 minutes, to minimize risk of adverse cardiac effects. Sometimes administered as continuous I.V. infusion. Use infusion pump if given in a total volume of 250 ml over 24 hours or less.
- I.V. solutions compatible for dilution with cimetidine include 0.9% sodium chloride solution, D_5W and $D_{10}W$ (and combinations of these), lactated Ringer's solution, and 5% sodium bicarbonate injection. Do not dilute with sterile water for injection.
- I.M. administration may be painful.
- Hemodialysis reduces blood levels of cimetidine. Schedule cimetidine dose at end of hemodialysis treatment. Adjust dosage as ordered in patients with renal failure.
- Up to 10 g overdosage has been reported without adverse reactions.
- Give tablets with meals to ensure a more consistent therapeutic effect.
- Remind patients taking cimetidine once daily to take it at bedtime for best results.
- Identify tablet strength when obtaining a drug history.
- Urge patients to avoid cigarette smoking because it may increase gastric acid secretion and worsen disease.
- Effectiveness in treatment of gastric ulceration not as great as in duodenal ulceration. Cimetidine may prove useful but is still unapproved in pancreatic insufficiency, short-bowel syndrome, psoriasis, prevention and treatment of GI bleeding, and prevention of gastric inactivation of oral enzyme preparations by gastric acid and pepsin.
- Although not recommended for children under 16 years, doses of 20 to 40 mg/kg/day have been used.
- Has been used investigationally before anesthesia for prophylaxis of aspiration pneumonitis and to treat hyperparathyroidism, herpes zoster, and chronic hives.

famotidine

Pepcid, Pepcidine‡

Pregnancy Risk Category: B

HOW SUPPLIED

Tablets: 20 mg, 40 mg
Powder for oral suspension: 40 mg/5 ml after reconstitution
Injection: 10 mg/ml

ACTION

Mechanism: Competitively inhibits the action of histamine (H_2) at receptor sites of the parietal cells, decreasing gastric acid secretion.
Onset: within 1 hour. **Peak:** Peak effects occur within 20 minutes of I.V. injection, 1 to 3 hours after oral administration. **Duration:** up to 12 hours; half-life, 2½ to 3½ hours.

INDICATIONS & DOSAGE

Duodenal ulceration –
Adults: For acute therapy, 40 mg P.O. once daily h.s. For maintenance therapy, give 20 mg P.O. once daily h.s.
Benign gastric ulceration –
Adults: 40 mg P.O. daily h.s. for 8 weeks.
Pathologic hypersecretory conditions (such as Zollinger-Ellison syndrome) –
Adults: 20 mg P.O. q 6 hours. May administer up to 160 mg q 6 hours.
Hospitalized patients with intractable ulcerations or hypersecretory conditions or patients who cannot take oral medication –
Adults: 20 mg I.V. q 12 hours.
Gastroesophageal reflux disease (GERD) –
Adults: 20 mg P.O. b.i.d. for up to 6 weeks. For esophagitis caused by GERD, give 20 to 40 mg b.i.d. for up to 12 weeks.

ADVERSE REACTIONS

CNS: *headache,* dizziness, hallucinations.
GI: diarrhea, constipation, nausea, flatulence.
GU: increased BUN and creatinine levels.
Hematologic: ***thrombocytopenia*** (rare).
Skin: acne, pruritus, rash.
Other: transient irritation at I.V. site.

INTERACTIONS

None significant.

CONTRAINDICATIONS

- Contraindicated in patients hypersensitive to the drug.

NURSING CONSIDERATIONS

- Advise the patient not to take drug for longer than 8 weeks unless the doctor specifically orders it.
- With doctor's knowledge, the patient may take antacids concomitantly, especially at the beginning of therapy when pain is severe.
- Urge the patient to avoid cigarette smoking because it may increase gastric acid secretion and worsen disease.
- Tell the patient to take famotidine with a snack if desired.
- Remind the patient that drug is most effective if taken at bedtime.
- Tell patients taking famotidine 20 mg b.i.d. to take at least one dose at bedtime.
- **I.V. use:** To prepare I.V. injection, dilute 2 ml (20 mg) famotidine with compatible I.V. solution to a total volume of either 5 or 10 ml and inject over at least 2 minutes. Compatible solutions include sterile water for injection, 0.9% sodium chloride injection, D_5W or $D_{10}W$ injection, 5% sodium bicarbonate injection, and lactated Ringer's injection.
- Alternatively, give famotidine by intermittent I.V. infusion. Dilute 20 mg (2 ml) famotidine in 100 ml of compatible solution and infuse over 15 to 30 minutes. Solution is stable for 48 hours at room temperature after dilution.
- Store I.V. injection in refrigerator at 36° to 46° F (2° to 8° C).
- Store reconstituted suspension below 86° F (30° C). Discard after 30 days.

misoprostol

Cytotec

Pregnancy Risk Category: X

HOW SUPPLIED

Tablets: 100 mcg, 200 mcg

ACTION

Mechanism: A synthetic prostaglandin E_1 analogue that replaces gastric prostaglandins depleted by NSAID therapy. Misoprostol also decreases basal and stimulated gastric acid secretion and may increase gastric mucus and bicarbonate production.
Onset: 30 minutes. **Peak:** Plasma levels peak within 10 to 15 minutes.
Duration: about 3 hours.

INDICATIONS & DOSAGE

Prevention of NSAID-induced gastric ulcerations in elderly or debilitated patients at high risk for complications from gastric ulceration and patients with a history of NSAID-induced ulcerations –
Adults: 200 mcg P.O. q.i.d. with food. If dosage isn't tolerated, decrease to 100 mcg P.O. q.i.d.

ADVERSE REACTIONS

CNS: headache.
GI: *diarrhea, abdominal pain,* nausea, flatulence, dyspepsia, vomiting, constipation.
Other: hypermenorrhea, dysmenorrhea, spotting, cramps, menstrual disorders.

INTERACTIONS

Antacids: reduced plasma levels when administered concomitantly. Not considered significant.

CONTRAINDICATIONS

• Contraindicated in patients hypersensitive to prostaglandins and in pregnant patients.
• Don't routinely administer to women of childbearing age unless they are at high risk for developing ulcerations or complications from NSAID-induced ulcerations.

NURSING CONSIDERATIONS

• Take special precautions to prevent use of drug during pregnancy. Make sure the patient is fully aware of the dangers of misoprostol to a fetus and that she receives both oral and written warnings regarding these dangers. Also ensure that the patient can comply with effective contraceptive means and that she has a negative serum pregnancy test within 2 weeks of initiating therapy.
• Do not begin misoprostol therapy until the second or third day of the next normal menstrual period.
• Instruct all patients not to share misoprostol. Remind them that when taken by a pregnant patient this drug may cause miscarriage, often with potentially life-threatening bleeding.
• Used investigationally for the prophylaxis and treatment of gastric ulceration, reflux esophagitis, ethanol-induced gastritis, hemorrhagic gastritis, and fat malabsorption in patients with cystic fibrosis.

nizatidine

Axid, Tazac‡

Pregnancy Risk Category: C

HOW SUPPLIED

Capsules: 150 mg, 300 mg

ACTION

Mechanism: Competitively inhibits the action of histamine (H_2) at receptor sites of the parietal cells, decreasing gastric acid secretion.
Onset: within 30 minutes. **Peak:** Peak levels occur in ½ to 3 hours.
Duration: up to 12 hours.

INDICATIONS & DOSAGE
Active duodenal ulceration –
Adults: 300 mg P.O. daily h.s. Alternatively, give 150 mg b.i.d.
Maintenance therapy of duodenal ulceration –
Adults: 150 mg daily h.s.
Benign gastric ulceration –
Adults: 150 mg P.O. b.i.d. or 300 mg h.s. for 8 weeks.
Gastroesophageal reflux disease –
Adults: 150 mg P.O. b.i.d.
In patients with impaired renal function: If creatinine clearance is 20 to 50 ml/minute/1.73 m^2, give 150 mg daily for treatment of active duodenal ulceration or 150 mg every other day for maintenance therapy; if creatinine clearance is below 20 ml/minute/1.73 m^2, give 150 mg every other day for treatment or 150 mg every third day for maintenance.

ADVERSE REACTIONS
CNS: *somnolence.*
CV: arrhythmias.
Hematologic: ***thrombocytopenia.***
Skin: *diaphoresis,* rash, urticaria, ***exfoliative dermatitis.***
Other: liver damage, hyperuricemia, fever.

INTERACTIONS
Aspirin: possibly elevated serum salicylate levels (high-dose).
Tomato-based mixed-vegetable juices: may decrease potency of the drug when used concomitantly. Monitor diet.

CONTRAINDICATIONS
- Contraindicated in patients hypersensitive to H_2-receptor antagonists and in pregnant patients.
- Use cautiously and in reduced dosages in patients with impaired renal function.

NURSING CONSIDERATIONS
- False-positive test results for urobilinogen may occur.
- Nizatidine has not been associated with antiandrogenic activity and does not appear to affect hepatic drug-metabolizing enzyme systems.
- Urge patients to avoid cigarette smoking because it may increase gastric acid secretion and worsen disease.
- Capsules may be opened and contents mixed with apple juice. However, drug has been shown to lose some potency when combined with tomato-based mixed-vegetable juices. Check with pharmacist for compatibility.

omeprazole
Prilosec, Losec†‡

Pregnancy Risk Category: C

HOW SUPPLIED
Capsules (delayed-release): 20 mg

ACTION
Mechanism: Inhibits the activity of the acid (proton) pump, and binds to hydrogen/potassium adenosine triphosphatase, located at the secretory surface of the gastric parietal cell to block the formation of gastric acid.
Onset: within 1 hour. **Peak:** Peak effects occur within 2 hours. **Duration:** 3 days or more; may take 4 days for gastric acid production to return to normal.

INDICATIONS & DOSAGE
Severe erosive esophagitis; symptomatic, poorly responsive gastroesophageal reflux disease (GERD) –
Adults: 20 mg P.O. daily for 4 to 8 weeks. Patients with GERD should have failed initial therapy with a histamine H_2 antagonist.
Pathologic hypersecretory conditions (such as Zollinger-Ellison syndrome) –
Adults: initially, 60 mg P.O. daily; titrate dosage according to patient response. If daily dosage exceeds 80 mg, administer in divided doses. Dos-

ages up to 120 mg t.i.d. have been given. Continue therapy as long as clinically indicated.
Duodenal ulceration –
Adults: 20 mg P.O. daily for 4 to 8 weeks.

ADVERSE REACTIONS
CNS: headache, dizziness.
GI: diarrhea, abdominal pain, nausea, vomiting, constipation, flatulence.
Respiratory: cough.
Skin: rash.
Other: back pain.

INTERACTIONS
Ampicillin esters, iron derivatives, ketoconazole: may exhibit poor bioavailability in patients taking omeprazole because optimal absorption of these drugs requires a low gastric pH.
Diazepam, phenytoin, warfarin: decreased hepatic clearance, possibly leading to increased serum levels. Monitor closely.

CONTRAINDICATIONS
• Contraindicated in patients hypersensitive to the drug or any component of the formulation.
• Prolonged (2-year) studies in rats revealed a dose-related increase in gastric carcinoid tumors; studies in humans have not detected a risk from short-term exposure. Further study is needed to assess the impact of sustained hypergastrinemia and hypochlorhydria. The manufacturer recommends that therapy with omeprazole not exceed the indicated duration.

NURSING CONSIDERATIONS
• Tell the patient to swallow capsules whole and not to open or crush.
• Omeprazole increases its own bioavailability with repeated administration. Drug is labile in gastric acid; less drug is lost to hydrolysis because the drug increases gastric pH.
• Dosage adjustments are not required for renal or hepatic impairment.
• Most patients with duodenal ulcers heal within 4 weeks. Don't use omeprazole for maintenance therapy.

ranitidine hydrochloride
Apo-Ranitidine†, Zantac*, Zantac-C†

Pregnancy Risk Category: B

HOW SUPPLIED
Tablets: 150 mg, 300 mg
Dispersible tablets: 150 mg‡
Effervescent tablets: 150 mg
Effervescent granules: 150 mg
Syrup: 15 mg/ml*
Injection: 25 mg/ml
Infusion: 0.5 mg/ml in 100-ml containers

ACTION
Mechanism: Competitively inhibits the action of histamine (H_2) at receptor sites of the parietal cells, decreasing gastric acid secretion.
Onset: within 1 hour. **Peak:** Peak effects occur in 1 to 3 hours. **Duration:** up to 13 hours.

INDICATIONS & DOSAGE
Duodenal and gastric ulceration (short-term treatment); pathological hypersecretory conditions, such as Zollinger-Ellison syndrome –
Adults: 150 mg P.O., b.i.d. or 300 mg daily h.s. Alternatively, give 50 mg I.V. or I.M. q 6 to 8 hours. Patients with Zollinger-Ellison syndrome may require dosages up to 6 g daily.
Maintenance therapy of duodenal ulceration –
Adults: 150 mg P.O., h.s.
Gastroesophageal reflux disease (GERD) –
Adults: 150 mg P.O. b.i.d.
Erosive esophagitis –
Adults: 150 mg P.O. q.i.d.

ADVERSE REACTIONS
CNS: headache, malaise, dizziness, confusion.
CV: bradycardia.
GI: nausea, constipation.
Hematologic: ***neutropenia, thrombocytopenia.***
Hepatic: elevated liver enzymes, jaundice.
Skin: rash.
Other: burning and itching at injection site.

INTERACTIONS
Antacids: possible interference with ranitidine absorption. Stagger doses if possible.
Diazepam: decreased absorption of diazepam.
Glipizide: possible increased hypoglycemic effect. Adjust glipizide dosage as necessary.
Procainamide: possible decreased renal clearance of procainamide.
Warfarin: possible interference with warfarin clearance.

CONTRAINDICATIONS
- Contraindicated in patients hypersensitive to the drug.
- Use cautiously in patients with hepatic dysfunction. Adjust dosage in patients with impaired renal function.

NURSING CONSIDERATIONS
- Take without regard to meals; absorption not affected by food.
- Drug is incompatible with aluminum. Avoid using aluminum-based needles or other equipment when mixing or administering drug.
- Remind patients taking ranitidine once daily to take it at bedtime for best results.
- Urge patients to avoid cigarette smoking because it may increase gastric acid secretion and worsen disease.
- **I.V. use:** When administering by I.V. push, dilute to a total volume of 20 ml and inject over a period of 5 minutes. No dilution is necessary when administering I.M. May also be administered by intermittent I.V. infusion: dilute 50 mg ranitidine in 100 ml of D_5W and infuse over 15 to 20 minutes. Alternatively, give by continuous I.V. infusion: 150 mg in 250 ml of compatible solution. Administer at 6.25 mg/hour using an infusion pump. When administering premixed I.V. infusion, give by slow I.V. drip (over 15 to 20 minutes). Do not add other drugs to the solution. If used with a primary I.V. fluid system, discontinue the primary solution during the infusion.
- To prepare I.V. injection, dilute 50 mg (2 ml) in 100 ml of compatible solution and infuse over 15 to 20 minutes. Compatible solutions include 0.9% sodium chloride injection, D_5W or $D_{10}W$ injection, 5% sodium bicarbonate injection, or lactated Ringer's injection.

sucralfate
Carafate, SCF‡, Sulcrate†

Pregnancy Risk Category: B

HOW SUPPLIED
Tablets: 1 g

ACTION
Mechanism: Adheres to and protects the ulceration surface by forming a barrier.
Duration: up to 6 hours.

INDICATIONS & DOSAGE
Short-term (up to 8 weeks) treatment of duodenal ulceration –
Adults: 1 g P.O. q.i.d. 1 hour before meals and h.s.
Maintenance therapy of duodenal ulceration –
Adults: 1 g P.O. b.i.d.

ADVERSE REACTIONS
CNS: dizziness, sleepiness.
GI: *constipation,* nausea, gastric discomfort, diarrhea, bezoar formation.

INTERACTIONS
Antacids: may decrease binding of drug to gastroduodenal mucosa, impairing effectiveness. Don't administer within 30 minutes of each other. *Cimetidine, ciprofloxacin, digoxin, norfloxacin, phenytoin, ranitidine, tetracycline, theophylline:* decreased absorption. Separate administration times by at least 2 hours.

CONTRAINDICATIONS
None reported.

NURSING CONSIDERATIONS
- Drug is minimally absorbed. Low incidence of adverse reactions.
- Tell patient for best results to take sucralfate on an empty stomach (1 hour before each meal and at bedtime).
- Pain and ulcerative symptoms may subside within first few weeks of therapy. Tell patients to continue on prescribed regimen to ensure complete healing.
- Monitor for severe, persistent constipation.
- Studies suggest that sucralfate is as effective as cimetidine in healing duodenal ulcerations.
- Drug has been used to treat gastric ulcerations, but effectiveness of this use is still under investigation.
- Drug contains aluminum but isn't classified as an antacid.
- Urge patients to avoid cigarette smoking because it may increase gastric acid secretion and worsen disease.

52

Corticosteroids

betamethasone
betamethasone acetate and betamethasone sodium phosphate
betamethasone sodium phosphate
cortisone acetate
dexamethasone
dexamethasone acetate
dexamethasone sodium phosphate
fludrocortisone acetate
hydrocortisone
hydrocortisone acetate
hydrocortisone cypionate
hydrocortisone sodium phosphate
hydrocortisone sodium succinate
methylprednisolone
methylprednisolone acetate
methylprednisolone sodium succinate
paramethasone acetate
prednisolone
prednisolone acetate
prednisolone acetate and prednisolone sodium phosphate
prednisolone sodium phosphate
prednisolone steaglate
prednisolone tebutate
prednisone
triamcinolone
triamcinolone acetonide
triamcinolone diacetate
triamcinolone hexacetonide

COMBINATION PRODUCTS

DECADRON WITH XYLOCAINE: dexamethasone phosphate 4 mg and lidocaine hydrochloride 10 mg/ml.

betamethasone

Betnelan†, Betnesol†, Celestone*

betamethasone acetate and betamethasone sodium phosphate

Celestone Chronodose‡, Celestone Soluspan

betamethasone sodium phosphate

Celestone Phosphate, Selestoject

Pregnancy Risk Category: C

HOW SUPPLIED

betamethasone
Tablets: 600 mcg
Tablets (extended-release): 1 mg
Tablets (effervescent): 500 mcg†
Syrup: 600 mcg/5 ml
betamethasone acetate and betamethasone sodium phosphate
Injection (suspension): betamethasone acetate 3 mg and betamethasone sodium phosphate (equivalent to 3-mg base)/ml
betamethasone sodium phosphate
Tablets (effervescent): 500 mcg*
Injection: 4 mg (3-mg base)/ml in 5-ml vials

ACTION

Mechanism: Decreases inflammation, mainly by stabilizing leukocyte lysosomal membranes; suppresses the immune response; stimulates bone marrow; and influences protein, fat, and carbohydrate metabolism.
Onset: 1 to 3 hours after I.M. injection. **Duration:** 3 days after oral or I.M. use; 1 to 2 weeks after intra-articular or intralesional use of suspension.

INDICATIONS & DOSAGE

Severe inflammation or immunosuppression –
Adults: 0.6 to 7.2 mg P.O. daily; or 0.5 to 9 mg (sodium phosphate) I.M.,

I.V., or into joint or soft tissue daily; or 1.5 to 12 mg of sodium phosphate-acetate suspension into joint or soft tissue q 1 to 2 weeks, p.r.n.
Prevention of neonatal respiratory distress syndrome –
Adults (pregnant women): 12 mg I.M. of betamethasone acetate or betamethasone sodium phosphate-acetate suspension 36 to 48 hours before premature delivery. Repeat in 24 hours.

ADVERSE REACTIONS
Most adverse reactions to corticosteroids are dose- or duration-dependent.
CNS: *euphoria, insomnia,* psychotic behavior, pseudotumor cerebri.
CV: ***CHF,*** hypertension, edema.
EENT: cataracts, glaucoma.
GI: *peptic ulceration,* GI irritation, increased appetite, pancreatitis.
Skin: delayed wound healing, acne, various skin eruptions.
Other: muscle weakness, osteoporosis, hirsutism, susceptibility to infections; hypokalemia, hyperglycemia, and carbohydrate intolerance; growth suppression in children, ***acute adrenal insufficiency may follow increased stress (infection, surgery, or trauma) or abrupt withdrawal after long-term therapy***.
After abrupt withdrawal: rebound inflammation, fatigue, weakness, arthralgia, fever, dizziness, lethargy, depression, fainting, orthostatic hypotension, dyspnea, anorexia, hypoglycemia. ***After prolonged use, sudden withdrawal may be fatal.***

INTERACTIONS
Aspirin, indomethacin, and other NSAIDs: increased risk of GI distress and bleeding. Give together cautiously.
Barbiturates, phenytoin, rifampin: decreased corticosteroid effect. Corticosteroid dose may need to be increased.
Oral anticoagulants: altered dosage requirements. Monitor PT closely.
Potassium-depleting drugs such as thiazide diuretics: enhanced potassium-wasting effects of betamethasone. Monitor serum potassium levels.
Skin-test antigens: decreased response. Defer skin testing until therapy is completed.
Toxoids and vaccines: decreased antibody response and increased risk of neurologic complications. Avoid concomitant use.

CONTRAINDICATIONS
- Contraindicated in patients hypersensitive to the drug and in those with systemic fungal infections.
- Use cautiously in patients with GI ulceration or renal disease, hypertension, osteoporosis, varicella, vaccinia, exanthema, diabetes mellitus, Cushing's syndrome, thromboembolic disorders, seizures, myasthenia gravis, CHF, tuberculosis, ocular herpes simplex, hypoalbuminemia, emotional instability, and psychotic tendencies. Because some formulations contain sulfite preservatives, also use cautiously in patients sensitive to sulfites.

NURSING CONSIDERATIONS
- Elderly patients may be more susceptible to osteoporosis. Advise patients receiving long-term therapy to consider exercise or physical therapy. Give vitamin D or calcium supplements as ordered.
- Don't use for alternate-day therapy.
- Always titrate to lowest effective dose.
- Gradually reduce drug dosage after long-term therapy. Tell patients not to stop drug abruptly or without the doctor's consent.
- Adrenal suppression may last up to 1 year after drug is stopped.
- A calorie- or sodium-restricted diet with protein supplementation may be

necessary for patients receiving long-term therapy.
• Watch for additional potassium depletion from diuretics and amphotericin B. Potassium supplements may be necessary for patients receiving long-term therapy.
• Make sure patients understand to contact the doctor if symptoms are worsening or the medication is no longer effective. Tell patients not to increase dosage without the doctor's consent.
• Teach patients about the drug's effects. Warn those on long-term therapy about cushingoid symptoms and to report sudden weight gain or swelling to the doctor.
• Make sure patients report symptoms associated with corticosteroid withdrawal, including fatigue, weakness, arthralgia, orthostatic hypotension, and dyspnea.
• Observe for signs of infection, especially after steroid withdrawal. Tell patients to report slow healing.
• Instruct patients to carry a card indicating their need for supplemental glucocorticoids during stress.
• Obtain baseline weight before starting therapy, and weigh patients daily; report any sudden weight gain to the doctor.
• Monitor blood glucose and serum potassium levels regularly. Diabetic patients may require adjustments in insulin dosage.
• Advise patients receiving prolonged therapy to have periodic ophthalmic examinations.
• Periodic measurement of growth and development may be necessary during high-dose or prolonged therapy in children.
• Monitor for depression or mood changes, especially in patients receiving long-term therapy.
• For better results and less toxicity, give a daily dose in the morning.
• To reduce GI irritation, give with milk or food.
• Tell patients using the effervescent tablets to dissolve them in water immediately before ingestion.
• To prevent muscle atrophy, give I.M. injection deeply. Rotate injection sites.
• **I.V. use:** Compatible with 0.9% sodium chloride, D_5W, lactated Ringer's injection, dextrose 5% in lactated Ringer's injection, and dextrose 5% in Ringer's injection.

cortisone acetate

Cortate‡, Cortone Acetate

Pregnancy Risk Category: D

HOW SUPPLIED

Tablets: 5 mg, 10 mg, 25 mg
Injection (suspension): 25 mg/ml, 50 mg/ml

ACTION

Mechanism: Decreases inflammation, mainly by stabilizing leukocyte lysosomal membranes; suppresses the immune response; stimulates bone marrow; and influences protein, fat, and carbohydrate metabolism.
Onset: rapid after oral administration, slow after I.M. injection. **Peak:** Peak effects occur within 2 hours of oral dose or within 20 to 48 hours after I.M. injection. **Duration:** 30 to 36 hours.

INDICATIONS & DOSAGE

Adrenal insufficiency, allergy, inflammation –
Adults: 25 to 300 mg P.O. or I.M. daily or on alternate days. Dosages are highly individualized, depending on severity of disease.

ADVERSE REACTIONS

Most adverse reactions to corticosteroids are dose- or duration-dependent.
CNS: *euphoria, insomnia,* psychotic behavior, pseudotumor cerebri.
CV: ***CHF,*** hypertension, edema.

EENT: cataracts, glaucoma.
GI: *peptic ulceration,* GI irritation, increased appetite, pancreatitis.
Skin: delayed wound healing, acne, various skin eruptions; atrophy at I.M. injection sites.
Other: muscle weakness, osteoporosis, hirsutism, susceptibility to infections; possible hypokalemia, hyperglycemia, and carbohydrate intolerance; growth suppression in children, ***acute adrenal insufficiency may follow increased stress (infection, surgery, or trauma) or abrupt withdrawal after long-term therapy.***
After abrupt withdrawal: rebound inflammation, fatigue, weakness, arthralgia, fever, dizziness, lethargy, depression, fainting, orthostatic hypotension, dyspnea, anorexia, hypoglycemia. ***After prolonged use, sudden withdrawal may be fatal.***

INTERACTIONS
Aspirin, indomethacin, and other NSAIDS: increased risk of GI distress and bleeding. Give together cautiously.
Barbiturates, phenytoin, rifampin: decreased corticosteroid effect. Increase corticosteroid dose as ordered.
Live attenuated virus vaccines, other toxoids and vaccines: decreased antibody response and increased risk of neurologic complications. Avoid concomitant use.
Oral anticoagulants: altered dosage requirements. Monitor PT closely.
Potassium-depleting drugs such as thiazide diuretics: enhanced potassium-wasting effects of cortisone. Monitor serum potassium levels.
Skin-test antigens: decreased response. Defer skin testing until therapy is completed.

CONTRAINDICATIONS
- Contraindicated in patients with systemic fungal infections. Injection is contraindicated in patients sensitive to sulfites.
- Use cautiously in patients with GI ulceration or renal disease, hypertension, osteoporosis, varicella, vaccinia, exanthema, diabetes mellitus, Cushing's syndrome, thromboembolic disorders, seizures, myasthenia gravis, CHF, tuberculosis, ocular herpes simplex, hypoalbuminemia, emotional instability, and psychotic tendencies.

NURSING CONSIDERATIONS
- Elderly patients may be more susceptible to osteoporosis. Advise patients receiving long-term therapy to consider exercise or physical therapy. Give vitamin D or calcium supplements as ordered.
- Gradually reduce drug dosage after long-term therapy. Tell patients not to discontinue drug abruptly or without the doctor's consent.
- Always titrate to lowest effective dose.
- Patients may need low-sodium diet and potassium supplements.
- Drug of choice for replacement therapy in adrenal insufficiency.
- Observe for signs of infection, especially after steroid withdrawal. Tell patients to report slow healing.
- Immunizations may show decreased antibody response.
- Monitor serum electrolyte and blood glucose levels.
- Watch for additional potassium depletion from diuretics and amphotericin B.
- Warn patients on long-term therapy about cushingoid symptoms and to report sudden weight gain or swelling to the doctor.
- Instruct patients to carry a card indicating their need for supplemental glucocorticoids during stress.
- To reduce GI irritation, give with milk or food.
- For better results and less toxicity, give a daily dose in the morning.
- Not for I.V. use.
- I.M. route causes slow onset of ac-

tion. Don't use in acute conditions where a rapid effect is required. May use on a twice-daily schedule matching diurnal variation. Rotate injection sites to prevent muscle atrophy.

• Mixing or diluting parenteral suspension may alter absorption rate and decrease the drug's effectiveness.

dexamethasone

Decadron*, Deronil†, Dexamethasone Intensol*, Dexasone†, Dexone 0.5, Dexone 0.75, Dexone 1.5, Dexone 4, Hexadrol*, Mymethasone*

dexamethasone acetate

Dalalone D.P., Dalalone L.A., Decadron L.A., Decaject-L.A., Dexacen LA-8, Dexasone-LA, Dexone LA, Solurex-LA

dexamethasone sodium phosphate

Ak-Dex, Dalalone, Decadrol, Decadron Phosphate, Decaject, Dexacen-4, Dexone, Hexadrol Phosphate, Solurex

Pregnancy Risk Category: C

HOW SUPPLIED

dexamethasone

Tablets: 0.25 mg, 0.5 mg, 0.75 mg, 1 mg, 1.5 mg, 2 mg, 4 mg, 6 mg

Oral solution: 0.5 mg/5 ml, 1 mg/ml

Elixir: 0.5 mg/5 ml*

dexamethasone acetate

Injection: 8 mg/ml, 16 mg/ml suspension

dexamethasone sodium phosphate

Injection: 4 mg/ml, 10 mg/ml, 20 mg/ml, 24 mg/ml

ACTION

Mechanism: Decreases inflammation, mainly by stabilizing leukocyte lysosomal membranes; suppresses the immune response; stimulates bone marrow; and influences protein, fat, and carbohydrate metabolism.

Onset: within 1 hour after I.M. or I.V. administration; 1 to 2 hours after oral administration. **Peak:** Peak effects occur within 1 hour after I.M. or I.V. administration, within 1 to 2 hours after oral administration, or within 8 hours after use of the injectable suspension (acetate). **Duration:** about 2½ days after oral use, 6 days after I.M. use (acetate), and up to 3 weeks after intralesional or intra-articular use (acetate or sodium phosphate).

INDICATIONS & DOSAGE

Cerebral edema –

Adults: initially, 10 mg (phosphate) I.V.; then 4 to 6 mg I.M. q 6 hours for 2 to 4 days; then tapered over 5 to 7 days.

Children: initially, 0.5 to 1.5 mg/kg I.V. daily; then 0.2 to 0.5 mg/kg I.V. daily in divided doses q 6 hours.

Inflammatory conditions, allergic reactions, neoplasias –

Adults: 0.25 to 4 mg P.O. b.i.d., t.i.d., or q.i.d.; or 4 to 16 mg (acetate) I.M. into joint or soft tissue q 1 to 3 weeks; or 0.8 to 1.6 mg (acetate) into lesions q 1 to 3 weeks.

Shock –

Adults: 1 to 6 mg/kg (phosphate) I.V. as a single dose; or 40 mg q 2 to 6 hours, p.r.n.

Dexamethasone suppression test for Cushing's syndrome –

Adults: after determining 24-hour urine levels of 17-hydroxycorticosteroids, give 0.5 mg P.O. q 6 hours for 48 hours.

Adjunct for bacterial meningitis –

Infants and children: 0.15 mg/kg I.V. (phosphate) q.i.d. for the first 4 days of anti-infective therapy.

Prevention of hyaline membrane disease in neonates –

Adults: 4 mg I.M. (phosphate) b.i.d. for 2 days before delivery.

To prevent chemotherapy-induced nausea and vomiting –

Adults: 10 to 20 mg I.V. (phosphate)

at least 30 minutes before administering emetogenic chemotherapy.

ADVERSE REACTIONS

Most adverse reactions to corticosteroids are dose- or duration-dependent.

CNS: *euphoria, insomnia,* psychotic behavior, pseudotumor cerebri.

CV: ***CHF,*** hypertension, edema.

EENT: cataracts, glaucoma.

GI: *peptic ulceration,* GI irritation, increased appetite, pancreatitis.

Skin: delayed wound healing, acne, various skin eruptions; atrophy at I.M. injection sites.

Other: muscle weakness, osteoporosis, hirsutism, susceptibility to infections; hypokalemia, hyperglycemia, and carbohydrate intolerance; growth suppression in children, ***acute adrenal insufficiency may follow increased stress (infection, surgery, or trauma) or abrupt withdrawal after long-term therapy.***

After abrupt withdrawal: rebound inflammation, fatigue, weakness, arthralgia, fever, dizziness, lethargy, depression, fainting, orthostatic hypotension, dyspnea, anorexia, hypoglycemia. ***After prolonged use, sudden withdrawal may be fatal.***

INTERACTIONS

Aspirin, indomethacin, and other NSAIDs: increased risk of GI distress and bleeding. Give together cautiously.

Barbiturates, phenytoin, rifampin: decreased corticosteroid effect. Increase corticosteroid dose as ordered.

Oral anticoagulants: altered dosage requirements. Monitor PT closely.

Potassium-depleting drugs such as thiazide diuretics: enhanced potassium-wasting effects of dexamethasone. Monitor serum potassium levels.

Skin-test antigens: decreased response. Defer skin testing until therapy is completed.

Toxoids and vaccines: decreased antibody response and increased risk of neurologic complications. Avoid concomitant use.

CONTRAINDICATIONS

- Contraindicated in patients hypersensitive to any component of the drug; in those with systemic fungal infections, and for alternate-day therapy. Injectable forms may contain sulfites, which can cause an allergic reaction in sensitive patients.
- Use cautiously in patients with GI ulceration or renal disease, hypertension, osteoporosis, varicella, vaccinia, exanthema, diabetes mellitus, Cushing's syndrome, thromboembolic disorders, seizures, myasthenia gravis, metastatic cancer, CHF, tuberculosis, ocular herpes simplex, hypoalbuminemia, emotional instability, and psychotic tendencies, and in children.

NURSING CONSIDERATIONS

- Elderly patients may be more susceptible to osteoporosis. Advise patients receiving long-term therapy to consider exercise or physical therapy. Give vitamin D or calcium supplements as ordered.
- Gradually reduce drug dosage after long-term therapy. Tell patients not to discontinue drug abruptly or without the doctor's consent.
- Always titrate to lowest effective dose.
- For better results and less toxicity, give a daily dose in the morning.
- Dexamethasone most recently used in the diagnosis of depression.
- Monitor patients' weight, blood pressure, and serum electrolyte levels.
- Instruct patients to carry a card indicating their need for supplemental systemic glucocorticoids during stress, especially as dosage is decreased.
- Warn patients on long-term therapy about cushingoid symptoms and to re-

port sudden weight gain or swelling to the doctor.
- Watch for additional potassium depletion from diuretics and amphotericin B. Potassium supplements may be necessary.
- Teach patients signs of early adrenal insufficiency: fatigue, muscular weakness, joint pain, fever, anorexia, nausea, dyspnea, dizziness, and fainting.
- May mask or exacerbate infections, including latent amebiasis.
- Watch for depression or psychotic episodes, especially in high-dose therapy.
- Inspect patients' skin for petechiae. Warn patients about easy bruising.
- Diabetic patients may need increased insulin; monitor blood glucose levels.
- Monitor growth in infants and children on long-term therapy.
- Advise patients receiving long-term therapy to have periodic ophthalmic examinations.
- Give P.O. dose with food when possible.
- Give I.M. injection deep into gluteal muscle. Rotate injection sites to prevent muscle atrophy. Avoid S.C. injection because atrophy and sterile abscesses may occur.
- **I.V. use:** When administering as direct injection, inject undiluted over at least 1 minute. When administering as an intermittent or continuous infusion, dilute solution according to the manufacturer's instructions and give over the prescribed duration. If used for continuous infusion, change solution every 24 hours.

---

fludrocortisone acetate

Florinef

Pregnancy Risk Category: C

HOW SUPPLIED

Tablets: 0.1 mg

ACTION

Mechanism: Increases sodium reabsorption and potassium and hydrogen secretion at the nephron's distal convoluted tubule.

Duration: 1 to 2 days; biological half-life, 18 to 36 hours.

INDICATIONS & DOSAGE

Adrenal insufficiency (partial replacement), adrenogenital syndrome –

Adults: 0.1 to 0.2 mg P.O. daily.

ADVERSE REACTIONS

CV: *sodium and water retention,* hypertension, cardiac hypertrophy, edema.

Other: hypokalemia.

INTERACTIONS

Potassium-depleting drugs such as thiazide diuretics: enhanced potassium-wasting effects of fludrocortisone. Monitor serum potassium levels.

CONTRAINDICATIONS

- Contraindicated in patients with hypertension, CHF, or cardiac disease.
- Use cautiously in patients with Addison's disease.

NURSING CONSIDERATIONS

- Monitor patients' blood pressure and serum electrolyte levels. If hypertension occurs, decrease dosage by 50%.
- Weigh patients daily; report sudden weight gain to the doctor.
- Tell patients to report worsening symptoms, such as hypotension, weakness, cramping, and palpitations, to the doctor.
- Warn patients that mild peripheral edema is common.
- Unless contraindicated, give low-sodium diet high in potassium and protein. Potassium supplements may be needed.
- Watch for additional potassium de-

pletion from diuretics and amphotericin B.

- Used with cortisone or hydrocortisone in adrenal insufficiency.
- Also prescribed to treat chronic severe orthostatic hypotension caused by levodopa therapy or diabetes mellitus.

hydrocortisone
Cortef, Cortenema, Hydrocortone

hydrocortisone acetate
Cortifoam, Hydrocortone Acetate

hydrocortisone cypionate
Cortef

hydrocortisone sodium phosphate
Hydrocortone Phosphate

hydrocortisone sodium succinate
A-HydroCort, Solu-Cortef

Pregnancy Risk Category: C

HOW SUPPLIED
hydrocortisone
Tablets: 5 mg, 10 mg, 20 mg
Injection: 25 mg/ml*, 50 mg/ml* suspension
Enema: 100 mg/60 ml
hydrocortisone acetate
Injection: 25 mg/ml*, 50 mg/ml* suspension
Enema: 10% aerosol foam (provides 90 mg/application)
Suppositories: 25 mg
hydrocortisone cypionate
Oral suspension: 10 mg/5 ml
hydrocortisone sodium phosphate
Injection: 50 mg/ml solution
hydrocortisone sodium succinate
Injection: 100 mg/vial*, 250 mg/vial*, 500 mg/vial*, 1,000 mg/vial*

ACTION
Mechanism: Decreases inflammation, mainly by stabilizing leukocyte lysosomal membranes; suppresses the immune response; stimulates bone marrow; and influences protein, fat, and carbohydrate metabolism.
Peak: Peak levels occur within 1 hour of oral or I.M. injection or immediately after an I.V. injection. **Duration:** plasma half-life, 80 to 118 minutes; biological half-life, 8 to 12 hours; anti-inflammatory action, 30 to 48 hours after single dose.

INDICATIONS & DOSAGE
Severe inflammation, adrenal insufficiency–
Adults: 5 to 30 mg P.O. b.i.d., t.i.d., or q.i.d. (as much as 80 mg q.i.d. may be given in acute situations); or initially, 100 to 250 mg (succinate) I.M. or I.V., and then 50 to 100 mg I.M., as indicated; or 15 to 240 mg (phosphate) I.M. or I.V. q 12 hours; or 5 to 75 mg (acetate) into joints or soft tissue. Dosage varies with size of joint. Local anesthetics are often injected with dose.
Shock–
Adults: initially, 50 mg/kg I.V. (succinate), repeated in 4 hours. Repeat dosage q 24 hours as needed. Alternatively, give 500 mg to 2 g q 2 to 6 hours.
Children: 0.16 to 1 mg/kg (phosphate or succinate) I.M. or I.V., b.i.d. or t.i.d.
Adjunct for ulcerative colitis and proctitis–
Adults: 1 enema (100 mg) P.R. nightly for 21 days.

ADVERSE REACTIONS
Most adverse reactions to corticosteroids are dose- or duration-dependent.
CNS: *euphoria, insomnia,* psychotic behavior, pseudotumor cerebri.
CV: ***CHF,*** hypertension, edema.
EENT: cataracts, glaucoma.
GI: *peptic ulceration,* GI irritation, increased appetite, pancreatitis.

Skin: delayed wound healing, acne, various skin eruptions, easy bruising.
Other: muscle weakness, osteoporosis, hirsutism, susceptibility to infections; possible hypokalemia, hyperglycemia, and carbohydrate intolerance; growth suppression in children, ***acute adrenal insufficiency may occur with increased stress (infection, surgery, or trauma) or abrupt withdrawal after long-term therapy.***
After abrupt withdrawal: rebound inflammation, fatigue, weakness, arthralgia, fever, dizziness, lethargy, depression, fainting, orthostatic hypotension, dyspnea, anorexia, hypoglycemia. ***After prolonged use, sudden withdrawal may be fatal.***

INTERACTIONS

Aspirin, indomethacin, and other NSAIDs: increased risk of GI distress and bleeding. Give together cautiously.
Barbiturates, phenytoin, rifampin: decreased corticosteroid effect. Increase corticosteroid dose as ordered.
Live attenuated virus vaccines, other toxoids and vaccines: decreased antibody response and increased risk of neurologic complications. Avoid concomitant use.
Oral anticoagulants: altered dosage requirements. Monitor PT closely.
Potassium-depleting drugs such as thiazide diuretics: enhanced potassium-wasting effects of hydrocortisone. Monitor serum potassium levels.
Skin-test antigens: decreased response. Defer skin testing until therapy is completed.

CONTRAINDICATIONS

- Contraindicated in patients allergic to any component of the formulation, and in those with systemic fungal infections. Certain injectable forms contain sulfites, which can cause an allergic reaction in sensitive patients.
- Use cautiously in patients with GI ulceration or renal disease, hypertension, osteoporosis, varicella, vaccinia, exanthema, diabetes mellitus, Cushing's syndrome, thromboembolic disorders, seizures, myasthenia gravis, metastatic cancer, CHF, tuberculosis, ocular herpes simplex, hypoalbuminemia, emotional instability, and psychotic tendencies, and in children.

NURSING CONSIDERATIONS

- Elderly patients may be more susceptible to osteoporosis. Advise patients receiving long-term therapy to consider exercise or physical therapy. Give vitamin D or calcium supplements as ordered.
- High-dose therapy is usually not continued beyond 48 hours.
- Always titrate to lowest effective dose.
- Gradually reduce drug dosage after long-term therapy. Tell patients not to discontinue the drug abruptly or without the doctor's consent.
- Unless contraindicated, give low-sodium diet high in potassium and protein. Administer potassium supplements as needed. Watch for additional potassium depletion from diuretics and amphotericin B.
- Warn patients on long-term therapy about cushingoid symptoms and to report sudden weight gain or swelling to the doctor.
- Monitor patients' weight, blood pressure, and serum electrolyte levels.
- May mask or exacerbate infections, including latent amebiasis.
- Instruct patients to carry a card identifying their need for supplemental systemic glucocorticoids during stress.
- Stress (fever, trauma, surgery, and emotional problems) may increase adrenal insufficiency. Increase dose as ordered.
- Teach patients signs of early adrenal insufficiency: fatigue, muscular weakness, joint pain, fever, anorexia,

nausea, dyspnea, dizziness, and fainting.
- Watch for depression or psychotic episodes, especially during high-dose therapy.
- Inspect patients' skin for petechiae. Warn patients about easy bruising.
- Diabetic patients may need increased insulin; monitor blood glucose levels.
- Advise patients receiving prolonged therapy to have periodic ophthalmic examinations.
- Periodic measurement of growth and development may be necessary during high-dose or prolonged therapy in children.
- For better results and less toxicity, give a daily dose in the morning.
- **I.V. use:** Do not use the acetate or suspension form for I.V. use. When administering as direct injection, inject directly into vein or an I.V. line containing a free-flowing compatible solution over 30 seconds to several minutes. When administering as an intermittent or continuous infusion, dilute solution according to manufacturer's instructions and give over the prescribed duration. If used for continuous infusion, change solution every 24 hours.
- Hydrocortisone sodium phosphate may be added directly to D_5W or 0.9% sodium chloride for I.V. administration.
- Reconstitute hydrocortisone sodium succinate with bacteriostatic water or bacteriostatic sodium chloride solution before adding to I.V. solutions. When giving by direct I.V. injection, inject over at least 30 seconds. For infusion, dilute with D_5W, 0.9% sodium chloride, or 5% dextrose in 0.9% sodium chloride to a concentration of 1 mg/ml or less.
- Give I.M. injection deep into gluteal muscle. Rotate injection sites to prevent muscle atrophy. Avoid S.C. injection because atrophy and sterile abscesses may occur.
- Do not confuse Solu-Cortef with Solu-Medrol (methyl prednisolone sodium succinate).
- Injectable forms not used for alternate-day therapy.
- Give P.O. dose with food when possible.
- Enema may produce same systemic effects as other forms of hydrocortisone. If enema therapy must exceed 21 days, discontinue gradually by reducing administration to every other night for 2 or 3 weeks.

methylprednisolone
Medrol**, Meprolone

methylprednisolone acetate
depMedalone-40, depMedalone-80, Depoject-40, Depoject-80, Depo-Medrol, Depopred-40, Depopred-80, Depo-Predate 40, Depo-Predate 80, Duralone-40, Duralone-80, Medralone-40, Medralone-80, Medrol Enpak

methylprednisolone sodium succinate
A-Metha-pred, Solu-Medrol

Pregnancy Risk Category: C

HOW SUPPLIED

methylprednisolone

Tablets: 2 mg, 4 mg, 8 mg, 16 mg, 24 mg, 32 mg

methylprednisolone acetate

Injection (suspension): 20 mg/ml, 40 mg/ml, 80 mg/ml

Enema: 40 mg

methylprednisolone sodium succinate

Injection: 40 mg/vial, 125 mg/vial, 500 mg/vial, 1,000 mg/vial, 2,000 mg/vial

ACTION

Mechanism: Decreases inflammation, mainly by stabilizing leukocyte lysosomal membranes; suppresses the

immune response; stimulates bone marrow; and influences protein, fat, and carbohydrate metabolism.
Onset: rapid after I.V. or oral administration; slow (6 to 48 hours) after I.M. injection of acetate suspension.
Peak: Peak effects ocur immediately after I.V. injection, within 1 to 2 hours after oral administration, 4 to 8 days after I.M. use, or 7 days after intralesional or intra-articular administration. **Duration:** 30 to 36 hours after oral administration, 1 to 4 weeks after I.M. use, or 1 to 5 weeks after intralesional or intra-articular administration.

INDICATIONS & DOSAGE
Severe inflammation or immunosuppression –
Adults: 2 to 60 mg P.O. daily in four divided doses; or 40 to 80 mg (acetate) I.M. daily, or 10 to 250 mg (succinate) I.M. or I.V. q 4 hours; or 4 to 30 mg (acetate) into joint or soft tissue, p.r.n.
Children: 117 mcg to 1.66 mg/kg (succinate) daily I.V. in three or four divided doses.
Shock –
Adults: 100 to 250 mg (succinate) I.V. at 2- to 6-hour intervals; or 30 mg/kg I.V. initially, repeated q 4 to 6 hours p.r.n. Continue therapy for 2 to 3 days or until the patient is stable.
To decrease residual damage after spinal cord trauma –
Adults: 30 mg/kg (succinate) I.V. as a bolus injection within 8 hours of the injury, followed by a continuous infusion of 5.4 mg/kg/hour for the next 23 hours.
Adjunct for Pneumocystis carinii *pneumonia –*
Adults and children 12 years and older: initiate treatment within 1 to 3 days of starting anti-infective therapy. Initially, 30 mg I.V. (succinate) b.i.d. for 5 days; then 30 mg daily for 5 days. Finally, give 15 mg I.V. daily for 11 days or until anti-infective treatment is stopped.
Proctitis –
Adults: 40 mg P.R. as a retention enema or treatment by continuous I.V. drip three to seven times a week for at least 2 weeks.
Children: 500 mcg to 1 mg/kg or 15 to 30 mg/m² P.R. q 1 to 2 days for at least 2 weeks.

ADVERSE REACTIONS
Most adverse reactions to corticosteroids are dose- or duration-dependent.
CNS: *euphoria, insomnia,* psychotic behavior, pseudotumor cerebri.
CV: ***CHF,*** hypertension, edema.
EENT: cataracts, glaucoma.
GI: *peptic ulceration,* GI irritation, increased appetite, pancreatitis.
Skin: delayed wound healing, acne, various skin eruptions.
Other: muscle weakness, osteoporosis, hirsutism, susceptibility to infections; hypokalemia, hyperglycemia, and carbohydrate intolerance; growth suppression in children, ***acute adrenal insufficiency may occur with increased stress (infection, surgery, or trauma) or abrupt withdrawal after long-term therapy.***
After abrupt withdrawal: rebound inflammation, fatigue, weakness, arthralgia, fever, dizziness, lethargy, depression, fainting, orthostatic hypotension, dyspnea, anorexia, hypoglycemia. ***After prolonged use, sudden withdrawal may be fatal.***

INTERACTIONS
Aspirin, indomethacin, and other NSAIDs: increased risk of GI distress and bleeding. Give together cautiously.
Barbiturates, phenytoin, rifampin: decreased corticosteroid effect. Increase corticosteroid dose as ordered.
Oral anticoagulants: altered dosage requirements. Monitor PT closely.
Potassium-depleting drugs such as

thiazide diuretics: enhanced potassium-wasting effects of methylprednisolone. Monitor serum potassium levels.
Skin-test antigens: decreased response. Defer skin testing until therapy is completed.
Toxoids and vaccines: decreased antibody response and increased risk of neurologic complications. Avoid concomitant use.

CONTRAINDICATIONS
• Contraindicated in patients allergic to any component of the formulation and in those with systemic fungal infections. Certain injectable forms contain sulfites, which can cause an allergic reaction in sensitive patients.
• Use cautiously in patients with GI ulceration or renal disease, hypertension, osteoporosis, varicella, vaccinia, exanthema, diabetes mellitus, Cushing's syndrome, thromboembolic disorders, seizures, myasthenia gravis, metastatic cancer, CHF, tuberculosis, ocular herpes simplex, hypoalbuminemia, emotional instability, and psychotic tendencies.

NURSING CONSIDERATIONS
• Elderly patients may be more susceptible to osteoporosis. Advise patients receiving long-term therapy to consider exercise or physical therapy. Give vitamin D or calcium supplements as ordered.
• Gradually reduce drug dosage after long-term therapy. Tell patients not to discontinue drug abruptly or without the doctor's consent.
• Always titrate to lowest effective dose.
• Monitor patients' weight, blood pressure, serum electrolyte levels, and sleep patterns. Euphoria may initially interfere with sleep, but patients generally adjust to the medication after 1 to 3 weeks.
• Warn patients on long-term therapy about cushingoid symptoms and to report sudden weight gain or swelling to the doctor.
• May mask or exacerbate infections, including latent amebiasis.
• Instruct patients to carry a card identifying their need for supplemental systemic glucocorticoids during stress.
• Teach patients signs of early adrenal insufficiency: fatigue, muscular weakness, joint pain, fever, anorexia, nausea, dyspnea, dizziness, and fainting.
• Watch for depression or psychotic episodes, especially in high-dose therapy.
• Diabetic patients may need increased insulin; monitor blood glucose levels.
• Watch for an enhanced response to drug in patients with hypothyroidism or cirrhosis.
• Unless contraindicated, give low-sodium diet high in potassium and protein. Administer potassium supplements as needed. Watch for additional potassium depletion from diuretics and amphotericin B.
• May be used for alternate-day therapy.
• For better results and less toxicity, give a daily dose in the morning.
• Give P.O. dose with food when possible. Critically ill patients may require concomitant antacid or histamine$_2$-receptor antagonist therapy.
• **I.V. use:** Use only methylprednisolone sodium succinate; never use acetate form for I.V. use. Reconstitute according to the manufacturer's directions using the supplied diluent, or use bacteriostatic water for injection with benzyl alcohol.
• When administering as direct injection, inject diluted drug into a vein or free-flowing compatible I.V. solution over at least 1 minute. For treatment of shock, give massive doses over at least 10 minutes to prevent arrhythmias and circulatory collapse. When

administering as an intermittent or continuous infusion, dilute solution according to the manufacturer's instructions and give over the prescribed duration. If used for continuous infusion, change solution every 24 hours.

- Compatible solutions include D_5W, 0.9% sodium chloride, and dextrose 5% in 0.9% sodium chloride.
- Give I.M. injection deep into gluteal muscle. Avoid S.C. injection because atrophy and sterile abscesses may occur.
- Dermal atrophy may occur with large doses of acetate salt. Use multiple small injections rather than a single large dose and rotate injection sites.
- Don't use acetate salt when immediate onset of action is needed.
- Discard reconstituted solutions after 48 hours.
- The manufacturers of Solu-Medrol state that the drug should not be given intrathecally because severe adverse reactions have been reported.
- Do not confuse Solu-Medrol with Solu-Cortef (hydrocortisone sodium succinate).

paramethasone acetate

Haldrone

Pregnancy Risk Category: C

HOW SUPPLIED

Tablets: 2 mg

ACTION

Mechanism: Decreases inflammation, mainly by stabilizing leukocyte lysosomal membranes; suppresses the immune response; stimulates bone marrow; and influences protein, fat, and carbohydrate metabolism.

Onset: 1 to 2 hours. **Duration:** 2 days.

INDICATIONS & DOSAGE

Inflammatory conditions –

Adults: 0.5 to 6 mg P.O. t.i.d. or q.i.d.

Children: 58 to 800 mcg/kg P.O. daily in divided doses t.i.d. or q.i.d.

ADVERSE REACTIONS

Most adverse reactions to corticosteroids are dose- or duration-dependent.

CNS: *euphoria, insomnia,* psychotic behavior, pseudotumor cerebri.

CV: ***CHF,*** hypertension, edema.

EENT: cataracts, glaucoma.

GI: *peptic ulceration,* GI irritation, increased appetite, pancreatitis.

Skin: delayed wound healing, acne, various skin eruptions.

Other: muscle weakness, osteoporosis, hirsutism, susceptibility to infections; hypokalemia, hyperglycemia, and carbohydrate intolerance; growth suppression in children, ***acute adrenal insufficiency may occur with increased stress (infection, surgery, or trauma) or abrupt withdrawal after long-term therapy.***

After abrupt withdrawal: rebound inflammation, fatigue, weakness, arthralgia, fever, dizziness, lethargy, depression, fainting, orthostatic hypotension, dyspnea, anorexia, hypoglycemia. ***After prolonged use, sudden withdrawal may be fatal.***

INTERACTIONS

Aspirin, indomethacin, and other NSAIDs: increased risk of GI distress and bleeding. Give together cautiously.

Barbiturates, phenytoin, rifampin: decreased corticosteroid effect. Increase corticosteroid dose as ordered.

Oral anticoagulants: altered dosage requirements. Monitor PT closely.

Potassium-depleting drugs such as thiazide diuretics: enhanced potassium-wasting effects of paramethasone. Monitor serum potassium levels.

Skin-test antigens: decreased response. Defer skin testing until therapy is completed.
Toxoids and vaccines: decreased antibody response and increased risk of neurologic complications. Avoid concomitant use.

CONTRAINDICATIONS

- Contraindicated in patients with systemic fungal infections and during alternate-day therapy.
- Use cautiously in patients with GI ulceration or renal disease, hypertension, osteoporosis, varicella, vaccinia, exanthema, diabetes mellitus, Cushing's syndrome, thromboembolic disorders, seizures, myasthenia gravis, metastatic cancer, CHF, tuberculosis, ocular herpes simplex, hypoalbuminemia, emotional instability, and psychotic tendencies.

NURSING CONSIDERATIONS

- Elderly patients may be more susceptible to osteoporosis. Advise patients receiving long-term therapy to consider exercise or physical therapy. Give vitamin D or calcium supplements as ordered.
- Gradually reduce drug dosage after long-term therapy. Tell patients not to discontinue drug abruptly or without the doctor's consent.
- Titrate to lowest effective dose.
- Monitor patients' weight, blood pressure, and serum electrolyte levels.
- May mask or exacerbate infections, including latent amebiasis.
- Instruct patients to carry a card identifying their need for supplemental systemic glucocorticoids during stress.
- For better results and less toxicity, give a daily dose in the morning.
- Teach patients signs of early adrenal insufficiency: fatigue, muscular weakness, joint pain, fever, anorexia, nausea, dyspnea, dizziness, and fainting.
- Warn patients on long-term therapy about cushingoid symptoms and to report sudden weight gain or swelling to the doctor.
- Watch for depression or psychotic episodes with high-dose therapy.
- Diabetic patients may need increased insulin; monitor blood glucose levels.
- Monitor growth in infants and children on long-term therapy.
- Advise patients receiving long-term therapy to have periodic ophthalmic examinations.
- Unless contraindicated, give low-sodium diet high in potassium and protein. Administer potassium supplements as needed. Watch for additional hypokalemia from diuretics and amphotericin B.
- Give P.O. dose with food when possible, especially if GI irritation occurs.

prednisolone
Delta-Cortef, Deltasolone‡, Panafcortelone‡, Prelone, Solone‡

prednisolone acetate
Articulose-50, Key-Pred 25, Key-Pred 50, Predaject-50, Predalone-50, Predate-50, Predcor-50, Predicort-50

prednisolone acetate and prednisolone sodium phosphate

prednisolone sodium phosphate
Hydeltrasol, Key-Pred-SP, Pediapred, Predate-S, Predicort RP, Predsol Retention Enema‡, Predsol Suppositories‡

prednisolone steaglate
Sintisone‡

prednisolone tebutate

Hydeltra-TBA, Nor-Pred TBA, Predalone TBA, Predate TBA, Predcor TBA

Pregnancy Risk Category: B

HOW SUPPLIED

prednisolone
Tablets: 1 mg‡, 5 mg, 25 mg‡
Syrup: 15 mg/5 ml
prednisolone acetate
Injection (suspension): 25 mg/ml, 50 mg/ml, 100 mg/ml
prednisolone acetate and prednisolone sodium phosphate
Injection (suspension): 80 mg acetate and 20 mg sodium phosphate/ml
prednisolone sodium phosphate
Oral solution: 5 mg/5 ml
Injection: 20 mg/ml
Retention enema: 20 mg/100 ml‡
Suppositories: 5 mg‡
prednisolone steaglate
Tablets: 6.65 mg (equal to 3.5 mg prednisolone)‡
prednisolone tebutate
Injection (suspension): 20 mg/ml

ACTION

Mechanism: Decreases inflammation, mainly by stabilizing leukocyte lysosomal membranes; suppresses the immune response; stimulates bone marrow; and influences protein, fat, and carbohydrate metabolism.
Onset: rapid after I.V., I.M., or oral administration; 1 to 2 days after intralesional or intra-articular use of tebutate suspension. **Peak:** Peak levels occur within 1 hour of I.M. or I.V. injection or within 1 to 2 hours of oral administration. **Duration:** 30 to 36 hours after oral use; up to 4 weeks after I.M. use, or 3 days to 4 weeks after intralesional or intra-articular use.

INDICATIONS & DOSAGE

Severe inflammation or immunosuppression –
Adults: 2.5 to 15 mg P.O. b.i.d., t.i.d., or q.i.d.; 2 to 30 mg I.M. (acetate, phosphate) or I.V. (phosphate) q 12 hours; or 2 to 30 mg (phosphate) into joints, lesions, or soft tissue; or 4 to 40 mg (tebutate) into joints and lesions; or 0.25 to 1 ml (sodium phosphate-acetate suspension) into joints weekly, p.r.n.
Proctitis‡ –
Adults: 1 suppository b.i.d., preferably in the morning and h.s.
Ulcerative colitis‡ –
Adults: 1 retention enema h.s. nightly for 2 to 4 weeks. The contents of the enema should be retained overnight.

ADVERSE REACTIONS

Most adverse reactions to corticosteroids are dose- or duration-dependent.
CNS: *euphoria, insomnia,* psychotic behavior, pseudotumor cerebri.
CV: ***CHF,*** hypertension, edema.
EENT: cataracts, glaucoma.
GI: *peptic ulceration,* GI irritation, increased appetite, pancreatitis.
Skin: delayed wound healing, acne, various skin eruptions.
Other: muscle weakness, osteoporosis, hirsutism, susceptibility to infections; hypokalemia, hyperglycemia, and carbohydrate intolerance; growth suppression in children, ***acute adrenal insufficiency may occur with increased stress (infection, surgery, or trauma) or abrupt withdrawal after long-term therapy.***
After abrupt withdrawal: rebound inflammation, fatigue, weakness, arthralgia, fever, dizziness, lethargy, depression, fainting, orthostatic hypotension, dyspnea, anorexia, hypoglycemia. ***After prolonged use, sudden withdrawal may be fatal.***

INTERACTIONS

Aspirin, indomethacin, and other NSAIDs: increased risk of GI distress and bleeding. Give together cautiously.
Barbiturates, phenytoin, rifampin: de-

*Liquid form contains alcohol. *Common* reactions are in italics; ***life-threatening,*** in bold italics.
**May contain tartrazine.

creased corticosteroid effect. Increase corticosteroid dose as ordered.
Oral anticoagulants: altered dosage requirements. Monitor PT closely.
Potassium-depleting drugs such as thiazide diuretics: enhanced potassium-wasting effects of prednisolone. Monitor serum potassium levels.
Skin-test antigens: decreased response. Defer skin testing until therapy is completed.
Toxoids and vaccines: decreased antibody response and increased risk of neurologic complications. Avoid concomitant use.

CONTRAINDICATIONS

- Contraindicated in patients with systemic fungal infections.
- Use cautiously in patients with GI ulceration or renal disease, hypertension, osteoporosis, varicella, vaccinia, exanthema, diabetes mellitus, Cushing's syndrome, thromboembolic disorders, seizures, myasthenia gravis, metastatic cancer, CHF, tuberculosis, ocular herpes simplex, hypoalbuminemia, emotional instability, and psychotic tendencies.

NURSING CONSIDERATIONS

- Don't confuse with prednisone.
- Elderly patients may be more susceptible to osteoporosis. Advise patients receiving long-term therapy to consider exercise or physical therapy. Give vitamin D or calcium supplements as ordered.
- Gradually reduce drug dosage after long-term therapy. Tell patients not to discontinue drug abruptly or without the doctor's consent.
- Always titrate to lowest effective dose.
- Prednisolone salts (acetate, sodium phosphate, and tebutate) are used parenterally less often than other corticosteroids that have more potent anti-inflammatory action.
- May be used for alternate-day therapy.
- Monitor patients' weight, blood pressure, and serum electrolyte levels.
- May mask or exacerbate infections, including latent amebiasis. Tell patients to report slow healing.
- Instruct patients to carry a card identifying their need for supplemental systemic glucocorticoids during stress.
- Teach patients signs of early adrenal insufficiency: fatigue, muscular weakness, joint pain, fever, anorexia, nausea, dyspnea, dizziness, and fainting.
- Warn patients on long-term therapy about cushingoid symptoms and to report sudden weight gain or swelling to the doctor.
- Watch for depression or psychotic episodes, especially in high-dose therapy.
- Diabetic patients may need increased insulin; monitor blood glucose levels.
- Unless contraindicated, give low-sodium diet high in potassium and protein. Administer potassium supplements as needed. Watch for additional potassium depletion from diuretics and amphotericin B.
- **I.V. use:** Use only prednisolone sodium phosphate; never give acetate form I.V. When administering as direct injection, inject undiluted over at least 1 minute. When administering as an intermittent or continuous infusion, dilute solution according to the manufacturer's instructions and give over the prescribed duration. D_5W or 0.9% sodium chloride are recommended as diluents for I.V. infusions.
- Give I.M. injection deep into gluteal muscle. Rotate injection sites to prevent muscle atrophy. Avoid S.C. injection because atrophy and sterile abscesses may occur.
- Give P.O. dose with food when possible to reduce GI irritation.

prednisone

Apo-Prednisone†, Deltasone, Liquid Pred*, Meticorten, Novo-prednisone†, Orasone, Panafcort‡, Panasol, Prednicen-M, Prednisone Intensol*, Sone‡, Sterapred, Winpred†

Pregnancy Risk Category: B

HOW SUPPLIED

Tablets: 1 mg, 2.5 mg, 5 mg, 10 mg, 20 mg, 25 mg, 50 mg
Oral solution: 5 mg/5 ml*, 5 mg/ml (concentrate)*
Syrup: 5 mg/5 ml*

ACTION

Mechanism: Decreases inflammation, mainly by stabilizing leukocyte lysosomal membranes; suppresses the immune response; stimulates bone marrow; and influences protein, fat, and carbohydrate metabolism.
Peak: Peak effect occurs in 1 to 2 hours. **Duration:** 30 to 36 hours.

INDICATIONS & DOSAGE

Severe inflammation or immunosuppression –
Adults: 2.5 to 15 mg P.O. b.i.d., t.i.d., or q.i.d. Give maintenance dosage once daily or every other day. Dosage must be individualized.
Children: 0.14 to 2 mg/kg P.O. daily in divided doses q.i.d.
Acute exacerbations of multiple sclerosis –
Adults: 200 mg P.O. daily for 1 week; then 80 mg every other day for 1 month.
Adjunct for Pneumocystis carinii *pneumonia –*
Adults and children over age 12: initiate therapy within 1 to 3 days of anti-infective therapy. Start treatment with 40 mg P.O. b.i.d. for 5 days; then 40 mg for 5 days. Finally, give 20 mg for 11 days or until anti-infective therapy is stopped.

ADVERSE REACTIONS

Most adverse reactions to corticosteroids are dose- or duration-dependent.
CNS: *euphoria, insomnia,* psychotic behavior, pseudotumor cerebri.
CV: ***CHF,*** hypertension, edema.
EENT: cataracts, glaucoma.
GI: *peptic ulceration,* GI irritation, increased appetite, pancreatitis.
Skin: delayed wound healing, acne, various skin eruptions.
Other: muscle weakness, osteoporosis, hirsutism, susceptibility to infections; hypokalemia, hyperglycemia, and carbohydrate intolerance; growth suppression in children, ***acute adrenal insufficiency may occur with increased stress (infection, surgery, or trauma) or abrupt withdrawal after long-term therapy.***
After abrupt withdrawal: rebound inflammation, fatigue, weakness, arthralgia, fever, dizziness, lethargy, depression, fainting, orthostatic hypotension, dyspnea, anorexia, hypoglycemia. ***After prolonged use, sudden withdrawal may be fatal.***

INTERACTIONS

Aspirin, indomethacin, and other NSAIDs: increased risk of GI distress and bleeding. Give together cautiously.
Barbiturates, phenytoin, rifampin: decreased corticosteroid effect. Increase corticosteroid dose as ordered.
Oral anticoagulants: altered dosage requirements. Monitor PT closely.
Potassium-depleting drugs such as thiazide diuretics: enhanced potassium-wasting effects of prednisone. Monitor serum potassium levels.
Skin-test antigens: decreased response. Defer skin testing until therapy is completed.
Toxoids and vaccines: decreased antibody response and increased risk of neurologic complications. Avoid concomitant use.

CONTRAINDICATIONS

• Contraindicated in patients with systemic fungal infections.

• Use cautiously in patients with GI ulceration or renal disease, hypertension, osteoporosis, varicella, vaccinia, exanthema, diabetes mellitus, Cushing's syndrome, thromboembolic disorders, seizures, myasthenia gravis, metastatic cancer, CHF, tuberculosis, ocular herpes simplex, hypoalbuminemia, emotional instability, and psychotic tendencies.

NURSING CONSIDERATIONS

• Don't confuse with prednisolone.

• Elderly patients may be more susceptible to osteoporosis. Advise patients receiving long-term therapy to consider exercise or physical therapy. Give vitamin D or calcium supplements as ordered.

• Gradually reduce drug dosage after long-term therapy. Tell patients not to discontinue drug abruptly or without the doctor's consent.

• Always titrate to lowest effective dose.

• May be used for alternate-day therapy.

• Monitor patients' blood pressure, sleep patterns, and serum potassium levels.

• Weigh patients daily; report sudden weight gain to the doctor.

• May mask or exacerbate infections, including latent amebiasis. Tell patients to report slow healing.

• Instruct patients to carry a card identifying their need for supplemental systemic glucocorticoids during stress.

• For better results and less toxicity, give a daily dose in the morning.

• Teach patients signs of early adrenal insufficiency: fatigue, muscular weakness, joint pain, fever, anorexia, nausea, dyspnea, dizziness, and fainting.

• Warn patients on long-term therapy about cushingoid symptoms and to report sudden weight gain or swelling to the doctor.

• Watch for depression or psychotic episodes, especially in high-dose therapy.

• Diabetic patients may need increased insulin; monitor blood glucose levels.

• Monitor growth in infants and children on long-term therapy.

• Advise patients receiving long-term therapy to have periodic opththalmic examinations.

• Unless contraindicated, give low-sodium diet high in potassium and protein. Administer potassium supplements as needed. Watch for additional potassium depletion from diuretics and amphotericin B.

• Unless contraindicated, give P.O. dose with food when possible to reduce GI irritation.

triamcinolone

Aristocort, Atolone, Kenacort**

triamcinolone acetonide

Cenocort A-40, Cinonide-40, Kenaject-40, Kenalog, Kenalog-40, Tac-3, Triam-A, Triamonide-40, Tri-Kort, Trilog

triamcinolone diacetate

Amcort, Aristocort, Aristocort Forte, Aristocort Intralesional, Articulose-L.A., Cenocort Forte, Cinalone-40, Kenacort Diacetate, Triam-Forte, Triamolone-40, Trilone, Tristoject

triamcinolone hexacetonide

Aristospan Intra-articular, Aristospan Intralesional

Pregnancy Risk Category: C

HOW SUPPLIED

triamcinolone

Tablets: 1 mg, 2 mg, 4 mg, 8 mg
Syrup: 2 mg/ml, 4 mg/ml

triamcinolone acetonide
Injection (suspension): 3 mg/ml, 10 mg/ml, 40 mg/ml
triamcinolone diacetate
Injection (suspension): 25 mg/ml, 40 mg/ml
triamcinolone hexacetonide
Injection (suspension): 5 mg/ml, 20 mg/ml

ACTION

Mechanism: Decreases inflammation, mainly by stabilizing leukocyte lysosomal membranes; suppresses the immune response; stimulates bone marrow; and influences protein, fat, and carbohydrate metabolism.
Onset: 1 to 2 days after I.M. injection. **Peak:** Peak effects occur within 1 to 2 hours after oral administration.
Duration: about 2 days after oral use, 1 to 6 weeks after I.M. use, or 1 to 8 weeks after intralesional or intra-articular use.

INDICATIONS & DOSAGE

Severe inflammation or immunosuppression–
Adults: 4 to 48 mg P.O. daily in divided doses b.i.d., t.i.d., or q.i.d.; 40 mg I.M. (diacetate, acetonide) weekly; 5 to 48 mg (diacetate, acetonide) into lesions; 2 to 40 mg (diacetate, acetonide) into joints or soft tissue; up to 0.5 mg (hexacetonide) per square inch of affected skin intralesionally; or 2 to 20 mg (hexacetonide) by intra-articular or intrasynovial use into soft tissue or into joint or lesion. A local anesthetic is often injected along with triamcinolone into the joint.

ADVERSE REACTIONS

Most adverse reactions to corticosteroids are dose- or duration-dependent.
CNS: *euphoria, insomnia,* psychotic behavior, pseudotumor cerebri.
CV: ***CHF,*** hypertension, edema.
EENT: cataracts, glaucoma.
GI: *peptic ulceration,* GI irritation, increased appetite, pancreatitis.
Skin: delayed wound healing, acne, various skin eruptions.
Other: muscle weakness, osteoporosis, hirsutism, susceptibility to infections; hypokalemia, hyperglycemia, and carbohydrate intolerance; growth suppression in children, ***acute adrenal insufficiency may occur with increased stress (infection, surgery, or trauma) or abrupt withdrawal after long-term therapy.***
After abrupt withdrawal: rebound inflammation, fatigue, weakness, arthralgia, fever, dizziness, lethargy, depression, fainting, orthostatic hypotension, dyspnea, anorexia, hypoglycemia. ***After prolonged use, sudden withdrawal may be fatal.***

INTERACTIONS

Aspirin, indomethacin, and other NSAIDs: increased risk of GI distress and bleeding. Give together cautiously.
Barbiturates, phenytoin, rifampin: decreased corticosteroid effect. Increase corticosteroid dose as ordered.
Oral anticoagulants: altered dosage requirements. Monitor PT closely.
Potassium-depleting drugs such as thiazide diuretics: enhanced potassium-wasting effects of triamcinolone. Monitor serum potassium levels.
Skin-test antigens: decreased response. Defer skin testing until therapy is completed.
Toxoids and vaccines: decreased antibody response and increased risk of neurologic complications. Avoid concomitant use.

CONTRAINDICATIONS

• Contraindicated in patients hypersensitive to any component of the formulation or in those with systemic fungal infections. Injectable form may contain sulfites, which can cause an allergic response in sensitive pa-

tients. Also, do not use to treat adrenocortical insufficiency.
• Use cautiously in patients with GI ulceration or renal disease, hypertension, osteoporosis, varicella, vaccinia, exanthema, diabetes mellitus, Cushing's syndrome, thromboembolic disorders, seizures, myasthenia gravis, metastatic cancer, CHF, tuberculosis, ocular herpes simplex, hypoalbuminemia, emotional instability, and psychotic tendencies.

NURSING CONSIDERATIONS
• Elderly patients may be more susceptible to osteoporosis. Advise patients receiving long-term therapy to consider exercise or physical therapy. Give vitamin D or calcium supplements as ordered.
• Gradually reduce drug dosage after long-term therapy. Tell patients not to discontinue drug abruptly or without the doctor's consent.
• Always titrate to lowest effective dose.
• Monitor patients' weight, blood pressure, and serum electrolyte levels.
• May mask or exacerbate infections, including latent amebiasis. Tell patients to report slow healing.
• Instruct patients to carry a card identifying their need for supplemental systemic glucocorticoids during stress.
• For better results and less toxicity, give a daily dose in the morning.
• Teach patients signs of early adrenal insufficiency: fatigue, muscular weakness, joint pain, fever, anorexia, nausea, dyspnea, dizziness, and fainting.
• Warn patients on long-term therapy about cushingoid symptoms and to report sudden weight gain and swelling to the doctor.
• Watch for depression or psychotic episodes, especially in high-dose therapy.
• Diabetic patients may need increased insulin; monitor blood glucose levels.
• Unless contraindicated, give low-sodium diet high in potassium and protein. Administer potassium supplements as needed. Watch for additional potassium depletion from diuretics and amphotericin B.
• Give P.O. dose with food when possible to reduce GI irritation.
• Not used for alternate-day therapy.
• Parenteral form is *not* for I.V. use.
• Don't use diluents that contain preservatives; flocculation may occur.
• Give I.M. injection deep into gluteal muscle. Rotate injection sites to prevent muscle atrophy.

53

Androgens and anabolic steroids

danazol
fluoxymesterone
methyltestosterone
nandrolone decanoate
nandrolone phenpropionate
oxandrolone
oxymetholone
stanozolol
testosterone
testosterone cypionate
testosterone enanthate
testosterone propionate
testosterone transdermal system

COMBINATION PRODUCTS
ANDRO-ESTRO 90-4, DEPANDROGEN, DEPO-TESTADIOL, DEPOTESTOGEN, DUO-CYP, DURATESTRIN, MENOJECT-L.A., TEST EST CYP (oil): testosterone cypionate 50 mg and estradiol cypionate 2 mg.
ANDROGYN L.A., DELADUMONE, VALERTEST NO. 1: testosterone enanthate 90 mg/ml and estradiol valerate 4 mg/ml in sesame oil.
ESTRATEST: esterified estrogens 1.25 mg and methyltestosterone 2.5 mg.
ESTRATEST H.S.: esterified estrogens 0.625 mg and methyltestosterone 1.25 mg.
HALODRIN: fluoxymesterone 1 mg with ethinyl estradiol 0.02 mg.
PREMARIN WITH METHYLTESTOSTERONE: conjugated estrogens 0.625 mg and methyltestosterone 5 mg; or conjugated estrogens 1.25 mg and methyltestosterone 10 mg.
VALERTEST NO. 2: estradiol valerate 8 mg and testosterone enanthate 180 mg.

danazol

Cycloment†, Danocrine
Pregnancy Risk Category: X

HOW SUPPLIED
Capsules: 50 mg, 100 mg, 200 mg

ACTION
Mechanism: Gonadotropin inhibitor that suppresses the pituitary-ovarian axis and inhibits estrogenic effects.
Onset: pain relief for fibrocystic breast disease, within 1 month. **Peak:** Peak effects occur in 6 to 8 weeks when treating endometriosis and in 2 to 3 months when treating fibrocystic breast disease. **Duration:** half-life, about 4½ hours.

INDICATIONS & DOSAGE
Mild endometriosis –
Women: initially, 100 to 200 mg P.O. b.i.d. Base subsequent dosage on patient response.
Moderate to severe endometriosis –
Women: 400 mg P.O. b.i.d. uninterrupted for 3 to 6 months; may continue for 9 months.
Fibrocystic breast disease –
Women: 100 to 400 mg P.O. daily in two divided doses uninterrupted for 2 to 6 months.
Prevention of hereditary angioedema –
Adults: 200 mg P.O. b.i.d to t.i.d., continued until favorable response is achieved. Then decrease dosage 50% at 1- to 3-month intervals.

ADVERSE REACTIONS
CNS: dizziness, headache, sleep disorders, fatigue, tremor, irritability, excitation, lethargy, mental depression, chills, paresthesia.
CV: elevated blood pressure.
EENT: visual disturbances.
GI: gastric irritation, nausea, vomiting, diarrhea, constipation, change in appetite.
GU: hematuria.

Hematologic: thrombocytopenia, elevated serum lipid levels.
Hepatic: reversible jaundice, peliosis hepatis, elevated liver enzyme levels, ***liver cell tumors.***
Other: muscle cramps or spasms; androgenic effects in women *(weight gain, hirsutism,* hoarseness, clitoral enlargement, *decrease in breast size,* changes in libido, *oily skin or hair); hypoestrogenic effects (flushing, diaphoresis, vaginitis, including itching, dryness, and burning; vaginal bleeding, nervousness, emotional lability, menstrual irregularities).*

INTERACTIONS
None significant.

CONTRAINDICATIONS
- Contraindicated in patients with undiagnosed abnormal genital bleeding or impaired renal, cardiac, or hepatic function; during pregnancy; and in breast-feeding patients.
- Use cautiously in patients with seizure disorder or migraine headaches.

NURSING CONSIDERATIONS
- Avoid use in women of childbearing age until pregnancy is ruled out. Make sure they understand the importance of using an effective nonhormonal contraceptive during therapy.
- Unless contraindicated, use with diet high in calories and protein.
- Monitor closely for signs of virilization. Some androgenic effects, such as deepening of voice, may not be reversible upon discontinuation of drug.
- Periodically evaluate hepatic function. Semen evaluation is routinely performed every 3 to 4 months, especially in adolescent males.
- Consider periodic dosage decreases or gradual drug withdrawal.
- After withdrawal of treatment, ovulation and cyclic bleeding usually return in 2 to 3 months; fibrocystic disease symptoms return to 50% of patients within 1 year.
- Advise patients taking danazol for fibrocystic breast disease to examine breasts regularly and to call the doctor immediately if breast nodule enlarges during treatment.
- Advise washing after intercourse to decrease the risk of vaginitis. Instruct patients to wear cotton underwear.
- Has been used investigationally with impressive results in treating hemophilia and Christmas disease; also used to decrease symptoms of systemic lupus erythematosus in women and to treat gynecomastia in men.

fluoxymesterone
Android F, Halotestin**
Controlled Substance Schedule III
Pregnancy Risk Category: X

HOW SUPPLIED
Tablets: 2 mg, 5 mg, 10 mg

ACTION
Mechanism: Stimulates target tissues to develop normally in androgen-deficient men.
Duration: half-life, about 9 hours.

INDICATIONS & DOSAGE
Hypogonadism and impotence caused by testicular deficiency –
Adults: 2 to 20 mg P.O. daily. Most patients respond to 2.5 to 10 mg daily.
Palliation of breast cancer in women –
Adults: 10 to 40 mg P.O. daily in divided doses. Individualize all dosages and reduce to minimum when effect is noted.
Postpartum breast engorgement –
Adults: 2.5 mg P.O., followed by 5 to 10 mg daily for 5 days.

ADVERSE REACTIONS
CV: edema.
GI: gastroenteritis, nausea, vomiting, constipation, change in appetite.
GU: bladder irritability.

Hematologic: thrombocytopenia, elevated serum lipid levels.
Hepatic: reversible jaundice, peliosis hepatis, elevated liver enzyme levels, ***liver cell tumors***.
Other: hypercalcemia; androgenic effects in women (acne, edema, *weight gain, hirsutism,* hoarseness, clitoral enlargement, *decrease in breast size,* changes in libido, male pattern baldness, *oily skin or hair); hypoestrogenic effects in women (flushing; diaphoresis; vaginitis, including itching, dryness, and burning; vaginal bleeding; nervousness; emotional lability; menstrual irregularities); excessive hormonal effects in men (prepubertal – premature epiphyseal closure, acne,* priapism, *growth of body and facial hair,* phallic enlargement; postpubertal – testicular atrophy, oligospermia, decreased ejaculatory volume, impotence, gynecomastia, epididymitis).

INTERACTIONS

Hepatotoxic medications: increased risk of hepatotoxicity. Monitor closely.
Insulin, oral antidiabetic agents: altered dosage requirements. Monitor blood glucose levels in diabetic patients.
Oral anticoagulants: altered dosage requirements. Monitor PT.

CONTRAINDICATIONS

- Contraindicated in patients with benign prostatic hyperplasia with obstruction; males with breast cancer, prostate cancer, nephrosis, hypercalcemia, and cardiac, hepatic, or renal decompensation; during pregnancy; in breast-feeding patients; and in premature infants.
- Use cautiously in prepubertal males, diabetic patients, those with coronary disease, and those taking corticotropin, corticosteroids, or anticoagulants.

NURSING CONSIDERATIONS

- Avoid use in women of childbearing age until pregnancy is ruled out. Make sure they understand the importance of using an effective nonhormonal contraceptive during therapy.
- Advise washing after intercourse to decrease the risk of vaginitis. Instruct patients to wear only cotton underwear.
- Hypercalcemia symptoms may be difficult to distinguish from symptoms associated with condition being treated, unless anticipated and thought of as a symptom cluster. Hypercalcemia is particularly likely to occur in patients with metastatic breast cancer and may indicate bone metastases.
- Explain to patients taking drug for palliation of breast cancer that virilization usually occurs at dosage used. Give emotional support. Tell patients to report androgenic effects immediately. Stopping drug will prevent further androgenic changes but will probably not reverse existing effects.
- When used in breast cancer, subjective effects may not occur for about 1 month; objective effects on clinical symptoms may take 3 months.
- Tell women to report menstrual irregularities and to discontinue therapy pending etiologic determination.
- Monitor male patients for signs of excessive sexual stimulation or priapism.
- Semen evaluation is routinely performed every 3 to 4 months, especially in adolescent males.
- Edema is generally controllable with sodium restriction or diuretics. Monitor weight routinely.
- Watch for symptoms of jaundice and periodically evaluate hepatic function. Dosage adjustment may reverse condition. If liver function tests are abnormal, therapy should be stopped.
- Observe patients on concomitant anticoagulant therapy for ecchymotic

areas, petechiae, or abnormal bleeding. Monitor PT.
• Watch for symptoms of hypoglycemia in diabetic patients. Check blood glucose levels. Dosage of antidiabetic drug may need adjustment.
• Unless contraindicated, use with diet high in calories and protein. Give small, frequent feedings.
• If GI upset occurs, tell patients to take drug with food or meals.

methyltestosterone

Android, Metandren**, Metandren Linguets, Oreton Methyl, Testomet‡, Testred, Virilon
Controlled Substance Schedule III
Pregnancy Risk Category: X

HOW SUPPLIED
Tablets: 5 mg‡, 10 mg, 25 mg, 50 mg‡
Tablets (buccal): 5 mg, 10 mg
Capsules: 10 mg

ACTION
Mechanism: Stimulates target tissues to develop normally in androgen-deficient men.
Duration: half-life, 2½ to 3½ hours.

INDICATIONS & DOSAGE
Postpartum breast engorgement in non-breast-feeding women –
Adults: 80 mg P.O. daily, or 40 mg buccally daily for 3 to 5 days.
Breast cancer in women 1 to 5 years postmenopausal –
Adults: 200 mg P.O. daily; or 100 mg buccally daily.
Eunuchoidism and eunuchism, male climacteric symptoms –
Adults: 10 to 50 mg P.O. daily; or 5 to 25 mg buccally daily.
Postpubertal cryptorchidism –
Adults: 30 mg P.O. daily; or 15 mg buccally daily.

ADVERSE REACTIONS
CV: edema.
EENT: irritation of oral mucosa with buccal administration.
GI: gastroenteritis, constipation, nausea, vomiting, diarrhea, change in appetite.
GU: bladder irritability.
Hepatic: reversible jaundice, cholestatic hepatitis, abnormal liver enzyme levels.
Other: hypercalcemia, muscle cramps or spasms; androgenic effects in women (acne, edema, *weight gain, hirsutism,* hoarseness, clitoral enlargement, *decrease in breast size,* changes in libido, male pattern baldness, *oily skin or hair); hypoestrogenic effects in women (flushing; diaphoresis; vaginitis, including itching, dryness, and burning; vaginal bleeding; nervousness; emotional lability; menstrual irregularities); excessive hormonal effects in men (prepubertal – premature epiphyseal closure, acne,* priapism, *growth of body and facial hair,* phallic enlargement; postpubertal – testicular atrophy, oligospermia, decreased ejaculatory volume, impotence, gynecomastia, epididymitis).

INTERACTIONS
Hepatotoxic medications: increased risk of hepatotoxicity. Monitor closely.
Insulin, oral antidiabetic agents: altered dosage requirements. Monitor blood glucose levels in diabetic patients.
Oral anticoagulants: altered dosage requirements. Monitor PT.

CONTRAINDICATIONS
• Contraindicated in pregnant and breast-feeding patients; elderly, asthenic men who may react adversely to androgen overstimulation; males with breast cancer, prostate cancer, or benign prostatic hyperplasia with obstruction; patients with hypercalcemia, conditions aggravated by fluid

retention, hypertension, or cardiac, hepatic, or renal decompensation; and in premature infants.
• Use cautiously in patients with MI or coronary artery disease.

NURSING CONSIDERATIONS
• Avoid use in women of childbearing age until pregnancy is ruled out. Make sure they understand the importance of using an effective nonhormonal contraceptive during therapy.
• Treatment of breast cancer usually restricted to patients 1 to 5 years postmenopausal.
• Edema is generally controllable with sodium restriction or diuretics. Check weight regularly.
• Periodically check hemoglobin and hematocrit values, serum cholesterol and calcium levels, and cardiac and liver function tests.
• In children, X-rays of the wrist bones should be taken before therapy to establish the level of bone maturation. During treatment, bone maturation may proceed more rapidly than linear growth; ensure intermittent dosage and periodically review X-ray results to monitor bone maturation.
• Semen evaluation is routinely performed every 3 to 4 months, especially in adolescent males.
• Typically used only for intermittent therapy. Because of potential hepatotoxicity, watch closely for jaundice.
• In metastatic breast cancer, hypercalcemia may indicate progression of bone metastases. Report signs of hypercalcemia.
• Therapeutic response in breast cancer is usually apparent within 3 months. Therapy should be stopped if signs of disease progression appear.
• Enhances hypoglycemia; teach patient signs of hypoglycemia and method for checking blood glucose level. Instruct patients to report hypoglycemia immediately.
• Watch for ecchymoses, petechiae, and abnormal bleeding in patients receiving concomitant anticoagulants.
• Advise washing after intercourse to decrease the risk of vaginitis. Instruct patients to wear only cotton underwear.
• Promptly report signs of virilization in women.
• Unless contraindicated, use with diet high in calories and protein. Give small, frequent feedings.
• Buccal tablets are twice as potent as oral tablets. Tell patients to avoid eating, drinking, chewing, or smoking while buccal tablet is in place and not to swallow tablet. Place in upper or lower buccal pouch between cheek and gum; tablet requires 30 to 60 minutes to dissolve. Instruct patients to change tablet absorption site with each dose to minimize risk of buccal irritation.
• Has been abused to enhance athletic ability.

nandrolone decanoate
Anabolin LA, Androlone-D, Deca-Durabolin, Decolone, Hybolin Decanoate, Kabolin, Nandrobolic L.A., Neo-Durabolic

nandrolone phenpropionate
Anabolin IM, Androlone, Durabolin, Hybolin Improved, Nandrobolic
Controlled Substance Schedule III

Pregnancy Risk Category: X

HOW SUPPLIED
decanoate
Injection (in oil): 50 mg/ml, 100 mg/ml, 200 mg/ml
phenpropionate
Injection (in oil): 25 mg/ml, 50 mg/ml

ACTION
Mechanism: Anabolic steroid that promotes tissue-building processes,

reverses catabolism, and stimulates erythropoiesis.
Peak: Serum levels peak in 1 to 2 days.

INDICATIONS & DOSAGE
Severe debility or disease states, refractory anemias –
Adults: 100 to 200 mg (decanoate) I.M. weekly. Therapy should be intermittent.
Tissue-building –
Adults: 50 to 100 mg (decanoate) I.M. q 3 to 4 weeks.
Children 2 to 13 years: 25 to 50 mg (decanoate) I.M. q 3 to 4 weeks.
Control of metastatic breast cancer –
Adults: 25 to 50 mg (phenpropionate) I.M. weekly.
Children 2 to 13 years: 12.5 to 25 mg (phenpropionate) I.M. q 2 to 4 weeks.

ADVERSE REACTIONS
CV: edema.
GI: gastroenteritis, nausea, vomiting, diarrhea, change in appetite.
GU: bladder irritability.
Hematologic: thrombocytopenia, elevated serum lipid levels.
Hepatic: reversible jaundice, peliosis hepatis, elevated liver enzyme levels, ***liver cell tumors.***
Skin: pain and induration at injection site.
Other: hypercalcemia; muscle cramps or spasms; androgenic effects in women (acne, edema, *weight gain, hirsutism,* hoarseness, clitoral enlargement, *decrease in breast size,* changes in libido, male pattern baldness, *oily skin or hair); hypoestrogenic effects in women (flushing; diaphoresis; vaginitis, including itching, dryness, and burning; vaginal bleeding; nervousness; emotional lability; menstrual irregularities); excessive hormonal effects in men (prepubertal – premature epiphyseal closure, acne,* priapism, *growth of body and facial hair,* phallic enlargement; postpubertal – testicular atrophy, oligospermia, decreased ejaculatory volume, impotence, gynecomastia, epididymitis).

INTERACTIONS
Hepatotoxic medications: increased risk of hepatotoxicity. Monitor closely.
Insulin, oral antidiabetic agents: altered dosage requirements. Monitor blood glucose levels in diabetic patients.
Oral anticoagulants: altered dosage requirements. Monitor PT.

CONTRAINDICATIONS
- Contraindicated in patients with prostatic hyperplasia with obstruction, males with breast cancer, and patients with prostate cancer, nephrosis, and cardiac, hepatic, or renal decompensation; during pregnancy; in breast-feeding patients; and in premature infants.
- Use cautiously in prepubertal males, diabetic patients, those with coronary disease, and those taking corticotropin, corticosteroids, or anticoagulants.

NURSING CONSIDERATIONS
- Avoid use in women of childbearing age until pregnancy is ruled out. Make sure they understand the importance of using an effective nonhormonal contraceptive during therapy.
- Advise washing after intercourse to decrease the risk of vaginitis. Instruct patients to wear only cotton underwear.
- When used to promote erythropoiesis in refractory anemias, make sure patients have adequate daily iron intake.
- Hypercalcemia is most likely to occur in patients with breast cancer; check quantitative urine and serum calcium levels.
- Tell women to report menstrual irregularities and to discontinue therapy pending etiologic determination.

• Watch for signs of virilization, which may be irreversible despite prompt discontinuation of therapy.
• In children, X-rays of the wrist bones should be taken before surgery to establish the level of bone maturation. During treatment, bone maturation may proceed more rapidly than linear growth; ensure intermittent dosage and review X-ray results periodically.
• Closely observe boys under 7 years for precocious development of male sexual characteristics.
• Semen evaluation is routinely performed every 3 to 4 months, especially in adolescent males.
• Periodically evaluate hepatic function. Watch for jaundice; dosage adjustment may reverse condition. If liver function tests are abnormal, therapy should be stopped.
• Edema is generally controllable with sodium restrictions or diuretics. Check weight regularly.
• Observe patients receiving concomitant anticoagulant therapy for ecchymotic areas, petechiae, or abnormal bleeding. Monitor PT.
• Watch for symptoms of hypoglycemia in diabetic patients. Check blood glucose levels. Adjust dosage of antidiabetic drug as necessary.
• Inject drug deep I.M., preferably into upper outer quadrant of gluteal muscle in adults. Rotate injection sites to prevent muscle atrophy.
• Unless contraindicated, use with diet high in calories and protein. Give small, frequent feedings.
• Has been abused to enhance athletic ability.
• Anabolic steroids may alter results of laboratory studies performed during therapy and for 2 to 3 weeks after therapy ends.

oxandrolone

Anavar, Lonavar‡, Oxandrin
Controlled Substance Schedule III
Pregnancy Risk Category: X

HOW SUPPLIED
Tablets: 2.5 mg

ACTION
Mechanism: Anabolic steroid that promotes tissue-building processes, reverses catabolism, and stimulates erythropoiesis.
Duration: terminal elimination half-life, 9 hours.

INDICATIONS & DOSAGE
To combat catabolic effects of corticosteroid therapy, osteoporosis, prolonged immobilization, and debilitated states –
Adults: 2.5 mg P.O. b.i.d., t.i.d., or q.i.d., up to 20 mg daily for 2 to 4 weeks.
Children: 0.25 mg/kg daily P.O. for 2 to 4 weeks.

Continuous therapy should not exceed 3 months.
Turner's syndrome –
Children: 50 to 125 mcg/kg P.O. daily.

ADVERSE REACTIONS
CV: edema.
GI: gastroenteritis, nausea, vomiting, constipation or diarrhea, change in appetite.
GU: bladder irritability.
Hematologic: thrombocytopenia, elevated serum lipid levels.
Hepatic: reversible jaundice, peliosis hepatis, elevated liver enzyme levels, ***liver cell tumors***.
Other: hypercalcemia, muscle cramps or spasms; androgenic effects in women (acne, edema, *weight gain, hirsutism,* hoarseness, clitoral enlargement, *decrease in breast size,* changes in libido, male pattern baldness, *oily skin or hair); hypoestro-*

*Liquid form contains alcohol.
**May contain tartrazine.
Common reactions are in italics; ***life-threatening,*** in bold italics.

genic effects in women (flushing; diaphoresis; vaginitis, including itching, dryness, and burning; vaginal bleeding; nervousness; emotional lability; menstrual irregularities); excessive hormonal effects in men (prepubertal – premature epiphyseal closure, acne, priapism, *growth of body and facial hair,* phallic enlargement; postpubertal – testicular atrophy, oligospermia, decreased ejaculatory volume, impotence, gynecomastia, epididymitis).

INTERACTIONS
Hepatotoxic medications: increased risk of hepatotoxicity. Monitor closely.
Insulin, oral antidiabetic agents: altered dosage requirements. Monitor blood glucose levels in diabetic patients.
Oral anticoagulants: altered dosage requirements. Monitor PT.

CONTRAINDICATIONS
• Contraindicated in patients with prostatic hyperplasia with obstruction, males with breast cancer, and patients with prostate cancer, nephrosis, and cardiac, hepatic, or renal decompensation; during pregnancy; in breast-feeding patients; and in premature infants.
• Use cautiously in prepubertal males, diabetic patients, those with coronary disease, and those taking corticotropin, corticosteroids, or anticoagulants.

NURSING CONSIDERATIONS
• Avoid use in women of childbearing age until pregnancy is ruled out. Make sure they understand the importance of using an effective nonhormonal contraceptive during therapy.
• When used to promote erythropoiesis, make sure patients have adequate daily iron intake.
• Advise washing after intercourse to decrease the risk of vaginitis. Instruct patients to wear only cotton underwear.
• Hypercalcemia symptoms may be difficult to distinguish from symptoms of condition being treated, unless anticipated and thought of as a cluster. Hypercalcemia is most likely to occur with metastatic breast cancer and may indicate bone metastases.
• Tell women to report menstrual irregularities and to discontinue therapy pending etiologic determination.
• Watch for signs of virilization, which may be irreversible despite prompt discontinuation of therapy. Doctor must decide if benefits outweigh adverse effects.
• Semen evaluation is routinely performed every 3 to 4 months, especially in adolescent males.
• Closely observe boys under 7 years for precocious development of male sexual characteristics.
• In children, X-rays of the wrist bones should be taken before therapy to establish the level of bone maturation. During treatment, bone maturation may proceed more rapidly than linear growth; ensure intermittent dosage and review X-ray results periodically.
• Edema is generally controllable with sodium restriction or diuretics. Monitor weight routinely.
• Periodically monitor hepatic function. Watch for jaundice. Dosage adjustment may reverse condition. Periodically check liver function tests.
• Observe patients on concomitant anticoagulant therapy for ecchymotic areas, petechiae, or abnormal bleeding. Monitor PT.
• Watch for symptoms of hypoglycemia in diabetic patients. Check blood glucose levels. Adjust dosage of antidiabetic drug as necessary.
• Unless contraindicated, use with diet high in calories and protein. Give small, frequent feedings.
• If GI upset occurs, tell patients to take drug with food or meals.

• Has been abused to enhance athletic ability.
• Anabolic steroids may alter results of laboratory studies performed during therapy and for 2 to 3 weeks after therapy ends.

oxymetholone

Anadrol, Anapolon 50†‡
Controlled Substance Schedule III
Pregnancy Risk Category: X

HOW SUPPLIED

Tablets: 50 mg

ACTION

Mechanism: Anabolic steroid that promotes tissue-building processes, reverses catabolism, and stimulates erythropoiesis.
Onset: 3 to 6 months.

INDICATIONS & DOSAGE

Aplastic anemia; prophylaxis and treatment of hereditary angioedema –
Adults and children: 1 to 5 mg/kg P.O. daily. Dosage is highly individualized; and response is not immediate. A trial of 3 to 6 months is required.

ADVERSE REACTIONS

CV: edema.
GI: gastroenteritis, nausea, vomiting, constipation, diarrhea, change in appetite.
GU: bladder irritability.
Hematologic: thrombocytopenia, elevated serum lipid levels.
Hepatic: reversible jaundice, peliosis hepatis, elevated liver enzyme levels, ***liver cell tumors.***
Other: hypercalcemia; muscle cramps or spasms; androgenic effects in women (acne, edema, *weight gain, hirsutism,* hoarseness, clitoral enlargement, *decrease in breast size,* changes in libido, male pattern baldness, *oily skin or hair); hypoestrogenic effects in women (flushing; diaphoresis; vaginitis, including itching, dryness, and burning; vaginal bleeding; nervousness; emotional lability; menstrual irregularities); excessive hormonal effects in men (prepubertal – premature epiphyseal closure, acne,* priapism, *growth of body and facial hair,* phallic enlargement; postpubertal – testicular atrophy, oligospermia, decreased ejaculatory volume, impotence, gynecomastia, epididymitis).

INTERACTIONS

Hepatotoxic medications: increased risk of hepatotoxicity. Monitor closely.
Insulin, oral antidiabetic agents: altered dosage requirements. Monitor blood glucose levels in diabetic patients.
Oral anticoagulants: altered dosage requirements. Monitor PT.

CONTRAINDICATIONS

• Contraindicated in patients with prostatic hyperplasia with obstruction, males with breast cancer, and patients with prostate cancer, nephrosis, or cardiac, hepatic, or renal decompensation; during pregnancy; in breast-feeding patients; and in premature infants.
• Use cautiously in prepubertal males, diabetic patients, those with coronary diseases, and those taking corticotropin, corticosteroids, or anticoagulants.

NURSING CONSIDERATIONS

• Avoid use in women of childbearing age until pregnancy is ruled out. Make sure they understand the importance of using an effective nonhormonal contraceptive during therapy.
• Advise washing after intercourse to decrease the risk of vaginitis. Instruct patients to wear only cotton underwear.
• When used to promote erythropoiesis, make sure patients have adequate daily iron intake.
• Hypercalcemia symptoms may be

difficult to distinguish from symptoms of condition being treated, unless anticipated and thought of as a cluster. Hypercalcemia is most likely to occur in metastatic breast cancer and may indicate bone metastases.

- Used for supportive treatment of anemias (transfusions; correction of iron, folic acid, vitamin B_{12}, or pyridoxine deficiency). Give 3 to 6 months for response.
- Tell women to report menstrual irregularities and to discontinue therapy pending etiologic determination.
- Watch for signs of virilization, which may be irreversible despite prompt discontinuation of therapy. Doctor must decide if benefits outweigh adverse effects.
- Closely observe boys under 7 years for precocious development of male sexual characteristics.
- Semen evaluation is routinely performed every 3 to 4 months, especially in adolescent males.
- In children, X-rays of the wrist bones should be taken before therapy to establish the level of bone maturation. During treatment, bone maturation may proceed more rapidly than linear growth; ensure intermittent dosage and review X-ray results periodically. Epiphyseal development may continue 6 months after stopping therapy.
- Edema is generally controllable with sodium restriction or diuretics. Monitor weight routinely.
- Periodically evaluate hepatic function. Watch for symptoms of jaundice; dosage adjustment may reverse condition. If liver function tests are abnormal, therapy should be stopped.
- Observe patients on concomitant anticoagulant therapy for ecchymotic areas, petechiae, or abnormal bleeding. Monitor PT.
- Watch for symptoms of hypoglycemia in diabetic patients. Check blood glucose levels. Adjust dosage of antidiabetic drug as necessary.
- Unless contraindicated, use with diet high in calories and protein. Give small, frequent feedings.
- If GI upset occurs, tell patients to take with food or meals.
- Has been abused to enhance athletic ability.
- Anabolic steroids may alter results of laboratory studies performed during therapy and for 2 to 3 weeks after therapy ends.

stanozolol

Winstrol

Controlled Substance Schedule III

Pregnancy Risk Category: X

HOW SUPPLIED

Tablets: 2 mg

ACTION

Mechanism: Anabolic steroid that promotes tissue-building processes, reverses catabolism, and stimulates erythropoiesis.

Onset: 1 to 2 months.

INDICATIONS & DOSAGE

Prevention of hereditary angioedema –

Adults: initially, 2 mg P.O. t.i.d. to 4 mg q.i.d for 5 days. Gradually reduce dosage at 1- to 3-month intervals to a dosage of 2 mg daily.

Children under age 6: 1 mg P.O. daily.

Children ages 6 to 12: up to 2 mg P.O. daily.

Note: Use stanozolol in children only during an acute attack.

ADVERSE REACTIONS

CV: edema.

GI: gastroenteritis, nausea, vomiting, constipation, diarrhea, change in appetite.

GU: bladder irritability.

Hematologic: thrombocytopenia, elevated serum lipid levels.

Hepatic: reversible jaundice, peliosis

hepatis, elevated liver enzyme levels, ***liver cell tumors.***
Other: hypercalcemia; muscle cramps or spasms; androgenic effects in women (acne, edema, *weight gain, hirsutism,* hoarseness, clitoral enlargement, *decrease in breast size,* changes in libido, male pattern baldness, *oily skin or hair); hypoestrogenic effects in women (flushing; diaphoresis; vaginitis, including itching, dryness, and burning; vaginal bleeding; nervousness; emotional lability; menstrual irregularities); excessive hormonal effects in men (prepubertal – premature epiphyseal closure, acne,* priapism, *growth of body and facial hair,* phallic enlargement; postpubertal – testicular atrophy, oligospermia, decreased ejaculatory volume, impotence, gynecomastia, epididymitis).

INTERACTIONS

Hepatotoxic medications: increased risk of hepatotoxicity. Monitor closely.
Insulin, oral antidiabetic agents: altered dosage requirements. Monitor blood glucose levels in diabetic patients.
Oral anticoagulants: altered dosage requirements. Monitor PT.

CONTRAINDICATIONS

- Contraindicated in patients with prostatic hyperplasia with obstruction, males with breast cancer, and patients with prostate cancer, nephrosis, or cardiac, hepatic, or renal decompensation; during pregnancy; in breast-feeding patients; and in premature infants.
- Use cautiously in prepubertal males; diabetic patients, those with coronary disease, and those taking corticotropin, corticosteroids, or anticoagulants.

NURSING CONSIDERATIONS

- Avoid use in women of childbearing age until pregnancy is ruled out. Make sure they understand the importance of using an effective nonhormonal contraceptive during therapy.
- A lower dosage in young women (2 mg b.i.d.) is recommended to avoid virilization. Watch for signs of virilization, which may be irreversible despite prompt discontinuation of therapy. Doctor must decide if benefits of therapy outweigh adverse effects.
- Tell women to report menstrual irregularities and to discontinue therapy pending etiologic determination.
- Closely observe boys under 7 years for precocious development of male sexual characteristics.
- Semen evaluation is routinely performed every 3 to 4 months, especially in adolescent males.
- In children, X-rays of the wrist bones should be taken before therapy to establish the level of bone maturation. During treatment, bone maturation may proceed more rapidly than linear growth; ensure intermittent dosage and review X-ray results periodically.
- Edema is generally controllable with sodium restriction or diuretics. Monitor weight routinely.
- Periodically evaluate hepatic function. Watch for symptoms of jaundice; dosage adjustment may reverse condition. Check liver function tests regularly; if abnormal, therapy should be discontinued.
- Observe patients on concomitant anticoagulant therapy for ecchymotic areas, petechiae, or abnormal bleeding. Monitor PT.
- Watch for symptoms of hypoglycemia in diabetic patients. Check blood glucose levels. Adjust dosage of antidiabetic drug as necessary.
- Monitor serum cholesterol levels.
- Unless contraindicated, use with diet high in calories and protein. Give small, frequent feedings.
- To minimize GI distress, administer before or with meals.
- Advise washing after intercourse to

decrease the risk of vaginitis. Instruct patients to wear only cotton underwear.

- Has been abused to enhance athletic ability.
- Anabolic steroids may alter results of laboratory studies performed during therapy and for 2 to 3 weeks after therapy ends.

testosterone

Andro-100, Andronaq-50, Histerone-50, Histerone-100, Testamone 100, Testaqua, Testoject-50

testosterone cypionate

Andro-Cyp 100, Andro-Cyp 200, Andronaq-LA, Andronate 100, Andronate 200, dep Andro 100, dep Andro 200, Depotest, Depo-Testosterone, Duratest-100, Duratest-200, T-Cypionate, Testa-C, Testoject-LA, Testred Cypionate 200, Virilon IM

testosterone enanthate

Andro-LA, Andropository 100, Andryl 200, Delatest, Delatestryl, Durathate-200, Everone, Malogex†, Testone L.A. 200, Testrin-P.A.

testosterone propionate

Malogen†, Testex

Controlled Substance Schedule III

Pregnancy Risk Category: X

HOW SUPPLIED

testosterone
Injection (aqueous suspension): 25 mg/ml, 50 mg/ml, 100 mg/ml
testosterone cypionate
Injection (in oil): 50 mg/ml, 100 mg/ml, 200 mg/ml
testosterone enanthate
Injection (in oil): 100 mg/ml, 200 mg/ml
testosterone propionate
Injection (in oil): 25 mg/ml, 50 mg/ml, 100 mg/ml

ACTION

Mechanism: Stimulates target tissues to develop normally in androgen-deficient men. Testosterone may have some antiestrogen properties, making it useful to treat certain estrogen-dependent breast cancers. Its action in postpartum breast engorgement is not known because testosterone does not suppress lactation.
Duration: 2 to 4 weeks for suspensions (cypionate, enanthate, or propionate).

INDICATIONS & DOSAGE

Eunuchism, eunuchoidism, deficiency after castration and male climacteric –
Adults: 10 to 25 mg I.M. two to five times weekly, or 50 to 400 mg (cypionate, enanthate) I.M. q 2 to 4 weeks, or 10 to 25 mg (propionate) I.M. two to four times weekly.
Oligospermia –
Adults: 100 to 200 mg (cypionate, enanthate) I.M. q 4 to 6 weeks for development and maintenance of testicular function.
Breast engorgement in non-breast-feeding patients –
Adults: 25 to 50 mg I.M. daily for 3 to 4 days, starting at delivery.
Metastatic breast cancer in women –
Adults: 50 to 100 mg (propionate) I.M. three times weekly; or 200 to 400 mg (cypionate, enanthate) I.M. q 2 to 4 weeks.
Breast cancer in women 1 to 5 years postmenopausal –
Adults: 100 mg I.M. three times weekly as long as improvement is maintained.
Postmenopausal or primary osteoporosis –
Adults: 200 to 400 mg (enanthate) I.M. q 4 weeks.

ADVERSE REACTIONS

CV: edema.
GI: gastroenteritis, nausea, vomiting, constipation, diarrhea, change in appetite.
GU: bladder irritability.
Hepatic: reversible jaundice, cholestatic hepatitis, abnormal liver enzyme levels.
Skin: pain and induration at injection site, local edema.
Other: hypercalcemia; androgenic effects in women (*acne, edema, oily skin, weight gain, hirsutism, hoarseness,* clitoral enlargement, decreased or increased libido); hypoestrogenic effects in women (flushing; diaphoresis; vaginitis, including itching, drying, and burning; vaginal bleeding; menstrual irregularities); excessive hormonal effects in men (prepubertal – premature epiphyseal closure, *acne,* priapism, *growth of body and facial hair,* phallic enlargement; postpubertal – testicular atrophy, oligospermia, decreased ejaculatory volume, impotence, gynecomastia, epididymitis).

INTERACTIONS

Hepatotoxic medications: increased risk of hepatotoxicity. Monitor closely.
Insulin, oral antidiabetic agents: altered dosage requirements. Monitor blood glucose levels in diabetic patients.
Oral anticoagulants: altered dosage requirements. Monitor PT.

CONTRAINDICATIONS

- Contraindicated in elderly, asthenic men, who may react adversely to androgen overstimulation, and males with breast cancer; in patients with hypercalcemia; in those with cardiac, hepatic, or renal decompensation; in males with prostatic or breast cancer; in benign prostatic hyperplasia with obstruction; in conditions aggravated by fluid retention and hypertension; in women of childbearing potential (possible masculization of female infant); during pregnancy; in breast-feeding patients and in premature infants.
- Use cautiously in patients with MI or coronary artery disease and in prepubertal males.

NURSING CONSIDERATIONS

- Avoid use in women of childbearing age until pregnancy is ruled out. Make sure they understand the importance of using an effective nonhormonal contraceptive during therapy.
- Monitor periodic liver function tests.
- In metastatic breast cancer, hypercalcemia usually indicates progression of bone metastases. Report signs of hypercalcemia.
- Therapeutic response in breast cancer is usually apparent within 3 months. Stop therapy if signs of disease progression appear.
- Enhances hypoglycemia; teach patients to recognize signs of hypoglycemia and immediately report them.
- Instruct men to report priapism, reduced ejaculatory volume, and gynecomastia. Withdraw drug if these occur.
- Inject deep into upper outer quadrant of gluteal muscle. Rotate injection sites to prevent muscle atrophy. Report soreness at site because of the possibility of postinfection furunculosis.
- Watch for ecchymotic areas, petechiae, or abnormal bleeding in patients on concomitant anticoagulant therapy. Monitor PT.
- Report signs of virilization in females; reevaluate treatment.
- Monitor prepubertal males by X-ray for rate of bone maturation.
- Edema is generally controllable with sodium restriction or diuretics. Monitor weight routinely.
- Unless contraindicated, use with diet high in calories and protein. Give small, frequent feedings.

• Advise washing after intercourse to decrease the risk of vaginitis. Instruct patients to wear only cotton underwear.
• Administer daily dosage requirement in divided doses for best results.
• Store I.M. preparations at room temperature. If crystals appear, warm and shake the bottle to disperse them.
• Androgens may alter results of laboratory studies during therapy and for 2 to 3 weeks after therapy ends.

testosterone transdermal system

Testoderm
Controlled Substance Schedule III

Pregnancy Risk Category: X

HOW SUPPLIED
Transdermal system: 4 mg/day, 6 mg/day

ACTION
Mechanism: Releases testosterone, which stimulates target tissues to develop normally in androgen-deficient men.
Peak: Serum levels peak within 2 to 4 hours after application. Steady-state levels are reached after 3 to 4 weeks of therapy. **Duration:** testosterone levels decline toward baseline within 2 hours after removal.

INDICATIONS & DOSAGE
Primary or hypogonadotropic hypogonadism in men ages 18 and older –
Adults: apply one 6 mg/day patch to the scrotal area daily. If scrotal area is too small for the 6 mg/day patch, start therapy with a (smaller sized) 4 mg/day patch.

ADVERSE REACTIONS
CV: *CVA.*
GU: *gynecomastia,* prostatitis, urinary tract infection, breast tenderness.
Skin: acne.
Other: *itching,* discomfort, irritation.

INTERACTIONS
Antidiabetic agents: altered antidiabetic agent dosage requirements. Monitor blood glucose levels.
Oral anticoagulants: altered anticoagulant dosage requirements. Monitor PT.
Oxyphenbutazone: may elevate serum levels of oxyphenbutazone. Monitor patients for adverse reactions.

CONTRAINDICATIONS
• Contraindicated in patients hypersensitive to the drug, in women, and men with known or suspected breast or prostate cancer.
• Use cautiously in elderly men because they may be at greater risk for developing prostatic hyperplasia or prostate cancer. Also use cautiously in patients with preexisting renal, hepatic, or cardiac disease.

NURSING CONSIDERATIONS
• Because chronic use of systemic androgens is associated with polycythemia, monitor hematocrit and hemoglobin levels periodically in patients on long-term therapy.
• Periodically assess liver function tests, serum lipid profiles, and prostatic acid phosphatase and prostate-specific antigen levels.
• Advise patients to report persistent erections, nausea, vomiting, changes in skin color, or ankle edema to the doctor.
• Topical testosterone preparations used by men have caused virilization in female partners. These women should report acne or changes in body hair distribution.
• Teach patients how to apply the transdermal system. Warn patients that adequate serum levels will not be attained if the patch is not applied to genital skin.

54

Estrogens and progestins

chlorotrianisene
dienestrol
diethylstilbestrol
diethylstilbestrol diphosphate
esterified estrogens
estradiol
estradiol cypionate
estradiol valerate
estrogens, conjugated
estrone
estropipate
ethinyl estradiol
ethinyl estradiol and desogestrel
ethinyl estradiol and ethynodiol diacetate
ethinyl estradiol and levonorgestrel
ethinyl estradiol and norethindrone
ethinyl estradiol and norethindrone acetate
ethinyl estradiol and norgestimate
ethinyl estradiol and norgestrel
ethinyl estradiol, norethindrone acetate, and ferrous fumarate
mestranol and norethindrone
hydroxyprogesterone caproate
levonorgestrel
medroxyprogesterone acetate
norethindrone
norethindrone acetate
norgestrel
progesterone
quinestrol

COMBINATION PRODUCTS

MENRIUM 5-2: chlordiazepoxide 5 mg and esterified estrogens 0.2 mg.
MENRIUM 5-4: chlordiazepoxide 5 mg and esterified estrogens 0.4 mg.
MENRIUM 10-4: chlordiazepoxide 10 mg and esterified estrogens 0.4 mg.
PMB 200: conjugated estrogens 0.45 mg and meprobamate 200 mg.

chlorotrianisene

TACE**

Pregnancy Risk Category: X

HOW SUPPLIED

Capsules: 12 mg, 25 mg

ACTION

Mechanism: Increases the synthesis of DNA, RNA, and protein in responsive tissues and reduces release of follicle-stimulating hormone and luteinizing hormone from the pituitary.
Duration: about 24 hours.

INDICATIONS & DOSAGE

Prostate cancer –
Adults: 12 to 25 mg P.O. daily.
Atrophic vaginitis –
Adults: 12 to 25 mg P.O. daily for 30 to 60 days.
Female hypogonadism –
Adults: 12 to 25 mg P.O. for 21 days, followed by one dose of progesterone 100 mg I.M. or 5 days of oral progestogen concurrently with last 5 days of chlorotrianisene (for example, medroxyprogesterone 5 to 10 mg).
Menopausal symptoms –
Adults: 12 to 25 mg P.O. daily for 30 days or cyclic (3 weeks on, 1 week off).
Vulvar squamous hyperplasia –
Adults: 12 to 25 mg P.O. daily.

ADVERSE REACTIONS

CNS: headache, dizziness, chorea, migraine, depression.
CV: thrombophlebitis; ***thromboembolism;*** hypertension; edema; ***increased risk of CVA, pulmonary embolism, and MI.***

*Liquid form contains alcohol.
**May contain tartrazine.

Common reactions are in italics; ***life-threatening,*** in bold italics.

EENT: worsening of myopia or astigmatism, intolerance of contact lenses.
GI: *nausea,* vomiting, abdominal cramps, bloating, diarrhea, constipation, anorexia, increased appetite, excessive thirst, weight changes, pancreatitis.
GU: in women – breakthrough bleeding, altered menstrual flow, dysmenorrhea, amenorrhea, cervical erosion or abnormal secretions, enlargement of uterine fibromas, vaginal candidiasis; in men – *gynecomastia, testicular atrophy, impotence.*
Hepatic: cholestatic jaundice.
Skin: melasma, urticaria, acne, seborrhea, oily skin, hirsutism or hair loss.
Other: leg cramps, purpura, breast changes (tenderness, enlargement, secretion), hyperglycemia, hypercalcemia, folic acid deficiency, libido changes.

INTERACTIONS

Bromocriptine: may cause amenorrhea, interfering with bromocriptine's effects. Avoid concomitant use.
Carbamazepine, phenobarbital, rifampin: decreased effectiveness of estrogen therapy. Monitor closely.
Corticosteroids: possible enhanced effects. Monitor closely.
Cyclosporine: increased risk of toxicity. Use together with caution and frequently monitor cyclosporine levels.
Dantrolene, other hepatotoxic medications: increased risk of hepatotoxicity. Monitor closely.
Oral anticoagulants: dosage adjustments may be necessary. Monitor PT.
Tamoxifen: estrogens may interfere with effectiveness of tamoxifen. Avoid concomitant use.

CONTRAINDICATIONS

- Contraindicated in patients with thrombophlebitis or thromboembolic disorders; in those with breast, reproductive organ, or genital cancer; in those with undiagnosed abnormal genital bleeding; and during pregnancy.
- Use cautiously in patients with hypertension, asthma, mental depression, bone diseases, blood dyscrasias, gallbladder disease, migraine, seizures, diabetes mellitus, amenorrhea, heart failure, hepatic or renal dysfunction, uterine fibroids, hypercalcemia from metastatic breast disease, and family history (mother, grandmother, sister) of breast or genital tract cancer. Development or worsening of these conditions may require discontinuation of drug.

NURSING CONSIDERATIONS

- Studies suggest that postmenopausal women who use estrogen replacement for more than 5 years to treat menopausal symptoms may be at increased risk for endometrial carcinoma. This risk is reduced by using cyclic rather than continuous therapy and the lowest possible dosages of estrogen. Adding progestins to the regimen decreases the incidence of endometrial hyperplasia; however, it isn't known if progestins affect the incidence of endometrial carcinoma. Most studies show no increased risk of breast cancer. Emphasize the importance of regular physical examinations.
- Ensure that patients have a thorough physical examination before initiating estrogen therapy. Advise patients receiving long-term therapy to have repeat examinations yearly. Periodically monitor blood pressure, hepatic function, and serum lipid levels.
- Patient package insert that describes estrogen's adverse effects is available; however, also provide verbal explanation.
- Warn patients to immediately report suspected pregnancy; abdominal pain; pain, numbness, or stiffness in legs or buttocks; pressure or pain in chest; shortness of breath; severe headaches; visual disturbances, such as blind

spots, flashing lights, or blurriness; vaginal bleeding or discharge; breast lumps; swelling of hands or feet; yellow skin and sclera; dark urine; and light-colored stools.

- Not used for menstrual disorders because duration of action is very long.
- Notify the pathologist about any patients receiving estrogen therapy.
- Tell diabetic patients to report elevated blood glucose test results so antidiabetic medication dose can be adjusted.
- Teach women how to perform routine breast self-examination.
- Explain to patients on cyclic therapy for postmenopausal symptoms that, although withdrawal bleeding may occur during week off drug, fertility has not been restored. Pregnancy cannot occur because patients have not ovulated.
- May cause fluid retention and edema. Monitor weight regularly and recommend sodium restriction, as needed.
- Because of the risk of thromboembolism, discontinue therapy at least 1 month before procedures associated with prolonged immobilization or thromboembolism, such as knee or hip surgery.

dienestrol (dienoestrol)

DV, Ortho Dienestrol

Pregnancy Risk Category: X

HOW SUPPLIED

Vaginal cream: 0.01%

ACTION

Mechanism: Increases the synthesis of DNA, RNA, and protein in responsive tissues. Also reduces release of follicle-stimulating hormone and luteinizing hormone from the pituitary.
Duration: 24 to 48 hours.

INDICATIONS & DOSAGE

Atrophic vaginitis and kraurosis vulvae –
Postmenopausal women: 1 to 2 intravaginal applications of vaginal cream daily for 1 to 2 weeks (as directed); then half that dose for the same period. Doctor may prescribe a maintenance dosage of 1 applicatorful one to three times a week.

ADVERSE REACTIONS

GU: vaginal discharge, increased intravaginal discomfort, uterine bleeding with excessive use, burning sensation.
Other: systemic effects (breast tenderness, peripheral edema).

INTERACTIONS

Bromocriptine: may cause amenorrhea, interfering with bromocriptine's effects. Avoid concomitant use.
Carbamazepine, phenobarbital, rifampin: decreased effectiveness of estrogen therapy. Monitor closely.
Corticosteroids: possible enhanced effects. Monitor closely.
Cyclosporine: increased risk of toxicity. Use together with caution and frequently monitor cyclosporine levels.
Dantrolene, other hepatotoxic medications: increased risk of hepatotoxicity. Monitor closely.
Oral anticoagulants: dosage adjustments may be necessary. Monitor PT.
Tamoxifen: estrogens may interfere with effectiveness of tamoxifen. Avoid concomitant use.

CONTRAINDICATIONS

- Contraindicated in patients with thrombophlebitis or thromboembolic disorders; in those with breast, reproductive organ, or genital cancer; or in those with undiagnosed abnormal genital bleeding; and during pregnancy.
- Use cautiously in patients with menstrual irregularities or endometriosis.

NURSING CONSIDERATIONS

- Ensure that patients have a thorough physical examination before initiating estrogen therapy. Patients receiving long-term therapy should have repeat examinations yearly. Periodically monitor body weight, blood pressure, hepatic function, and serum lipid levels.
- Instruct patients to apply drug at bedtime to increase effectiveness.
- Patient package insert that describes estrogen's adverse effects is available; however, also provide verbal explanation.
- Systemic reactions are possible with normal intravaginal use. Monitor closely.
- Warn patients not to exceed the prescribed dose.
- Withdrawal bleeding may occur if estrogen is suddenly stopped.
- Patients should not wear a tampon while receiving vaginal therapy. They may need to wear a sanitary pad to protect clothing.
- Teach patients how to insert suppositories or cream and tell them to wash vaginal area with soap and water before application.
- Instruct patients to remain recumbent for 30 minutes after administration to prevent loss of drug.
- Instruct patients to report systemic reactions (breast pain or tenderness, swelling of the hands or feet) or vaginal discharge or bleeding.
- Teach women how to perform routine breast self-examination.

diethylstilbestrol (stilboestrol)

DES

diethylstilbestrol diphosphate

DES, Honvol†, Stilphostrol

Pregnancy Risk Category: X

HOW SUPPLIED

diethylstilbestrol

Tablets: 1 mg, 5 mg

diethylstilbestrol diphosphate

Tablets: 50 mg, 83 mg†

Injection: 50 mg/ml†

ACTION

Mechanism: Increases the synthesis of DNA, RNA, and protein in responsive tissues. Also reduces release of follicle-stimulating hormone and luteinizing hormone from the pituitary.

Duration: about 24 hours.

INDICATIONS & DOSAGE

Postcoital contraception ("morning-after pill") –

Women: 25 mg P.O. b.i.d. for 5 days. Start therapy within 24 hours after coitus.

Prostate cancer –

Men: initially, 1 to 3 mg P.O. daily; may be reduced to 1 mg daily, or 50 to 200 mg (diphosphate) t.i.d. Or, give 250 to 1,000 mg I.V. daily for 5 days; then once or twice weekly.

Breast cancer –

Men and postmenopausal women: 15 mg P.O. daily.

ADVERSE REACTIONS

CNS: headache, dizziness, chorea, depression, lethargy.

CV: thrombophlebitis; ***thromboembolism;*** hypertension; edema; ***increased risk of CVA, pulmonary embolism, and MI.***

EENT: worsening of myopia or astigmatism, intolerance of contact lenses.

GI: *nausea,* vomiting, abdominal cramps, bloating, diarrhea, constipation, anorexia, increased appetite, excessive thirst, weight changes, pancreatitis.

GU: in women – breakthrough bleeding, altered menstrual flow, dysmenorrhea, amenorrhea, cervical erosion, altered cervical secretions, enlargement of uterine fibromas, vaginal candidiasis, loss of libido; in men – gyne-

comastia, testicular atrophy, impotence.
Hepatic: cholestatic jaundice.
Skin: melasma, urticaria, acne, seborrhea, oily skin, hirsutism or hair loss.
Other: leg cramps, breast tenderness or enlargement, hyperglycemia, hypercalcemia, folic acid deficiency.

INTERACTIONS

Bromocriptine: may cause amenorrhea, interfering with bromocriptine's effects. Avoid concomitant use.
Carbamazepine, phenobarbital, rifampin: decreased effectiveness of estrogen therapy. Monitor closely.
Corticosteroids: possible enhanced effects. Monitor closely.
Cyclosporine: increased risk of toxicity. Use together with caution and frequently monitor cyclosporine levels.
Dantrolene, other hepatotoxic medications: increased risk of hepatotoxicity. Monitor closely.
Oral anticoagulants: dosage adjustments may be necessary. Monitor PT.
Tamoxifen: estrogens may interfere with effectiveness of tamoxifen. Avoid concomitant use.

CONTRAINDICATIONS

- Contraindicated in patients with thrombophlebitis or thromboembolic disorders and undiagnosed abnormal genital bleeding and during pregnancy.
- Use cautiously in patients with hypertension, asthma, mental depression, bone disease, migraine, seizures, blood dyscrasias, diabetes mellitus, gallbladder disease, amenorrhea, heart failure, hepatic or renal dysfunction, and family history (mother, grandmother, sister) of breast or genital tract cancer. Development or worsening of these conditions may require discontinuation of drug.

NURSING CONSIDERATIONS

- Ensure that patients have a thorough physical examination before initiating estrogen therapy. Patients receiving long-term therapy should have repeat examinations yearly. Periodically monitor body weight, blood pressure, hepatic function, and serum lipid levels.
- Patient package insert that describes estrogen's adverse effects is available; however, also provide verbal explanation.
- Warn patients to stop taking drug immediately if they become pregnant because drug can adversely affect the fetus.
- Warn patients to immediately report abdominal pain; pain, numbness, or stiffness in legs or buttocks; pressure or pain in chest; shortness of breath; severe headache; visual disturbances, such as blind spots, flashing lights, or blurriness; vaginal bleeding or discharge; breast lumps; sudden weight gain; swelling of hands or feet; yellow sclera or skin; dark urine; or light-colored stools.
- Notify the pathologist about any patients receiving estrogen therapy.
- Tell diabetic patients to report elevated blood glucose test results so antidiabetic medication dose can be adjusted.
- High incidence of gross nonmalignant genital changes may occur in offspring of women taking drug during pregnancy. Female offspring have a higher than normal risk of developing cervical and vaginal adenocarcinoma. Male offspring may have a higher than normal risk of developing testicular tumors, epididymal cysts, and impaired fertility.
- Increased number of CV deaths reported in men taking diethylstilbestrol tablet (5 mg daily) for prostate cancer over long time period. This effect is not associated with 1-mg daily dose.
- **I.V. use:** Mix ordered dose in 250 to

500 ml of D_5W or 0.9% sodium chloride. Infuse at 1 to 2 ml/minute for the first 15 minutes; if no adverse reactions occur, increase infusion rate to administer entire dose within 1 hour.
- To administer I.M., give by deep injection. Rotate injection sites to prevent muscle atrophy.
- If patients experience GI upset, give drug with or immediately after meals.
- Do not crush, break, or chew enteric-coated tablets.
- Because of the risk of thromboembolism, discontinue therapy at least 1 month before procedures associated with prolonged immobilization or thromboembolism, such as knee or hip surgery.
- Teach women how to perform routine breast self-examination.

esterified estrogens
Estratab, Menest, Neo-Estrone†

Pregnancy Risk Category: X

HOW SUPPLIED
Tablets: 0.3 mg, 0.625 mg, 1.25 mg, 2.5 mg

ACTION
Mechanism: Increases the synthesis of DNA, RNA, and protein in responsive tissues. Also reduces release of follicle-stimulating hormone and luteinizing hormone from the pituitary.
Duration: about 24 hours.

INDICATIONS & DOSAGE
Inoperable prostate cancer –
Men: 1.25 to 2.5 mg P.O. t.i.d.
Breast cancer –
Men and postmenopausal women: 10 mg P.O. t.i.d. for 3 or more months.
Hypogonadism, castration, primary ovarian failure –
Women: 2.5 mg P.O. daily to t.i.d. in cycles of 3 weeks on, 1 week off.
Menopausal symptoms –
Women: average dosage is 0.3 to 3.75 mg P.O. daily in cycles of 3 weeks on, 1 week off.

ADVERSE REACTIONS
CNS: headache, dizziness, chorea, depression, lethargy.
CV: thrombophlebitis; ***thromboembolism;*** hypertension; edema; ***increased risk of CVA, pulmonary embolism, and MI.***
EENT: worsening of myopia or astigmatism, intolerance of contact lenses.
GI: *nausea,* vomiting, abdominal cramps, bloating, diarrhea, constipation, anorexia, increased appetite, weight changes, pancreatitis.
GU: in women – breakthrough bleeding, altered menstrual flow, dysmenorrhea, amenorrhea, cervical erosion, altered cervical secretions, enlargement of uterine fibromas, vaginal candidiasis; in men – gynecomastia, testicular atrophy, impotence.
Hepatic: cholestatic jaundice.
Skin: melasma, rash, acne, hirsutism or hair loss, seborrhea, oily skin.
Other: breast changes (tenderness, enlargement, secretion), hyperglycemia, hypercalcemia, folic acid deficiency, libido changes.

INTERACTIONS
Bromocriptine: may cause amenorrhea, interfering with bromocriptine's effects. Avoid concomitant use.
Carbamazepine, phenobarbital, rifampin: decreased effectiveness of estrogen therapy. Monitor closely.
Corticosteroids: possible enhanced effects. Monitor closely.
Cyclosporine: increased risk of toxicity. Use together with caution and frequently monitor cyclosporine levels.
Dantrolene, other hepatotoxic medications: increased risk of hepatotoxicity. Monitor closely.
Oral anticoagulants: dosage adjustments may be necessary. Monitor PT.
Tamoxifen: estrogens may interfere with effectiveness of tamoxifen. Avoid concomitant use.

CONTRAINDICATIONS

• Contraindicated in patients with thrombophlebitis or thromboembolic disorders and undiagnosed abnormal genital bleeding, and during pregnancy.

• Use cautiously in patients with history of hypertension, mental depression, gallbladder disease, migraine, seizures, diabetes mellitus, amenorrhea, or family history (mother, grandmother, sister) of breast or genital tract cancer. Development or worsening of these conditions may require discontinuation of drug.

NURSING CONSIDERATIONS

• Ensure that patients have a thorough physical examination before initiating estrogen therapy. Patients receiving long-term therapy should have repeat examinations yearly. Periodically monitor body weight, blood pressure, serum lipid levels, and hepatic function.

• Patient package insert that describes estrogen's adverse effects is available; however, also provide verbal explanation.

• Studies suggest that postmenopausal women who use estrogen replacement for more than 5 years to treat menopausal symptoms may be at increased risk for endometrial carcinoma. This risk is reduced by using cyclic rather than continuous therapy and the lowest possible dosages of estrogen. Adding progestins to the regimen decreases the incidence of endometrial hyperplasia; however, it isn't known if progestins affect the incidence of endometrial carcinoma. Most studies show no increased risk of breast cancer. Emphasize the importance of regular physical examinations.

• Warn patients to immediately report abdominal pain; pain, numbness, or stiffness in legs or buttocks; pressure or pain in chest; shortness of breath; severe headaches; visual disturbances, such as blind spots, flashing lights, or blurriness; vaginal bleeding or discharge; breast lumps; swelling of hands or feet; yellow skin or sclera; dark urine; or light-colored stools.

• Notify the pathologist about any patients receiving estrogen therapy.

• Tell diabetic patients to report elevated blood glucose test results so antidiabetic medication dosage can be adjusted.

• Explain to patients on cyclic therapy for postmenopausal symptoms that, although they may experience withdrawal bleeding during week off drug, fertility has not been restored. Pregnancy cannot occur because patients have not ovulated.

• Because of the risk of thromboembolism, discontinue therapy at least one month before procedures associated with prolonged immobilization or thromboembolism, such as knee or hip surgery.

• Teach women how to perform routine breast self-examination.

estradiol (oestradiol)

Estrace**, Estrace Vaginal Cream, Estraderm

estradiol cypionate

depGynogen, Depo-Estradiol, Dura-Estrin, E-Cypionate, Estro-Cyp, Estrofem, Estroject-L.A.

estradiol valerate (oestradiol valerate)

Delestrogen, Dioval, Duragen 10, Duragen 20, Duragen 40, Estradiol L.A., Estraval, Estraval P.A., Estra-L 20, Estra-L 40, Feminate, Femogex, Gynogen L.A., L.A.E., Menaval, Primogyn Depot‡, Ru-Est-Span 20, Ru-Est-Span 40, Valergen 10, Valergen 20, Valergen 40

Pregnancy Risk Category: X

HOW SUPPLIED
estradiol
Tablets (micronized): 0.5 mg, 1 mg, 2 mg
Transdermal: 4 mg/10 cm² (delivers 0.05 mg/24 hours); 8 mg/20 cm² (delivers 0.1 mg/24 hours)
Vaginal cream (in nonliquefying base): 0.1 mg/g
estradiol cypionate
Injection (in oil): 1 mg/ml, 5 mg/ml
estradiol valerate
Injection (in oil): 10 mg/ml, 20 mg/ml, 40 mg/ml

ACTION
Mechanism: Increases the synthesis of DNA, RNA, and protein in responsive tissues. Also reduces release of follicle-stimulating hormone and luteinizing hormone from the pituitary.
Duration: about 24 hours.

INDICATIONS & DOSAGE
Menopausal symptoms, female hypogonadism, female castration, primary ovarian failure –
Adults: 1 to 2 mg P.O. daily, in cycles of 21 days on and 7 days off or cycles of 5 days on and 2 days off; or 0.2 to 1 mg I.M. weekly.
Kraurosis vulvae –
Adults: 1 to 1.5 mg I.M. once or more per week.
Atrophic vaginitis –
Adults: 2 to 4 g intravaginal applications of cream daily for 1 to 2 weeks. When vaginal mucosa is restored, begin maintenance dosage of 1 g one to three times weekly.
Menopausal symptoms –
Adults: 1 to 5 mg (cypionate) I.M. q 3 to 4 weeks; or 5 to 20 mg (valerate) I.M., repeated once after 2 to 3 weeks.
Postpartum breast engorgement –
Adults: 10 to 25 mg (valerate) I.M. at end of first stage of labor.
Inoperable breast cancer in women –
Adults: 10 mg P.O. (estradiol) t.i.d. for 3 months.
Moderate to severe menopausal symptoms, female hypogonadism, female castration, primary ovarian failure, and atrophic conditions caused by deficient endogenous estrogen production –
Adults: place 1 Estraderm transdermal patch on trunk of body twice weekly on cycles of 3 weeks on and 1 week off.
Inoperable prostate cancer –
Adults: 30 mg (valerate) I.M. q 1 to 2 weeks, or 1 to 2 mg P.O. (estradiol) t.i.d.

ADVERSE REACTIONS
CV: thrombophlebitis, ***thromboembolism,*** hypertension, edema.
EENT: worsening of myopia or astigmatism, intolerance of contact lenses.
GI: *nausea,* vomiting, abdominal cramps, bloating, diarrhea, constipation, anorexia, increased appetite, weight changes, pancreatitis.
GU: in women – breakthrough bleeding, altered menstrual flow, dysmenorrhea, amenorrhea, cervical erosion, altered cervical secretions, enlargement of uterine fibromas, vaginal candidiasis; in men – gynecomastia, testicular atrophy, impotence.
Hepatic: cholestatic jaundice.
Skin: melasma, urticaria, acne, seborrhea, oily skin, hirsutism or hair loss.
Other: breast changes (tenderness, enlargement, secretion), leg cramps, hyperglycemia, hypercalcemia, folic acid deficiency.

INTERACTIONS
Bromocriptine: may cause amenorrhea, interfering with bromocriptine's effects. Avoid concomitant use.
Carbamazepine, phenobarbital, rifampin: decreased effectiveness of estrogen therapy. Monitor closely.
Corticosteroids: possible enhanced effects. Monitor closely.
Cyclosporine: increased risk of toxic-

ity. Use together with caution and frequently monitor cyclosporine levels.
Dantrolene, other hepatotoxic medications: increased risk of hepatotoxicity. Monitor closely.
Oral anticoagulants: dosage adjustments may be necessary. Monitor PT.
Tamoxifen: estrogens may interfere with effectiveness of tamoxifen. Avoid concomitant use.

CONTRAINDICATIONS

- Contraindicated in patients with thrombophlebitis or thromboembolic disorders, breast or reproductive organ cancer, and undiagnosed abnormal genital bleeding, and during pregnancy.
- Use cautiously in patients with hypertension, mental depression, bone diseases, blood dyscrasias, migraine, seizures, diabetes mellitus, amenorrhea, heart failure, hepatic or renal dysfunction, or family history (mother, grandmother, sister) of breast or genital tract cancer. Development or worsening of these conditions may require discontinuation of drug.

NURSING CONSIDERATIONS

- Studies suggest that postmenopausal women who use estrogen replacement for more than 5 years to treat menopausal symptoms may be at increased risk for endometrial carcinoma. This risk is reduced by using cyclic rather than continuous therapy and the lowest possible dosages of estrogen. Adding progestins to the regimen decreases the incidence of endometrial hyperplasia; however, it isn't known if progestins affect the incidence of endometrial carcinoma. Most studies show no increased risk of breast cancer. Emphasize the importance of regular physical examinations.
- Ensure that patients have a thorough physical examination before initiating estrogen therapy. Patients receiving long-term therapy should have repeat examinations yearly. Periodically monitor serum lipid levels, blood pressure, body weight, and hepatic function.
- Patient package insert that describes estrogen's adverse effects is available; however, also provide verbal explanation.
- Warn patients to immediately report abdominal pain; pain, numbness, or stiffness in legs or buttocks; pressure or pain in chest; shortness of breath; severe headaches; visual disturbances, such as blind spots, flashing lights, or blurriness; vaginal bleeding or discharge; breast lumps; swelling of hands or feet; yellow skin or sclera; dark urine; or light-colored stools.
- Tell diabetic patients to report elevated blood glucose test results so antidiabetic medication dosage can be adjusted.
- Notify the pathologist about any patients receiving estrogen therapy.
- Ask patients about allergies, especially to foods or plants. Estradiol is available as an aqueous solution or as a solution in peanut oil; estradiol cypionate, as a solution in cottonseed oil or vegetable oil; estradiol valerate, as a solution in castor oil, sesame oil, or vegetable oil.
- Teach patients how to use vaginal cream. Patients should wash vaginal area with soap and water before applying. Tell them to take drug at bedtime or to lie flat for 30 minutes after instillation to minimize drug loss.
- To administer as an injection, make sure drug is well dispersed in solution by rolling vial between palms. Inject deep I.M. into large muscle. Rotate injection sites to prevent muscle atrophy. Never give drug I.V.
- Apply the transdermal patch to clean, dry, hairless, intact skin on abdomen or buttocks. Do not apply to breasts, waistline, or other areas where clothing can loosen the patch. When applying, ensure good contact

with the skin, especially around the edges, and hold in place with the palm for about 10 seconds. Rotate application sites.

- In women who are currently taking oral estrogen, treatment with the Estraderm transdermal patch can begin 1 week after withdrawal of oral therapy or sooner if menopausal symptoms appear before the end of the week.
- Teach women how to perform routine breast self-examination.
- Explain to patients on cyclic therapy for postmenopausal symptoms that, although withdrawal bleeding may occur during week off drug, fertility has not been restored. Pregnancy cannot occur because patients have not ovulated.
- Because of the risk of thromboembolism, discontinue therapy at least 1 month before procedures associated with prolonged immobilization or thromboembolism, such as knee or hip surgery.

estrogens, conjugated (estrogenic substances, conjugated; oestrogens, conjugated)

C.E.S.†, Premarin, Premarin Intravenous

Pregnancy Risk Category: X

HOW SUPPLIED

Tablets: 0.3 mg, 0.625 mg, 0.9 mg, 1.25 mg, 2.5 mg
Injection: 25 mg/5 ml
Vaginal cream: 0.625 mg/g

ACTION

Mechanism: Increases the synthesis of DNA, RNA, and protein in responsive tissues. Also reduces release of follicle-stimulating hormone and luteinizing hormone from the pituitary.
Duration: about 24 hours.

INDICATIONS & DOSAGE

Abnormal uterine bleeding (hormonal imbalance) –
Women: 25 mg I.V. or I.M. Repeat in 6 to 12 hours.
Breast cancer (at least 5 years after menopause) –
Postmenopausal women: 10 mg P.O. t.i.d. for 3 months or more.
Castration, primary ovarian failure, osteoporosis –
Women: 1.25 mg P.O. daily in cycles of 3 weeks on and 1 week off.
Hypogonadism –
Women: 2.5 mg P.O. b.i.d. or t.i.d. for 20 consecutive days each month.
Menopausal symptoms –
Women: 0.3 to 1.25 mg P.O. daily in cycles of 3 weeks on and 1 week off.
Postpartum breast engorgement –
Women: 3.75 mg P.O. q 4 hours for five doses or 1.25 mg q 4 hours for 5 days.
Atrophic vaginitis, kraurosis vulvae associated with menopause –
Women: 2 to 4 g intravaginally on a cyclical basis (3 weeks on and 1 week off).
Inoperable prostate cancer –
Men: 1.25 to 2.5 mg P.O. t.i.d.

ADVERSE REACTIONS

CNS: headache, dizziness, chorea, depression, lethargy.
CV: thrombophlebitis; ***thromboembolism;*** hypertension; edema; ***increased risk of CVA, pulmonary embolism, and MI.***
EENT: worsening of myopia or astigmatism, intolerance of contact lenses.
GI: *nausea,* vomiting, abdominal cramps, bloating, diarrhea, constipation, anorexia, increased appetite, weight changes, pancreatitis.
GU: in women – breakthrough bleeding, altered menstrual flow, dysmenorrhea, amenorrhea, cervical erosion, altered cervical secretions, enlargement of uterine fibromas, vaginal candidiasis; in men – gynecomastia, testicular atrophy, impotence.

Hepatic: cholestatic jaundice.
Skin: melasma, urticaria, acne, seborrhea, oily skin, flushing (when given rapidly I.V.), hirsutism or hair loss.
Other: breast changes (tenderness, enlargement, secretion), leg cramps, hyperglycemia, hypercalcemia, folic acid deficiency, libido changes.

INTERACTIONS

Bromocriptine: may cause amenorrhea, interfering with bromocriptine's effects. Avoid concomitant use.
Carbamazepine, phenobarbital, rifampin: decreased effectiveness of estrogen therapy. Monitor closely.
Corticosteroids: possible enhanced effects. Monitor closely.
Cyclosporine: increased risk of toxicity. Use together with caution and frequently monitor cyclosporine levels.
Dantrolene, other hepatotoxic medications: increased risk of hepatotoxicity. Monitor closely.
Oral anticoagulants: dosage adjustments may be necessary. Monitor PT.
Tamoxifen: estrogens may interfere with effectiveness of tamoxifen. Avoid concomitant use.

CONTRAINDICATIONS

- Contraindicated in patients with thrombophlebitis or thromboembolic disorders and undiagnosed abnormal genital bleeding, and during pregnancy.
- Use cautiously in patients with hypertension, gallbladder disease, bone diseases, blood dyscrasias, migraine, seizures, diabetes mellitus, amenorrhea, heart failure, hepatic or renal dysfunction, or family history (mother, grandmother, sister) of breast or genital tract cancer. Development or worsening of these conditions may require discontinuation of drug.

NURSING CONSIDERATIONS

- Studies suggest that postmenopausal women who use estrogen replacement for more than 5 years to treat menopausal symptoms may be at increased risk for endometrial carcinoma. This risk is reduced by using cyclic rather than continuous therapy and the lowest possible dosages of estrogen. Adding progestins to the regimen decreases the incidence of endometrial hyperplasia; however, it isn't known if progestins affect the incidence of endometrial carcinoma. Most studies show no increased risk of breast cancer. Emphasize the importance of regular physical examinations.
- Ensure that patients have a thorough physical examination before initiating estrogen therapy. Patients receiving long-term therapy should have repeat examinations yearly. Periodically monitor serum lipid levels, blood pressure, body weight, and hepatic function.
- Patient package insert that describes estrogen's adverse effects is available; however, also provide verbal explanation.
- Warn patients to immediately report abdominal pain; pain, numbness, or stiffness in legs or buttocks; pressure or pain in chest; shortness of breath; severe headaches; visual disturbances, such as blind spots, flashing lights, or blurriness; vaginal bleeding or discharge; breast lumps; swelling of hands or feet; yellow skin or sclera; dark urine; or light-colored stools.
- Teach patients how to use vaginal cream. Patients should wash the vaginal area with soap and water before applying. Tell them to use drug at bedtime or to lie flat for 30 minutes after instillation to minimize drug loss.
- I.M. or I.V. use preferred for rapid treatment of dysfunctional uterine bleeding or reduction of surgical bleeding.
- **I.V. use:** When giving by direct I.V.

injection, administer slowly to avoid flushing reaction. For infusion, mix with D_5W, 0.9% sodium chloride injection, or invert sugar solutions. Avoid mixing with solutions of acidic pH to prevent incompatibility.

- Refrigerate before reconstituting. Agitate gently after adding diluent.
- When administering by I.M. injection, inject deep into large muscle. Rotate injection sites to prevent muscle atrophy.
- Notify the pathologist about any patients receiving estrogen therapy.
- Tell diabetic patients to report elevated blood glucose test results so antidiabetic medication dosage can be adjusted.
- Teach women how to perform routine breast self-examination.
- Explain to patients on cyclic therapy for postmenopausal symptoms that, although withdrawal bleeding may occur during week off drug, fertility has not been restored. Pregnancy cannot occur because they have not ovulated.
- Because of the risk of thromboembolism, discontinue therapy at least 1 month before procedures associated with prolonged immobilization or thromboembolism, such as knee or hip surgery.

estrone (oestrone)

Estrone "5", Estroject-2, Estrone A, Femogen Forte†, Gynogen, Kestrin Aqueous, Kestrone-5, Theelin Aqueous, Unigen, Wehgen

Pregnancy Risk Category: X

HOW SUPPLIED

Injection (aqueous suspension): 2 mg/ml, 5 mg/ml

ACTION

Mechanism: Increases the synthesis of DNA, RNA, and protein in responsive tissues. Also reduces release of follicle-stimulating hormone and luteinizing hormone from the pituitary.
Duration: 48 to 72 hours.

INDICATIONS & DOSAGE

Atrophic vaginitis and menopausal symptoms –
Adults: 0.1 to 0.5 mg I.M. two or three times weekly.
Female hypogonadism and primary ovarian failure –
Adults: 0.1 to 1 mg I.M. weekly as a single dose or in divided doses.
Inoperable prostate cancer –
Adults: 2 to 4 mg I.M. two to three times weekly.

ADVERSE REACTIONS

CNS: headache, dizziness, chorea, depression, lethargy.
CV: thrombophlebitis, ***thromboembolism,*** hypertension, edema.
EENT: worsening of myopia or astigmatism, intolerance of contact lenses.
GI: *nausea,* vomiting, abdominal cramps, bloating, diarrhea, constipation, anorexia, increased appetite, weight changes, pancreatitis.
GU: in women – breakthrough bleeding, altered menstrual flow, dysmenorrhea, amenorrhea, cervical erosion, altered cervical secretions, enlargement of uterine fibromas, vaginal candidiasis; in men – gynecomastia, testicular atrophy, impotence.
Hepatic: cholestatic jaundice.
Skin: melasma, urticaria, acne, seborrhea, oily skin, hirsutism or hair loss.
Other: breast changes (tenderness, enlargement, secretion), leg cramps, hyperglycemia, hypercalcemia, folic acid deficiency, libido changes.

INTERACTIONS

Bromocriptine: may cause amenorrhea, interfering with bromocriptine's effects. Avoid concomitant use.
Carbamazepine, phenobarbital, rifampin: decreased effectiveness of estrogen therapy. Monitor closely.

Corticosteroids: possible enhanced effects. Monitor closely.
Cyclosporine: increased risk of toxicity. Use together with caution and frequently monitor cyclosporine levels.
Dantrolene, other hepatotoxic medications: increased risk of hepatotoxicity. Monitor closely.
Oral anticoagulants: dosage adjustments may be necessary. Monitor PT.
Tamoxifen: estrogens may interfere with effectiveness of tamoxifen. Avoid concomitant use.

CONTRAINDICATIONS

• Contraindicated in patients with thrombophlebitis or thromboembolic disorders, breast or reproductive organ cancer, and undiagnosed abnormal genital bleeding, and during pregnancy.

• Use cautiously in patients with hypertension, mental depression, migraine, seizures, diabetes mellitus, amenorrhea, hepatic or renal dysfunction, or family history (mother, grandmother, sister) of breast or genital tract cancer. Development or worsening of these conditions may require discontinuation of drug.

NURSING CONSIDERATIONS

• Studies suggest that postmenopausal women who use estrogen replacement for more than 5 years to treat menopausal symptoms may be at increased risk for endometrial carcinoma. This risk is reduced by using cyclic rather than continuous therapy and the lowest possible dosages of estrogen. Adding progestins to the regimen decreases the incidence of endometrial hyperplasia; however, it isn't known if progestins affect the incidence of endometrial carcinoma. Most studies show no increased risk of breast cancer. Emphasize the importance of regular physical examinations.

• Ensure that patients have a thorough physical examination before initiating estrogen therapy. Patients receiving long-term therapy should have repeat examinations yearly. Periodically monitor serum lipid levels, blood pressure, body weight, and hepatic function.

• Patient package insert that describes estrogen's adverse effects is available; however, also provide verbal explanation.

• Administer estrone I.M. Rotate injection sites to prevent muscle atrophy.

• Warn patients to immediately report abdominal pain; pain, numbness, or stiffness in legs or buttocks; pressure or pain in chest; shortness of breath; severe headaches; visual disturbances, such as blind spots, flashing lights, or blurriness; vaginal bleeding or discharge; breast lumps; swelling of hands or feet; yellow skin and sclera; dark urine; or light-colored stools.

• Notify the pathologist about any patients receiving estrogen therapy.

• Tell diabetic patients to report elevated blood glucose test results so antidiabetic medication dosage can be adjusted.

• Teach women how to perform routine breast self-examination.

• Explain to patients on cyclic therapy for postmenopausal symptoms that, although withdrawal bleeding may occur during week off drug, fertility has not been restored. Pregnancy cannot occur because patients have not ovulated.

• Because of the risk of thromboembolism, discontinue therapy at least 1 month before procedures associated with prolonged immobilization or thromboembolism, such as knee or hip surgery.

estropipate (piperazine estrone sulfate)

Ogen, OrthoEST

Pregnancy Risk Category: X

HOW SUPPLIED

Tablets: 0.75 mg, 1.5 mg, 3 mg, 5 mg
Vaginal cream: 1.5 mg/g

ACTION

Mechanism: Increases the synthesis of DNA, RNA, and proteins in responsive tissues. Also reduces release of follicle-stimulating hormone and luteinizing hormone from the pituitary.
Duration: 24 hours.

INDICATIONS & DOSAGE

Atrophic vaginitis or kraurosis vulvae –
Adults: 0.625 to 5 mg P.O. daily; or 2 to 4 g of vaginal cream daily. Typically, give dosage on a cyclical, short-term basis.
Primary ovarian failure, female castration, female hypogonadism, or moderate to severe vasomotor symptoms associated with menopause –
Adults: administer on a cyclical basis – 1.25 to 7.5 mg P.O. daily for the first 3 weeks, followed by a rest period of 8 to 10 days. If bleeding does not occur by the end of the rest period, repeat cycle.
Prevention of osteoporosis in women –
Adults: 0.625 mg P.O. daily for 25 days of a 31-day cycle each month.

ADVERSE REACTIONS

CNS: depression, headache, dizziness, migraine.
CV: edema, thrombophlebitis; ***increased risk of CVA, pulmonary embolism, and MI.***
GI: nausea, vomiting, abdominal cramps, bloating, weight changes.
GU: increased size of uterine fibromyomata, vaginal candidiasis, cystitis-like syndrome, dysmenorrhea, amenorrhea, breakthrough bleeding, premenstrual-like syndrome.
Hepatic: cholestatic jaundice.
Skin: hemorrhagic eruption, erythema nodosum, ***erythema multiforme,*** hirsutism, chloasma, hair loss.
Other: breast engorgement or enlargement, aggravation of porphyria, libido changes.

INTERACTIONS

Bromocriptine: may cause amenorrhea, interfering with bromocriptine's effects. Avoid concomitant use.
Carbamazepine, phenobarbital, rifampin: decreased effectiveness of estrogen therapy. Monitor closely.
Corticosteroids: possible enhanced effects. Monitor closely.
Cyclosporine: increased risk of toxicity. Use together with caution and frequently monitor cyclosporine levels.
Dantrolene, other hepatotoxic medications: increased risk of hepatotoxicity. Monitor closely.
Oral anticoagulants: dosage adjustments may be necessary. Monitor PT.
Tamoxifen: estrogens may interfere with effectiveness of tamoxifen. Avoid concomitant use.

CONTRAINDICATIONS

• Contraindicated in patients with thrombophlebitis or thromboembolic disorders; breast, reproductive organ, or genital cancer; and undiagnosed genital bleeding; and during pregnancy.
• Use cautiously in patients with hypertension, asthma, mental depression, bone diseases, blood dyscrasias, gallbladder disease, migraine, seizures, diabetes mellitus, amenorrhea, heart failure, hepatic or renal dysfunction, and a family history (mother, grandmother, sister) of breast or genital cancer. Development or worsening of any of these conditions may require discontinuation of drug.

NURSING CONSIDERATIONS

- Studies suggest that postmenopausal women who use estrogen replacement for more than 5 years to treat menopausal symptoms may be at increased risk for endometrial carcinoma. This risk is reduced by using cyclic rather than continuous therapy and the lowest possible dosages of estrogen. Adding progestins to the regimen decreases the incidence of endometrial hyperplasia; however, it isn't known if progestins affect the incidence of endometrial carcinoma. Most studies show no increased risk of breast cancer. Stress the importance of regular physical examinations.
- Ensure that patients have a thorough physical examination before initiating estrogen therapy. Patients receiving long-term therapy should have repeat examinations yearly. Periodically monitor serum lipid levels, blood pressure, body weight, and hepatic function.
- Patient package insert that describes estrogen's adverse effects is available; however, also provide verbal explanation.
- Warn patients to immediately report abdominal pain; pain, stiffness, or numbness in the legs or buttocks; pressure or pain in the chest; shortness of breath; severe headaches; visual disturbances, such as blind spots or flashing lights; vaginal bleeding or discharge; breast lumps; swelling of the hands or feet; yellow skin or sclera; dark urine; or light-colored stools.
- Teach women how to perform routine breast self-examination.
- When used to treat hypogonadism, the duration of therapy necessary to produce withdrawal bleeding depends on the patient's endometrial response to the drug. If satisfactory withdrawal bleeding does not occur, add an oral progestin to the regimen, as ordered. Explain to the patient that, despite the return of withdrawal bleeding, pregnancy cannot occur because she is not ovulating.
- Because of the risk of thromboembolism, discontinue therapy at least 1 month before procedures associated with prolonged immobilization or thromboembolism, such as knee or hip surgery.

---

ethinyl estradiol (ethinyloestradiol)

Estinyl**, Feminone

Pregnancy Risk Category: X

HOW SUPPLIED

Tablets: 0.02 mg, 0.05 mg, 0.5 mg

ACTION

Mechanism: Increases the synthesis of DNA, RNA, and protein in responsive tissues. Also reduces release of follicle-stimulating hormone and luteinizing hormone from the pituitary.
Duration: about 24 hours.

INDICATIONS & DOSAGE

Breast cancer (at least 5 years after menopause) –
Postmenopausal women: 1 mg P.O. t.i.d. for at least 3 months.
Hypogonadism –
Women: 0.05 mg P.O. once daily to t.i.d. 2 weeks a month, followed by 2 weeks of progesterone therapy; continue for three to six monthly dosing cycles, followed by 2 months off.
Menopausal symptoms –
Women: 0.02 to 0.05 mg P.O. daily for cycles of 3 weeks on and 1 week off.
Inoperable prostate cancer –
Men: 0.15 to 2 mg P.O. daily.

ADVERSE REACTIONS

CNS: headache, dizziness, chorea, depression, lethargy.
CV: thrombophlebitis, ***thromboembolism,*** hypertension, edema.

*Liquid form contains alcohol.
**May contain tartrazine.

Common reactions are in italics; ***life-threatening,*** in bold italics.

EENT: worsening of myopia or astigmatism, intolerance to contact lenses.
GI: *nausea,* vomiting, abdominal cramps, bloating, diarrhea, constipation, anorexia, increased appetite, weight changes.
GU: in women – breakthrough bleeding, altered menstrual flow, dysmenorrhea, amenorrhea, cervical erosion, altered cervical secretions, enlargement of uterine fibromas, vaginal candidiasis; in men – gynecomastia, testicular atrophy, impotence.
Hepatic: cholestatic jaundice.
Skin: melasma, urticaria, acne, seborrhea, oily skin, hirsutism or hair loss.
Other: breast changes (tenderness, enlargement, secretion), leg cramps, hyperglycemia, hypercalcemia, folic acid deficiency, libido changes.

INTERACTIONS

Bromocriptine: may cause amenorrhea, interfering with bromocriptine's effects. Avoid concomitant use.
Carbamazepine, phenobarbital, rifampin: decreased effectiveness of estrogen therapy. Monitor closely.
Corticosteroids: possible enhanced effects. Monitor closely.
Cyclosporine: increased risk of toxicity. Use together with caution and frequently monitor cyclosporine levels.
Dantrolene, other hepatotoxic medications: increased risk of hepatotoxicity. Monitor closely.
Oral anticoagulants: dosage adjustments may be necessary. Monitor PT.
Tamoxifen: estrogens may interfere with effectiveness of tamoxifen. Avoid concomitant use.

CONTRAINDICATIONS

- Contraindicated in patients with thrombophlebitis or thromboembolic disorders and undiagnosed abnormal genital bleeding, and during pregnancy.
- Use cautiously in patients with hypertension, mental depression, bone diseases, migraine, seizures, blood dyscrasias, diabetes mellitus, amenorrhea, heart failure, hepatic or renal dysfunction, or family history (mother, grandmother, sister) of breast or genital tract cancer. Development or worsening of these conditions may require discontinuation of drug.

NURSING CONSIDERATIONS

- Studies suggest that postmenopausal women who use estrogen replacement for more than 5 years to treat menopausal symptoms may be at increased risk for endometrial carcinoma. This risk is reduced by using cyclic rather than continuous therapy and the lowest possible dosages of estrogen. Adding progestins to the regimen decreases the incidence of endometrial hyperplasia; however, it isn't known if progestins affect the incidence of endometrial carcinoma. Most studies show no increased risk of breast cancer. Emphasize the importance of regular physical examinations.
- Ensure that patients have a thorough physical examination before initiating estrogen therapy. Patients receiving long-term therapy should have repeat examinations yearly. Periodically monitor serum lipid levels, blood pressure, body weight, and hepatic function.
- Patient package insert that describes estrogen's adverse effects is available; however, also provide verbal explanation.
- Warn patients to immediately report abdominal pain; pain, numbness, or stiffness in legs or buttocks; pressure or pain in chest; shortness of breath; severe headaches; visual disturbances, such as blind spots, flashing lights, or blurriness; vaginal bleeding or discharge; breast lumps; swelling of hands or feet; yellow skin or sclera; dark urine; or light-colored stools.

• Notify the pathologist about any patients receiving estrogen therapy.
• Tell diabetic patients to report elevated blood glucose test results so antidiabetic medication dosage can be adjusted.
• Teach women how to perform routine breast self-examination.
• Explain to patients on cyclic therapy for postmenopausal symptoms that, although withdrawal bleeding may occur during week off drug, fertility has not been restored. Pregnancy cannot occur because patients have not ovulated.
• Because of the risk of thromboembolism, discontinue therapy at least 1 month before procedures associated with prolonged immobilization or thromboembolism, such as knee or hip surgery.

---

ethinyl estradiol and desogestrel
monophasic: Desogen

ethinyl estradiol and ethynodiol diacetate
monophasic: Demulen 1/35, Demulen 1/50

ethinyl estradiol and levonorgestrel
monophasic: Levlen, Nordette
triphasic: Tri-Levlen, Triphasil

ethinyl estradiol and norethindrone
monophasic: Brevicon, Genora 0.5/35, Genora 1/35, Modicon, N.E.E. 1/35, Nelova 0.5/35 E, Nelova 1/35 E, Norcept-E 1/35, Norethin 1/35 E, Norinyl 1 + 35, Ortho-Novum 1/35, Ovcon-35, Ovcon-50
biphasic: Nelova 10/11, Ortho-Novum 10/11
triphasic: Ortho-Novum 7/7/7, Tri-Norinyl

ethinyl estradiol and norethindrone acetate
monophasic: Loestrin 21 1/20, Loestrin 21 1.5/30, Norlestrin 21 1/50, Norlestrin 21 2.5/50

ethinyl estradiol and norgestimate
monophasic: Ortho Cyclen

ethinyl estradiol and norgestrel
monophasic: Lo/Ovral, Ovral

ethinyl estradiol, norethindrone acetate, and ferrous fumarate
monophasic: Loestrin Fe 1/20, Loestrin Fe 1.5/30, Norlestrin Fe 1/50, Norlestrin Fe 2.5/50

mestranol and norethindrone
monophasic: Genora 1/50, Nelova 1/50 M, Norethin 1/50 M, Norinyl 1 + 50, Ortho-Novum 1/50

Pregnancy Risk Category: X

HOW SUPPLIED
Monophasic oral contraceptives
ethinyl estradiol and desogestrel
Tablets: ethinyl estradiol 30 mcg and desogestrel 0.15 mg (Desogen)
ethinyl estradiol and ethynodiol diacetate
Tablets: ethinyl estradiol 35 mcg and ethynodiol diacetate 1 mg (Demulen 1/35); ethinyl estradiol 50 mcg and ethynodiol diacetate 1 mg (Demulen 1/50)
ethinyl estradiol and levonorgestrel
Tablets: ethinyl estradiol 30 mcg and levonorgestrel 0.15 mg (Levlen, Nordette)
ethinyl estradiol and norethindrone
Tablets: ethinyl estradiol 35 mcg and norethindrone 0.4 mg (Ovcon-35); ethinyl estradiol 35 mcg and norethindrone 0.5 mg (Brevicon, Genora 0.5/35, Modicon, Nelova 0.5/35 E); ethinyl estradiol 35 mcg and norethin-

drone 1 mg (Genora 1/35, N.E.E. 1/35, Nelova 1/35 E, Norcept-E 1/35, Norethin 1/35 E, Norinyl 1 + 35, Ortho-Novum 1/35), ethinyl estradiol 50 mcg and norethindrone 1 mg (Ovcon-50)

ethinyl estradiol and norethindrone acetate
Tablets: ethinyl estradiol 20 mcg and norethindrone acetate 1 mg (Loestrin 21 1/20); ethinyl estradiol 30 mcg and norethindrone acetate 1.5 mg (Loestrin 21 1.5/30); ethinyl estradiol 50 mcg and norethindrone acetate 1 mg (Norlestrin 21 1/50); ethinyl estradiol 50 mcg and norethindrone acetate 2.5 mg (Norlestrin 21 2.5/50)

ethinyl estradiol and norgestimate
Tablets: ethinyl estradiol 35 mcg and norgestimate 0.25 mg (Ortho Cyclen)

ethinyl estradiol and norgestrel
Tablets: ethinyl estradiol 30 mcg and norgestrel 0.3 mg (Lo/Ovral); ethinyl estradiol 50 mcg and norgestrel 0.5 mg (Ovral)

ethinyl estradiol, norethindrone acetate, and ferrous fumarate
Tablets: ethinyl estradiol 20 mcg, norethindrone acetate 1 mg, and ferrous fumarate 75 mg (Loestrin Fe 1/20); ethinyl estradiol 30 mcg, norethindrone acetate 1.5 mg, and ferrous fumarate 75 mg (Loestrin Fe 1.5/30); ethinyl estradiol 50 mcg, norethindrone acetate 1 mg, and ferrous fumarate 75 mg (Norlestrin Fe 1/50); ethinyl estradiol 50 mcg, norethindrone acetate 2.5 mg, and ferrous fumarate 75 mg (Norlestrin Fe 2.5/50)

mestranol and norethindrone
Tablets: mestranol 50 mcg and norethindrone 1 mg (Genora 1/50, Nelova 1/50 M, Norethin 1/50 M, Norinyl 1 + 50, Ortho-Novum 1/50)

mestranol and norethynodrel
Tablets: mestranol 75 mg and norethynodrel 5 mg (Enovid 5 mg); mestranol 150 mg and norethynodrel 9.85 mg (Enovid 10 mg).

Biphasic oral contraceptives
ethinyl estradiol and norethindrone
Tablets: ethinyl estradiol 35 mcg and norethindrone 0.5 mg during phase 1 [10 days]; ethinyl estradiol 35 mcg and norethindrone 1 mg during phase 2 [11 days] (Nelova 10/11, Ortho-Novum 10/11)

Triphasic oral contraceptives
ethinyl estradiol and levonorgestrel
Tablets: (Tri-Levlen, Triphasil) ethinyl estradiol 35 mcg and levonorgestrel 0.05 mg during phase 1 [6 days]; ethinyl estradiol 35 mcg and levonorgestrel 0.075 mg during phase 2 [5 days]; ethinyl estradiol 35 mcg and levonorgestrel 0.125 mg during phase 3 [10 days]

ethinyl estradiol and norethindrone
Tablets: (Tri-Norinyl) ethinyl estradiol 35 mcg and norethindrone 0.5 mg during phase 1 [7 days]; ethinyl estradiol 35 mcg and norethindrone 1 mg during phase 2 [9 days]; ethinyl estradiol 35 mcg and norethindrone 0.5 mg during phase 3 [5 days]; (Ortho-Novum 7/7/7) ethinyl estradiol 35 mcg and norethindrone 0.5 mg during phase 1 [7 days]; ethinyl estradiol 35 mcg and norethindrone 0.75 mg during phase 2 [7 days]; ethinyl estradiol 35 mcg and norethindrone 1 mg during phase 3 [7 days]

ACTION

Mechanism: Oral contraceptives inhibit ovulation through a negative feedback mechanism directed at the hypothalamus. They may also prevent transport of the ovum through the fallopian tubes.

Estrogen suppresses secretion of follicle-stimulating hormone, blocking follicular development and ovulation.

Progestin suppresses secretion of luteinizing hormone so ovulation cannot occur even if the follicle develops. Progestin thickens cervical mucus, which interferes with sperm migration, and also causes endometrial changes that prevent implantation of the fertilized ovum.

Peak: Plasma levels of ethinyl estradiol peak within 1 to 2 hours; of norethindrone, within ½ to 4 hours.
Duration: half-life of ethinyl estradiol 6 to 20 hours; levonorgestrel, 11 to 45 hours; norethindrone, 5 to 14 hours.

INDICATIONS & DOSAGE

Contraception –
Adults: 1 tablet P.O. daily, beginning on day 5 of menstrual cycle (first day of menstrual flow is day 1). With 20- and 21-tablet packages, new dosing cycle begins 7 days after last tablet taken. With 28-tablet packages, dosage is 1 tablet daily without interruption; extra tablets are placebos or contain iron. Biphasic oral contraceptives – 1 color tablet P.O. daily for 10 days; then next color tablet for 11 days.
Triphasic oral contraceptives – 1 tablet P.O. daily in the sequence specified by the brand.
Endometriosis –
Adults: Enovid 5 mg or 10 mg – 1 tablet P.O. daily for 2 weeks starting on day 5 of menstrual cycle. Continue without interruption for 6 to 9 months, increasing dosage by 5 to 10 mg q 2 weeks, up to 20 mg daily. Give up to 40 mg daily as needed and ordered if breakthrough bleeding occurs.

ADVERSE REACTIONS

CNS: *headache, dizziness,* depression, lethargy, migraine.
CV: ***thromboembolism,*** hypertension, edema.
EENT: worsening of myopia or astigmatism, intolerance of contact lenses.
GI: *nausea,* vomiting, abdominal cramps, bloating, diarrhea, constipation, anorexia, changes in appetite, weight gain, *bowel ischemia,* pancreatitis.
GU: *breakthrough bleeding,* granulomatous colitis, dysmenorrhea, amenorrhea, cervical erosion or abnormal secretions, enlargement of uterine fibromas, vaginal candidiasis.
Hepatic: gallbladder disease, cholestatic jaundice, liver tumors.
Skin: rash, acne, seborrhea, oily skin, ***erythema multiforme,*** hyperpigmentation.
Other: *breast tenderness,* enlargement, secretion; hyperglycemia, hypercalcemia, folic acid deficiency; libido changes.

INTERACTIONS

Bromocriptine: may cause amenorrhea, interfering with bromocriptine's effects. Avoid concomitant use.
Carbamazepine, phenobarbital, rifampin: decreased effectiveness of estrogen therapy. Monitor closely.
Corticosteroids: possible enhanced effects. Monitor closely.
Cyclosporine: increased risk of toxicity. Use together with caution and frequently monitor cyclosporine levels.
Dantrolene, other hepatotoxic medications: increased risk of hepatotoxicity. Monitor closely.
Oral anticoagulants: dosage adjustments may be necessary. Monitor PT.
Tamoxifen: estrogens may interfere with effectiveness of tamoxifen. Avoid concomitant use.

CONTRAINDICATIONS

- Contraindicated in patients with thromboembolic disorders, cerebrovascular or coronary artery disease, MI, known or suspected breast or reproductive organ cancer, benign or malignant liver tumors, and undiagnosed abnormal vaginal bleeding; in known or suspected pregnancy; in breast-feeding patients; and in adolescents with incomplete epiphyseal closure. Also contraindicated in women ages 35 or older who smoke more than 15 cigarettes a day and in all women over age 40.
- Use cautiously in patients with systemic lupus erythematosus, hypertension, mental depression, migraine,

seizure disorders, asthma, diabetes mellitus, amenorrhea, scanty or irregular periods, fibrocystic breast disease, family history (mother, grandmother, sister) of breast or genital tract cancer, and renal or gallbladder disease. Report development or worsening of these conditions to the doctor. Prolonged therapy is inadvisable in women who plan to become pregnant.

NURSING CONSIDERATIONS

- Discontinue if patients develop granulomatous colitis while on oral contraceptives.
- Discontinue at least 1 week before surgery to decrease risk of thromboembolism. Use an alternative method of birth control.
- If one menstrual period is missed and tablets have been taken on schedule, tell patients to continue taking them. If two consecutive menstrual periods are missed, tell patients to stop drug and have pregnancy test. Progestins may cause birth defects if taken early in pregnancy.
- Missed doses in midcycle greatly increase likelihood of pregnancy.
- If one tablet is missed, tell patients to take it as soon as remembered or to take two tablets the next day and continue regular schedule. If patients miss 2 consecutive days, instruct them to take two tablets daily for 2 days and then resume normal schedule. Also advise them to use an additional method of birth control for 7 days after two missed doses. If three or more doses are missed, tell patients to discard remaining tablets in monthly package and to substitute another contraceptive method. If next menstrual period doesn't begin on schedule, warn patients to rule out pregnancy before starting new dosing cycle. If menstrual period begins, have patients start new dosing cycle 7 days after last tablet was taken.
- Warn patients that headache, nausea, dizziness, breast tenderness, spotting, and breakthrough bleeding are common at first. These effects should diminish after three to six dosing cycles (months).
- Warn patients to immediately report abdominal pain; numbness, stiffness, or pain in legs or buttocks; pressure or pain in chest; shortness of breath; severe headache; visual disturbances, such as blind spots, blurriness, or flashing lights; undiagnosed vaginal bleeding or discharge; two consecutive missed menstrual periods; lumps in the breast; swelling of hands or feet; or severe pain in the abdomen (tumor rupture in the liver).
- Advise patients to use an additional method of birth control, such as condoms or a diaphragm with spermicide, for the first week of administration in the initial cycle.
- Tell patients to take tablets at same time each day; nighttime dosing may reduce nausea and headaches.
- Advise patients not to take same drug for longer than 12 months without consulting the doctor. Stress importance of Papanicolaou tests and annual gynecologic examinations.
- Warn patients of possible delay in achieving pregnancy when drug is discontinued.
- Many doctors recommend that women not become pregnant within 2 months after stopping drug. Advise patients to check with the doctor about how soon pregnancy may be attempted after hormonal therapy is stopped.
- Teach patients how to perform routine breast self-examination.
- Advise patients of increased risks associated with simultaneous use of cigarettes and oral contraceptives.
- Periodically monitor serum lipid levels, blood pressure, body weight, and hepatic function.
- Know that many laboratory tests are affected by oral contraceptives.
- Estrogens and progestins may alter

glucose tolerance, thus changing requirements for antidiabetic drugs. Monitor blood glucose levels.
• Instruct patients to weigh themselves at least twice a week and to report any sudden weight gain or edema to the doctor.
• Warn patients to avoid exposure to ultraviolet light or prolonged exposure to sunlight.
• Many doctors advise women on prolonged therapy (5 years or longer) to stop drug and use other birth control methods. Periodically reassess patients while off hormone therapy.
• The Centers for Disease Control and Prevention reports that the use of oral contraceptives *may decrease* the incidence of ovarian and endometrial cancers. Also, oral contraceptives do not appear to increase a woman's risk of breast cancer. However, the FDA reports that oral contraceptives may be linked to an increased risk of cervical cancer.
• Ovral has been prescribed as a postcoital contraceptive ("morning-after pill"). Give patients two tablets at the initial visit and two tablets 12 hours later.
• Triphasic oral contraceptives may cause fewer adverse reactions, such as breakthrough bleeding and spotting.

hydroxyprogesterone caproate

Delta-Lutin, Duralutin, Gesterol L.A. 250, Hy/Gesterone, Hylutin, Hyprogest 250, Pro-Depo, Prodrox, Pro-Span

Pregnancy Risk Category: X

HOW SUPPLIED

Injection: 125 mg/ml, 250 mg/ml

ACTION

Mechanism: Suppresses ovulation, possibly by inhibiting pituitary gonadotropin secretion, and forms thick cervical mucus.
Duration: 7 to 14 days.

INDICATIONS & DOSAGE

Menstrual disorders –
Adults: 125 to 375 mg I.M. q 4 weeks. Stop after four cycles.
Uterine cancer –
Adults: 1 to 5 g I.M. weekly.

ADVERSE REACTIONS

CNS: dizziness, migraine headache, lethargy, depression.
CV: hypertension, thrombophlebitis, ***pulmonary embolism,*** edema.
GI: nausea, vomiting, abdominal cramps.
GU: breakthrough bleeding, dysmenorrhea, amenorrhea, cervical erosion, abnormal secretions, uterine fibromas, vaginal candidiasis.
Hepatic: cholestatic jaundice.
Skin: melasma, rash.
Local: irritation and pain at injection site.
Other: breast tenderness, enlargement, or secretion; decreased libido; hyperglycemia.

INTERACTIONS

Barbiturates, carbamazepine, rifampin: decreased progestin effects. Monitor for diminished therapeutic response.
Bromocriptine: may cause amenorrhea, interfering with bromocriptine's effects. Avoid concomitant use.
Corticosteroids: possible enhanced effects. Monitor closely.
Dantrolene, other hepatotoxic medications: increased risk of hepatotoxicity. Monitor closely.
Oral anticoagulants: dosage adjustments may be necessary. Monitor PT.

CONTRAINDICATIONS

• Contraindicated in patients with thromboembolic disorders, breast cancer, undiagnosed abnormal vaginal bleeding, severe hepatic disease, and missed abortion, and during pregnancy.

• Use cautiously in patients with diabetes mellitus, seizure disorder, migraine, cardiac or renal disease, asthma, and mental illness.

NURSING CONSIDERATIONS

• FDA regulations require that, before receiving first dose, patients read package insert explaining possible adverse effects of progestin. Also provide verbal explanation.
• Tell patients to report any unusual symptoms immediately and to stop drug and call the doctor if visual disturbances or migraine occur.
• Do not use hydroxyprogesterone to induce withdrawal bleeding or as a test for pregnancy; drug may cause birth defects and masculinization of female fetus.
• Warn patients that edema and weight gain are likely. Monitor weight routinely and recommend sodium-restricted diet as needed.
• Instruct patients to report breast pain or tenderness, vaginal discharge or bleeding, and swelling of the hands or feet.
• Give oil solutions (sesame oil and castor oil) deep I.M. in gluteal muscle. Rotate injection sites to prevent muscle atrophy.
• Teach patients how to perform routine breast self-examination.
• Instruct patients that normal menstrual cycles may not resume for 2 to 3 months after drug is stopped.

levonorgestrel

Norplant System

Pregnancy Risk Category: X

HOW SUPPLIED

Implants: 36 mg per capsule; each kit contains six capsules

ACTION

Mechanism: Slowly releases the synthetic progestin levonorgestrel into the bloodstream. How progestins provide contraception is not fully understood, but they alter the mucus covering the cervix, prevent implantation of the egg, and in some patients prevent ovulation.
Peak: Peak levels occur within 24 hours. **Duration:** about 5 years.

INDICATIONS & DOSAGE

Prevention of pregnancy –
Women: six capsules implanted subdermally in the midportion of the upper arm, about 8 cm above the elbow crease, during the first 7 days of the onset of menses. Capsules should be placed fanlike, 15 degrees apart (total of 75 degrees). Contraceptive efficacy lasts for 5 years.

ADVERSE REACTIONS

CNS: headache, nervousness, dizziness.
GI: nausea, *abdominal discomfort,* appetite change.
GU: *amenorrhea, many bleeding days or prolonged bleeding, spotting, irregular onset of bleeding, frequent onset of bleeding, scanty bleeding, cervicitis, vaginitis, leukorrhea.*
Skin: dermatitis, acne, hirsutism, hypertrichosis, scalp hair loss, infection at implant site, transient pain or itching at implant site.
Other: adnexal enlargement, mastalgia, weight gain, *musculoskeletal pain, removal difficulty, breast discharge.*

INTERACTIONS

Carbamazepine, phenytoin, rifampin: may reduce the contraceptive efficacy of levonorgestrel implants.

CONTRAINDICATIONS

• Contraindicated in patients with thrombophlebitis or thromboembolic disorders, undiagnosed abnormal genital bleeding, acute liver disease, malignant or benign liver tumors, and breast cancer, and in known or suspected pregnancy.

• Use cautiously in patients with a history of depression because progestins can worsen depression and in diabetic and prediabetic patients because progestins may alter carbohydrate metabolism (patients using oral contraceptives containing progestins may show a decreased glucose tolerance; this has yet to be demonstrated with the implant system). Also use cautiously in patients with hyperlipidemia because progestins may alter lipid metabolism (in clinical trials of the implant, patients experienced decreased cholesterol, low-density lipoprotein, and triglyceride levels, but both increased and decreased high-density lipoprotein levels; the long-term effects of these changes are not known).

NURSING CONSIDERATIONS

• Most patients develop variations in menstrual bleeding patterns, including irregular bleeding, prolonged bleeding, spotting, and amenorrhea. In most patients, these irregularities diminish over time.
• Be aware that irregular bleeding may mask symptoms of cervical or endometrial cancer.
• Warn patients that missed menstrual periods are not an accurate indicator of early pregnancy because drug may induce amenorrhea. Advise patients that 6 weeks or more of amenorrhea (after a pattern of regular menstrual periods) could indicate pregnancy. If pregnancy is confirmed, the implants must be removed.
• Expect implants to be removed if patients develop active thrombophlebitis or thromboembolic disease or will be immobilized for a significant length of time because of illness or some other factor.
• If jaundice develops, expect implants to be removed because steroid hormone metabolism is impaired in patients with liver failure.
• Closely monitor patients with conditions that may be aggravated by fluid retention because steroid hormones may cause fluid retention.
• Encourage regular (at least annual) physical examinations.
• Tell patients to report to the doctor immediately if one of the implant capsules falls out (before the skin heals over the implant). Contraceptive efficacy may be impaired.
• Although retinal thrombosis after use of oral contraceptives has been reported, no similar incidents have been documented after use of the implant system. However, patients with sudden unexplained vision problems, including users of contact lenses who develop vision changes or changes in lens tolerance, should be immediately evaluated by an ophthalmologist.
• Laboratory tests for sex hormone-binding globulin and thyroxine concentrations may show decreased values; for triiodothyronine uptake, increased values.
• Implants do not contain estrogen. Levonorgestrel is a totally synthetic progestin.

medroxyprogesterone acetate

Amen, Curretab, Cycrin, Depo-Provera, Provera

Pregnancy Risk Category: X

HOW SUPPLIED

Tablets: 2.5 mg, 5 mg, 10 mg
Injection (suspension): 100 mg/ml, 150 mg/ml, 400 mg/ml

ACTION

Mechanism: Suppresses ovulation, possibly by inhibiting pituitary gonadotropin secretion, and forms thick cervical mucus.
Peak: Absorbed slowly after I.M. injection; peak levels occur within 3 weeks of injection. **Duration:** half-life about 50 days; usually undetectable after 4 to 6 months.

INDICATIONS & DOSAGE
Abnormal uterine bleeding caused by hormonal imbalance –
Adults: 5 to 10 mg P.O. daily for 5 to 10 days beginning on sixteenth day of menstrual cycle. If the patient has received estrogen – 10 mg P.O. daily for 10 days beginning on sixteenth day of cycle.
Secondary amenorrhea –
Adults: 5 to 10 mg P.O. daily for 5 to 10 days.
Endometrial or renal carcinoma –
Adults: 400 to 1,000 mg/week I.M.
Contraception in women –
Adults: 150 mg I.M. once q 3 months.

ADVERSE REACTIONS
CNS: dizziness, migraine headache, lethargy, depression.
CV: hypertension, thrombophlebitis, ***pulmonary embolism,*** edema.
GI: nausea, vomiting, abdominal cramps.
GU: breakthrough bleeding, dysmenorrhea, amenorrhea, cervical erosion, abnormal secretions, uterine fibromas, vaginal candidiasis.
Hepatic: cholestatic jaundice.
Skin: melasma, rash, pain, induration, sterile abscesses.
Other: hyperglycemia; breast tenderness, enlargement, or secretion; decreased libido.

INTERACTIONS
Aminoglutethimide, rifampin: decreased progestin effects. Monitor for diminished therapeutic response. Patient should use a nonhormonal contraceptive during therapy with these drugs.
Bromocriptine: may cause amenorrhea, interfering with bromocriptine's effects. Avoid concomitant use.

CONTRAINDICATIONS
- Contraindicated in patients with thromboembolic disorders, breast cancer, undiagnosed abnormal vaginal bleeding, missed abortion, and hepatic dysfunction, and during pregnancy.
- Use cautiously in patients with diabetes mellitus, seizure disorder, migraine, cardiac or renal disease, asthma, and mental illness.

NURSING CONSIDERATIONS
- FDA regulations require that, before receiving first dose, patients read package insert explaining possible adverse effects of progestins. Also, provide verbal explanation.
- Tell patients to report any unusual symptoms immediately and to stop drug and call the doctor if visual disturbances or migraine occurs.
- Don't use as test for pregnancy; drug may cause birth defects and masculinization of female fetus.
- I.M. injection may be painful. Monitor sites for evidence of sterile abscess. Rotate injection sites to prevent muscle atrophy.
- Teach women how to perform routine monthly breast self-examination.
- Has been used effectively to treat obstructive sleep apnea.
- Drug has a prolonged but reversible contraceptive effect. Studies have shown that the median time to conception after discontinuation of drug is 10 months (range 4 to 31 months) in 93% of women; median time to conception is not related to duration of drug use.

norethindrone
Micronor, Norlutin, Nor-Q.D.

norethindrone acetate
Aygestin, Aygestin Cycle Pack, Norlutate

Pregnancy Risk Category: X

HOW SUPPLIED
norethindrone
Tablets: 0.35 mg, 5 mg

norethindrone acetate
Tablets: 5 mg

ACTION

Mechanism: Suppresses ovulation, possibly by inhibiting pituitary gonadotropin secretion, and forms thick cervical mucus.
Duration: elimination half-life, 5 to 14 hours.

INDICATIONS & DOSAGE

Amenorrhea, abnormal uterine bleeding –
Adults: 5 to 20 mg (norethindrone) or 2.5 to 10 mg (norethindrone acetate) P.O. daily on days 5 to 25 of menstrual cycle.
Endometriosis –
Adults: give 10 mg (norethindrone) P.O. daily for 14 days; then increase by 5 mg daily q 2 weeks up to 30 mg daily. Or give 5 mg (norethindrone acetate) P.O. daily for 14 days; then increase by 2.5 mg daily q 2 weeks up to 15 mg daily.
Contraception in women –
Adults: initially, 0.35 mg (norethindrone) P.O. on the first day of menstruation; then 0.35 mg daily.

ADVERSE REACTIONS

CNS: dizziness, migraine headache, lethargy, depression.
CV: hypertension, thrombophlebitis, ***pulmonary embolism,*** edema.
GI: nausea, vomiting, abdominal cramps.
GU: breakthrough bleeding, dysmenorrhea, amenorrhea, cervical erosion, abnormal secretions, uterine fibromas, vaginal candidiasis.
Hepatic: cholestatic jaundice.
Skin: melasma, rash.
Other: breast tenderness, enlargement, or secretion; decreased libido; hyperglycemia.

INTERACTIONS

Barbiturates, carbamazepine, rifampin: decreased progestin effects. Monitor for diminished therapeutic response.
Bromocriptine: may cause amenorrhea, interfering with bromocriptine effects. Avoid concomitant use.

CONTRAINDICATIONS

- Contraindicated in patients with thromboembolic disorders, breast cancer, undiagnosed abnormal vaginal bleeding, severe hepatic disease, and missed abortion, and during pregnancy.
- Use cautiously in patients with diabetes mellitus, seizure disorder, migraine, cardiac or renal disease, asthma, and mental illness.

NURSING CONSIDERATIONS

- Norethindrone acetate is twice as potent as norethindrone. Don't use norethindrone acetate for contraception.
- Preliminary estrogen treatment is usually needed in menstrual disorders.
- FDA regulations require that, before receiving first dose, patients read package insert explaining possible adverse effects of progestin. Also provide verbal explanation.
- Tell patients to report any unusual symptoms immediately and to stop drug and call the doctor if visual disturbances or migraine occurs.
- Don't use as test for pregnancy; drug may cause birth defects and masculinization of female fetus.
- Teach patients how to perform routine monthly breast self-examination.
- Watch patients carefully for signs of edema.

norgestrel

Ovrette**

Pregnancy Risk Category: X

HOW SUPPLIED

Tablets: 0.075 mg

ACTION

Mechanism: Suppresses ovulation, possibly by inhibiting pituitary gonadotropin secretion, and forms thick cervical mucus.
Duration: up to 24 hours.

INDICATIONS & DOSAGE

Contraception in women–
Adults: 0.075 mg P.O. daily.

ADVERSE REACTIONS

CNS: cerebral thrombosis or hemorrhage, migraine headache, lethargy, depression.
CV: hypertension, thrombophlebitis, ***pulmonary embolism,*** edema.
GI: nausea, vomiting, abdominal cramps, gallbladder disease.
GU: *breakthrough bleeding, change in menstrual flow,* dysmenorrhea, spotting, amenorrhea, cervical erosion, vaginal candidiasis.
Hepatic: cholestatic jaundice.
Skin: melasma, rash.
Other: breast tenderness, enlargement, or secretion.

INTERACTIONS

Barbiturates, carbamazepine, rifampin: decreased progestin effects. Monitor for diminished therapeutic response.
Bromocriptine: may cause amenorrhea, interfering with bromocriptine's effects. Avoid concomitant use.

CONTRAINDICATIONS

- Contraindicated in patients with thromboembolic disorders, breast cancer, undiagnosed abnormal vaginal bleeding, severe hepatic disease, and missed abortion, and during pregnancy.
- Use cautiously in patients with diabetes mellitus, seizure disorder, migraine, cardiac or renal disease, asthma, and mental illness.

NURSING CONSIDERATIONS

- FDA regulations require that, before receiving first dose, patients read package insert explaining possible adverse effects of progestins. Also provide verbal explanation.
- Tell patients to report any unusual symptoms immediately and to stop drug and call the doctor if visual disturbances, migraine, or numbness or tingling in limbs occurs.
- Tell patients to take pill every day, at the same time, even if menstruating.
- Norgestrel is a progestin-only oral contraceptive known as the "minipill."
- Risk of pregnancy increases with each tablet missed. Tell patients who miss one tablet to take it as soon as remembered and then take the next tablet at the regular time. Advise patients who miss two tablets to take one as soon as remembered and then take the next regular dose at the usual time and to use a nonhormonal method of contraception in addition to norgestrel until 14 tablets have been taken. Instruct patients who miss three or more tablets to discontinue drug and use a nonhormonal method of contraception until after menses. If menstrual period does not occur within 45 days, pregnancy testing is necessary.
- Teach patients how to perform routine breast self-examination.
- Advise women using oral contraceptives of the increased risk of serious adverse CV reactions associated with heavy cigarette smoking (15 or more cigarettes per day). These risks are quite marked in women over age 35.
- Instruct patients to immediately report excessive bleeding or bleeding between menstrual cycles, breast pain or tenderness, vaginal discharge, or swelling of the hands or feet.

progesterone

Gesterol 50, Progestilin†

Pregnancy Risk Category: X

HOW SUPPLIED

Injection (in oil): 50 mg/ml

ACTION

Mechanism: Suppresses ovulation, possibly by inhibiting pituitary gonadotropin secretion, and forms thick cervical mucus.

Duration: plasma half-life, less than 60 minutes.

INDICATIONS & DOSAGE

Amenorrhea –

Adults: 5 to 10 mg I.M. daily for 6 to 8 days.

Dysfunctional uterine bleeding –

Adults: 5 to 10 mg I.M. daily for six doses.

Corpus luteum insufficiency –

Adults: 25 mg as a suppository (prepared by the pharmacist) either P.R. or vaginally b.i.d. Start treatment at the onset of ovulation and continue through week 11 of gestation.

ADVERSE REACTIONS

CNS: dizziness, migraine headache, lethargy, depression.

CV: hypertension, thrombophlebitis, ***pulmonary embolism,*** edema.

GI: nausea, vomiting, abdominal cramps.

GU: breakthrough bleeding, dysmenorrhea, amenorrhea, cervical erosion, abnormal secretions, uterine fibromas, vaginal candidiasis.

Hepatic: cholestatic jaundice.

Local: pain at injection site.

Skin: melasma, rash.

Other: breast tenderness, enlargement, or secretion; decreased libido; hyperglycemia.

INTERACTIONS

Barbiturates, carbamazepine, rifampin: decreased progestin effects. Monitor for diminished therapeutic response.

Bromocriptine: may cause amenorrhea, interfering with bromocriptine's effects. Avoid concomitant use.

CONTRAINDICATIONS

- Contraindicated in patients with thromboembolic disorders, breast cancer, undiagnosed abnormal vaginal bleeding, severe hepatic disease, and missed abortion.
- Use cautiously in patients with diabetes mellitus, seizure disorder, migraine, cardiac or renal disease, asthma, and mental illness.

NURSING CONSIDERATIONS

- FDA regulations require that, before receiving first dose, patients read package insert explaining possible adverse effects of progestins. Also provide verbal explanation.
- Tell patients to report any unusual symptoms immediately and to stop drug and call the doctor if visual disturbances or migraine occurs.
- Preliminary estrogen treatment is usually needed in menstrual disorders.
- Give oil solutions (peanut oil or sesame oil) deep I.M. Check sites frequently for irritation. Rotate injection sites.
- Progesterone suppositories are not commercially available and must be prepared by the pharmacist.
- Teach patients how to perform routine breast self-examination.
- Progesterone has been used during the first trimester of pregnancy to treat habitual abortion or pending spontaneous abortion.

quinestrol

Estrovis

Pregnancy Risk Category: X

HOW SUPPLIED

Tablets: 100 mcg

ACTION

Mechanism: Increases the synthesis of DNA, RNA, and protein in responsive tissues. Also reduces release of follicle-stimulating hormone and luteinizing hormone from the pituitary.
Duration: plasma half-life, about 5 days.

INDICATIONS & DOSAGE

Moderate to severe vasomotor symptoms associated with menopause, atrophic vaginitis, kraurosis vulvae, female hypogonadism, female castration, primary ovarian failure –
Adults: 100 mcg P.O. once daily for 7 days, followed by 100 mcg weekly as maintenance dosage beginning 2 weeks after start of treatment. Increase dosage to 200 mcg weekly if necessary.

ADVERSE REACTIONS

CNS: headache, dizziness, chorea, migraine, depression.
CV: thrombophlebitis; ***thromboembolism;*** hypertension; edema; ***increased risk of CVA, pulmonary embolism, and MI.***
EENT: worsening of myopia or astigmatism, intolerance of contact lenses.
GI: *nausea,* vomiting, abdominal cramps, bloating, diarrhea, constipation, anorexia, increased appetite, excessive thirst, weight changes.
GU: breakthrough bleeding, altered menstrual flow, dysmenorrhea, amenorrhea, cervical erosion or abnormal secretions, enlargement of uterine fibromas, vaginal candidiasis.
Hepatic: cholestatic jaundice.
Skin: melasma, urticaria, acne, seborrhea, oily skin, hirsutism or hair loss.
Other: leg cramps, purpura, breast changes (tenderness, enlargement, secretion), hyperglycemia, hypercalcemia, folic acid deficiency, libido changes.

INTERACTIONS

Bromocriptine: may cause amenorrhea, interfering with bromocriptine's effects. Avoid concomitant use.
Carbamazepine, phenobarbital, rifampin: decreased effectiveness of estrogen therapy. Monitor closely.
Corticosteroids: possible enhanced effects. Monitor closely.
Cyclosporine: increased risk of toxicity. Use together with caution and frequently monitor cyclosporine levels.
Dantrolene, other hepatotoxic medications: increased risk of hepatotoxicity. Monitor closely.
Oral anticoagulants: dosage adjustments may be necessary. Monitor PT.
Tamoxifen: estrogens may interfere with effectiveness of tamoxifen. Avoid concomitant use.

CONTRAINDICATIONS

- Contraindicated in patients with thrombophlebitis or thromboembolic disorders, breast or reproductive organ cancer, and undiagnosed abnormal genital bleeding, and during pregnancy.
- Use cautiously in patients with hypertension, mental depression, migraine, seizures, diabetes mellitus, amenorrhea, hepatic or renal dysfunction, or family history (mother, grandmother, sister) of breast or genital tract cancer. Development or worsening of these conditions may require discontinuation of drug.

NURSING CONSIDERATIONS

- Studies suggest that postmenopausal women who use estrogen replacement for more than 5 years to treat menopausal symptoms may be at increased risk for endometrial carcinoma. This risk is reduced by using cyclic rather than continuous therapy and the lowest possible dosages of estrogen. Adding progestins to the regimen decreases the incidence of endometrial hyperplasia; however, it isn't known if progestins affect the incidence of endometrial carcinoma. Most studies show no increased risk of breast cancer. Emphasize the importance of regular physical examinations.

- Ensure that patients have a thorough physical examination before initiating estrogen therapy. Patients receiving long-term therapy should have repeat examinations yearly. Periodically monitor body weight, blood pressure, hepatic function, and serum lipid levels.
- Patient package insert that describes estrogen's adverse effects is available; however, also provide verbal explanation.
- Attempts to discontinue medication should be made at 3- to 6-month intervals.
- Similar in effectiveness to conjugated estrogens in treating postmenopausal symptoms. Biggest advantage is that quinestrol can be taken once a week.
- Warn patients to immediately report abdominal pain; pain, numbness, or stiffness in legs or buttocks; pressure or pain in chest; shortness of breath; severe headaches; visual disturbances, such as blind spots, flashing lights, or blurriness; vaginal bleeding or discharge; breast lumps; swelling of hands or feet; yellow skin or sclera; dark urine; or light-colored stools.
- Notify the pathologist about any patients receiving estrogen therapy.
- Tell diabetic patients to report elevated blood glucose test results so antidiabetic medication dosage can be adjusted.
- Explain to patients on replacement therapy for postmenopausal symptoms that, although menstrual-like bleeding or spotting may occur, fertility has not been restored. Pregnancy cannot occur because patients have not ovulated.
- Teach women how to perform routine breast self-examination.

55

Gonadotropins

gonadorelin acetate
gonadorelin hydrochloride
gonadotropin, chorionic
histrelin acetate
menotropins
nafarelin acetate

COMBINATION PRODUCTS

None.

gonadorelin acetate

Lutrepulse

Pregnancy Risk Category: B

HOW SUPPLIED

Injection: 0.8 mg/10 ml, 3.2 mg/10 ml vials; supplied as a kit with I.V. supplies and ambulatory infusion pump

ACTION

Mechanism: Mimics the action of gonadotropin releasing hormone (GnRH), which results in the synthesis and release of luteinizing hormone (LH) from the anterior pituitary. LH subsequently acts upon the reproductive organs to regulate hormone synthesis.

Peak: Peak levels occur immediately after I.V. injection. **Duration:** terminal elimination half-life, about 40 minutes.

INDICATIONS & DOSAGE

Induction of ovulation in women with primary hypothalamic amenorrhea – **Adults:** 5 mcg I.V. q 90 minutes for 21 days. If no response follows three treatment intervals, increase dosage as ordered.

ADVERSE REACTIONS

Skin: hematoma, local infection, inflammation, mild phlebitis.

Other: multiple pregnancy, ovarian hyperstimulation.

INTERACTIONS

None significant.

CONTRAINDICATIONS

- Contraindicated in patients hypersensitive to the drug, in women with conditions that could be complicated by pregnancy (such as pituitary prolactinoma), in those who are anovulatory from any cause other than a hypothalamic disorder, and in those with ovarian cysts.

NURSING CONSIDERATIONS

- Ensure that patients understand a multiple pregnancy is possible (incidence about 12%). Close monitoring of dosage, as well as ovarian ultrasonography to monitor drug response, is necessary.
- Patients usually require pelvic ultrasound on days 7 and 14 after establishment of a baseline scan. Some clinicians prefer shorter intervals between scans.
- Encourage patients to adhere to the close monitoring schedule required by the therapy. Regular pelvic examinations, midluteal phase serum progesterone determinations, and multiple ovarian ultrasound scans are necessary. Inspect the I.V. site at each visit.
- **I.V. use:** To mimic the naturally occurring hormone, administer gonadorelin in a pulsatile fashion with the available ambulatory infusion pump. Set the pulse period at 1 minute (infuse drug over 1 minute) and the pulse interval at 90 minutes.
- To administer 2.5 mcg/pulse, reconstitute the 0.8-mg vial with 8 ml of supplied diluent and set the pump to deliver 25 microliters/pulse. To ad-

minister 5 mcg/pulse, use the same dosage strength and dilution but set the pump to deliver 50 microliters/pulse.

- Some patients may require higher I.V. doses. To administer 10 mcg/pulse, reconstitute the 3.2-mg vial with 8 ml of supplied diluent and set the pump to deliver 25 microliters/pulse. To administer 20 mcg/pulse, use the same dosage strength and dilution but set the pump to deliver 50 microliters/pulse.
- Instruct patients about proper aseptic technique and care of the I.V. site. Cannula and I.V. site should be changed every 48 hours. Written instructions are available for patients.
- Anaphylaxis has been reported with similar drugs. Teach patients how to recognize signs and symptoms of hypersensitivity reactions (hives, wheezing, difficulty breathing) and encourage them to report these as soon as possible.
- Advise patients to report signs of infection, hematoma, inflammation, or phlebitis at the injection site. Patients should also immediately report severe abdominal pain, bloating, swelling of the hands or feet, nausea, vomiting, diarrhea, substantial weight gain, or shortness of breath.

gonadorelin hydrochloride (luteinizing hormone-releasing hormone, LHRH; gonadotropin releasing hormone, GnRH)

Factrel

Pregnancy Risk Category: B

HOW SUPPLIED

Injection: 100 mcg, 500 mcg

ACTION

Mechanism: A synthetic luteinizing hormone that releases LHRH.
Duration: half-life, 10 to 40 minutes; action, 3 to 5 hours.

INDICATIONS & DOSAGE

Evaluation of the functional capacity and response of gonadotropic hormones –

Adults: 100 mcg S.C. or I.V. In women for whom the menstrual cycle phase can be established, perform test between day 1 and day 7.

ADVERSE REACTIONS

CNS: headache, flushing, light-headedness.
GI: nausea, abdominal discomfort.
Skin: local swelling, occasionally with pain and pruritus when administered S.C.; rash after long-term S.C. administration.

INTERACTIONS

Digoxin, oral contraceptives: may depress gonadotropin levels. Monitor results carefully.
Levodopa, spironolactone: may elevate gonadotropin levels. Monitor results carefully.

CONTRAINDICATIONS

- Contraindicated in patients hypersensitive to the drug.
- Use cautiously in patients allergic to other drugs. Keep epinephrine readily available.

NURSING CONSIDERATIONS

- The gonadorelin test can be performed concomitantly with other post-treatment evaluations.
- For specific test methodology and interpretation of test results, refer to the manufacturer's full product information. Ask the pharmacist for a copy.
- Keep epinephrine readily available when administering gonadorelin to patients allergic to other drugs.
- **I.V. use:** Reconstitute vial with 1 to 2 ml of accompanying sterile diluent. Inject drug directly into vein over 3 to 5 minutes. Alternatively, inject into an I.V. line containing a free-flowing compatible solution. Prepare solution

immediately before use. After reconstitution, store at room temperature and use within 1 day. Discard unused reconstituted solution and diluent.
• As a single injection, gonadorelin can be used to evaluate the functional capacity and response of the gonadotropins of the anterior pituitary. Prolonged or repeated administration may be necessary to measure pituitary gonadotropic reserve.

gonadotropin, chorionic (HCG)

A.P.L., Pregnyl, Profasi, Profasi HP†

Pregnancy Risk Category: C

HOW SUPPLIED

Injection: 200 units/ml, 500 units/ml, 1,000 units/ml, 2,000 units/ml (after reconstitution)

ACTION

Mechanism: Serves as a substitute for luteinizing hormone to stimulate ovulation of human menopausal gonadotropin-prepared follicle. Also promotes secretion of gonadal steroid hormones by stimulating production of androgen by the interstitial cells of the testes (Leydig's cells).
Onset: within 2 hours. **Peak:** Serum levels peak within 6 hours. **Duration:** at least 36 hours.

INDICATIONS & DOSAGE

Anovulation and infertility in women –
Adults: 5,000 to 10,000 units I.M. 1 day after last dose of menotropins.
Hypogonadism –
Adults: 500 to 1,000 units I.M. three times weekly for 3 weeks; then twice weekly for 3 weeks. Or 4,000 units I.M. three times weekly for 6 to 9 months; then 2,000 units three times weekly for 3 more months.
Nonobstructive cryptorchidism –
Boys 4 to 9 years: 1,000 to 5,000 units I.M. two to three times a week for a maximum of 10 doses or until response occurs.
Corpus luteum insufficiency –
Adults: 1,500 units I.M. every other day beginning on the day of ovulation through expected menses or confirmed pregnancy. Some clinicians continue therapy through 10 weeks of gestation.

ADVERSE REACTIONS

CNS: headache, fatigue, irritability, restlessness, depression.
CV: edema.
Skin: *pain at injection site.*
Other: gynecomastia, early puberty (growth of testes, penis, pubic and axillary hair; voice change; down on upper lip; growth of body hair).

INTERACTIONS

None significant.

CONTRAINDICATIONS

• Contraindicated in patients with pituitary hypertrophy or tumor, prostate cancer, early puberty (usual onset between ages 10 and 13), undiagnosed vaginal bleeding, uterine fibroids, ovarian cyst, history of thrombophlebitis, and during pregnancy.
• Use cautiously in patients with seizure disorders, migraine headache, asthma, and cardiac or renal disease.

NURSING CONSIDERATIONS

• When used with menotropins to induce ovulation, multiple births are possible.
• Usually used only after failure of clomiphene in anovulatory patients.
• In infertility, encourage daily intercourse from day before chorionic gonadotropin is given until ovulation occurs.
• Inspect genitalia of boys for signs of early puberty.
• Be alert for symptoms of ectopic pregnancy, which is typically evident between weeks 8 to 12 of gestation.

• Reconstitute with 1 to 2 ml of supplied diluent just before use. Use reconstituted solutions within 24 hours.
• For I.M. use only. Don't inject I.V. Rotate injection sites to prevent muscle atrophy.
• Instruct patients to immediately report severe abdominal pain, bloating, swelling of the hands or feet, nausea, vomiting, diarrhea, substantial weight gain, or shortness of breath.

histrelin acetate

Supprelin

Pregnancy Risk Category: X

HOW SUPPLIED

Injection: 120 mcg/0.6 ml, 300 mcg/0.6 ml, 600 mcg/0.6 ml

ACTION

Mechanism: An agonist that mimics the effects of gonadotropin releasing hormone (GnRH; also called luteinizing hormone-releasing hormone, or LHRH) but is more potent than the naturally occurring hormone. Chronic administration desensitizes responsiveness of the pituitary gonadotropin, decreasing sex hormone production by the testes or ovaries.

Onset: decreased levels of luteinizing hormone (LH), follicle-stimulating hormone (FSH), and sex hormones, within 3 months.

INDICATIONS & DOSAGE

Centrally mediated (idiopathic or neurogenic) precocious puberty –

Children (girls 2 to 8 years; boys 2 to 9½ years): 10 mg/kg S.C. daily.

ADVERSE REACTIONS

CNS: migraine headache, *headache, visual disturbances, mood changes, nervousness, dizziness, depression, libido changes, insomnia, anxiety,* paresthesia, cognitive changes, syncope, somnolence, lethargy, impaired consciousness, tremor, hyperkinesia, ***seizures,*** hot flashes, conduct disorder.

CV: *vasodilation,* edema, palpitations, tachycardia, hypertension.

EENT: epistaxis, ear congestion, abnormal pupillary function, otalgia, hearing loss, polyopia, pharyngitis, photophobia, rhinorrhea, sinusitis.

GI: *abdominal pain, nausea, vomiting, diarrhea, flatulence, decreased appetite, dyspepsia,* cramps, constipation, thirst, gastritis.

GU: *menstrual changes, vaginal dryness, leukorrhea, menorrhagia,* tenderness of female genitalia, glycosuria.

Hematologic: hyperlipidemia, anemia.

Respiratory: *upper respiratory infection, respiratory congestion, cough,* asthma, breathing disorder, bronchitis, hyperventilation.

Skin: pallor.

Other: urticaria, *pyrexia, arthralgia, muscle stiffness, muscle cramps, breast pain or edema,* breast discharge, decreased breast size, muscle pain, hypotonia, goiter, ***acute hypersensitivity reactions (anaphylaxis, angioedema).***

INTERACTIONS

None significant.

CONTRAINDICATIONS

• Contraindicated in patients hypersensitive to any component of the drug and in pregnant or breast-feeding patients.
• Safety and efficacy have not been established in children under 2 years.

NURSING CONSIDERATIONS

• Drug is indicated only for patients who will comply with the daily administration schedule. Noncompliance or inadequate dosing may result in inadequate control of the pubertal process, which can result in recurrence of symptoms, including onset of menses, breast development, or testic-

ular growth; long-term consequences may involve decreased adult height.
• A complete physical and endocrinologic evaluation should be performed before initiating drug therapy; several indices should be reexamined at 3 months, then every 6 to 12 months thereafter. Such evaluations should include determinations of height and weight, hand and wrist X-ray for bone age determination, sex steroid (estradiol or testosterone) levels, and GnRH stimulation test. Monitor these tests periodically to determine effectiveness of therapy.
• Additional tests to rule out other causes of precocious puberty include beta human chorionic gonadotropin levels (to detect chorionic gonadotropin-secreting tumor); pelvic/adrenal/testicular ultrasound (to detect steroid-secreting tumor); and computed tomography scan of the head (to detect any previously undiagnosed intracranial tumor). Workup also establishes baseline of gonad size for serial monitoring.
• Decreases in FSH, LH, and sex steroid levels occur within 3 months.
• Reevaluate patients if prepubertal levels of sex steroids or GnRH test responses are not achieved within 3 months of therapy.
• Because drug is a peptide, it's destroyed in the GI tract and therefore must be administered parenterally. Give S.C. and rotate injection site to minimize local reactions.
• Explain to patients the importance of rotating injection sites daily. Sites should include upper arms, thighs, and abdomen.
• Store drug in the refrigerator (36° to 46° F [2° to 8° C]) protected from light and in its original container. Use vials only once because drug does not contain preservatives. Allow medication to reach room temperature before giving.
• Drug is dispensed as a 7-day kit that contains a patient information leaflet. Ensure that caregivers read and understand the leaflet.
• Before initiating therapy, make sure that patients and their parents understand the importance of adhering to the daily administration schedules. Tell them to give drug at about the same time each day to facilitate compliance and ensure adequate dosing.
• Warn patients of the potential risks of therapy and potential adverse effects. During the first month of treatment, girls commonly experience a slight menstrual flow, which is probably related to decreasing estrogen levels brought on by treatment. As estrogen levels drop, menses begins because estrogens support the endometrium.
• Advise patients to seek immediate medical attention if they have any signs of hypersensitivity reactions: sudden development of skin rash, difficulty in breathing or swallowing, or rapid heartbeat. Notify the doctor if severe or persistent swelling, redness, or irritation is present at the injection site.

menotropins

Pergonal

Pregnancy Risk Category: C

HOW SUPPLIED

Injection: 75 international units (IU) of luteinizing hormone (LH) and 75 units of follicle-stimulating hormone (FSH) activity/ampule; 150 units of LH and 150 units of FSH activity/ampule

ACTION

Mechanism: When administered to women who have not had primary ovarian failure, mimics FSH in inducing follicular growth and LH in aiding follicular maturation.
Onset: for follicular growth and maturation, 9 to 12 days.

INDICATIONS & DOSAGE

Anovulation –

Adults: 75 units each of FSH and LH I.M. daily for 9 to 12 days, followed by 10,000 units of human chorionic gonadotropin (HCG) I.M. 1 day after last dose of menotropins. Repeat for one to three menstrual cycles until ovulation occurs.

Infertility with ovulation –

Adults: 75 units each of FSH and LH I.M. daily for 9 to 12 days, followed by 10,000 units of HCG I.M. 1 day after last dose of menotropins. Repeat for two menstrual cycles and then increase to 150 units each of FSH and LH daily for 9 to 12 days, followed by 10,000 units of HCG I.M. 1 day after last dose of menotropins. Repeat for two menstrual cycles.

Infertility in men –

Adults: 75 units each of FSH and LH I.M. three times weekly (given concomitantly with 2,000 units of HCG twice weekly) for at least 4 months. If increased spermatogenesis does not occur, increase dosage to 150 units each of FSH and LH three times weekly (do not increase dosage of HCG).

ADVERSE REACTIONS

GI: nausea, vomiting, diarrhea.

GU: *ovarian enlargement with pain and abdominal distention,* multiple births, ovarian hyperstimulation syndrome (sudden ovarian enlargement, ascites with or without pain, or pleural effusion).

Hematologic: hemoconcentration with fluid loss into abdomen.

Other: fever, *gynecomastia.*

INTERACTIONS

None significant.

CONTRAINDICATIONS

- Contraindicated in patients hypersensitive to the drug; in those with ovarian failure, high urinary gonadotropin levels, thyroid or adrenal dysfunction, pituitary tumor, abnormal uterine bleeding, uterine fibroids, or ovarian cysts or enlargement; and in pregnant patients.
- Use cautiously in patients with cardiac, renal, or pulmonary disease; seizure disorder; migraine headache; history of thrombophlebitis; or polycystic ovary syndrome.

NURSING CONSIDERATIONS

- Close monitoring of patient response is critical to ensure adequate ovarian stimulation without hyperstimulation.
- Tell patients about possibility of multiple births.
- In infertility, encourage daily intercourse from day before HCG is given until ovulation occurs.
- Pregnancy usually occurs 4 to 6 weeks after therapy.
- Reconstitute with 1 to 2 ml of sterile saline injection. Use immediately.
- Rotate injection sites to prevent muscle atrophy.
- Instruct patients to immediately report severe abdominal pain, bloating, swelling of the hands or feet, nausea, vomiting, diarrhea, substantial weight gain, or shortness of breath.

nafarelin acetate

Synarel

Pregnancy Risk Category: X

HOW SUPPLIED

Nasal solution: 200 mcg/spray in metered-dose spray bottle (2 mg/ml)

ACTION

Mechanism: A gonadotropin-releasing hormone (GnRH) analog that acts on the pituitary to decrease release of follicle-stimulating hormone (FSH) and luteinizing hormone (LH), thus decreasing ovarian stimulation, lowering circulating estrogens, and improving symptoms associated with endometriosis.

Onset: decreased levels of sex hormones after 4 weeks. **Peak:** Serum levels peak 10 to 45 minutes after dose.

INDICATIONS & DOSAGE

Management of endometriosis –
Women 18 years and older: 1 spray in one nostril b.i.d. Begin treatment between days 2 and 4 of the menstrual cycle. Maximum duration of therapy is 6 months.

Central precocious puberty –
Children: 2 sprays in each nostril in the morning and evening. Total daily dosage is 8 sprays (1,600 mcg).

ADVERSE REACTIONS

CNS: *headaches, emotional lability, insomnia,* depression.
CV: edema.
EENT: *nasal irritation.*
Skin: *acne,* seborrhea, hirsutism.
Other: *hot flashes, decreased libido, myalgia,* reduced breast size, weight gain or loss, increased libido, decreased bone density, *vaginal dryness.*

INTERACTIONS

None significant.

CONTRAINDICATIONS

- Contraindicated in patients hypersensitive to GnRH analogs or any components of the formulation (benzalkonium chloride, sorbitol, purified water, glacial acetic acid, hydrochloric acid, or sodium hydroxide), in those with undiagnosed vaginal bleeding, in breast-feeding patients, and during pregnancy (because it may harm the fetus).

NURSING CONSIDERATIONS

- Studies have confirmed a small loss in bone density after 6 months of therapy, probably caused by drug-induced hypoestrogenic state. Patients with major risk factors for osteoporosis (chronic alcohol or tobacco use, strong family history of osteoporosis, or use of drugs that may reduce bone mass such as anticonvulsants or corticosteroids) should not receive additional courses of therapy and should strongly weigh the risks and benefits before an initial trial of the drug.
- Tell patients who develop a cold or rhinitis during therapy to notify the doctor. If a topical nasal decongestant is required, the manufacturer suggests that it be used at least 30 minutes after nafarelin treatment to reduce possible interference with nafarelin absorption.
- Advise patients to use a nonhormonal form of contraception (such as barrier contraception). Although drug will usually inhibit ovulation and stop menstruation, it's not a reliable contraceptive, particularly if patients miss a few doses. Tell patients to stop the drug immediately and contact the doctor if they believe that they are pregnant.
- Teach patients that menstruation will stop with regular use of drug and to contact the doctor if menstruation persists or breakthrough bleeding occurs.
- Instruct patients to immediately report severe abdominal pain, bloating, swelling of the hands or feet, nausea, vomiting, diarrhea, substantial weight gain, or shortness of breath.

56
Antidiabetic agents and glucagon

acetohexamide
chlorpropamide
glipizide
glucagon
glyburide
insulins
tolazamide
tolbutamide

COMBINATION PRODUCTS
HUMULIN 50/50◇: isophane insulin suspension (human) 50% and insulin injection (human) 50%, 100 units/ml
HUMULIN 70/30◇, MIXTARD HUMAN‡, NOVOLIN 70/30◇): isophane insulin suspension (human) 70% and insulin injection (human) 30%, 100 units/ml

acetohexamide
Dimelor†, Dymelor
Pregnancy Risk Category: D

HOW SUPPLIED
Tablets: 250 mg, 500 mg

ACTION
Mechanism: A sulfonylurea that stimulates insulin release from the pancreatic beta cells and reduces glucose output by the liver. An extrapancreatic effect increases peripheral sensitivity to insulin.
Peak: Plasma levels of acetohexamide peak within 2 hours; plasma levels of insulin, within 1 to 2 hours.
Duration: 12 to 24 hours.

INDICATIONS & DOSAGE
Adjunct to diet to lower blood glucose level in patients with type II diabetes (non-insulin-dependent) –
Adults: initially, 250 mg P.O. daily before breakfast; increase dosage q 5 to 7 days (by 250 to 500 mg) as needed to maximum of 1.5 g daily in divided doses b.i.d. to t.i.d. before meals.
To replace insulin therapy –
Adults: if insulin dosage is less than 20 units daily, stop insulin and start oral therapy with 250 mg P.O. daily, before breakfast, increased as above if needed. If insulin dosage is 20 to 40 units daily, start oral therapy with 250 mg P.O. daily, before breakfast, while reducing insulin dosage 25% to 30% daily or every other day, depending on response to oral therapy.

ADVERSE REACTIONS
GI: nausea, heartburn, vomiting.
Skin: rash, pruritus, facial flushing.
Other: ***hypersensitivity reactions,*** sodium loss, ***hypoglycemia.***

INTERACTIONS
Anabolic steroids, chloramphenicol, clofibrate, guanethidine, MAO inhibitors, phenylbutazone, salicylates, sulfonamides: increased hypoglycemic activity. Monitor blood glucose level.
Beta blockers, clonidine: prolonged hypoglycemic effect and masked symptoms of hypoglycemia. Use together cautiously.
Corticosteroids, glucagon, rifampin, thiazide diuretics: decreased hypoglycemic response. Monitor blood glucose level.
Ethanol: possible disulfiram-like reaction. Avoid concomitant use.
Hydantoins: increased blood levels of hydantoins. Monitor blood levels closely.
Oral anticoagulants: increased hypoglycemic activity or enhanced anticoagulant effect. Monitor blood glucose level and PT.

CONTRAINDICATIONS

• Contraindicated for treating patients with type I diabetes (insulin-dependent) or diabetes that can be adequately controlled by diet. Also contraindicated in patients with type II diabetes (non-insulin-dependent) complicated by ketosis, acidosis, diabetic coma, Raynaud's disease, gangrene, renal or hepatic impairment, or thyroid or other endocrine dysfunction, and during pregnancy or breast-feeding.

• Use cautiously in patients hypersensitive to sulfonamides and in those with a history of porphyria.

NURSING CONSIDERATIONS

• Instruct patients about nature of disease, importance of following therapeutic regimen, adhering to specific diet, weight reduction, exercise, and personal hygiene programs and about avoiding infection. Explain how and when to perform self-monitoring of blood glucose level and teach recognition of and intervention for hypoglycemia and hyperglycemia.

• Make sure patients understand that therapy relieves symptoms but doesn't cure disease.

• Patients transferring from another oral agent usually need no transition period.

• Patients transferring from insulin therapy to an oral antidiabetic agent requires blood glucose monitoring at least three times a day before meals. Patients may require hospitalization during transition.

• During periods of increased stress, such as infection, fever, surgery, or trauma, patients may require insulin therapy. Monitor patients closely for hyperglycemia in these situations.

• Advise patients to avoid moderate to large intake of alcohol because of possible disulfiram-like reaction.

• Tell patients not to change drug dosage without the doctor's consent. Report abnormal blood or urine glucose test results.

• Advise patients not to take any other medication, including OTC drugs, without first checking with the doctor.

• Advise patients to carry medical identification identifying them as diabetic patients.

• Teach patients to carry candy or other simple sugars to treat mild hypoglycemic episodes. Severe episodes may require hospital treatment.

chlorpropamide

Apo-Chlorpropamide†, Diabinese, Glucamide, Novopropamide†

Pregnancy Risk Category: D

HOW SUPPLIED

Tablets: 100 mg, 250 mg

ACTION

Mechanism: A sulfonylurea that stimulates insulin release from the pancreatic beta cells and reduces glucose output by the liver. An extrapancreatic effect increases peripheral sensitivity to insulin. Also exerts an antidiuretic effect in patients with pituitary-deficient diabetes insipidus.
Onset: within 1 hour. **Peak:** Peak levels occur in 2 to 4 hours; peak hypoglycemic effect, within 3 to 6 hours.
Duration: 24 to 48 hours.

INDICATIONS & DOSAGE

Adjunct to diet to lower blood glucose level in patients with type II diabetes (non-insulin-dependent) –
Adults: 250 mg P.O. daily with breakfast or in divided doses if GI disturbances occur. Give first dosage increase after 5 to 7 days because of extended duration of action; then increase dosage q 3 to 5 days by 50 to 125 mg, if needed, to a maximum of 750 mg daily.
Adults over 65 years: initially, 100 to 125 mg P.O. daily.

To change from insulin to oral therapy –

Adults: if insulin dosage is less than 40 units daily, stop insulin and start oral therapy as above. If insulin dosage is 40 units or more daily, start oral therapy as above with insulin reduced 50%. Reduce insulin dosage further according to patient response.

ADVERSE REACTIONS

GI: nausea, heartburn, vomiting.
GU: tea-colored urine.
Skin: rash, pruritus, facial flushing.
Other: ***hypersensitivity reactions; prolonged hypoglycemia, dilutional hyponatremia.***

INTERACTIONS

Anabolic steroids, chloramphenicol, clofibrate, guanethidine, MAO inhibitors, phenylbutazone, salicylates, sulfonamides: increased hypoglycemic activity. Monitor blood glucose level.
Beta blockers, clonidine: prolonged hypoglycemic effect and masked symptoms of hypoglycemia. Use together cautiously.
Corticosteroids, glucagon, rifampin, thiazide diuretics: decreased hypoglycemic response. Monitor blood glucose level.
Ethanol: possible disulfiram-like reaction. Avoid concomitant use.
Hydantoins: increased blood levels of hydantoins. Monitor blood levels closely.
Oral anticoagulants: increased hypoglycemic activity or enhanced anticoagulant effect. Monitor blood glucose level and PT.

CONTRAINDICATIONS

- Contraindicated for treating type I diabetes (insulin-dependent) or diabetes that can be adequately controlled by diet. Also contraindicated in patients with type II diabetes (non-insulin-dependent) complicated by fever, ketosis, acidosis, diabetic coma, major surgery, severe trauma, Raynaud's disease, gangrene, renal or hepatic impairment, or thyroid or other endocrine dysfunction, and during pregnancy or breast-feeding.
- Use cautiously in patients hypersensitive to sulfonamides.

NURSING CONSIDERATIONS

- Elderly patients may be more sensitive to drug's adverse effects.
- Instruct patients about nature of the disease, importance of following therapeutic regimen, adhering to specific diet, weight reduction, exercise, and personal hygiene programs, and avoiding infection. Explain how and when to perform self-monitoring of blood glucose level and teach recognition of and intervention for hypoglycemia and hyperglycemia.
- Make sure patients understand that therapy relieves symptoms but doesn't cure disease.
- Adverse effects of chlorpropamide, especially hypoglycemia, may be more frequent or severe than with some other sulfonylureas (acetohexamide, tolazamide, and tolbutamide) because of its long duration of action.
- If hypoglycemia occurs, monitor patients closely for a minimum of 3 to 5 days.
- Patients transferring from another oral antidiabetic agent usually need no transition period.
- Patients may require hospitalization during transition from insulin therapy to an oral antidiabetic agent. Monitor patients' blood glucose levels at least three times a day before meals. If performing both urine glucose and urine ketone testing, emphasize the need for a double-voided specimen.
- Drug may accumulate in patients with renal insufficiency.
- Advise patients to avoid intake of alcohol. Chlorpropamide-alcohol flush is characterized by facial flushing, light-headedness, headache, and occasional breathlessness. Even very

small amounts of alcohol can produce this reaction.
- Monitor serum alkaline phosphatase levels routinely. Progressive increases may indicate the need to discontinue drug.
- Watch for signs of impending renal insufficiency, such as dysuria, anuria, and hematuria, and report them to the doctor immediately.
- May potentiate ADH. Sometimes used to treat diabetes insipidus.
- Tell patients not to change drug dosage without the doctor's consent. Report abnormal blood or urine glucose test results.
- Advise patients not to take any other medication, including OTC drugs, without first checking with the doctor.
- Advise patients to carry medical identification identifying them as diabetic patients.
- Teach patients to carry candy or other simple sugars to treat mild hypoglycemic episodes. Severe episodes may require hospital treatment.

glipizide

Glucotrol, Minidiab‡

Pregnancy Risk Category: C

HOW SUPPLIED

Tablets: 5 mg, 10 mg

ACTION

Mechanism: A sulfonylurea that stimulates insulin release from the pancreatic beta cells and reduces glucose output by the liver. An extrapancreatic effect increases peripheral sensitivity to insulin.
Onset: within 10 to 30 minutes.
Peak: Serum drug levels peak 1 to 3 hours after oral dose; peak insulin levels occur in ½ to 2 hours. **Duration:** about 24 hours.

INDICATIONS & DOSAGE

Adjunct to diet to lower blood glucose level in patients with type II diabetes (non-insulin-dependent) –
Adults: initially, 5 mg P.O. daily before breakfast. Elderly patients or those with liver disease may be started on 2.5 mg. Usual maintenance dosage is 10 to 15 mg. Maximum recommended daily dosage is 40 mg.
To replace insulin therapy –
Adults: if insulin dosage is more than 20 units daily, start the patient at usual dosage in addition to 50% of the insulin. If insulin dosage is less than 20 units, insulin may be discontinued.

ADVERSE REACTIONS

CNS: dizziness.
GI: nausea, vomiting, constipation.
Hepatic: cholestatic jaundice.
Skin: rash, pruritus, facial flushing.
Other: ***hypoglycemia.***

INTERACTIONS

Anabolic steroids, chloramphenicol, clofibrate, guanethidine, MAO inhibitors, phenylbutazone, probenecid, salicylates, sulfonamides: increased hypoglycemic activity. Monitor blood glucose level.
Beta blockers, clonidine: prolonged hypoglycemic effect and masked symptoms of hypoglycemia. Use together cautiously.
Corticosteroids, glucagon, rifampin, thiazide diuretics: decreased hypoglycemic response. Monitor blood glucose level.
Ethanol: possible disulfiram-like reaction. Avoid concomitant use.
Hydantoins: increased blood levels of hydantoins. Monitor blood levels closely.
Oral anticoagulants: increased hypoglycemic activity or enhanced anticoagulant effect. Monitor blood glucose levels and PT.

CONTRAINDICATIONS

- Contraindicated in patients with diabetic ketoacidosis, with or without coma, and during pregnancy or breast-feeding.
- Use cautiously in patients hypersensitive to sulfonamides and in those with renal and hepatic disease.

NURSING CONSIDERATIONS

- Elderly patients may be more sensitive to drug's adverse effects.
- Patients transferring from insulin therapy to an oral antidiabetic agent require blood glucose monitoring at least three times daily before meals. Patients may require hospitalization during transition.
- During periods of increased stress, such as infection, fever, surgery, or trauma, patients may require insulin therapy. Monitor patients closely for hyperglycemia in these situations.
- Instruct patients about nature of disease, importance of following therapeutic regimen, adhering to specific diet, weight reduction, exercise, personal hygiene programs, and avoiding infection. Explain how and when to perform self-monitoring of blood glucose level, and teach recognition of hypoglycemia and hyperglycemia.
- Some patients taking glipizide may attain effective control on a once-daily regimen, whereas others show a better response with divided dosing.
- Give approximately 30 minutes before meals.
- Glipizide is a second-generation sulfonylurea. The frequency of adverse reactions appears to be lower than with first-generation drugs such as chlorpropamide and tolbutamide.
- Glipizide has a mild diuretic effect. May be useful in patients with CHF or cirrhosis.
- Tell patients not to change drug dosage without the doctor's consent. Report abnormal blood or urine glucose test results.
- Advise patients not to take any other medication, including OTC drugs, without first checking with the doctor.
- Advise patients to carry medical identification identifying them as diabetic patients.

glucagon

Pregnancy Risk Category: B

HOW SUPPLIED

Powder for injection: 1 mg (1 unit)/vial, 10 mg (10 units)/vial

ACTION

Mechanism: Raises blood glucose level by promoting catalytic depolymerization of hepatic glycogen to glucose.

Peak: Peak hyperglycemic effect occurs within 30 minutes. **Duration:** 1 to 2 hours.

INDICATIONS & DOSAGE

Coma of insulin-shock therapy –
Adults: 0.5 to 1 mg S.C., I.M., or I.V. 1 hour after coma develops; may repeat within 25 minutes, if necessary. In very deep coma, also give glucose 10% to 50% I.V. for faster response. When patient responds, give additional carbohydrate immediately.

Severe insulin-induced hypoglycemia during diabetic therapy –
Adults and children: 0.5 to 1 mg S.C., I.M., or I.V.; may repeat q 20 minutes for two doses, if necessary. If coma persists, give glucose 10% to 50% I.V.

Diagnostic aid for radiologic examination –
Adults: 0.25 to 2 mg I.V. or I.M. before initiation of radiologic procedure.

ADVERSE REACTIONS

GI: nausea, vomiting.

Other: hypersensitivity reactions (***bronchospasm,*** rash, dizziness, light-headedness).

INTERACTIONS

Phenytoin: inhibited glucagon-induced insulin release. Use cautiously.

CONTRAINDICATIONS

- Use cautiously in patients with insulinoma pheochromocytoma.

NURSING CONSIDERATIONS

- Unstable hypoglycemic diabetic patients may not respond to glucagon; give dextrose I.V. instead.
- It is vital to arouse patients from coma as quickly as possible and to give additional carbohydrates orally to prevent secondary hypoglycemic reactions.
- Instruct patients and their family members in proper glucagon administration, recognition of hypoglycemia, and urgency of calling the doctor immediately in emergencies.
- Has a positive inotropic and chronotropic action on the heart. May be used to treat overdosage of beta-adrenergic blockers.
- **I.V. use:** Reconstitute 1-unit vial with 1 ml of diluent; reconstitute 10-unit vial with 10 ml of diluent. Use only the diluent supplied by the manufacturer when preparing doses of 2 mg or less. For larger doses, dilute with sterile water for injection.
- For I.V. drip infusion, use dextrose solution, which is compatible with glucagon; drug forms a precipitate in chloride solutions. Give directly into vein or into I.V. tubing of a free-flowing compatible solution over 2 to 5 minutes. Interrupt primary infusion during glucagon injection if you're using the same I.V. line.

---

glyburide (glibenclamide)

DiaBeta**, Euglucon†, Glynase Prestab, Micronase

Pregnancy Risk Category: B

HOW SUPPLIED

Tablets: 1.25 mg, 2.5 mg, 5 mg
Tablets (micronized): 1.5 mg, 3 mg

ACTION

Mechanism: A sulfonylurea that stimulates insulin release from the pancreatic beta cells and reduces glucose output by the liver. An extrapancreatic effect increases peripheral sensitivity to insulin and causes a mild diuretic effect.
Onset: 15 minutes to 1 hour. **Peak:** Peak levels of glyburide occur in 2 to 4 hours; maximum increases in insulin levels are seen in 1 to 2 hours.
Duration: 24 hours.

INDICATIONS & DOSAGE

Adjunct to diet to lower blood glucose level in patients with type II diabetes (non-insulin-dependent) –
Adults: initially, 2.5 to 5 mg P.O. (regular tablets) daily with breakfast. Patients who are more sensitive to antidiabetic agents should be started at 1.25 mg daily. Usual maintenance dosage is 1.25 to 20 mg daily as a single dose or in divided doses.

Alternatively, use micronized formulation. Initial dosage is 1.5 to 3 mg daily. Patients who are more sensitive to antidiabetic agents should be started at 0.75 mg daily.
To replace insulin therapy –
Adults: if insulin dosage is more than 40 units daily, start patient on 5 mg of glyburide (regular tablets) or 3 mg of glyburide (micronized formulation) daily in addition to 50% of the insulin dosage.

ADVERSE REACTIONS

GI: nausea, epigastric fullness, heartburn.
Hepatic: cholestatic jaundice.
Skin: rash, pruritus, facial flushing.
Other: ***hypoglycemia.***

INTERACTIONS

Anabolic steroids, chloramphenicol, clofibrate, guanethidine, MAO inhibitors, phenylbutazone, salicylates, sulfonamides: increased hypoglycemic activity. Monitor blood glucose level.
Beta blockers, clonidine: prolonged hypoglycemic effect and masked symptoms of hypoglycemia. Use together cautiously.
Corticosteroids, glucagon, rifampin, thiazide diuretics: decreased hypoglycemic response. Monitor blood glucose level.
Ethanol: possible disulfiram-like reaction. Avoid concomitant use.
Hydantoins: increased blood levels of hydantoins. Monitor blood levels closely.
Oral anticoagulants: increased hypoglycemic activity or enhanced anticoagulant effect. Monitor blood glucose level and PT.

CONTRAINDICATIONS

- Contraindicated in patients with diabetic ketoacidosis, with or without coma, and during pregnancy or breast-feeding.
- Use cautiously in patients hypersensitive to sulfonamides and in those with severe renal impairment.

NURSING CONSIDERATIONS

- Elderly patients may be more sensitive to drug's adverse effects.
- Micronized glyburide (Glynase Prestab) contains drug in a smaller particle size and is not bioequivalent to regular glyburide tablets. Retitrate patients who have been taking Micronase or DiaBeta.
- Patients transferring from insulin therapy to an oral antidiabetic agent require blood glucose monitoring at least three times a day before meals. Patients may require hospitalization during transition.
- During periods of increased stress, such as infection, fever, surgery, or trauma, patients may require insulin therapy. Monitor patients closely for hyperglycemia in these situations.
- Instruct patients about nature of disease, importance of following therapeutic regimen, adhering to specific diet, weight reduction, exercise, personal hygiene programs, and avoiding infection. Explain how and when to perform self-monitoring of blood glucose levels and teach recognition of and intervention for hypoglycemia and hyperglycemia.
- A maintenance dosage of 5 mg of glyburide (regular tablets) provides approximately the same degree of blood glucose control as 250 to 375 mg of chlorpropamide, 250 to 375 mg of tolazamide, 500 to 750 mg of acetohexamide, or 1,000 to 1,500 mg of tolbutamide.
- Although most patients may take glyburide once daily, patients taking more than 10 mg daily may achieve better results with twice-daily dosage.
- Glyburide is a second-generation sulfonylurea. The frequency of adverse effects appears to be lower than with first-generation drugs, such as chlorpropamide and tolbutamide.
- Glyburide exerts a mild diuretic effect. May be useful in patients with CHF or cirrhosis.
- Tell patients not to change drug dosage without the doctor's consent. Report abnormal blood or urine glucose test results.
- Advise patients not to take any other medication, including OTC drugs, without first checking with the doctor.
- Advise patients to carry medical identification identifying them as diabetic patients.
- Teach patients to carry candy or other simple sugars to treat mild hypoglycemic episodes. Severe episodes may require hospital treatment.

insulins

insulin injection (regular insulin, crystalline zinc insulin)

Actrapid HM‡, Actrapid HM Penfill‡, Actrapid MC‡, Actrapid MC Penfill‡, Humulin R◇, Hypurin Neutral‡, Insulin 2‡, Novolin R◇, Novolin R Penfill◇, Pork Regular Iletin II◇, Regular (Concentrated) Iletin II, Regular Iletin I◇, Regular Purified Pork Insulin◇, Velosulin Human‡, Velosulin Insuject‡

insulin zinc suspension, prompt (semilente)

Semilente MC‡, Semilente Purified Pork◇

isophane insulin suspension (neutral protamine Hagedorn insulin, NPH)

Humulin N◇, Humulin NPH‡, Hypurin Isophane‡, Insulatard‡, Insulatard Human†, Isotard MC‡, Novolin N◇, NPH Insulin◇, NPH Purified Pork◇, Pork NPH Iletin II◇, Protaphane HM‡, Protaphane HM Penfill‡, Protaphane MC‡

isophane insulin suspension with insulin injection

Actraphane HM‡, Actraphane HM Penfill‡, Actraphane MC‡, Humulin 50/50◇, Humulin 70/30◇, Novolin 70/30

insulin zinc suspension (lente)

Humulin L◇, Lente Insulin◇, Lente MC‡, Lente Purified Pork Insulin◇, Monotard HM‡, Monotard MC‡, Novolin L◇

protamine zinc suspension (PZI)

Protamine Zinc Insulin MC‡

insulin zinc suspension, extended (ultralente)

Ultralente Insulin◇, Ultralente Purified Beef◇, Ultratard HM‡, Ultratard MC‡

Pregnancy Risk Category: B

HOW SUPPLIED

insulin injection

Injection (human): 100 units/ml (Actrapid HM‡, Humulin R◇, Novolin R◇, Velosulin Human‡); 100 units/ml in 1.5-ml cartridge system◇ (Actrapid HM Penfill‡, Novolin R Penfill◇)

Injection (from pork): 100 units/ml◇

Injection (purified beef): 100 units/ml (Hypurin Neutral‡, Insulin 2‡)

Injection (purified pork): 100 units/ml (Actrapid MC‡, Pork Regular Iletin II◇, Regular Purified Pork Insulin◇); 100 units/ml in 1.5-ml cartridge system‡ (Actrapid MC Penfill‡); 100 units/ml in 2-ml cartridge system‡; 500 units/ml (Regular [Concentrated] Iletin II)

insulin zinc suspension, prompt

Injection (purified pork): 100 units/ml◇ (Semilente MC‡, Semilente Purified Pork◇)

isophane insulin suspension

Injection (from beef): 100 units/ml◇ (NPH Insulin◇)

Injection (human, recombinant): 100 units/ml (Humulin N◇, Humulin NPH‡, Insulatard Human†, Novolin N◇, Protaphane HM‡); 100 units/ml in 1.5-ml cartridge system‡ (Protaphane HM Penfill‡)

Injection (purified beef): 100 units/ml (Hypurin Isophane‡, Isotard MC‡)

Injection (purified pork): 100 units/ml (Insulatard‡, NPH Purified Pork◇, Pork NPH Iletin II, Protaphane MC‡)

isophane insulin suspension 50% with insulin injection 50%

Injection (human): 100 units/ml (Humulin 50/50◇)

isophane insulin suspension 70% with insulin injection 30%

Injection (human): 100 units/ml (Actraphane HM‡, Humulin 70/30◇, No-

volin 70/30◇); 100 units/ml in 1.5-ml cartridge system‡ (Actraphane HM Penfill‡)
Injection (purified pork): 100 units/ml (Actraphane MC‡)
insulin zinc suspension
Injection (from beef): 100 units/ml (Lente Insulin◇, Lente MC‡)
Injection (purified beef): 100 units/ml (Lente MC‡)
Injection (purified pork): 100 units/ml (Monotard MC‡, Lente Purified Pork Insulin◇)
Injection (human): 100 units/ml◇ (Humulin L◇, Monotard HM‡, Novolin I◇)
protamine zinc suspension
Injection (purified pork): Protamine Zinc Insulin MC‡
insulin zinc suspension, extended
Injection (from beef): 100 units/ml◇ (Ultralente Purified Beef◇)
Injection (human): 100 units/ml‡ (Ultratard HM‡)
Injection (purified pork): 100 units/ml‡ (Ultratard MC‡)

ACTION

Mechanism: Increases glucose transport across muscle and fat cell membranes to reduce blood glucose level. Promotes conversion of glucose to its storage form, glycogen; triggers amino acid uptake and conversion to protein in muscle cells and inhibits protein degradation; stimulates triglyceride formation and inhibits release of free fatty acids from adipose tissue; and stimulates lipoprotein lipase activity, which converts circulating lipoproteins to fatty acids.

INDICATIONS & DOSAGE

Diabetic ketoacidosis (use regular insulin only) –
Adults: 25 to 150 units I.V. immediately; then additional doses q 1 hour based on blood glucose level until patient is out of acidosis; thereafter, give S.C. q 6 hours.

Alternatively, give 50 to 100 units I.V. and 50 to 100 units S.C. stat; then additional doses q 2 to 6 hours based on blood glucose levels. Or 0.33 units/kg as an I.V. bolus, followed by 7 to 10 units/hour by continuous infusion. Continue infusion until blood glucose level drops to 250 mg/dl; then start S.C. insulin q 6 hours.
Children: 0.5 to 1 unit/kg in two divided doses, one I.V. and the other S.C., followed by 0.5 to 1 unit/kg I.V. q 1 to 2 hours. Or 0.1 unit/kg as an I.V. bolus; then 0.1 unit/kg hourly by continuous infusion until blood glucose level drops to 250 mg/dl; then start S.C. insulin. To prepare infusion, add 100 units of regular insulin and 1 g of albumin to 100 ml of 0.9% sodium chloride solution. Insulin concentration will be 1 unit/ml. (The albumin will adsorb to plastic, preventing loss of the insulin to plastic.)
Type I diabetes (insulin-dependent), ketosis-prone diabetics patients, diabetes mellitus inadequately controlled by diet and oral antidiabetic agents –
Adults and children: therapeutic reg-

Insulin types	Onset (hours)	Peak (hours)	Duration (hours)
Rapid-acting			
insulin injection	½ to 1	2 to 3	5 to 7
insulin zinc suspension, prompt	1 to 1½	4 to 7	12 to 16
Intermediate-acting			
isophane insulin suspension with insulin injection	1 to 2	4 to 12	18 to 24
insulin zinc suspension	1 to 2½	7 to 15	18 to 24
Long-acting			
protamine zinc suspension	4 to 8	14 to 24	36
insulin zinc suspension, extended	4 to 8	10 to 30	>36

*Liquid form contains alcohol.
**May contain tartrazine.
Common reactions are in italics; ***life-threatening,*** in bold italics.

imen is prescribed by the doctor and adjusted according to patient's blood and urine glucose concentrations.

ADVERSE REACTIONS
Skin: urticaria, itching, swelling, redness, stinging, warmth at injection site.
Other: *lipoatrophy, lipohypertrophy,* hypersensitivity reaction (***anaphylaxis,*** rash); ***hypoglycemia,*** hyperglycemia (rebound, or Somogyi, effect).

INTERACTIONS
Anabolic steroids, beta blockers, clofibrate, ethanol, fenfluramine, guanethidine, MAO inhibitors, salicylates, tetracycline: prolonged hypoglycemic effect. Monitor blood glucose level carefully.
Corticosteroids, dextrothyroxine, epinephrine, thiazide diuretics: diminished insulin response. Monitor for hyperglycemia.
Diazoxide, phenytoin (high doses): may inhibit endogenous insulin secretion and may cause hypoglycemia in diabetic patients. Carefully adjust insulin dosage when using with these drugs.
Oral contraceptives: may decrease glucose tolerance in diabetic patients. Monitor blood glucose levels and adjust insulin dosage carefully.

CONTRAINDICATIONS
- Use cautiously in surgery and in patients with high fever, thyroid disease, severe infections, trauma, impaired hepatic or renal function, eating disorders, nausea, vomiting, or diarrhea.

NURSING CONSIDERATIONS
- Use only regular insulin in patients with circulatory collapse, diabetic ketoacidosis, or hyperkalemia. Do not use regular insulin concentrated (500 units/ml) I.V. Do not use intermediate or long-acting insulins for coma or other emergency requiring rapid drug action.
- Accuracy of measurement is very important, especially with regular insulin concentrated. Aids, such as magnifying sleeve, dose magnifier, or cornwall syringe, may improve accuracy.
- Dosage is always expressed in USP units. Remember to use only the syringes calibrated for the particular concentration of insulin administered. U-500 insulin must be administered with a U-100 syringe because no syringes are made for this drug.
- Don't interchange single-source beef or pork insulins; dosage adjustment may be required.
- Lente, semilente, and ultralente insulins may be mixed in any proportion.
- Regular insulin may be mixed with NPH or lente insulins in any proportion.
- Advise patient not to alter the order of mixing insulins or change the model or brand of syringe or needle.
- Note that switching from separate injections to a prepared mixture may alter patient response. Whenever NPH or lente is mixed with regular insulin in the same syringe, be sure to administer immediately to avoid binding.
- Store insulin in cool area. Refrigeration is desirable but not essential, except with regular insulin concentrated.
- Don't use insulin that changes color or becomes clumped or granular in appearance.
- Check expiration date on vial before using contents.
- **I.V. use:** Only administer regular insulin I.V. Inject directly at ordered rate into vein, through an intermittent infusion device, or into a port close to I.V. access site. Intermittent infusion is not recommended. If given by continuous infusion, infuse drug diluted in 0.9% sodium chloride at a rate sufficient to reverse ketoacidosis.

• Usual administration route is S.C. because absorption rate and pain are less than with I.M. injections. For proper S.C. administration, remember to pinch a fold of skin with the fingers at least 3 inches apart and insert the needle at a 45- to 90-degree angle. Aspirate to check for inadvertent I.V. or I.M. administration.
• Ketosis-prone type I, severely ill, and newly diagnosed diabetic patients with very high blood glucose levels may require hospitalization and I.V. treatment with regular fast-acting insulin.
• Ketosis-resistant diabetic patients may be treated as outpatients with intermediate-acting insulin and instructions on how to alter dosage according to self-performed blood glucose determinations.
• Instruct patients on proper use of equipment for performing self-monitoring of blood glucose levels.
• Press but do not rub site after injection. Rotate injection sites and chart to avoid overuse of one area. However, unstable diabetic patients may achieve better control if injection site is rotated within same anatomic region.
• To mix insulin suspension, swirl vial gently or rotate between palms or between palm and thigh. Don't shake vigorously: this causes bubbling and air in syringe.
• Insulin requirements increase, sometimes drastically, in pregnant diabetic patients, and then decline immediately postpartum.
• Make sure patients know that therapy relieves symptoms but doesn't cure disease.
• Instruct patients about nature of disease, importance of following the therapeutic regimen, adhering to specific diet, weight reduction, exercise, personal hygiene program, and avoiding infection. Emphasize the importance of the timing of injections and eating and that meals must not be omitted.
• Teach that self-monitoring of blood glucose levels and urine ketone tests are essential guides to dosage and success of therapy. It's important to recognize hypoglycemic symptoms because insulin-induced hypoglycemia is hazardous and may cause brain damage if prolonged; most adverse effects are self-limiting and temporary.
• Advise patients to wear a medical identification bracelet at all times, to carry ample insulin supply and syringes on trips, to have carbohydrates (lump of sugar or candy) on hand for emergencies, and to take note of time zone changes for dose schedule when traveling.
• Marijuana use may increase insulin requirements.
• Cigarette smoking decreases the amount of absorption of insulin administered subcutaneously. Advise patients not to smoke within 30 minutes after insulin injection.
• Some patients may develop insulin resistance and require large insulin doses to control symptoms of diabetes. U-500 insulin is available as Regular (Concentrated) Iletin II for such patients. Although every pharmacy may not normally stock it, it is readily available. Tell patients to notify the pharmacist several days before refill of prescription is needed. Nurses should give the hospital pharmacy sufficient notice before needing to refill in-house prescription. Never store U-500 insulin in same area with other insulin preparations because of danger of severe overdose if given accidentally to other patients.
• Humulin is synthesized by a strain of *Escherichia coli* that has been genetically altered. Novolin is derived from enzymatic alteration of pork insulin.

tolazamide

Tolamide, Tolinase

Pregnancy Risk Category: C

HOW SUPPLIED

Tablets: 100 mg, 250 mg, 500 mg

ACTION

Mechanism: A sulfonylurea that stimulates insulin release from the pancreatic beta cells and reduces glucose output by the liver. An extrapancreatic effect increases peripheral sensitivity to insulin.
Onset: 15 minutes to 1 hour. **Peak:** Peak levels occur in 3 to 4 hours.
Duration: 10 hours.

INDICATIONS & DOSAGE

Adjunct to diet to lower blood glucose levels in patients with type II diabetes (non-insulin-dependent) –
Adults: initially, 100 mg P.O. daily with breakfast if fasting blood sugar (FBS) is under 200 mg/dl or 250 mg if FBS is over 200 mg/dl. May adjust dosage at weekly intervals by 100 to 250 mg. Maximum daily dosage is 500 mg b.i.d. before meals.
Adults over age 65: 100 mg P.O. once daily.
To change from insulin to oral therapy –
Adults: if insulin dosage is under 20 units daily, stop insulin and start oral therapy at 100 mg P.O. daily with breakfast. If insulin dosage is 20 to 40 units daily, stop insulin and start oral therapy at 250 mg P.O. daily with breakfast. If insulin dosage is over 40 units daily, decrease insulin 50% and start oral therapy at 250 mg P.O. daily with breakfast. May adjust dosages by 100 to 250 mg.

ADVERSE REACTIONS

GI: nausea, vomiting.
Skin: rash, urticaria, facial flushing.
Other: ***hypersensitivity reactions, hypoglycemia.***

INTERACTIONS

Anabolic steroids, chloramphenicol, clofibrate, guanethidine, MAO inhibitors, phenylbutazone, salicylates, sulfonamides: increased hypoglycemic activity. Monitor blood glucose level.
Beta blockers, clonidine: prolonged hypoglycemic effect and masked symptoms of hypoglycemia. Use together cautiously.
Corticosteroids, glucagon, rifampin, thiazide diuretics: decreased hypoglycemic response. Monitor blood glucose level.
Ethanol: possible disulfiram-like reaction. Avoid concomitant use of moderate to large amounts of ethanol.
Hydantoins: increased blood levels of hydantoins. Monitor blood levels closely.
Oral anticoagulants: increased hypoglycemic activity or enhanced anticoagulant effect. Monitor blood glucose levels and PT.

CONTRAINDICATIONS

- Contraindicated for treating type I diabetes (insulin-dependent) or diabetes that can be adequately controlled by diet. Also contraindicated in patients with type II diabetes (non-insulin-dependent) complicated by fever, ketosis, acidosis, coma, major surgery, severe trauma, Raynaud's disease, renal or hepatic impairment, or thyroid or other endocrine dysfunction, and during pregnancy or breast-feeding.
- Use cautiously in patients hypersensitive to sulfonamides and in elderly, debilitated, or malnourished patients.

NURSING CONSIDERATIONS

- Elderly patients may be more sensitive to drug's adverse effects.
- Instruct patients about nature of disease, importance of following therapeutic regimen, adhering to specific diet, weight reduction, exercise, personal hygiene programs, and avoiding infection. Explain how and when to

perform self-monitoring of blood glucose levels and teach recognition, of and intervention for hypoglycemia and hyperglycemia.

- Make sure patients know that therapy relieves symptoms but doesn't cure disease.
- Patients transferring from another oral antidiabetic agent usually need no transition period.
- Patients transferring from insulin therapy to an oral antidiabetic agent require blood glucose level testing at least three times a day before meals. Hospitalization may be required during the transition.
- Advise patients to avoid moderate to large intake of alcohol because of possible disulfiram-like reaction.
- Tell patients not to change drug dosage without the doctor's consent. Report abnormal blood or urine glucose test results.
- Advise patients not to take any other medication, including OTC drugs, without first checking with the doctor.
- Advise patients to carry medical identification identifying them as diabetic patients.
- Teach patients to carry candy or other simple sugars to treat mild hypoglycemic episodes. Severe episodes may require hospital treatment.

tolbutamide

Apo-Tolbutamide, Mobenol†, Novobutamide†, Oramide, Orinase

Pregnancy Risk Category: C

HOW SUPPLIED

Tablets: 250 mg, 500 mg

ACTION

Mechanism: A sulfonylurea that stimulates insulin release from the pancreatic beta cells and reduces glucose output by the liver. An extrapancreatic effect increases peripheral sensitivity to insulin.

Onset: 30 to 60 minutes. **Peak:** Plasma levels peak in 3 to 5 hours.
Duration: 6 to 12 hours.

INDICATIONS & DOSAGE

Stable, nonketotic, maturity-onset (type II) diabetes mellitus uncontrolled by diet alone and previously untreated –

Adults: initially, 1 to 2 g P.O. daily as a single dose or in divided doses b.i.d. to t.i.d. Adjust dosage, if necessary, to maximum of 3 g daily; however, the manufacturer states that little benefit occurs with doses greater than 2 g/day.

To change from insulin to oral therapy –

Adults: if insulin dosage is under 20 units daily, stop insulin and start oral therapy at 1 to 2 g P.O. daily. If insulin dosage is 20 to 40 units daily, reduce insulin 30% to 50% and start oral therapy as above. If insulin dosage is over 40 units daily, decrease insulin 20% and start oral therapy as above. Further reductions in insulin are based on the patient's response to oral therapy.

ADVERSE REACTIONS

GI: nausea, heartburn.
Skin: rash, pruritus, facial flushing.
Other: ***hypersensitivity reactions, hypoglycemia, dilutional hyponatremia.***

INTERACTIONS

Anabolic steroids, chloramphenicol, clofibrate, guanethidine, MAO inhibitors, phenylbutazone, salicylates, sulfonamides: increased hypoglycemic activity. Monitor blood glucose level.
Beta blockers, clonidine: prolonged hypoglycemic effect and masked symptoms of hypoglycemia. Use together cautiously.
Corticosteroids, glucagon, rifampin, thiazide diuretics: decreased hypoglycemic response. Monitor blood glucose level.

Ethanol: possible disulfiram-like reaction. Avoid concomitant use of moderate to large amount of ethanol.
Hydantoins: increased blood levels of hydantoins. Monitor blood levels closely.
Oral anticoagulants: increased hypoglycemic activity or enhanced anticoagulant effect. Monitor blood glucose levels and PT.

CONTRAINDICATIONS

- Contraindicated for treating type I diabetes (insulin-dependent) or diabetes that can be adequately controlled by diet. Also contraindicated in patients with type II diabetes (non-insulin-dependent) complicated by fever, ketosis, acidosis, coma, major surgery, severe trauma, Raynaud's disease, renal or hepatic impairment, or thyroid or other endocrine dysfunction, and during pregnancy or breast-feeding.
- Use cautiously in patients hypersensitive to sulfonamides.

NURSING CONSIDERATIONS

- Elderly patients may be more sensitive to drug's adverse effects.
- Instruct patients about nature of disease, importance of following therapeutic regimen, adhering to specific diet, weight reduction, exercise, personal hygiene program, and avoiding infection. Explain how and when to perform self-monitoring of blood glucose levels and teach recognition of and intervention for hypoglycemia and hyperglycemia.
- Make sure patients know that therapy relieves symptoms but doesn't cure disease.
- Patients transferring from another oral antidiabetic agent usually need no transition period.
- Patients transferring from insulin therapy to an oral antidiabetic agent require blood glucose level testing at least three times a day before meals. Hospitalization may be required during the transition.
- Advise patients to avoid moderate to large intake of alcohol because of possible disulfiram-like reaction.
- Tell patients not to change drug dosage without the doctor's consent. Report abnormal blood or urine glucose test results.
- Advise patients not to take any other medication, including OTC drugs, without first checking with the doctor.
- Advise patients to carry medical identification identifying them as diabetic patients.
- Teach patients to carry candy or other simple sugars to treat mild hypoglycemic episodes. Severe episodes may require hospital treatment.

57

Thyroid hormones

levothyroxine sodium
liothyronine sodium
liotrix
thyroid
thyrotropin

COMBINATION PRODUCTS
None.

levothyroxine sodium (T_4 or L-thyroxine sodium)

Eltroxin†, Levoid, Levothroid, Levoxine, Oroxine‡, Synthroid**

Pregnancy Risk Category: A

HOW SUPPLIED

Tablets: 25 mcg, 50 mcg, 75 mcg, 88 mcg, 100 mcg, 112 mcg, 125 mcg, 150 mcg, 175 mcg, 200 mcg, 300 mcg

Injection: 200 mcg/vial, 500 mcg/vial

ACTION

Mechanism: Stimulates metabolism of all body tissues by accelerating the rate of cellular oxidation.

Duration: half-life, normally 6 to 7 days; in patients with hyperthyroidism, 3 to 4 days; in patients with myxedema, 9 to 10 days.

INDICATIONS & DOSAGE

Cretinism –

Children under 1 year: initially, 25 to 50 mcg P.O. daily, increased by 50 mcg P.O. q 2 to 3 weeks to total daily dosage of 100 to 400 mcg.

Myxedema coma –

Adults: 400 mcg I.V.; then 100 to 300 mcg daily. After condition is stabilized, gradually decrease dosage to 50 to 100 mcg daily. Switch to oral maintenance as soon as possible.

Thyroid hormone replacement –

Adults: initially, 25 to 100 mcg P.O. daily, increased by 50 to 100 mcg P.O. q 1 to 4 weeks until desired response occurs. Maintenance dosage is 100 to 400 mcg daily. May administer I.V. or I.M. when P.O. ingestion is precluded for long periods.

Adults over 65 years: 25 mcg P.O. daily. May increase by 25 mcg at 3- to 4-week intervals depending on response.

Children: initially, maximum 50 mcg P.O. daily, gradually increased by 25 to 50 mcg q 1 to 4 weeks until desired response occurs.

ADVERSE REACTIONS

Adverse reactions to thyroid hormones are extensions of their pharmacologic properties and reflect patient sensitivity to them.

CNS: *nervousness, insomnia, tremor.*

CV: *tachycardia, palpitations,* ***arrhythmias,*** *angina pectoris,* hypertension.

GI: appetite change, nausea, diarrhea.

Other: headache, leg cramps, weight loss, diaphoresis, heat intolerance, fever, menstrual irregularities.

INTERACTIONS

Cholestyramine and colestipol: impaired levothyroxine absorption. Separate doses by 4 to 5 hours.

Insulin, oral antidiabetic agents: altered serum glucose levels. Monitor blood glucose levels. Dosage adjustments may be necessary.

I.V. phenytoin: free thyroid released. Monitor for tachycardia.

Oral anticoagulants: altered PT. Monitor PT. Dosage adjustments may be necessary.

Sympathomimetics such as epinephrine: increased risk of coronary insufficiency. Monitor closely.

*Liquid form contains alcohol.
**May contain tartrazine.

Common reactions are in italics; ***life-threatening,*** in bold italics.

CONTRAINDICATIONS

- Contraindicated in patients with MI, thyrotoxicosis (except with antithyroid drugs), or uncorrected adrenal insufficiency (thyroid hormones increase tissue demand for adrenocortical hormone and may cause acute adrenal crisis).
- Use with extreme caution in patients with angina pectoris, hypertension, or other CV disorders; renal insufficiency; and ischemic states.
- Use cautiously in patients with myxedema because these patients are unusually sensitive to thyroid hormone.

NURSING CONSIDERATIONS

- Thyroid hormone replacement requirements are about 25% lower in patients over age 60 than in young adults.
- Patients with adult hypothyroidism are unusually sensitive to thyroid hormone. Start at lowest dose and titrate to higher doses according to patients' symptoms and laboratory data until euthyroid state is reached.
- High initial I.V dosage is usually well tolerated by patients in myxedema coma; however, monitor blood pressure and heart rate closely. Normal serum levels of T_4 should occur within 24 hours, followed by a threefold increase in serum T_3 in 3 days.
- Rapid replacement in patients with arteriosclerosis may precipitate angina, coronary occlusion, or CVA. Use cautiously in these patients.
- In patients with coronary artery disease who must receive thyroid hormone, observe carefully for possible coronary insufficiency.
- Potentially dangerous; not indicated to relieve such vague symptoms as sluggishness, irritability, depression, and ill-defined pains; to treat obesity in euthyroid persons; to treat metabolic insufficiency not associated with thyroid insufficiency; or to treat menstrual disorders or male infertility unless associated with hypothyroidism.
- When changing from levothyroxine to liothyronine, stop levothyroxine and begin liothyronine. Increase in small increments after residual effects of levothyroxine have disappeared. When changing from liothyronine to levothyroxine, start levothyroxine several days before withdrawing liothyronine to avoid relapse.
- **I.V. use:** Prepare I.V. dose immediately before injection. Do not mix with other solutions. Inject into vein over 1 to 2 minutes.
- Thyroid hormones alter thyroid function test results. Monitor PT; patients taking these hormones usually require less anticoagulant. Alert patients to report unusual bleeding and bruising.
- To avoid problems with bioequivalence, advise patients who have achieved a stable response not to change product brands.
- Warn patients (especially elderly patients) to tell the doctor at once if chest pain, palpitations, sweating, nervousness, shortness of breath, or other signs of overdosage or aggravated CV disease occur.
- Make sure patients understand the importance of compliance. Tell patients to take thyroid hormones at the same time each day, preferably before breakfast, to maintain constant hormone levels. Suggest morning dosage to prevent insomnia.
- Monitor pulse and blood pressure.
- Patients taking levothyroxine who need to have radioactive iodine uptake studies performed must discontinue drug 4 weeks before test.

liothyronine sodium (T_3)

Cyronine, Cytomel, Tertroxin‡

Pregnancy Risk Category: A

HOW SUPPLIED
Tablets: 5 mcg, 25 mcg, 50 mcg

ACTION
Mechanism: Stimulates the metabolism of all body tissues by accelerating the rate of cellular oxidation.
Peak: Peak effect occurs within 2 to 3 days. **Duration:** about 3 days.

INDICATIONS & DOSAGE
Myxedema–
Adults: initially, 5 mcg P.O. daily, increased by 5 to 10 mcg q 1 or 2 weeks. Maintenance dosage is 50 to 100 mcg daily.
Nontoxic goiter–
Adults: initially, 5 mcg P.O. daily; may increase by 5 to 10 mcg daily q 1 to 2 weeks, until daily dosage reaches 25 mcg. Then, increase by 12.5 to 25 mcg daily q 1 to 2 weeks. Usual maintenance dosage is 75 mcg daily.
Adults over 65 years: initially, 5 mcg P.O. daily, increased by 5-mcg increments at weekly intervals until desired response occurs.
Children: initially, 5 mcg P.O. daily, increased by 5-mcg increments at weekly intervals until desired response occurs.
Thyroid hormone replacement–
Adults: initially, 25 mcg P.O. daily, increased by 12.5 to 25 mcg q 1 to 2 weeks until satisfactory response. Usual maintenance dosage is 25 to 75 mcg daily.
T_3 suppression test to differentiate hyperthyroidism from euthyroidism–
Adults: 75 to 100 mcg P.O. daily for 7 days.

ADVERSE REACTIONS
Adverse reactions to thyroid hormones are extensions of their pharmacologic properties and reflect patient sensitivity to them.
CNS: hyperirritability, *nervousness, insomnia,* twitching, *tremor,* headache.
CV: increased cardiac output, *tachycardia,* ***arrhythmias,*** angina pectoris, increased blood pressure, ***cardiac decompensation and collapse.***
GI: diarrhea, abdominal cramps, vomiting.
Other: weight loss, heat intolerance, diaphoresis; accelerated rate of bone maturation in infants and children, menstrual irregularities.

INTERACTIONS
Cholestyramine and colestipol: impaired liothyronine absorption. Separate doses by 4 to 5 hours.
Insulin, oral antidiabetic agents: altered serum glucose levels. Monitor blood glucose levels. Dosage adjustments may be necessary.
I.V. phenytoin: free thyroid released. Monitor for tachycardia.
Oral anticoagulants: altered PT. Monitor PT. Dosage adjustments may be necessary.
Sympathomimetics such as epinephrine: increased risk of coronary insufficiency. Monitor closely.

CONTRAINDICATIONS
- Contraindicated in patients with MI, thyrotoxicosis (except with antithyroid drugs), or uncorrected adrenal insufficiency (thyroid hormones increase tissue demand for adrenocortical hormone and may cause acute adrenal crisis).
- Use with extreme caution in patients with angina pectoris, hypertension, or other CV disorders; renal insufficiency; and ischemic states. Adverse cardiac effects are more common with liothyronine than with levothyroxine.
- Use cautiously in patients with myxedema because these patients are unusually sensitive to thyroid hormone.
- Liothyronine is not recommended for treating cretinism because drug crosses the blood-brain barrier poorly.

NURSING CONSIDERATIONS

- Levothyroxine is usually the preferred agent for thyroid hormone replacement therapy. Liothyronine may be used when a rapid onset or a rapidly reversible agent is desirable or in patients with impaired peripheral conversion of levothyroxine to liothyronine.
- In most patients, regulation of liothyronine dosage is difficult.
- Thyroid hormone replacement requirements are about 25% lower in patients over age 60 than in young adults.
- Rapid replacement in patients with arteriosclerosis may precipitate angina, coronary occlusion, or CVA. Use cautiously in these patients.
- In patients with coronary artery disease who must receive thyroid hormones, observe carefully for possible coronary insufficiency.
- Potentially dangerous; not indicated to relieve vague symptoms, such as sluggishness, irritability, depression, and ill-defined aches and pains; to treat obesity in euthyroid persons; to treat metabolic insufficiency; or to treat menstrual disorders or male infertility unless associated with hypothyroidism.
- When changing from levothyroxine to liothyronine, stop levothyroxine and begin liothyronine. Increase in small increments after residual effects of levothyroxine have disappeared. When changing from liothyronine to levothyroxine, start levothyroxine several days before withdrawing liothyronine to avoid relapse.
- To avoid problems with bioequivalence, advise patients who have achieved a stable response not to change product brands.
- Warn patients (especially elderly patients) to tell the doctor at once if chest pain, palpitations, sweating, nervousness, or other signs of overdosage occur and to notify the doctor immediately if any signs of aggravated CV disease (chest pain, dyspnea, and tachycardia) develop.
- Make sure patients understand the importance of compliance. Tell patients to take thyroid hormones at the same time each day, preferably before breakfast, to maintain constant hormone levels. Suggest morning dosage to prevent insomnia.
- Monitor pulse and blood pressure.
- Thyroid hormones alter thyroid function tests. Monitor PT; patients taking these hormones usually require less anticoagulant. Alert patients to report unusual bleeding and bruising.
- Patients taking liothyronine who need to have radioactive iodine uptake studies performed must discontinue drug 7 to 10 days before test.

liotrix

Euthroid**, Thyrolar

Pregnancy Risk Category: A

HOW SUPPLIED

Tablets: levothyroxine sodium 12.5 mcg and liothyronine sodium 3.1 mcg (Thyrolar-¼); levothyroxine sodium 25 mcg and liothyronine sodium 6.25 mcg (Thyrolar-½); levothyroxine sodium 50 mcg and liothyronine sodium 12.5 mcg (Thyrolar-1); levothyroxine sodium 100 mcg and liothyronine sodium 25 mcg (Thyrolar-2); levothyroxine sodium 150 mcg and liothyronine sodium 37.5 mcg (Thyrolar-3)

ACTION

Mechanism: Stimulates metabolism of all body tissues by accelerating the rate of cellular oxidation and provides both T_3 and T_4 to the tissues.

Onset: variable. **Duration:** up to 3 weeks.

INDICATIONS & DOSAGE

Dosages are expressed in thyroid equivalents and must be individualized to approximate the deficit in the patient's thyroid secretion.

Hypothyroidism–
Adults and children: initially, 50 mcg of levothyroxine and 12.5 mcg of liothyronine P.O. daily or 60 mcg of levothyroxine and 15 mcg of liothyronine daily. Increase dosage in increments of the initial dose at monthly intervals to desired response.
Adults over 65 years: initially, give one-fourth to one-half of the initial adult dosage; increase at intervals of 6 to 8 weeks.

ADVERSE REACTIONS

Adverse reactions to thyroid hormones are extensions of their pharmacologic properties and reflect patient sensitivity to them.
CNS: hyperirritability, *nervousness, insomnia,* twitching, *tremor.*
CV: increased cardiac output, *tachycardia,* ***arrhythmias,*** angina pectoris, increased blood pressure, ***cardiac decompensation and collapse.***
GI: diarrhea, abdominal cramps, vomiting.
Other: weight loss, heat intolerance, diaphoresis; accelerated rate of bone maturation in infants and children, menstrual irregularities.

INTERACTIONS

Cholestyramine and colestipol: impaired liotrix absorption. Separate doses by 4 to 5 hours.
Insulin, oral antidiabetic agents: altered serum glucose levels. Monitor blood glucose levels. Dosage adjustments may be necessary.
I.V. phenytoin: free thyroid released. Monitor for tachycardia.
Oral anticoagulants: altered PT. Monitor PT. Dosage adjustments may be necessary.
Sympathomimetics such as epinephrine: increased risk of coronary insufficiency. Monitor closely.

CONTRAINDICATIONS

- Contraindicated in patients with MI, thyrotoxicosis (except with antithyroid drugs), or uncorrected adrenal insufficiency (thyroid hormones increase tissue demand for adrenocortical hormone and may cause acute adrenal crisis).
- Use with extreme caution in patients with angina pectoris, hypertension, or other CV disorders; renal insufficiency; and ischemic states.
- Use cautiously in patients with myxedema because these patients are unusually sensitive to thyroid hormone.

NURSING CONSIDERATIONS

- In most patients, levothyroxine (T_4) is the preferred agent for thyroid replacement therapy. Because peripheral tissues convert T_4 to T_3, using liotrix offers no advantage.
- Thyroid hormone replacement requirements are about 25% lower in patients over age 60 than in young adults.
- Rapid replacement in arteriosclerosis may precipitate angina, coronary occlusion, or CVA. Use cautiously in these patients.
- In patients with coronary artery disease who must receive thyroid hormones, observe carefully for possible coronary insufficiency. Also observe carefully during surgery because cardiac arrhythmias can be precipitated.
- Potentially dangerous; not indicated to relieve vague symptoms, such as sluggishness, irritability, depression, and ill-defined pains; to treat obesity in euthyroid persons; to treat metabolic insufficiency not associated with thyroid insufficiency; or to treat menstrual disorders or male infertility unless associated with hypothyroidism.
- Make sure patients understand the importance of compliance. Tell patients to take thyroid hormones at the same time each day, preferably before breakfast, to maintain constant hormone levels. Suggest morning dosage to prevent insomnia.
- To avoid problems with bioequiva-

lence, advise patients who have achieved a stable response not to change product brands.

• Warn patients (especially elderly patients) to tell the doctor at once if chest pain, palpitations, sweating, nervousness, or other signs of overdosage occur. Also notify the doctor immediately if any signs of aggravated CV disease develop (chest pain, dyspnea, and tachycardia).

• The two commercially prepared liotrix drugs contain different amounts of each ingredient; do not change from one brand to the other without considering the differences in potency: Thyrolar-½ contains 25 mcg of T_4 and 6.25 mcg of T_3; Euthroid-½ contains 30 mcg of T_4 and 7.5 mcg of T_3.

• Monitor pulse and blood pressure.

• Thyroid hormones alter thyroid function test results. Monitor PT; patients taking these hormones usually require less anticoagulant. Alert patients to report unusual bleeding and bruising.

thyroid

Armour Thyroid, S-P-T, Thyrar, Thyroid Strong, Thyroid USP Enseals, Thyro-Teric

Pregnancy Risk Category: A

HOW SUPPLIED

Tablets: 16 mg, 32 mg, 65 mg, 98 mg, 130 mg, 195 mg, 260 mg, 325 mg
Tablets (bovine origin): 32 mg, 65 mg, 130 mg
Tablets (enteric-coated): 32 mg, 65 mg, 130 mg
Strong tablets (50% stronger than thyroid USP, and containing 0.3% iodine): 32 mg, 65 mg, 130 mg, 195 mg
Capsules (porcine origin): 65 mg, 130 mg, 195 mg, 325 mg

ACTION

Mechanism: Stimulates metabolism of all body tissues by accelerating the rate of cellular oxidation.
Duration: 1 to 3 weeks.

INDICATIONS & DOSAGE

Hypothyroidism –
Adults: initially, 60 mg P.O. daily, increased by 60 mg q 30 days until desired response occurs. Usual maintenance dosage is 60 to 180 mg daily as a single dose.
Adults over 65 years: 7.5 to 15 mg P.O. daily; double dosage at 6- to 8-week intervals.
Myxedema –
Adults: 16 mg P.O. daily. May double dosage q 2 weeks to maximum 120 mg.
Cretinism and juvenile hypothyroidism –
Children 0 to 6 months: 4.8 to 6 mg/kg or 15 to 30 mg/day P.O.
Children 6 to 12 months: 3.6 to 4.8 mg/kg or 30 to 45 mg/day P.O.
Children 1 to 5 years: 3 to 3.6 mg/kg or 45 to 60 mg/day P.O.
Children 6 to 11 years: 2.4 to 3 mg/kg or 60 to 90 mg/day P.O.
Children 12 years and older: 1.2 to 1.8 mg/kg or 90 mg/day P.O.

ADVERSE REACTIONS

Adverse reactions to thyroid hormones are extensions of their pharmacologic properties and reflect patient sensitivity to them.
CNS: *hyperirritability, nervousness, insomnia,* twitching, tremor, headache.
CV: increased cardiac output, *tachycardia,* ***arrhythmias,*** angina pectoris, increased blood pressure, ***cardiac decompensation and collapse.***
GI: diarrhea, abdominal cramps, vomiting.
Other: weight loss, heat intolerance, diaphoresis; accelerated rate of bone maturation in infants and children, menstrual irregularities.

INTERACTIONS

Cholestyramine: impaired thyroid absorption. Separate doses by 4 to 5 hours.
Insulin, oral antidiabetic agents: altered serum glucose levels. Monitor blood glucose levels. Dosage adjustments may be necessary.
I.V. phenytoin: free thyroid released. Monitor for tachycardia.
Oral anticoagulants: altered PT. Monitor PT. Dosage adjustments may be necessary.
Sympathomimetics such as epinephrine: increased risk of coronary insufficiency. Monitor closely.

CONTRAINDICATIONS

- Contraindicated in patients with MI, thyrotoxicosis (except with antithyroid drugs), or uncorrected adrenal insufficiency (thyroid hormones increase tissue demand for adrenocortical hormone and may cause acute adrenal crisis).
- Use with extreme caution in patients with angina pectoris, hypertension, or other CV disorders; renal insufficiency; and ischemic states.
- Use cautiously in patients with myxedema because these patients are unusually sensitive to thyroid hormone.

NURSING CONSIDERATIONS

- In most patients, levothyroxine (T_4) is the preferred agent for thyroid replacement therapy. Brand name products contain different ratios of T_3 and T_4.
- Thyroid hormone replacement requirements are about 25% lower in patients over age 60 than in young adults.
- In patients with coronary artery disease who must receive thyroid hormones, observe carefully for possible coronary insufficiency.
- Potentially dangerous; not indicated to relieve vague symptoms, such as sluggishness, irritability, depression, and ill-defined pains; to treat obesity in euthyroid persons; to treat metabolic insufficiency not associated with thyroid insufficiency; or to treat menstrual disorders or male infertility unless caused by hypothyroidism.
- Tell patients to take thyroid hormones at the same time each day to maintain constant hormone levels.
- To avoid problems with bioequivalence, advise patients who have achieved a stable response not to change product brands.
- Warn patients (especially elderly patients) to tell the doctor at once if chest pain, palpitations, sweating, nervousness, or other signs of overdosage occur and to notify the doctor immediately if any signs of aggravated CV disease develop (chest pain, dyspnea, and tachycardia).
- Suggest morning dosage to prevent insomnia.
- Monitor pulse and blood pressure.
- In children, sleeping pulse rate and basal morning temperature are guides to treatment.
- Thyroid hormones alter thyroid function test results. Monitor PT; patients taking these hormones usually require less anticoagulant. Alert patients to report unusual bleeding and bruising.

thyrotropin (thyroid-stimulating hormone, or TSH)

Thytropar

Pregnancy Risk Category: C

HOW SUPPLIED

Powder for injection: 10 IU/vial

ACTION

Mechanism: Stimulates uptake of radioactive iodine in patients with thyroid carcinoma and promotes thyroid hormone production by the anterior pituitary.
Onset: minutes. **Peak:** Hypertrophy

*Liquid form contains alcohol.
**May contain tartrazine.

Common reactions are in italics; ***life-threatening,*** in bold italics.

and hyperplasia of the thyroid gland occur within 24 hours.

INDICATIONS & DOSAGE

Diagnosis of thyroid cancer remnant with ^{131}I after surgery –
Adults: 10 IU I.M. or S.C. for 3 to 7 days.
Differential diagnosis of primary and secondary hypothyroidism –
Adults: 10 IU I.M. or S.C. for 1 to 3 days.
In protein-bound iodine or ^{131}I uptake determinations for differential diagnosis of subclinical hypothyroidism or low thyroid reserve –
Adults: 10 IU I.M. or S.C.
Therapy for thyroid carcinoma (local or metastatic) with ^{131}I –
Adults: 10 IU I.M. or S.C. for 3 to 8 days.
To determine thyroid status of patient receiving thyroid hormone –
Adults: 10 units I.M. or S.C. for 1 to 3 days.

ADVERSE REACTIONS

CNS: headache.
CV: *tachycardia,* atrial fibrillation, angina pectoris, ***CHF,*** hypotension.
GI: nausea, vomiting.
Other: thyroid hyperplasia (large doses), fever, hypersensitivity reactions (postinjection flare, urticaria, ***anaphylaxis***), menstrual irregularities.

INTERACTIONS

Insulin, oral antidiabetic agents: altered serum glucose levels. Monitor blood glucose levels. Dosage adjustments may be necessary.
Oral anticoagulants: altered PT. Monitor PT. Dosage adjustments may be necessary.
Sympathomimetics such as epinephrine: increased risk of coronary insufficiency. Monitor closely.

CONTRAINDICATIONS

- Contraindicated in patients hypersensitive to the drug and in those with coronary thrombosis and untreated Addison's disease.
- Use cautiously in patients with angina pectoris, CHF, hypopituitarism, and adrenocortical suppression.

NURSING CONSIDERATIONS

- Three-day dosage schedule may be used in long-standing pituitary myxedema or with prolonged use of thyroid medication.

58

Thyroid hormone antagonists

methimazole
potassium iodide
potassium iodide, saturated solution
strong iodine solution
propylthiouracil
radioactive iodine (sodium iodide) ^{131}I

COMBINATION PRODUCTS
None.

methimazole

Tapazole

Pregnancy Risk Category: D

HOW SUPPLIED
Tablets: 5 mg, 10 mg

ACTION
Mechanism: Inhibits oxidation of iodine in the thyroid gland, blocking iodine's ability to combine with tyrosine to form thyroxine. May also prevent the coupling of monoiodotyrosine and diiodotyrosine to form thyroxine and triiodothyronine.
Onset: within 5 days (for serum levels of T_3 and T_4 to drop). **Peak:** Plasma levels peak in ½ to 1 hour.
Duration: elimination half-life, 5 to 6 hours.

INDICATIONS & DOSAGE
Hyperthyroidism –
Adults: if mild, 15 mg P.O. daily as a single dose or in two divided doses; if moderately severe, 30 to 45 mg daily as a single dose or in two divided doses; if severe, 60 mg daily as a single dose or in two divided doses. Continue until the patient is euthyroid; then start maintenance dosage of 5 mg daily to t.i.d. Maximum daily dosage is 150 mg.
Children: 0.4 mg/kg P.O. daily in divided doses q 8 hours. Continue until the patient is euthyroid; then start maintenance dosage of 0.2 mg/kg daily in divided doses q 8 hours.
Adjunct for treatment of thyrotoxic crisis –
Adults: 15 to 20 mg P.R. on the first day. Adjust dosage according to patient response.
Children: 400 mcg P.R. as a single dose or in two equally divided doses. Adjust subsequent dosage based on patient response.

ADVERSE REACTIONS
CNS: headache, drowsiness, vertigo.
EENT: loss of taste.
GI: diarrhea, nausea, vomiting (may be dose-related); salivary gland enlargement.
Hematologic: ***agranulocytosis,*** leukopenia, granulopenia, thrombocytopenia (appear to be dose-related).
Hepatic: jaundice; hepatic dysfunction (anorexia, pruritus, right upper quadrant pain, yellow skin or sclera).
Skin: rash, urticaria, skin discoloration.
Other: arthralgia, myalgia, drug fever, lymphadenopathy; hypothyroidism (mental depression; cold intolerance; hard, nonpitting edema).

INTERACTIONS
None significant.

CONTRAINDICATIONS
• Use cautiously in pregnant and breast-feeding patients.

NURSING CONSIDERATIONS
• Watch for signs of hypothyroidism (mental depression; cold intolerance; hard, nonpitting edema); adjust dosage as necessary.

• Rectal suppositories are not commercially available and must be compounded by a pharmacist.
• Monitor CBC periodically to detect impending leukopenia, thrombocytopenia, and agranulocytosis. Also monitor hepatic function.
• Doses of over 30 mg/day increase the risk of agranulocytosis.
• Warn patients to immediately report fever, sore throat, or mouth sores (possible signs of developing agranulocytosis). Agranulocytosis can develop too rapidly to be detected by periodic blood cell counts. Tell patients also to immediately report skin eruptions (sign of hypersensitivity).
• Teach patients to recognize and immediately report signs and symptoms of hepatic dysfunction (anorexia, pruritus, right upper quadrant pain, yellow skin or sclera).
• Discontinue drug if severe rash or enlarged cervical lymph nodes develop.
• Pregnant women may require less drug as pregnancy progresses. Monitor thyroid function studies closely. Thyroid may be added to regimen. Drug may be stopped during last few weeks of pregnancy.
• Although drug is excreted in breast milk, small doses given to breast-feeding patients (15 mg/day or less) do not pose a major risk to infants if infants' thyroid function tests are monitored frequently (at biweekly or weekly intervals).
• Tell patients to ask the doctor about using iodized salt and eating shellfish during treatment.
• Warn patients against OTC cough medicines; many contain iodine.
• Give with meals to reduce adverse GI reactions.
• Store in light-resistant container.

potassium iodide

Iostat, Pima, Thyro-Block

potassium iodide, saturated solution (SSKI)

strong iodine solution (Lugol's solution)

Pregnancy Risk Category: D

HOW SUPPLIED

potassium iodide
Tablets: 130 mg
Tablets (enteric-coated): 300 mg
Oral solution: 500 mg/15 ml
Syrup: 325 mg/5 ml
potassium iodide, saturated solution
Oral solution: 1 g/ml
strong iodine solution
Oral solution: iodine 50 mg/ml and potassium iodide 100 mg/ml

ACTION

Mechanism: Inhibits thyroid hormone formation by blocking iodotyrosine and iodothyronine synthesis, limits iodide transport into the thyroid gland, and blocks thyroid hormone release.
Onset: within 24 hours. **Peak:** Peak effect on thyroid function occurs within 10 to 15 days.

INDICATIONS & DOSAGE

Preparation for thyroidectomy –
Adults and children: strong iodine solution, USP, 0.1 to 0.3 ml P.O. t.i.d., or potassium iodide, saturated solution (SSKI), 1 to 5 drops in water P.O. t.i.d., after meals for 10 to 14 days before surgery.
Thyrotoxic crisis –
Adults and children: 500 mg P.O. q 4 hours (approximately 10 drops of SSKI).
Radiation protectant for thyroid gland –
Adults: 100 to 150 mg P.O. 24 hours before and for 3 to 10 days after radiation exposure.

ADVERSE REACTIONS

CNS: frontal headache.
EENT: acute rhinitis, inflammation of salivary glands, tooth discoloration, periorbital edema, conjunctivitis, hyperemia.
GI: burning, irritation, *nausea,* vomiting, diarrhea (sometimes bloody), *metallic taste.*
Skin: acneiform rash, mucous membrane ulceration.
Other: fever, ***hypersensitivity reactions, including symptoms resembling serum sickness.***

INTERACTIONS

ACE inhibitors, potassium-sparing diuretics: risk of hyperkalemia. Avoid concomitant use.
Antithyroid medications: potassium iodide may potentiate hypothyroid or goitrogenic effects. Monitor closely.
Lithium carbonate: hypothyroidism may occur. Use with caution.

CONTRAINDICATIONS

• Contraindicated in patients with tuberculosis, iodide hypersensitivity, or hyperkalemia; after meals that contain excessive starch; and in patients with laryngeal edema or swelling of salivary glands. Some formulations contain sulfites, which may precipitate allergic reactions in certain hypersensitive individuals.

NURSING CONSIDERATIONS

• Earliest signs of delayed hypersensitivity reactions caused by iodides are irritation and swelling of the eyelids.
• Dilute oral doses in water, milk, or fruit juice, and give after meals to prevent gastric irritation, to hydrate the patient, and to mask the very salty taste.
• Store in light-resistant container.
• Give iodides through straw to avoid tooth discoloration.
• Usually given with other antithyroid drugs.
• Tell patients to ask the doctor about using iodized salt and eating shellfish during treatment. Iodine-rich foods may not be permitted.
• Warn patients that sudden withdrawal may precipitate thyroid storm.
• Avoid using enteric-coated tablets, which have been associated with small bowel lesions and can lead to serious complications, including perforation, hemorrhage, or obstruction.
• Although drug was once commonly used as an expectorant, clinical studies have failed to demonstrate a clinically significant action.

propylthiouracil (PTU)

Propyl-Thyracil†

Pregnancy Risk Category: D

HOW SUPPLIED

Tablets: 50 mg, 100 mg†

ACTION

Mechanism: Inhibits oxidation of iodine in the thyroid gland, blocking iodine's ability to combine with tyrosine to form thyroxine, and may prevent the coupling of monoiodotyrosine and diiodotyrosine to form thyroxine and triiodothyronine.
Peak: Plasma levels peak 1 to 1.5 hours after oral administration. **Duration:** half-life, 1 to 2 hours.

INDICATIONS & DOSAGE

Hyperthyroidism –
Adults: 100 mg P.O. t.i.d.; up to 300 mg q 8 hours have been used in severe cases. Continue until the patient is euthyroid; then start maintenance dosage of 100 mg daily to t.i.d.
Children over 10 years: 100 mg P.O. t.i.d. Continue until the patient is euthyroid; then start maintenance dosage of 25 mg t.i.d. to 100 mg b.i.d.
Children 6 to 10 years: 50 to 150 mg P.O. in divided doses q 8 hours.
Preparation for thyroidectomy –
Adults and children: same doses as

for hyperthyroidism; then iodine may be added 10 days before surgery.
Thyrotoxic crisis –
Adults and children: same doses as for hyperthyroidism, with concomitant iodine therapy and propranolol.

ADVERSE REACTIONS
CNS: headache, drowsiness, vertigo.
CV: vasculitis.
EENT: visual disturbances.
GI: diarrhea, *nausea, vomiting* (may be dose-related), salivary gland enlargement, loss of taste.
Hematologic: ***agranulocytosis,*** leukopenia, thrombocytopenia (appear to be dose-related).
Hepatic: jaundice, ***hepatotoxicity.***
Skin: rash, urticaria, skin discoloration, pruritus.
Other: arthralgia, myalgia, drug fever, lymphadenopathy; dose-related hypothyroidism (mental depression; cold intolerance; hard, nonpitting edema).

INTERACTIONS
None significant.

CONTRAINDICATIONS
• Use cautiously in pregnant and breast-feeding patients.

NURSING CONSIDERATIONS
• Watch for signs of hypothyroidism (mental depression; cold intolerance; hard, nonpitting edema); adjust dosage as necessary.
• Monitor CBC periodically to detect impending leukopenia, thrombocytopenia, and agranulocytosis.
• Warn patients to immediately report fever, sore throat, or mouth sores (possible signs of developing agranulocytosis). Agranulocytosis can develop too rapidly to be detected by periodic blood cell counts. Tell patients to also report skin eruptions (sign of hypersensitivity) immediately.
• Discontinue drug if severe rash or enlarged cervical lymph nodes develop.
• Pregnant women may require less drug as pregnancy progresses. Monitor thyroid function studies closely. Thyroid may be added to regimen. Drug may be stopped during last few weeks of pregnancy.
• Although small amounts of drug are excreted in breast milk, it appears safe for use by breast-feeding women if the infant's thyroid function is monitored at weekly or biweekly intervals.
• Tell patients to ask the doctor about using iodized salt and eating shellfish during treatment.
• Warn patients against OTC cough medicines; many contain iodine.
• Give with meals to reduce adverse GI reactions.
• Store in light-resistant container.

radioactive iodine (sodium iodide) ^{131}I

Iodotope Therapeutic, Sodium Iodide ^{131}I Therapeutic

Pregnancy Risk Category: X

HOW SUPPLIED
All radioactivity concentrations are determined at the time of calibration.
Iodotope Therapeutic
Capsules: radioactivity range is 1 to 50 millicuries (mCi)/capsule at time of calibration
Oral solution: radioactivity concentration is 7.05 mCi/ml at time of calibration; in vials containing approximately 7, 14, 28, 70, or 106 mCi at time of calibration
Sodium Iodide ^{131}I Therapeutic
Capsules: radioactivity range is 0.8 to 100 mCi/capsule at the time of calibration
Oral solution: radioactivity range is 3.5 to 150 mCi/vial at the time of calibration

ACTION

Mechanism: Limits thyroid hormone secretion by destroying thyroid tissue. The affinity of thyroid tissue for radioactive iodine facilitates uptake of drug by cancerous thyroid tissue that has metastasized to other sites in the body.

Onset: 2 to 4 weeks. **Peak:** Peak effect occurs in 2 to 4 months. **Duration:** biological half-life, 90 days in euthyroid patients; 20 to 40 days in hyperthyroid patients; radionuclide half-life, about 8 days.

INDICATIONS & DOSAGE

Hyperthyroidism –

Adults: usual dosage is 4 to 10 mCi P.O. Dosage is based on estimated weight of thyroid gland and thyroid uptake. Repeat treatment after 6 weeks, according to serum thyroxine level.

Thyroid cancer –

Adults: 50 to 150 mCi P.O. Dosage is based on estimated malignant thyroid tissue and metastatic tissue as determined by total body scan. Repeat treatment according to clinical status.

ADVERSE REACTIONS

EENT: *feeling of fullness in neck,* metallic taste, "radiation mumps."

Other: hypothyroidism, radiation thyroiditis; possible increased risk of developing ***leukemia*** later in life after sufficient ^{131}I dose for thyroid ablation following cancer surgery; possible increased risk of birth defects in offspring after sufficient ^{131}I dose for thyroid ablation after cancer surgery.

INTERACTIONS

Lithium carbonate: hypothyroidism may occur. Use with caution.

The following drugs can interfere with the action of ^{131}I and should be withheld the specified time before administering the ^{131}I dose:

Adrenocorticoids: 1 week.

Benzodiazepines: 1 month.

Cholecystographic agents: 6 to 9 months.

Contrast media containing iodine: 1 to 2 months.

Iodine-containing products, including vitamins, expectorants, antitussives, and topical agents: 2 weeks.

Salicylates: 1 to 2 weeks.

CONTRAINDICATIONS

- Contraindicated in pregnant patients except to treat thyroid cancer and contraindicated during breast-feeding.

NURSING CONSIDERATIONS

- Stop all antithyroid medications and thyroid preparations 1 week before ^{131}I dose. If medications are not stopped, patients may receive thyroid-stimulating hormone for 3 days before ^{131}I dose. When treating women of childbearing age, give dose during menstruation or within 7 days after menstruation.
- Food may delay absorption; tell patients to fast overnight before administration.
- After therapy for hyperthyroidism, patients should not resume antithyroid drugs, but should continue propranolol or other drugs used to treat symptoms of hyperthyroidism until onset of full ^{131}I effect occurs (usually 6 weeks).
- Monitor thyroid function with serum thyroxine levels.
- After dose for hyperthyroidism, patients' urine and saliva are slightly radioactive for 24 hours; vomitus is highly radioactive for 6 to 8 hours. Institute full radiation precautions during this time. Instruct patients to use appropriate disposal methods when coughing and expectorating.
- After dose for thyroid cancer, patients' urine, saliva, and perspiration remain radioactive for 3 days. Isolate patients and observe the following precautions: do not allow pregnant personnel to care for patients, use dis-

posable eating utensils and linens; instruct patients to save all urine in lead containers for 24 to 48 hours so amount of radioactive material excreted can be determined. Tell patients to drink as much fluid as possible for 48 hours after drug administration to facilitate excretion. Limit contact with patients to 30 minutes per shift per person the first day and increase time, as necessary, to 1 hour second day and longer on third day.

• Warn patients who are discharged less than 7 days after ^{131}I dose for thyroid cancer to avoid close, prolonged contact with small children (for example, holding children on lap) and not to sleep in the same room with spouse for 7 days after treatment because of increased risk of thyroid cancer in persons exposed to ^{131}I. Tell patients it's okay to use the same bathroom facilities as the rest of the family.

59
Pituitary hormones

corticotropin
cosyntropin
desmopressin acetate
leuprolide acetate
(See Chapter 72, ANTINEOPLASTICS THAT ALTER HORMONE BALANCE.)
lypressin
sermorelin acetate
somatrem
vasopressin

COMBINATION PRODUCTS
None.

corticotropin (adrenocorticotropic hormone, ACTH)
ACTH, Acthar

repository corticotropin
Acthar Gel (H.P.)†, ACTH Gel, H.P. Acthar Gel

Pregnancy Risk Category: C

HOW SUPPLIED
Aqueous injection: 25 units/vial, 40 units/vial
Repository injection: 40 units/ml, 80 units/ml

ACTION
Mechanism: By replacing the body's own tropic hormone, stimulates the adrenal cortex to secrete its entire spectrum of hormones.
Onset: rapid. **Peak:** Plasma levels peak within 1 hour of administration.
Duration: plasma half-life, about 15 minutes; repository forms, up to 3 days.

INDICATIONS & DOSAGE
Diagnostic test of adrenocortical function –
Adults: up to 80 units I.M. or S.C. in divided doses or as a single dose (repository form); or 10 to 25 units (aqueous form) in 500 ml of D_5W I.V. over 8 hours, between blood samplings.

Individual dosages generally vary with adrenal glands' sensitivity to stimulation as well as with specific disease. Infants and younger children require larger doses per kilogram than do older children and adults.
For therapeutic use –
Adults: 40 units S.C. or I.M. in four divided doses (aqueous); or 40 units q 12 to 24 hours (gel or repository form).

ADVERSE REACTIONS
CNS: ***seizures,*** *dizziness,* papilledema, headache, *euphoria, insomnia,* mood swings, personality changes, depression, psychosis.
EENT: cataracts, glaucoma.
GI: peptic ulceration with perforation and hemorrhage, pancreatitis, abdominal distention, ulcerative esophagitis, nausea, vomiting.
Skin: impaired wound healing, thin fragile skin, petechiae, ecchymoses, facial erythema, diaphoresis, acne, hyperpigmentation, allergic skin reactions, hirsutism.
Other: muscle weakness, steroid myopathy, loss of muscle mass, osteoporosis, vertebral compression fractures, cushingoid state, suppression of growth in children, activation of latent diabetes mellitus, progressive increase in antibodies, loss of corticotropin stimulatory effect, hypersensitivity reactions (rash, ***bronchospasm***), *sodium and fluid retention,* calcium and potassium loss, hypokalemic alkalosis, negative nitrogen balance, menstrual irregularities.

INTERACTIONS

Anticonvulsants, barbiturates, rifampin: increased metabolism of corticotropin and decreased effectiveness. Monitor for lack of effect.
Estrogens: may potentiate the effects of cortisol. Dosage adjustments may be necessary.
NSAIDs, salicylates: increased risk of GI bleeding. Avoid concomitant use.
Oral anticoagulants: altered PT. Monitor PT. Dosage adjustments may be necessary.
Potassium-wasting diuretics: increased risk of hypokalemia. Monitor serum potassium levels.

CONTRAINDICATIONS

- Contraindicated in patients with scleroderma, osteoporosis, systemic fungal infections, ocular herpes simplex, recent surgery, peptic ulceration, CHF, hypertension, sensitivity to pork and pork products, concomitant smallpox vaccination, adrenocortical hyperfunction or primary insufficiency, or Cushing's syndrome.
- Use cautiously in pregnant or breast-feeding patients and in women of childbearing age. Also use cautiously in patients being immunized and in those patients with latent tuberculosis or tuberculin reactivity, hypothyroidism, cirrhosis, infection (use anti-infective therapy during and after corticotropin treatment), acute gouty arthritis (limit corticotropin treatment to a few days, and use conventional therapy during and for several days after corticotropin treatment), emotional instability or psychotic tendencies, diabetes, abscess, pyogenic infections, or renal insufficiency, or myasthenia gravis.

NURSING CONSIDERATIONS

- Corticotropin treatment should be preceded by verification of adrenal responsiveness and test for hypersensitivity and allergic reactions.
- Corticotropin should be adjunctive, not sole, therapy. Oral agents are preferred for long-term therapy.
- Unusual stress may require additional use of rapidly acting corticosteroids. When possible, gradually reduce corticotropin dosage to smallest effective dose to minimize induced adrenocortical insufficiency. Reinstitute therapy if stressful situation (trauma, surgery, severe illness) occurs shortly after stopping drug.
- Watch neonates of corticotropin-treated mothers for signs of hypoadrenalism.
- Counteract edema by low-sodium, high-potassium intake; nitrogen loss by high-protein diet; and psychotic changes by reducing corticotropin dosage or administering sedatives.
- Corticotropin may mask signs of chronic disease and decrease host resistance and ability to localize infection.
- Note and record weight changes, fluid exchange, and resting blood pressures until minimal effective dose is achieved.
- Refrigerate reconstituted solution and use within 24 hours.
- **I.V. use:** Use only the aqueous form for I.V. administration. Dilute in 500 ml of D_5W and infuse over 8 hours.
- If administering gel, warm it to room temperature, draw into large needle, and give slowly deep I.M. with 21G or 22G needle. Warn patients that injection is painful.

---

cosyntropin

Cortrosyn

Pregnancy Risk Category: C

HOW SUPPLIED

Injection: 0.25 mg/vial

ACTION

Mechanism: By replacing the body's own tropic hormone, stimulates the adrenal cortex to secrete its entire spectrum of hormones.

Onset: within 5 minutes of I.V. use.
Peak: Peak cortisol levels occur within 1 hour of I.M. or I.V. use.

INDICATIONS & DOSAGE
Diagnostic test of adrenocortical function –
Adults and children: 0.25 to 1 mg I.M. or I.V. (unless label prohibits I.V. administration) between blood samplings.
Children under 2 years: 0.125 mg I.M. or I.V.

ADVERSE REACTIONS
Skin: pruritus.
Other: flushing, hypersensitivity reactions (***anaphylaxis,*** [rare]).

INTERACTIONS
Spironolactone: may interfere with fluorometric analysis of cortisol levels. Avoid concomitant use.

CONTRAINDICATIONS
• Use cautiously in patients hypersensitive to natural corticotropin.

NURSING CONSIDERATIONS
• Drug is synthetic duplication of the biologically active part of the corticotropin molecule. It is less likely to produce sensitivity than natural corticotropin from animal sources.
• Monitor patients for allergic reactions, rashes, dyspnea, wheezing, or evidence of anaphylaxis.
• **I.V. use:** Reconstitute with 1 ml of supplied diluent. For direct injection, administer over at least 2 minutes. May be further diluted with D_5W or 0.9% sodium chloride and infused over 6 hours. Solution is stable for 12 hours at room temperature.

desmopressin acetate
DDAVP, Minirin‡, Stimate
Pregnancy Risk Category: B

HOW SUPPLIED
Nasal solution: 0.1 mg/ml
Injection: 4 mcg/ml

ACTION
Mechanism: Increases the permeability of the renal tubular epithelium to adenosine monophosphate and water; the epithelium promotes reabsorption of water and produces a concentrated urine (ADH effect). Desmopressin also increases factor VIII activity by releasing endogenous factor VIII from plasma storage sites.
Onset: 15 to 60 minutes. **Peak:** Peak antidiuretic effects occur within 1 to 5 hours. **Duration:** 5 to 21 hours.

INDICATIONS & DOSAGE
Nonnephrogenic diabetes insipidus, temporary polyuria and polydipsia associated with pituitary trauma –
Adults: 0.1 to 0.4 ml intranasally daily in one to three doses. Adjust morning and evening doses separately for adequate diurnal rhythm of water turnover. Alternatively, may administer injectable form in dosage of 0.5 to 1 ml I.V. or S.C. daily, usually in two divided doses.
Children 3 months to 12 years: 0.05 to 0.3 ml intranasally daily in one or two doses.
Hemophilia A and von Willebrand's disease –
Adults and children: 0.3 mcg/kg diluted in 0.9% sodium chloride and infused I.V. over 15 to 30 minutes. May repeat dose if necessary as indicated by laboratory response and the patient's clinical condition.
Primary nocturnal enuresis –
Children 5 years and over: initially, 20 mcg intranasally h.s. Adjust dose according to response. Maximum recommended dosage is 40 mcg daily.

ADVERSE REACTIONS
CNS: headache.
CV: slight rise in blood pressure at high dosage.

EENT: nasal congestion, rhinitis.
GI: nausea, abdominal cramps.
GU: vulval pain.
Other: flushing.

INTERACTIONS

Clofibrate: enhanced and prolonged effects of desmopressin. Monitor carefully.
Demeclocycline, ethanol, epinephrine, heparin, lithium: increased risk of adverse effects. Monitor closely.

CONTRAINDICATIONS

- Contraindicated in patients hypersensitive to the drug, patients with type IIb von Willebrand's disease, and children under age 3 months.
- Use cautiously in patients with coronary artery insufficiency or hypertensive CV disease.

NURSING CONSIDERATIONS

- Adjust fluid intake to reduce risk of water intoxication and sodium depletion, especially in children or elderly patients. Warn these patients to drink only enough water to satisfy thirst.
- Overdose may cause oxytocic or vasopressor activity. Withhold drug until effects subside. Use furosemide if fluid retention is excessive.
- Some patients may have difficulty measuring and inhaling drug into nostrils. Teach patients and caregivers correct method of administration.
- Instruct patients to clear nasal passages before administering drug.
- Nasal congestion, allergic rhinitis, or upper respiratory infections may impair drug absorption. Advise patients to report such conditions to the doctor; they may require a dosage adjustment.
- For treating nocturnal enuresis, the recommended method of administration is one-half of the calculated dose in each nostril.
- Intranasal use can cause changes in the nasal mucosa resulting in erratic, unreliable absorption. Report a worsening condition to the doctor, who may prescribe injectable DDAVP.
- Teach patients using S.C. desmopressin to rotate injection sites to prevent tissue damage.
- Don't use desmopressin injection to treat hemophilia A with factor VIII levels of 0% to 5% or severe cases of von Willebrand's disease.
- In treating patients for hemophilia A and von Willebrand's disease, giving desmopressin may avoid the hazards of using blood products.
- Advise patients to wear a medical alert identification bracelet identifying their use of agent.
- Has been used successfully to reduce blood loss during cardiac surgery.

lypressin

Diapid

Pregnancy Risk Category: B

HOW SUPPLIED

Nasal spray: 0.185 mg/ml

ACTION

Mechanism: Increases the permeability of the renal tubular epithelium to adenosine monophosphate and water; the epithelium promotes reabsorption of water and produces a concentrated urine (ADH effect).
Onset: rapid. **Peak:** Peak effects occur within ½ to 2 hours. **Duration:** 3 to 8 hours.

INDICATIONS & DOSAGE

Nonnephrogenic diabetes insipidus – **Adults and children:** 1 or 2 sprays (approximately 2 USP posterior pituitary pressor units/spray) in either or both nostrils q.i.d. and an additional dose h.s., if needed, to prevent nocturia. If usual dosage is inadequate, increase frequency rather than number of sprays.

ADVERSE REACTIONS

CNS: headache, dizziness.
EENT: nasal congestion or ulceration, irritation or pruritus of nasal passages, rhinorrhea, conjunctivitis.
GI: heartburn because of drip of excess spray into pharynx, abdominal cramps, frequent bowel movements.
GU: possible transient fluid retention from overdose.
Skin: hypersensitivity reaction.

INTERACTIONS

None significant.

CONTRAINDICATIONS

- Contraindicated in patients hypersensitive to the drug.
- Use cautiously in patients with coronary artery disease, hypertension, allergic rhinitis, or upper airway infection.

NURSING CONSIDERATIONS

- Ensure that patients understand drug is for topical application to the nasal mucosa and should not be inhaled.
- Instruct patients to clear nasal passage before administering drug.
- Inadvertent inhalation of spray may cause tightness in chest, coughing, and transient dyspnea.
- To administer a uniform, well-diffused spray, hold bottle upright with patient in vertical position holding head upright.
- Particularly useful if diabetes insipidus is unresponsive to other therapy or if ADHs of animal origin cause adverse reactions.
- Nasal congestion, allergic rhinitis, or upper respiratory infections may diminish drug absorption and require larger dose or adjunctive therapy.
- Test patients sensitive to ADH for sensitivity to lypressin.
- Instruct patients to wear a medical identification bracelet identifying their condition.

sermorelin acetate

Geref

Pregnancy Risk Category: C

HOW SUPPLIED

Powder for injection: 50 mcg/ampule

ACTION

Mechanism: A synthetic polypeptide that mimics the aminoterminal segment of the naturally occurring human growth hormone (GH).
Peak: Peak levels of GH occur in about 30 minutes after injection in children; 35 minutes after injection in adults.

INDICATIONS & DOSAGE

Diagnostic aid to determine the pituitary gland's ability to secrete GH–
Adults and children: 1 mcg/kg as a single I.V. injection.

ADVERSE REACTIONS

CNS: headache.
EENT: unusual taste in mouth.
GI: nausea.
Skin: pain, redness, or swelling at injection site.
Other: transient warmth or flushing of face, antibody formation, paleness, tightness in chest.

INTERACTIONS

Anticholinergics, antithyroid medications (such as propylthiouracil): decreased response to sermorelin.
Clonidine, insulin-induced hypoglycemia, levodopa: may elevate somatotropin levels.
Corticosteroids, cyclooxygenase inhibitors (for example, acetaminophen, aspirin, or NSAIDs), insulin: altered pituitary secretion of somatotropin. Don't perform the test in patients receiving these drugs.

CONTRAINDICATIONS
• Contraindicated in patients with hypersensitivity to the drug or any components of the formulation.

NURSING CONSIDERATIONS
• Response to drug may be blunted in hypothyroid patients.
• Although hypersensitivity reactions have been reported with the administration of other polypeptide hormones, none have been reported with sermorelin. About 25% of patients develop antibody formation with prolonged use; however, no symptomatic allergic reactions have been reported.
• In clinical trials, GH peak plasma levels of 13 to 43 ng/ml occurred 3 to 57 minutes after the injection.
• Discontinue GH therapy 1 week before the test.
• Baseline GH levels are generally low (< 4 ng/ml). Provocative tests such as sermorelin are useful in determining that the pituitary somatotroph can respond. However, a normal response doesn't rule out GH deficiency if the deficit is caused by hypothalamic dysfunction. This test is most easily interpreted if patients have had a subnormal response to conventional provocative testing (such as clonidine, levodopa, or arginine) and a normal response to sermorelin, suggesting that the cause of GH deficiency is hypothalamic dysfunction. Abnormal results from both conventional tests and sermorelin can't locate the dysfunction.
• Make sure patients understand that the test must be performed in the morning after an overnight fast. They shouldn't take anything by mouth after midnight.
• **I.V. use:** Reconstitute each ampule with a minimum of 0.5 ml of the supplied diluent. One ampule contains 50 mcg of drug, which is sufficient to test a 110-lb (50-kg) subject. Larger subjects require the use of multiple ampules.
• Draw venous blood samples for GH determinations 15 minutes before and immediately before injection. Administer bolus injection (1 mcg/kg I.V.) and follow with 3-ml of 0.9% sodium chloride injection flush. Venous samples for GH determinations should be drawn at 15-minute intervals after injection (15 minutes, 30 minutes, 45 minutes, and 60 minutes).

somatrem
Protropin

Pregnancy Risk Category: C

HOW SUPPLIED
Injectable lyophilized powder: 5 mg (10 IU)/vial

ACTION
Mechanism: Purified growth hormone (GH) of recombinant DNA origin that stimulates linear, skeletal muscle, and organ growth.
Duration: 12 to 48 hours; half-life, 3 to 5 hours after I.M. or S.C. dose.

INDICATIONS & DOSAGE
Long-term treatment of children who have growth failure because of lack of adequate endogenous GH secretion –
Children (prepuberty): 0.1 mg/kg I.M. or S.C. three times weekly.

ADVERSE REACTIONS
Other: hypothyroidism, hyperglycemia; antibodies to GH.

INTERACTIONS
Glucocorticoids: may inhibit growth-promoting action of somatrem. Adjust glucocorticoid dose as necessary.

CONTRAINDICATIONS
• Contraindicated in patients with closed epiphyses, or an active underlying intracranial lesion.
• Use cautiously in patients with hypothyroidism and in those whose GH deficiency results from an intracranial

lesion. Examine patients frequently for progression or recurrence of the underlying disease.

NURSING CONSIDERATIONS

- Regular checkups with monitoring of height and of blood and radiologic studies are necessary.
- Observe patients for signs of glucose intolerance and hyperglycemia.
- Monitor periodic thyroid function tests for hypothyroidism, which may require treatment with a thyroid hormone.
- Drug replaces pituitary-derived human GH, which was removed from the market in 1985 because of an association with a rare but fatal viral infection (Jakob-Creutzfeldt disease). Reassure patients and their family members that somatrem is *pure* and *safe*.
- To prepare the solution, inject the supplied bacteriostatic water for injection into the vial containing the drug. Then swirl the vial with a gentle rotary motion until the contents are completely dissolved. *Don't shake* the vial.
- After reconstitution, vial solution should be clear. Don't inject into the patient if the solution is cloudy or contains any particles.
- Store reconstituted vial in refrigerator; use within 7 days.
- If drug is used in neonates, reconstitute immediately before use with sterile water for injection (without bacteriostat). Use the vial once; then discard.
- Be sure to check this product's expiration date.

vasopressin (ADH)

Pitressin

Pregnancy Risk Category: B

HOW SUPPLIED

Injection: 0.5-ml and 1-ml ampules, 20 units/ml

ACTION

Mechanism: Increases the permeability of the renal tubular epithelium to adenosine monophosphate and water; the epithelium promotes reabsorption of water and produces a concentrated urine (ADH effect).
Duration: 2 to 8 hours.

INDICATIONS & DOSAGE

Nonnephrogenic, nonpsychogenic diabetes insipidus –
Adults: 5 to 10 units I.M. or S.C. b.i.d. to q.i.d., p.r.n.; or intranasally (aqueous solution used as spray or applied to cotton balls) in individualized doses, based on response.
Children: 2.5 to 10 units I.M. or S.C. b.i.d. to q.i.d., p.r.n.; or intranasally (aqueous solution used as spray or applied to cotton balls) in individualized doses.
Postoperative abdominal distention –
Adults: initially, 5 units (aqueous) I.M.; then q 3 to 4 hours, increasing dose to 10 units, if needed. Reduce dose proportionately for children.
To expel gas before abdominal X-ray –
Adults: inject 10 units S.C. at 2 hours; then again at 30 minutes before X-ray. Enema before first dose may also help to eliminate gas.
Upper GI tract hemorrhage –
Adults: 0.2 to 0.4 units/minute by intra-arterial injection.

ADVERSE REACTIONS

CNS: tremor, dizziness, headache.
CV: angina in patients with vascular disease, vasoconstriction; large doses may cause hypertension, ECG changes (with intra-arterial infusion – ***bradycardia, cardiac arrhythmias, pulmonary edema.***)
GI: abdominal cramps, nausea, vomiting, diarrhea, intestinal hyperactivity.
GU: anuria.
Skin: circumoral pallor.
Other: uterine cramps, water intoxi-

cation (drowsiness, listlessness, headache, confusion, weight gain, ***seizures, coma)***, hypersensitivity reactions (urticaria, angioedema, ***bronchoconstriction***, fever, rash, wheezing, dyspnea, ***anaphylaxis***), diaphoresis.

INTERACTIONS

Carbamazepine, chlorpropamide, clofibrate, fludrocortisone, tricyclic antidepressants: increased antidiuretic response. Use together cautiously.

Demeclocycline, ethanol, heparin, lithium, norepinephrine: reduced antidiuretic activity. Use together cautiously.

CONTRAINDICATIONS

- Contraindicated in patients with chronic nephritis with nitrogen retention.
- Use cautiously in children, elderly patients, pregnant patients, and those with seizure disorders, migraine headache, asthma, CV disease, or fluid overload.

NURSING CONSIDERATIONS

- Never inject during first stage of labor; may cause ruptured uterus.
- Monitor specific gravity of urine and fluid intake and output to aid evaluation of drug effectiveness.
- Instruct patients to rotate injection sites to prevent tissue damage.
- Give with 1 to 2 glasses of water to reduce adverse reactions and to improve therapeutic response.
- To prevent possible seizures, coma, and death, observe patients closely for early signs of water intoxication.
- Use minimum effective dosage to reduce adverse reactions.
- May be used for transient polyuria resulting from ADH deficiency related to neurosurgery or head injury.
- Synthetic desmopressin is sometimes preferred because of longer duration of action and less frequent adverse reactions. Desmopressin is also commercially available as a nasal solution.
- Monitor blood pressure of patients on vasopressin twice daily. Watch for excessively elevated blood pressure or lack of response to drug, which may be indicated by hypotension. Also monitor fluid intake and output and daily weight.
- A rectal tube will facilitate gas expulsion after vasopressin injection.

60

Parathyroid-like agents

calcifediol
calcitonin (human)
calcitonin (salmon)
calcitriol
dihydrotachysterol
etidronate disodium

COMBINATION PRODUCTS
None.

calcifediol

Calderol

Pregnancy Risk Category: A

HOW SUPPLIED
Capsules: 20 mcg, 50 mcg

ACTION
Mechanism: A vitamin-D analogue that stimulates calcium absorption from the GI tract and promotes secretion of calcium from bone to blood.
Peak: Peak levels occur in 4 hours.
Duration: 15 to 20 days; plasma half-life, 16 to 22 days.

INDICATIONS & DOSAGE
Metabolic bone disease associated with chronic renal failure –
Adults: initially, 300 to 350 mcg P.O. weekly. Increase dosage at 4-week intervals. Carefully determine optimal dosage for each patient.

ADVERSE REACTIONS
Vitamin D intoxication associated with hypercalcemia:
CNS: headache, somnolence.
EENT: conjunctivitis, photosensitivity reactions, rhinorrhea.
GI: nausea, vomiting, constipation, metallic taste, dry mouth, anorexia, diarrhea.
GU: polyuria.
Other: weakness, bone and muscle pain.

INTERACTIONS
Cholestyramine, colestipol: decreased absorption of orally administered vitamin D analogues. Avoid concomitant use.
Corticosteroids: counteracted vitamin D analogue effects. Don't use together.
Digitalis glycosides: increased risk of cardiac arrhythmias. Avoid concomitant use.
Magnesium-containing antacids: possible hypermagnesemia, especially in patients with chronic renal failure. Avoid concomitant use.
Other vitamin D analogues: increased toxicity. Avoid concomitant use.

CONTRAINDICATIONS
- Contraindicated in patients with hypercalcemia or vitamin D toxicity. Withhold all preparations containing vitamin D.

NURSING CONSIDERATIONS
- Monitor serum calcium level; serum calcium level multiplied by serum phosphate level should not exceed 70. During titration, serum calcium level should be determined at least weekly. If hypercalcemia occurs, discontinue calcifediol but resume after serum calcium level returns to normal.
- Provide the patient with adequate daily intake of calcium.
- Teach the patient to report signs and symptoms of hypercalcemia.

calcitonin (human)

Cibacalcin

calcitonin (salmon)

Calcimar, Miacalcin

Pregnancy Risk Category: B

HOW SUPPLIED

human

Injection: 0.5 mg/vial

salmon

Injection: 100 IU/ml, 1-ml ampules; 200 IU/ml, 2-ml ampules

ACTION

Mechanism: Decreases osteoclastic activity by inhibiting osteocytic osteolysis and decreases mineral release and matrix or collagen breakdown in bone.

Onset: immediately after I.V. injection, within 15 minutes after I.M. or S.C. injection. **Peak:** Plasma levels peak immediately after I.V. injection, within 4 hours after I.M. or S.C. injection. **Duration:** effects persist 30 minutes to 12 hours after I.V. administration, 8 to 24 hours after I.M. or S.C. injection.

INDICATIONS & DOSAGE

Paget's disease of bone (osteitis deformans) –

Adults: initially, 100 IU of calcitonin (salmon) daily S.C. or I.M. Maintenance dosage is 50 to 100 IU daily or every other day. Alternatively, give calcitonin (human) 0.5 mg S.C. daily. If the patient improves sufficiently, reduce dosage to 0.25 mg. daily 2 or 3 times per week. Some patients may need as much as 1 mg daily.

Hypercalcemia –

Adults: 4 IU/kg of calcitonin (salmon) q 12 hours I.M.

Postmenopausal osteoporosis –

Adults: 100 IU of calcitonin (salmon) daily I.M. or S.C.

ADVERSE REACTIONS

CNS: headache.

GI: transient nausea, unusual taste, diarrhea, anorexia.

GU: transient diuresis.

Local: inflammation at injection site, rash.

Other: *facial flushing;* hypocalcemia; hyperglycemia; hand swelling, tingling, and tenderness; hypersensitivity reactions ***(anaphylaxis)***.

INTERACTIONS

None significant.

CONTRAINDICATIONS

- Contraindicated in patients allergic to gelatin diluent used to prepare drug. Not recommended for breast-feeding patients, or those who are or may become pregnant. Safe use in children not established.

NURSING CONSIDERATIONS

- Monitor periodic serum alkaline phosphatase and 24-hour urine hydroxyproline levels to evaluate drug effect.
- Examinations of urine sediment are advisable periodically.
- Skin test is usually done before therapy.
- Systemic allergic reactions possible since hormone is protein. Keep epinephrine handy.
- In patients with good initial clinical response to calcitonin who suffer relapse, evaluate for antibody response to the hormone protein.
- Tell the patient in whom calcitonin loses its hypocalcemic activity that further medication or increased dosages will be of no value.
- Facial flushing and warmth occur in 20% to 30% of all patients within minutes of injection and usually last about 1 hour. Reassure the patient that this is a transient effect.
- Observe the patient for signs of hypocalcemic tetany during therapy (muscle twitching, tetanic spasms, and seizures if hypocalcemia is severe).
- Monitor serum calcium level closely. Watch for signs of hypercalcemic relapse: bone pain, renal cal-

culi, polyuria, anorexia, nausea, vomiting, thirst, constipation, lethargy, bradycardia, muscle hypotonicity, pathologic fracture, psychosis, and coma.

• Calcitonin (human) is especially indicated in patients who have developed resistance to calcitonin (salmon). Calcitonin (human) is associated with risk of diminishing efficacy caused by antibody formation or hypersensitivity reactions.
• Administer h.s. when possible to minimize nausea and vomiting.
• If symptoms have been relieved after 6 months, treatment may be discontinued until symptoms or radiologic signs recur.
• I.M. route is preferred if the volume of the dose to be administered exceeds 2 ml.
• When administered for postmenopausal osteoporosis, remind the patient to take adequate calcium and vitamin D supplements.
• Store calcitonin (human) at room temperature (77° F [25° C]); refrigerate calcitonin (salmon) at 36° to 46° F (2° to 8° C).
• Use freshly reconstituted solution within 2 hours.

calcitriol (1,25-dihydroxycholecalciferol)

Rocaltrol

Pregnancy Risk Category: A (D in doses > RDA)

HOW SUPPLIED

Capsules: 0.25 mcg, 0.5 mcg

ACTION

Mechanism: A vitamin D analogue that stimulates calcium absorption from the GI tract and promotes secretion of calcium from bone to blood.
Onset: 2 to 6 hours. **Peak:** Plasma levels peak in 3 to 6 hours. **Duration:** 3 to 5 days; plasma half-life, 3 to 6 hours.

INDICATIONS & DOSAGE

Hypocalcemia in patients undergoing chronic dialysis –
Adults: initially, 0.25 mcg P.O. daily. Dosage may be increased by 0.25 mcg daily at 2- to 4-week intervals. Maintenance dosage is 0.25 mcg every other day up to 1.25 mcg daily.
Hypoparathyroidism and pseudohypoparathyroidism –
Adults and children over 1 year: initially, 0.25 mcg P.O. daily. Dosage may be increased at 2- to 4-week intervals. Maintenance dosage is 0.25 to 2 mcg daily.

ADVERSE REACTIONS

Vitamin D intoxication associated with hypercalcemia:
CNS: headache, somnolence.
EENT: conjunctivitis, photophobia, rhinorrhea.
GI: nausea, vomiting, constipation, metallic taste, dry mouth, anorexia.
GU: polyuria.
Other: weakness, bone and muscle pain.

INTERACTIONS

Cholestyramine, colestipol, excessive use of mineral oil: decreased absorption of orally administered vitamin D analogues. Avoid concomitant use.
Corticosteroids: counteracted vitamin D analogue effects. Don't use together.
Digitalis glycosides: increased risk of cardiac arrhythmias. Avoid concomitant use.
Magnesium-containing antacids: may induce hypermagnesemia, especially in patients with chronic renal failure. Avoid concomitant use.

CONTRAINDICATIONS

• Contraindicated in patients with hypercalcemia or vitamin D toxicity. Withhold all preparations containing vitamin D. Not recommended in breast-feeding patients.

NURSING CONSIDERATIONS

- Monitor serum calcium level; serum calcium level multiplied by the serum phosphate level should not exceed 70. During titration, determine serum calcium twice weekly. Discontinue if hypercalcemia occurs, but resume after serum calcium level returns to normal. The patient should receive adequate daily intake of calcium – 1,000 mg.
- Protect from heat and light.
- Instruct the patient to adhere to diet and calcium supplementation and to avoid unapproved OTC drugs and magnesium-containing antacids.
- Tell the patient to immediately report early symptoms of vitamin D intoxication: weakness, nausea, vomiting, dry mouth, constipation, muscle or bone pain, or metallic taste.
- Tell the patient that this drug must not be taken by anyone for whom it was not prescribed because of its potentially serious toxicities. It is the most potent form of vitamin D available.

dihydrotachysterol

AT-10‡, DHT Intensol*, Hytakerol

Pregnancy Risk Category: A (D if used in doses > RDA)

HOW SUPPLIED

Tablets: 0.125 mg, 0.2 mg, 0.4 mg
Capsules: 0.125 mg
Oral solution: 0.2 mg/5 ml, 0.2 mg/ml* (DHT Intensol*), 0.25 mg/ml (in sesame oil)

ACTION

Mechanism: A vitamin D analogue that stimulates calcium absorption from the GI tract and promotes secretion of calcium from bone to blood.
Onset: several hours. **Peak:** Peak effects occur in 1 to 2 weeks. **Duration:** up to 9 weeks.

INDICATIONS & DOSAGE

1 mg of dihydrotachysterol is equal to 120,000 units ergocalciferol (vitamin D_2)

Familial hypophosphatemia –
Adults and children: 0.5 to 2 mg P.O. daily. Maintenance dosage is 0.3 to 1.5 mg daily.

Hypocalcemia associated with hypoparathyroidism and pseudohypoparathyroidism –
Adults: initially, 0.8 to 2.4 mg P.O. daily for several days. Maintenance dosage is 0.2 to 2 mg daily. Average dosage is 0.6 mg daily.
Children: initially, 1 to 5 mg P.O. for several days. Maintenance dosage is 0.2 to 1 mg daily.

Renal osteodystrophy in chronic uremia –
Adults: 0.1 to 0.6 mg P.O. daily.

Prophylaxis of hypocalcemic tetany following thyroid surgery –
Adults: 0.25 mg P.O. daily (with calcium supplements).

ADVERSE REACTIONS

Vitamin D intoxication associated with hypercalcemia:
CNS: headache, somnolence.
EENT: conjunctivitis, photophobia, rhinorrhea.
GI: nausea, vomiting, constipation, metallic taste, dry mouth, anorexia, diarrhea.
GU: polyuria.
Other: weakness, bone and muscle pain.

INTERACTIONS

Cholestyramine, colestipol, excessive use of mineral oil: decreased absorption of orally administered vitamin D analogues. Avoid concomitant use.
Corticosteroids: counteracted vitamin D analogue effects. Don't use together.
Digitalis glycosides: increased risk of cardiac arrhythmias. Avoid concomitant use.
Magnesium-containing antacids: pos-

sible hypermagnesemia, especially in patients with chronic renal failure. Avoid concomitant use.
Other vitamin D analogues: increased toxicity. Avoid concomitant use.

CONTRAINDICATIONS
• Contraindicated in patients with hypercalcemia, hypocalcemia associated with renal insufficiency and hyperphosphatemia, renal stones, hypersensitivity to vitamin D, and in breast-feeding patients.

NURSING CONSIDERATIONS
• Monitor serum calcium level; the serum calcium level multiplied by serum phosphate level should not exceed 70. During titration, determine serum calcium twice weekly. Discontinue if hypercalcemia occurs, but resume after serum calcium level returns to normal. Adequate daily intake of calcium – 1,000 mg.
• Monitor urine calcium.
• Report any early signs of hypercalcemia: thirst, headache, vertigo, tinnitus, or anorexia.
• Store in tightly closed, light-resistant container. Don't refrigerate.

etidronate disodium
Didronel
Pregnancy Risk Category: B

HOW SUPPLIED
Tablets: 200 mg, 400 mg
Injection: 50 mg/ml

ACTION
Mechanism: Decreases osteoclastic activity by inhibiting osteocytic osteolysis and decreases mineral release and matrix or collagen breakdown in bone.
Onset: in Paget's disease, within 1 month; in hypercalemia, decreased urinary calcium excretion within 24 hours. **Peak:** In hypercalcemia, peak effects occur within 24 hours after the third I.V. infusion. **Duration:** in hypercalcemia, effects persist up to 11 days after treatment; in heterotopic ossification, effects persist several months after therapy; in Paget's disease, effects persist up to 1 year after therapy.

INDICATIONS & DOSAGE
Symptomatic Paget's disease –
Adults: 5 mg/kg P.O. daily in single dose 2 hours before a meal with water or juice. Tell the patient not to eat for 2 hours after dose. Give up to 10 mg/kg daily in severe cases; maximum dosage is 20 mg/kg daily.
Heterotopic ossification in spinal cord injuries –
Adults: 20 mg/kg P.O. daily for 2 weeks, then 10 mg/kg daily for 10 weeks. Total treatment period is 12 weeks.
Heterotopic ossification after total hip replacement –
Adults: 20 mg/kg P.O. daily for 1 month before total hip replacement and for 3 months afterward.
Hypercalcemia –
Adults: 7.5 mg/kg I.V. daily for 3 consecutive days. Maintenance dosage is 20 mg/kg P.O. daily for 30 days. May be used for a maximum of 90 days.

ADVERSE REACTIONS
GI: seen most frequently at 20 mg/kg daily – diarrhea, increased frequency of bowel movements, nausea.
Other: increased or recurrent bone pain, pain at previously asymptomatic sites, increased risk of fracture, *elevated serum phosphate.*

INTERACTIONS
None significant.

CONTRAINDICATIONS
• Use cautiously in patients with enterocolitis and in those with impaired renal function.

NURSING CONSIDERATIONS

- Don't give longer than 3 months at doses above 10 mg/kg daily; resume after 3 months, if needed. Therapy should not exceed 6 months.
- Don't give drug with food, milk, or antacids; may reduce absorption.
- Monitor renal function before and during therapy.
- Elevated serum phosphate level may occur, especially in patients receiving higher doses. However, serum phosphate level usually returns to normal 2 to 4 weeks after drug is discontinued.
- To monitor drug effect, review serum alkaline phosphatase and urinary hydroxyproline excretion; both will decrease if therapy is effective.
- Tell the patient that improvement may not occur for up to 3 months but may continue for months after drug is stopped.
- Stress importance of a diet high in calcium and vitamin D.
- Has been used investigationally to prevent or treat osteoporosis.
- **I.V. use:** Dilute daily dose in at least 250 ml 0.9% sodium chloride solution or D_5W., and infuse over at least 2 hours.
- Some patients may receive I.V. etidronate for up to 7 days. However, the risk of hypokalemia increases after 3 days of treatment.

61
Diuretics

acetazolamide
acetazolamide sodium
amiloride hydrochloride
bendroflumethiazide
benzthiazide
bumetanide
chlorothiazide
chlorothiazide sodium
chlorthalidone
dichlorphenamide
ethacrynate sodium
ethacrynic acid
furosemide
hydrochlorothiazide
hydroflumethiazide
indapamide
mannitol
methazolamide
methyclothiazide
metolazone
polythiazide
quinethazone
spironolactone
torsemide
triamterene
trichlormethiazide
urea

COMBINATION PRODUCTS

ALDACTAZIDE: spironolactone 25 mg and hydrochlorothiazide 25 mg.
ALDACTAZIDE 50/50: spironolactone 50 mg and hydrochlorothiazide 50 mg.
DYAZIDE: triamterene 50 mg and hydrochlorothiazide 25 mg.
MAXZIDE: triamterene 75 mg and hydrochlorothiazide 50 mg.
MAXZIDE-25MG: triamterene 37.5 mg and hydrochlorothiazide 25 mg.
MODURETIC: amiloride hydrochloride 5 mg and hydrochlorothiazide 50 mg.
SPIROZIDE: spironolactone 25 mg and hydrochlorothiazide 25 mg.
ZIAC 2.5: bisoprolol fumarate 2.5 mg and hydrochlorthiazide 6.25 mg.
ZIAC 5: bisoprolol fumarate 5 mg and hydrochlorthiazide 6.25 mg.
ZIAC 10: bisoprolol fumarate 10 mg and hydrochlorthiazide 6.25 mg.

acetazolamide
Acetazolam†, Apo-Acetazolamide†, Dazamide, Diamox, Diamox Sequels, Storzolamide

acetazolamide sodium
Diamox Parenteral, Diamox Sodium†

Pregnancy Risk Category: C

HOW SUPPLIED

acetazolamide
Tablets: 125 mg, 250 mg
Capsules (extended-release): 500 mg
acetazolamide sodium
Injection: 500 mg/vial

ACTION

Mechanism: Blocks the action of carbonic anhydrase, promoting renal excretion of sodium, potassium, bicarbonate, and water, and decreases secretion of aqueous humor in the eye, thereby lowering intraocular pressure. As an anticonvulsant, may inhibit carbonic anhydrase in the CNS and decrease abnormal paroxysmal or excessive neuronal discharge. In acute mountain sickness, carbonic anhydrase inhibitors produce a respiratory and metabolic acidosis that may stimulate ventilation, increase cerebral blood flow, promote the release of oxygen from hemoglobin, and increase ventilation.
Onset: 1 to 1½ hours after tablets, 2 hours after capsules, 2 minutes after

I.V. injection. **Peak:** Peak effects occur 2 to 4 hours after tablets, 8 to 12 hours after capsules, 15 minutes after I.V. injection. **Duration:** 8 to 12 hours after tablets, 18 to 24 hours after capsules, 4 to 5 hours after injection.

INDICATIONS & DOSAGE

Secondary glaucoma and preoperative treatment of acute angle-closure glaucoma –

Adults: 250 mg P.O. q 4 hours; or 250 mg P.O. b.i.d. for short-term therapy. To rapidly lower intraocular pressure, give 500 mg I.V. or I.M. q 2 to 4 hours.

Children: 10 to 15 mg/kg/day P.O.in divided doses q 6 to 8 hours; or 5 to 10 mg/kg I.M. or I.V. q 6 hours.

Edema in CHF –

Adults: 250 to 375 mg P.O., I.M., or I.V. daily in a.m.

Chronic open-angle glaucoma –

Adults: 250 mg to 1 g P.O. daily in divided doses q.i.d., or 500 mg (extended-release) P.O. b.i.d.

Prevention or amelioration of acute mountain sickness –

Adults: 500 mg to 1 g P.O. daily in divided doses q 8 to 12 hours, or 500 mg (extended-release) P.O. b.i.d. Start treatment 24 to 48 hours before ascent, and continue for 48 hours while at high altitude.

Adjunctive treatment of myoclonic, refractory generalized tonic-clonic, absence, or mixed seizures –

Adults and children: 8 to 30 mg/kg P.O. daily in 1 to 4 divided doses. For adults, the optimum dosage range is 375 mg to 1 g daily. Usually given with other anticonvulsants.

ADVERSE REACTIONS

CNS: drowsiness, paresthesia, confusion.

EENT: transient myopia.

GI: nausea, vomiting, anorexia, altered taste.

GU: crystalluria, renal calculi, hematuria.

Hematologic: ***aplastic anemia,*** hemolytic anemia, leukopenia.

Skin: rash.

Other: *pain at injection site,* sterile abscesses, hyperchloremic acidosis, hypokalemia, asymptomatic hyperuricemia.

INTERACTIONS

Amphetamines, anticholinergics, mecamylamine, quinidine: decreased renal clearance of these agents, increasing toxicity. Monitor closely.

Methenamine: reduced effectiveness of acetazolamide. Avoid concomitant use.

CONTRAINDICATIONS

• Contraindicated in long-term therapy for chronic noncongestive acute angle-closure glaucoma; also contraindicated in hyponatremia or hypokalemia, renal or hepatic disease or dysfunction, adrenal gland failure, or hyperchloremic acidosis.

• Use cautiously in patients with respiratory acidosis, emphysema, or chronic pulmonary disease, and in patients receiving other diuretics.

NURSING CONSIDERATIONS

• Monitor fluid intake and output and electrolytes, especially serum potassium, bicarbonate, and chloride. When used in diuretic therapy, consult the doctor and dietitian to provide high-potassium diet.

• Elderly patients are especially susceptible to excessive diuresis.

• Weigh the patient daily. Rapid or excessive fluid loss causes weight loss and hypotension.

• Diuretic effect decreases when acidosis occurs but can be reestablished by withdrawing drug for several days and then restarting, or by using intermittent administration schedules.

• Reconstitute 500-mg vial with at least 5 ml of sterile water for injection. Use within 24 hours of reconstitution.

- I.M. injection is painful because of alkalinity of solution.
- **I.V. use:** Inject 100 to 500 mg/minute into a large vein using a 21G or 23G needle. Intermittent or continuous infusion is not recommended.
- Bicarbonate ion excretion makes the patient's urine alkaline; may cause false-positive urine protein tests.
- If the patient is unable to swallow oral forms, check with a pharmacist. He may make a suspension using crushed acetazolamide tablets in a highly flavored syrup, such as cherry, raspberry, or chocolate. Although concentrations up to 500 mg/5 ml are feasible, concentrations of 250 mg/5 ml are more palatable. Refrigeration improves palatability but doesn't improve stability. Suspensions are stable for 1 week.

amiloride hydrochloride

Kaluril‡, Midamor

Pregnancy Risk Category: B

HOW SUPPLIED

Tablets: 5 mg

ACTION

Mechanism: A potassium-sparing diuretic that inhibits sodium reabsorption and potassium excretion in the distal tubule.

Onset: 2 hours. **Peak:** Peak effects occur in 6 to 10 hours. **Duration:** 24 hours.

INDICATIONS & DOSAGE

Hypertension; edema associated with CHF, usually in patients also taking thiazide or other potassium-wasting diuretics –

Adults: usual dosage is 5 mg P.O. daily. Increase to 10 mg daily, if necessary. Maximum dosage is 20 mg daily.

ADVERSE REACTIONS

CNS: *headache,* weakness, dizziness.
CV: orthostatic hypotension.
GI: *nausea, anorexia, diarrhea, vomiting,* abdominal pain, constipation.
GU: impotence.
Other: hyperkalemia.

INTERACTIONS

ACE inhibitors, potassium-containing salt substitutes, potassium-sparing diuretics, potassium supplements: possible hyperkalemia. Avoid concomitant use.
Lithium: decreased lithium clearance, increasing risk of lithium toxicity. Monitor lithium level.
NSAIDs: decreased diuretic effectiveness. Avoid concomitant use.

CONTRAINDICATIONS

- Contraindicated in patients with elevated serum potassium level (greater than 5.5 mEq/L). Don't administer to patients receiving other potassium-sparing diuretics, such as spironolactone and triamterene.
- Also contraindicated in patients with anuria and acute or chronic renal insufficiency because potassium retention is increased.

NURSING CONSIDERATIONS

- If amiloride is not taken concurrently with a potassium-wasting drug, monitor potassium level daily because of increased risk of hyperkalemia. Discontinue drug immediately if potassium level exceeds 6.5 mEq/L.
- Advise the patient to avoid sudden posture changes and to rise slowly to avoid orthostatic hypotension.
- Warn the patient to avoid excessive ingestion of potassium-rich foods, potassium-containing salt substitutes, or potassium supplements to prevent serious hyperkalemia.
- To prevent nausea, administer amiloride with meals.

bendroflumethiazide (bendrofluazide)

Aprinox‡, Aprinox-M‡, Benzide‡, Naturetin

Pregnancy Risk Category: C

HOW SUPPLIED

Tablets: 2.5 mg, 5 mg, 10 mg

ACTION

Mechanism: A thiazide diuretic that increases sodium and water excretion by inhibiting sodium and chloride reabsorption in the nephron's distal segment.
Onset: 1 to 2 hours. **Peak:** Peak effects occur in 4 hours. **Duration:** 6 to 12 hours.

INDICATIONS & DOSAGE

Edema, hypertension –
Adults: initially, 5 to 20 mg P.O. daily or divided b.i.d. Maintenance dosage is 2.5 to 15 mg P.O. daily.
Children: initially, 0.1 to 0.4 mg/kg (3 to 12 mg/m^2) P.O. daily or divided b.i.d. Maintenance dosage is 0.05 to 0.1 mg/kg (1.5 to 3 mg/m^2) P.O. daily or divided b.i.d.

ADVERSE REACTIONS

CV: volume depletion and dehydration, orthostatic hypotension.
GI: anorexia, nausea, pancreatitis.
GU: nocturia, polyuria, frequent urination.
Hematologic: ***aplastic anemia, agranulocytosis,*** leukopenia, thrombocytopenia.
Hepatic: hepatic encephalopathy.
Skin: dermatitis, photosensitivity, rash.
Other: hypokalemia; asymptomatic hyperuricemia; hyperglycemia and impairment of glucose tolerance; fluid and electrolyte imbalances, including dilutional hyponatremia and hypochloremia, metabolic alkalosis, hypercalcemia; gout; hypersensitivity reactions, such as pneumonitis and vasculitis.

INTERACTIONS

Cholestyramine, colestipol: decreased intestinal absorption of thiazides. Separate doses.
Diazoxide: increased antihypertensive, hyperglycemic, and hyperuricemic effects. Use together cau-
Digitalis gycosides: increased risk of digitalis toxicity from bendroflumethiazide-induced hypokalemia. Monitor potassium and digitalis levels.
Lithium: decreased lithium clearance, increasing risk of lithium toxicity. Monitor lithium level.
NSAIDs: increased risk of NSAID-induced renal failure. Monitor closely.

CONTRAINDICATIONS

- Contraindicated in patients with anuria or hypersensitivity to other thiazides or other sulfonamide-derived drugs.
- Use cautiously in patients with severe renal disease and impaired hepatic function.

NURSING CONSIDERATIONS

- Monitor fluid intake and output, weight, serum electrolyte levels, serum creatinine, and BUN regularly. Drug is not as effective if serum creatinine and BUN are more than twice normal.
- Watch for signs of hypokalemia, such as muscle weakness and cramps. Drug may be used with potassium-sparing diuretic to prevent potassium loss.
- Consult the doctor and dietitian to provide high-potassium diet. Foods rich in potassium include citrus fruits, bananas, tomatoes, dates, and apricots.
- Monitor blood glucose levels, and check insulin requirements in diabetic patients.
- Monitor blood uric acid levels, es-

pecially in patients with a history of gout.
- Elderly patients are especially susceptible to excessive diuresis.
- To prevent nocturia, give in the morning.
- In hypertension, therapeutic response may be delayed several days.
- Thiazides and thiazide-like diuretics should be discontinued before parathyroid function tests are performed.
- Advise the patient to avoid sudden posture changes and to rise slowly to avoid orthostatic hypotension.
- Advise the patient to use a sunblock to prevent photosensitivity reactions.
- May produce false-negative results in phentolamine, phenolsulfonphthalein, and tyramine tests.

benzthiazide

Exna**, Hydrex

Pregnancy Risk Category: D

HOW SUPPLIED

Tablets: 50 mg

ACTION

Mechanism: A thiazide diuretic that increases sodium and water excretion by inhibiting sodium and chloride reabsorption in the nephron's distal segment.
Onset: 2 hours. **Peak:** Peak effects occur in 4 to 6 hours. **Duration:** 12 to 18 hours.

INDICATIONS & DOSAGE

Edema, hypertension –
Adults: 50 to 200 mg P.O. daily or in divided doses.
Children: 1 to 4 mg/kg P.O. daily in three divided doses.

ADVERSE REACTIONS

CV: volume depletion and dehydration, orthostatic hypotension.
GI: anorexia, nausea, pancreatitis.
GU: nocturia, polyuria, frequent urination.
Hematologic: ***aplastic anemia, agranulocytosis,*** leukopenia, thrombocytopenia.
Hepatic: hepatic encephalopathy.
Skin: dermatitis, photosensitivity, rash.
Other: hypokalemia; asymptomatic hyperuricemia; hyperglycemia and impairment of glucose tolerance; fluid and electrolyte imbalances, including dilutional hyponatremia and hypochloremia, metabolic alkalosis, hypercalcemia; gout; hypersensitivity reactions, such as pneumonitis and vasculitis.

INTERACTIONS

Cholestyramine, colestipol: decreased intestinal absorption of thiazides. Separate doses.
Diazoxide: increased antihypertensive, hyperglycemic, and hyperuricemic effects. Use together cautiously.
Digitalis glycosides: increased risk of digitalis toxicity from benzthiazide-induced hypokalemia. Monitor potassium and digitalis levels.
Lithium: decreased lithium clearance, increasing risk of lithium toxicity. Monitor lithium level.
NSAIDs: increased risk of NSAID-induced renal failure. Monitor closely.

CONTRAINDICATIONS

- Contraindicated in patients with anuria or hypersensitivity to other thiazides or other sulfonamide-derived drugs.
- Use cautiously in patients with severe renal disease and impaired hepatic function.

NURSING CONSIDERATIONS

- Monitor fluid intake and output, weight, and serum electrolyte levels regularly. Watch for signs of hypokalemia, such as muscle weakness and cramps. Drug may be used with po-

tassium-sparing diuretic to prevent potassium loss.
- Consult the doctor and dietitian to provide high-potassium diet. Foods rich in potassium include citrus fruits, bananas, tomatoes, dates, and apricots.
- Monitor blood pressure routinely. If possible, teach the patient or family how to check blood pressure.
- Monitor serum creatinine and BUN levels regularly. Drug is not as effective if these levels are more than twice normal.
- Monitor blood glucose levels, and check insulin requirements in diabetic patients.
- Monitor blood uric acid levels, especially in patients with a history of gout.
- To prevent nocturia, give in the morning.
- Elderly patients are especially susceptible to excessive diuresis.
- In patients with hypertension, therapeutic response may be delayed several days.
- Thiazides and thiazide-like diuretics should be discontinued before parathyroid function tests are performed.
- Advise the patient to avoid sudden posture changes and to rise slowly to avoid orthostatic hypotension.
- Advise the patient to use a sunblock to avoid photosensitivity reactions.

bumetanide

Bumex, Burinex‡

Pregnancy Risk Category: C

HOW SUPPLIED

Tablets: 0.5 mg, 1 mg, 2 mg
Injection: 0.25 mg/ml

ACTION

Mechanism: A potent loop diuretic that inhibits sodium and chloride reabsorption at the ascending portion of the loop of Henle.
Onset: 10 minutes after I.V. injection, 40 minutes after I.M. injection, 30 to 60 minutes after oral use. **Peak:** Peak effects occur 15 to 45 minutes after I.V. injection, 1 to 2 hours after oral use. **Duration:** 4 to 6 hours.

INDICATIONS & DOSAGE

Edema in CHF, or hepatic or renal disease –
Adults: 0.5 to 2 mg P.O. once daily. If diuretic response is not adequate, a second or third dose may be given at 4- to 5-hour intervals. Maximum dosage is 10 mg/day. May be administered parenterally if P.O. not feasible. Usual initial dose is 0.5 to 1 mg given I.V. or I.M. If response is not adequate, a second or third dose may be given at 2- to 3-hour intervals. Maximum dosage is 10 mg/day.

ADVERSE REACTIONS

CNS: dizziness, headache.
CV: volume depletion and dehydration, orthostatic hypotension, ECG changes.
EENT: transient deafness.
GI: nausea.
GU: nocturia, polyuria, frequent urination, oliguria.
Hematologic: azotemia.
Skin: rash.
Other: hypokalemia; hypochloremic alkalosis; asymptomatic hyperuricemia; fluid and electrolyte imbalances, including dilutional hyponatremia, hypocalcemia, hypomagnesemia; hyperglycemia and glucose intolerance impairment; muscle pain and tenderness.

INTERACTIONS

Aminoglycoside antibiotics: potentiated ototoxicity. Use together cautiously.
Antihypertensives: increased risk of hypotension. Use together cautiously.
Digitalis glycosides: increased risk of digitalis toxicity from bumetanide-in-

duced hypokalemia. Monitor potassium and digitalis levels.
Indomethacin, NSAIDs, probenicid: inhibited diuretic response. Use together cautiously.
Lithium: decreased lithium clearance, increasing risk of lithium toxicity. Monitor lithium level.
Metolazone: profound diuresis and potential electrolyte loss. Monitor the patient for fluid and electrolyte disorders.
Other potassium-wasting drugs: increased risk of hyperkalemia. Use together cautiously.

CONTRAINDICATIONS
- Contraindicated in patients experiencing anuria, hepatic coma, or in states of severe electrolyte depletion.
- Contraindicated in children and neonates.
- Use cautiously in patients hypersensitive to the drug or to sulfonamides (possible cross-sensitivity).
- Use cautiously in patients with hepatic cirrhosis and ascites. Supplemental potassium or potassium-sparing diuretics may be used to prevent hypokalemia and metabolic alkalosis in these patients. Also use cautiously in patients with depressed renal function.

NURSING CONSIDERATIONS
- Use in children is not FDA-approved; however, dosage of 0.015 mg/kg on alternate days to 0.1 mg/kg daily have been used in children with CHF. Do not use injection in neonates; drug contains benzyl alcohol.
- Bumentanide can lead to profound water and electrolyte depletion. Monitor blood pressure and pulse rate during rapid diuresis.
- If oliguria or azotemia develops or increases, the doctor may stop drug.
- Monitor fluid intake and output, weight, and serum electrolyte, BUN, and carbon dioxide levels frequently.
- Watch for signs of hypokalemia, such as muscle weakness and cramps.
- Consult the doctor and dietitian to provide high-potassium diet. Foods rich in potassium include citrus fruits, tomatoes, bananas, dates, and apricots.
- Monitor blood glucose levels in diabetic patients.
- Monitor blood uric acid levels, especially in patients with a history of gout.
- **I.V. use:** Give I.V. doses directly using a 21G or 23G needle over 1 to 2 minutes. For intermittent infusion, give diluted drug through an intermittent infusion device or piggybank into an I.V. line containing a free-flowing, compatible solution. Infuse at ordered rate. Continuous infusion not recommended.
- Advise patients to stand up slowly to prevent dizziness, and to limit alcohol intake and strenuous exercise in hot weather to avoid exacerbating orthostatic hypotension.
- Bumetanide can be safely used in patients allergic to furosemide; 1 mg of bumetanide equals 40 mg of furosemide. May be less ototoxic than furosemide, but the clinical relevance of this has not been determined.
- To prevent nocturia, give in the morning. If second dose is necessary, give in early afternoon.
- The safest and most effective dosage schedule for control of edema is intermittent dosage given on alternate days, or for 3 to 4 days with 1 or 2 days intervening.

chlorothiazide
Azide‡, Chlotride‡, Diachlor, Diuret‡, Diurigen, Diuril

chlorothiazide sodium
Diuril Sodium

Pregnancy Risk Category: D

HOW SUPPLIED

Tablets: 250 mg, 500 mg
Oral suspension: 250 mg/5 ml
Injection: 500-mg vial

ACTION

Mechanism: A thiazide diuretic that increases sodium and water excretion by inhibiting sodium reabsorption in the nephron's cortical diluting site.
Onset: 2 hours. **Peak:** Peak effects occur in about 4 hours. **Duration:** 6 to 12 hours.

INDICATIONS & DOSAGE

Edema, hypertension –
Adults: 500 mg to 2 g P.O. or I.V. daily or in divided doses.
Diuresis –
Children over 6 months: 10 to 20 mg/kg P.O. daily in divided doses.
Children under 6 months: 10 to 30 mg/kg P.O. daily in two divided doses.

ADVERSE REACTIONS

CV: volume depletion and dehydration, orthostatic hypotension.
GI: anorexia, nausea, pancreatitis.
GU: nocturia, polyuria, frequent urination.
Hematologic: ***aplastic anemia, agranulocytosis,*** leukopenia, thrombocytopenia.
Hepatic: hepatic encephalopathy.
Skin: dermatitis, photosensitivity, rash.
Other: hypersensitivity reactions, such as pneumonitis and vasculitis; hypokalemia; asymptomatic hyperuricemia; hyperglycemia and impairment of glucose tolerance; fluid and electrolyte imbalances, including dilutional hyponatremia and hypochloremia, metabolic alkalosis, hypercalcemia; gout.

INTERACTIONS

Cholestyramine, colestipol: decreased intestinal absorption of thiazides. Separate doses.
Diazoxide: increased antihypertensive, hyperglycemic, and hyperuricemic effects. Use together cautiously.
Digitalis glycosides: increased risk of digitalis toxicity from chlorothiazide-induced hypokalemia. Monitor potassium and digitalis levels.
Lithium: decreased lithium clearance, increasing risk of lithium toxicity. Monitor lithium level.
NSAIDs: increased risk of NSAID-induced renal failure. Monitor the patient for renal failure.

CONTRAINDICATIONS

- Contraindicated in patients with anuria, hypersensitivity to other thiazides or other sulfonamide-derived drugs, impaired hepatic function, or progressive hepatic disease.
- Use cautiously in patients with severe renal disease.

NURSING CONSIDERATIONS

- Monitor fluid intake and output, weight, blood pressure, and serum electrolyte levels.
- Watch for signs of hypokalemia, such as muscle weakness and cramps. Drug may be used with potassium-sparing diuretic to prevent potassium loss.
- Consult the doctor and dietitian to provide high-potassium diet. Foods rich in potassium include citrus fruits, tomatoes, bananas, dates, and apricots.
- Monitor blood glucose levels, and check insulin requirements in diabetic patients.
- Monitor serum creatinine and BUN regularly. Drug not as effective if these levels are more than twice normal.
- Monitor blood uric acid level, especially in patients with a history of gout.
- Monitor serum calcium and watch for progressive renal impairment.

• To prevent nocturia, give in the morning.
• Administering oral form with food may enhance absorption.
• Bioavailability studies show that 250 mg P.O. every 6 hours is better absorbed than a single dose of 1 g. Don't give more than 250 mg P.O. at any one time.
• In patients with hypertension, therapeutic response may be delayed several days.
• Elderly patients are especially susceptible to excessive diuresis.
• Thiazides and thiazide-like diuretics should be discontinued before parathyroid function tests are performed.
• Advise the patient to avoid sudden posture changes and to rise slowly to avoid orthostatic hypotension.
• Advise the patient to use a sunblock to prevent photosensitivity reactions.
• **I.V. use:** Reconstitute 500 mg with 18 ml of sterile water for injection. Inject reconstituted drug directly into vein, through an I.V. line containing a free-flowing, compatible solution, or through an intermittent infusion device. Store reconstituted solutions at room temperature up to 24 hours. Compatible with I.V. dextrose or sodium chloride solutions.
• Never inject I.M. or S.C.
• Avoid I.V. infiltration; can be very painful.
• Avoid simultaneous administration with whole blood and its derivatives.

chlorthalidone

Apo-Chlorthalidone†, Hygroton, Novo-Thalidone†, Thalitone, Uridon†

Pregnancy Risk Category: D

HOW SUPPLIED

Tablets: 25 mg, 50 mg, 100 mg

ACTION

Mechanism: Although not a thiazide, chlorthalidone acts similarly, increasing sodium and water excretion by inhibiting sodium and chloride reabsorption in the nephron's distal segment.
Onset: 2 hours. **Peak:** Peak effects occur in 2 to 6 hours. **Duration:** 2 to 3 days.

INDICATIONS & DOSAGE

Edema, hypertension –
Adults: initially, 50 to 100 mg P.O. daily, or up to 200 mg P.O. on alternate days.
Children: 2 mg/kg or 60 mg/m^2 P.O. 3 times weekly.

ADVERSE REACTIONS

CV: volume depletion and dehydration, orthostatic hypotension.
GI: anorexia, nausea, pancreatitis.
GU: impotence, nocturia, polyuria, frequent urination.
Hematologic: ***aplastic anemia, agranulocytosis,*** leukopenia, thrombocytopenia.
Hepatic: hepatic encephalopathy.
Skin: dermatitis, photosensitivity, rash.
Other: hypersensitivity reactions, such as pneumonitis and vasculitis; hypokalemia; asymptomatic hyperuricemia; hyperglycemia and impairment of glucose tolerance; fluid and electrolyte imbalances, including dilutional hyponatremia and hypochloremia, metabolic alkalosis, hypercalcemia; gout.

INTERACTIONS

Cholestyramine, colestipol: decreased intestinal absorption of thiazides. Separate doses.
Diazoxide: increased antihypertensive, hyperglycemic, and hyperuricemic effects. Use together cautiously.
Digitalis glycosides: increased risk of digitalis toxicity from chlorthalidone-

induced hypokalemia. Monitor potassium and digitalis levels.
Lithium: decreased lithium clearance, increasing risk of lithium toxicity. Monitor lithium level.
NSAIDs: increased risk of NSAID-induced renal failure. Monitor closely.

CONTRAINDICATIONS
- Contraindicated in patients with anuria or hypersensitivity to thiazides or other sulfonamide-derived drugs.
- Use cautiously in patients with severe renal disease, progressive hepatic disease, and impaired hepatic function.

NURSING CONSIDERATIONS
- Monitor fluid intake and output, weight, blood pressure, and serum electrolyte levels.
- Watch for signs of hypokalemia, such as muscle weakness, and cramps. Drug may be used with potassium-sparing diuretic to prevent potassium loss.
- Consult the doctor and dietitian to provide high-potassium diet. Foods rich in potassium include citrus fruits, tomatoes, bananas, dates, and apricots.
- Monitor serum creatinine and BUN levels regularly. Drug is not as effective if these levels are more than twice normal.
- Monitor blood uric acid levels, especially in patients with a history of gout.
- Monitor blood glucose levels, and check insulin requirements in diabetic patients.
- In patients with hypertension, therapeutic response may be delayed several days.
- To prevent nocturia, give in the morning.
- Elderly patients are especially susceptible to excessive diuresis.
- Thiazides and thiazide-like diuretics should be discontinued before parathyroid function tests are performed.
- Advise the patient to avoid sudden posture changes and to rise slowly to avoid orthostatic hypotension.
- Advise the patient to use a sunblock to prevent photosensitivity reactions.
- Do not confuse Uridon tablets (available in Canada only) with the urinary anti-infective Uridon Modified (available in the United States).

dichlorphenamide
Daranide
Pregnancy Risk Category: C

HOW SUPPLIED
Tablets: 50 mg

ACTION
Mechanism: A carbonic anhydrase inhibitor that decreases secretion of aqueous humor, lowering intraocular pressure.
Onset: ½ to 1 hour. **Peak:** Peak effects occur in 2 to 4 hours. **Duration:** 6 to 12 hours.

INDICATIONS & DOSAGE
Adjunct in glaucoma –
Adults: initially, 100 to 200 mg P.O., followed by 100 mg q12 hours until desired response obtained. Maintenance dosage is 25 to 50 mg P.O. daily b.i.d. or t.i.d., given concomitantly with miotics.

ADVERSE REACTIONS
CNS: drowsiness, paresthesia.
EENT: transient myopia.
GI: nausea, vomiting, anorexia, altered taste.
GU: crystalluria, renal calculi.
Hematologic: ***aplastic anemia, hemolytic anemia,*** leukopenia.
Skin: rash.
Other: hyperchloremic acidosis, hypokalemia, asymptomatic hyperuricemia.

INTERACTIONS

Amphetamines, anticholinergics, mecamylamine, quinidine: decreased renal clearance of these agents, increasing toxicity. Avoid concomitant use.
Methenamine: reduced effectiveness of dichlorphenamide. Avoid concomitant use.

CONTRAINDICATIONS

- Contraindicated in patients with hepatic insufficiency, renal failure, adrenocortical insufficiency, hyperchloremic acidosis, depressed sodium or potassium level, severe pulmonary obstruction with inability to increase alveolar ventilation, or Addison's disease. Long-term use contraindicated in patients with severe, absolute, or chronic noncongestive acute angle-closure glaucoma.
- Use cautiously in patients with respiratory acidosis.

NURSING CONSIDERATIONS

- Monitor electrolyte levels, especially serum potassium, in initial treatment; potassium supplements may be necessary.
- In patients with respiratory acidosis, monitor blood pH and blood gases.
- May cause false-positive results in urine protein tests.
- Evaluate patients for eye pain to determine if drug is effective.

---

ethacrynate sodium

Edecrin Sodium

ethacrynic acid

Edecril‡, Edecrin

Pregnancy Risk Category: D

HOW SUPPLIED

Tablets: 25 mg, 50 mg
Injection: 50 mg (with 62.5 mg of mannitol and 0.1 mg of thimerosal)

ACTION

Mechanism: A potent loop diuretic that inhibits sodium and chloride reabsorption at the proximal and distal tubules and the ascending loop of Henle.
Onset: 5 minutes after I.V. use, 30 minutes after oral use. **Peak:** Peak effects occur 15 to 30 minutes after I.V. use, 2 hours after oral use. **Duration:** 2 hours after I.V use, 6 to 8 hours after oral use.

INDICATIONS & DOSAGE

Acute pulmonary edema –
Adults: 50 mg or 0.5 to 1 mg/kg I.V. May be repeated in 2 to 4 hours, then q 4 to 6 hours if the patient responds. May be administered every hour in emergencies.
Edema –
Adults: 50 to 200 mg P.O. daily. Refractory cases may require up to 200 mg b.i.d.
Children: initial dose is 25 mg P.O., increased cautiously in 25-mg increments daily until desired effect is achieved.

ADVERSE REACTIONS

CV: volume depletion and dehydration, orthostatic hypotension.
EENT: transient deafness with too-rapid I.V. injection.
GI: abdominal discomfort and pain, diarrhea.
GU: nocturia, polyuria, frequent urination, oliguria.
Hematologic: ***agranulocytosis,*** neutropenia, thrombocytopenia, azotemia.
Skin: dermatitis.
Other: hypokalemia; hypochloremic alkalosis; asymptomatic hyperuricemia; fluid and electrolyte imbalances, including dilutional hyponatremia, hypocalcemia, hypomagnesemia; hyperglycemia and impairment of glucose tolerance.

INTERACTIONS

Aminoglycoside antibiotics: potentiated ototoxic adverse reactions of both drugs. Use together cautiously.
Antihypertensives: increased risk of hypotension. Use together cautiously.
Cisplatin: increased risk of ototoxicity. Avoid concomitant use.
Digitalis glycosides: increased risk of digitalis toxicity from ethacrynate-induced hypokalemia. Monitor potassium and digitalis levels.
Lithium: decreased lithium clearance, increasing risk of lithium toxicity. Monitor lithium level.
Metolazone: profound diuresis and enhanced electrolyte loss. Use together cautiously.
NSAIDs: decreased diuretic effectiveness. Use together cautiously.
Warfarin: potentiated anticoagulant effect. Use together cautiously.

CONTRAINDICATIONS

- Contraindicated in patients with anuria and in infants.
- Use cautiously in patients with electrolyte abnormalities. If electrolyte imbalance, azotemia, or oliguria develops, may require discontinuing drug.

NURSING CONSIDERATIONS

- Monitor fluid intake and output, weight, blood pressure, and serum electrolyte levels.
- Watch for signs of hypokalemia, such as muscle weakness and cramps.
- Consult the doctor and dietitian to provide high-potassium diet. Foods rich in potassium include citrus fruits, tomatoes, bananas, dates, and apricots. Potassium chloride and sodium supplements may be needed.
- Oral use may cause GI upset. Give with food or milk.
- Elderly patients are especially susceptible to excessive diuresis.
- Advise diabetic patients to closely monitor blood glucose levels.
- To prevent nocturia, give oral doses in the morning.
- Severe diarrhea may necessitate discontinuing drug.
- Monitor blood uric acid levels, especially in patients with a history of gout.
- Advise patients to avoid sudden posture changes and to rise slowly to avoid orthostatic hypotension.
- **I.V. use:** Reconstitute vacuum vial with 50 ml of D_5W or 0.9% sodium chloride solution. Give slowly through tubing of running infusion over several minutes. Discard unused solution after 24 hours. Don't use cloudy or opalescent solutions.
- Don't mix with whole blood or its derivatives.
- Don't give S.C. or I.M.

furosemide (frusemide)

Apo-Furosemide†, Furoside†, Lasix*, Lasix Special†, Myrosemide*, Novosemide†, Urex‡, Urex-M‡, Uritol†

Pregnancy Risk Category: C

HOW SUPPLIED

Tablets: 20 mg, 40 mg, 80 mg, 500 mg†
Oral solution: 8 mg/ml, 10 mg/ml, 50 mg/ml
Injection: 10 mg/ml

ACTION

Mechanism: A potent loop diuretic that inhibits sodium and chloride reabsorption at the proximal portion of the ascending loop of Henle.
Onset: about 5 minutes after I.V. injection, about 60 minutes after oral administration. **Peak:** Peak effect occurs within 30 minutes of I.V. injection, within 1 to 2 hours of oral administration. **Duration:** about 2 hours after I.V. use, 6 to 8 hours after oral administration.

INDICATIONS & DOSAGE

Acute pulmonary edema –
Adults: 40 mg I.V. injected slowly; then 80 mg I.V. in 1 to 1½ hours if needed.
Infants and children: 1 mg/kg I.V. or I.M., increased by 1 mg/kg q 2 hours until desired effect is obtained. The recommended maximum single parenteral dose is 6 mg/kg.
Edema –
Adults: 20 to 80 mg P.O. daily in a.m., second dose in 6 to 8 hours; carefully titrate up to 600 mg daily if needed. Or, 20 to 40 mg I.M. or I.V., increased by 20 mg q 2 hours until desired response is achieved. Give I.V. dose slowly over 1 to 2 minutes.
Infants and children: 1 mg/kg P.O daily, increased by 1 to 2 mg/kg in 6 to 8 hours if needed; carefully titrate up to 6 mg/kg daily if needed.
Hypertension –
Adults: 40 mg P.O. b.i.d. Adjust dosage according to response.
Hypertensive crisis, acute renal failure –
Adults: 100 to 200 mg I.V. over 1 to 2 minutes.
Chronic renal failure –
Adults: initially, 80 mg P.O. daily. Increase by 80 to 120 mg daily until desired response is achieved.
Infants and children: 1 mg/kg I.V. or I.M.; increased by 1 mg/kg q 2 hours until desired effect is obtained. The recommended maximum single parenteral dose is 6 mg/kg.
Hypercalcemia –
Adults: 80 to 100 mg I.V. q 2 hours as needed and tolerated.

ADVERSE REACTIONS

CV: volume depletion and dehydration, orthostatic hypotension.
EENT: transient deafness with too rapid I.V. injection.
GI: abdominal discomfort and pain, diarrhea (with oral solution).
GU: nocturia, polyuria, frequent urination, oliguria.
Hematologic: ***agranulocytosis,*** leukopenia, thrombocytopenia, azotemia.
Skin: dermatitis.
Other: hypokalemia; hypochloremic alkalosis; asymptomatic hyperuricemia; fluid and electrolyte imbalances, including dilutional hyponatremia, hypocalcemia, hypomagnesemia; hyperglycemia and impairment of glucose tolerance.

INTERACTIONS

Aminoglycoside antibiotics, cisplatin: potentiated ototoxicity. Use together cautiously.
Antidiabetic agents: decreased hypoglycemic effects. Monitor blood glucose levels.
Antihypertensives: increased risk of hypotension. Use together cautiously.
Corticosteroids, corticotropin, amphotericin B, metolazone: increased risk of hypokalemia. Monitor potassium levels closely.
Digitalis glycosides, neuromuscular blocking agents: increased toxicity of these agents from furosemide-induced hypokalemia. Monitor potassium levels closely.
Lithium: decreased lithium excretion, resulting in lithium toxicity. Monitor lithium level.
NSAIDs: inhibited diuretic response. Use together cautiously.

CONTRAINDICATIONS

- Contraindicated in patients with anuria or in patients with a history of hypersensitivity to the drug or sulfonamides (possible cross-sensitivity).
- Use cautiously in patients experiencing cardiogenic shock complicated by pulmonary edema, anuria, hepatic coma, or electrolyte imbalances. Drug is not routinely administered to patients of childbearing age because its safety in pregnancy hasn't been established.

NURSING CONSIDERATIONS

- Furosemide can lead to profound water and electrolyte depletion. Monitor weight, blood pressure, and pulse rate routinely with chronic use and during rapid diuresis.
- If oliguria or azotemia develops or increases, may require stopping drug.
- Monitor fluid intake and output, serum electrolytes, BUN, and carbon dioxide frequently.
- Watch for signs of hypokalemia, such as muscle weakness and cramps.
- Consult the doctor and dietitian to provide high-potassium diet. Foods rich in potassium include citrus fruits, tomatoes, bananas, dates, and apricots.
- Monitor blood glucose levels in diabetic patients.
- Monitor blood uric acid, especially in patients with a history of gout.
- To prevent nocturia, give P.O. and I.M. preparations in the morning. Give second doses in early afternoon. Advise patients to take the drug with food to prevent GI upset.
- Elderly patients are especially susceptible to excessive diuresis, with potential for circulatory collapse and thromboembolic complications.
- Store tablets in light-resistant container to prevent discoloration (doesn't affect potency). Don't use discolored (yellow) injectable preparation. Refrigreate oral furosemide solution to ensure drug stability.
- Advise patients to stand slowly to prevent dizziness, and to limit alcohol intake and strenuous exercise in hot weather to avoid exacerbating orthostatic hypotension.
- Advise patients to immediately report ringing in ears, severe abdominal pain, or sore throat and fever; may indicate furosemide toxicity.
- Discourage patients taking furosemide at home from storing different types of medication in the same container, increasing the risk of drug errors. The most popular strengths of furosemide and digoxin are white tablets approximately equal in size.
- Tell patients to check with the doctor or pharmacist before taking any OTC medications.
- **I.V. use:** Given by direct injection over 1 to 2 minutes. Alternatively, dilute with D_5W, 0.9% sodium chloride solution, or lactated Ringer's solution and infuse no faster than 4 mg/minute to avoid ototoxicity. Use prepared infusion solution within 24 hours.
- Don't use parenteral route in infants and children unless oral form is not practical.

hydrochlorothiazide

Apo-Hydro†, Dichlotride‡, Diuchlor H†, Esidrix, Hydro-chlor, Hydro-D, HydroDIURIL, Neo-Codema†, Novo-Hydrazide†, Oretic, Urozide†

Pregnancy Risk Category: D

HOW SUPPLIED

Tablets: 25 mg, 50 mg, 100 mg
Oral solution: 10 mg/ml, 100 mg/ml

ACTION

Mechanism: A thiazide diuretic that increases sodium and water excretion by inhibiting sodium and chloride reabsorption in the nephron's distal segment.
Onset: 2 hours. **Peak:** Peak effects occur within 4 to 6 hours. **Duration:** 6 to 12 hours.

INDICATIONS & DOSAGE

Edema –
Adults: initially, 25 to 200 mg P.O. daily or intermittently. Maintenance dosage is 25 to 100 mg daily or intermittently.
Children over 6 months: 2 to 2.2 mg/kg or 60 mg/m^2 P.O. divided b.i.d. Total daily dosage may range from 37.5 to 100 mg.
Children under 6 months: up to 3.3 mg/kg P.O. daily divided b.i.d. Total

daily dosage may range from 12.5 to 37.5 mg.
Hypertension –
Adults: 25 to 100 mg P.O. daily as a single dose or divided b.i.d. Daily dosage increased or decreased according to blood pressure.

ADVERSE REACTIONS
CV: volume depletion and dehydration, orthostatic hypotension.
GI: anorexia, nausea, pancreatitis.
GU: nocturia, polyuria, frequent urination.
Hematologic: ***aplastic anemia, agranulocytosis,*** leukopenia, thrombocytopenia.
Hepatic: hepatic encephalopathy.
Skin: dermatitis, photosensitivity, rash.
Other: hypersensitivity reactions, such as pneumonitis and vasculitis; hypokalemia; asymptomatic hyperuricemia; hyperglycemia and impairment of glucose tolerance; fluid and electrolyte imbalances, including dilutional hyponatremia and hypochloremia, metabolic alkalosis, hypercalcemia; gout.

INTERACTIONS
Antidiabetic agents: decreased effectiveness of hypoglycemic agents; dosage adjustments may be necessary. Monitor blood glucose levels.
Cholestyramine, colestipol: decreased intestinal absorption of thiazides. Separate doses.
Diazoxide: increased antihypertensive, hyperglycemic, and hyperuricemic effects. Use together cautiously.
Digitalis glycosides: increased risk of digitalis toxicity from hydrochlorothiazide-induced hypokalemia. Monitor potassium and digitalis levels.
Lithium: decreased lithium excretion, increasing risk of lithium toxicity. Monitor lithium level.
NSAIDs: increased risk of NSAID-induced renal failure. Monitor closely.

CONTRAINDICATIONS
- Contraindicated in patients with anuria or hypersensitivity to other thiazides or other sulfonamide derivatives.
- Use cautiously in patients with severe renal disease, impaired hepatic function, and progressive hepatic disease.

NURSING CONSIDERATIONS
- Monitor fluid intake and output, weight, blood pressure, and serum electrolyte levels.
- Watch for signs of hypokalemia, such as muscle weakness and cramps. Drug may be used with potassium-sparing diuretic to prevent potassium loss.
- Consult the doctor and dietitian to provide high-potassium diet. Foods rich in potassium include citrus fruits, tomatoes, bananas, dates, and apricots.
- Monitor serum creatinine and BUN levels regularly. Drug is not as effective if these levels are more than twice normal.
- Monitor blood uric acid levels, especially in patients with a history of gout.
- Check insulin requirements in diabetic patients.
- In patients with hypertension, therapeutic response may be delayed several days.
- Tell the patient to check with the doctor or pharmacist before taking any OTC medications.
- Advise the patient to take the drug with food to minimize GI upset.
- To prevent nocturia, give in the morning.
- Elderly patients are especially susceptible to excessive diuresis.
- Thiazides and thiazide-like diuretics should be discontinued before parathyroid function tests are performed.
- Advise the patient to avoid sudden

*Liquid form contains alcohol.
**May contain tartrazine.

Common reactions are in italics; ***life-threatening,*** in bold italics.

posture changes and to rise slowly to avoid orthostatic hypotension.

• Advise the patient to use a sunsblock to prevent photosensitivity reactions.

hydroflumethiazide

Diucardin, Saluron

Pregnancy Risk Category: B

HOW SUPPLIED

Tablets: 50 mg

ACTION

Mechanism: A thiazide diuretic that increases sodium and water excretion by inhibiting sodium and chloride reabsorption in the nephron's distal segment.

Onset: 1 to 2 hours. **Peak:** Peak effects occur in 3 to 4 hours. **Duration:** 18 to 24 hours.

INDICATIONS & DOSAGE

Edema –

Adults: 25 to 100 mg P.O. daily or b.i.d. Maintenance dosages may be on intermittent or alternate-day schedule.

Children: 1 mg/kg or 30 mg/m^2 P.O. daily.

Hypertension –

Adults: 50 to 100 mg P.O. daily or b.i.d.

ADVERSE REACTIONS

CV: volume depletion and dehydration, orthostatic hypotension.

GI: anorexia, nausea, pancreatitis.

GU: nocturia, polyuria, frequent urination.

Hematologic: ***aplastic anemia, agranulocytosis,*** leukopenia, thrombocytopenia.

Hepatic: hepatic encephalopathy.

Skin: dermatitis, photosensitivity, rash.

Other: hypersensitivity reactions, such as pneumonitis and vasculitis; hypokalemia; asymptomatic hyperuricemia; hyperglycemia and impairment of glucose tolerance; fluid and electrolyte imbalances, including dilutional hyponatremia and hypochloremia, metabolic alkalosis, hypercalcemia; gout.

INTERACTIONS

Cholestyramine, colestipol: decreased intestinal absorption of thiazides. Separate doses.

Diazoxide: increased antihypertensive, hyperglycemic, and hyperuricemic effects. Use together cautiously.

Digitalis glycosides: increased risk of digitalis toxicity from hydroflumethiazide-induced hypokalemia. Monitor potassium and digitalis levels.

Lithium: decreased lithium clearance, increasing risk of lithium toxicity. Monitor lithium level.

NSAIDs: increased risk of NSAID-induced renal failure. Monitor the patient for signs of renal failure.

CONTRAINDICATIONS

• Contraindicated in patients with anuria or hypersensitivity to thiazides or other sulfonamide-derived drugs.

• Use cautiously in patients with severe renal disease, impaired hepatic function, and progressive hepatic disease.

NURSING CONSIDERATIONS

• Monitor fluid intake and output, weight, blood pressure, and serum electrolyte levels.

• Watch for signs of hypokalemia, such as muscle weakness and cramps. Drug may be used with potassium-sparing diuretic to prevent potassium loss.

• Consult the doctor and dietitian to provide high-potassium diet. Foods rich in potassium include citrus fruits, tomatoes, bananas, dates, and apricots.

• To minimize GI upset, give drug with food or milk.

- Monitor serum creatinine and BUN levels regularly. Drug is not as effective if these levels are more than twice normal.
- Monitor blood uric acid levels, especially in patients with a history of gout.
- Check insulin requirements in diabetic patients.
- To prevent nocturia, give in the morning.
- In patients with hypertension, therapeutic response may be delayed several days.
- Elderly patients are especially susceptible to excessive diuresis.
- Thiazides and thiazide-like diuretics should be discontinued before parathyroid function tests are performed.
- Advise the patient to avoid sudden posture changes and to rise slowly to avoid orthostatic hypotension.
- Advise the patient to use a sunblock to prevent photosensitivity reactions.

indapamide

Lozide†, Lozol, Natrilix‡

Pregnancy Risk Category: B

HOW SUPPLIED

Tablets: 1.25 mg, 2.5 mg

ACTION

Mechanism: A thiazide-like diuretic that inhibits sodium reabsorption in the nephron's distal segment. Also has a direct vasodilating effect that may be a result of calcium channel-blocking action.

Onset: 1 to 2 hours. **Peak:** Peak effects occur within 24 hours. **Duration:** up to 36 hours.

INDICATIONS & DOSAGE

Edema, hypertension –

Adults: 1.25 to 2.5 mg P.O. as a single daily dose taken in a.m. Dosage may be increased to 5 mg daily.

ADVERSE REACTIONS

CNS: headache, irritability, nervousness.

CV: volume depletion and dehydration, orthostatic hypotension.

GI: anorexia, nausea, pancreatitis.

GU: nocturia, polyuria, frequent urination.

Skin: dermatitis, photosensitivity, rash.

Other: muscle cramps and spasms; hypokalemia; asymptomatic hyperuricemia; fluid and electrolyte imbalances, including dilutional hyponatremia and hypochloremia, metabolic alkalosis; gout.

INTERACTIONS

Diazoxide: increased antihypertensive, hyperglycemic, and hyperuricemic effects. Use together cautiously.

Digitalis glycosides: increased risk of digitalis toxicity from indapamide-induced hypokalemia. Monitor potassium and digitalis levels.

NSAIDs: increased risk of NSAID-induced renal failure. Monitor the patient for signs of renal failure.

CONTRAINDICATIONS

- Contraindicated in patients with anuria or hypersensitivity to other sulfonamide-derived drugs.
- Use cautiously in patients with severe renal disease, impaired hepatic function, and progressive hepatic disease.

NURSING CONSIDERATIONS

- Monitor fluid intake and output, weight, blood pressure, and serum electrolyte levels.
- Watch for signs of hypokalemia, such as muscle weakness and cramps. Drug may be used with potassium-sparing diuretic to prevent potassium loss.
- Consult the doctor and dietitian to provide high-potassium diet. Foods rich in potassium include citrus fruits,

tomatoes, bananas, dates, and apricots.

- Monitor serum creatinine and BUN levels regularly. Drug is not as effective if these levels are more than twice normal.
- Monitor blood uric acid levels, especially in patients with a history of gout.
- Check insulin requirements in diabetic patients.
- To prevent nocturia, give in the morning.
- In patients with hypertension, therapeutic response may be delayed several days.
- Elderly patients are especially susceptible to excessive diuresis.
- Thiazides and thiazide-like diuretics should be discontinued before parathyroid function tests are performed.
- Advise the patient to avoid sudden posture changes and to rise slowly to avoid orthostatic hypotension.
- Advise the patient to use a sunblock to prevent photosensitivity reactions.

mannitol

Osmitrol†

Pregnancy Risk Category: C

HOW SUPPLIED

Injection: 5%, 10%, 15%, 20%, 25%

ACTION

Mechanism: An osmotic diuretic that increases the osmotic pressure of glomerular filtrate, inhibiting tubular reabsorption of water and electrolytes, and that elevates blood plasma osmolality, resulting in enhanced water flow into extracellular fluid.
Onset: 30 to 60 minutes **Peak:** Peak effects occur within 1 hour. **Duration:** 6 to 8 hours.

INDICATIONS & DOSAGE

Test dose for marked oliguria or suspected inadequate renal function –
Adults and children over 12 years: 200 mg/kg or 12.5 g as a 15% or 20% I.V. solution over 3 to 5 minutes. Response adequate if 30 to 50 ml urine/hour is excreted over 2 to 3 hours; if response is inadequate, give a second test dose. If still no response after the second dose, do not use mannitol.
Oliguria –
Adults and children over 12 years: 50 to 100 g I.V. as a 15% to 20% solution over 90 minutes to several hours.
Prevention of oliguria or acute renal failure –
Adults and children over 12 years: 50 to 100 g I.V. of a concentrated solution (5% to 25%). Exact concentration determined by fluid requirements.
Edema; ascites caused by renal, hepatic, or cardiac failure –
Adults and children over 12 years: 100 g I.V. as a 10% to 20% solution over 2 to 6 hours.
Reduction of intraocular or intracranial pressure –
Adults and children over 12 years: 1.5 to 2 g/kg as a 15% to 25% I.V. solution over 30 to 60 minutes.
Diuresis in drug intoxication –
Adults and children over 12 years: 5% to 10% solution continuously up to 200 g I.V., while maintaining 100 to 500 ml urine output/hour and a positive fluid balance.
Irrigating solution during transurethral resection of the prostate –
Adults: 2.5% to 5% solution as needed.

ADVERSE REACTIONS

CNS: rebound increase in intracranial pressure 8 to 12 hours after diuresis; headache, confusion.
CV: transient expansion of plasma volume during infusion causing circulatory overload and ***pulmonary***

edema, tachycardia, angina-like chest pain.
EENT: blurred vision, rhinitis.
GI: thirst, nausea, vomiting.
GU: urine retention.
Other: fluid and electrolyte imbalance, water intoxication, cellular dehydration.

INTERACTIONS
None significant.

CONTRAINDICATIONS
- Contraindicated in patients with anuria, severe pulmonary congestion, frank pulmonary edema, severe CHF, severe dehydration, metabolic edema, progressive renal disease or dysfunction, or active intracranial bleeding except during craniotomy.

NURSING CONSIDERATIONS
- Monitor vital signs,including central venous pressure, and fluid intake and output hourly. Report increasing oliguria. Monitor weight, renal function, fluid balance, and serum and urine sodium and potassium levels daily.
- To redisolve crystallized solution (occurs at low temperatures or in concentrations greater than 15%), warm bottle in hot water bath and shake vigorously. Cool to body temperature before giving. Do not use solution with undissolved crystals.
- For maximum intraocular pressure reduction before surgery, give 1 to 1½ hours preoperatively.
- Can be used to measure glomerular filtration rate.
- To relieve thirst, give frequent mouth care or fluids as permitted.
- Urethral catheter is inserted in comatose or incontinent patients because therapy is based on strict evaluation of fluid intake and output. In patients with urethral catheters, use an hourly urometer collection bag to facilitate accurate evaluation of output.
- When used as an irrigating solution for prostate surgery, concentrations of 3.5% or greater are needed to avoid hemolysis.
- **I.V. use:** Administer as intermittent or continuous infusion at prescribed rate, using an in-line filter and an infusion pump. Direct injection is not recommended. Check I.V. line patency at infusion site before and during administration.
- Avoid infiltration; if it occurs, observe for inflammation, edema, and necrosis.

---

methazolamide
Neptazane
Pregnancy Risk Category: C

HOW SUPPLIED
Tablets: 25 mg, 50 mg

ACTION
Mechanism: A carbonic anhydrase inhibitor that decreases secretion of aqueous humor, lowering intraocular pressure.
Onset: 2 to 4 hours. **Peak:** Peak effects occur in 6 to 8 hours. **Duration:** 10 to 18 hours.

INDICATIONS & DOSAGE
Glaucoma (chronic open-angle, or preoperatively in obstructive or acute angle-closure) –
Adults: 50 to 100 mg b.i.d. or t.i.d.

ADVERSE REACTIONS
CNS: drowsiness, paresthesia.
EENT: transient myopia.
GI: nausea, vomiting, anorexia.
GU: crystalluria, renal calculi.
Hematologic: ***aplastic anemia, hemolytic anemia,*** leukopenia.
Skin: rash.
Other: hyperchloremic acidosis, hypokalemia, asymptomatic hyperuricemia.

INTERACTIONS
Amphetamines, anticholinergics, mecamylamine, quinidine: decreased renal clearance of these agents, increasing the risk of toxicity. Avoid concomitant use.
Methenamine compounds: reduced methenamine effectiveness. Avoid concomitant use.

CONTRAINDICATIONS
- Contraindicated in patients with severe or absolute glaucoma; for long-term use in chronic noncongestive acute angle-closure glaucoma; in patients with depressed serum sodium or potassium levels, renal or hepatic disease or dysfunction, adrenal gland dysfunction, or hyperchloremic acidosis.
- Use cautiously in patients with respiratory acidosis, emphysema, and chronic pulmonary disease.

NURSING CONSIDERATIONS
- Monitor fluid intake and output, weight, and serum electrolyte levels.
- May cause false-positive urine protein tests by alkalinizing urine.
- Elderly patients are especially susceptible to excessive diuresis.
- Anticipate that drug will be given every day for glaucoma but intermittently for edema. Caution the patient to comply with prescribed dosage to lessen risk of metabolic acidosis. Effects may decrease in acidosis.
- Evaluate the patient for eye pain to ensure drug is effective in decreasing intraocular pressure.

methyclothiazide
Aquatensen, Duretic†, Enduron, Enduron M‡

Pregnancy Risk Category: D

HOW SUPPLIED
Tablets: 2.5 mg, 5 mg

ACTION
Mechanism: A thiazide diuretic that increases sodium and water excretion by inhibiting sodium and chloride reabsorption in the nephron's distal segment.
Onset: 2 hours. **Peak:** Peak effects occur in 4 to 6 hours. **Duration:** 24 or more hours.

INDICATIONS & DOSAGE
Edema, hypertension –
Adults: 2.5 to 10 mg P.O daily.
Children: 0.05 to 2 mg/kg or 1.5 to 6 mg/m² P.O. as a single dose.

ADVERSE REACTIONS
CV: volume depletion and dehydration, orthostatic hypotension.
GI: anorexia, nausea, pancreatitis.
GU: nocturia, polyuria, frequent urination.
Hematologic: ***aplastic anemia, agranulocytosis,*** leukopenia, thrombocytopenia.
Hepatic: hepatic encephalopathy.
Skin: dermatitis, photosensitivity, rash.
Other: asymptomatic hyperuricemia; gout; hyperglycemia and glucose tolerance impairment; fluid and electrolyte imbalances, including hypokalemia, dilutional hyponatremia and hypochloremia, metabolic alkalosis, hypercalcemia; hypersensitivity reactions, such as pneumonitis and vasculitis.

INTERACTIONS
Cholestyramine, colestipol: decreased intestinal absorption of thiazides. Separate doses.
Diazoxide: increased antihypertensive, hyperglycemic, and hyperuricemic effects. Use together cautiously.
Digitalis glycosides: increased risk of digitalis toxicity from methyclothiazide-induced hypokalemia. Monitor potassium and digitalis levels.
Lithium: decreased lithium clearance,

†Available in Canada only. ‡Available in Australia only. ◇Available OTC.

increasing risk of lithium toxicity. Monitor lithium levels.
NSAIDs: increased risk of NSAID-induced renal failure. Monitor closely.

CONTRAINDICATIONS
• Contraindicated in patients with renal decompensation, anuria, or hypersensitivity to other thiazides or other sulfonamide-derived drugs.
• Use cautiously in patients with potassium depletion, renal disease or dysfunction, impaired hepatic function, and progressive hepatic disease.

NURSING CONSIDERATIONS
• Monitor fluid intake and output, weight, blood pressure, and serum electrolyte levels.
• Watch for signs of hypokalemia, such as muscle weakness and cramps. Drug may also be used with potassium-sparing diuretic to prevent potassium loss.
• Consult the doctor and dietitian to provide high-potassium diet. Foods rich in potassium include citrus fruits, tomatoes, bananas, dates, and apricots.
• Monitor blood glucose levels.
• Monitor serum creatinine and BUN levels regularly. Drug is not as effective if these levels are more than twice normal.
• Monitor blood uric acid levels, especially in patients with a history of gout.
• In patients with hypertension, therapeutic response may be delayed several days.
• To prevent nocturia, give in the morning.
• Elderly patients are especially susceptible to excessive diuresis.
• Thiazides and thiazide-like diuretics should be discontinued before parathyroid function tests are performed.
• Advise the patient to avoid sudden posture changes and to rise slowly to avoid orthostatic hypotension.
• Advise the patient to use a sunblock to prevent photosensitivity reactions.

metolazone
Diulo, Mykrox, Zaroxolyn**
Pregnancy Risk Category: D

HOW SUPPLIED
Tablets (extended): 2.5 mg, 5 mg, 10 mg
Tablets (prompt): 0.5 mg

ACTION
Mechanism: Increases sodium and water excretion by inhibiting sodium reabsorption in the cortical diluting site of the ascending loop of Henle.
Onset: 1 hour. **Peak:** Peak effects occur in about 2 hours. **Duration:** 12 to 24 hours.

INDICATIONS & DOSAGE
Edema in CHF –
Adults: 5 to 10 mg (prompt) P.O. daily.
Edema in renal disease –
Adults: 5 to 20 mg (prompt) P.O. daily.
Hypertension –
Adults: 2.5 to 5 mg (prompt) P.O. daily. Maintenance dosage determined by patient's blood pressure. Or 0.5 mg (extended) P.O. once daily in a.m., increased to 1 mg P.O. daily as needed. If response is inadequate, add another antihypertensive agent.

ADVERSE REACTIONS
CNS: dizziness, headache, fatigue.
CV: volume depletion and dehydration, orthostatic hypotension.
GI: anorexia, nausea, pancreatitis.
GU: nocturia, polyuria, frequent urination.
Hematologic: ***aplastic anemia, agranulocytosis,*** leukopenia, thrombocytopenia.
Hepatic: hepatic encephalopathy.
Skin: dermatitis, photosensitivity, rash.

Other: asymptomatic hyperuricemia; hyperglycemia and glucose tolerance impairment; fluid and electrolyte imbalances, including hypokalemia, dilutional hyponatremia and hypochloremia, metabolic alkalosis, hypercalcemia; gout; muscle cramps, swelling; hypersensitivity reactions, such as pneumonitis and vasculitis.

INTERACTIONS

Cholestyramine, colestipol: decreased intestinal absorption of thiazides. Separate doses.
Diazoxide: increased antihypertensive, hyperglycemic, and hyperuricemic effects. Use together cautiously.
Digitalis glycosides: increased risk of digitalis toxicity from metolazone-induced hypokalemia. Monitor potassium and digitalis levels.
Lithium: decreased lithium clearance, increasing risk of lithium toxicity. Monitor lithium level.
NSAIDs: increased risk of NSAID-induced renal failure. Monitor the patient for signs of renal failure.

CONTRAINDICATIONS

- Contraindicated in patients with anuria, hepatic coma or precoma, or hypersensitivity to thiazides or other sulfonamide-derived drugs.
- Use cautiously in patients with hyperuricemia, gout, and impaired renal or hepatic function.

NURSING CONSIDERATIONS

- Mykrox (prompt) tablets are more rapidly and completely absorbed than other brands mimicking an oral solution. Do not interchange Mykrox with Diulo (extended) or Zaroxolyn (extended) tablets.
- Monitor fluid intake and output, weight, blood pressure, and serum electrolyte levels.
- Watch for signs of hypokalemia, such as muscle weakness and cramps. Drug may be used with potassium-sparing diuretic to prevent potassium loss.
- Consult the doctor and dietitian to provide high-potassium diet. Foods rich in potassium include citrus fruits, tomatoes, bananas, dates, and apricots.
- Monitor blood glucose levels.
- Monitor blood uric acid levels, especially in patients with a history of gout.
- In patients with hypertension, therapeutic response may be delayed several days.
- To prevent nocturia, give in the morning.
- Elderly patients are especially susceptible to excessive diuresis.
- Unlike thiazide diuretics, metolazone is effective in patients with decreased renal function.
- Used as an adjunct in furosemide-resistant edema.
- Thiazides and thiazide-like diuretics should be discontinued before parathyroid function tests are performed.
- Advise the patient to avoid sudden posture changes and to rise slowly to avoid orthostatic hypotension.
- Advise the patient to use a sunblock to prevent photosensitivity reactions.

polythiazide

Renese

Pregnancy Risk Category: D

HOW SUPPLIED

Tablets: 1 mg, 2 mg, 4 mg

ACTION

Mechanism: A thiazide diuretic that increases sodium and water excretion by inhibiting sodium and chloride reabsorption in the nephron's distal segment.
Onset: 2 hours. **Peak:** Peak effects occur in about 6 hours. **Duration:** 24 to 48 hours.

INDICATIONS & DOSAGE

Hypertension –

Adults: 2 to 4 mg P.O. daily.

Edema in heart or renal failure –

Adults: 1 to 4 mg P.O. daily.

Children: 0.02 to 0.08 mg/kg P.O. daily.

ADVERSE REACTIONS

CV: volume depletion and dehydration, orthostatic hypotension.

GI: anorexia, nausea, pancreatitis.

GU: nocturia, polyuria, frequent urination.

Hematologic: ***aplastic anemia, agranulocytosis,*** leukopenia, thrombocytopenia.

Hepatic: hepatic encephalopathy.

Skin: dermatitis, photosensitivity, rash.

Other: hypokalemia; asymptomatic hyperuricemia; hyperglycemia and glucose tolerance impairment; fluid and electrolyte imbalances, including dilutional hyponatremia and hypochloremia, metabolic alkalosis, hypercalcemia; gout; hypersensitivity reactions, such as pneumonitis and vasculitis.

INTERACTIONS

Cholestyramine, colestipol: decreased intestinal absorption of thiazides. Separate doses.

Diazoxide: increased antihypertensive, hyperglycemic, and hyperuricemic effects. Use together cautiously.

Digitalis glycosides: increased risk of digitalis toxicity from polythiazide-induced hypokalemia.

Lithium: decreased lithium clearance, increasing risk of toxicity. Monitor lithium levels.

NSAIDs: increased risk of NSAID-induced renal failure. Monitor the patient for signs of renal failure.

CONTRAINDICATIONS

- Contraindicated in patients wtih anuria or hypersensitivity to thiazides or other sulfonamide-derived drugs.
- Use cautiously in patients with severe renal disease, impaired hepatic function, and allergies.

NURSING CONSIDERATIONS

- Monitor fluid intake and output, weight, blood pressure, and serum electrolytes.
- Watch for signs of hypokalemia, such as muscle weakness and cramps. Drug may be used with potassium-sparing diuretic to prevent potassium loss.
- Consult the doctor and dietitian to provide high-potassium diet. Foods rich in potassium include citrus fruits, tomatoes, bananas, dates, and apricots.
- Monitor blood uric acid levels, especially in patients with a history of gout.
- Check insulin requirements in diabetic patients.
- In patients with hypertension, therapeutic response may be delayed several days.
- To prevent nocturia, give in the morning.
- Elderly patients are especially susceptible to excessive diuresis.
- Thiazides and thiazide-like diuretics should be discontinued before tests for parathyroid function tests are performed.
- Advise the patient to avoid sudden posture changes and to rise slowly to avoid orthostatic hypotension.
- Advise the patient to use a sunblock to prevent photosensitivity reactions.

quinethazone

Aquamox‡, Hydromox

Pregnancy Risk Category: D

HOW SUPPLIED

Tablets: 50 mg

ACTION

Mechanism: Although not a thiazide diuretic, quinethazone acts similarly, increasing sodium and water excretion by inhibiting sodium reabsorption in the nephron's cortical diluting site.
Onset: 2 hours. **Peak:** Peak effects occur in 6 hours. **Duration:** 24 hours.

INDICATIONS & DOSAGE

Management of edema or hypertension –
Adults: 50 to 100 mg P.O. daily or 50 mg P.O. b.i.d. Occasionally, up to 150 to 200 mg P.O. daily may be needed.

ADVERSE REACTIONS

CV: volume depletion and dehydration, orthostatic hypotension.
GI: anorexia, nausea, pancreatitis.
GU: nocturia, polyuria, frequent urination.
Hematologic: ***aplastic anemia, agranulocytosis,*** leukopenia, thrombocytopenia.
Hepatic: hepatic encephalopathy.
Skin: dermatitis, photosensitivity, rash.
Other: hypokalemia; asymptomatic hyperuricemia; hyperglycemia and glucose tolerance impairment; fluid and electrolyte imbalances, including dilutional hyponatremia and hypochloremia, metabolic alkalosis, hypercalcemia; gout; hypersensitivity reactions, such as pneumonitis and vasculitis.

INTERACTIONS

Cholestyramine, colestipol: decreased intestinal absorption of thiazides. Separate doses.
Diazoxide: increased antihypertensive, hyperglycemic, and hyperuricemic effects. Use together cautiously.
Digitalis glycosides: increased risk of digitalis toxicity from quinethazone-induced hypokalemia. Monitor potassium and digitalis levels.
Lithium: decreased lithium clearance, increasing risk of lithium toxicity. Monitor lithium level.
NSAIDs: increased risk of NSAID-induced renal failure. Monitor the patient for signs of renal failure.

CONTRAINDICATIONS

- Contraindicated in patients with anuria or hypersensitivity to quinethazones, thiazides, or other sulfonamide-derived drugs.
- Use cautiously in patients with severe renal disease, impaired hepatic function, and allergies.

NURSING CONSIDERATIONS

- Monitor fluid intake and output, weight, blood pressure, and serum electrolytes.
- Watch for signs of hypokalemia, such as muscle weakness and cramps. Drug may be used with potassium-sparing diuretic to prevent potassium loss.
- Consult the doctor and dietitian to provide high-potassium diet. Foods rich in potassium include citrus fruits, tomatoes, bananas, dates, and apricots.
- Monitor serum creatinine, BUN, and blood glucose levels regularly.
- Monitor blood uric acid levels, especially in patients with a history of gout.
- In patients with hypertension, therapeutic response may be delayed several days.
- To prevent nocturia, give in the morning.
- Elderly patients are especially susceptible to excessive diuresis.
- Thiazides and thiazide-like diuretics should be discontinued before parathyroid function tests are performed.
- Advise the patient to avoid sudden posture changes and to rise slowly to avoid orthostatic hypotension.
- Advise the patient to use a sunblock to prevent photosensitivity reactions.

spironolactone

Aldactone, Novospiroton†, Spirotone‡
Pregnancy Risk Category: D

HOW SUPPLIED

Tablets: 25 mg, 50 mg, 100 mg

ACTION

Mechanism: A potassium-sparing diuretic that antagonizes aldosterone in the distal tubule, increasing sodium and water excretion.
Onset: 1 to 2 days. **Peak:** Peak effects occur within 2 to 3 days. **Duration:** 2 to 3 days.

INDICATIONS & DOSAGE

Edema –
Adults: 25 to 200 mg P.O. daily in divided doses.
Children: 3.3 mg/kg P.O. daily in divided doses.
Hypertension –
Adults: 50 to 100 mg P.O. daily in divided doses.
Diuretic-induced hypokalemia –
Adults: 25 to 100 mg P.O. daily when oral potassium supplements are contraindicated.
Detection of primary hyperaldosteronism –
Adults: 400 mg P.O. daily for 4 days (short test) or 3 to 4 weeks (long test). If hypokalemia and hypertension are corrected, a presumptive diagnosis of primary hyperaldosteronism is made.

ADVERSE REACTIONS

CNS: headache.
GI: anorexia, nausea, diarrhea.
Skin: urticaria.
Other: ***hyperkalemia,*** dehydration, hyponatremia, transient elevation in BUN, metabolic acidosis, gynecomastia, breast soreness and menstrual disturbances in women.

INTERACTIONS

ACE inhibitors, potassium-containing salt substitutes, potassium-rich foods, potassium supplements: increased risk of hyperkalemia. Don't use together, especially in patients with renal impairment.
Aspirin: possible blocked spironolactone effect. Watch for diminished spironolactone response.
Digoxin: may alter digoxin clearance, increasing risk of digoxin toxicity. Monitor digoxin levels.

CONTRAINDICATIONS

- Contraindicated in patients with anuria, acute or progressive renal insufficiency, or hyperkalemia.
- Use cautiously in patients with fluid or electrolyte imbalances, impaired renal function, and hepatic disease.

NURSING CONSIDERATIONS

- Less potent than thiazide and loop diuretics; useful as an adjunct to other diuretic therapy. Diuretic effect delayed 2 to 3 days when used alone.
- Monitor serum electrolytes, fluid intake and output, weight, and blood pressure.
- Maximum antihypertensive response may be delayed up to 2 weeks.
- Warn the patient to avoid excessive ingestion of potassium-rich foods, potassium-containing salt substitutes, and potassium supplements to prevent serious hyperkalemia.
- Elderly patients are more susceptible to excessive diuresis.
- Mild acidosis, which may occur during therapy, is dangerous in patients with hepatic cirrhosis.
- Protect drug from light.
- Breast cancer reported in some patients taking spironolactone.
- To enhance absorption, give drug with meals.
- Because of its antiandrogenic properties, 200 mg spironolactone daily has been prescribed to treat hirsutism.
- May interfere with some laboratory

tests that measure digoxin levels. Inform laboratory that the patient is taking spironolactone.

torsemide

Demadex

Pregnancy Risk Category: B

HOW SUPPLIED

Injection: 10 mg/ml
Tablets: 5 mg, 10 mg, 20 mg, 100 mg

ACTION

Mechanism: A loop diuretic that enhances excretion of sodium, chloride, and water by acting on the ascending portion of the loop of Henle.
Onset: within 10 minutes of I.V. use, 1 hour after oral use. **Peak:** Peak effects occur within 1 hour of I.V. use, 1 to 2 hours after oral use. **Duration:** 6 to 8 hours.

INDICATIONS & DOSAGE

Diuresis in patients with CHF –
Adults: initially, 10 to 20 mg P.O. or I.V. once daily. If response is inadequate, double the dose until a response is obtained. Maximum dosage is 200 mg daily.
Diuresis in patients with chronic renal failure –
Adults: initially, 20 mg P.O. or I.V. once daily. If response is inadequate, double the dose until a response is obtained. Maximum dosage is 200 mg daily.
Diuresis in patients with hepatic cirrhosis –
Adults: initially, 5 to 10 mg P.O. or I.V. once daily with an aldosterone antagonist or a potassium-sparing diuretic. If response is inadequate, double the dose until a response is obtained. Maximum dosage is 40 mg daily.
Hypertension –
Adults: initially, 5 mg P.O. daily. Increase to 10 mg if needed and tolerated. If response is still inadequate, add another antihypertensive agent.

ADVERSE REACTIONS

CNS: dizziness, headache, nervousness, insomnia.
CV: ECG abnormalitites, chest pain, edema.
EENT: rhinitis, cough, sore throat.
GI: diarrhea, constipation, nausea, dyspepsia.
GU: *excessive urination.*
Other: asthenia, arthralgia, myalgia.

INTERACTIONS

Cholestyramine: decreased absorption of torsemide. Separate administration times by at least 3 hours.
Digoxin: decreased torsemide clearance. No dosage adjustments are necessary.
Indomethacin: decreased diuretic effectiveness in sodium-restricted patients. Avoid concomitant use.
Lithium, ototoxic drugs such as aminoglycosides or ethacrynic acid: possible increased toxicity of these agents. Avoid concomitant use.
NSAIDs: may potentiate nephrotoxicity of NSAIDs. Use together cautiously.
Probenecid: decreased diuretic effectiveness. Avoid concomitant use.
Salicylates: decreased excretion, possibly leading to salicylate toxicity. Avoid concomitant use.
Spironolactone: decreased renal clearance of spironolactone. No dosage adjustments are necessary.

CONTRAINDICATIONS

- Contraindicated in patients hypersensitive to the drug or other sulfonylurea derivatives.
- Use cautiously in patients with hepatic disease and associated cirrhosis and ascites; sudden changes in fluid and electrolyte balance may precipitate hepatic coma in these patients.

NURSING CONSIDERATIONS

- Drug can cause profound diuresis and water and electrolyte depletion. Monitor fluid intake and output, serum electrolyte levels, blood pressure, weight, and pulse rate during rapid diuresis and routinely with chronic use.
- Watch for signs of hypokalemia, such as muscle weakness and cramps.
- Consult the doctor and dietitian to provide high-potassium diet. Foods rich in potassium include citrus fruits, tomatoes, bananas, dates, and apricots.
- To prevent nocturia, give in the morning.
- Elderly patients are especially susceptible to excessive diuresis, with potential for circulatory collapse and thromboembolic complications.
- Advise the patient to change positions slowly to prevent dizziness, and to limit alcohol intake and strenuous exercise in hot weather to prevent orthostatic hypotension.
- Advise the patient to immediately report ringing in ears. May indicate toxicity.
- Tell the patient to check with the doctor or pharmacist before taking any OTC medications.
- **I.V. use:** May be given by direct injection over at least 2 minutes. Rapid injection may cause ototoxicity. Don't give more than 200 mg at a time.
- Inspect ampules for precipitate or discoloration before use.

triamterene

Dyrenium, Dytac‡

Pregnancy Risk Category: D

HOW SUPPLIED

Tablets†: 50 mg, 100 mg
Capsules: 50 mg, 100 mg

ACTION

Mechanism: A potassium-sparing diuretic that inhibits sodium reabsorption and potassium excretion by direct action on the distal tubule.
Onset: 2 to 4 hours. **Peak:** Peak effects occur after 1 to several days.
Duration: 7 to 9 hours.

INDICATIONS & DOSAGE

Edema –
Adults: initially, 100 mg P.O. b.i.d. after meals. Total dosage should not exceed 300 mg daily.

ADVERSE REACTIONS

CNS: dizziness.
CV: hypotension, dehydration.
EENT: sore throat.
GI: dry mouth, nausea, vomiting.
Hematologic: megaloblastic anemia related to low folic acid levels.
Skin: photosensitivity, rash.
Other: ***anaphylaxis, hyperkalemia,*** muscle cramps, dehydration, hyponatremia, transient elevation in BUN, acidosis.

INTERACTIONS

ACE inhibitors, potassium-containing salt subtitutes, potassium-rich foods, potassium supplements: increased risk of hyperkalemia. Don't use together.
Amantadine: increased risk of amantadine toxicity. Don't use together.
Indomethacin, NSAIDs: may enhance risk of nephrotoxicity. Avoid concomitant use.
Quinidine: may interfere with some laboratory tests that measure quinidine levels. Inform laboratory that patient is taking triamterene.

CONTRAINDICATIONS

- Contraindicated in patients with anuria, severe or progressive renal disease or dysfunction, severe hepatic disease, or hyperkalemia.
- Use cautiously in patients with impaired hepatic function, diabetes mellitus, or during pregnancy or lactation.

NURSING CONSIDERATIONS

- Watch for blood dyscrasia.
- Monitor blood pressure, BUN, and serum electrolyte levels.
- Less potent than thiazides and loop diuretics; useful as an adjunct to other diuretic therapy. Usually used with potassium-wasting diuretics. Full effect delayed 2 to 3 days when used alone.
- Warn patients to avoid excessive ingestion of potassium-rich foods, potassium-containing salt substitutes, and potassium supplements to prevent serious hyperkalemia.
- To prevent nausea, give medication after meals.
- To prevent excessive rebound potassium excretion, withdraw drug gradually.
- Teach the patient to avoid direct sunlight, wear protective clothing, and use a sunblock to prevent photosensitivity reactions.

trichlormethiazide

Metahydrin**, Naqua, Trichlorex

Pregnancy Risk Category: D

HOW SUPPLIED

Tablets: 2 mg, 4 mg

ACTION

Mechanism: A thiazide diuretic that increases sodium and water excretion by inhibiting sodium and chloride reabsorption in the nephron's distal segment.

Onset: 2 hours. **Peak:** Peak effects occur in about 6 hours. **Duration:** 24 hours.

INDICATIONS & DOSAGE

Edema –

Adults: 1 to 4 mg P.O. daily or b.i.d.

Children over 6 months: 0.07 mg/kg (2 mg/m²) P.O. daily or b.i.d.

Hypertension –

Adults: 2 to 4 mg P.O. daily.

Children over 6 months: 0.07 mg/kg (2 mg/m²) P.O. daily or b.i.d.

ADVERSE REACTIONS

CV: volume depletion and dehydration, orthostatic hypotension.

GI: anorexia, nausea, pancreatitis.

GU: nocturia, polyuria, frequent urination.

Hematologic: ***aplastic anemia, agranulocytosis,*** leukopenia, thrombocytopenia.

Hepatic: hepatic encephalopathy.

Skin: dermatitis, photosensitivity, rash.

Other: hypokalemia; asymptomatic hyperuricemia; hyperglycemia and glucose tolerance impairment; fluid and electrolyte imbalances, including dilutional hyponatremia and hypochloremia, metabolic alkalosis, hypercalcemia; gout; hypersensitivity reactions, such as pneumonitis and vasculitis.

INTERACTIONS

Cholestyramine, colestipol: decreased intestinal absorption of thiazides. Separate doses.

Diazoxide: increased antihypertensive, hyperglycemic, and hyperuricemic effects. Use together cautiously.

Digitalis glycosides: increased risk of digitalis toxicity from trichlormethiazide-induced hypokalemia. Monitor potassium and digitalis levels.

Lithium: decreased lithium clearance, increasing risk of lithium toxicity. Monitor lithium level.

NSAIDs: increased risk of NSAID-induced renal failure. Monitor the patient for signs of renal failure.

CONTRAINDICATIONS

- Contraindicated in patients with anuria or hypersensitivity to thiazides or other sulfonamide-derived drugs.
- Use cautiously in patients with severe renal disease and impaired hepatic function.

NURSING CONSIDERATIONS

- Monitor fluid intake and output, weight, blood pressure, and serum electrolyte levels.
- Watch for signs of hypokalemia, such as muscle weakness and cramps. Drug may be used with potassium-sparing diuretic to prevent hypokalemia.
- Consult the doctor and dietitian to provide high-potassium diet. Foods rich in potassium include citrus fruits, tomatoes, bananas, dates, and apricots.
- Monitor serum creatinine, BUN, and blood glucose levels regularly. Drug is not as effective if these levels are more than twice normal.
- Monitor blood glucose levels and check insulin requirements in patients with diabetes. Treat severe hyperglycemia with oral antidiabetics.
- Monitor blood uric acid levels, especially in patients with a history of gout.
- In patients with hypertension, therapeutic response may be delayed several days.
- To prevent nocturia, give in the morning.
- Elderly patients are especially susceptible to excessive diuresis.
- Thiazides and thiazide-like diuretics should be discontinued before parathyroid function tests are performed.
- Advise the patient to avoid sudden posture changes and to rise slowly to avoid orthostatic hypotension.
- Advise the patient to use a sunblock to prevent photosensitivity reactions.

urea (carbamide)

Ureaphil

Pregnancy Risk Category: C

HOW SUPPLIED

Injection: 40 g/150 ml

ACTION

Mechanism: An osmotic diuretic that increases the osmotic pressure of glomerular filtrate, inhibiting tubular reabsorption of water and electrolytes. Also elevates blood plasma osmolality, resulting in enhanced water flow into extracellular fluid.

Onset: 10 minutes. **Peak:** Peak effects occur in 1 to 2 hours. **Duration:** diuresis and decreased CSF pressure last for 3 to 10 hours; decreased intraocular pressure lasts 5 to 6 hours.

INDICATIONS & DOSAGE

Elevated intracranial or intraocular pressure –

Adults: 1 to 1.5 g/kg as a 30% solution by slow I.V. infusion over 1 to 2.5 hours. Maximum dosage is 120 g daily.

Children over 2 years: 0.5 to 1.5 g/kg slow I.V. infusion.

Children under 2 years: as little as 0.1 g/kg slow I.V. infusion.

ADVERSE REACTIONS

CNS: *headache.*

CV: tachycardia, ***CHF.***

GI: *nausea, vomiting.*

Respiratory: *pulmonary edema*

Other: sodium and potassium depletion; irritation or necrotic sloughing with extravasation.

INTERACTIONS

Lithium: increased lithium clearance and decreased lithium effectiveness. Monitor lithium level.

CONTRAINDICATIONS

- Contraindicated in patients with severely impaired renal function, marked dehydration, frank hepatic failure, or active intracranial bleeding.
- Use cautiously in patients with cardiac disease, hepatic impairment, and sickle-cell disease with CNS involvement, and during pregnancy and lactation.

NURSING CONSIDERATIONS

- Watch for signs of hyponatremia (nausea, vomiting, tachycardia) or hypokalemia (muscle weakness, lethargy); may indicate electrolyte depletion before serum levels are reduced.
- Maintain adequate hydration; monitor blood pressure, fluid intake and output, and serum electrolyte levels.
- In patients with renal disease, monitor BUN level.
- To ensure bladder emptying in comatose patients, use an indwelling urinary catheter, and use an hourly urometer collection bag for accurate evaluation of diuresis.
- If satisfactory diuresis does not occur in 6 to 12 hours, urea should be discontinued and renal function reevaluated.
- Assess breath sounds for crackles, indicating pulmonary edema.
- **I.V. use:** Avoid rapid I.V. infusion; may cause hemolysis or increased capillary bleeding. Maximum infusion rate is 4 ml/minute. Avoid extravasation; may cause reactions ranging from mild irritation to necrosis.
- To prepare 135 ml of 30% solution, mix contents of 40-g vial of urea with 105 ml of D_5W or dextrose 10% in water or 10% invert sugar in water. Each ml of 30% solution provides 300 mg urea.
- Don't give through the same infusion set as blood or blood derivatives.
- Use freshly reconstituted urea only for I.V. infusion; solution becomes ammonia upon standing. Use within minutes of reconstitution and discard within 24 hours.
- Don't infuse into leg veins; may cause phlebitis or thrombosis, especially in elderly patients.

62

Electrolytes and replacement solutions

calcium acetate
calcium carbonate
calcium chloride
calcium citrate
calcium glubionate
calcium gluceptate
calcium gluconate
calcium lactate
calcium phosphate, dibasic
calcium phosphate, tribasic
dextran, low molecular weight
dextran, high molecular weight
hetastarch
magnesium chloride
magnesium sulfate
potassium acetate
potassium bicarbonate
potassium chloride
potassium gluconate
Ringer's injection
Ringer's injection, lactated
sodium chloride

COMBINATION PRODUCTS

KLORVESS*: 20 mEq each potassium and chloride (from potassium chloride, potassium bicarbonate, and l-lysine monohydrochloride).
K-LYTE-CL: 25 mEq potassium, 25 mEq chloride (from potassium chloride, potassium bicarbonate, and lysine hydrochloride).
NEUTRA-PHOS: phosphorus 250 mg, sodium 164 mg, potassium 278 mg (from dibasic and monobasic sodium and potassium phosphate).
TWIN-K: 15 ml supplies 20 mEq of potassium ions as a combination of potassium gluconate and potassium citrate.

calcium acetate
Phos-Ex◊, Phos-Lo

calcium carbonate
Apo-Cal†◊, BioCal◊, Calcarb 600◊, Calci-Chew◊, Calciday 667◊, Calcilac◊, Calcite 500†◊, Calcium 500†◊, Calcium 600◊, Calglycine◊, Calsan†◊, Caltrate 300†◊, Caltrate 600†◊, Caltrate Chewable†◊, Chooz◊, Dicarbosil◊, Gencalc◊, Mega-Cal†◊, Mellamint◊, Nephro-Calci◊, Nu-Cal†◊, Os-Cal†◊, Os-Cal 500◊, Os-Cal Chewable†◊, Oysco◊, Oysco 500 Chewable◊, Oyst-Cal 500◊, Oyst-Cal 500 Chewable◊, Oystercal 500◊, Rolaids Calcium Rich◊, Super Calcium 1200◊, Titralac◊, Tums◊, Tums E-X◊

calcium chloride◊
Calciject†

calcium citrate◊
Citrical◊, Citrical Liquitabs†◊

calcium glubionate◊
Calcium-Sandoz†, Neo-Calglucon

calcium gluceptate◊

calcium gluconate
Kalcinate

calcium lactate◊

calcium phosphate, dibasic◊

calcium phosphate, tribasic
Posture◊

Pregnancy Risk Category: C

HOW SUPPLIED

acetate
Contains 253 mg or 12.7 mEq of elemental calcium/g

*Liquid form contains alcohol.
**May contain tartrazine.

Common reactions are in italics; ***life-threatening,*** in bold italics.

Tablets: 250 mg◊, 500 mg◊, 667 mg, 668 mg◊, 1,000 mg◊
Injection: 0.5 mEq Ca^{++} per ml
carbonate
Contains 400 mg or 20 mEq of elemental calcium/g
Tablets: 650 mg◊, 667 mg◊, 750 mg◊, 1.25 g◊, 1.5 g◊
Tablets (chewable): 350 mg◊, 420 mg◊, 500 mg◊, 625 mg◊, 750 mg◊, 850 mg◊, 1.25 g◊
Capsules: 1.512 g◊
Oral suspension: 1.25 g/5 ml◊
Squares (chewable): 1.5 g◊
Powder packets: 6.5 g (2,400 mg calcium) per packet◊
chloride
Contains 270 mg or 13.5 mEq of elemental calcium/g
Injection: 10% solution in 10-ml ampules, vials, and syringes
citrate
Contains 211 mg or 10.6 mEq of elemental calcium/g
Tablets: 950 mg◊
glubionate
Contains 64 mg or 3.2 mEq elemental calcium/g
Syrup: 1.8 g/5 ml
gluceptate
Contains 82 mg or 4.1 mEq elemental calcium/g
Injection: 1.1 g/5 ml in 5-ml ampules or 50-ml vials
gluconate
Contains 90 mg or 4.5 mEq of elemental calcium/g
Tablets: 500 mg◊, 650 mg◊, 975 mg◊, 1 g◊
Injection: 10% solution in 10-ml ampules and vials, 10-ml or 20-ml vials
lactate
Contains 130 mg or 6.5 mEq of elemental calcium/g
Tablets: 325 mg, 650 mg
phosphate, dibasic
Contains 230 mg or 11.5 mEq of elemental calcium/g
Tablets: 468 mg◊
phosphate, tribasic
Contains 400 mg or 20 mEq of elemental calcium/g
Tablets: 300 mg◊, 600 mg◊

ACTION

Mechanism: Replaces and maintains calcium.
Peak: Serum levels peak immediately after I.V. injection, and return to normal within ½ to 2 hours.

INDICATIONS & DOSAGE

Hypocalcemic emergency –
Adults: 7 to 10 mEq calcium I.V. May be given as a 10% calcium gluconate solution, 2 to 10% calcium chloride solution, or a 22% calcium gluceptate solution.
Children: 1 to 7 mEq calcium I.V.
Infants: up to 1 mEq calcium I.V.
Hypocalcemic tetany –
Adults: 4.5 to 16 mEq calcium I.V. Repeat until tetany is controlled.
Children: 0.5 to 0.7 mEq calcium I.V. 3 to 4 times a day until tetany is controlled.
Neonates: 2.4 mEq I.V. daily in divided doses.
Adjunctive treatment of cardiac arrest –
Adults: 2.7 mEq calcium chloride I.V., 4.5 to 6.3 mEq calcium gluceptate I.V., or 2.3 to 3.7 mEq calcium gluconate I.V.
Children: 0.27 mEq/kg calcium chloride I.V. Repeat in 10 minutes if necessary; determine serum calcium levels before administering further doses.
Adjunctive treatment of magnesium intoxication –
Adults: initially, 7 mEq I.V. Subsequent doses must be based upon the patient's response.
During exchange transfusions –
Adults: 1.35 mEq concurrently with each 100 ml citrated blood.
Neonates: 0.45 mEq after each 100 ml citrated blood.
Hyperphosphatemia –
Adults: 1,334 to 2,000 mg P.O. cal-

cium acetate t.i.d. with meals. Most dialysis patients will require 3 to 4 tablets with each meal.
Calcium supplementation during total parenteral nutrition –
Adults: 10 to 15 mEq calcium chloride I.V. daily.
Children: 5 to 20 mEq calcium chloride I.V. daily.
Neonates: 0.5 to 3 mEq/kg calcium chloride I.V. daily.

ADVERSE REACTIONS
CNS: with I.V. use, tingling sensations, sense of oppression or heat waves; with rapid I.V. injection, syncope.
CV: mild fall in blood pressure; with rapid I.V. injection, vasodilation, bradycardia, ***arrhythmias, cardiac arrest.***
GI: with oral use, irritation, hemorrhage, *constipation;* with I.V. use, chalky taste; with oral calcium chloride, hemorrhage, nausea, vomiting, thirst, abdominal pain.
GU: hypercalcemia, polyuria, renal calculi.
Skin: with I.M. use, local reactions including burning, necrosis, tissue sloughing, cellulitis, soft tissue calcification.
Other: with S.C. injection, pain and irritation; with I.V. use, *vein irritation.*

INTERACTIONS
Atenolol, tetracyclines, fluoroquinolones: decreased bioavailability of these agents and calcium when oral preparations are taken together. Separate administration times.
Calcium channel blockers: decreased calcium effectiveness. Avoid concomitant use.
Digitalis glycosides: increased digitalis toxicity; administer calcium cautiously (if at all) to digitalized patients.
Sodium polystyrene sulfonate: risk of metabolic acidosis in patients with renal disease. Avoid concomitant use.
Thiazide diuretics: risk of hypercalcemia. Avoid concomitant use.
Foods containing oxalic acid (found in rhubarb and spinach), phytic acid (bran and whole cereals), and phosphorus (milk and dairy products): may interfere with calcium absorption.

CONTRAINDICATIONS
- Contraindicated in patients with ventricular fibrillation, hypercalcemia, or renal calculi.
- Use all calcium products cautiously in patients with sarcoidosis and renal or cardiac disease, and in digitalized patients. Use calcium chloride cautiously in patients with cor pulmonale, respiratory acidosis, and respiratory failure.

NURSING CONSIDERATIONS
- Monitor blood calcium levels frequently. Hypercalcemia may result after large doses in chronic renal failure. Report abnormalities.
- Warm solutions to body temperature before administration.
- Severe necrosis and tissue sloughing follow extravasation. Calcium gluconate is less irritating to veins and tissues than calcium chloride.
- If GI upset occurs, give oral calcium products 1 to 1½ hours after meals.
- **I.V. use (direct injection):** Administer slowly through a small needle into a large vein or through an I.V. line containing a free-flowing, compatible solution at a rate not exceeding 1 ml/minute (1.5 mEq/minute) for calcium chloride, 1.5 to 5 ml/minute for calcium gluconate, and 2 ml/minute for calcium gluceptate. Do not use scalp veins in children.
- **I.V. use (intermittent infusion):** Infuse diluted solution through an I.V. line containing a compatible solution. Maximum rate of 200 mg/minute sug-

gested for calcium gluceptate and calcium gluconate.

• Monitor ECG when giving calcium I.V. Stop if the patient complains of discomfort. Following I.V. injection, the patient should remain recumbent for 15 minutes.

• Give calcium chloride I.V. only. When adding to parenteral solutions that contain other additives (especially phosphorus or phosphate), observe closely for precipitate. Use an in-line filter.

• Give I.M. injection in the gluteal region in adults; lateral thigh in infants. I.M. route used only in emergencies when no I.V. route available.

• Crash carts usually contain both calcium gluconate and calcium chloride. Ensure that the doctor specifies form he wants administered.

dextran, low molecular weight (dextran 40)

Gentran 40, Rheomacrodex LMD, 10% LMD, Dextran 40

Pregnancy Risk Category: C

HOW SUPPLIED

Injection: 10% dextran in D_5W or 0.9% sodium chloride solution

ACTION

Mechanism: Expands plasma volume via colloidal osmotic effect, drawing fluid from insterstitial to intravascular space, providing fluid replacement.

Peak: Serum levels peak immediately after an I.V. infusion.

INDICATIONS & DOSAGE

Plasma volume expansion –

Adults: dosage by I.V. infusion depends on amount of fluid loss. Infuse first 500 ml of dextran rapidly with central venous pressure monitoring, remaining dose slowly. Total dosage not to exceed 2 g/kg body weight daily. If therapy continued past 24 hours, do not exceed 1 g/kg daily. Continue for no longer than 5 days.

Reduction of blood sludging –

Adults: 500 ml by I.V. infusion.

Prophylaxis of venous thrombosis –

Adults: 10 ml/kg (500 to 1,000 ml) I.V. on the day of the procedure; 500 ml on days 2 and 3.

ADVERSE REACTIONS

GI: nausea, vomiting.

GU: tubular stasis and blocking, increased urine viscosity.

Hematologic: *decreased hemoglobin and hematocrit levels;* with higher doses, increased bleeding time.

Hepatic: increased AST and ALT levels.

Skin: hypersensitivity reactions, urticaria.

Other: ***anaphylaxis.***

INTERACTIONS

None significant.

CONTRAINDICATIONS

• Contraindicated in patients with marked hemostatic defects; marked cardiac decompensation, heart failure, or pulmonary edema; renal disease with severe oliguria or anuria; or extreme dehydration.

• Use cautiously in patients with active hemorrhage; may cause additional blood loss. Evaluate the patient's hydration status before administration.

NURSING CONSIDERATIONS

• The doctor may order dextran 1 to protect against dextran-induced anaphylaxis. Administer 20 ml of dextran (containing 150 mg/ml) I.V. over 60 seconds, 1 to 2 minutes before the I.V. infusion of dextran.

• **I.V. use:** Observe the patient closely during early phase of infusion, when most anaphylactic reactions occur.

• Hazardous for patients with heart failure, especially when given in

0.9% sodium chloride solution. Use dextrose in water solution instead.

- Provides plasma expansion slightly greater than volume infused. Watch for circulatory overload and a rise in central venous pressure.
- Monitor urine flow rate during administration. If oliguria or anuria occurs or is not relieved by infusion, stop dextran and give loop diuretic as ordered.
- Assess hydration before starting therapy; otherwise, use urine or serum osmolarity because urine specific gravity is affected by urine dextran concentration.
- Check hemoglobin and hematocrit levels; if values fall below 30% by volume, notify the doctor.
- May interfere with analyses of blood grouping, crossmatching, bilirubin, blood glucose, and protein.
- Store at constant 77° F (25° C). May precipitate in storage, but can be heated to dissolve if necessary.

dextran, high molecular weight (dextran 70, dextran 75)

Dextran 75, Gentran 75, Macrodex

Pregnancy Risk Category: C

HOW SUPPLIED

Injection: 6% dextran 70 in 0.9% sodium chloride solution or dextrose 5%; 6% dextran 75 in 0.9% sodium chloride solution or dextrose 5%

ACTION

Mechanism: Expands plasma volume via colloidal osmotic effect, drawing fluid from interstitial to intravascular space, providing fluid replacement.

Peak: Serum levels peak immediately after I.V. infusion.

INDICATIONS & DOSAGE

Plasma expander–

Adults: 30 g (500 ml of 6% solution) I.V. In emergencies, may be administered at rate of 1.2 to 2.4 g (20 to 40 ml) per minute. In normovolemic or nearly normovolemic patients, rate of infusion should not exceed 240 mg (4 ml)/minute.

Total dosage during first 24 hours not to exceed 1.2 g/kg; actual dosage depends on amount of fluid loss and resultant hemoconcentration, and must be determined for each patient.

ADVERSE REACTIONS

GI: nausea, vomiting.

GU: increased specific gravity and viscosity of urine, tubular stasis and blocking. oliguria, anuria.

Hematologic: *decreased level of hemoglobin and hematocrit;* with doses of 15 ml/kg body weight, prolonged bleeding time and significant suppression of platelet function.

Hepatic: increased AST and ALT levels.

Skin: hypersensitivity reactions, urticaria.

Other: fever, arthralgia, nasal congestion, ***anaphylaxis***.

INTERACTIONS

None significant.

CONTRAINDICATIONS

- Contraindicated in patients with marked hemostatic defects; marked cardiac decompensation, heart failure, or pulmonary edema; renal disease with severe oliguria or anuria; or extreme dehydration.
- Use cautiously in patients with active hemorrhage; may cause additional blood loss.

NURSING CONSIDERATIONS

- Doctor may order dextran 1 to protect against dextran-induced anaphylaxis. Administer 20 ml of dextran 1 (containing 150 mg/ml) I.V. over 60 seconds, 1 to 2 minutes before the I.V. infusion of dextran 70.
- **I.V. use:** Observe the patient closely

during early phase of infusion, when most anaphylactic reactions occur.

- Hazardous for patients with heart failure, especially if given in 0.9% sodium chloride solution. Use D_5W solution instead.
- Provides plasma expansion slightly greater than volume infused. Watch for circulatory overload.
- Monitor urine flow rate during administration. If oliguria or anuria occurs or is not relieved by infusion, stop dextran and give loop diuretic.
- Assess hydration before starting therapy; otherwise, use urine or serum osmolarity because urine specific gravity is affected by the urine dextran concentration.
- Monitor hemoglobin and hematocrit levels; if values fall below 30% by volume, notify the doctor.
- Have blood samples drawn *before* starting infusion.
- May interfere with analyses of blood grouping, crossmatching, bilirubin, blood glucose, and protein.
- May precipitate in storage, but can be heated to dissolve if necessary.

hetastarch

Hespan

Pregnancy Risk Category: C

HOW SUPPLIED

Injection: 500 ml (6 g/100 ml in 0.9% sodium chloride solution)

ACTION

Mechanism: Expands plasma volume and provides fluid replacement.
Peak: Serum levels peak immediately after I.V. infusion.

INDICATIONS & DOSAGE

Plasma expander –
Adults: 500 to 1,000 ml I.V., depending on amount of blood lost and resultant hemoconcentration. Total dosage usually not to exceed 1,500 ml/day. Up to 20 ml/kg hourly may be used in hemorrhagic shock.

ADVERSE REACTIONS

CNS: headaches.
CV: peripheral edema of lower extremities.
EENT: periorbital edema.
GI: nausea, vomiting.
Skin: urticaria.
Other: wheezing, mild fever.

INTERACTIONS

None significant.

CONTRAINDICATIONS

- Contraindicated in patients with severe bleeding disorders, severe CHF, or renal failure with oliguria and anuria.

NURSING CONSIDERATIONS

- To avoid circulatory overload, monitor patients with impaired renal function carefully.
- Discontinue if allergic or sensitivity reactions occur. If necessary, administer an antihistamine as ordered.
- When used in continuous-flow centrifugation, leukapheresis ratio is usually 1 part hetastarch to 8 parts venous whole blood.
- Hetastarch is *not* a substitute for blood or plasma.
- Discard partially used bottles.

magnesium chloride

Slow-Mag◇

magnesium sulfate

Pregnancy Risk Category: B

HOW SUPPLIED

chloride
Tablets (delayed-release): 64 mg
sulfate
Injectable solutions: 10%, 12.5%, 25%, 50% in 2-ml, 5-ml, 10-ml, 20-ml, and 30-ml ampules, vials, and prefilled syringes

ACTION

Mechanism: Replaces and maintains magnesium levels; as an anticonvulsant, reduces muscle contractions by interfering with release of acetylcholine at myoneural junction.

Peak: Serum levels peak within 4 hours of oral dose. **Duration:** 4 to 6 hours.

INDICATIONS & DOSAGE

Hypomagnesemia –

Adults: 1 g, or 8.12 mEq, of 50% solution (2 ml) I.M. every 6 hours for 4 doses, depending on serum magnesium level.

Severe hypomagnesemia (serum magnesium 0.8 mEq/L or less, with symptoms) –

Adults: 6 g, or 50 mEq, of 50% solution I.V. in 1 liter of solution over 4 hours.

Subsequent doses depend on serum magnesium levels.

Magnesium supplementation –

Adults: 64 mg (1 tablet) P.O. t.i.d.

Magnesium supplementation in total parenteral nutrition (TPN) –

Adults: 8 to 24 mEq I.V. daily added to TPN solution.

Children over 6 years: 2 to 10 mEq I.V. daily added to TPN solution.

Each 2 ml of 50% solution contains 1 g, or 8.12 mEq, magnesium sulfate.

Acute treatment of preeclampsia and eclampsia –

Adults: loading dose: 2 to 4 g (4 to 8 ml of 50% solution) given by slow I.V. bolus (over 5 minutes). Maintenance dosage is 1 to 2 g hourly by constant infusion. Prepare by adding 8 ml of 50% solution to 250 ml D_5W.

Hypomagnesemic seizures –

Adults: 1 to 2 g of 10% solution I.V. over 15 minutes, then 1 g I.M. q 4 to 6 hours, based on the patient's response and magnesium blood level.

Seizures secondary to hypomagnesemia in acute nephritis –

Adults: 0.2 ml/kg of 50% solution I.M. q 4 to 6 hours, p.r.n. or 100 mg/kg of 10% solution I.V. very slowly. Titrate dosage according to magnesium blood level and seizure response.

Paroxysmal atrial tachycardia unresponsive to other treatments –

Adults: 3 to 4 g I.V. of 10% solution over 30 seconds, with close monitoring of ECG.

ADVERSE REACTIONS

CNS: toxicity – *weak or absent deep tendon reflexes,* flaccid paralysis, hypothermia, drowsiness, hypocalcemia (perioral paresthesia, twitching carpopedal spasm, tetany, and seizures).

CV: slow, weak pulse; arrhythmias (caused by hypocalcemia); *hypotension.*

Respiratory: *respiratory paraylsis*

Skin: flushing, diaphoresis.

Other: hypocalcemia.

INTERACTIONS

Neuromuscular blocking agents: possible increased neuromuscular blockage. Use cautiously.

Nitrofurantoin, tetracyclines, penicillamine: decreased bioavailability with oral magnesium supplements. Separate administration times by 2 to 3 hours.

CONTRAINDICATIONS

- Contraindicated in patients with impaired renal function, myocardial damage, or heart block, and in actively progressing labor.
- Use parenteral magnesium with extreme caution in patients receiving digitalis glycosides. Treating magnesium toxicity with calcium in such patients could cause serious alterations in cardiac conduction; heart block may result.

NURSING CONSIDERATIONS

- Monitor fluid intake and output. Output should be 100 ml or more during 4-hour period before dose.
- Keep I.V. calcium available to reverse magnesium intoxication.

- Test knee-jerk and patellar reflexes before each additional dose. If absent, give no more magnesium until reflexes return; otherwise, the patient may develop temporary respiratory failure and need cardiopulmonary resuscitation or I.V. administration of calcium.
- Check magnesium level after repeated doses.
- After giving to toxemic patients within 24 hours before delivery, watch neonate for signs of magnesium toxicity, including neuromuscular and respiratory depression.
- **I.V. use:** Inject I.V. bolus dose slowly, using infusion pump for contineous infusion if available, to avoid respiratory or cardiac arrest. Maximum infusion rate is 150 mg/minute. Rapid drip causes feeling of heat.
- When giving I.V. for severe hypomagnesemia, watch for respiratory depression and signs of heart block. Respirations should be more than 16/minute before dose is given.
- Undiluted 50% solutions may be given by deep I.M. injection to adults. Dilute solutions to 20% or less for use in children.
- Magnesium sulfate may form a precipitate when mixed with solutions containing ethanol, arsenates, barium, calcium, clindamycin, heavy metals, hydrocortisone sodium succinate, phosphates, polymyxin B sulfate, procaine, salicylates, or tartrates. Drug is also incompatible with alkalis, including carbonates and bicarbonates.

potassium acetate

Pregnancy Risk Category: C

HOW SUPPLIED
Injection: 2 mEq/ml in 20-ml, 30-ml vials.

ACTION
Mechanism: Replaces and maintains potassium level.
Peak: Serum levels peak immediately after I.V. infusion.

INDICATIONS & DOSAGE
Treatment of hypokalemia –
Adults: No more than 20 mEq hourly in concentration of 40 mEq/L or less. Total 24-hour dosage should not exceed 150 mEq (3 mEq/kg in children). Potassium replacement should be done with ECG monitoring and frequent serum potassium determinations. I.V. should be used only for life-threatening hypokalemia or when oral replacement not feasible.
Prevention of hypokalemia –
Adults: dosage is individualized to the patient's needs, not to exceed 150 mEq/day. Administer as an additive to I.V. infusions. Usual dose is 40 mEq/L infused at a rate not to exceed 20 mEq/hour.
Children: individualized dosage not to exceed 3 mEq/kg/day. Administer as an additive to I.V. infusions.

ADVERSE REACTIONS
Signs of hyperkalemia:
CNS: paresthesia of the extremities, listlessness, mental confusion, weakness or heaviness of legs, flaccid paralysis.
CV: ***peripheral vascular collapse with fall in blood pressure, arrhythmias,*** heart block, possible cardiac arrest, ECG changes (prolonged PR intervals; widened QRS complex; ST-segment depression; tall, tented T waves).
GI: nausea, vomiting, abdominal pain, diarrhea, bowel ulceration.
GU: oliguria.
Skin: cold skin, gray pallor.
Other: pain and redness at infusion site.

INTERACTIONS
ACE inhibitors, potassium-sparing diuretics: increased risk of hyperkalemia. Use with extreme caution.

CONTRAINDICATIONS
- Contraindicated in patients with severe renal impairment with oliguria, anuria, azotemia; untreated Addison's disease; or in patients with acute dehydration, hyperkalemia, hyperkalemic form of familial periodic paralysis, and conditions associated with extensive tissue breakdown.
- Use cautiously in patients with cardiac disease, in patients receiving potassium-sparing diuretics, and in those with renal impairment.

NURSING CONSIDERATIONS
- During therapy, monitor ECG, renal function, fluid intake and output, and serum potassium, serum creatinine, and BUN levels. Never give potassium postoperatively until urine flow is established.
- Give slowly as diluted solution; potentially fatal hyperkalemia may result from too-rapid infusion.
- **I.V. use:** Give by I.V. infusion only; never I.V. push or I.M. Observe for pain and redness at infusion site. Large-bore needle reduces local irritation.
- Watch for signs of GI ulceration: obstruction, pain, distention, severe vomiting, and bleeding.
- Reconstitute potassium acetate powder with liquids; give after meals with a full glass of water or fruit juice to minimize GI irritation.

potassium bicarbonate
K+Care ET, K-Ide, Klor-Con/EF, K-Lyte

Pregnancy Risk Category: A

HOW SUPPLIED
Effervescent tablets: 25 mEq

ACTION
Mechanism: Replaces and maintains potassium.

Peak: Peak levels occur within 4 hours.

INDICATIONS & DOSAGE
Hypokalemia –

Adults: 25 to 50 mEq dissolved in one-half to a full glass of water (120 to 240 ml) once daily to q.i.d.

ADVERSE REACTIONS
CNS: paresthesia of the extremities, listlessness, mental confusion, weakness or heaviness of legs, flaccid paralysis.

CV: ***arrhythmias,*** ECG changes (prolonged PR interval; widened QRS complex; ST-segment depression; tall, tented T waves).

GI: *nausea, vomiting, abdominal pain,* diarrhea, ulcerations, hemorrhage, obstruction, perforation.

INTERACTIONS
ACE inhibitors, potassium-sparing diuretics: risk of hyperkalemia. Use with extreme caution.

CONTRAINDICATIONS
- Contraindicated in patients with severe renal impairment with oliguria, anuria, azotemia, and untreated Addison's disease; also in patients with acute dehydration, hyperkalemia, hyperkalemic form of familial periodic paralysis, and other conditions associated with extensive tissue breakdown.
- Use cautiously in patients with cardiac disease and in those receiving potassium-sparing diuretics.

NURSING CONSIDERATIONS
- Monitor BUN, serum potassium, and creatinine levels, and monitor fluid intake and output.
- Never switch potassium products without a doctor's order. Potassium bicarbonate cannot be given instead of potassium chloride.

- Dissolve potassium bicarbonate tablets completely in 6 to 8 ounces of cold water to minimize GI irritation.
- Don't administer potassium supplements postoperatively until urine flow has been established.
- Have the patient take with meals and sip slowly over 5 to 10 minutes.
- Potassium bicarbonate does not correct hypochloremic alkalosis.
- Ask the patient's flavor preference. Available in lime and orange flavors.

potassium chloride

Cena-K, K+10, K+Care, Kaochlor 10%*, Kaochlor S-F 10%*, Kaon-Cl, Kaon-Cl 20%*, Kato Powder, Kay Ciel*, K-Dur, K-Lease, K-Lor, Klor-10%*, Klor-Con, Klorvess, Klotrix, K-Lyte/Cl, K-Norm, K-Tab, Micro-K Extencaps, Rum-K, Slow-K, Ten-K

Pregnancy Risk Category: A

HOW SUPPLIED

Tablets: 1.22 mEq (99 mg), 8 mEq (600 mg), 10 mEq (750 mg), 20 mEq (1,500 mg), 25 mEq (1,875 mg)
Tablets (controlled-release): 6.7 mEq (500 mg), 8 mEq (600 mg), 10 mEq (750 mg), 20 mEq (1,500 mg)
Tablets (enteric-coated): 4 mEq (300 mg), 13.4 mEq (1,000 mg)
Capsules (controlled-release): 8 mEq (600 mg), 10 mEq (750 mg)
Oral liquid: 5% (10 mEq/15 ml), 7.5% (15 mEq/15 ml), 10% (20 mEq/15 ml), 15% (30 mEq/15 ml), 20% (40 mEq/15 ml)
Powder for oral use: 15 mEq/packet, 20 mEq/packet, 25 mEq/packet, 25 mEq/dose
Injection: 20 mEq, 40 mEq ampules; additive syringes containing 30 mEq or 40 mEq; 10 mEq, 20 mEq, 30 mEq, 40 mEq, 45 mEq, 60 mEq, 100 mEq, 200 mEq, 400 mEq, or 1,000 mEq vials

ACTION

Mechanism: Replaces and maintains potassium level.
Peak: Serum levels peak immediately after I.V. infusion.

INDICATIONS & DOSAGE

Hypokalemia –
Adults: 40 to 100 mEq P.O. daily in three or four divided doses for treatment; 20 mEq for prevention. Further dosage based on serum potassium level.
Children: 3 mEq/kg daily.
Total dosage not to exceed 150 mEq daily or 40 mEq/m².

Use I.V. route only when oral replacement is not feasible or when hypokalemia is life-threatening. If serum potassium is less than 2 mEq/ml, maximum infusion rate is 40 mEq/hour; maximum infusion concentration is 80 mEq/L; and maximum 24-hour dose is 400 mEq. If serum potassium level is greater than 2 mEq/ml, maximum infusion rate is 10 mEq/hour; maximum infusion concentration is 40 mEq/L; and maximum 24-hour dose is 200 mEq. For routine supplementation, the usual dose 20 mEq hourly in concentration of 40 mEq/L or less.

ADVERSE REACTIONS

Signs of hyperkalemia –
CNS: paresthesia of the extremities, listlessness, mental confusion, weakness or heaviness of limbs, flaccid paralysis.
CV: ***peripheral vascular collapse with fall in blood pressure, arrhythmias, heart block, possible cardiac arrest,*** ECG changes (prolonged PR interval; widened QRS complex; ST-segment depression; tall, tented T waves).
GI: *nausea, vomiting, abdominal pain,* diarrhea, GI ulcerations (possible stenosis, hemorrhage, obstruction, perforation).
GU: oliguria.

Skin: cold skin, gray pallor.
Other: *postinfusion phlebitis.*

INTERACTIONS

ACE inhibitors, potassium-sparing diuretics: risk of hyperkalemia. Use with extreme caution.

CONTRAINDICATIONS

- Contraindicated in patients with severe renal impairment with oliguria, anuria, azotemia, and untreated Addison's disease; also in patients with acute dehydration, hyperkalemia, hyperkalemic form of familial periodic paralysis, and other conditions associated with extensive tissue breakdown.
- Use cautiously in patients with cardiac disease, in postoperative patients, and in those receiving potassium-sparing diuretics.

NURSING CONSIDERATIONS

- Potassium should not be given during immediate postoperative period until urine flow is established.
- Give oral potassium supplements with extreme caution because its many forms deliver varying amounts of potassium. Never switch products without a doctor's order.
- Sugar-free liquid available (Kaochlor S-F 10%); use if tablet or capsule passage is likely to be delayed, such as in GI obstruction. Have patients sip slowly to minimize GI irritation.
- Give with or after meals with full glass of water or fruit juice to lessen GI distress.
- Make sure powders are completely dissolved before administering.
- Enteric-coated tablets not recommended because of increased potential for GI bleeding and small-bowel ulcerations.
- Tablets in wax matrix sometimes lodge in esophagus and cause ulceration in cardiac patients who have esophageal compression from enlarged left atrium. Use liquid form in such patients and in those with esophageal stasis or obstruction.
- Microencapsulated form (Micro-K) was indicated in one study to cause less GI bleeding than the wax matrix tablets. (Not confirmed).
- Often used orally with potassium-wasting diuretics to maintain potassium levels.
- Monitor ECG and serum electrolyte levels during therapy.
- Don't crush sustained-release potassium products.
- **I.V. use:** Give by infusion only; never I.V. push or I.M. Give slowly as dilute solution; potentially fatal hyperkalemia may result from too-rapid infusion.
- Small amounts of lidocaine injection (1 to 3 ml of the 1% strength) may be added directly to the potassium chloride solution to reverse postinfusion phlebitis.

potassium gluconate

Glu-K, Kaon Liquid*, Kaon Tablets, Kaylixer*, K-G Elixir*, Potassium Rougier†

Pregnancy Risk Category: A

HOW SUPPLIED

Tablets: 500 mg (2 mEq K^+), 1,170 mg (5 mEq K^+)
Elixir: 4.68 g (20 mEq K^+)/15 ml*

ACTION

Mechanism: Replaces and maintains potassium.
Peak: Peak levels occur within 4 hours of oral dose.

INDICATIONS & DOSAGE

Hypokalemia –
Adults: 40 to 100 mEq P.O. daily in three or four divided doses for treatment; 20 mEq daily for prevention. Further dosage based on serum potassium determinations.

ADVERSE REACTIONS
CNS: paresthesia of the extremities, listlessness, mental confusion, weakness or heaviness of legs, flaccid paralysis.
CV: ***arrhythmias,*** ECG changes (prolonged PR interval; widened QRS complex; ST-segment depression; tall, tented T waves).
GI: *nausea, vomiting, abdominal pain,* diarrhea, GI ulcerations with oral products (especially enteric-coated tablets); ulcerations may be accompanied by stenosis, hemorrhage, obstruction, perforation.

INTERACTIONS
ACE inhibitors, potassium-sparing diuretics: risk of hyperkalemia. Use with extreme caution.

CONTRAINDICATIONS
• Contraindicated in patients with severe renal impairment with oliguria, anuria, azotemia, and untreated Addison's disease; also in patients with acute dehydration, hyperkalemia, hyperkalemic form of familial periodic paralysis, and other conditions associated with extensive tissue breakdown.
• Use cautiously in patients with cardiac disease, postoperative patients, and in those receiving potassium-sparing diuretics.

NURSING CONSIDERATIONS
• Monitor ECG, serum potassium and creatinine levels, BUN, and fluid intake and output.
• Give oral potassium supplements with extreme caution because their many forms deliver varying amounts of potassium. Never switch products without a doctor's order.
• Don't administer potassium supplements postoperatively until urine flow has been established.
• Have the patient sip liquid potassium slowly to minimize GI irritation.
• To lessen GI distress, give with or after meals with full glass of water or fruit juice.
• Potassium gluconate does not correct hypokalemic hypochloremic alkalosis.
• Enteric-coated tablets not recommended because of increased potential for GI bleeding and small-bowel ulcerations.

Ringer's injection

Pregnancy Risk Category: C

HOW SUPPLIED
Injection: 250 ml, 500 ml, 1,000 ml

ACTION
Mechanism: Replaces fluids and electrolytes.
Peak: Serum levels peak immediately after I.V. infusion.

INDICATIONS & DOSAGE
Fluid and electrolyte replacement –
Adults and children: dose highly individualized, but usually 1.5 to 3 liters (2% to 6% body weight) infused I.V. over 18 to 24 hours.

ADVERSE REACTIONS
CV: fluid overload.

INTERACTIONS
None significant.

CONTRAINDICATIONS
• Contraindicated in patients with renal failure, except as emergency volume expander.
• Use cautiously in patients with CHF, circulatory insufficiency, renal dysfunction, hypoproteinemia, and pulmonary edema.

NURSING CONSIDERATIONS
• Ringer's injection contains sodium, 147 mEq/L; potassium, 4 mEq/L; calcium, 4.5 mEq/L; and chloride, 155.5 mEq/L.
• Electrolyte content is insufficient

for treating severe electrolyte deficiencies, but it does provide electrolytes in levels approximately equal to those of the blood.

Ringer's injection, lactated (Hartmann's solution, Ringer's lactate solution)

Pregnancy Risk Category: C

HOW SUPPLIED

Injection: 250 ml, 500 ml, 1,000 ml

ACTION

Mechanism: Replaces fluids and electrolytes.

Peak: Serum levels peak immediately after I.V. infusion.

INDICATIONS & DOSAGE

Fluid and electrolyte replacement – **Adults and children:** dosage highly individualized, but usually 1.5 to 3 liters (2% to 6% body weight) infused I.V. over 18 to 24 hours.

ADVERSE REACTIONS

CV: fluid overload.

INTERACTIONS

None significant.

CONTRAINDICATIONS

- Contraindicated in patients with renal failure, except as emergency volume expander.
- Use cautiously in patients with CHF, circulatory insufficiency, renal dysfunction, hypoproteinemia, and pulmonary edema.

NURSING CONSIDERATIONS

- Lactated Ringer's injection contains sodium, 130 mEq/L; potassium, 4 mEq/L; calcium, 3 mEq/L; chloride, 109.7 mEq/L; and lactate, 28 mEq/L.
- Lactated Ringer's injection more closely approximates the electrolyte concentration in blood plasma.

sodium chloride

Pregnancy Risk Category: C

HOW SUPPLIED

Tablets (enteric-coated): 1 g
Tablets (slow-release): 600 mg
Injection: 0.45% sodium chloride solution 500 ml, 1,000 ml; 0.9% sodium chloride solution 50 ml, 100 ml, 150 ml, 250 ml, 500 ml, 1,000 ml; 3% sodium chloride solution 500 ml; 5% sodium chloride solution 500 ml; 14.6% sodium chloride solution 20 ml, 40 ml, 200 ml; 23.4% sodium chloride solution 30 ml, 50 ml, and 200 ml.

ACTION

Mechanism: Replaces and maintains sodium and chloride levels.

Peak: Serum levels peak immediately after I.V. infusion.

INDICATIONS & DOSAGE

Fluid and electrolyte replacement in hyponatremia caused by electrolyte loss or in severe salt depletion – **Adults:** dosage is highly individualized. Use 3% or 5% solution only with frequent electrolyte determination and give only slow I.V. With 0.45% solution: 3% to 8% of body weight, according to deficiencies, over 18 to 24 hours; with 0.9% solution: 2% to 6% of body weight, according to deficiencies, over 18 to 24 hours.

Management of heat cramp caused by excessive perspiration – **Adults:** 1 g P.O. with every glass of water.

ADVERSE REACTIONS

CV: aggravation of CHF; edema if given too rapidly or in excess.

Respiratory: ***pulmonary edema*** if given too rapidly or in excess.

Other: hypernatremia and aggravation of existing metabolic acidosis with excessive infusion; serious electrolyte disturbances, loss of potassium.

INTERACTIONS
None significant.

CONTRAINDICATIONS
• Use cautiously in patients with CHF, circulatory insufficiency, renal dysfunction, and hypoproteinemia.

NURSING CONSIDERATIONS
• Monitor serum electrolyte levels.
• **I.V. use:** Infuse 3% and 5% solutions very slowly and cautiously to avoid pulmonary edema. Use only for critical situations, and observe the patient continually.
• Concentrates (14.6%, 23.4%) available to add to parenteral nutrient solutions. Don't confuse these parenteral soutions with 0.9% sodium chloride injection, and never administer without diluting. Read label carefully.

63

Acidifier and alkalinizers

ammonium chloride
sodium bicarbonate
sodium lactate
tromethamine

COMBINATION PRODUCTS
BICITRA: sodium citrate 500 mg and citric acid 334 mg/5ml

ammonium chloride◇

Pregnancy Risk Category: B

HOW SUPPLIED
Tablets: 500 mg◇
Tablets (enteric-coated): 500 mg◇, 1,000 mg◇
Injection: 2.14% (0.4 mEq/ml), 26.75% (5 mEq/ml)

ACTION
Mechanism: Increases free hydrogen ion concentration and acts as an expectorant by causing reflex stimulation of bronchial mucous glands.
Peak: Serum levels peak immediately after I.V. infusion.

INDICATIONS & DOSAGE
Metabolic alkalosis; chloride replacement–
Adults and children: I.V. dose (in mEq) is equal to the serum chloride deficit (in mEq/ml) multiplied by the extracellular fluid volume (estimated as 20% of the body weight in kilograms). One-half the calculated volume should be given, then the patient reassessed.
Acidifier–
Adults: 4 to 12 g P.O. daily in divided doses.
Children: 75 mg/kg P.O. daily in four divided doses.
Expectorant–
Adults: 250 to 500 mg P.O. every 2 to 4 hours.

ADVERSE REACTIONS
Adverse reactions usually result from ammonia toxicity or too-rapid I.V. administration.
CNS: headache, confusion, progressive drowsiness, excitement alternating with ***coma,*** hyperventilation, ***calcium-deficient tetany, twitching,*** hyperreflexia, EEG abnormalities.
CV: bradycardia.
GI: with oral dose–*gastric irritation, nausea, vomiting,* thirst, anorexia, retching.
GU: glycosuria.
Skin: rash, pallor.
Other: ***metabolic acidosis, hyperchloremia, hypokalemia,*** hyperglycemia, pain at injection site, irregular respirations with periods of apnea.

INTERACTIONS
Spironolactone: increased systemic acidosis. Use together cautiously.

CONTRAINDICATIONS
- Contraindicated in patients with severe hepatic or renal dysfunction.
- Use cautiously in patients with pulmonary insufficiency or cardiac edema and in infants.

NURSING CONSIDERATIONS
- To decrease GI adverse reactions, give oral form after meals. Enteric-coated tablets may also minimize GI symptoms but are absorbed erratically.
- Do not administer drug with milk or other alkaline solutions; they are not compatible.
- Determine carbon dioxide (CO_2) combining power and serum electro-

lytes before and during therapy to prevent acidosis. Each gram of ammonium chloride will reduce the CO_2 combining power by 1.1 volume percent.

- Monitor urine pH and output. Diuresis is normal for first 2 days.
- Monitor rate and depth of respirations frequently.
- When using as an expectorant, give with full glass of water.
- **I.V. use:** Dilute concentrated form (26.75%) before administration. Add 100 to 200 mEq (20 to 40 ml of the 26.75% solution) to 500 or 1,000 ml of 0.9% sodium chloride injection. Administer via infusion pump, not exceeding 5 ml/min in adults.
- Lessen pain of I.V. injection by decreasing infusion rate.

sodium bicarbonate◇

Arm and Hammer Pure Baking Soda, Bell/ans, Citrocarbonate, Soda Mint

Pregnancy Risk Category: C

HOW SUPPLIED

Tablets: 300 mg◇, 325 mg◇, 600 mg◇, 650 mg◇
Injection: 4% (2.4 mEq/5 ml), 4.2% (5 mEq/10 ml), 5% (297.5 mEq/500 ml), 7.5% (8.92 mEq/10 ml and 44.6 mEq/50 ml), 8.4% (10 mEq/10 ml and 50 mEq/50 ml)

ACTION

Mechanism: Restores body's buffering capacity of the body and neutralizes excess acid.
Peak: Peak serum levels occur immediately after I.V. infusion.

INDICATIONS & DOSAGE

Cardiac arrest –
Adults and children: 1 mEq/kg I.V. of 7.5% or 8.4% solution followed by 0.5 mEq/kg I.V. every 10 minutes, depending on blood gases. Further dosages based on results of blood gas analysis. If blood gases unavailable, use 0.5 mEq/kg I.V. every 10 minutes until spontaneous circulation returns.
Infants up to 2 years: not to exceed 8 mEq/kg I.V. daily of 4.2% solution.
Metabolic acidosis –
Adults and children: dosage depends on blood CO_2 content, pH, and the patient's clinical condition. Generally, 2 to 5 mEq/kg I.V. infused over 4- to 8-hour period.
Systemic or urinary alkalinization –
Adults: 325 mg to 2 g P.O. q.i.d.
Children: 12 to 120 mg/kg P.O. daily.
Antacid –
Adults: 300 mg to 2 g P.O. chewed and taken with glass of water.

ADVERSE REACTIONS

GI: gastric distention, belching, flatulence.
GU: renal calculi or crystals.
Other: with overdose – ***metabolic alkalosis,*** hypernatremia, ***hyperkalemia,*** hyperosmolarity.

INTERACTIONS

Anorexients, flecainide, quinidine, sympathomimetics: increased urine alkalinization causes increased renal clearance of these drugs and reduced effectiveness. Monitor closely.
Chlorpropamide, lithium, methotrexate, salicylates, tetracycline: urine alkalinization causes decreased renal clearance of these drugs and increased risk of toxicity. Monitor closely.
Enteric-coated drugs: may be released prematurely in stomach. Avoid concomitant use.

CONTRAINDICATIONS

- Contraindicated in patients with hypertension, in those with tendency toward edema, or who are losing chlorides by vomiting or from continuous GI suction, in patients receiving diuretics known to produce hypochloremic alkalosis, and in those on sodium-restricted diets or with renal disease.

NURSING CONSIDERATIONS

• To avoid risk of alkalosis, determine blood pH, PaO_2, $PaCO_2$, and serum electrolytes. Keep the doctor informed of serum laboratory results.
• Tell the patient not to take with milk. May cause hypercalcemia, alkalosis, and possibly renal calculi.
• Discourage use as an antacid. Offer a nonabsorbable alternative antacid if it is to be used repeatedly.
• Sodium bicarbonate is not routinely recommended for use in cardiac arrest because it may produce a paradoxical acidosis from CO_2 production. It should not be routinely administered during the early stages of resuscitation unless preexisting acidosis is clearly present. May be used at team leader's discretion after such interventions as defibrillation, cardiac compression, and administration of first-line drugs.
• If sodium bicarbonate is being used to produce an alkaline urine, monitor urine pH every 4 to 6 hours (should be > 7.0).
• **I.V. use:** May be added to other I.V. fluids. Sodium bicarbonate inactivates such catecholamines as norepinephrine and dopamine, and forms precipitate with calcium. Do not mix sodium bicarbonate with I.V. solutions of these agents, and flush I.V. line adequately.

sodium lactate

Pregnancy Risk Category: C

HOW SUPPLIED

Injection: ⅙ molar solution
Injection: 2.5 mEq/ml

ACTION

Mechanism: Metabolized to sodium bicarbonate, producing buffering effect.
Peak: Serum levels peak immediately after I.V. infusion.

INDICATIONS & DOSAGE

Alkalinize urine –
Adults: 30 ml of ⅙ molar solution/kg of body weight I.V. given in divided doses over 24 hours.
Metabolic acidosis –
Adults: ⅙ molar injection (167 mEq lactate/L I.V.); dosage depends on degree of bicarbonate deficit.

ADVERSE REACTIONS

Other: with overdose – ***metabolic alkalosis,*** hypernatremia, hyperosmolarity.

INTERACTIONS

None significant.

CONTRAINDICATIONS

• Contraindicated in patients with severe hepatic and renal disease, respiratory alkalosis, or acidosis associated with congenital heart disease with persistent cyanosis.
• Do not use in patients with severe acidosis because rapid replacement of serum bicarbonate is required. Sodium lactate is slowly metabolized to bicarbonate by the liver; serum bicarbonate levels may not rise for 1 to 2 hours after administration.

NURSING CONSIDERATIONS

• Monitor serum electrolyte levels to avoid alkalosis.
• **I.V. use:** Add sodium lactate to other I.V. solutions, or give as an isotonic ⅙ molar solution. Drug is compatible with most common I.V. solutions.

tromethamine

Tham

Pregnancy Risk Category: C

HOW SUPPLIED

Injection: 18 g/500 ml

ACTION

Mechanism: Combines with hydrogen ions and associated acid anions; resulting salts are excreted. Also has osmotic diuretic effect.
Peak: Serum levels peak immediately after I.V. infusion.

INDICATIONS & DOSAGE

Metabolic acidosis associated with cardiac bypass surgery or with cardiac arrest –
Adults: dosage depends on bicarbonate deficit. Calculate as follows: each ml of 0.3 M tromethamine solution required = weight in kg × bicarbonate deficit (mEq/L). Additional therapy based on serial determinations of existing bicarbonate deficit.
Children: calculate dosage as above. Give slowly over 3 to 6 hours. Additional therapy based on degree of acidosis. Total 24-hour dosage should not exceed 33 to 40 ml/kg.

ADVERSE REACTIONS

Respiratory: ***respiratory depression.***
Other: hypoglycemia, ***hyperkalemia*** (with decreased urine output), venospasm; I.V. thrombosis; inflammation, necrosis, and sloughing if extravasation occurs.

INTERACTIONS

None significant.

CONTRAINDICATIONS

- Contraindicated in patients with anuria, uremia, or chronic respiratory acidosis, or during pregnancy (except in acute, life-threatening situations).
- Use cautiously in patients with renal disease and poor urine output. Monitor ECG and serum potassium levels in these patients.

NURSING CONSIDERATIONS

- To prevent blood pH from rising above normal, adjust dosage carefully.
- Make the following determinations before, during and after therapy: blood pH; carbon dioxide tension; bicarbonate, glucose, and electrolyte levels.
- In patients with associated respiratory acidosis, mechanical ventilation should be available.
- Do not use longer than 1 day except in life-threatening situations.
- **I.V. use:** Give slowly through 18G to 20G needle into largest antecubital vein, or by indwelling I.V. catheter.
- If extravasation occurs, infiltrate area with 1% procaine and 150 units hyaluronidase; may reduce vasospasm and dilute remaining drug locally.

Hematinics

ferrous fumarate
ferrous gluconate
ferrous sulfate
iron dextran

COMBINATION PRODUCTS

FERGON PLUS: ferrous gluconate 58 mg, vitamin B_{12} ½ NF unit with intrinsic factor, and vitamin C 75 mg.
FERMALOX: ferrous sulfate 200 mg, magnesium hydroxide 100 mg, and aluminium hydroxide 100 mg.
FEROCYL◇: ferrous fumarate 50 mg and docusate sodium 100 mg.
FERRO-SEQUELS◇: ferrous fumarate 50 mg and docusate sodium 100 mg.
FERRO-DOCUSATE-T.R., FERRO-DOK TR, FERRO-DSS S.R.: ferrous fumarate 150 mg and docusate sodium 100 mg.

ferrous fumarate

Femiron◇, Feostat◇, Feostat Drops◇, Fumasorb◇, Fumerin◇, Hemocyte◇, Ircon◇, Nephro-Fer◇, Novofumar†, Palafer†, Palafer Pediatric Drops†, Span-FF◇

Pregnancy Risk Category: A

HOW SUPPLIED

Each 100 mg of ferrous fumarate provides 33 mg of elemental iron.
Tablets◇*:* 63 mg, 195 mg, 200 mg, 324 mg, 325 mg
Tablets (chewable): 100 mg◇
Capsules (extended-release): 325 mg◇
Oral suspension: 100 mg/5 ml◇
Drops: 45 mg/0.6 ml◇

ACTION

Mechanism: Provides elemental iron, an essential component in the formation of hemoglobin.
Onset: 4 days. **Peak:** 7 to 10 days.
Duration: 2 to 4 months.

INDICATIONS & DOSAGE

Iron deficiency –
Adults: 200 mg P.O. t.i.d. or q.i.d.
Children: 3 mg/kg P.O. t.i.d., increased to 6 mg/kg P.O. t.i.d. as needed and tolerated.

ADVERSE REACTIONS

GI: *nausea,* vomiting, *constipation, black stools.*
Other: suspension and drops may stain teeth.

INTERACTIONS

Antacids, levodopa, penicillamine, quinolones, tetracycline, vitamin E: decreased iron absorption. Separate doses by 2 to 4 hours.
Chloramphenicol: delayed response to iron therapy. Watch patient carefully.
Vitamin C: may increase iron absorption. Beneficial drug interaction.

CONTRAINDICATIONS

- Contraindicated in patients with hemosiderosis; also contraindicated in patients with hemochromatosis and hemolytic anemia unless an iron deficiency anemia is also present.
- Use cautiously in patients with peptic ulceration, regional enteritis, and ulcerative colitis. Also use cautiously on long-term basis.

NURSING CONSIDERATIONS

- GI upset may be related to dose. Between-meal dosing preferable, but can be given with some foods, although absorption may be decreased. Enteric-coated products reduce GI upset but also reduce amount of iron absorbed.
- Parents should be aware that doses

as small as 60 mg have been fatal in children.

- Tablets may be given with juice (preferably orange juice) or water, but not with milk or antacids.
- To avoid staining teeth, give suspension with straw and place drops at back of throat.
- Check for constipation; record color and amount of stool. Teach dietary measures for preventing constipation.
- Oral iron may turn stools black. Although this unabsorbed iron is harmless, it could mask the presence of melena.
- Monitor hemoglobin and hematocrit levels and reticulocyte counts during therapy.
- Do not crush or allow the patient to chew extended-release iron preparations.
- If the patient misses a dose, tell him to take it as soon as he remembers but not to double-dose.
- Combination products, such as Ferro-Sequels and Ferocyl, contain stool softeners, which help prevent constipation, a common adverse reaction.
- Certain foods may impair oral iron absorption, including yogurt, cheese, eggs, milk, whole-grain breads and cereals, tea, and coffee.

ferrous gluconate

Fergon*◇, Ferralet◇, Fertinic†, Novoferrogluc†

Pregnancy Risk Category: A

HOW SUPPLIED

Each 100 mg of ferrous gluconate provides 11.6 mg of elemental iron.
Tablets: 300 mg◇, 320 mg◇ (contains 37 mg Fe^{+}), 325 mg◇
Capsules: 86 mg◇, 325 mg◇, 435 mg◇
Elixir: 300 mg/5 ml (contains 35 mg Fe^{+})*◇

ACTION

Mechanism: Provides elemental iron, an essential component in the formation of hemoglobin.
Onset: 4 days. **Peak:** 7 to 10 days.
Duration: 2 to 4 months.

INDICATIONS & DOSAGE

Iron deficiency –
Adults: 300 to 325 mg P.O. q.i.d., increased to 650 mg q.i.d. as needed and tolerated.
Children 2 years or older: 8 mg/kg P.O. t.i.d., increased to 16 mg P.O. t.i.d. as needed and tolerated.

ADVERSE REACTIONS

GI: *nausea,* vomiting, *constipation, black stools.*
Other: elixir may stain teeth.

INTERACTIONS

Antacids, levodopa, penicillamine, quinolones, tetracycline, vitamin E: decreased iron absorption. Separate doses if possible.
Chloramphenicol: delayed response to iron therapy. Watch the patient carefully.
Vitamin C: may increase iron absorption. Beneficial drug interaction.

CONTRAINDICATIONS

- Contraindicated in patients with peptic ulceration, regional enteritis, ulcerative colitis, hemosiderosis, and hemochromatosis. Also contraindicated in patients with hemolytic anemia unless an iron deficiency anemia is also present.
- Use cautiously on long-term basis.

NURSING CONSIDERATIONS

- GI upset may be related to dose. Between-meal dosing preferable, but can be given with some foods, although absorption may be decreased. Enteric-coated products reduce GI upset but also reduce amount of iron absorbed.
- Parents should be aware that 3 or 4

tablets can cause serious iron poisoning in children.

- Dilute liquid preparations in juice (preferably orange juice) or water, but not in milk or antacids. To promote absorption, give tablets with orange juice.
- To avoid staining teeth, give elixirs with straw; the patient may take with water or fruit juice.
- Check for constipation; record color and amount of stool. Teach dietary measures for preventing constipation.
- Oral iron may turn stools black. This unabsorbed iron is harmless; however, it could mask melena.
- Monitor hemoglobin and hematocrit levels and reticulocyte counts during therapy.
- If the patient misses a dose, tell him to take it as soon as he remembers but not to double-dose.
- Certain foods may impair oral iron absorption, including yogurt, cheese, eggs, milk, whole-grain breads and cereals, tea, and coffee.

ferrous sulfate

Apo-Ferrous Sulfate†, Feosol*◊, Fer-In-Sol*◊, Fer-In-Sol Drops*◊, Fer-In-Sol Syrup*◊, Fer-Iron Drops◊, Feritard‡, Fero-Grad†, Fero-Gradumet◊, Ferospace◊, Ferralyn Lanacaps◊, Ferra-TD‡

ferrous sulfate, dried

Mol-Iron*◊, Novoferrosulfa†, PMS Ferrous Sulfate†, Slow-Fe◊

Pregnancy Risk Category: A

HOW SUPPLIED

Ferrous sulfate is 20% elemental iron; dried and powdered, about 32% elemental iron.
Tablets: 195 mg◊, 300 mg◊, 325 mg◊; 200 mg (dried)
Tablets (extended-release): 160 mg (dried)◊, 525 mg
Capsules: 150 mg◊, 159 mg (dried), 190 mg (dried), 250 mg◊, 390 mg◊
Capsules (extended-release): 159 mg (dried)◊, 525 mg◊
Elixir: 220 mg/5 ml* ◊
Liquid: 75 mg/0.6 ml◊, 125 mg/ml
Syrup: 90 mg/5 ml◊
Solution: 300 mg/5 ml
Drops: 125 mg/ml

ACTION

Mechanism: Provides elemental iron, an essential component in the formation of hemoglobin.
Onset: 4 days. **Peak:** 7 to 10 days.
Duration: 2 to 4 months.

INDICATIONS & DOSAGE

Iron deficiency –
Adults: 325 mg P.O. t.i.d. or q.i.d. Alternatively, give 1 extended-release capsule (160 or 525 mg) P.O. twice daily.
Children: 4 to 6 mg/kg daily in 3 divided doses.
Prophylaxis for iron deficiency anemia –
Pregnant patients: 150 mg P.O. daily during the last 2 trimesters.
Premature or undernourished infants: 1 to 2 mg/kg P.O. daily in divided doses.

ADVERSE REACTIONS

GI: *nausea,* vomiting, *constipation, black stools.*
Other: liquid forms may stain teeth.

INTERACTIONS

Antacids, levodopa, penicillamine, quinolones, tetracycline, vitamin E: decreased iron absorption. Separate doses if possible.
Chloramphenicol: delayed response to iron therapy. Watch patient carefully.
Vitamin C: may increase iron absorption. Beneficial drug interaction.

CONTRAINDICATIONS

- Contraindicated in patients with hemosiderosis and hemochromatosis. Also contraindicated in patients with

*Liquid form contains alcohol.
**May contain tartrazine.

Common reactions are in italics; ***life-threatening,*** in bold italics.

hemolytic anemia unless iron deficiency anemia is also present.
• Use cautiously in patients with peptic ulceration, ulcerative colitis, and regional enteritis. Also use cautiously on long-term basis.

NURSING CONSIDERATIONS
• Rate and extent of iron absorption varies with need; normal patients absorb only 5% to 10% of dietary iron, whereas patients with iron deficiency can absorb 30% or more of dietary iron.
• GI upset may be related to dose. Between-meal dosing preferable, but can be given with some foods, although absorption may be decreased. Enteric-coated products reduce GI upset but also reduce amount of iron absorbed.
• Parents should be aware that 3 to 4 tablets can cause serious iron poisoning in children.
• Dilute liquid preparations in juice (preferably orange juice) or water, but not in milk or antacids. To promote iron absorption, give tablets with orange juice.
• To avoid staining teeth, give elixirs with straw and place in back of throat.
• Check for constipation; record color and amount of stool. Teach dietary measures for preventing constipation.
• Oral iron may turn stools black. Although this unabsorbed iron is harmless, it could mask melena.
• Monitor hemoglobin and hematocrit levels and reticulocyte counts during therapy.
• Do not crush or allow the patient to chew extended-release preparations.
• If the patient misses a dose, tell him to take it as soon as he remembers, but not to double-dose.
• Certain foods may impair oral iron absorption, including yogurt, cheese, eggs, milk, whole-grain breads and cereals, tea, and coffee.

iron dextran
Hydextran, Imferon, InFeD, K-FeRON, Proferdex
Pregnancy Risk Category: C

HOW SUPPLIED
1 ml iron dextran provides 50 mg elemental iron.
Injection: 50 mg elemental iron/ml

ACTION
Mechanism: Provides elemental iron, an essential component in the formation of hemoglobin. **Onset:** 3 days. **Peak:** Peak levels occur within 2 hours.

INDICATIONS & DOSAGE
Iron deficiency anemia –
Adults: I.M. or I.V. test dose required before administration.
I.M. (by Z-track): inject 0.5 ml test dose. If no reactions occur, daily dosage should ordinarily not exceed 0.5 ml (25 mg) for infants under 5 kg; 1 ml (50 mg) for children under 9 kg; 2 ml (100 mg) for patients under 50 kg; 5 ml (250 mg) for patients over 50 kg.
I.V. push: inject 0.5 ml test dose. If no reactions occur, raise dosage within 2 to 3 days to 2 ml daily I.V. Single dose should not exceed 100 mg. Give slowly (1 ml/minute).
I.V. infusion: dosages are expressed in terms of elemental iron. Dilute in 250 to 1,000 ml of 0.9% sodium chloride solution; dextrose increases local vein irritation. Infuse test dose of 25 mg slowly over 5 minutes. If no reactions occur in 5 minutes, start infusion. Infuse total dose slowly over 6 to 12 hours.

ADVERSE REACTIONS
CNS: headache, transitory paresthesia, arthralgia, myalgia, dizziness, malaise, syncope.
CV: *hypotensive reaction, peripheral vascular flushing with overly rapid I.V. administration, tachycardia.*

GI: nausea, vomiting, metallic taste, transient loss of taste.
Respiratory: ***bronchospasm.***
Skin: rash, urticaria.
Other: *soreness and inflammation at I.M. injection site; brown skin discoloration at I.M. injection site; local phlebitis at I.V. injection site,* sterile abscess, necrosis, atrophy, fibrosis, ***anaphylaxis,*** delayed sensitivity reactions.

INTERACTIONS

None significant.

CONTRAINDICATIONS

- Contraindicated in patients wtih all anemias except iron deficiency anemia.
- Use with extreme caution in patients with impaired hepatic function or rheumatoid arthritis and in infants.

NURSING CONSIDERATIONS

- Patients with certain inflammatory diseases, such as rheumatoid arthritis or ankylosing spondylitis, may be at higher risk for certain delayed reactions.
- Monitor the patient's vital signs for drug reactions, which range from pain, inflammation, and myalgia to hypotension, shock, and death.
- Monitor hemoglobin and hematocrit levels and reticulocyte count.
- **I.V. use:** Check hospital policy before administering I.V. Some do not permit infusion because its safety is controversial.
- I.M. or I.V. injections of iron are advisable only for patients for whom oral administration is impossible or ineffective. Use I.V. in these situations: Insufficient muscle mass for deep I.M. injection; impaired absorption from muscle due to stasis or edema; possibility of uncontrolled I.M. bleeding from trauma (as may occur in hemophilia); and with massive and prolonged parenteral therapy (as may be necessary in cases of chronic substantial blood loss).
- Upon completion of I.V. infusion, flush the vein with 10 ml of 0.9% sodium chloride solution. The patient should rest 15 to 30 minutes after I.V. administration.
- Inject deeply into upper outer quadrant of buttock – never into arm or other exposed area – with a 2- to 3-inch, 19G or 20G needle. Use Z-track technique to avoid leakage into S.C. tissue and staining of skin.
- Not removed by hemodialysis.
- Minimize skin staining by using a separate needle to withdraw the drug from its container.

Anticoagulants

dicumarol
enoxaparin
heparin calcium
heparin sodium
warfarin sodium

COMBINATION PRODUCTS
None.

dicumarol (bishydroxycoumarin)

Pregnancy Risk Category: D

HOW SUPPLIED
Tablets: 25 mg, 50 mg

ACTION
Mechanism: Inhibits vitamin K-dependent activation of clotting factors II, VII, IX, and X, formed in the liver.
Onset: ½ to 3 days. **Duration:** 2 to 5 days.

INDICATIONS & DOSAGE
Pulmonary embolism associated with chronic atrial fibrillation, deep vein thrombosis, MI, rheumatic heart disease with heart valve damage, and prosthetic heart valves –
Adults: 200 to 300 mg P.O. on first day, 25 to 200 mg P.O. daily thereafter depending on PT.

ADVERSE REACTIONS
GI: anorexia, nausea, vomiting, cramps, *diarrhea,* mouth ulcerations.
GU: hematuria.
Hematologic: ***hemorrhage with excessive dosage,*** leukopenia, ***agranulocytosis.***
Hepatic: hepatitis, elevated liver function tests, jaundice.
Skin: dermatitis, urticaria, necrosis, gangrene, alopecia, *rash.*
Other: *fever.*

INTERACTIONS
Acetaminophen: may increase bleeding with chronic (greater than 2 weeks) therapy with high doses (> 2 g/day) of acetaminophen. Monitor very carefully.
Allopurinol, amiodarone, anabolic steroids, cephalosporins, chloramphenicol, cimetidine, ciprofloxacin, clofibrate, diflunisal, disulfiram, glucagon, heparin, methimazole, metronidazole, propylthiouracil, sulfinpyrazone, sulfonamides, sulindac, thyroid drugs, tricyclic antidepressants, vitamin E: increased PT. Monitor the patient carefully for bleeding. Consider anticoagulant dosage reduction.
Barbiturates: inhibited hypoprothrombinemic effect of dicumarol. If barbiturates are withdrawn, reduce anticoagulant dosage; inhibition may last weeks after barbiturate is withdrawn, but fatal hemorrhage can occur when inhibiting effect disappears.
Carbamazepine, ethchlorvynol, griseofulvin, rifampin: decreased PT with reduced anticoagulant effect. Monitor patient carefully.
Chloral hydrate, glutethimide, sulfinpyrazone, triclofos sodium: increased or decreased PT. Avoid use if possible, and monitor the patient carefully.
Cholestyramine: decreased response when administered too close together. Administer 6 hours after oral anticoagulants.
Hydantoins: increased serum levels of hydantoin. Monitor closely.
Indomethacin, mefenamic acid, oxyphenbutazone, phenylbutazone, salicylates: increased PT; ulcerogenic effects. Don't use together.
Sulfonylureas (oral antidiabetic

agents): increased hypoglycemic response. Monitor blood glucose levels. *Foods or enteral products containing vitamin K:* may impair anticoagulation. Patient should maintain consistent daily intake of leafy green vegetables.

CONTRAINDICATIONS

- Contraindicated in patients with hemophilia, thrombocytopenic purpura, polycythemia vera, leukemia with pronounced bleeding tendency, open wounds or ulcerations, cerebrovascular hemorrhage, aneurysms, pericarditis, pericardial effusions, vasculitis, diverticulitis, impaired hepatic or renal function, severe hypertension, acute nephritis, subacute bacterial endocarditis, and GI, GU, or respiratory tract ulcerations. Also contraindicated during pregnancy and in patients with recent eye, CNS, or spinal cord surgery.
- Use with extreme caution in psychiatric, debilitated, or cachectic patients. Also use cautiously in breast-feeding patients. Monitor infants carefully; may easily bruise or bleed.
- Use cautiously during menses, during use of any drainage tube, and in any patient in whom slight bleeding is dangerous.
- Use caution when adding or stopping any drug for patients receiving anticoagulants. May change the patient's clotting status and result in hemorrhage.

NURSING CONSIDERATIONS

- Fever and skin rash signal severe adverse reactions. Withhold drug and call the doctor.
- Give drug at same time daily. Stress importance of complying with recommended dosage and follow-up appointments. The patient should carry a card identifying him as a potential bleeder.
- Regularly inspect the patient for bleeding gums, bruises on arms or legs, petechiae, nosebleeds, melena, tarry stools, hematuria, and hematemesis. Tell the patient and his family to watch for these signs and notify the doctor immediately.
- Warn the patient to avoid OTC products containing aspirin, other salicylates, or drugs that may interact with dicumarol.
- Dose given depends on PT. Doctors typically try to maintain PT at one and one-half to two times normal. PT values depend on procedure and reagents used in individual laboratory.
- Tell patients to notify their doctor if menses is heavier than usual; may require dosage adjustment.
- Tell patients to use electric razor when shaving to avoid scratching skin and to use a soft toothbrush.
- May turn alkaline urine red-orange.
- Light to moderate alcohol intake does not significantly affect PT.
- Tell patients to eat a consistent amount of leafy green vegetables every day. These contain vitamin K, and eating different amounts daily may alter anticoagulant effect.

enoxaparin sodium

Lovenox

Pregnancy Risk Category: B

HOW SUPPLIED

Injection: 30 mg per 0.3 ml

ACTION

Mechanism: A low-molecular weight heparin derivative that accelerates formation of antithrombin III-thrombin complex and deactivates thrombin, preventing conversion of fibrinogen to fibrin. Enoxaparin has a higher anti-factor Xa-to anti-factor IIa-activity ratio.

Peak: Peak effects occur 3 to 5 hours after S.C. injection. **Duration:** up to 24 hours.

INDICATIONS & DOSAGE
Pulmonary embolism and deep vein thrombosis –
Adults: 30 mg S.C. b.i.d. for 7 to 10 days. Give the initial dose as soon as possible after surgery, but no later than 24 hours postoperatively.

ADVERSE REACTIONS
CNS: confusion.
CV: edema, peripheral edema.
GI: nausea.
Hematologic: hypochromic anemia, moderate thrombocytopenia.
Other: irritation, pain, hematoma, or erythema at the injection site; fever; pain; hemorrhage; ecchymosis; bleeding complications.

INTERACTIONS
Anticoagulants, antiplatelet agents: increased risk of bleeding. Don't use together.

CONTRAINDICATIONS
- Contraindicated in patients hypersensitive to the drug; in patients with active, major bleeding; and in patients who demonstrate antiplatelet antibodies in the presence of the drug.
- Never administer I.M.
- Use cautiously in patients with conditions that put them at increased risk for hemorrhage, such as bacterial endocarditis; congenital or acquired bleeding disorders; ulcer disease; angiodysplastic GI disease; hemorrhagic stroke; or recent spinal, eye, or brain surgery.

NURSING CONSIDERATIONS
- Draw blood to establish baseline coagulation parameters before therapy. Monitor platelet counts regularly. Patients with normal coagulation will not require regular monitoring of PT or PTT.
- Regularly inspect the patient for bleeding gums, bruises on arms or legs, petechiae, nosebleeds, melena, tarry stools, hematuria, hematemesis. Tell the patient and his family to watch for these signs and notify the doctor immediately.
- Tell the patient to avoid OTC medications containing aspirin or other salicylates.
- Don't massage after S.C. injection. Watch for signs of bleeding at injection site. Rotate sites and keep accurate record.
- Avoid excessive I.M. injections of other drugs to prevent or minimize hematomas. If possible, don't give I.M. injections at all.
- To treat severe overdose, give protamine sulfate (a heparin antagonist) by slow I.V. infusion at a concentration of 1% to equal the dosage of enoxaparin injected.

heparin calcium
Calcilean†, Calciparine, Caprin‡, Uniparin-Ca‡

heparin sodium
Hepalean†, Heparin Lock Flush Solution (Tubex), Hep Lock, Heparin Leo†, Liquaemin Sodium, Uniparin‡

Pregnancy Risk Category: C

HOW SUPPLIED
Products are derived from beef lung or porcine intestinal mucosa.
calcium
Ampule: 12,500 units/0.5 ml; 20,000 units/0.8 ml
Syringe: 5,000 units/0.2 ml
sodium
Carpuject: 5,000 units/ml
Disposable syringes: 1,000 units/ml, 2,500 units/ml, 5,000 units/ml, 7,500 units/ml, 10,000 units/ml, 15,000 units/ml, 20,000 units/ml, 40,000 units/ml
Premixed I.V. solutions: 1,000 units in 500 ml of 0.9% sodium chloride solution; 2,000 units in 1,000 ml of 0.9% sodium chloride solution; 12,500 units in 250 ml of 0.45% so-

dium chloride solution; 25,000 units in 250 ml of 0.45% sodium chloride solution; 25,000 units in 500 ml of 0.45% sodium chloride solution; 10,000 units in 100 ml of D_5W; 12,500 units in 250 ml of D_5W; 25,000 units in 250 ml D_5W; 25,000 units in 500 ml D_5W; 20,000 units in 500 ml of D_5W
Unit-dose ampules: 1,000 units/ml, 5,000 units/ml, 10,000 units/ml
Vials: 1,000 units/ml, 2,500 units/ml, 5,000 units/ml, 7,500 units/ml, 10,000 units/ml, 15,000 units/ml, 20,000 units/ml, 40,000 units/ml
heparin sodium flush
Disposable syringes: 10 units/ml, 100 units/ml
Vials: 10 units/ml, 100 units/ml

ACTION

Mechanism: Accelerates formation of antithrombin III-thrombin complex and deactivates thrombin, preventing conversion of fibrinogen to fibrin.
Onset: 20 to 60 minutes after S.C. administration, immediately after I.V. injection. **Peak:** Plasma levels peak 2 to 4 hours after S.C. injection. **Duration:** poor correlation between plasma level and drug effect; heparin is rapidly cleared from plasma within ½ to 3 hours, but its duration of action is dose-dependent.

INDICATIONS & DOSAGE

Heparin dosing is highly individualized, depending upon disease state, age, renal and hepatic status.
Deep vein thrombosis, MI–
Adults: initially, 5,000 to 7,500 units I.V. push, then adjusted according to PTT and given I.V. q 4 hours (usually 4,000 to 5,000 units); or 5,000 to 7,500 units I.V. bolus, then 1,000 units/hour by I.V. infusion pump. Wait 8 hours after bolus dose, and adjust hourly rate according to PTT.
Pulmonary embolism; consumptive coagulopathy (such as disseminated intravascular coagulation)–
Adults: initially, 7,500 to 10,000 units I.V. push, then adjusted according to PTT and given I.V. q 4 hours (usually 4,000 to 5,000 units); or 7,500 to 10,000 units I.V. bolus, then 1,000 units/hour by I.V. infusion pump. Wait 8 hours after bolus dose, and adjust hourly rate according to PTT.
Children: initially, 50 units/kg I.V. drip. Maintenance dosage is 100 units/kg I.V. drip q 4 hours. Constant infusion: 20,000 units/m^2 daily. Adjust dosages according to PTT.
Embolism, venous thrombosis, pulmonary embolism, atrial fibrillation with embolism; postoperative deep vein thrombosis–
Adults: 5,000 units S.C. q 12 hours. In surgical patients, give first dose 2 hours before procedure; follow with 5,000 units S.C. q 8 to 12 hours for 5 to 7 days or until patient is fully ambulatory.
Open-heart surgery–
Adults: (total body perfusion) 150 to 300 units/kg continuous I.V infusion.
Patency maintenance of I.V. indwelling catheters–
Adults: 10 to 100 units I.V. flush. Use sufficient volume to fill the device. Not intended for therapeutic use.

ADVERSE REACTIONS

Hematologic: ***hemorrhage with excessive dosage,*** *overly prolonged clotting time,* ***thrombocytopenia.***
Other: irritation; mild pain; hematoma; ulceration; cutaneous or subcutaneous necrosis; ***"white clot" syndrome;*** hypersensitivity reactions, including chills, fever, pruritus, rhinitis, burning of feet, conjunctivitis, lacrimation, arthralgia, urticaria.

INTERACTIONS

Anticoagulants, oral: increased additive anticoagulation. Monitor PT and PTT.
Salicylates, other antiplatelet agents:

increased anticoagulant effect. Don't use together.
Thrombolytics: increased risk of hemorrhage. Monitor closely.

CONTRAINDICATIONS

• Contraindicated in patients hypersensitive to the drug. Conditionally contraindicated in patients with active bleeding; blood dyscrasia; or bleeding tendencies, such as hemophilia, thrombocytopenia, or hepatic disease with hypoprothrombinemia; suspected intracranial hemorrhage; suppurative thrombophlebitis; inaccessible ulcerative lesions (especially of GI tract) and open ulcerative wounds; extensive denudation of skin; ascorbic acid deficiency and other conditions causing increased capillary permeability; during or after brain, eye, or spinal cord surgery; during spinal tap or spinal anesthesia; during continuous tube drainage of stomach or small intestine; in subacute bacterial endocarditis; shock; advanced renal disease; threatened abortion; severe hypertension.

Although use of heparin is clearly hazardous in these conditions, its risk versus benefit must be evaluated.

• Use cautiously during menses; in patients with mild hepatic or renal disease, alcoholism, occupations with the risk of physical injury; immediately postpartum; and in patients with history of allergies, asthma, or GI ulcerations.

NURSING CONSIDERATIONS

• When the patient requires anticoagulation during pregnancy, most clinicians use heparin.

• Monitor platelet counts regularly. Thrombocytopenia caused by heparin may be associated with a type of arterial thrombosis known as "white clot" syndrome.

• Measure PTT carefully and regularly. Anticoagulation present when PTT values are one and one-half to two times control values.

• Drug requirements are higher in early phases of thrombogenic diseases and febrile states; lower when the patient's condition stabilizes.

• Regularly inspect the patient for bleeding gums, bruises on arms or legs, petechiae, nosebleeds, melena, tarry stools, hematuria, hematemesis. Tell the patient and his family to watch for these signs and notify the doctor immediately.

• Tell the patient to avoid OTC medications containing aspirin, other salicylates, or drugs that may interact with heparin.

• Heparin comes in various concentrations. Check order and vial carefully.

• Give low-dose injections sequentially between iliac crests in lower abdomen deep into S.C. fat. Inject drug S.C. slowly into fat pad. Leave needle in place for 10 seconds after injection; then withdraw needle. Don't massage after S.C. injection, and watch for signs of bleeding at injection site. Alternate sites every 12 hours – right for morning, left for evening.

• Avoid excessive I.M. injections of other drugs to prevent or minimize hematomas. If possible, don't give I.M. injections at all.

• **I.V. use:** I.V. administration using infusion pump to provide maximum safety preferred because of long-term effect and irregular absorption when given S.C. Check constant I.V. infusions regularly, even when pumps are in good working order, to prevent overdosage or underdosage. Place notice above the patient's bed to inform I.V. team or laboratory personnel to apply pressure dressings after taking blood.

• During intermittent I.V. therapy, always draw blood ½ hour before next scheduled dose to avoid falsely elevated PTT. Blood for PTT may be drawn any time after 8 hours of initiation of continuous I.V. heparin therapy. Blood for PTT should never be drawn from the I.V. tubing of the heparin infusion, or from the infused vein. Falsely elevated PTT will result. Always draw blood from the opposite arm.

- Do not skip a dose or "catch up" with an I.V. containing heparin. If I.V. is out, restart it as soon as possible and reschedule bolus dose immediately.
- Concentrated heparin solutions (greater than 100 units/ml) can irritate blood vessels.
- Elderly patients should usually start at lower doses.
- Never piggyback other drugs into an infusion line while the heparin infusion is running. Many antibiotics and other drugs deactivate heparin. Never mix any drug with heparin in syringe when bolus therapy is used.
- Abrupt withdrawal may cause increased coagulability, and heparin therapy is usually followed by oral anticoagulants for prophylaxis.
- To treat severe heparin calcium or heparin sodium overdose, use protamine sulfate, a heparin antagonist. Dosage is based on the dose of heparin, its route of administration, and the time elapsed since it was given. As a general rule, give 1 to 1.5 units of protamine/100 units of heparin if only a few minutes have elapsed; 0.5 to 0.75 mg protamine/100 units heparin if 30 to 60 minutes have elapsed, 0.25 to 0.375 mg protamine/100 units heparin if 2 hours or more have elapsed.

warfarin sodium

Coumadin, Sofarin, Warfilone Sodium†

Pregnancy Risk Category: D

HOW SUPPLIED

Tablets: 1 mg, 2 mg, 2.5 mg, 4 mg, 5 mg, 7.5 mg, 10 mg

ACTION

Mechanism: Inhibits vitamin K-dependent activation of clotting factors II, VII, IX, and X, formed in the liver.

Onset: 2 to 7 days. **Duration:** 3 to 7 days after discontinuation.

INDICATIONS & DOSAGE

Pulmonary embolism associated with deep vein thrombosis, M.I., rheumatic heart disease with heart valve damage, prosthetic heart valves, chronic atrial fibrillation –

Adults: 10 to 15 mg P.O. for 3 days, then based on daily PT. Usual maintenance dosage is 2 to 10 mg P.O. daily. Alternative regimen: initially, 40 to 60 mg P.O. as a single dose, or 20 to 30 mg for elderly or debilitated patients; then 2 to 10 mg daily based on PT.

ADVERSE REACTIONS

GI: paralytic ileus, intestinal obstruction (both resulting from hemorrhage), diarrhea, vomiting, cramps, nausea.

GU: excessive uterine bleeding.

Hematologic: ***hemorrhage with excessive dosage,*** eosinophilia, leukopenia.

Skin: dermatitis, urticaria, *rash,* necrosis, gangrene, alopecia.

Other: *fever,* hepatitis, jaundice.

INTERACTIONS

Acetaminophen: increased bleeding possible with chronic (greater than 2 weeks) high-dose acetaminophen therapy. Monitor very carefully.

Amiodarone, anabolic steroids, cephalosporins, chloramphenicol, cimetidine, ciprofloxacin, clofibrate, diflunisal, disulfiram, glucagon, heparin, methimazole, metronidazole, propylthiouracil, sulfinpyrazone, sulfonamides, sulindac, thyroid drugs, vitamin E: increased PT. Monitor the patient carefully for bleeding. Consider anticoagulant dosage reduction.

Barbiturates: inhibited hypoprothrombinemic effect of anticoagulants. If barbiturates are withdrawn, reduce anticoagulant dose; inhibition may last weeks after barbiturate is withdrawn, but fatal hemorrhage can occur when inhibition disappears.
Carbamazepine, ethchlorvynol, griseofulvin, paraldehyde, rifampin: decreased PT with reduced anticoagulant effect. Monitor the patient carefully.
Cholestyramine: decreased response when used too close together. Administer 6 hours after oral anticoagulants.
Chloral hydrate, glutethimide, triclofos sodium: increased or decreased PT. Avoid use if possible, or monitor the patient carefully.
Hydantoins: increased serum levels of hydantoins. Monitor closely.
Indomethacin, mefenamic acid, oxyphenbutazone, phenylbutazone, salicylates: increased PT; ulcerogenic effects. Don't use together.
Sulfonylureas (oral antidiabetic agents): increased hypoglycemic response. Monitor blood glucose levels.
Food and enteral products containing vitamin K: may impair anticoagulation. The patient should maintain consistent daily intake of leafy green vegetables.

CONTRAINDICATIONS

- Contraindicated in patients with bleeding or hemorrhagic tendencies resulting from open wounds, visceral cancer, GI ulcerations, severe hepatic or renal disease, severe uncontrolled hypertension, subacute bacterial endocarditis, polycythemia vera, vitamin K deficiency; and after recent eye, brain, or spinal cord surgery.
- Use cautiously in patients with diverticulitis, colitis, mild or moderate hypertension, mild or moderate hepatic or renal disease, with drainage tubes in any orifice; with regional or lumbar block anesthesia; or in any condition increasing risk of hemorrhage and during lactation.

NURSING CONSIDERATIONS

- Observe breast-feeding infants of patients on drug for unexpected bleeding.
- PT determinations essential for proper control. Doctors typically try to maintain PT at 1.5 to 2 times normal; high incidence of bleeding when PT exceeds 2.5 times control values.
- Give warfarin at same time daily. Stress importance of complying with prescribed dosage and follow-up appointments. The patient should carry a card that identifies him as a potential bleeder.
- Elderly patients and patients with renal or hepatic failure are especially sensitive to warfarin effect.
- Half-life of warfarin's anticoagulant effect is 36 to 44 hours. Effect can be neutralized by vitamin K injections.
- Regularly inspect the patient for bleeding gums, bruises on arms or legs, petechiae, nosebleeds, melena, tarry stools, hematuria, and hematemesis. Tell the patient and his family to watch for these signs and notify the doctor immediately if they occur.
- Warn the patient to avoid OTC products containing aspirin, other salicylates, or drugs that may interact with warfarin.
- Because onset of action is delayed, heparin sodium is often given during first few days of treatment. When heparin is being given simultaneously, blood for PT should not be drawn within 5 hours of intermittent I.V. heparin administration. However, blood for PT may be drawn at any time during continuous heparin infusion.
- Fever and skin rash signal severe adverse reactions. Withhold drug and call the doctor immediately.
- Tell the patient to notify the doctor if menses is heavier than usual; may require dosage adjustment.

• Tell the patient to use electric razor when shaving to avoid scratching skin and to use a soft toothbrush.
• Best oral anticoagulant for the patient taking antacids or phenytoin.
• Light to moderate alcohol intake does not significantly affect PT.
• Possibly effective in treatment of transient cerebral ischemic attacks.
• Food and enteral feedings that contain vitamin K may impair anticoagulation. Warn the patient to read labels.
• Tell the patient to eat a daily, consistent amount of leafy green vegetables, which contain vitamin K. Eating different amounts daily may alter anticoagulant effects.
• **I.V. use:** I.V. form rarely used and may be in periodic short supply. Reconstitute with sterile water for injection. Use immediately after reconstitution and discard any unused solution.

Hemostatics

absorbable gelatin sponge
microfibrillar collagen hemostat
oxidized cellulose
thrombin

COMBINATION PRODUCTS
None.

absorbable gelatin sponge

Gelfoam

Pregnancy Risk Category: C

HOW SUPPLIED
Sponges: 20 mm × 60 mm × 3 mm, 20 mm × 60 mm × 7 mm, 80 mm × 62.5 mm × 10 mm, 80 mm × 125 mm × 10 mm, 80 mm × 250 mm × 10 mm, 80 mm × 125 mm (compressed)
Packs: 40 cm × 2 cm, 40 cm × 6 cm
Dental packs: 10 mm × 20 mm × 7 mm, 20 mm × 20 mm × 7 mm
Prostatectomy cones: 13 cm (5″) diameter, 18 cm (7″) diameter

ACTION
Mechanism: Absorbs and holds many times its weight in blood, providing a framework for growth of granulation tissue.
Onset: immediate.

INDICATIONS & DOSAGE
Pressure ulcers –
Adults: place aseptically deep into wound. Don't disturb or remove; add extra p.r.n.
Hemostasis in surgery (adjunct) –
Adults: apply saturated with 0.9% sodium chloride or thrombin solution. Hold in place for 10 to 15 seconds. When oozing is controlled, allow material to remain in place.

ADVERSE REACTIONS
CNS: ***compression of brain or spinal cord,*** neurologic symptoms, headache, hearing loss.
Other: infection, giant cell granuloma, fever, ***toxic shock syndrome.***

INTERACTIONS
None significant.

CONTRAINDICATIONS
- Contraindicated in patients with frank infection, or postpartum bleeding or hemorrhage; also contraindicated as a sole hemostatic agent in abnormal bleeding.

NURSING CONSIDERATIONS
- Do not use to close skin incisions.
- Avoid overpacking when placed into body cavities or closed tissue spaces.
- Systemically absorbed within 4 to 6 weeks; no need to remove except when used in laminectomy procedures or when used to pack foramen in bone.

microfibrillar collagen hemostat

Avitene

Pregnancy Risk Category: C

HOW SUPPLIED
Nonwoven web: 70 mm × 70 mm × 1 mm, 70 mm × 35 mm × 1 mm
Fibrous form: 1-g, 5-g jars

ACTION
Mechanism: Attracts and aggregates platelets.
Onset: immediate.

INDICATIONS & DOSAGE
Hemostasis in surgery (adjunct) –
Adults and children: amount de-

pends on severity of bleeding. Compress area with dry sponges. Apply web or fibrous form directly to bleeding site for 1 to 5 minutes, gently removing excess. Reapply if needed.

ADVERSE REACTIONS
Hematologic: hematoma.
Other: exacerbation of wound dehiscence, abscess formation, foreign body reaction, adhesion formation, enhanced infection in contaminated wounds, mediastinitis, hypersensitivity reactions, allergic reactions.

INTERACTIONS
None significant.

CONTRAINDICATIONS
- Contraindicated in patients with closure of skin incisions; hemostat may interfere with healing. Do not use on bone surfaces where cement is needed to attach prostheses.

NURSING CONSIDERATIONS
- Don't spill on nonbleeding surfaces.
- Don't dilute. Always apply dry.
- Adheres to wet gloves, instruments, or tissue surfaces. Handle and apply with smooth, dry forceps. Apply directly to source of bleeding.
- Autoclaving inactivates product. Avoid ethylene oxide sterilization.

oxidized cellulose
Oxycel, Surgicel

Pregnancy Risk Category: C

HOW SUPPLIED
Pads: 3″ × 3″, 8 ply
Pledgets: 2″ × 1″ × 1″
Strips: ½ × 2″, ½ × 5″, ½ × 36″; 2″ × 3″, 2″ × 14″, 2″ × 18″; 4″ × 8″

ACTION
Mechanism: Absorbs and holds many times its weight in blood.
Onset: immediately on contact with blood.

INDICATIONS & DOSAGE
Hemostasis in surgery (adjunct); external bleeding at tumor sites –
Adults and children: apply loosely against bleeding surface with sterile technique, p.r.n. Remove after hemostasis, if possible, with dry sterile forceps. Leave in place if necessary.

ADVERSE REACTIONS
CNS: headache when used as packing for epistaxis, or after rhinologic procedures or application to surface wounds.
EENT: sneezing, epistaxis, stinging, or burning when used as packing for rhinologic procedures; nasal membrane necrosis or septal perforation.
GI: intestinal obstruction (when used in GI procedures).
GU: difficult urination (when used in GU procedures).
Other: encapsulation of fluid, foreign body reaction, burning or stinging after application to surface wounds, possible prolongation of drainage, ***intestinal obstruction following cholecystectomy.***

INTERACTIONS
Thrombin: may decrease blood clotting effectiveness.

CONTRAINDICATIONS
- Contraindicated in controlling hemorrhage from large arteries; for use on nonhemorrhagic, serous, oozing surfaces; in implantation in bone defects.

NURSING CONSIDERATIONS
- Don't pack or wad unless cellulose will be removed after hemostasis. Don't apply too tightly when used as wrap sheet in vascular surgery.
- Don't use for permanent packing in fractures because it may result in cyst formation.
- Always remove after hemostasis when used in laminectomies or near optic nerve chiasm.
- Don't autoclave this product.

• Use only amount needed to produce hemostasis, removing excess before surgical closure.
• Use minimal amounts in urologic procedures.
• In large wounds, don't overlap skin edges.
• Use sterile technique to remove from open wounds after hemostasis. Don't remove without irrigating material first; otherwise, fresh bleeding may occur.
• Don't moisten. Hemostatic effect is greater when applied dry.

thrombin

Thrombinar, Thrombostat‡

Pregnancy Risk Category: C

HOW SUPPLIED

Powder: 1,000-, 5,000-, 10,000-, and 20,000-unit vials
Kit: 10,000-unit or 20,000-unit with sprayer assembly

ACTION

Mechanism: Converts fibrinogen to fibrin.
Onset: immediate.

INDICATIONS & DOSAGE

Bleeding from parenchymatous tissue, cancellous bone, dental sockets, nasal and laryngeal surgery, and in plastic surgery and skin-grafting procedures –
Adults: apply 100 units/ml of sterile isotonic sodium chloride solution or sterile distilled water to area where clotting needed (or may apply dry powder in bone surgery); in major bleeding, apply 1,000 to 2,000 units/ml of sterile 0.9% sodium chloride solution. Sponge blood from area before application, but avoid sponging area after application.

ADVERSE REACTIONS

Other: hypersensitivity reactions and fever from systemic absorption.

INTERACTIONS

None significant.

CONTRAINDICATIONS

• Contraindicated in patients with hypersensitivity to thrombin or bovine products.
• Contraindicated as I.V. injection (of topical thrombin).

NURSING CONSIDERATIONS

• Obtain a patient history of reactions to thrombin or bovine products.
• Observe patient for allergic reactions, and monitor vital signs regularly.
• Have blood typed and crossmatched to treat possible hemorrhage.
• Injecting topical thrombin or allowing it to enter large blood vessels may cause death because of severe intravascular clotting.
• May be used with absorbable gelatin sponge but not with oxidized cellulose. Check sponge labeling before use.
• Neutralize stomach acids before oral use in GI hemorrhage.
• Keep refrigerated (preferably frozen) until ready to use. Unstable in solution. Store away from heat. Use solutions within 3 hours. Refrigerate excess solution at 2° to 8° C or freeze for up to 48 hours.
• Broken down by diluted acid, alkali, and salts of heavy metals.

67
Blood derivatives

albumin 5%
albumin 25%
antihemophilic factor
antithrombin III, human
factor IX complex
factor IX (human)
intravascular perfluorochemical emulsion
plasma protein fraction

COMBINATION PRODUCTS
None.

albumin 5%
Albuminar 5%, Albutein 5%, Buminate 5%, Plasbumin 5%

albumin 25%
Albuminar 25%, Albumisol 25%, Buminate 25%, Plasbumin 25%
Pregnancy Risk Category: C

HOW SUPPLIED
albumin 5%
Injection: 50-ml, 250-ml, 500-ml, 1,000-ml vials
albumin 25%
Injection: 10-ml, 20-ml, 50-ml, 100-ml vials

ACTION
Mechanism: Albumin 5% supplies colloid to the blood and expands plasma volume. Albumin 25% provides intravascular oncotic pressure in a 5:1 ratio, causing a fluid shift from interstitial spaces to the circulation and slightly increasing plasma protein concentration.
Peak: Serum levels peak immediately after I.V. infusion.

INDICATIONS & DOSAGE
Shock–
Adults: initially, 500 ml 5% solution by I.V. infusion, repeated q 30 minutes, p.r.n. Dosage varies with the patient's condition and response.
Children: 25% to 50% adult dose in nonemergency.
Burns–
Adults: 1,000 to 1,500 ml 5% solution by I.V. infusion daily, maximum rate 5 to 10 ml/minute; or 25 to 100 g 25% solution by I.V. infusion daily, maximum rate 3 ml/minute. Dosage varies with the patient's condition and response.
Hyperbilirubinemia–
Infants: 1 g albumin (4 ml 25%)/kg before transfusion.

ADVERSE REACTIONS
CV: ***vascular overload after rapid infusion,*** hypotension, altered pulse rate.
GI: increased salivation, nausea, vomiting.
Respiratory: altered respiration.
Skin: urticaria, rash.
Other: chills, fever.

INTERACTIONS
None significant.

CONTRAINDICATIONS
- Contraindicated in patients hypersensitive to the drug, and in patients with severe anemia or renal or heart failure.
- Use cautiously in patients with low cardiac reserve, no albumin deficiency, and on sodium restriction.

NURSING CONSIDERATIONS
- Do not give more than 250 g in 48 hours.
- Watch for hemorrhage or shock after surgery or injury. Rapid rise in blood pressure may cause bleeding

*Liquid form contains alcohol.
**May contain tartrazine.

Common reactions are in italics; ***life-threatening,*** in bold italics.

from sites that are not apparent at lower pressures.
- Monitor vital signs carefully.
- Watch for signs of vascular overload (heart failure or pulmonary edema).
- Properly hydrate the patient before solution infusion.
- This product is very expensive, and random supply shortages occur often. Take care when preparing and administering drug to minimize waste.
- Monitor fluid intake and output, hemoglobin, hematocrit, and serum protein and electrolytes during therapy.
- **I.V. use:** Avoid rapid I.V. infusion. Specific rate is individualized according to the patient's age, condition, and diagnosis. Dilute with sterile water for injection, 0.9% sodium chloride solution, or D_5W injection. Use solution promptly; contains no preservatives. Discard unused solution. Don't use cloudy solutions or those containing sediment. Solution should be clear amber color.
- Freezing may cause bottle to break. Follow storage instructions on bottle.
- One volume of 25% albumin is equivalent to five volumes of 5% albumin in producing hemodilution and relative anemia.

antihemophilic factor (AHF)

Hemofil M, Humate P, Hyate:C, Koate-HP, Koate-HS, Monoclate, Monoclate P, Profilate SD

Pregnancy Risk Category: C

HOW SUPPLIED
Injection: vials, with diluent. Units specified on label.

ACTION
Mechanism: Directly replaces deficient clotting factor.
Onset: coagulant levels rise immediately after I.V. infusion. **Duration:** plasma half-life, 9 to 15 hours in hemophiliacs.

INDICATIONS & DOSAGE
Spontaneous hemorrhage in patients with hemophilia A (factor VIII deficiency) –
Adults and children: calculate dosage using this formula:

$$\text{AHF required (IU)} = \text{body weight (kg)} \times \text{desired factor VIII increase (\% of normal)} \times 0.5$$

To prevent spontaneous hemorrhage, the desired level of factor VIII is 5% of normal; for mild hemorrhage, 30% of normal; for moderate hemorrhage and minor surgery, 30% to 50% of normal; for severe hemorrhage, 80% to 100% of normal.
Treatment of bleeding in patients with hemophilia A (factor VIII deficiency) –
Adults and children: For minor hemorrhage into muscle and joints, 8 to 10 IU/kg I.V q 8 to 12 hours for 1 or more days. For overt bleeding, give an initial dose of 15 to 25 IU/kg I.V., followed by 8 to 15 IU/kg q 8 to 12 hours for 3 to 4 days. To treat massive bleeding or hemorrhage involving major organs, follow an initial dose of 40 to 50 IU/kg I.V. by 20 to 25 IU/kg I.V. q 8 to 12 hours.
Prevention of bleeding in hemophilic patients requiring surgery –
Adults: 25 to 30 IU/kg I.V. one hour before surgery, followed by one-half of the initial dosage 5 hours later. Dosage should be adjusted to achieve a level of AHF 80% to 100% of normal during surgery.

ADVERSE REACTIONS
CNS: headache, paresthesia, clouding or loss of consciousness, somnolence, lethargy.
CV: tachycardia, hypotension, ***hemolysis*** in patients with blood type A, B, or AB.
EENT: visual disturbances.
GI: nausea, vomiting.
Skin: erythema, *urticaria.*
Other: *chills, fever, backache, flush-*

ing, chest constriction, ***hypersensitivity reactions,*** rigor, stinging at injection site.

INTERACTIONS
None significant.

CONTRAINDICATIONS
• Use cautiously in neonates, infants, and patients with hepatic disease because of susceptibility to hepatitis, which may be transmitted in antihemophilic factor.
• Some patients develop inhibitors to factor VIII, resulting in decreased response to the drug.

NURSING CONSIDERATIONS
• Monitor vital signs regularly.
• A new porcine product is now available for patients with congenital hemophilia A who have antibodies to human factor VIII:C.
• **I.V. use:** Use plastic syringe; drug may interact with glass syringe and bind to its surface. Take baseline pulse rate before I.V. administration. If pulse rate increases significantly, flow rate should be reduced or administration stopped.
• Do not use S.C. or I.M.
• Monitor the patient for allergic reactions.
• Refrigerate concentrate until ready to use. Warm concentrate and diluent bottles to room temperature before reconstituting. To mix drug, gently roll vial between hands.
• Reconstituted solution unstable; use within 3 hours. Store away from heat and do not refrigerate. Refrgeration after reconstitution may cause the active ingredient to precipitate. Don't shake or mix with other I.V. solutions.
• Monitor coagulation studies before and during therapy.
• As ordered, administer hepatitis B vaccine before administering antihemophilic factor.
• Risk of hepatitis, including non-A and non-B hepatitis, must be weighed against risk of the patient not receiving the drug.
• Because of the manufacturing process, the risk of HIV transmission is extremely low.

antithrombin III, human (AT-III, heparin cofactor I)

ATnativ

Pregnancy Risk Category: C

HOW SUPPLIED
Injection: 500 IU

ACTION
Mechanism: Replaces deficient AT-III in patients with hereditary AT-III deficiency, normalizing coagulation inhibition and inhibiting thromboembolism formation. Also deactivates plasmin (to lesser extent than the clotting factor).
Duration: about 4 days.

INDICATIONS & DOSAGE
Thromboembolism associated with hereditary AT-III deficiency –
Adults and children: initial dose is individualized to quantity required to increase AT-III activity to 120% of normal activity as determined 30 minutes after administration. Usual dose is 50 to 100 IU/minute I.V., not to exceed 100 IU/minute. Dose is calculated based on anticipated 1% increase in plasma AT-III activity produced by 1 IU/kg of body weight using the formula:

$$\text{Dose (Units)} = \frac{(\text{desired activity [\%]} - \text{baseline activity [\%]}) \times \text{weight (kg)}}{1\%\ (\text{IU/kg})}$$

Maintenance dosage is individualized to quantity required to increase AT-III activity to 80% of normal activity and is administered at 24-hour intervals.

To calculate the dosage, multiply the desired AT-III activity (as % of normal) minus the baseline AT-III activity (as % of normal) by body weight (in kg). Divide by actual increase in AT-III activity (in %) produced by 1 IU/kg as determined 30 minutes after administration of initial dose.

Treatment is usually continued for 2 to 8 days but may be prolonged in pregnancy or when used with surgery or immobilization.

ADVERSE REACTIONS
CV: vasodilation, lowered blood pressure.
GU: diuresis.

INTERACTIONS
Heparin: increased anticoagulant effect of both drugs. Heparin dosage reduction may be necessary.

CONTRAINDICATIONS
- Use with extreme caution in children and neonates because safety and efficacy have not been established.
- Use drug cautiously. It is prepared from pooled plasma from human donors, and carries with it a minimal risk of transmission of viruses, including hepatitis and HIV.

NURSING CONSIDERATIONS
- Not recommended for long-term prophylaxis of thrombotic episodes.
- Because of the risk of neonatal thromboembolism (sometimes fatal) in children of parents with hereditary AT-III deficiency, AT-III levels should be measured immediately after birth.
- Determinations of AT-III activity should be performed twice daily until the dosage requirement has stabilized, then daily immediately before dose. Functional assays are preferred because quantitative immunologic test results may be normal despite decreased AT-III activity.
- One IU is equivalent to the quantity of endogenous AT-III present in 1 ml of normal human plasma.
- Dyspnea and increased blood pressure may occur if administration rate is too rapid (1,500 IU in 5 minutes).
- Heparin binds to AT-III lysine binding sites, resulting in increased efficacy of heparin.
- **I.V. use:** Reconstitute using 10 ml of sterile water (provided), 0.9% sodium chloride solution, or D_5W. *Do not shake vial.* Dilute further in same diluent solution if desired.
- Store at 36° to 46° F (2° to 8° C).

factor IX complex
Bebulin VH Immuno, Konyne-80, Proplex T

factor IX (human)
AlphaNine, AlphaNine-SD, Mononine

Pregnancy Risk Category: C

HOW SUPPLIED
Injection: vials, with diluent. Units specified on label.

ACTION
Mechanism: Directly replaces deficient clotting factor.
Duration: half-life, 23 to 31 hours.

INDICATIONS & DOSAGE
Factor IX deficiency (hemophilia B or Christmas disease), anticoagulant overdosage –
Adults and children: units required equal 0.8 to 1 × body weight in kg × percentage of desired increase of factor IX level, by slow I.V. infusion or I.V. push. Dosage is highly individualized, depending on degree of deficiency, level of factor IX desired, weight of the patient, and severity of bleeding.

ADVERSE REACTIONS
CNS: somnolence, lethargy, headache.
CV: ***thromboembolic reactions; MI; disseminated intravascular coagulation; pulmonary embolism;*** possible

hemolysis in patients with blood types A, B, or AB; changes in blood pressure or heart rate.
GI: nausea, vomiting.
Skin: urticaria.
Other: *transient fever, chills, flushing, tingling, hypersensitivity reactions **(anaphylaxis)**.*

INTERACTIONS

Aminocaproic acid: increased risk of thrombosis. Avoid concomitant use.

CONTRAINDICATIONS

- Contraindicated in patients with hepatic disease, intravascular coagulation, or fibrinolysis.
- Use cautiously in neonates and infants because of susceptibility to hepatitis, which may be transmitted with factor IX complex.

NURSING CONSIDERATIONS

- Observe the patient for allergic reactions, and monitor vital signs regularly.
- Risk of hepatitis, including non-A and non-B hepatitis, must be weighed against risk of not receiving the drug.
- Because of the manufacturing process, the risk of HIV transmission is extremely low.
- As ordered, administer hepatitis B vaccine before administering factor IX complex.
- **I.V. use:** Avoid rapid infusion. If tingling sensation, fever, chills, or headache develops, decrease flow rate and notify the doctor.
- Reconstitute with 20 ml of sterile water for injection for each vial of lyophilized drug. Keep refrigerated until ready to use; warm to room temperature before reconstituting. Use within 3 hours of reconstitution. Unstable in solution. Don't shake, refrigerate, or mix solution with other I.V. solutions. Store away from heat.

intravascular perfluorochemical emulsion

Fluosol

Pregnancy Risk Category: B

HOW SUPPLIED

Injection: 20% emulsion; supplied in kit form with additive solutions (1 and 2) and materials to provide continuous oxygenation

ACTION

Mechanism: An emulsion of synthetic perfluorochemicals that acts as an oxygen carrier.
Duration: half-life, dose dependant; traces of perfluochemicals can persist for 3 months or longer.

INDICATIONS & DOSAGE

To prevent or decrease myocardial ischemia during percutaneous transluminal coronary angioplasty (PTCA) in patients at high risk for ischemic complications of angioplasty (including patients with a low baseline ejection fraction, patients with large areas of the myocardium at risk, patients with recent MI, and patients with unstable angina or refractory angina requiring hospitalization) –
Adults: withdraw a test dose of 0.5 ml from the prepared solution and injected into a peripheral vein. If no adverse reactions occur within 10 minutes, warmed, oxygenated emulsion may be administered by intracoronary injection at a rate of 60 to 90 ml/minute. Administer through the central lumen of an angioplasty balloon catheter without removing the guide wire. Use an angiographic power injector with a warming jacket.

ADVERSE REACTIONS

CV: ***ventricular tachycardia or fibrillation,*** bradycardia, chest discomfort, hypotension.

Respiratory: dyspnea, increased respiratory rate, coughing.
Skin: mild pruritus.

INTERACTIONS

Anesthetics: may prolong action of lipid-soluble anesthetics. Monitor the patient carefully.
Hepatotoxic agents: may enhance hepatotoxic effects of hepatotoxic agents. Monitor the patient closely.

CONTRAINDICATIONS

- Contraindicated in patients with hypersensitivity to any components of the compound and in those with functionally critical secondary stenosis in areas distal to the site of the lesion being treated.
- Use cautiously in asplenic patients because drug may accumulate.

NURSING CONSIDERATIONS

- Because this drug reportedly accumulates in the body after repeated dosage, it should not be given more than once every 6 months.
- Drug should be administered only by doctors familiar with PTCA. Follow institutional policy regarding emergency surgical procedures for coronary artery bypass graft surgery.
- Do not add anything other than solutions 1 and 2 or carbogen gas (95% oxygen, 5% carbon dioxide) to the emulsion. Do not oxygenate with 100% oxygen because this will adversely affect the solution's final pH.
- Allow more than 4 minutes of perfusion time when used with an angiographic power injector reservoir of 260 ml and a flow rate of 60 ml/minute. Perfusion time should be limited by the patient's tolerance and the doctor's judgment.
- In the unlikely event that the patient reacts adversely to the test dose (1.2% of patients in clinical trials reacted), do not give the drug. Severe reactions can be managed with methylprednisolone or diphenhydramine.
- Breast-feeding is not recommended because drug is excreted in breast milk.
- **I.V. use:** Do not use an in-line filter when administering because it may damage the emulsion. Never administer any solution that shows evidence of emulsion separation.
- Oxygenate the emulsion and warm to approximately 98.6° F (37° C) before administration. Infusion of solutions at room temperature has been associated with ventricular fibrillation.
- Store the container of intravascular perfluorochemical emulsion in the freezer (between 23° and −22° F [−5° and −30° C]). Do not use emulsions that appear to have partially thawed during storage. Use a warming cabinet or water bath set at 98.6° F to thaw the solution, not a microwave oven, because this may cause uneven heating of the solution. Allow at least 30 minutes for thawing of the solution. Do not refreeze thawed solutions, and use within 8 hours.
- The additive solutions (solutions 1 and 2) should not be frozen; store at room temperature not exceeding 86° F (30° C).

plasma protein fraction

Plasmanate, Plasma-Plex, Plasmatein, Protenate

Pregnancy Risk Category: C

HOW SUPPLIED

Injection: 5% solution in 50-ml, 250-ml, 500-ml vials

ACTION

Mechanism: Supplies colloid to the blood and expands plasma volume.
Peak: Serum levels peak immediately after I.V. infusion.

INDICATIONS & DOSAGE

Shock –
Adults: varies with the patient's con-

dition and response, but usual dose is 250 to 500 ml I.V. (12.5 to 25 g protein), usually no faster than 10 ml/minute.
Children: 22 to 33 ml/kg I.V., 5 to 10 ml/minute.
Hypoproteinemia –
Adults: 1,000 to 1,500 ml I.V. daily. Maximum infusion rate is 8 ml/minute.

ADVERSE REACTIONS

CNS: headache.
CV: various effects on blood pressure after rapid infusion or intraarterial administration; ***vascular overload after rapid infusion.***
GI: nausea, vomiting, hypersalivation.
Skin: erythema, urticaria.
Other: flushing, chills, fever, back pain, dyspnea.

INTERACTIONS

None significant.

CONTRAINDICATIONS

- Contraindicated in patients with severe anemia or heart failure, and in those undergoing cardiac bypass.
- Use cautiously in patients with hepatic or renal failure, low cardiac reserve, and restricted sodium intake.

NURSING CONSIDERATIONS

- Monitor blood pressure. Infusion should be slowed or stopped if hypotension suddenly occurs. Vital signs should return to normal gradually; monitor hourly.
- Watch for signs of vascular overload (heart failure or pulmonary edema).
- Monitor intake and output. Watch for and report decreased urine output.
- **I.V. use:** Check expiration date before using. Don't use solutions that are cloudy, contain sediment, or have been frozen. Discard solutions in containers opened for more than 4 hours because it contains no preservatives.
- If the patient is dehydrated, give additional fluids either P.O. or I.V.
- Do not give more than 250 g or 5,000 mls in 48 hours.
- Contains 130 to 160 mEq sodium/L.

*Liquid form contains alcohol.
**May contain tartrazine.

Common reactions are in italics; ***life-threatening,*** in bold italics.

68
Thrombolytic enzymes

alteplase
anistreplase
streptokinase
urokinase

COMBINATION PRODUCTS
None.

alteplase (tissue plasminogen activator, recombinant; t-PA)
Actilyse‡, Activase

Pregnancy Risk Category: C

HOW SUPPLIED
Injection: 20-mg (11.6 million-IU), 50-mg (29 million-IU) vials

ACTION
Mechanism: Binds to fibrin in a thrombus, and locally converts plasminogen to plasmin, which initiates local fibrinolysis.
Peak: Peak effects occur in about 45 minutes. **Duration:** 6 hours to 2 days.

INDICATIONS & DOSAGE
Lysis of thrombi obstructing coronary arteries in acute MI –
Adults: 100 mg I.V. infusion over 3 hours as follows: 60 mg in the first hour, of which 6 to 10 mg is given as a bolus over the first 1 to 2 minutes. Then 20 mg/hr infusion for 2 hours. Smaller adults (< 65 kg) should receive 1.25 mg/kg in a similar fashion (60% in the first hour, 10% as a bolus; then 20% of the total dose per hour for 2 hours).
Management of acute massive pulmonary embolism –
Adults: 100 mg I.V. infusion over 2 hours. Begin heparin at the end of the infusion when PTT or PT returns to twice normal or less.

Do not exceed 100-mg dose. Higher doses may increase risk of intracranial bleeding.

ADVERSE REACTIONS
CNS: ***cerebral hemorrhage,*** fever.
CV: hypotension, arrhythmias, edema.
GI: nausea, vomiting.
Hematologic: ***severe, spontaneous bleeding (cerebral, retroperitoneal, GU, GI).***
Other: bleeding at puncture sites, hypersensitivity reactions ***(anaphylaxis),*** urticaria, arthralgias.

INTERACTIONS
Aspirin, coumarin anticoagulants, dipyridamole, heparin: increased risk of bleeding. Monitor the patient carefully.

CONTRAINDICATIONS
- Contraindicated in patients with active internal bleeding, intracranial neoplasm, arteriovenous malformation, aneurysm, and severe uncontrolled hypertension. Also contraindicated in patients with a history of CVA, recent (within 2 months) intraspinal or intracranial trauma or surgery, or known bleeding diathesis.
- Use cautiously in patients with recent (within 10 days) major surgery; in pregnancy and first 10 days postpartum; organ biopsy; trauma (including cardiopulmonary resuscitation); GI or GU bleeding; cerebrovascular disease; hypertension (systolic ≥ 180 mm Hg or diastolic ≥ 110 mm Hg); mitral stenosis, atrial fibrillation, or other condition that may lead to left heart thrombus; acute pericarditis or subacute bacterial endocarditis; septic thrombophlebitis; diabetic hemorrhagic retinopathy; in

patients receiving anticoagulants; and in patients age 75 and older.

NURSING CONSIDERATIONS

- Coronary thrombolysis is associated with arrhythmias induced by reperfusion of ischemic myocardium. Such arrhythmias do not differ from those commonly associated with MI. Have antiarrhythmic agents readily available, and carefully monitor ECG.
- Recanalization of occluded coronary arteries and improvement of heart function require initiation of treatment with alteplase as soon as possible after the onset of symptoms.
- Bleeding is the most common adverse effect and may occur internally and at external puncture sites. Avoid invasive procedures during thrombolytic therapy. Carefully monitor the patient for signs of internal bleeding and frequently check all puncture sites.
- Heparin therapy is frequently initiated after treatment with alteplase to decrease the risk of rethrombosis.
- **I.V. use:** Reconstitute drug with sterile water for injection (without preservatives) only. Do not use vial if the vacuum is not present. Reconstitute with a large-bore (18G) needle, directing the stream of sterile water at the lyophilized cake. Do not shake. Slight foaming is common, and solution should be clear or pale yellow.
- Drug may be administered as reconstituted (1 mg/ml) or diluted with an equal volume of 0.9% sodium chloride solution or D_5W to make a 0.5 mg/ml solution. Adding other drugs to the infusion is not recommended.
- Reconstitute alteplase solution immediately before use, and administer it within 8 hours because it contains no preservatives. The drug may be temporarily stored at 35° to 86° F (2° to 30° C), but it is only stable for 8 hours at room temperature. Discard any unused solution.
- Studies are underway to determine the best dosage regimen. Accelerated infusion revealed that a modified alteplase regimen was superior to streptokinase or streptokinase plus alteplase in reducing mortality following MI. In this modified regimen, the 100-mg dose is administered over 90 minutes, with two-thirds of the dose given in the first 30 minutes. Because of a slightly higher incidence of stroke, it is too early to recommend this protocol for all patients.

anistreplase (anisoylated plasminogen-streptokinase activator complex; APSAC)

Eminase

Pregnancy Risk Category: C

HOW SUPPLIED

Injection: 30 units/vial

ACTION

Mechanism: Anistreplase, derived from Lys-plasminogen and streptokinase, is formulated into a fibrinolytic enzyme plus activator complex with the activator temporarily blocked by an anisoyl group. The drug is activated in vivo by a nonenzymatic process that removes the anisoyl group. The active Lys-plasminogen-streptokinase activator complex is progressively formed in the bloodstream or within the thrombus.

Peak: Peak effects occur in about 45 minutes. **Duration:** 6 hours to 2 days.

INDICATIONS & DOSAGE

Lysis of cornary artery thrombi following acute MI –

Adults: 30 units I.V. over 2 to 5 minutes. Administer by direct injection.

ADVERSE REACTIONS

CNS: ***intracranial hemorrhage.***

CV: arrhythmias, conduction disorders, hypotension, edema.

EENT: hemoptysis, gum or mouth hemorrhage.

GI: ***bleeding.***
GU: hematuria.
Hematologic: ***bleeding tendency,*** eosinophilia.
Skin: hematomas, urticaria, itching, flushing, delayed (2 weeks after therapy) purpuric rash.
Other: bleeding at puncture sites, ***anaphylaxis or anaphylactoid reactions (rare),*** arthralgias.

INTERACTIONS

Heparin, oral anticoagulants, drugs that alter platelet function (including aspirin and dipyridamole): may increase the risk of bleeding. Use together cautiously.

CONTRAINDICATIONS

• Contraindicated in patients with a history of severe allergic reaction to anistreplase or streptokinase; active internal bleeding, CVA, recent (within the past 2 months) intraspinal or intracranial surgery or trauma, aneurysm, arteriovenous malformation, intracranial neoplasm, uncontrolled hypertension, or known bleeding diathesis.
• Use cautiously in patients with recent (within 10 days) major surgery; trauma (including cardiopulmonary resuscitation); GI or GU bleeding; cerebrovascular disease; hypertension (systolic ≥180 mm Hg or diastolic ≥110 mm Hg); mitral stenosis, atrial fibrillation, or other conditions that may lead to left heart thrombus; acute pericarditis or subacute bacterial endocarditis; septic thrombophlebitis; diabetic hemorrhagic retinopathy; in pregnancy and first 10 days postpartum; in patients receiving anticoagulants; and in patients 75 years and older.

NURSING CONSIDERATIONS

• Thrombolytic therapy is associated with reperfusion arrhythmias that may signify successful thrombolysis. These arrhythmias are similar to those seen in the course of an acute MI and may include sinus bradycardia, accelerated idioventricular rhythm, ventricular tachycardia, or premature ventricular depolarizations. Be prepared to treat bradycardia or ventricular irritability during anistreplase therapy. Carefully monitor ECG during treatment with anistreplase.
• Anistreplase is derived from human plasma. No cases of hepatitis or HIV infection have been reported to date. The manufacturing process is designed to purify the plasma used in the preparation of the drug.
• Bleeding is the most common adverse reaction and may occur internally and at external puncture sites. Carefully monitor the patient.
• Heparin therapy is frequently initiated after treatment with anistreplase to decrease the risk of rethrombosis.
• Teach the patient signs of internal bleeding, and tell him to report these immediately. Advise the patient about proper dental care to avoid excessive gum trauma.
• **I.V. use:** Unlike other thrombolytics that must be infused, anistreplase is given by direct injection over 2 to 5 minutes.
• Reconstitute the drug by slowly adding 5 ml of sterile water for injection. Direct the stream against the side of the vial, not at the drug itself. Gently roll the vial to mix the dry powder and water. To avoid excessive foaming, don't shake the vial. The reconstituted solution should be colorless to pale yellow. Inspect for precipitate. If the drug is not administered within 30 minutes of reconstituting, discard the vial.
• Do not mix the drug with other medications; do not dilute the solution after reconstitution.
• In-vitro coagulation tests will be affected by the presence of anistreplase. This can be attenuated if blood sam-

ples are collected in the presence of aprotinin (150 to 200 units/ml).
• Efficacy of drug may be limited if atistreptokinase antibodies are present. Antibody levels may be elevated if more than 5 days has elapsed since previous treatment with anistreplase or streptokinase, or if the patient has had a recent streptococcal infection.

streptokinase

Kabikinase, Streptase

Pregnancy Risk Category: C

HOW SUPPLIED

Injection: 100,000 IU, 250,000 IU, 600,000 IU, 750,000 IU, 1,500,000 IU in vials for reconstitution

ACTION

Mechanism: Activates plasminogen in two steps: Plasminogen and streptokinase form a complex that exposes the plasminogen-activating site; plasminogen is then converted to plasmin by cleavage of the peptide bond.
Peak: Peak effects occur in 20 minutes to 2 hours. **Duration:** 6 to 24 hours; half-life of activator complex, 23 minutes.

INDICATIONS & DOSAGE

Arteriovenous cannula occlusion –
Adults: 250,000 IU in 2 ml I.V. solution by I.V. pump infusion into each occluded limb of the cannula over 25 to 35 minutes. Clamp off cannula for 2 hours. Then aspirate contents of cannula; flush with sodium chloride solution and reconnect.
Venous thrombosis, pulmonary embolism, and arterial thrombosis and embolism –
Adults: loading dose is 250,000 IU I.V. infusion over 30 minutes. Sustaining dose is 100,000 IU/hour I.V. infusion for 72 hours for deep vein thrombosis and 100,000 IU/hour over 24 to 72 hours by I.V. infusion pump for pulmonary embolism.
Lysis of coronary artery thrombi following acute MI –
Adults: 140,000 units administered as a loading dose followed by maintenance infusion. Loading dose is 20,000 IU via coronary catheter, followed by infusion of maintenance dose of 2,000 IU/minute for 60 minutes. Alternatively, may be administered as an I.V. infusion. Usual adult dose is 1.5 million units infused over 60 minutes.

ADVERSE REACTIONS

CNS: polyradiculoneuropathy.
CV: transient lowering or elevation of blood pressure, reperfusion arrhythmias.
EENT: periorbital edema.
Hematologic: ***bleeding,*** low hematocrit.
Respiratory: minor breathing difficulty, ***bronchospasm.***
Skin: urticaria, pruritus, flushing.
Other: phlebitis at injection site, hypersensitivity reactions ***(anaphylaxis),*** delayed hypersensitivity reactions (interstitial nephritis, vasculitits, serum sickness-like reactions), musculoskeletal pain, ***angioedema,*** fever.

INTERACTIONS

Anticoagulants: increased risk of bleeding. Monitor the patient closely.
Aspirin, dipyridamole, indomethacin, phenylbutazone, drugs affecting platelet activity: increased risk of bleeding. Monitor patients closely. Combined therapy with low-dose aspirin (162.5 mg) or dipyridamole has improved acute and long-term results.

CONTRAINDICATIONS

• Contraindicated in patients with ulcerative wounds, active internal bleeding, and recent CVA; recent trauma with possible internal injuries; visceral or intracranial malignant neoplasms; ulcerative colitis; diverticulitis; severe hypertension; acute or chronic hepatic or renal insufficiency;

uncontrolled hypocoagulation; chronic pulmonary disease with cavitation; subacute bacterial endocarditis or rheumatic valvular disease; recent cerebral embolism, thrombosis, or hemorrhage.

• Also contraindicated within 10 days after intra-arterial diagnostic procedure or any surgery, including liver or kidney biopsy, lumbar puncture, thoracentesis, paracentesis, or extensive or multiple cutdowns.

• I.M. injections and other invasive procedures are contraindicated during streptokinase therapy.

• Use cautiously when treating arterial embolism that originates from left side of heart because of danger of cerebral infarction.

NURSING CONSIDERATIONS

• Before initiating therapy, draw blood to determine PTT and PT. Rate of I.V. infusion depends on thrombin time and streptokinase resistance.

• If the patient has had either a recent streptococcal infection or recent treatment with streptokinase, a higher loading dose may be necessary.

• **I.V. use:** Reconstitute each vial with 5 ml of 0.9% sodium chloride solution for injection. Further dilute to 45 ml. Don't shake; roll gently to mix. Some flocculation may be present after reconstituting; discard if large amounts are present. Filter solution with 0.8 micron or larger filter. Use within 24 hours. Store powder at room temperature and refrigerate after reconstitution.

• Monitor the patient for excessive bleeding every 15 minutes for the first hour, every 30 minutes for the second through eighth hours, then once every shift. If bleeding is evident, stop therapy. Pretreatment with heparin or drugs affecting platelets causes high risk of bleeding, but may improve long-term results. Monitor closely.

• Monitor pulses, color, and sensation of extremities every hour.

• Have typed and crossmatched packed red cells and whole blood ready to treat possible hemorrhage.

• Keep aminocaproic acid available to treat bleeding, and corticosteroids to treat allergic reactions.

• Before using streptokinase to clear an occluded arteriovenous cannula, try flushing with heparinized sodium chloride solution.

• Bruising more likely during therapy; avoid unnecessary handling of patients. Side rails should be padded.

• Maintain the involved extremity in straight alignment to prevent bleeding from the infusion site.

• Keep venipuncture sites to a minimum; use pressure dressing on puncture sites for at least 15 minutes.

• Keep a laboratory flow sheet on the patient's chart to monitor PTT, PT, and hemoglobin and hematocrit levels.

• To check for hypersensitivity reactions, give 100 IU intradermally; a wheal and flare response within 20 minutes means the patient is probably allergic. Monitor vital signs frequently.

• Watch for signs of hypersensitivity. Notify the doctor immediately. Antihistamines or corticosteroids may be used to treat mild allergic reactions. If a severe reaction occurs, the infusion should be stopped immediately.

• Heparin by continuous infusion is usually started within an hour after stopping streptokinase. Use infusion pump to administer heparin.

• Only doctors with wide experience in thrombotic disease management where clinical and laboratory monitoring can be performed should use streptokinase.

• Thrombolytic therapy in patients with acute MI may decrease infarct size, improve ventricular function, and decrease incidence of CHF. Streptokinase must be administered within 6 hours of the onset of symptoms for optimal effect.

urokinase

Abbokinase, Open-Cath, Ukidan‡, Win-Kinase

Pregnancy Risk Category: B

HOW SUPPLIED

Injection: 5,000 units (IU) per unit-dose vial; 9,000 units (IU) per unit-dose vial; 250,000-IU vial

ACTION

Mechanism: Activates plasminogen by directly cleaving peptide bonds at two different sites.
Peak: Peak effects occur in 20 minutes to 2 hours. **Duration:** 6 to 24 hours.

INDICATIONS & DOSAGE

Lysis of acute massive pulmonary embolism and lysis of pulmonary embolism accompanied by unstable hemodynamics –
Adults: for I.V. infusion only by constant infusion pump delivering total volume of 195 ml.
Priming dose: 4,400 IU/kg of urokinase-0.9% sodium chloride solution admixture given over 10 minutes. Follow with 4,400 IU/kg hourly for 12 to 24 hours. Total volume should not exceed 200 ml. Follow therapy with continuous I.V. infusion of heparin, then oral anticoagulants.
Coronary artery thrombosis –
Adults: after a bolus dose of heparin ranging from 2,500 to 10,000 units, infuse 6,000 IU/minute of urokinase into the occluded artery for up to 2 hours. Average total dosage is 500,000 IU.
Venous catheter occlusion –
Adults: Instill 5,000 IU into occluded line, wait 5 minutes, then aspirate. Repeat aspiration attempts q 5 minutes for 30 minutes. If not patent after 30 minutes, cap line and let urokinase work for 30 to 60 minutes before aspirating again. May require second instillation.

ADVERSE REACTIONS

Hematologic: ***bleeding,*** low hematocrit.
Respiratory: bronchospasm.
Other: phlebitis at injection site, hypersensitivity reactions ***(anaphylaxis),*** musculoskeletal pain, fever.

INTERACTIONS

Anticoagulants: increased risk of bleeding. Monitor the patient closely.
Aspirin, dipyridamole, indomethacin, phenylbutazone, other drugs affecting platelet activity: increased risk of bleeding.

CONTRAINDICATIONS

- Contraindicated in patients with ulcerative wounds, active internal bleeding, and cerebrovascular accident; aneurysm; arteriovenous malformation; known bleeding diathesis, recent trauma with possible internal injuries; visceral or intracranial malignancy; pregnancy and first 10 days postpartum; ulcerative colitis; diverticulitis; severe hypertension; acute or chronic hepatic or renal insufficiency; uncontrolled hypocoagulation; chronic pulmonary disease with cavitation; subacute bacterial endocarditis or rheumatic valvular disease; and recent cerebral embolism, thrombosis, or hemorrhage.
- Also contraindicated within 10 days after intra-arterial diagnostic procedure or any surgery (liver or kidney biopsy, lumbar puncture, thoracentesis, paracentesis, or extensive or multiple cutdowns); intracranial or intraspinal surgery in the past 2 months.
- I.M. injections and other invasive procedures are contraindicated during urokinase therapy.

NURSING CONSIDERATIONS

- Maintain the involved extremity in straight alignment to prevent bleeding from the infusion site.
- Monitor the patient for excessive bleeding every 15 minutes for the first

hour; every 30 minutes for the second through eighth hours; then once every shift. Pretreatment with drugs affecting platelets places patient at high risk of bleeding.

• Instruct the patient to report symptoms of bleeding.
• Although the incidence of hypersensitivity reactions is low, watch for signs of this reaction.
• Monitor pulses, color, and sensation of extremities every hour.
• Have typed and crossmatched red cells, whole blood, and aminocaproic acid available to treat bleeding, and corticosteroids to treat allergic reactions.
• Keep a laboratory flow sheet on the patient's chart to monitor PTT, PT, and hemoglobin and hematocrit levels.
• Monitor vital signs.
• Keep venipuncture sites to a minimum; use pressure dressing on puncture sites for at least 15 minutes.
• Heparin by continuous infusion is usually started within an hour after urokinase has been stopped to prevent recurrent thrombosis.
• Bruising is more likely during therapy; avoid unnecessary handling of the patient. Side rails should be padded.
• **I.V. use:** Add 5 ml of sterile water for injection to vial. Dilute further with 0.9% sodium chloride solution or D_5W solution before infusion. The total volume of fluid administered should not exceed 200 ml. Don't use bacteriostatic water for injection to reconstitute; it contains preservatives.

69
Alkylating agents

busulfan
carboplatin
carmustine
chlorambucil
cisplatin
cyclophosphamide
dacarbazine
ifosfamide
lomustine
mechlorethamine hydrochloride
melphalan
pipobroman
streptozocin
thiotepa
uracil mustard

COMBINATION PRODUCTS
None.

busulfan
Myleran
Pregnancy Risk Category: D

HOW SUPPLIED
Tablets: 2 mg

ACTION
Mechanism: Cross-links strands of cellular DNA and interferes with RNA transcription, causing an imbalance of growth that leads to cell death. Cell cycle-nonspecific.
Onset: 1 to 2 weeks. **Duration:** half-life, about 2½ hours.

INDICATIONS & DOSAGE
Chronic myelocytic (granulocytic) leukemia –
Adults: 4 to 8 mg P.O. daily up to 12 mg P.O. daily until WBC count falls to 15,000/mm³; stop drug until WBC count rises to 50,000/mm³, and then resume treatment as before; or 4 to 8 mg P.O. daily until WBC count falls to 10,000 to 20,000/mm³, and then reduce daily dosage as needed to maintain WBC count at this level (usually 2 mg daily).
Children: 0.06 to 0.12 mg/kg/day or 1.8 to 4.6 mg/m²/day P.O.; adjust dosage to maintain WBC count at 20,000/mm³, but never less than 10,000/mm³.

ADVERSE REACTIONS
CNS: ***seizures,*** unusual tiredness or weakness.
GI: nausea, vomiting, diarrhea, cheilosis, glossitis.
GU: amenorrhea, testicular atrophy, impotence.
Hematologic: WBC count falling after about 10 days and continuing to fall for 2 weeks after stopping drug; ***thrombocytopenia, anemia.***
Respiratory: persistent cough; dyspnea; ***irreversible pulmonary fibrosis, commonly termed "busulfan lung."***
Skin: transient hyperpigmentation, rash, urticaria, anhidrosis.
Other: gynecomastia, alopecia, Addison-like wasting syndrome, profound hyperuricemia caused by increased cell lysis.

INTERACTIONS
Anticoagulants, aspirin: increased risk of bleeding. Avoid concomitant use.
Thioguanine: may cause hepatotoxicity, esophageal varices, or portal hypertension. Use together cautiously.

CONTRAINDICATIONS
- Contraindicated in patients with chronic myelogenous leukemia, which is known to be resistant to the drug.
- Use cautiously in patients recently given other myelosuppressive drugs or radiation treatment and in those with

depressed neutrophil or platelet count. Because high-dose therapy has been associated with seizures, use such therapy cautiously in patients with a history of head trauma or seizures or in patients receiving other drugs that lower the seizure threshold.

NURSING CONSIDERATIONS
- Therapeutic effects are often accompanied by toxicity.
- Warn patients to watch for signs of infection (fever, sore throat, fatigue) and bleeding (easy bruising, nosebleeds, bleeding gums, melena). Take temperature daily.
- Pulmonary fibrosis may occur as late as 4 to 6 months after treatment with busulfan.
- Persistent cough and progressive dyspnea with alveolar exudate, suggestive of pneumonia, may be the result of drug toxicity. Instruct patients to report symptoms so dosage adjustments can be made.
- To prevent hyperuricemia with resulting uric acid nephropathy, allopurinol may be used with adequate hydration. Monitor serum uric acid.
- Patient response (increased appetite and sense of well-being, decreased total WBC count, reduced size of spleen) usually begins within 1 to 2 weeks.
- Instruct patients to avoid any OTC product containing aspirin.
- To prevent bleeding, avoid all I.M. injections when platelet count is below 100,000/mm³.

carboplatin
Paraplatin, Paraplatin-AQ†

Pregnancy Risk Category: D

HOW SUPPLIED
Injection: 50-mg, 150-mg, 450-mg vials

ACTION
Mechanism: An alkylating agent that produces cross-linking of DNA strands. Cell cycle-nonspecific.
Duration: terminal half-life, 2½ to 6 hours.

INDICATIONS & DOSAGE
Palliative treatment of ovarian cancer –
Adults: 360 mg/m² I.V. on day 1 q 4 weeks; doses should not be repeated until platelet count exceeds 100,000/mm³ and neutrophil count exceeds 2,000/mm³. Subsequent doses are based on blood counts. Clinical trials have suggested the following dosage adjustments: if platelet count is above 100,000/mm³ and neutrophil count is above 2,000/mm³, dose administered should be 125% of the recommended starting dose. Dose should be reduced to 75% if platelet count falls below 50,000/mm³ or neutrophil count is below 500/mm³.

ADVERSE REACTIONS
CNS: dizziness, confusion, peripheral neuropathy, ototoxicity, central neurotoxicity.
GI: constipation, diarrhea, *nausea, vomiting.*
Hematologic: ***thrombocytopenia, leukopenia, neutropenia, anemia, bone marrow suppression.***
Hepatic: hepatotoxicity.
Other: alopecia; hypersensitivity reactions; *increased BUN, creatinine, AST, or alkaline phosphatase levels.*

INTERACTIONS
Bone marrow depressants (including radiation therapy): increased hematologic toxicity.
Nephrotoxic agents: enhanced nephrotoxicity of carboplatin.

CONTRAINDICATIONS
- Contraindicated in patients with a history of hypersensitivity to cisplatin, platinum-containing compounds,

or mannitol. Should be avoided in patients with severe bone marrow suppression or bleeding.

NURSING CONSIDERATIONS

- Determine serum electrolyte, creatinine, and BUN levels; CBC; and creatinine clearance before the first infusion and before each course of treatment.
- Hydration or diuresis before or after treatment is not necessary.
- Blood transfusions may be necessary during treatment because of cumulative anemia.
- Bone marrow suppression may be more severe in patients with creatinine clearance below 60 ml/minute; dosage adjustments are recommended for such patients. Patients with a creatinine clearance of 41 to 59 ml/minute should receive a starting dose of 250 mg/m²; patients with a creatinine clearance of 16 to 40 ml/minute should receive a starting dose of 200 mg/m². Recommended dosage adjustments are not available for patients with a creatinine clearance of 15 ml/minute or less.
- Patients over age 65 are at greater risk for neurotoxicity.
- Carboplatin can produce severe vomiting. Administer antiemetic therapy as ordered.
- Monitor vital signs during infusion.
- Monitor CBC and platelet count frequently during therapy and, when indicated, until recovery. WBC and platelet count nadirs usually occur by day 21. Levels usually return to baseline by day 28. Don't repeat dose unless platelet count exceeds 100,000/mm³.
- Preparation and administration of parenteral form of this drug is associated with mutagenic, teratogenic, and carcinogenic risks for personnel. Follow your institutional policy to reduce risks.
- Check ordered dose against laboratory test results carefully. Only one increase in dosage is recommended. Subsequent doses should not exceed 125% of starting dose.
- Because of the possibility of infant toxicity, breast-feeding patients taking carboplatin should discontinue breast-feeding.
- Have epinephrine, corticosteroids, and antihistamines available when administering carboplatin because anaphylactoid reactions may occur within minutes of administration.
- **I.V. use:** Reconstitute with D_5W, 0.9% sodium chloride solution, or sterile water for injection to make a concentration of 10 mg/ml. Add 5 ml of diluent to the 50-mg vial, 15 ml of diluent to the 150-mg vial, or 45 ml of diluent to the 450-mg vial. It can then be further diluted for infusion with 0.9% sodium chloride solution or D_5W. A concentration as low as 0.5 mg/ml can be prepared. Give drug by continuous or intermittent infusion over at least 15 minutes.
- Do not use needles or I.V. administration sets containing aluminum to administer carboplatin; precipitation and loss of drug's potency may occur.
- Store unopened vials at room temperature. Once reconstituted and diluted as directed, drug is stable at room temperature for 8 hours. Because the drug does not contain antibacterial preservatives, discard unused drug after 8 hours.
- Advise women of childbearing age to avoid becoming pregnant during therapy. Also recommend consulting with the doctor before becoming pregnant.

carmustine (BCNU)

BiCNU, Biodel

Pregnancy Risk Category: D

HOW SUPPLIED

Injection: 100-mg vial (lyophilized), with a 3-ml vial of absolute alcohol supplied as a diluent

ACTION

Mechanism: Cross-links strands of cellular DNA and interferes with RNA transcription, causing an imbalance of growth that leads to cell death. Cell cycle-nonspecific.
Duration: half-life of parent drug, 15 to 30 minutes; of metabolites, several days.

INDICATIONS & DOSAGE

Brain, colon, and stomach cancers; Hodgkin's disease; non-Hodgkin's lymphoma; melanoma; multiple myeloma; and hepatoma –
Adults: 75 to 100 mg/m² I.V. by slow infusion daily for 2 days; repeat q 6 weeks if platelet count is above 100,000/mm³ and WBC count is above 4,000/mm³. Dosage is reduced by 30% when WBC count is 2,000 to 3,000/mm³ and platelet count is 25,000 to 75,000/mm³. Dosage is reduced by 50% when WBC count is less than 2,000/mm³ and platelet count is less than 25,000/mm³.

Alternative therapy: 200 mg/m² I.V. by slow infusion as a single dose, repeated q 6 to 8 weeks; or 40 mg/m² I.V. by slow infusion for 5 consecutive days, repeated q 6 weeks.

ADVERSE REACTIONS

CNS: ataxia, drowsiness.
GI: *nausea beginning in 2 to 6 hours (can be severe), vomiting, anorexia, dysphagia, esophagitis, diarrhea.*
GU: nephrotoxicity.
Hematologic: ***cumulative bone marrow suppression,*** delayed 4 to 6 weeks, lasting 1 to 2 weeks; ***leukopenia; thrombocytopenia; acute leukemia or bone marrow dysplasia*** may occur after long-term use.
Hepatic: hepatotoxicity.
Respiratory: ***pulmonary fibrosis.***
Skin: facial flushing, hyperpigmentation (if drug contacts skin).
Other: *intense pain at infusion site from venous spasm;* possible hyperuricemia in lymphoma patients when rapid cell lysis occurs.

INTERACTIONS

Anticoagulants, aspirin: increased risk of bleeding. Avoid concomitant use.
Cimetidine: may increase carmustine's bone marrow toxicity. Avoid combination if possible.

CONTRAINDICATIONS

- Contraindicated in patients hypersensitive to drug. Either avoid use or reduce dosage in patients with hepatic or renal impairment or compromised hematologic status or in those recently exposed to cytotoxic or radiation therapy.

NURSING CONSIDERATIONS

- Therapeutic effects are often accompanied by toxicity.
- Because carmustine crosses the blood-brain barrier, it may be used to treat primary brain tumors.
- Pulmonary toxicity appears to be dose-related. Baseline pulmonary function tests should be performed before therapy and periodically thereafter.
- Perform liver and renal function tests periodically.
- Monitor CBC.
- Warn patients to watch for signs of infection (fever, sore throat, fatigue) and bleeding (easy bruising, nosebleeds, bleeding gums, melena). Take temperature daily.
- To reduce nausea, give antiemetic before administering drug.
- To prevent hyperuricemia with resulting uric acid nephropathy, allopurinol may be used with adequate hydration. Monitor serum uric acid level.
- Instruct patients to avoid any OTC product containing aspirin.
- To prevent bleeding, avoid all I.M. injections when platelet count is below 100,000/mm³.

• Don't mix with other drugs during administration.
• Preparation and administration of parenteral form of this drug is associated with carcinogenic, mutagenic, and teratogenic risks for personnel. Follow institutional policy to reduce risks.
• Avoid contact with skin because carmustine will cause a brown stain. If drug comes into contact with skin, wash off thoroughly.
• **I.V. use:** To reconstitute, dissolve 100 mg of carmustine in the 3 ml of absolute alcohol provided by the manufacturer. Dilute solution with 27 ml of sterile water for injection. Resultant solution contains 3.3 mg of carmustine/ml in 10% alcohol. Dilute in 0.9% sodium chloride solution or D_5W for I.V. infusion. Give at least 250 ml over 1 to 2 hours. To reduce pain on infusion, dilute further or slow infusion rate.
• If powder liquefies or appears oily, decomposition has occurred; discard drug.
• Solution is unstable in plastic I.V. bags. Administer only in glass containers.
• Reconstituted solution may be stored in refrigerator for 48 hours. May decompose at temperatures above 80° F (26.6° C).

chlorambucil

Leukeran

Pregnancy Risk Category: D

HOW SUPPLIED

Tablets: 2 mg

ACTION

Mechanism: Cross-links strands of cellular DNA and interferes with RNA transcription, causing an imbalance of growth that leads to cell death. Cell cycle-nonspecific.
Onset: 3 to 4 weeks. **Duration:** half-life, about 1½ hours.

INDICATIONS & DOSAGE

Chronic lymphocytic leukemia, diffuse lymphocytic lymphoma, nodular lymphocytic lymphoma, Hodgkin's disease, macroglobulinemia, mycosis fungoides, nephrotic syndrome, ovarian carcinoma, polycythemia vera, testicular cancer–
Adults: 0.1 to 0.2 mg/kg P.O. daily for 3 to 6 weeks; then adjust for maintenance (usually 4 to 10 mg daily).
Children: 0.1 to 0.2 mg/kg P.O. daily or 4.5 mg/m² daily as a single dose or in divided doses.

ADVERSE REACTIONS

CNS: seizures (with overdose).
GI: *nausea, vomiting, stomatitis.*
GU: *azoospermia, infertility.*
Hematologic: ***neutropenia,*** delayed up to 3 weeks, lasting up to 10 days after last dose; ***thrombocytopenia; anemia;*** myelosuppression (usually moderate, gradual, and rapidly reversible).
Hepatic: hepatotoxicity (rare).
Respiratory: interstitial pneumonitis, ***pulmonary fibrosis*** (rare).
Skin: ***exfoliative dermatitis,*** rash.
Other: allergic febrile reaction, hyperuricemia.

INTERACTIONS

Anticoagulants, aspirin: increased risk of bleeding. Avoid concomitant use.

CONTRAINDICATIONS

• Contraindicated in patients with hypersensitivity or resistance to previous therapy. Patients hypersensitive to melphalan may also be hypersensitive to chlorambucil. Dosage adjustment is recommended in patients with hematologic impairment.
• Use cautiously in patients with a history of head trauma or seizures or in patients receiving other drugs that lower the seizure threshold.

NURSING CONSIDERATIONS

- Therapeutic effects are often accompanied by toxicity.
- Severe neutropenia is reversible up to cumulative dosage of 6.5 mg/kg in a single course. If WBC count falls below 2,000/mm³ or granulocyte count falls below 1,000/mm³, follow institutional policy for infection control in immunocompromised patients.
- Warn patients to watch for signs of infection (fever, sore throat, fatigue) and bleeding (easy bruising, nosebleeds, bleeding gums, melena). Take temperature daily.
- Monitor CBC.
- To prevent hyperuricemia with resulting uric acid nephropathy, allopurinol may be used with adequate hydration. Monitor serum uric acid level.
- To prevent bleeding, avoid all I.M. injections when platelet count is below 100,000/mm³.
- Instruct patients to avoid OTC products containing aspirin.

cisplatin (cis-platinum)

Platamine‡, Platinol, Platinol AQ

Pregnancy Risk Category: D

HOW SUPPLIED

Injection: 0.5 mg/ml†, 1 mg/ml
Powder for injection: 10 mg, 50 mg

ACTION

Mechanism: Cross-links strands of cellular DNA and interferes with RNA transcription, causing an imbalance of growth that leads to cell death. Cell cycle-nonspecific.
Duration: half-life, 2½ to 3 days; inhibition of DNA, several days.

INDICATIONS & DOSAGE

Adjunctive therapy in metastatic testicular cancer–
Adults: 20 mg/m² I.V. daily for 5 days. Repeat q 3 weeks for three cycles or longer.
Adjunctive therapy in metastatic ovarian cancer–
Adults: 100 mg/m² I.V. Repeat q 4 weeks; or 50 mg/m² I.V. q 3 weeks with concurrent doxorubicin therapy.
Advanced bladder cancer–
Adults: 50 to 70 mg/m² I.V. q 3 to 4 weeks. Patients who have received other antineoplastic agents or radiation therapy should receive 50 mg/m² q 4 weeks.

Note: Prehydration and mannitol diuresis may reduce renal toxicity and ototoxicity significantly.

ADVERSE REACTIONS

CNS: peripheral neuritis, loss of taste, ***seizures.***
EENT: *tinnitus, hearing loss.*
GI: *nausea, vomiting, beginning 1 to 4 hours after dose and lasting 24 hours;* diarrhea; metallic taste.
GU: *more prolonged and severe renal toxicity with repeated courses of therapy.*
Hematologic: *mild myelosuppression in 25% to 30% of patients;* ***leukopenia, thrombocytopenia, anemia;*** nadirs in circulating platelet and WBC counts on days 18 to 23, with recovery by day 39.
Other: ***anaphylactoid reaction,*** hypomagnesemia, hypokalemia, hypocalcemia.

INTERACTIONS

Aminoglycoside antibiotics: additive nephrotoxicity. Monitor renal function studies very carefully.
Bumetanide, ethacrynic acid, furosemide: additive ototoxicity. Avoid concomitant use.
Phenytoin: decreased serum phenytoin levels. Monitor serum levels.

CONTRAINDICATIONS

- Contraindicated in patients hypersensitive to the drug or to carboplatin and in those with severe renal disease, hearing impairment, or myelosuppression.

• Use cautiously and with dosage modification as needed in patients with mild to moderate renal impairment, myelosuppression, or hearing impairment.

NURSING CONSIDERATIONS

• Therapeutic effects are often accompanied by toxicity.
• Hydrate patient with 0.9% sodium chloride solution before giving drug. Maintain urine output of 100 ml/hour for 4 consecutive hours before therapy and for 24 hours after therapy.
• Investigational protocols may include intense hydration of patients with 0.9% sodium chloride. The cisplatin dose is then administered in 3% sodium chloride.
• Mannitol may be given as 12.5-g I.V. bolus before starting cisplatin infusion. Follow, if ordered, by infusion of mannitol at rate of up to 10 g/hour p.r.n. to maintain urine output during and 6 to 24 hours after cisplatin infusion.
• Some clinicians use I.V. sodium thiosulfate to minimize toxicity. Check current protocol.
• Do not repeat dosage unless platelet count is over 100,000/mm^3, WBC count is over 4,000/mm^3, creatinine level is under 1.5 mg/dl, or BUN level is under 25 mg/dl.
• Warn patients to watch for signs of infection (fever, sore throat, fatigue) and bleeding (easy bruising, nosebleeds, bleeding gums, melena). Take temperature daily.
• Monitor CBC, electrolyte levels (especially potassium and magnesium), platelet count, and renal function studies before initial and subsequent dosages.
• To prevent hypokalemia, potassium chloride (10 to 20 mEq/L) is frequently added to I.V. fluids before and after cisplatin therapy.
• To prevent permanent hearing loss, perform audiometry before initial dosage and subsequent courses, and tell patients to report tinnitus immediately.
• Nausea and vomiting may be severe and protracted (up to 24 hours). Administer antiemetics as ordered. Monitor intake and output. Continue I.V. hydration until patient can tolerate adequate oral intake.
• Ondansetron or high-dose metoclopramide has been used very effectively to treat and prevent nausea and vomiting. Some clinicians combine metoclopramide with dexamethasone and antihistamines.
• Delayed-onset vomiting (3 to 5 days after treatment) has been reported. Patients may need prolonged antiemetic treatment.
• Is given with bleomycin and vinblastine for testicular cancer and with doxorubicin for ovarian cancer.
• Renal toxicity is cumulative. Renal function must return to normal before next dose can be given.
• Anaphylactoid reaction usually responds to immediate treatment with epinephrine, corticosteroids, or antihistamines.
• To prevent bleeding, avoid all I.M. injections when platelet counts are below 100,000/mm^3.
• Preparation and administration of parenteral form of this drug is associated with carcinogenic, mutagenic, and teratogenic risks for personnel. Follow institutional policy to reduce risks.
• **I.V. use:** Reconstitute powder using sterile water for injection. Add 10 ml to the 10-mg vial or 50 ml to the 50-mg vial to make a solution containing 1 mg/ml. If necessary, further dilute with dextrose 5% in 0.3% sodium chloride injection or dextrose 5% in 0.45% sodium chloride injection. Solutions are stable for 20 hours at room temperature. Don't refrigerate.
• Infusions are most stable in chloride-containing solutions (such as 0.9% sodium chloride, 0.45% sodium

chloride, and 0.22% sodium chloride).
• The manufacturer recommends administering the drug as an I.V. infusion in 2 liters of 0.9% sodium chloride solution with 37.5 g of mannitol over 6 to 8 hours.
• Do not use needles or I.V. administration sets that contain aluminum because it will displace the platinum, causing a loss of potency and formation of a black precipitate.

cyclophosphamide

Cycoblastin‡, Cytoxan**, Cytoxan Lyophilized, Endoxan-Asta‡, Neosar, Procytox†

Pregnancy Risk Category: D

HOW SUPPLIED

Tablets: 25 mg, 50 mg
Injection: 100-mg, 200-mg, 500-mg, 1-g, 2-g vials

ACTION

Mechanism: Cross-links strands of cellular DNA and interferes with RNA transcription, causing an imbalance of growth that leads to cell death. Cell cycle-nonspecific.
Peak: Plasma concentrations of metabolites peak 2 to 3 hours after I.V. dose. **Duration:** half-life, 3 to 12 hours.

INDICATIONS & DOSAGE

Breast, head, neck, prostate, lung, and ovarian cancers; Hodgkin's disease; chronic lymphocytic leukemia; chronic myelocytic leukemia; acute lymphoblastic leukemia; acute myelocytic leukemia; neuroblastoma; retinoblastoma; non-Hodgkin's lymphoma; multiple myeloma; mycosis fungoides; sarcoma; nephrotic syndrome –
Adults: initially, 40 to 50 mg/kg I.V. in divided doses over 2 to 5 days; then adjust for maintenance. Or 1 to 5 mg/kg P.O. daily, depending on patient tolerance. Maintenance dosage is 1 to 5 mg/kg P.O. daily; or 10 to 15 mg/kg I.V. q 7 to 10 days; or 3 to 5 mg/kg I.V. twice weekly.
Children: 2 to 8 mg/kg daily or 60 to 250 mg/m² daily P.O. or I.V. for 6 days (dosage depends on susceptibility of neoplasm). Maintenance dosage is 2 to 5 mg/kg or 50 to 150 mg/m² P.O. twice weekly.

ADVERSE REACTIONS

CV: ***cardiotoxicity*** (with very high doses and in combination with doxorubicin).
GI: anorexia; *nausea and vomiting beginning within 6 hours, lasting 4 hours;* stomatitis; mucositis.
GU: gonadal suppression (may be irreversible), ***hemorrhagic cystitis,*** bladder fibrosis, nephrotoxicity.
Hematologic: ***leukopenia,*** nadir between days 8 to 15, recovery in 17 to 28 days; ***thrombocytopenia; anemia.***
Respiratory: ***pulmonary fibrosis*** (high doses).
Other: *reversible alopecia in 50% of patients, especially with high doses;* secondary malignancies, ***anaphylaxis,*** hyperuricemia, SIADH (with high doses).

INTERACTIONS

Barbiturates: increased pharmacologic effect and enhanced cyclophosphamide toxicity due to induction of hepatic enzymes.
Cardiotoxic drugs: additive adverse cardiac effects.
Chloramphenicol, corticosteroids: reduced activity of cyclophosphamide. Use cautiously.
Digoxin: may decrease serum digoxin levels. Monitor levels closely.
Succinylcholine: prolonged neuromuscular blockade. Don't use together.

CONTRAINDICATIONS

• Contraindicated in patients hypersensitive to the drug. Repeat courses

are contraindicated in patients in whom it causes hemorrhagic cystitis.
• Use cautiously in patients with severe leukopenia, thrombocytopenia, malignant cell infiltration of bone marrow, or hepatic or renal disease, and in those who have recently undergone radiation therapy or chemotherapy.

NURSING CONSIDERATIONS
• Therapeutic effects are often accompanied by toxicity.
• Advise both male and female patients to practice contraception while taking this drug and for 4 months after; drug is potentially teratogenic.
• Monitor CBC and renal and liver function tests.
• To minimize the risk of hemorrhagic cystitis, encourage patients to void every 1 to 2 hours while awake and to drink at least 3 liters of fluid daily. Don't give the drug at bedtime; infrequent urination during the night may increase the possibility of cystitis. If cystitis occurs, discontinue drug. Cystitis can occur months after therapy ceases. Mesna may be given to lower the incidence and severity of bladder toxicity.
• To prevent hyperuricemia with resulting uric acid nephropathy, allopurinol may be used with adequate hydration. Monitor serum uric acid level.
• Warn patients that alopecia is likely to occur, but that it is reversible.
• Monitor for cyclophosphamide toxicity if patient's corticosteroid therapy is discontinued.
• To prevent bleeding, avoid all I.M. injections when platelet count is below 100,000/mm³.
• Preparation and administration of parenteral form of this drug is associated with carcinogenic, mutagenic, and teratogenic risks for personnel. Follow institutional policy to reduce risks.
• **I.V. use:** Reconstitute powder using sterile water for injection or bacteriostatic water for injection containing only parabens. For the nonlyophilized product, add 5 ml to the 100-mg vial, 10 ml to the 200-mg vial, 25 ml to the 500-mg vial, 50 ml to the 1-g vial, or 100 ml to the 2-g vial to produce a solution containing 20 mg/ml. Shake to dissolve; this may take up to 6 minutes and it may be difficult to completely dissolve drug. Lyophilized preparation is much easier to reconstitute; check package insert for quantity of diluent needed to reconstitute drug.
• After reconstitution, drug may be given by direct I.V. injection. For I.V. infusion, further dilute with D_5W, dextrose 5% in 0.9% sodium chloride injection, dextrose 5% in Ringer's injection, lactated Ringer's injection, sodium lactate injection, or 0.45% sodium chloride injection.
• Reconstituted solution is stable for 6 days refrigerated or 24 hours at room temperature. However, use stored solutions cautiously because the drug contains no preservatives.
• Check reconstituted solution for small particles. Filter solution if necessary.

dacarbazine (DTIC)
DTIC†, DTIC-Dome

Pregnancy Risk Category: C

HOW SUPPLIED
Injection: 100-mg, 200-mg vials

ACTION
Mechanism: Cross-links strands of cellular DNA and interferes with RNA transcription, causing an imbalance of growth that leads to cell death. Cell cycle-nonspecific.
Peak: Serum levels peak immediately after I.V. infusion. **Duration:** terminal elimination half-life, about 5 hours.

INDICATIONS & DOSAGE

Metastatic malignant melanoma –
Adults: 2 to 4.5 mg/kg or 70 to 160 mg/m^2 I.V. daily for 10 days; then repeat q 4 weeks as tolerated. Or 250 mg/m^2 I.V. daily for 5 days, repeated at 3-week intervals.
Hodgkin's disease –
Adults: 150 mg/m^2 I.V. daily (in combination with other agents) for 5 days, repeated q 4 weeks; or 375 mg/m^2 on the first day of a combination regimen, repeated q 15 days.

ADVERSE REACTIONS

GI: *severe nausea and vomiting, beginning within 1 to 3 hours in 90% of patients, and lasting 1 to 12 hours; anorexia.*
Hematologic: ***leukopenia and thrombocytopenia,*** nadir between 3 and 4 weeks.
Hepatic: increased liver enzyme levels, hepatotoxicity (rare).
Skin: phototoxicity.
Other: *flulike syndrome* (fever, malaise, myalgia beginning 7 days after treatment stopped and possibly lasting 7 to 21 days), alopecia, ***anaphylaxis;*** severe pain if I.V. solution infiltrates or if solution is too concentrated; tissue damage; hyperuricemia.

INTERACTIONS

Allopurinol: additive hypouricemic effects. Monitor closely.
Anticoagulants, aspirin: increased risk of bleeding. Avoid concomitant use.
Bone marrow suppressants: additive toxicity. Monitor closely.
Phenobarbital, phenytoin, other drugs that induce hepatic metabolism: enhanced dacarbazine activation and risk of toxicity. Monitor closely.

CONTRAINDICATIONS

- Contraindicated in patients hypersensitive to the drug.
- Use cautiously at lower dosage if renal or bone marrow function is impaired. Stop drug if WBC count falls to $3,000/mm^3$ or platelet count drops to $100,000/mm^3$. Monitor CBC.

NURSING CONSIDERATIONS

- Therapeutic effects are often accompanied by toxicity.
- Warn patients to watch for signs of infection (fever, sore throat, fatigue) and bleeding (easy bruising, nosebleeds, bleeding gums, melena). Take temperature daily.
- For Hodgkin's disease, drug is usually given with bleomycin, vinblastine, and doxorubicin.
- Advise patients to avoid sunlight and sunlamps for first 2 days after treatment.
- Administering antiemetics before giving dacarbazine may help decrease nausea. Nausea and vomiting may sometimes subside after several doses.
- Instruct patients to avoid OTC products containing aspirin.
- Reassure patients that flulike syndrome may be treated with mild antipyretics, such as acetaminophen.
- To prevent bleeding, avoid all I.M. injections when platelet count is below $100,000/mm^3$.
- Preparation and administration of parenteral form of this drug is associated with carcinogenic, mutagenic, and teratogenic risks for personnel. Follow institutional policy to reduce risks.
- **I.V. use:** Reconstitute drug using sterile water for injection. Add 9.9 ml to the 100-mg vial or 19.7 ml to the 200-mg vial. The resulting solution will be colorless to clear yellow. For infusion, further dilute using up to 250 ml of 0.9% sodium chloride injection or D_5W; infuse over 30 minutes.
- During infusion, protect bag from direct sunlight to avoid possible drug breakdown. May dilute further or slow infusion to decrease pain at infusion site.

• Take care not to allow extravasation during infusion. If I.V. solution infiltrates, discontinue immediately and apply ice to area for 24 to 48 hours.
• Reconstituted solutions are stable for 8 hours at room temperature and normal lighting conditions, or up to 3 days if refrigerated. Diluted solutions are stable for 8 hours at normal room temperature and light, or up to 24 hours if refrigerated. If solutions turn pink, decomposition has occurred; discard drug.
• Discard refrigerated solution after 72 hours and room temperature solution after 8 hours.

ifosfamide

IFEX

Pregnancy Risk Category: D

HOW SUPPLIED

Injection: 1 g (supplied with 200-mg ampule of mesna), 2 g†, 3 g†

ACTION

Mechanism: Cross-links strands of cellular DNA and interferes with RNA transcription, causing an imbalance of growth that leads to cell death. Cell cycle-nonspecific.
Peak: Serum levels peak immediately after I.V. infusion. **Duration:** half-life about 7 hours, in patients receiving up to 2.4 g/m²/day; terminal half-life, about 15 hours in patients receiving up to 5 g/m²/day.

INDICATIONS & DOSAGE

Testicular cancer–
Adults: 1.2 g/m²/day I.V. for 5 consecutive days. Treatment is repeated q 3 weeks or after the patient recovers from hematologic toxicity.

ADVERSE REACTIONS

CNS: *lethargy, somnolence, confusion, depressive psychosis,* ***coma.***
CV: supraventricular arrhythmias.
GI: *nausea, vomiting.*
GU: *hemorrhagic cystitis (dose-limiting, occurring in up to 50% of patients), hematuria,* nephrotoxicity.
Hematologic: ***leukopenia, thrombocytopenia, myelosuppression.***
Hepatic: elevated liver enzyme levels.
Other: *alopecia.*

INTERACTIONS

Allopurinol: may produce excessive ifosfamide effect by prolonging half-life. Monitor for enhanced toxicity.
Anticoagulants, aspirin: increased risk of bleeding. Avoid concomitant use.
Barbiturates, chloral hydrate, phenytoin: may increase ifosfamide toxicity by inducing hepatic enzymes that hasten the formation of toxic metabolites.
Corticosteroids: may inhibit hepatic enzymes, reducing ifosfamide's effect. Monitor for enhanced ifosfamide toxicity if concurrent steroid dosage is suddenly reduced or discontinued.
Myelosuppressants: enhanced hematologic toxicity. Dosage adjustment may be necessary.

CONTRAINDICATIONS

• Contraindicated in patients hypersensitive to the drug and in those with severely depressed bone marrow function.
• Use cautiously in patients with renal or hepatic impairment.

NURSING CONSIDERATIONS

• Administer ifosfamide with a protecting agent (mesna) to prevent hemorrhagic cystitis. Adequate fluid intake (2 liters/day, either P.O. or I.V.) is essential.
• Obtain urinalysis before each dose. If microscopic hematuria is present, patients should be evaluated for hemorrhagic cystitis. Dosage adjustments of mesna may be necessary.
• Bladder irrigation with 0.9% sodium chloride solution may decrease the possibility of cystitis.

• To minimize contact of ifosfamide and its metabolites with the bladder mucosa, remind patients to void frequently. Don't give the drug at bedtime; infrequent voiding during the night may increase the possibility of cystitis. If cystitis develops, discontinue drug.
• Warn patients to watch for signs of infection (fever, sore throat, fatigue) and bleeding (easy bruising, nosebleeds, bleeding gums, melena). Take temperature daily.
• Instruct patients to avoid OTC products containing aspirin.
• Administering antiemetics before giving ifosfamide may help decrease nausea.
• Monitor CBC and renal and liver function tests.
• Assess patients for mental status changes; dosage may have to be decreased.
• Has also been used for soft-tissue sarcomas, Ewing's sarcoma, non-Hodgkins lymphoma, and lung and pancreatic cancers.
• To prevent bleeding, avoid all I.M. injections when platelet count is below 100,000/mm³.
• Preparation and administration of parenteral form of this drug is associated with carcinogenic, mutagenic, and teratogenic risks for personnel. Follow institutional policy to reduce risks.
• **I.V. use:** Reconstitute each gram of drug with 20 ml of diluent to yield a solution of 50 mg/ml. Use sterile water for injection or bacteriostatic water for injection. Solutions may then be further diluted with sterile water, dextrose 2.5% or 5% in water, 0.45% or 0.9% sodium chloride injection, 5% dextrose and 0.9% sodium chloride injection, or lactated Ringer's injection.
• Infusing each dose over at least 30 minutes will decrease possibility of cystitis.
• Ifosfamide and mesna are physically compatible and may be mixed in the same I.V. solution.
• Reconstituted solution is stable for 1 week at room temperature or 6 weeks refrigerated. However, use solution within 6 hours if drug was reconstituted with sterile water without a preservative (such as benzyl alcohol or parabens).

lomustine (CCNU)

CeeNU

Pregnancy Risk Category: D

HOW SUPPLIED

Capsules: 10 mg, 40 mg, 100 mg, dose pack (two 10-mg, two 40-mg, two 100-mg capsules)

ACTION

Mechanism: Cross-links strands of cellular DNA and interferes with RNA transcription, causing an imbalance of growth that leads to cell death. Cell cycle-nonspecific.
Duration: half-life of parent drug, about 1½ hours; of metabolites, 16 to 48 hours.

INDICATIONS & DOSAGE

Brain tumors; GI, lung, breast, or renal cancers; malignant melanoma; multiple myeloma; Hodgkin's disease –
Adults and children: 100 to 130 mg/m² P.O. as a single dose q 6 weeks. Reduce dosage according to degree of bone marrow suppression. Repeat doses should not be given until WBC count is more than 4,000/mm³ and platelet count is more than 100,000/mm³.

ADVERSE REACTIONS

GI: *nausea and vomiting beginning within 4 to 5 hours and lasting 24 hours;* stomatitis.
GU: nephrotoxicity, progressive azotemia.
Hematologic: ***anemia, leukopenia,***

†Available in Canada only. ‡Available in Australia only. ◇Available OTC.

delayed up to 6 weeks, lasting 1 to 2 weeks; ***thrombocytopenia,*** delayed up to 4 weeks, lasting 1 to 2 weeks.

INTERACTIONS

Anticoagulants, aspirin: increased risk of bleeding. Avoid concomitant use.

CONTRAINDICATIONS

- Contraindicated in patients hypersensitive to the drug.
- Use cautiously in patients with decreased platelet, WBC, or RBC counts and in those receiving other myelosuppressant drugs.

NURSING CONSIDERATIONS

- Therapeutic effects are often accompanied by toxicity.
- Give 2 to 4 hours after meals. Lomustine will be more completely absorbed if taken when the stomach is empty. To avoid nausea, give antiemetic before administering.
- May be useful in cancer involving CNS because drug levels in the CSF equal 30% to 50% of plasma level 1 hour after administration.
- Monitor CBC weekly. Usually not administered more often than every 6 weeks; bone marrow toxicity is cumulative and delayed.
- Warn patients to watch for signs of infection (fever, sore throat, fatigue) and bleeding (easy bruising, nosebleeds, bleeding gums, melena). Take temperature daily.
- Periodically monitor liver function tests.
- To prevent bleeding, avoid all I.M. injections when platelet count is below 100,000/mm^3.
- Instruct patients to avoid OTC products containing aspirin.

mechlorethamine hydrochloride (nitrogen mustard)

Mustargen

Pregnancy Risk Category: D

HOW SUPPLIED

Injection: 10-mg vials

ACTION

Mechanism: Cross-links strands of cellular DNA and interferes with RNA transcription, causing an imbalance of growth that leads to cell death. Cell cycle-nonspecific.

Onset: seconds to minutes. **Peak:** Serum levels peak immediately after I.V. infusion.

INDICATIONS & DOSAGE

Polycythemia vera, chronic lymphocytic leukemia, chronic myelocytic leukemia, malignant effusions (pericardial, peritoneal, pleural), mycosis fungoides, Hodgkin's disease, non-Hodgkin's lymphoma, diffuse lymphocytic lymphoma –

Adults: 0.4 mg/kg or 10 mg/m^2 I.V. as a single dose or in divided doses q 3 to 6 weeks. Give through running I.V. infusion. Dosage reduced in prior radiation therapy or chemotherapy to 0.2 to 0.4 mg/kg. Dosage based on ideal or actual body weight, whichever is less.

Malignant effusions –

Adults: 0.2 to 0.4 mg/kg intracavitarily.

Mycosis fungoides –

Adults: topical solution or ointment applied to lesion. Topical preparations must be compounded by the pharmacist; drug concentration, frequency of application, and duration of therapy will vary according to patient tolerance and response. Ointments of 0.01% to 0.02% and topical solutions containing 10 mg/50 to 60 ml have been used.

ADVERSE REACTIONS

CNS: headache, weakness, drowsiness, vertigo, light-headedness, ***seizures,*** progressive paralysis, paresthesia, ***cerebral degeneration, coma.***
EENT: tinnitus, *metallic taste* (immediately after dose), deafness with high doses.
GI: *nausea, vomiting, and anorexia* beginning within minutes, lasting 8 to 24 hours.
Hematologic: ***thrombocytopenia, granulocytopenia, lymphocytopenia,*** nadir of myelosuppression occurring by days 4 to 10 and lasting 10 to 21 days; mild anemia begins in 2 to 3 weeks, possibly lasting 7 weeks.
Skin: rash, sloughing, severe irritation if drug extravasates or touches skin.
Other: *alopecia,* precipitation of herpes zoster, ***anaphylaxis,*** hyperuricemia; *thrombophlebitis.*

INTERACTIONS

Anticoagulants, aspirin: increased risk of bleeding. Avoid concomitant use.
Cyclophosphamide, procarbazine: possible increased risk of hepatotoxicity.

CONTRAINDICATIONS

- Contraindicated in patients hypersensitive to the drug. Drug should not be used in patients with acute or chronic suppurative inflammation because it may promote the rapid development of amyloidosis. The manufacturer states that the drug is contraindicated in patients with known infectious diseases.
- Use cautiously in patients with severe anemia, depressed neutrophil or platelet count, or in those who have recently undergone radiation therapy or chemotherapy. Monitor CBC.

NURSING CONSIDERATIONS

- Therapeutic effects are often accompanied by toxicity.
- Neurotoxicity increases with dose and patient age.
- To prevent hyperuricemia with resulting uric acid nephropathy, mechlorethamine may be used with adequate hydration. Monitor serum uric acid level.
- Warn patients to watch for signs of infection (fever, sore throat, fatigue) and bleeding (easy bruising, nosebleeds, bleeding gums, melena). Take temperature daily.
- Instruct patients to avoid OTC products containing aspirin.
- To prevent bleeding, avoid all I.M. injections when platelet count is below 100,000/mm³.
- Preparation and administration of parenteral form of this drug is associated with carcinogenic, mutagenic, and teratogenic risks for personnel. Follow institutional policy to reduce risks.
- **I.V. use:** Reconstitute the drug using 10 ml of sterile water for injection or 0.9% sodium chloride injection. The resulting solution contains 1 mg/ml of mechlorethamine. Give by direct injection into a vein or into the tubing of a free-flowing I.V. solution.
- Mechlorethamine is a potent vesicant. Make sure I.V. solution doesn't infiltrate. If drug extravasates, apply cold compresses and infiltrate the area with isotonic sodium thiosulfate.
- When given intracavitarily for sclerosing effect, dilute using up to 100 ml of 0.9% sodium chloride injection. Turn patient from side to side every 15 minutes to 1 hour to distribute drug.
- Very unstable solution. Prepare immediately before infusion. Visually inspect before using; use within 15 minutes, and discard unused solution.
- Do not use solutions that are discolored or contain particulate matter. Do not use vials that appear to contain droplets of water.
- Dispose of any equipment used in the preparation and administration of

mechlorethamine properly and according to institutional policy. Neutralize unused solution with an equal volume of 5% sodium bicarbonate and 5% sodium thiosulfate.

melphalan (L-phenylalanine mustard)

Alkeran

Pregnancy Risk Category: D

HOW SUPPLIED

Tablets (scored): 2 mg
Injection: 50 mg

ACTION

Mechanism: Cross-links strands of cellular DNA and interferes with RNA transcription, causing an imbalance of growth that leads to cell death. Cell cycle-nonspecific.
Duration: half-life, about 90 minutes.

INDICATIONS & DOSAGE

Multiple myeloma –
Adults: initially, 6 mg P.O. daily for 2 to 3 weeks; then stop drug for up to 4 weeks or until WBC and platelet counts stop dropping and begin to rise again; resume with maintenance dosage of 2 mg daily. Stop drug if WBC count is below 3,000/mm^3 or platelet count is below 100,000/mm^3. Alternative therapy: 0.15 mg/kg P.O. daily for 7 days, or 0.25 mg/kg for 4 days; repeat q 4 to 6 weeks.

Alternatively, administer I.V. to patients who can't tolerate oral therapy. Give 16 mg/m^2 by infusion over 15 to 20 minutes at 2-week intervals for four doses. After patient has recovered from toxicity, give drug at 4-week intervals.
Nonresectable advanced ovarian cancer –
Adults: 0.2 mg/kg P.O. daily for 5 days. Repeat q 4 to 5 weeks, depending on bone marrow recovery.

ADVERSE REACTIONS

Hematologic: ***thrombocytopenia, leukopenia, agranulocytosis.***
Respiratory: ***pneumonitis, pulmonary fibrosis.***
Skin: dermatitis, pruritus, rash.
Other: ***anaphylaxis,*** alopecia.

INTERACTIONS

Anticoagulants, aspirin: increased risk of bleeding. Avoid concomitant use.
Antigout agents: decreased effectiveness. Dosage adjustments may be necessary.
Bone marrow suppressants: additive toxicity. Monitor closely.
Vaccines: decreased effectiveness of killed-virus vaccines and increased risk of toxicity from live-virus vaccines. Postpone routine immunization for at least 3 months after last dose of melphalan.

CONTRAINDICATIONS

- Contraindicated in patients hypersensitive to the drug and in those whose disease is known to be resistant to the drug. Patients hypersensitive to chlorambucil may have cross-sensitivity to melphalan.

NURSING CONSIDERATIONS

- Therapeutic effects are often accompanied by toxicity.
- Not recommended in patients with severe leukopenia, thrombocytopenia, or anemia or in those with chronic lymphocytic leukemia.
- Monitor serum uric acid level and CBC.
- Dosage may need to be reduced in patients with renal impairment.
- Drug of choice in combination with prednisone in patients with multiple myeloma.
- Instruct patients to avoid OTC products containing aspirin.
- Absorption of drug is decreased by food; administer on empty stomach.
- Warn patients to watch for signs of

infection (fever, sore throat, fatigue) and bleeding (easy bruising, nosebleeds, bleeding gums, melena). Take temperature daily.

- To prevent bleeding, avoid all I.M. injections when platelet count is below 100,000/mm³.
- Preparation and administration of parenteral form of the drug is associated with carcinogenic, mutagenic, and teratogenic risks for personnel. Follow institutional policy to reduce risks.
- **I.V. use:** Because drug isn't stable in solution, reconstitute immediately before administering. Reconstitute drug with the 10 ml of sterile diluent supplied by the manufacturer. Shake vigorously until a clear solution is obtained. The resultant solution will contain 5 mg of melphalan/ml. Immediately dilute the required dose in 0.9% sodium chloride injection. Final concentration shouldn't exceed 0.45 mg/ml. Give I.V. infusion over 15 to 20 minutes.
- Prompt dilution and administration is very important; the reconstituted product begins to degrade within 30 minutes. After final dilution, nearly 1% of the drug degrades every 10 minutes. Don't refrigerate the reconstituted product because a precipitate will form.

pipobroman

Vercyte

Pregnancy Risk Category: D

HOW SUPPLIED

Tablets (scored): 25 mg

ACTION

Mechanism: An alkylating agent that has an unknown mechanism.

Peak: Peak levels occur within 2 hours.

INDICATIONS & DOSAGE

Polycythemia vera –

Adults and children over age 15: 1 mg/kg P.O. daily for 30 days; may increase to 1.5 to 3 mg/kg P.O. daily until hematocrit is reduced to 50% to 55%. Maintenance dosage is 0.1 to 0.2 mg/kg P.O. daily.

Chronic myelocytic leukemia –

Adults and children over age 15: 1.5 to 2.5 mg/kg P.O. daily until WBC count drops to 10,000/mm³. Maintenance dosage ranges from 7 to 175 mg daily. Stop drug if WBC count falls below 3,000/mm³ or platelet count falls below 150,000/mm³.

ADVERSE REACTIONS

GI: nausea, vomiting, abdominal cramps, diarrhea.

Hematologic: ***leukopenia, anemia, thrombocytopenia.***

Skin: rash.

INTERACTIONS

Anticoagulants, aspirin: increased risk of bleeding. Avoid concomitant use.

CONTRAINDICATIONS

- Contraindicated in patients hypersensitive to the drug. Also contraindicated in patients with bone marrow suppression following radiation therapy or cytotoxic drug therapy.

NURSING CONSIDERATIONS

- Periodically monitor renal and liver function tests.
- Monitor CBC once or twice a week and WBC counts every other day until therapeutic end-point is reached or toxicity becomes evident.
- Bone marrow studies should be performed before treatment and at the time of maximal hematologic response. Bone marrow suppression may not occur for 4 weeks or more after initiation of treatment. WBC count is the most reliable index of bone marrow response.

• Dose-dependent anemia frequently develops. Dose reductions may be necessary; transfusions may be used if anemia is severe. If hemoglobin drops rapidly and is accompanied by reticulocytosis and a rise in bilirubin levels, anemia may be caused by a hemolytic process. In such cases, discontinue drug.
• Advise patients to use contraception during therapy.
• Advise patients to avoid all products containing aspirin.

streptozocin

Zanosar

Pregnancy Risk Category: C

HOW SUPPLIED

Injection: 1-g vials

ACTION

Mechanism: Cross-links strands of cellular DNA and interferes with RNA transcription, causing an imbalance of growth that leads to cell death. Cell cycle-nonspecific.
Peak: Serum levels peak immediately after I.V. infusion. **Duration:** terminal elimination half-life of parent drug, about 35 minutes; of metabolites, 40 hours.

INDICATIONS & DOSAGE

Hodgkin's disease, metastatic islet and non-islet cell carcinoma of the pancreas, colon cancer, carcinoid tumors –
Adults and children: 500 mg/m² I.V. for 5 consecutive days q 6 weeks until maximum benefit or toxicity is observed. Alternatively, 1,000 mg/m² at weekly intervals for the first 2 weeks. Don't exceed a single dose of 1,500 mg/m².

ADVERSE REACTIONS

GI: *nausea, vomiting,* diarrhea.
GU: *renal toxicity* (evidenced by azotemia, glycosuria, and renal tubular acidosis), mild proteinuria.
Hematologic: ***anemia, leukopenia, thrombocytopenia.***
Hepatic: elevated liver enzyme levels.
Other: hyperglycemia, hypoglycemia, diabetes mellitus; *sloughing, severe irritation if extravasation occurs.*

INTERACTIONS

Doxorubicin: prolonged elimination half-life of doxorubicin. Dose of doxorubicin should be reduced.
Other potentially nephrotoxic drugs such as aminoglycosides: increased risk of renal toxicity. Use cautiously.
Phenytoin: may decrease the effectiveness of streptozocin in patients with pancreatic cancer. Monitor carefully.

CONTRAINDICATIONS

• Contraindicated in patients hypersensitive to the drug.
• Use cautiously. Dosage modification may be required in patients with preexisting renal or hepatic disease.

NURSING CONSIDERATIONS

• Therapeutic effects are often accompanied by toxicity.
• Renal toxicity resulting from streptozocin therapy is dose-related and cumulative. Monitor renal function tests before and after each course of therapy. Urinalysis; BUN, creatinine, and serum electrolyte levels; and creatinine clearance should be obtained before and at least weekly during drug administration. Weekly monitoring should continue for 4 weeks after each course.
• To minimize risk of renal toxicity, ensure adequate hydration using oral or parenteral fluids.
• Test urine for protein and glucose levels each nursing shift. Mild proteinuria is one of the first signs of renal toxicity; notify the doctor if this

occurs. Reduction of dosage may be necessary.

- Monitor CBC and liver function studies at least weekly.
- Warn patients to watch for signs of infection (fever, sore throat, fatigue) and bleeding (easy bruising, nosebleeds, bleeding gums, melena). Take temperature daily.
- Nausea and vomiting occur in most patients. Make sure patients are being treated with an antiemetic.
- Preparation and administration of parenteral form of this drug is associated with carcinogenic, mutagenic, and teratogenic risks for personnel. Follow institutional policy to reduce risks.
- **I.V. use:** Reconstitute streptozocin powder with 9.5 ml of D_5W or 0.9% sodium chloride injection. This will produce a pale gold solution. May be further diluted with D_5W or 0.9% sodium chloride injection. Infuse over at least 15 minutes to minimize the risk of phlebitis.
- If extravasation occurs, stop infusion immediately.
- The product contains no preservatives and is not intended as a multiple-dose vial. Use within 12 hours of reconstitution.
- Store unopened and unreconstituted vials of streptozocin in the refrigerator.

thiotepa

Thiotepa

Pregnancy Risk Category: D

HOW SUPPLIED

Injection: 15-mg vials

ACTION

Mechanism: Cross-links strands of cellular DNA and interferes with RNA transcription, causing an imbalance of growth that leads to cell death. Cell cycle-nonspecific.

Peak: Serum levels peak immediately after I.V. infusion. **Duration:** 60% of dose excreted in urine within 3 days.

INDICATIONS & DOSAGE

Breast and ovarian cancers, lymphoma, bronchogenic cancer –

Adults and children over 12 years: 0.2 mg/kg I.V. daily for 4 to 5 days at intervals of 2 to 4 weeks.

Bladder tumor –

Adults and children over 12 years: 60 mg in 60 ml of water instilled in bladder for 2 hours once weekly for 4 weeks.

Neoplastic effusions –

Adults and children over 12 years: 0.6 to 0.8 mg/kg intracavitarily.

Malignant meningeal neoplasms –

Adults: 1 to 10 mg/m² intrathecally once or twice weekly.

ADVERSE REACTIONS

CNS: headache, dizziness.

GI: *nausea, vomiting.*

GU: amenorrhea, decreased spermatogenesis.

Hematologic: ***leukopenia*** begins within 5 to 30 days; ***thrombocytopenia; neutropenia, anemia.***

Skin: hives, rash.

Other: fever, tightness of throat, alopecia, hyperuricemia, intense pain at administration site.

INTERACTIONS

Anticoagulants, aspirin: increased risk of bleeding. Avoid concomitant use.

CONTRAINDICATIONS

- Contraindicated in patients hypersensitive to the drug and in those with severe bone marrow, hepatic, or renal dysfunction.
- Use cautiously in patients with mild bone marrow suppression and renal or hepatic dysfunction.

NURSING CONSIDERATIONS

- Therapeutic effects are often accompanied by toxicity.

• Drug should be discontinued if WBC count is below 3,000/mm³ or if platelet count is below 150,000/mm³.
• Monitor CBC weekly for at least 3 weeks after last dose.
• Warn patients to watch for signs of infection (fever, sore throat, fatigue) and bleeding (easy bruising, nosebleeds, bleeding gums, melena). Take temperature daily. Tell patients to report even mild infections.
• Genitourinary adverse reactions are reversible in 6 to 8 months.
• May require use of local anesthetic at injection site if intense pain occurs.
• For bladder instillation: Dehydrate patients 8 to 10 hours before therapy. Instill drug into bladder by catheter; ask patients to retain solution for 2 hours. Volume may be reduced to 30 ml if discomfort is too great with 60 ml. Reposition patients every 15 minutes for maximum area contact.
• Toxicity is delayed and prolonged because drug binds to tissues and stays in body several hours.
• To prevent hyperuricemia with resulting uric acid nephropathy, allopurinol may be used with adequate hydration. Monitor serum uric acid levels.
• Can be given by all parenteral routes, including direct injection into the tumor.
• Instruct patients to avoid OTC products containing aspirin.
• To prevent bleeding, avoid all I.M. injections when platelet count is below 100,000/mm³.
• Preparation and administration of parenteral form of this drug is associated with mutagenic, teratogenic, and carcinogenic risks to personnel. Follow institutional policy to minimize risks.
• **I.V. use:** Reconstitute with 1.5 ml of sterile water for injection. Do not reconstitute with any other solution. Further dilute with 0.9% sodium chloride injection, D_5W, dextrose 5% in 0.9% sodium chloride injection, Ringer's injection, or lactated Ringer's injection. Solutions are stable for up to 5 days if refrigerated.
• If pain occurs at the insertion site, dilute the drug further or use a local anesthetic to reduce pain. Make sure drug does not infiltrate.
• Solutions should be clear to slightly opaque. Discard if solution appears grossly opaque or if a precipitate is present.
• For neoplastic effusions, drug may be mixed with 2% procaine hydrochloride or epinephrine hydrochloride 1:1,000.
• Refrigerate and protect dry powder from direct sunlight to avoid possible drug breakdown.

uracil mustard

Uracil Mustard Capsules**

Pregnancy Risk Category: X

HOW SUPPLIED

Capsules: 1 mg

ACTION

Mechanism: Cross-links strands of cellular DNA and interferes with RNA transcription, causing an imbalance of growth that leads to cell death. Cell cycle-nonspecific.
Duration: eliminated within 2 hours.

INDICATIONS & DOSAGE

Chronic lymphocytic and myelocytic leukemia; Hodgkin's disease; non-Hodgkin's lymphoma of the histiocytic and lymphocytic types; reticulum cell sarcoma; lymphoma; mycosis fungoides; polycythemia vera; ovarian, cervical, and lung cancers –
Adults: 1 to 2 mg P.O. daily for 3 months or until desired response or toxicity; maintenance dosage is 1 mg daily for 3 out of 4 weeks until optimum response or relapse; or 3 to 5 mg P.O. for 7 days not to exceed total dosage of 0.5 mg/kg, then 1 mg daily

until response, and then 1 mg daily 3 out of 4 weeks.

ADVERSE REACTIONS
CNS: irritability, nervousness, mental cloudiness, depression.
GI: *nausea, vomiting, diarrhea, epigastric distress,* abdominal pain, anorexia.
Hematologic: bone marrow suppression, delayed 2 to 4 weeks; ***thrombocytopenia; leukopenia; anemia.***
Skin: pruritus, dermatitis, hyperpigmentation.
Other: hyperuricemia, alopecia.

INTERACTIONS
Anticoagulants, aspirin: increased risk of bleeding. Avoid concomitant use.

CONTRAINDICATIONS
- Contraindicated in patients hypersensitive to the drug and in those with aplastic anemia, thrombocytopenia, or leukopenia.
- Use cautiously in patients with bone marrow suppression.
- Some commercially available capsules contain tartrazine dye, which may provoke hypersensitivity reactions in certain individuals. This reaction is rare but is more likely to occur in aspirin-sensitive persons.

NURSING CONSIDERATIONS
- Therapeutic effects are often accompanied by toxicity.
- Give at bedtime to reduce nausea.
- Warn patients to watch for signs of infection (fever, sore throat, fatigue) and bleeding (easy bruising, nosebleeds, bleeding gums, melena). Take temperature daily.
- Monitor platelet count. Check CBC once or twice weekly for 4 weeks; then 4 weeks after stopping drug.
- To prevent hyperuricemia and resulting uric acid nephropathy, allopurinol may be used with adequate hydration. Monitor serum uric acid level.
- To prevent bleeding, avoid all I.M. injections when platelet count is below 100,000/mm^3.
- Instruct patients to avoid OTC products containing aspirin.

70
Antimetabolites

cladribine
cytarabine
floxuridine
fludarabine phosphate
fluorouracil
hydroxyurea
mercaptopurine
methotrexate
methotrexate sodium
thioguanine
trimetrexate glucuronate

COMBINATION PRODUCTS
None.

cladribine (2-chlorodeoxyadenosine)
Leustatin

Pregnancy Risk Category: D

HOW SUPPLIED
Injection: 1 mg/ml

ACTION
Mechanism: A purine nucleoside analogue that enters tumor cells, is phosphorylated by deoxycytidine kinase, and is subsequently converted into an active triphosphate deoxynucleotide. This metabolite impairs synthesis of new DNA, inhibits repair of existing DNA, and disrupts cellular metabolism.
Onset: median time to response, 4 months. **Duration:** terminal elimination half-life, 5½ hours.

INDICATIONS & DOSAGE
Active hairy cell leukemia –
Adults: 0.09 mg/kg daily by continuous I.V. infusion for 7 days.

ADVERSE REACTIONS
CNS: *headache, fatigue, dizziness, insomnia, asthenia.*
CV: *tachycardia, edema.*
EENT: epistaxis.
GI: *nausea, decreased appetite, vomiting, diarrhea, constipation, abdominal pain.*
GU: acute renal insufficiency.
Hematologic: ***severe neutropenia, anemia, thrombocytopenia.***
Respiratory: *abnormal breath or chest sounds, cough, shortness of breath.*
Skin: *rash, pruritus, erythema,* purpura, petechiae.
Other: *fever,* ***infection,*** *local reactions at the injection site, chills, diaphoresis, malaise, trunk pain, myalgia, arthralgia,* hyperuricemia.

INTERACTIONS
None significant.

CONTRAINDICATIONS
- Contraindicated in patients hypersensitive to the drug.
- Use cautiously in patients with preexisting bone marrow suppression or renal or hepatic impairment. If possible, avoid using drug in patients with active infections.

NURSING CONSIDERATIONS
- Cladribine is a toxic drug, and some toxicity is expected during treatment. Monitor hematologic function closely, especially during the first 4 to 8 weeks of therapy. Severe bone marrow suppression, including neutropenia, anemia, and thrombocytopenia, commonly has been observed in patients treated with this drug; many patients also have preexisting hematologic impairment from their disease.
- Fever is commonly observed during the first month of therapy. In clinical

trials, virtually all patients received parenteral antibiotics.

- Because of the risk of hyperuricemia from tumor lysis, allopurinol should be administered during therapy.
- Because of the risk of fetal malformations, advise women of childbearing age to avoid becoming pregnant.
- Cladribine has also been used to treat advanced cutaneous T-cell lymphomas, chronic lymphocytic leukemia, malignant lymphomas, acute myeloid leukemias, mycosis fungoides, and Sézary syndrome.
- **I.V. use:** For a 24-hour infusion, add the calculated dose to a 500-ml infusion bag of 0.9% sodium chloride injection. Once diluted, administer promptly or begin administration within 8 hours. Don't use solutions that contain dextrose because studies have shown increased degradation of the drug. Because the drug product doesn't contain any bacteriostatic agents, use strict aseptic technique to prepare the admixture. Repeat daily for 7 consecutive days.
- Alternatively, prepare a 7-day infusion solution, using bacteriostatic sodium chloride injection, which contains 0.9% benzyl alcohol. Studies have shown acceptable physical and chemical stability using Pharmacia Deltec medication cassettes. First, pass the calculated amount of drug through a disposable 0.22-micron hydrophilic syringe filter into a sterile infusion reservoir. Next, add sufficient bacteriostatic sodium chloride injection to bring the total volume to 100 ml. Clamp off the line; then disconnect and discard the filter. If necessary, aseptically aspirate air bubbles from the reservoir using a new filter or a sterile vent filter assembly.
- Because the calculated dose dilutes the benzyl alcohol preservative, 7-day infusion solutions prepared for patients weighing more than 187 lb (85 kg) may have reduced preservative effectiveness.
- Refrigerate unopened vials at 36° to 46° F (2° to 8° C) and protect from light. Although freezing doesn't adversely affect the drug, a precipitate may form; this will disappear if the drug is allowed to warm to room temperature gradually and the vial is vigorously shaken. Don't heat or microwave; don't refreeze.

cytarabine (ara-C, cytosine arabinoside)

Alexan‡, Cytosar†, Cytosar-U

Pregnancy Risk Category: D

HOW SUPPLIED

Injection: 40-mg‡, 100-mg, 500-mg, 1-g, 2-g vials

ACTION

Mechanism: Inhibits DNA synthesis.
Peak: Levels peak 20 to 60 minutes after S.C. injection. **Duration:** half-life, 1 to 3 hours.

INDICATIONS & DOSAGE

Acute myelocytic and other acute leukemias, non-Hodgkin's lymphoma –
Adults and children: 200 mg/m² daily by continuous I.V. infusion for 5 days; repeat q 2 weeks. For maintenance, give 1 mg/kg S.C. once or twice a week.

Meningeal leukemias and meningeal neoplasms –
Adults and children: 10 to 30 mg/m² intrathecally q 4 days.

ADVERSE REACTIONS

CNS: neurotoxicity, including ataxia and cerebellar dysfunction, with high doses.
EENT: *keratitis, nystagmus.*
GI: *nausea, vomiting,* diarrhea, dysphagia; reddened area at juncture of lips, followed by sore mouth, oral ulcers in 5 to 10 days; high dose given

rapid I.V. may cause projectile vomiting.
Hematologic: ***leukopenia,*** with initial WBC count nadir 7 to 9 days after drug is stopped and a second (more severe) nadir 15 to 24 days after drug is stopped; anemia; reticulocytopenia; ***thrombocytopenia,*** with platelet count nadir occurring on day 10; *megaloblastosis.*
Hepatic: hepatotoxicity (usually mild and reversible).
Skin: rash.
Other: flulike syndrome, hyperuricemia, urate nephropathy.

INTERACTIONS
Digoxin: may decrease serum digoxin levels. Monitor closely.

CONTRAINDICATIONS
- Contraindicated in patients hypersensitive to the drug.
- Use cautiously in patients with thrombocytopenia, leukopenia, renal or hepatic disease, and after other chemotherapy or radiation therapy.

NURSING CONSIDERATIONS
- Diligent mouth care can help prevent stomatitis.
- Nausea and vomiting are more frequent when large doses are administered rapidly by I.V. push. These reactions are less frequent when given by infusion. To reduce nausea, give antiemetic before administering.
- Corticosteroid eye drops are prescribed to prevent drug-induced keratitis.
- Monitor fluid intake and output carefully. Maintain high fluid intake and give allopurinol, if ordered, to avoid urate nephropathy in leukemia induction therapy. Monitor serum uric acid level.
- Monitor hepatic and renal function studies and CBC.
- Warn patients to watch for signs of infection (fever, sore throat, fatigue) and bleeding (easy bruising, nosebleeds, bleeding gums, melena). Take temperature daily.
- Modify or discontinue therapy if granulocyte count is below 1,000/mm^3 or if platelet count is below 50,000/mm^3.
- Assess patients receiving high doses for neurotoxicity, which may first appear as nystagmus, but can progress to ataxia and cerebellar dysfunction.
- To prevent bleeding, avoid all I.M. injections when platelet count is below 100,000/mm^3.
- Preparation and administration of parenteral form of this drug is associated with carcinogenic, mutagenic, and teratogenic risks for personnel. Follow institutional policy to reduce risks.
- **I.V. use:** Reconstitute drug using the provided diluent, which is bacteriostatic water for injection containing benzyl alcohol. Avoid this diluent when preparing drug for neonates or for intrathecal use. Reconstitute 100-mg vial with 5 ml of diluent or 500-mg vial with 10 ml of diluent. Reconstituted solution is stable for 48 hours. Discard cloudy reconstituted solution.
- For I.V. infusion, further dilute using 0.9% sodium chloride injection, D_5W, or sterile water for injection.
- For intrathecal administration, use preservative-free 0.9% sodium chloride or Elliot's B solution. Add 5 ml to the 100-mg vial or 10 ml to the 500-mg vial. Use immediately after reconstitution. Discard unused drug.

floxuridine
FUDR
Pregnancy Risk Category: D

HOW SUPPLIED
Injection: 500-mg vials (50 mg/ml in 10-ml vials or 100 mg/ml in 5-ml vials)

ACTION

Mechanism: Inhibits DNA synthesis.
Onset: therapeutic effect, 1 to 6 weeks.

INDICATIONS & DOSAGE

Brain, breast, head, neck, liver, gallbladder, and bile duct cancers –
Adults: 0.1 to 0.6 mg/kg daily by intra-arterial infusion for 14 to 21 days or until toxicity occurs; or 0.4 to 0.6 mg/kg daily into hepatic artery.

ADVERSE REACTIONS

CNS: cerebellar ataxia, vertigo, nystagmus, seizures, depression, hemiplegia, hiccups, lethargy.
EENT: blurred vision.
GI: *anorexia, stomatitis, cramps, nausea, vomiting, diarrhea, bleeding, enteritis.*
Hematologic: ***leukopenia, anemia, thrombocytopenia.***
Hepatic: cholangitis, jaundice, elevated liver enzyme levels.
Skin: *erythema,* dermatitis, pruritus, rash.
Other: *alopecia.*

INTERACTIONS

None significant.

CONTRAINDICATIONS

- Contraindicated in patients with poor nutritional state, bone marrow suppression, or serious infection.
- Use cautiously following high-dose pelvic radiation therapy or use of alkylating agents, and in patients with impaired hepatic or renal function.

NURSING CONSIDERATIONS

- Severe skin and GI adverse reactions require stopping drug.
- Use of antacid eases but probably won't prevent GI distress.
- Diligent mouth care can help prevent stomatitis.
- Monitor fluid intake and output, CBC, and renal and hepatic function.
- Discontinue drug if WBC count falls below 3,500/mm³ or if platelet count falls below 100,000/mm³.
- Make sure patient knows that therapeutic effect may be delayed 1 to 6 weeks.
- To prevent bleeding, avoid all I.M. injections when platelet count is below 100,000/mm³.
- Preparation and administration of parenteral form of this drug is associated with carcinogenic, mutagenic, and teratogenic risks for personnel. Follow institutional policy to reduce risks.
- **IV use:** Reconstitute with sterile water for injection. To prepare infusion, dilute in D_5W or 0.9% sodium chloride solution.
- Use an infusion pump with intra-arterial infusions.
- Check line for bleeding, blockage, displacement, or leakage.
- Refrigerated solution is stable for no more than 2 weeks.

fludarabine phosphate

Fludara

Pregnancy Risk Category: D

HOW SUPPLIED

Powder for injection: 50 mg

ACTION

Mechanism: An antineoplastic antimetabolite; exact mechanism of action is not fully established and may be multifaceted. After conversion to its active metabolite, fludarabine interferes with DNA synthesis by inhibiting DNA polymerase alpha, ribonucleotide reductase, and DNA primase.
Onset: 7 to 21 weeks. **Peak:** Serum levels peak immediately after I.V. infusion. **Duration:** terminal half-life, 10 to 30 hours.

INDICATIONS & DOSAGE

B-cell chronic lymphocytic leukemia (CLL) in patients who have either not responded or responded inadequately

to at least one standard alkylating agent regimen –
Adults: 25 mg/m² I.V. over 30 minutes for 5 consecutive days. Repeat cycle q 28 days.

ADVERSE REACTIONS

CNS: *fatigue, malaise, weakness,* paresthesia, headache, sleep disorder, depression, cerebellar syndrome, ***CVA,*** transient ischemic attack, agitation, *confusion;* ***coma, death*** (with high doses).
CV: *edema,* angina, phlebitis, ***arrhythmias, CHF,*** supraventricular tachycardia, deep venous thrombosis, ***aneurysm,*** hemorrhage.
EENT: *visual disturbances,* hearing loss, delayed blindness (with high doses), sinusitis, pharyngitis, epistaxis.
GI: *nausea, vomiting,* diarrhea, constipation, *anorexia,* stomatitis, GI bleeding, esophagitis, mucositis.
GU: dysuria, urinary infection, urinary hesitancy, proteinuria, hematuria, ***renal failure.***
Hematologic: ***myelosuppression.***
Hepatic: liver failure, cholelithiasis.
Respiratory: cough, *pneumonia,* dyspnea, upper respiratory infection, allergic pneumonitis, hemoptysis, hypoxia, bronchitis.
Skin: rash, pruritus, seborrhea.
Other: *fever, chills, infection,* pain, myalgia, tumor lysis syndrome, alopecia, ***anaphylaxis,*** diaphoresis, hyperglycemia, dehydration, hyperuricemia, hyperphosphatemia.

INTERACTIONS

Other myelosuppressants: increased toxicity. Avoid concomitant use.

CONTRAINDICATIONS

- Contraindicated in patients hypersensitive to the drug or its components.
- Use cautiously in patients with renal insufficiency, hematologic impairment, or myelosuppression.

NURSING CONSIDERATIONS

- Advanced age, renal insufficiency, and bone marrow impairment may predispose patients to increased or excessive toxicity. Monitor patients closely and modify dosage based on toxicity. Most toxic effects are dose-dependent.
- Bone marrow suppression can be severe. Careful hematologic monitoring is required, especially of neutrophil and platelet counts.
- Severe neurologic effects occur when high doses are used to treat acute leukemia. Irreversible CNS toxicity characterized by delayed blindness, coma, and death is associated with high doses. No specific antidote exists.
- Optimal duration of therapy is not yet determined. Current recommendations suggest three additional cycles after achieving maximal response before discontinuing therapy.
- Used investigationally to treat non-Hodgkin's lymphoma, macroglobulinemic lymphoma, prolymphocytic leukemia or prolymphocytoid variant of CLL, mycosis fungoides, hairy-cell leukemia, and Hodgkin's disease.
- Preparation and administration of parenteral form of this drug is associated with mutagenic, teratogenic, and carcinogenic risks for personnel. Follow institutional policy to reduce risks.
- **I.V. use:** To prepare solution, add 2 ml of sterile water for injection to the solid cake of fludarabine. Dissolution should occur within 15 seconds; each milliliter will contain 25 mg of drug. Dilute further in 100 or 125 ml of D_5W or 0.9% sodium chloride injection. Use within 8 hours of reconstitution.
- Store drug in refrigerator at 36° to 46° F (2° to 8° C).

fluorouracil (5-fluorouracil, 5-FU)

Adrucil, Efudex, Fluoroplex

Pregnancy Risk Category: D

HOW SUPPLIED

Injection: 50 mg/ml
Cream: 1%, 5%
Topical solution: 1%, 2%, 5%

ACTION

Mechanism: Inhibits DNA synthesis.
Onset: 2 to 3 days after topical use, 2 to 6 weeks for actinic keratoses, 12 weeks for basal cell carcinoma.
Duration: terminal elimination half-life, about 20 hours.

INDICATIONS & DOSAGE

Colon, rectal, breast, ovarian, cervical, bladder, liver, and pancreatic cancers –
Adults: 12.5 mg/kg I.V. daily for 3 to 5 days q 4 weeks; or 15 mg/kg weekly for 6 weeks. (Dosages recommended based on lean body weight.) Maximum single recommended dose is 800 mg, although higher single doses (up to 1.5 g) have been used. The injectable form has been given orally but is not recommended.
Palliative treatment of advanced colorectal cancer –
Adults: 425 mg/m² I.V. daily for 5 consecutive days. Given with 20 mg/m² of leucovorin I.V. Repeat at 4-week intervals for two additional courses; then repeat at intervals of 4 to 5 weeks if tolerated.
Multiple actinic (solar) keratoses; superficial basal cell carcinoma –
Adults: apply cream or topical solution b.i.d.

ADVERSE REACTIONS

CNS: acute cerebellar syndrome, ataxia, confusion, disorientation, euphoria, headache, nystagmus, *weakness, malaise.*
GI: *stomatitis, GI ulcer* (may precede leukopenia), *nausea and vomiting in 30% to 50% of patients, diarrhea, anorexia.*
Hematologic: ***leukopenia, thrombocytopenia,*** anemia; WBC count nadir 9 to 14 days after first dose; platelet count nadir in 7 to 14 days.
Skin: *dermatitis,* hyperpigmentation (especially in blacks), nail changes, pigmented palmar creases; erythematous, desquamative rash of hands and feet with long-term use ("hand-foot syndrome").
Other: *reversible alopecia in 5% to 20% of patients; erythema, pain, burning, scaling, pruritus;* contact dermatitis, soreness, suppuration, swelling (with topical use).

INTERACTIONS

Leucovorin calcium, prior treatment with alkylating agents: increased toxicity of fluorouracil. Use with extreme caution.

CONTRAINDICATIONS

- Contraindicated in patients hypersensitive to the drug; patients who are in a poor nutritional state; patients with bone marrow suppression (WBC counts of 5,000/mm³ or less or platelet counts of 100,000/mm³ or less); patients with potentially serious infections; and in those who have had major surgery within the previous month.
- Use cautiously after high-dose pelvic radiation therapy or use of alkylating agents or in patients with impaired hepatic or renal function or widespread neoplastic infiltration of bone marrow.

NURSING CONSIDERATIONS

- Watch for stomatitis or diarrhea (signs of toxicity). May use topical oral anesthetic to soothe lesions. Discontinue drug if diarrhea occurs.
- Encourage diligent oral hygiene to prevent superinfection of denuded mucosa.

• Give antiemetic before administering drug to reduce nausea.
• Monitor WBC and platelet counts daily. Watch for ecchymoses, petechiae, easy bruising, and anemia.
• Consider protective isolation if WBC count is less than 2,000/mm³.
• Dermatologic adverse effects are reversible when drug is stopped. Patients should use highly protective sunblocks to avoid inflammatory erythematous dermatitis. Long-term use of the drug is associated with erythematous, desquamative rash of the hands and feet. May be treated with pyridoxine (50 to 150 mg P.O. daily) for 5 to 7 days.
• Therapeutic concentrations are not reached in CSF.
• Monitor fluid intake and output, CBC, and renal and hepatic function tests.
• Sometimes ordered as 5-fluorouracil or 5-FU. The numeral 5 is part of the drug name and should not be confused with dosage units.
• Warn patients that alopecia may occur, but that it's reversible.
• To prevent bleeding, avoid all I.M. injections when platelet count is below 100,000/mm³.
• Fluorouracil toxicity may be delayed for 1 to 3 weeks.
• Sometimes administered via hepatic arterial infusion in treatment of hepatic metastases.

For topical application:
• Avoid occlusive dressings because they increase the risk of inflammatory reactions in adjacent normal skin.
• Caution patients to avoid prolonged exposure to sunlight or ultraviolet light.
• Apply with caution near eyes, nose, and mouth.
• Warn patients that treated area may be unsightly during therapy and for several weeks after therapy. Complete healing may take 1 or 2 months.
• Ingestion and systemic absorption of topical form may cause leukopenia, thrombocytopenia, stomatitis, diarrhea, or GI ulceration, bleeding, and hemorrhage. Application to large ulcerated areas may cause systemic toxicity.
• Expect to use 1% concentration on the face. Higher concentrations are used for thicker-skinned areas or resistant lesions.
• Expect to use 5% strength for superficial basal cell carcinoma confirmed by biopsy.
• Wash hands immediately after handling medication.
• Preparation and administration of parenteral form of this drug is associated with carcinogenic, mutagenic, and teratogenic risks for personnel. Follow institutional policy to reduce risks.
• The manufacturer recommends using sodium hypochlorite 5% (household bleach) to inactivate the drug in the event of a spill.
• **I.V. use:** Drug may be administered by direct injection without dilution. For I.V. infusion, drug may be diluted with D_5W, sterile water for injection, or 0.9% sodium chloride injection. Infuse slowly over 2 to 8 hours.
• Don't use cloudy solution. If crystals form, redissolve by warming.
• Solution is more stable in plastic I.V. bags than in glass bottles. Use plastic I.V. containers for administering continuous infusions.
• Don't refrigerate fluorouracil.

hydroxyurea

Hydrea**

Pregnancy Risk Category: D

HOW SUPPLIED

Capsules: 500 mg

ACTION

Mechanism: Inhibits DNA synthesis.
Peak: Levels peak 2 hours after dose.
Duration: half-life, 3 to 4 hours.

*Liquid form contains alcohol.
**May contain tartrazine.

INDICATIONS & DOSAGE
Melanoma; resistant chronic myelocytic leukemia; recurrent, metastatic, or inoperable ovarian cancer; head and neck cancers –
Adults: 80 mg/kg P.O. as single dose q 3 days; or 20 to 30 mg/kg P.O. as a single daily dose.

ADVERSE REACTIONS
CNS: drowsiness, hallucinations.
GI: *anorexia, nausea, vomiting, diarrhea,* stomatitis.
GU: increased BUN and serum creatinine levels.
Hematologic: ***leukopenia, thrombocytopenia,*** anemia, *megaloblastosis; dose-limiting and dose-related* ***bone marrow suppression,*** with rapid recovery.
Skin: rash, pruritus.
Other: hyperuricemia.

INTERACTIONS
Cytotoxic drugs, radiation therapy: enhanced toxicity of hydroxyurea. Use together cautiously.

CONTRAINDICATIONS
- Contraindicated in patients hypersensitive to the drug.
- Use cautiously in patients with renal dysfunction. Discontinue if WBC count is less than 2,500/mm³ or if platelet count is less than 100,000/mm³.
- Dosage modification may be required after chemotherapy or radiation therapy.

NURSING CONSIDERATIONS
- Warn patients to watch for signs of infection (fever, sore throat, fatigue) and bleeding (easy bruising, nosebleeds, bleeding gums, melena). Take temperature daily.
- Tell patients who can't swallow capsules that they may empty contents into water and take immediately.
- Monitor fluid intake and output; keep patients hydrated.
- Routinely measure BUN, uric acid, and serum creatinine levels.
- Drug crosses blood-brain barrier.
- Auditory and visual hallucinations and hematologic toxicity increase when decreased renal function exists.
- Concomitant radiation therapy may increase incidence or severity of GI distress or stomatitis.
- To prevent bleeding, avoid all I.M. injections when platelet count is below 100,000/mm³.
- Has been used investigationally to relieve symptoms of sickle cell anemia. Dosage is highly variable; in early trials, the median dose was 20 mg/kg/day.

mercaptopurine (6-MP, 6-mercaptopurine)
Purinethol

Pregnancy Risk Category: D

HOW SUPPLIED
Tablets (scored): 50 mg

ACTION
Mechanism: Inhibits RNA and DNA synthesis.
Duration: terminal elimination half-life, about 10 hours.

INDICATIONS & DOSAGE
Acute myeloblastic leukemia, chronic myelocytic leukemia –
Adults: 80 to 100 mg/m² (rounded to the nearest 25 mg) P.O. daily as a single dose up to 5 mg/kg/day.
Children: 75 mg/m² (rounded to the nearest 25 mg) P.O. daily.
Acute lymphoblastic leukemia –
Children: 75 mg/m² (rounded to the nearest 25 mg) P.O. daily.

Usual maintenance for adults and children: 1.5 to 2.5 mg/kg/day.

ADVERSE REACTIONS
GI: *nausea, vomiting, and anorexia in 25% of patients;* painful oral ulcers.
Hematologic: ***leukopenia, thrombo-***

cytopenia, anemia; all may persist several days after drug is stopped.
Hepatic: biliary stasis, *jaundice, **hepatic necrosis.***
Skin: rash, hyperpigmentation.
Other: hyperuricemia.

INTERACTIONS
Allopurinol: slowed inactivation of mercaptopurine. Decrease mercaptopurine to ¼ or ⅓ normal dose.
Hepatotoxic drugs: may enhance hepatotoxicity of mercaptopurine.
Nondepolarizing neuromuscular blockers: antagonized muscle relaxant effect. Notify the anesthesiologist that the patient is receiving mercaptopurine.
Warfarin: enhanced anticoagulant effect.

CONTRAINDICATIONS
- Contraindicated in patients whose disease has shown resistance to the drug.
- Dosage modifications may be required after chemotherapy or radiation therapy, in patients with depressed neutrophil or platelet counts, and in those with impaired hepatic or renal function.

NURSING CONSIDERATIONS
- Observe for signs of bleeding and infection.
- Warn patients to watch for signs of infection (fever, sore throat, fatigue) and bleeding (easy bruising, nosebleeds, bleeding gums, melena). Take temperature daily.
- Hepatic dysfunction is reversible when drug is stopped. Watch for jaundice, clay-colored stools, and frothy dark urine. Drug should be stopped if hepatic tenderness occurs.
- Monitor blood counts and serum transaminase, alkaline phosphatase, and bilirubin levels weekly during induction and monthly during maintenance.
- Monitor fluid intake and output. Encourage adequate fluid intake (3 liters daily).
- Sometimes ordered as 6-mercaptopurine or 6-MP. The numeral 6 is part of drug name and does not signify number of dosage units.
- Warn patients that improvement may take 2 to 4 weeks or longer.
- GI adverse reactions are less common in children than in adults.
- To prevent bleeding, avoid all I.M. injections when platelet count is below 100,000/mm³.
- Monitor serum uric acid level. If allopurinol is necessary, use cautiously.

---

methotrexate

methotrexate sodium
Folex PFS, Mexate AQ, Rheumatrex

Pregnancy Risk Category: D

HOW SUPPLIED
Tablets (scored): 2.5 mg
Injection: 20-mg, 25-mg, 50-mg, 100-mg, 250-mg vials, lyophilized powder, preservative-free; 25-mg/ml vials, preservative-free solution; 2.5-mg/ml, 25-mg/ml vials, lyophilized powder, preserved

ACTION
Mechanism: Prevents reduction of folic acid to tetrahydrofolate by binding to dihydrofolate reductase.
Peak: Serum concentrations peak immediately after I.V. injection, within ½ to 1 hour after I.M. injection, or 1 to 2 hours after oral dose. **Duration:** half-life after low-dose therapy, 3 to 10 hours; after high-dose therapy, 8 to 15 hours.

INDICATIONS & DOSAGE
Trophoblastic tumors (choriocarcinoma, hydatidiform mole) –
Adults: 15 to 30 mg P.O. or I.M. daily for 5 days. Repeat after 1 or

*Liquid form contains alcohol.
**May contain tartrazine.

Common reactions are in italics; ***life-threatening,*** in bold italics.

more weeks, according to response or toxicity.
Acute lymphoblastic and lymphatic leukemia –
Adults and children: 3.3 mg/m²/day P.O., I.M., or I.V. for 4 to 6 weeks or until remission occurs; then 20 to 30 mg/m² P.O. or I.M. twice weekly.
Meningeal leukemia –
Adults and children: 10 to 15 mg/m² intrathecally q 2 to 5 days until CSF is normal. Use only 20-, 50-, or 100-mg vials of powder with no preservatives; dilute using 0.9% sodium chloride injection *without* preservatives or Elliot's B solution. Use only new vials of drug and diluent. Use immediately.
Burkitt's lymphoma (Stage I or Stage II) –
Adults: 10 to 25 mg P.O. daily for 4 to 8 days with 1-week rest intervals.
Lymphosarcoma (Stage III) –
Adults: 0.625 to 2.5 mg/kg daily P.O., I.M., or I.V.
Mycosis fungoides –
Adults: 2.5 to 10 mg P.O. daily, or 50 mg I.M. weekly, or 25 mg I.M. twice weekly.
Psoriasis –
Adults: 10 to 25 mg P.O., I.M., or I.V. as single weekly dose.
Rheumatoid arthritis –
Adults: initially, 7.5 mg P.O. weekly, either in a single dose or divided as 2.5 mg P.O. q 12 hours for three doses once a week. Dosage may be gradually increased to a maximum of 20 mg weekly.

ADVERSE REACTIONS

CNS: ***arachnoiditis*** within hours of intrathecal use; subacute neurotoxicity, which may begin a few weeks later; ***necrotizing demyelinating leukoencephalopathy*** a few years later.
EENT: pharyngitis, gingivitis.
GI: *stomatitis, diarrhea leading to* ***hemorrhagic enteritis and intestinal perforation,*** *nausea, vomiting.*
GU: nephropathy, *tubular necrosis.*
Hematologic: WBC and platelet count nadirs occurring on day 7; ***anemia, leukopenia, thrombocytopenia*** (all dose-related).
Hepatic: acute toxicity (elevated transaminase level), *chronic toxicity* (cirrhosis, ***hepatic fibrosis***).
Respiratory: ***pulmonary fibrosis, pulmonary interstitial infiltrates,*** pneumonitis.
Skin: *urticaria,* pruritus, hyperpigmentation; exposure to sun may aggravate psoriatic lesions, rash, photosensitivity.
Other: alopecia, osteoporosis (in children, with long-term use), hyperuricemia.

INTERACTIONS

Digoxin: may decrease serum digoxin levels. Monitor closely.
Folic acid derivatives: antagonized methotrexate effect.
NSAIDs, phenylbutazone, probenecid, salicylates, sulfonamides: increased methotrexate toxicity; don't use together if possible.
Phenytoin: may decrease serum phenytoin levels. Monitor closely.
Vaccines: immunizations may be ineffective; risk of disseminated infection with live-virus vaccines.

CONTRAINDICATIONS

- Contraindicated in patients hypersensitive to the drug.
- Use cautiously and at modified dosage in patients with impaired hepatic or renal function, bone marrow suppression, aplasia, leukopenia, thrombocytopenia, or anemia. Also use cautiously in patients with infection, peptic ulceration, and ulcerative colitis and in very young, elderly, or debilitated patients.

NURSING CONSIDERATIONS

- Rash, redness, or ulcerations in mouth or pulmonary adverse reactions may signal serious complications. Therapy may be discontinued if ulcerative stomatitis or other severe

GI adverse reaction occurs, or if pulmonary toxicity is detected.
• Teach and encourage diligent mouth care to reduce the risk of superinfection in the mouth.
• Perform baseline pulmonary function tests and monitor periodically.
• Warn patients to avoid conception during and immediately after therapy because of possible abortion or congenital anomalies.
• Monitor serum uric acid level.
• Monitor fluid intake and output daily. Encourage fluid intake of 2 to 3 liters daily.
• Alkalinize urine by giving sodium bicarbonate tablets to prevent precipitation of drug, especially with high doses. Maintain urine pH at more than 6.5. Reduce dosage if BUN level reaches 20 to 30 mg/dl or creatinine level reaches 1.2 to 2 mg/dl. Stop drug if BUN level is greater than 30 mg/dl or creatinine level is greater than 2 mg/dl.
• Watch for increases in AST, ALT, and alkaline phosphatase levels, which may signal hepatic dysfunction.
• Watch for signs of bleeding (especially GI) and infection.
• Warn patients to use highly protective sunblock when exposed to sunlight.
• Take temperature daily, and watch for cough, dyspnea, and cyanosis.
• Leucovorin rescue is necessary with high-dose (greater than 100 mg) protocols. Don't confuse with folic acid. This rescue technique is effective against systemic toxicity but does not interfere with the tumor cells' absorption of methotrexate.
• Advise patients not to discontinue leucovorin rescue if they experience severe nausea and vomiting. Parenteral leucovorin therapy may be necessary.
• To prevent bleeding, avoid all I.M. injections when platelet count is below 100,000/mm^3.
• Preparation and administration of parenteral form of this drug is associated with carcinogenic, mutagenic, and teratogenic risks for personnel. Follow institutional policy to reduce risks.
• **I.V. use:** May be administered undiluted by direct injection. Alternatively, dilute with up to 25 ml of 0.9% sodium chloride injection (for Folex) or 2 to 10 ml of sterile water for injection, 0.9% sodium chloride injection, or bacteriostatic water for injection containing parabens or benzyl alcohol (for Mexate).
• For intrathecal use, use preservative-free product. Reconstitute immediately before using with preservative-free 0.9% sodium chloride injection or Elliot's B solution. Dilute to a maximum concentration of 1 mg/ml.
• Reconstitute solutions without preservatives immediately before use, and discard any unused drug.

thioguanine (6-thioguanine, 6-TG)

Lanvis†

Pregnancy Risk Category: D

HOW SUPPLIED

Tablets (scored): 40 mg

ACTION

Mechanism: Inhibits purine synthesis.
Duration: half-life, ½ to 4 hours.

INDICATIONS & DOSAGE

Acute leukemia, chronic myelogenous leukemia –
Adults and children: initially, 2 mg/kg P.O. daily (usually calculated to nearest 20 mg). If necessary, dose is then increased gradually to 3 mg/kg/day as tolerated.

ADVERSE REACTIONS

GI: nausea, vomiting, stomatitis, diarrhea, anorexia.

*Liquid form contains alcohol.
**May contain tartrazine.

Common reactions are in italics; ***life-threatening,*** in bold italics.

Hematologic: ***leukopenia, anemia, thrombocytopenia*** (occurs slowly over 2 to 4 weeks).
Hepatic: ***hepatotoxicity,*** jaundice.
Other: hyperuricemia.

INTERACTIONS
Myelosuppressant drugs: increased risk of toxicity, especially myelosuppression and bleeding. Use together cautiously.

CONTRAINDICATIONS
- Contraindicated in patients whose disease has shown resistance to the drug.
- Use cautiously and with dosage modification in patients with renal or hepatic dysfunction.

NURSING CONSIDERATIONS
- Stop drug if hepatotoxicity or hepatic tenderness occurs. Watch for jaundice; may be reversible if drug is stopped promptly.
- Monitor CBC daily during induction, and then weekly during maintenance therapy.
- Monitor serum uric acid level.
- Sometimes ordered as 6-thioguanine. The numeral 6 is part of drug name and does not signify dosage units.
- To prevent bleeding, avoid all I.M. injections when platelet count is below 100,000/mm³.

trimetrexate glucuronate
Neutrexin

Pregnancy Risk Category: D

HOW SUPPLIED
Injection: 25-mg vials

ACTION
Mechanism: Prevents reduction of folic acid to tetrahydrofolate by binding to dihydrofolate reductase.
Peak: Peak levels occur immediately.
Duration: terminal elimination half-life, about 16 hours.

INDICATIONS & DOSAGE
Alternative treatment of Pneumocystis carinii *pneumonia in patients with AIDS –*
Adults: 45 mg/m² I.V. infusion over 60 to 90 minutes daily for 21 days, administered with 20 mg/m² of leucovorin I.V. or P.O. q 6 hours for 24 days.

ADVERSE REACTIONS
CNS: peripheral neuropathy.
GI: nausea, vomiting, stomatitis.
Hematologic: ***neutropenia, thrombocytopenia, anemia.***
Hepatic: hepatotoxicity.
Skin: rash.

INTERACTIONS
Acetaminophen, cimetidine, clotrimazole, erythromycin, fluconazole, ketoconazole, miconazole, rifampin, rifabutin: may interfere with trimetrexate metabolism and lead to toxicity. Monitor closely.
Chloride-containing solutions, leucovorin: precipitate will form if mixed with trimetrexate. Administer separately.
Hepatotoxic, myelosuppressive, or nephrotoxic drugs: enhanced toxicity. Use together cautiously and monitor closely.

CONTRAINDICATIONS
- Contraindicated in patients hypersensitive to trimetrexate, methotrexate, or leucovorin.
- Use cautiously in women of childbearing age because the drug may cause fetal harm. Avoid using during pregnancy.
- Leucovorin therapy must accompany trimetrexate treatments to avoid potentially life-threatening toxicity. Leucovorin therapy must extend for 3 days beyond trimetrexate treatment.

NURSING CONSIDERATIONS

- Many adverse effects may be decreased by adjusting the dosage of leucovorin. Monitor patients closely.
- Avoid I.M. injections in patients with thrombocytopenia.
- Warn patients to watch for signs of infection (fever, sore throat, fatigue) and bleeding (easy bruising, nosebleeds, bleeding gums, melena). Take temperature daily.
- When calculating the oral dose of leucovorin, round dosage up to the next increment of 25 mg.
- Preparation of parenteral form of this drug is associated with carcinogenic, mutagenic, and teratogenic risks for personnel. Follow institutional policy to reduce risks.
- **I.V. use:** Reconstitute 25-mg vial with 2 ml of D_5W or sterile water for injection to yield a solution of 12.5 mg/ml. Complete dissolution usually occurs within 30 seconds. Further dilute reconstituted solution with D_5W to yield a final concentration of 0.25 to 2 mg/ml. Infuse over 60 minutes. After reconstitution, the drug is stable at room temperature or refrigerated for 24 hours.
- Incompatible with chloride-containing solutions (including 0.9% sodium chloride solution) and leucovorin. Only D_5W is recommended for I.V. infusion.
- Flush the I.V. line with at least 10 ml of D_5W immediately before and after the trimetrexate infusion.
- Leucovorin may be administered either before or after trimetrexate. When giving I.V., be sure to flush the I.V. line with D_5W because the two drugs are incompatible. Leucovorin calcium may be infused over 5 to 10 minutes.

71

Antibiotic antineoplastic agents

bleomycin sulfate
dactinomycin
daunorubicin hydrochloride
doxorubicin hydrochloride
idarubicin hydrochloride
mitomycin
plicamycin
procarbazine hydrochloride

COMBINATION PRODUCTS
None.

bleomycin sulfate

Blenoxane

Pregnancy Risk Category: D

HOW SUPPLIED
Injection: 15-unit vials (1 unit = 1 mg)

ACTION
Mechanism: Inhibits DNA synthesis and causes scission of single- and double-stranded DNA.
Duration: half-life, about 2 hours.

INDICATIONS & DOSAGE
Dosage and indications may vary. Check the treatment protocol with the doctor.
Cervical, esophageal, head, neck, and testicular cancers; squamous cell carcinoma; lymphosarcoma; reticulum cell sarcoma –
Adults: 10 to 20 units/m² I.V., I.M., or S.C. 1 or 2 times weekly to total of 300 to 400 units.
Hodgkin's disease –
Adults: 10 to 20 units/m² I.V., I.M., or S.C. 1 or 2 times weekly. After 50% response, maintenance dosage is 1 unit I.M. or I.V. daily or 5 units I.M. or I.V. weekly.
Lymphoma –
Adults: first two doses should be 2 units or less, and the patient should be monitored for any allergic reaction. If no reaction occurs, then follow above dosing schedule.

ADVERSE REACTIONS
CNS: hyperesthesia of scalp and fingers, headache.
GI: *stomatitis, prolonged anorexia in 13% of patients, nausea, vomiting,* diarrhea.
Hematologic: *leukocytosis.*
Respiratory: ***pulmonary fibrosis*** in 10% of patients, *pulmonary adverse reactions (fine crackles, dyspnea), nonproductive cough.*
Skin: *erythema, vesiculation, and hardening and discoloration of palmar and plantar skin in 8% of patients;* desquamation of hands, feet, and pressure areas; *hyperpigmentation; acne.*
Other: *reversible alopecia,* swelling of interphalangeal joints, hypersensitivity reaction (*fever up to 106° F [41.1° C] with chills up to 5 hours after injection;* ***anaphylaxis*** in 1% to 6% of patients), fever.

INTERACTIONS
Digitalis glycosides: decreased serum digoxin levels. Monitor closely.
Phenytoin: decreased serum phenytoin levels. Monitor closely.

CONTRAINDICATIONS
- Contraindicated in patients hypersensitive to the drug.
- Use cautiously in patients with renal or pulmonary impairment.

NURSING CONSIDERATIONS
- Because of an increased risk of anaphylactoid reactions, the first two doses in patients with lymphoma should be limited to 2 units or less.

- Pulmonary adverse reactions are common in patients over age 70. Fatal pulmonary fibrosis occurs in 1% of patients, especially when cumulative dosage exceeds 400 units.
- Pulmonary function tests should be performed to establish pretreatment baseline. Drug should be stopped if pulmonary function test shows a marked decline.
- Monitor chest X-ray and listen to lungs.
- Monitor injection site for signs of irritation.
- Drug concentrates in keratin of squamous epithelium. To prevent linear streaking, don't use adhesive dressings on skin.
- Hypersensitivity reactions may be delayed for several hours, especially in patients with lymphoma.
- Warn patients that alopecia may occur, but that it's usually reversible.
- Bleomycin-induced fever is common and may be treated with antipyretics. This reaction usually occurs within 3 to 6 hours of administration.
- Preparation and administration of parenteral form of this drug is associated with carcinogenic, mutagenic, and teratogenic risks for personnel. Follow institutional policy to reduce risks.
- **I.V. use:** Reconstitute drug with 5 ml or more of D_5W or 0.9% sodium chloride injection. For I.V. infusion, dilute with 50 to 100 ml of D_5W or 0.9% sodium chloride injection.
- For I.M. use, dilute drug in 1 to 5 ml of sterile water for injection, bacteriostatic water for injection, 0.9% sodium chloride injection, or D_5W.
- Refrigerated, reconstituted solution is stable for 4 weeks; at room temperature, it's stable for 2 weeks. Bleomycin may adsorb to plastic I.V. bags. For prolonged stability, use glass containers.
- Refrigerate unopened vials containing dry powder.

dactinomycin (actinomycin D)

Cosmegen

Pregnancy Risk Category: C

HOW SUPPLIED

Injection: 500 mcg/vial

ACTION

Mechanism: Interferes with DNA-dependent RNA synthesis by intercalation.

Duration: half-life, 36 hours.

INDICATIONS & DOSAGE

Dosage and indications may vary. Check the treatment protocol with the doctor.

Sarcoma, trophoblastic tumors in women, testicular cancer –

Adults: 10 to 15 mcg/kg/day I.V. for 5 days. Repeat q 3 to 4 weeks. Alternatively, 500 mg/m² (maximum of 2 mg) once a week for 3 weeks. Maximum dosage is 15 mcg/kg or 400 to 600 mcg/m²/day for 5 days.

Wilms' tumor, rhabdomyosarcoma, Ewing's sarcoma –

Children: 10 to 15 mcg/kg or 450 mcg/m²/day I.V. for 5 days. Maximum dosage is 500 mcg/day. Or 2.5 mg/m² I.V. in equally divided daily doses over a 7-day period. Wait for bone marrow recovery (usually 6 to 7 weeks), and repeat course.

ADVERSE REACTIONS

GI: *anorexia, nausea, vomiting,* abdominal pain, diarrhea, *stomatitis,* ulceration, proctitis.

Hematologic: ***anemia, leukopenia, thrombocytopenia, pancytopenia.***

Hepatic: ***hepatotoxicity.***

Skin: *erythema;* desquamation; *hyperpigmentation of skin, especially in previously irradiated areas; acnelike eruptions (reversible).*

Other: phlebitis and severe damage to soft tissue at injection site; reversible alopecia.

INTERACTIONS

Bone marrow suppressants: additive toxicity. Monitor closely.
Doxorubicin: enhanced cardiotoxicity. Monitor closely.
Vitamin K derivatives: decreased effectiveness. Monitor closely.

CONTRAINDICATIONS

- Contraindicated in patients with renal, hepatic, or bone marrow impairment and in those with chicken pox or herpes zoster.
- Dosage must be reduced in patients who have recently been treated with, or who will receive concomitant treatment with, radiation therapy or other chemotherapy drugs.

NURSING CONSIDERATIONS

- Stomatitis, diarrhea, leukopenia, or thrombocytopenia may require modifying dosage and schedule.
- In obese or edematous patients, base dosage on body surface area.
- To reduce nausea, give antiemetic before administering drug.
- Monitor renal and hepatic functions.
- Monitor CBC daily and platelet counts frequently.
- Warn patients to watch for signs of infection (fever, sore throat, fatigue) and bleeding (easy bruising, nosebleeds, bleeding gums, melena). Take temperature daily.
- Warn patients that alopecia may occur, but that it's usually reversible.
- Preparation and administration of parenteral form of this drug is associated with carcinogenic, mutagenic, and teratogenic risks for personnel. Follow institutional policy to reduce risks.
- In the event of a spill, the manufacturer recommends using a solution of trisodium phosphate 5% to inactivate the drug.
- **I.V. use:** Use only sterile water (without preservatives) as diluent for reconstitution. Add 1.1 ml to the vial to yield a gold-colored solution containing 0.5 mg/ml. Give by direct injection into a vein or through the tubing of a free-flowing I.V. solution of 0.9% sodium chloride injection or D_5W.
- For I.V. infusion, drug may be diluted with up to 50 ml of D_5W or 0.9% sodium chloride injection and infused over 15 minutes.
- Dactinomycin is a vesicant. Administer through a running I.V. line with good blood return. If infiltration occurs, apply cold compresses to area.
- Discard unused portions of solutions because they do not contain a preservative.

daunorubicin hydrochloride (DNR)

Cerubidin‡, Cerubidine

Pregnancy Risk Category: D

HOW SUPPLIED

Injection: 20 mg/vial

ACTION

Mechanism: Interferes with DNA-dependent RNA synthesis by intercalation.
Duration: half-life of parent drug, 18½ hours; of active metabolite, 55 hours.

INDICATIONS & DOSAGE

Dosage and indications may vary. Check the treatment protocol with the doctor.
Remission induction in acute nonlymphocytic (myelogenous, monocytic, erythroid) leukemia, acute lymphocytic leukemia –
Adults: as a single agent, 60 mg/m²/day I.V. on days 1, 2, and 3 q 3 to 4 weeks; in combination, 45 mg/m²/day I.V. on days 1, 2, and 3 of the first course and on days 1 and 2 of subsequent courses with cytarabine infusions.

Note: Dosage should be reduced in

patients with hepatic or renal impairment.

ADVERSE REACTIONS

CV: ***irreversible cardiomyopathy*** (dose-related), ECG changes, arrhythmias, pericarditis, myocarditis.
GI: *nausea, vomiting, stomatitis, esophagitis,* anorexia, diarrhea.
GU: nephrotoxicity, red urine (transient).
Hematologic: ***bone marrow suppression*** (lowest blood counts 10 to 14 days after administration).
Hepatic: ***hepatotoxicity.***
Skin: rash, pigmentation of fingernails and toenails.
Other: *severe cellulitis or tissue sloughing if drug extravasates, generalized alopecia,* fever, chills, hyperuricemia.

INTERACTIONS

Dexamethasone, heparin: don't mix. May form a precipitate.
Doxorubicin: additive cardiotoxicity. Monitor closely.
Hepatotoxic drugs: increased risk of additive hepatotoxicity. Monitor closely.

CONTRAINDICATIONS

- Contraindicated in patients hypersensitive to the drug.
- Use cautiously in patients with myelosuppression and in those with impaired cardiac, renal, or hepatic function.

NURSING CONSIDERATIONS

- Limit cumulative dosage to 500 to 600 mg/m² (450 mg/m² when patients are also receiving or have received cyclophosphamide or radiation therapy to cardiac area).
- Stop drug immediately if signs of CHF or cardiomyopathy develop.
- Monitor ECG before treatment and monthly during therapy.
- Light resting pulse rate is a sign of cardiac adverse reactions. Notify the doctor if this occurs.
- Never give drug I.M. or S.C.
- Monitor CBC and hepatic function tests.
- Advise patients that red urine for 1 to 2 days is normal and does not indicate the presence of blood in urine.
- Advise patients that alopecia may occur, but that it's usually reversible.
- Nausea and vomiting may be very severe and may last 24 to 48 hours.
- Preparation and administration of parenteral form of this drug is associated with carcinogenic, mutagenic, and teratogenic risks for personnel. Follow institutional policy to reduce risks.
- **I.V. use:** Reconstitute drug using 4 ml of sterile water for injection to produce a 5 mg/ml solution.
- Withdraw the desired dose into a syringe containing 10 to 15 ml of 0.9% sodium chloride injection. Inject into the tubing of a free-flowing I.V. solution of D_5W or 0.9% sodium chloride injection over 2 to 3 minutes. Alternatively, dilute in 50 ml of 0.9% sodium chloride injection and infuse over 10 to 15 minutes, or dilute in 100 ml and infuse over 30 to 45 minutes.
- Avoid extravasation; inject into tubing of free-flowing I.V. line. If extravasation occurs, discontinue I.V. infusion immediately and apply ice to area for 24 to 48 hours. Local infiltration with hydrocortisone sodium succinate injection (50 to 100 mg) or sodium bicarbonate (5 ml of 8.4% injection) may be ordered.
- Reddish color is similar to that of doxorubicin. Take care to avoid confusing the two drugs.
- Reconstituted solution is stable for 24 hours at room temperature or 48 hours if refrigerated. Optimally, use within 8 hours of preparation.

doxorubicin hydrochloride

Adriamycin‡, Adriamycin PFS, Adriamycin RDF, Rubex

Pregnancy Risk Category: D

HOW SUPPLIED

Injection (preservative-free): 2 mg/ml
Powder for injection: 10-mg, 20-mg, 50-mg, 100-mg, 150-mg vials

ACTION

Mechanism: Interferes with DNA-dependent RNA synthesis by intercalation.
Duration: half-life of parent drug, about 16½ hours; of metabolite, about 31½ hours.

INDICATIONS & DOSAGE

Dosage and indications may vary. Check the treatment protocol with the doctor.
Bladder, breast, cervical, head, neck, liver, lung, ovarian, prostatic, stomach, testicular, and thyroid cancers; Hodgkin's disease; acute lymphoblastic and myeloblastic leukemia; Wilms' tumor; neuroblastoma; lymphoma; sarcoma –
Adults: 60 to 75 mg/m² I.V. as single dose q 3 weeks; or 30 mg/m² I.V. in single daily dose, days 1 to 3 of 4-week cycle. Alternatively, 20 mg/m² I.V. once weekly or 30 mg/m² I.V. on 3 successive days, repeated q 4 weeks. Maximum cumulative dosage is 550 mg/m².

ADVERSE REACTIONS

CV: cardiac depression, seen in such ECG changes as sinus tachycardia, T-wave flattening, ST-segment depression, voltage reduction; ***arrhythmias*** in 11% of patients; ***irreversible cardiomyopathy (sometimes with pulmonary edema) with mortality of 30% to 75%.***
GI: *nausea, vomiting,* diarrhea, *stomatitis,* esophagitis.
GU: enhancement of cyclophosphamide-induced bladder injury, red urine (transient).
Hematologic: ***leukopenia, especially agranulocytosis,*** during days 10 to 15, with recovery by day 21; ***thrombocytopenia.***
Skin: *hyperpigmentation of nails, dermal creases, or skin,* (especially in previously irradiated areas).
Other: *severe cellulitis or tissue sloughing if drug extravasates;* hyperuricemia; *complete alopecia within 3 to 4 weeks* (hair may regrow 2 to 5 months after drug is stopped).

INTERACTIONS

Aminophylline, cephalothin, dexamethasone, fluorouracil, heparin, hydrocortisone: may form a precipitate. Don't mix together.
Digoxin: may decrease serum digoxin levels. Monitor closely.
Streptozocin: increased and prolonged blood levels. Dosage may have to be adjusted.

CONTRAINDICATIONS

- Contraindicated in patients who have received lifetime cumulative dosage of 550 mg/m²; 30% of patients who exceed this dosage develop cardiac adverse reactions, which begin 2 weeks to 6 months after stopping drug.
- Dosage modification may be required in patients with myelosuppression and in those with impaired cardiac or hepatic function.

NURSING CONSIDERATIONS

- Stop drug or slow rate of infusion if tachycardia develops.
- Stop drug immediately if signs of CHF develop. In many instances, CHF can be prevented by limiting cumulative dosage to 550 mg/m² (400 mg/m² when patients are also receiving or have received cyclophosphamide or radiation therapy to cardiac area).

• Monitor ECG before treatment and monthly during therapy.
• Monitor CBC and hepatic function tests.
• Warn patients to watch for signs of infection (fever, sore throat, fatigue) and bleeding (easy bruising, nosebleeds, bleeding gums, melena). Take temperature daily.
• Advise patients that orange to red urine for 1 to 2 days is normal and does not indicate the presence of blood in urine.
• Warn patients that alopecia may occur, but that it's usually reversible.
• The alternative dosage schedule (once-weekly dosing) has been found to cause a lower incidence of cardiomyopathy.
• Decrease dosage if serum bilirubin is increased: 50% dosage when bilirubin is 1.2 to 3 mg/100 ml; 25% dosage when bilirubin is greater than 3 mg/100 ml.
• Esophagitis is very common in patients who have also received radiation therapy.
• Premedicate with antiemetic to reduce nausea.
• Reddish color is similar to that of daunorubicin. Take care to avoid confusing the two drugs.
• Never give this drug I.M. or S.C.
• Preparation and administration of parenteral form of this drug is associated with carcinogenic, mutagenic, and teratogenic risks for personnel. Follow institutional policy to reduce risks.
• In the event of a leak or spill, inactivate drug with 5% sodium hypochlorite solution (household bleach).
• **I.V. use:** Reconstitute using preservative-free 0.9% sodium chloride injection. Add 5 ml to the 10-mg vial, 10 ml to the 20-mg vial, or 25 ml to the 50-mg vial. Shake vial and allow drug to dissolve; final concentration will be 2 mg/ml. Give by direct injection into the tubing of a free-flowing I.V. solution containing D_5W or 0.9% sodium chloride injection.
• Avoid extravasation; don't place I.V. line over joints or in extremities with poor venous or lymphatic drainage. If extravasation occurs, discontinue I.V. infusion immediately and apply ice to area for 24 to 48 hours. Some clinicians will infiltrate the area with a parenteral corticosteroid. Monitor area closely because the extravasation reaction may be progressive. Early consultation with a plastic surgeon may be advisable.
• If vein streaking occurs, slow administration rate. However, if welts occur, stop administration and report this to the doctor.
• Refrigerated, reconstituted solution is stable for 48 hours; at room temperature, it's stable for 24 hours.

idarubicin hydrochloride
Idamycin

Pregnancy Risk Category: D

HOW SUPPLIED
Powder for injection: 5 mg, 10 mg

ACTION
Mechanism: An antineoplastic antibiotic that inhibits nucleic acid synthesis by intercalation and that interacts with the enzyme topoisomerase II. It is highly lipophilic, which results in an increased rate of cellular uptake.
Peak: Intracellular drug levels peak within a few minutes after injection.
Duration: half-life, 22 hours.

INDICATIONS & DOSAGE
Dosage and indications may vary. Check current literature for recommended protocol.
Acute myeloid leukemia, including FAB (French-American-British) classifications M1 through M7, in combination with other approved antileukemic agents–

Adults: 12 mg/m²/day for 3 days by slow I.V. injection (over 10 to 15 minutes) in combination with 100 mg/m²/day of cytarabine for 7 days by continuous I.V. infusion or as a 25 mg/m² bolus followed by 200 mg/m²/day for 5 days by continuous infusion.

A second course may be administered if needed. If patients experience severe mucositis, delay administration until recovery is complete and reduce dosage by 25%. Dosage should also be reduced in patients with hepatic or renal impairment. Idarubicin should not be given if bilirubin level is above 5 mg/dl.

ADVERSE REACTIONS

CNS: headache, changed mental status, peripheral neuropathy, ***seizures.***
CV: ***CHF,*** atrial fibrillation, chest pain, ***MI,*** asymptomatic decline in left ventricular ejection fraction, ***myocardial insufficiency, arrhythmias,*** *hemorrhage,* ***myocardial toxicity.***
GI: *nausea, vomiting,* cramps, diarrhea, *mucositis,* ***severe enterocolitis with perforation*** (rare).
GU: decreased renal function.
Hematologic: ***myelosuppression.***
Hepatic: changes in hepatic function.
Skin: rash, urticaria, bullous erythrodermatous rash on palms and soles, hives at injection site, erythema at previously irradiated sites, tissue necrosis at injection site (if extravasation occurs).
Other: *infection,* alopecia, fever, hyperuricemia, hypersensitivity reactions.

INTERACTIONS

Alkaline solutions, heparin: incompatible. Idarubicin should not be mixed with other drugs unless specific compatibility data is available.

CONTRAINDICATIONS

- Contraindicated in patients with severe myelosuppression, preexisting cardiac disease, and severe hemorrhagic conditions and in those with overwhelming infection.
- Use with extreme caution in patients with hepatic or renal function impairment; dosage reduction is necessary.

NURSING CONSIDERATIONS

- Monitor hepatic and renal function tests and CBC frequently.
- Hyperuricemia may result from rapid lysis of leukemic cells; take appropriate preventive measures (including adequate hydration) before starting treatment. Allopurinol may be ordered.
- Control systemic infections before therapy.
- Antiemetics may be used to prevent or treat nausea and vomiting.
- Advise patients that red urine for several days is normal and does not indicate the presence of blood in urine.
- Preparation and administration of parenteral form of this drug is associated with carcinogenic, mutagenic, and teratogenic risks for personnel. Follow institutional policy to reduce risks.
- **I.V. use:** Reconstitute to a final concentration of 1 mg/ml using 0.9% sodium chloride injection without preservatives. Add 5 ml to the 5-mg vial or 10 ml to the 10-ml vial. *Do not use bacteriostatic sodium chloride.* Vial is under negative pressure.
- Administer over 10 to 15 minutes into a free-flowing I.V. infusion of 0.9% sodium chloride or 5% dextrose solution that is running into a large vein.
- If extravasation occurs, discontinue infusion immediately and notify doctor. Treat with intermittent ice packs – ½ hour immediately, and then ½ hour four times daily for 4 days.
- Instruct patients to recognize signs and symptoms of extravasation and to call the doctor or nurse if these occur.

• Reconstituted solutions are stable for 3 days (72 hours) at room temperature (59° to 86° F [15° to 30° C]); 7 days if refrigerated. Label any unused solutions with CHEMOTHERAPY HAZARD label.

mitomycin (mitomycin-C)

Mutamycin

Pregnancy Risk Category: D

HOW SUPPLIED

Injection: 5-mg, 20-mg, 40-mg vials

ACTION

Mechanism: Acts like an alkylating agent, cross-linking strands of DNA. This causes an imbalance of cell growth, leading to cell death.
Duration: terminal half-life, about 50 minutes.

INDICATIONS & DOSAGE

Dosage and indications may vary. Check the treatment protocol with the doctor.

Breast, colon, head, neck, lung, pancreatic, and stomach cancers; malignant melanoma –

Adults: 2 mg/m²/day I.V. for 5 days. Stop drug for 2 days; then repeat dose for 5 more days. Or 20 mg/m² as a single dose. Repeat cycle after 6 to 8 weeks, when WBC count has returned to 3,000/mm³ and platelet count is 75,000/mm³.

ADVERSE REACTIONS

CNS: paresthesia.
GI: *nausea, vomiting,* anorexia, stomatitis.
Hematologic: ***thrombocytopenia, leukopenia*** (may be delayed up to 8 weeks and may be cumulative with successive doses).
Respiratory: ***interstitial pneumonitis.***
Other: desquamation, induration, pruritus, *pain at injection site;* cellulitis, ulceration, sloughing with extravasation; *reversible alopecia; purple coloration of nail beds;* fever; ***microangiopathic hemolytic anemia, characterized by thrombocytopenia, renal failure, and hypertension.***

INTERACTIONS

None significant.

CONTRAINDICATIONS

• Contraindicated in patients hypersensitive to the drug and in those with a platelet count of 75,000/mm³ or less or a WBC count of 3,000/mm³. Also contraindicated in patients with bleeding disorders, coagulopathy, serious infections, or impaired renal function. Because of the risk of generalized disease, do not give to patients who have recently had chicken pox or herpes zoster.

NURSING CONSIDERATIONS

• Continue CBC and blood studies at least 7 weeks after therapy is stopped.
• Warn patients to watch for signs of infection (fever, sore throat, fatigue) and bleeding (easy bruising, nosebleeds, bleeding gums, melena). Take temperature daily.
• Warn patients that alopecia may occur, but that it's usually reversible.
• Monitor renal function tests.
• Never administer this drug I.M. or S.C.
• Has been administered topically by bladder instillation and intra-arterially through the hepatic artery.
• Preparation and administration of parenteral form of this drug is associated with mutagenic, teratogenic, and carcinogenic risks to personnel. Follow institutional policy to reduce risks.
• **I.V. use:** Using sterile water for injection, reconstitute the 5-mg vials with 10 ml, the 20-mg vials with 40 ml, and the 40-mg vials with 80 ml.
• For infusion, dilute with 0.9% sodium chloride injection, D_5W, or sodium lactate for injection. After dilu-

tion, drug is stable for 3 hours in D_5W, 12 hours in 0.9% sodium chloride injection, and 24 hours in sodium lactate for injection at room temperature.

• Avoid extravasation. Stop infusion immediately if extravasation occurs because of the potential for severe ulceration and necrosis.

plicamycin (mithramycin)

Mithracin

Pregnancy Risk Category: X

HOW SUPPLIED

Injection: 2.5-mg vials

ACTION

Mechanism: Forms a complex with DNA, thus inhibiting RNA synthesis. Also inhibits osteocytic activity, blocking calcium and phosphorus resorption from bone.

Onset: 1 to 2 days. **Peak:** Effects peak 3 days after single dose. **Duration:** 7 to 10 days.

INDICATIONS & DOSAGE

Dosage and indications may vary. Check the treatment protocol with the doctor.

Hypercalcemia associated with advanced malignancy –

Adults: 15 to 25 mcg/kg/day I.V. for 3 to 4 days. Repeat dosage at weekly intervals until desired response is obtained.

Testicular cancer –

Adults: 25 to 30 mcg/kg/day I.V. for 8 to 10 days or until toxicity occurs. Dosage is based on ideal body weight or actual weight, whichever is less.

ADVERSE REACTIONS

CNS: drowsiness, weakness, lethargy, headache, dizziness, nervousness, depression.

GI: *nausea, vomiting,* anorexia, diarrhea, stomatitis, metallic taste.

GU: proteinuria; increased BUN and serum creatinine levels.

Hematologic: ***leukopenia, thrombocytopenia; bleeding syndrome from epistaxis to generalized hemorrhage;*** *facial flushing.*

Hepatic: ***elevated liver enzymes levels.***

Other: ***decreased serum calcium,*** potassium, and phosphorus levels; irritation, cellulitis with extravasation.

INTERACTIONS

None significant.

CONTRAINDICATIONS

• Contraindicated in patients with thrombocytopenia, bone marrow suppression, and in those with coagulation and bleeding disorders.

• Dosage modification may be required in patients with renal or hepatic impairment.

NURSING CONSIDERATIONS

• Monitor platelet count and PT before and during therapy. Discontinue drug if WBC count is less than 4,000/mm^3, platelet count falls to less than 150,000/mm^3, or if PT is prolonged more than 4 seconds longer than control.

• Warn patients to watch for signs of infection (fever, sore throat, fatigue) and bleeding (easy bruising, nosebleeds, bleeding gums, melena). Take temperature daily.

• Facial flushing is an early indicator of bleeding.

• Monitor lactate dehydrogenase, AST, ALT, alkaline phosphatase, BUN, creatinine, potassium, calcium, and phosphorus levels.

• To reduce nausea, give antiemetic before administering.

• Avoid contact with skin or mucous membranes.

• Therapeutic effect in hypercalcemia may not occur for 24 to 48 hours; may last 3 to 15 days.

• Precipitous drop in calcium level is

possible. Monitor patients for tetany, carpopedal spasm, Chvostek's sign, and muscle cramps; check serum calcium level.

- Preparation and administration of parenteral form of this drug is associated with carcinogenic, mutagenic, and teratogenic risks for personnel. Follow institutional policy to reduce risks.
- **I.V. use:** To prepare solution, add 4.9 ml of sterile water for injection to vial and shake to dissolve. Then dilute for I.V infusion in 1,000 ml of D_5W or 0.9% sodium chloride. Administer by infusion over 4 to 6 hours. Discard unused drug.
- Slow infusion reduces nausea that develops with I.V. push.
- Avoid extravasation. Plicamycin is a vesicant. If I.V. solution infiltrates, stop immediately and use ice packs. Restart I.V. line.
- Store lyophilized powder in refrigerator and protect from light.

procarbazine hydrochloride

Matulane, Natulan†‡

Pregnancy Risk Category: D

HOW SUPPLIED

Capsules: 50 mg

ACTION

Mechanism: Inhibits DNA, RNA, and protein synthesis.
Duration: half-life, 10 minutes.

INDICATIONS & DOSAGE

Dosage and indications may vary. Check the treatment protocol with the doctor.

Hodgkin's disease, lymphoma, brain and lung cancers –
Adults: 2 to 4 mg/kg P.O. daily in a single dose or divided doses for the first week. Then, 4 to 6 mg/kg/day until WBC count falls below 4,000/mm^3 or platelet count falls below 100,000/mm^3. After bone marrow recovers, resume maintenance dosage of 1 to 2 mg/kg/day.
Children: 50 mg/m^2 P.O. daily for first week; then 100 mg/m^2 until response or toxicity occurs. Maintenance dosage is 50 mg/m^2 P.O. daily after bone marrow recovery.

ADVERSE REACTIONS

CNS: nervousness, depression, insomnia, nightmares, paresthesia, neuropathy, *hallucinations,* confusion, ***seizures.***
EENT: retinal hemorrhage, nystagmus, photophobia.
GI: *nausea, vomiting, anorexia,* stomatitis, dry mouth, dysphagia, diarrhea, constipation.
Hematologic: ***bleeding tendency, thrombocytopenia, leukopenia, anemia.***
Respiratory: ***pleural effusion.***
Skin: dermatitis.
Other: reversible alopecia.

INTERACTIONS

CNS depressants: additive depressant effects. Avoid concomitant use.
Digoxin: may decrease serum digoxin levels. Monitor closely.
Drugs and foods high in tyramine (Chianti wine, cheese), local anesthetics, sympathomimetics, tricyclic antidepressants: possible tremors, palpitations, increased blood pressure. Monitor closely.
Ethanol: mild disulfiram-like reaction. Warn patients not to drink alcoholic beverages.
Meperidine: may cause severe hypotension and possible death. Don't give together.

CONTRAINDICATIONS

- Contraindicated in patients hypersensitive to the drug and in those with inadequate bone marrow reserve as documented by bone marrow aspiration.
- Use cautiously in patients with leukopenia, thrombocytopenia, or ane-

mia, and in those with impaired hepatic or renal function.

NURSING CONSIDERATIONS

- Warn patients to watch for signs of infection (fever, sore throat, fatigue) and bleeding (easy bruising, nosebleeds, bleeding gums, melena). Take temperature daily.
- Warn patients to avoid hazardous activities that require alertness and good motor coordination until the CNS effects are known.
- Discontinue drug if patients become confused, or if paresthesia or other neuropathies develop.
- To decrease nausea and vomiting, advise patients to take drug at bedtime and in divided doses.
- Warn patients to avoid alcohol while taking this drug. Instruct patients to stop medication and check with the doctor immediately if disulfiram-like reaction – chest pains, rapid or irregular heartbeat, severe headache, stiff neck – occurs.
- Monitor CBC and platelet counts.
- To prevent bleeding, avoid all I.M. injections when platelet count is below 100,000/mm^3.

Antineoplastics that alter hormone balance

aminoglutethimide
estramustine phosphate sodium
flutamide
goserelin acetate
leuprolide acetate
megestrol acetate
mitotane
tamoxifen citrate
testolactone
trilostane

COMBINATION PRODUCTS
None.

aminoglutethimide
Cytadren

Pregnancy Risk Category: D

HOW SUPPLIED
Tablets: 250 mg

ACTION
Mechanism: Blocks conversion of cholesterol to delta-5-pregnenolone in the adrenal cortex, inhibiting the synthesis of glucocorticoids, mineralocorticoids, and other steroids.
Onset: 3 to 5 days. **Peak:** Plasma levels peak in 1½ hours. **Duration:** adrenal function returns 1½ to 3 days after discontinuing drug.

INDICATIONS & DOSAGE
Suppression of adrenal function in Cushing's syndrome and adrenal cancer; metastatic breast cancer; prostate cancer –
Adults: initially, 250 mg P.O. b.i.d. or t.i.d. for 14 days. Drug is usually given with 40 mg of hydrocortisone P.O. daily (10 mg in the morning, 10 mg at 5 p.m., and 20 mg h.s.). Maintenance dosage is 250 mg q.i.d. at 6-hour intervals. Dosage may be increased in increments of 250 mg daily q 1 to 2 weeks to a maximum daily dosage of 2 g.

ADVERSE REACTIONS
CNS: *drowsiness,* headache, dizziness.
CV: hypotension, tachycardia.
GI: nausea, anorexia.
Hematologic: transient leukopenia, ***agranulocytosis.***
Skin: *morbilliform rash,* pruritus, urticaria.
Other: fever, myalgia, adrenal insufficiency, masculinization, hirsutism, hypothyroidism.

INTERACTIONS
Dexamethasone, medroxyprogesterone: increased hepatic metabolism of these agents.
Ethanol: may potentiate the effects of aminoglutethimide.
Oral anticoagulants: decreased anticoagulant effect.

CONTRAINDICATIONS
• Contraindicated in patients hypersensitive to the drug.

NURSING CONSIDERATIONS
• May cause adrenal hypofunction, especially under stressful conditions, such as surgery, trauma, or acute illness. Patients may need mineralocorticoid supplements to treat hyponatremia and orthostatic hypotension. Glucocorticoid replacement may also be necessary, especially in patients with breast cancer. Monitor such patients carefully.
• Monitor blood pressure frequently. Advise patients to stand up slowly to minimize orthostatic hypotension.
• May cause a decrease in thyroid hormone production. Monitor thyroid function studies.

• Perform baseline hematologic studies and monitor CBC periodically.
• Warn patients to watch for signs of infection (fever, sore throat, fatigue) and bleeding (easy bruising, nosebleeds, bleeding gums, melena). Take temperature daily.
• Warn patients to avoid activities that require alertness and good motor coordination until CNS effects of the drug are known.
• Tell patients to report if rash persists for more than 8 days. Reassure patients that drowsiness, nausea, and loss of appetite usually diminish within 2 weeks after start of aminoglutethimide therapy, but advise them to notify the doctor if these symptoms persist.

estramustine phosphate sodium

Emcyt, Estracyst‡

Pregnancy Risk Category: D

HOW SUPPLIED

Capsules: 140 mg

ACTION

Mechanism: A combination of estrogen and an alkylating agent; acts by its ability to bind selectively to a protein present in the human prostate.
Duration: terminal elimination half-life, 20 hours.

INDICATIONS & DOSAGE

Palliative treatment of metastatic or progressive prostate cancer –
Adults: 10 to 16 mg/kg P.O. in three to four divided doses. Usual dosage is 14 mg/kg daily. Therapy should continue for up to 3 months and, if successful, be maintained as long as the patient responds.

ADVERSE REACTIONS

CV: ***MI,*** sodium and fluid retention, thrombophlebitis, ***CHF,*** hypertension.
GI: *nausea, vomiting,* diarrhea.
GU: loss of libido.
Hematologic: ***leukopenia, thrombocytopenia.***
Respiratory: ***edema, pulmonary embolism.***
Skin: rash, pruritus.
Other: *painful gynecomastia and breast tenderness,* thinning of hair, hyperglycemia, fluid retention.

INTERACTIONS

Calcium-rich foods (milk and dairy products): impaired absorption of estramustine.

CONTRAINDICATIONS

• Contraindicated in patients hypersensitive to estradiol and nitrogen mustard. Also contraindicated in those with active thrombophlebitis or thromboembolic disorders, except when the actual tumor mass is the cause of the thromboembolic phenomenon.
• Use cautiously in patients with history of thrombophlebitis or thromboembolic disorders and cerebrovascular or coronary artery disease.

NURSING CONSIDERATIONS

• Tell patients to take this drug on an empty stomach (2 hours before or 1 hour after meals) and to avoid taking with milk or dairy products.
• Estramustine may exaggerate preexisting peripheral edema or CHF. Monitor weight regularly in these patients.
• Monitor blood pressure and glucose tolerance periodically throughout therapy.
• Each 140-mg capsule contains 12.5 mg of sodium.
• Because of the possibility of mutagenic effects, advise patients and their partners to use contraception if woman is of childbearing age.
• Estramustine is a combination of estrogen estradiol and a nitrogen mus-

tard, shown to be effective in patients refractory to estrogen therapy alone.
- Patients may continue estramustine as long as response is favorable. Some patients have taken the drug for more than 3 years.
- Store capsules in refrigerator.

flutamide
Euflex†, Eulexin
Pregnancy Risk Category: D

HOW SUPPLIED
Capsules: 125 mg, 250 mg†

ACTION
Mechanism: Inhibits androgen uptake or prevents binding of androgens in nucleus of cells within target tissues.
Peak: Plasma levels peak 2 hours after dose. **Duration:** half-life, 6 hours in adults; 8 to 9½ hours in elderly patients.

INDICATIONS & DOSAGE
Metastatic prostatic carcinoma (stage D_2) in combination with luteinizing hormone-releasing hormone analogues such as leuprolide acetate –
Adults: 250 mg P.O. q 8 hours.

ADVERSE REACTIONS
CNS: *drowsiness, confusion, numbness or tingling of hands or feet.*
CV: peripheral edema, hypertension.
GI: *diarrhea, nausea, vomiting.*
GU: *impotence, loss of libido.*
Hepatic: elevated liver enzyme levels, hepatitis.
Skin: rash, photosensitivity.
Other: *hot flashes,* gynecomastia.

INTERACTIONS
None significant.

CONTRAINDICATIONS
- Contraindicated in patients hypersensitive to the drug.

NURSING CONSIDERATIONS
- Monitor liver function tests periodically in patients receiving therapy with flutamide.
- Ensure that patients understand flutamide must be taken continuously with the agent used for medical castration (such as leuprolide acetate) to allow the full benefit of therapy. Leuprolide suppresses testosterone production while flutamide inhibits testosterone action at the cellular level. Together they can impair the growth of androgen-responsive tumors. Advise patients not to discontinue either drug without consulting their doctor.

goserelin acetate
Zoladex
Pregnancy Risk Category: X

HOW SUPPLIED
Implants: 3.6 mg

ACTION
Mechanism: A luteinizing hormone-releasing hormone (LHRH) analogue that acts on the pituitary to decrease the release of follicle-stimulating hormone and luteinizing hormone, resulting in dramatically lowered serum levels of sex hormones.
Onset: 2 to 4 weeks. **Peak:** Effects peak after 12 to 15 days. **Duration:** suppression of hormone production to castration levels persists throughout therapy.

INDICATIONS & DOSAGE
Palliative treatment of advanced carcinoma of the prostate; endometriosis –
Adults: 1 implant S.C. q 28 days into the upper abdominal wall. For endometriosis, maximum duration of therapy is 6 months.

ADVERSE REACTIONS
CNS: lethargy, pain (worsened in the first 30 days), dizziness, insomnia,

anxiety, depression, headache, chills, emotional lability.
CV: edema, ***CHF, arrhythmias, CVA,*** hypertension, ***MI,*** peripheral vascular disorder, chest pain.
GI: nausea, vomiting, diarrhea, constipation, ulcer.
GU: *impotence, sexual dysfunction, lower urinary tract symptoms,* renal insufficiency, urinary obstruction, urinary tract infection, amenorrhea, vaginal dryness.
Hematologic: anemia.
Respiratory: COPD, upper respiratory infection.
Skin: rash, diaphoresis.
Other: *hot flashes,* gout, hyperglycemia, weight increase, breast swelling and tenderness, changes in breast size, loss of bone mineral density in women, fever.

INTERACTIONS
None significant.

CONTRAINDICATIONS
- Contraindicated during pregnancy or breast-feeding.
- Because use of the drug is associated with a loss of bone mineral density in women, use cautiously in patients with other risk factors for osteoporosis, such as family history of osteoporosis, chronic alcohol or tobacco abuse, or the use of drugs such as corticosteroids or anticonvulsants that affect bone density.

NURSING CONSIDERATIONS
- When used for prostate cancer, LHRH analogues such as goserelin may initially cause a worsening of prostatic cancer symptoms because the drug initially increases testosterone serum levels. A few patients may experience increased bone pain. Rarely, disease exacerbation (either spinal cord compression or ureteral obstruction) has occurred.
- Advise patients to report every 28 days for a new implant. A delay of a couple of days is permissible.
- The implant comes in a preloaded syringe. If the package is damaged, do not use the syringe. Make sure that the drug is visible in the translucent chamber of the syringe.
- Administer drug into the upper abdominal wall using aspetic technique. After cleaning the area with an alcohol swab (and injecting a local anesthetic), stretch the patient's skin with one hand while grasping the barrel of the syringe with the other. Insert the needle into the subcutaneous fat; then change direction of the needle so that it parallels the abdominal wall. The needle should then be pushed in until the hub touches the patient's skin; then withdrawn about 1 cm (this creates a gap for the drug to be injected) before depressing the plunger completely.
- To avoid the need for a new syringe and injection site, do not aspirate after inserting the needle.
- Before administering to female patients, rule out pregnancy. Tell women to use a nonhormonal form of contraception during treatment. Caution patients about the significant risks to the fetus should pregnancy occur.
- Menstruation should stop during treatment; tell patients to call the doctor if menstruation persists or if breakthrough bleeding occurs.
- After therapy ends, some patients may experience a delayed return of menses. Persistent amenorrhea is rare.

leuprolide acetate

Lucrin‡, Lupron, Lupron Depot

Pregnancy Risk Category: X

HOW SUPPLIED
Injection: 1 mg/0.2 ml (5 mg/ml) in 2.8-ml multiple-dose vials
Depot injection: 7.5 mg/ml

ACTION

Mechanism: Initially stimulates but then inhibits the release of follicle-stimulating hormone and luteinizing hormone, resulting in testosterone suppression.
Onset: 2 to 4 weeks; in males, initial increase in testosterone levels may occur during first week of therapy.
Peak: Effects peak after 1 to 2 months of treatment. **Duration:** normal pituitary-gonadal function within 1 to 3 months.

INDICATIONS & DOSAGE

Advanced prostate cancer–
Adults: 1 mg S.C. daily. Alternatively, 7.5 mg I.M. (depot injection) monthly.
Endometriosis–
Adults: 3.75 mg I.M (depot injection only) as a single injection once a month for up to 6 months.

ADVERSE REACTIONS

CNS: dizziness, depression, headache.
CV: arrhythmias, angina, ***MI,*** peripheral edema.
GI: nausea, vomiting.
Hepatic: elevated liver enzyme levels.
Respiratory: pulmonary embolism.
Other: transient bone pain during first week of treatment, *hot flashes,* decreased libido, skin reactions at injection site.

INTERACTIONS

None significant.

CONTRAINDICATIONS

- Contraindicated in patients hypersensitive to the drug or other gonadotropin-releasing hormone analogues, during pregnancy, and in women with undiagnosed vaginal bleeding.
- Use cautiously in patients hypersensitive to benzyl alcohol.

NURSING CONSIDERATIONS

- Never administer by I.V. injection.
- Leuprolide is a nonsurgical alternative to orchiectomy for prostate cancer.
- Studies show leuprolide is therapeutically equivalent to diethylstilbestrol in "medical castration" palliation treatment but has significantly milder and fewer adverse reactions.
- Reassure patients with history of undesirable effects from other endocrine therapies that leuprolide is much easier to tolerate.
- Worsening of prostate cancer symptoms may occur when therapy is initiated. Reassure patients that these effects are transient and will disappear after about 1 week.
- Carefully instruct patients who will self-administer S.C. injection about proper administration techniques and advise them to use only the syringes provided by the manufacturer.
- If another syringe must be substituted, a low-dose insulin syringe (U-100, 0.5 ml) may be an appropriate choice.
- Advise patients to store the drug at room temperature, protected from light and sources of heat.
- Once-monthly depot injection should be administered under medical supervision. Use supplied diluent to reconstitute drug. Draw 1 ml into a syringe with a 22G needle (extra diluent is provided and should be discarded). Inject into vial; then shake well. Suspension will appear milky. Although the suspension is stable for 24 hours after reconstitution, it contains no bacteriostatic agent. Use immediately.

megestrol acetate

Megace, Megostat‡
Pregnancy Risk Category: X

HOW SUPPLIED
Tablets: 20 mg, 40 mg
Oral suspension: 40 mg/ml

ACTION
Mechanism: A progestin that changes the tumor's hormonal environment and alters the neoplastic process. Mechanism responsible for appetite stimulation is unknown.
Peak: Plasma levels peak within 1 to 3 hours.

INDICATIONS & DOSAGE
Breast cancer–
Adults: 40 mg P.O. q.i.d.
Endometrial cancer–
Adults: 40 to 320 mg P.O. daily in divided doses.
Treatment of anorexia, cachexia, or unexplained significant weight loss in patients with AIDS–
Adults: 800 mg P.O. (oral suspension) daily in divided doses.

ADVERSE REACTIONS
CV: hypertension, edema, thrombophlebitis.
GI: nausea, vomiting.
GU: breakthrough menstrual bleeding.
Other: weight gain, increased appetite, carpal tunnel syndrome, alopecia, hirsutism, breast tenderness.

INTERACTIONS
None significant.

CONTRAINDICATIONS
- Contraindicated in patients hypersensitive to the drug.
- Use cautiously in patients with history of thrombophlebitis.

NURSING CONSIDERATIONS
- Megestrol is a relatively nontoxic drug with a low incidence of adverse effects.
- Two months is an adequate trial when treating patients with cancer. Reassure patients that therapeutic response isn't immediate.

mitotane
Lysodren

Pregnancy Risk Category: C

HOW SUPPLIED
Tablets (scored): 500 mg

ACTION
Mechanism: Selectively destroys adrenocortical tissue and hinders extra-adrenal metabolism of cortisol.
Onset: steroid levels decrease within 2 to 3 days; tumor response, within 6 months. **Peak:** Levels peak 3 to 5 hours after dose. **Duration:** half-life, 18 to 159 days.

INDICATIONS & DOSAGE
Inoperable adrenocortical cancer–
Adults: initially, 1 to 6 g P.O. daily in divided doses t.i.d. or q.i.d.; increased to 9 to 10 g P.O. daily, in divided doses t.i.d. or q.i.d. Dosage is adjusted until maximum tolerated dosage is achieved (varies from 2 to 16 g/day but is usually 8 to 10 g/day).
Children: initially, 0.1 to 0.5 mg/kg P.O. (1 to 2 g daily) in divided doses. Increase dosage based on patient tolerance and response. Usual dosage is 5 to 7 g/day in divided doses.

ADVERSE REACTIONS
CNS: *depression, somnolence, lethargy, vertigo;* brain damage and dysfunction in long-term, high-dose therapy.
GI: *severe nausea, vomiting,* diarrhea, anorexia.
Skin: dermatitis, maculopapular rash.
Other: hypouricemia, increased serum cholesterol level, adrenal insufficiency.

INTERACTIONS
None significant.

CONTRAINDICATIONS

- Contraindicated in patients hypersensitive to the drug.
- Use cautiously in patients with hepatic disease; however, dosage need not be routinely reduced in such patients.
- Drug should not be used in patients in shock or who have suffered trauma. Use of corticosteroids may avoid acute adrenocorticoid insufficiency and is usually required. Glucocorticoid dosage should be increased in periods of physiologic stress such as infection or trauma.

NURSING CONSIDERATIONS

- Assess and record behavioral and neurologic signs daily throughout therapy. Prolonged therapy has been associated with significant neurologic impairment.
- To reduce nausea, give antiemetic before administering.
- Dosage may be reduced if GI or skin adverse reactions are severe.
- Because drug distributes mostly to body fat, obese patients may need higher dosage and may have longer-lasting adverse reactions.
- Warn ambulatory patients to avoid activities that require alertness and good motor coordination until CNS effects of the drug are known.
- Monitor effectiveness according to reduction in pain, weakness, and anorexia.
- An adequate therapeutic trial is at least 3 months, but treatment can continue if clinical benefits are observed.

tamoxifen citrate

Alpha-Tamoxifen†, Nolvadex, Nolvadex-D†‡, Novo-Tamoxifen†, Tamofen†, Tamone†, Tamoplex†

Pregnancy Risk Category: D

HOW SUPPLIED

Tablets: 10 mg, 20 mg
Tablets (enteric-coated)†: 10 mg, 20 mg

ACTION

Mechanism: Acts as an estrogen antagonist.
Onset: 4 to 10 weeks, but may take several months. **Duration:** estrogen antagonism may persist for several weeks after drug is discontinued; half-life, about 7 days.

INDICATIONS & DOSAGE

Advanced premenopausal and postmenopausal breast cancer –
Adults: 10 mg P.O. b.i.d. to t.i.d.

ADVERSE REACTIONS

GI: *nausea* in 10% of patients, vomiting, anorexia.
GU: vaginal discharge and bleeding.
Hematologic: transient fall in WBC or platelet counts.
Skin: rash.
Other: hypercalcemia, temporary bone or tumor pain, hot flashes in 7% of patients, brief exacerbation of pain from osseous metastases.

INTERACTIONS

None significant.

CONTRAINDICATIONS

- Contraindicated in patients hypersensitive to the drug.

NURSING CONSIDERATIONS

- Monitor CBC closely in patients with preexisting leukopenia or thrombocytopenia.
- Monitor serum lipid levels during long-term therapy in patients with preexisting hyperlipidemia.
- Monitor serum calcium levels. Drug may compound hypercalcemia related to bone metastases during initiation of therapy.
- Acts as an "antiestrogen." Best re-

sults have been reported in patients with positive estrogen receptors.
• Adverse reactions are usually minor and well tolerated.
• Reassure patients that acute exacerbation of bone pain during tamoxifen therapy usually indicates drug will produce good response. Use analgesic to relieve pain.
• Short-term therapy induces ovulation in premenopausal women. Barrier form of contraception is recommended.
• Tell patients taking enteric-coated tablets (Nolvadex-D†) to swallow the tablets whole without crushing or chewing. Tell them not to take antacids within 2 hours of a dose.
• Strongly encourage women who are taking or have taken tamoxifen to have regular gynecologic examinations because of increased risk of uterine cancer associated with its use.
• Also used to treat breast cancer in men and advanced ovarian cancer in women. Has been used to stimulate ovulation in women with oligomenorrhea or amenorrhea who previously used oral contraceptives.

testolactone

Teslac
Controlled Substance Schedule III
Pregnancy Risk Category: C

HOW SUPPLIED
Tablets: 50 mg

ACTION
Mechanism: An androgen that changes the tumor's hormonal environment and alters the neoplastic process.
Onset: 6 to 12 weeks.

INDICATIONS & DOSAGE
Advanced postmenopausal breast cancer–
Women: 250 mg P.O. q.i.d.

ADVERSE REACTIONS
CNS: paresthesia, peripheral neuropathy.
CV: increased blood pressure, edema.
GI: nausea, vomiting, diarrhea.
Other: hypercalcemia, alopecia.

INTERACTIONS
Oral anticoagulants: increased pharmacologic effects. Monitor carefully.

CONTRAINDICATIONS
• Contraindicated in patients hypersensitive to the drug and in males with breast cancer.
• Use cautiously in patients with cardiac or renal disease and in patients with hypercalcemia.

NURSING CONSIDERATIONS
• Three months is an adequate trial for this drug. Reassure patients that therapeutic response isn't immediate.
• Monitor fluid and electrolyte levels, especially calcium level.
• Immobilized patients are prone to hypercalcemia. Exercise may prevent it. Force fluids to aid calcium excretion.
• Higher-than-recommended doses do not increase incidence of remission.

trilostane

Modrastane
Pregnancy Risk Category: X

HOW SUPPLIED
Capsules: 30 mg, 60 mg

ACTION
Mechanism: Reversibly lowers elevated circulating levels of glucocorticoids by inhibiting the enzyme system essential for their production in the adrenal gland.
Onset: 2 weeks. **Duration:** elimination half-life, 8 hours.

INDICATIONS & DOSAGE
Adrenocortical hyperfunction in Cushing's syndrome –
Adults: 30 mg P.O. q.i.d. initially. May be increased at intervals of 3 to 4 days to maximum of 480 mg/day. Most patients respond to doses below 360 mg/day.

ADVERSE REACTIONS
CNS: headache, dizziness, lightheadedness.
CV: *orthostatic hypotension.*
EENT: burning of oral and nasal membranes.
GI: *diarrhea, upset stomach,* nausea, flatulence, cramps, bloating.
Skin: flushing, rash.
Other: fever, fatigue, hot flashes, muscle aches, hyperkalemia.

INTERACTIONS
Aminoglutethimide, mitotane: may cause severe adrenocortical hypofunction.
Loop diuretics, thiazides: decreased potassium loss because trilostane inhibits aldosterone production.

CONTRAINDICATIONS
- Contraindicated in patients with severe renal or hepatic disease.
- Use cautiously in patients who are receiving other drugs that suppress adrenal function.

NURSING CONSIDERATIONS
- Trilostane may prevent normal response to physiologically stressful situation. Therefore, patients who develop a severe illness or need surgery may need to have this drug temporarily discontinued. Supplemental corticosteroids may be necessary.
- Because the drug may cause orthostatic hypotension by suppressing aldosterone production, monitor blood pressure regularly in all patients.
- Trilostane is prescribed when surgery or pituitary radiation therapy is inappropriate or must be delayed. Explain to patients that the drug does not cure the underlying disease.

73

Miscellaneous antineoplastic agents

altretamine
asparaginase
***Erwinia* asparaginase**
bacillus Calmette-Guérin (BCG), live intravesical
etoposide
mitoxantrone hydrochloride
paclitaxel
pentostatin
teniposide
vinblastine sulfate
vincristine sulfate

COMBINATION PRODUCTS
None.

altretamine (hexamethylmelamine; HMM)

Hexalen

Pregnancy Risk Category: D

HOW SUPPLIED
Capsules: 50 mg

ACTION
Mechanism: Unknown. Structurally similar to the alkylating agent triethylenemelamine but not an alkylating agent. Metabolism is important for antitumor activity; metabolites of the drug are known alkylating agents.
Peak: Plasma levels peak in ½ to 3 hours. **Duration:** terminal elimination half-life, 5 to 10 hours; more than 90% of dose recovered from urine within 3 days.

INDICATIONS & DOSAGE
Palliative treatment of patients with persistent or recurrent ovarian cancer after first-line therapy with cisplatin or alkylating agent-based combination therapy –
Adults: 260 mg/m² P.O. daily in four divided doses with meals and h.s. for 14 or 21 consecutive days in a 28-day cycle.

ADVERSE REACTIONS
CNS: *sensory neuropathy,* anorexia, ataxia, paresthesia, hyporeflexia, fatigue, ***seizures.***
GI: *nausea and vomiting.*
Hematologic: ***leukopenia, thrombocytopenia, anemia.***
Skin: erythematous macropapular eczema.
Other: increased serum creatinine and BUN levels, alopecia.

INTERACTIONS
Cimetidine: may increase the half-life and toxicity of altretamine. Monitor closely for toxicity.
MAO inhibitors: severe orthostatic hypotension. Avoid concomitant use.

CONTRAINDICATIONS
- Contraindicated in patients hypersensitive to the drug and in those with preexisting bone marrow suppression or severe neurologic toxicity. However, patients with preexisting neuropathies caused by high-dose cisplatin therapy have been successfully treated with altretamine. Carefully monitor these patients for worsening neurologic function.

NURSING CONSIDERATIONS
- Perform a careful neurologic assessment before each course of therapy.
- Continuous high-dose daily treatment with altretamine is associated with a higher incidence of mild to moderate neurotoxicity. It appears to be reversible when therapy is discontinued.
- Unconfirmed reports suggest that

the severity and incidence of neurotoxicity may be decreased by concomitant administration of pyridoxine.
• Monitor CBC and platelet count before each course of therapy and monthly thereafter. Altretamine causes a mild to moderate dose-related myelosuppression. Nadirs of WBC and platelet counts are reached by 3 to 4 weeks. Normal counts are regained by 6 weeks.
• Discontinue drug temporarily for at least 14 days if laboratory tests show a platelet count below 75,000/mm³, WBC count below 2,000/mm³, or granulocyte count below 1,000/mm³. Also discontinue temporarily if patients experience severe GI distress that is unresponsive to symptomatic treatment or develop signs of progressive neuropathy. Drug should be discontinued if neurologic symptoms fail to stabilize.
• Continuous daily administration of this drug is associated with nausea and vomiting, which is usually treatable with antiemetics. To minimize this adverse effect, tell patients to take the drug with meals. If nausea and vomiting is severe, dosage reduction or temporary discontinuation of the drug may be necessary.
• Advise patients to use contraception; drug may harm a developing fetus.

asparaginase (L-asparaginase)

Elspar, Kidrolase†

Erwinia asparaginase (porton asparaginase)

Pregnancy Risk Category: C

HOW SUPPLIED

asparaginase
Injection: 10,000-unit vial
***Erwinia* asparaginase**
Available through National Cancer Institute
Injection: 10,000-unit vial

ACTION

Mechanism: Destroys the amino acid asparagine, which is needed for protein synthesis in acute lymphocytic leukemia. This leads to death of the leukemic cell.
Onset: immediate. **Duration:** plasma half-life, 8 to 30 hours; asparagine reappears in plasma within 23 to 33 days.

INDICATIONS & DOSAGE

Acute lymphocytic leukemia (in combination with other drugs) –
Adults and children: asparaginase – 1,000 IU/kg I.V. daily for 10 days, injected over 30 minutes or by slow I.V. push; or 6,000 IU/m² I.M. at intervals specified in protocol.
Adults: *Erwinia* asparaginase – 5,000 to 10,000 IU/m² daily for 7 days q 3 weeks or 10,000 to 40,000 IU/m² q 2 to 3 weeks. Doses may be given I.V. over 15 to 30 minutes or by I.M. injection.
Children: *Erwinia* asparaginase – 6,000 to 10,000 IU/m² I.V. or I.M. daily for 14 days; or 60,000 IU/m² every other day for a total of 12 doses; or 1,000 IU/kg for 10 days.
Sole induction agent for acute lymphocytic leukemia –
Adults: asparaginase – 200 IU/kg I.V. daily for 28 days.

ADVERSE REACTIONS

CNS: confusion, drowsiness, depression, hallucinations, nervousness, lethargy, somnolence.
GI: *vomiting* (may last up to 24 hours), *anorexia, nausea,* cramps, weight loss.
GU: *azotemia, **renal failure**,* uric acid nephropathy, glycosuria, polyuria, *increased blood ammonia level.*
Hematologic: ***anemia, hypofibrinogenemia,*** depression of other clotting factors, ***thrombocytopenia, leuko-***

*Liquid form contains alcohol.
**May contain tartrazine.

Common reactions are in italics; ***life-threatening,*** in bold italics.

penia, depression of serum albumin level.
Hepatic: elevated AST and ALT levels, ***hepatotoxicity.***
Skin: *rash, urticaria.*
Other: ***hemorrhagic pancreatitis and anaphylaxis*** *(common),* chills, fever, elevated alkaline phosphatase and bilirubin (direct and indirect levels), increase or decrease in total lipid level, *hyperuricemia, hyperglycemia.*

INTERACTIONS
Methotrexate: decreased methotrexate effectiveness.
Prednisone, vincristine: increased toxicity.

CONTRAINDICATIONS
- Contraindicated in patients with pancreatitis and previous hypersensitivity unless desensitized.
- Use cautiously in patients with preexisting hepatic dysfunction. Because of the unpredictability of adverse reactions, drug should be administered in hospital setting with close supervision.

NURSING CONSIDERATIONS
- Keep epinephrine, diphenhydramine, and I.V. corticosteroids available for treating anaphylaxis.
- Some patients may develop hypersensitivity to asparaginase, which is derived from cultures of *Escherichia coli. Erwinia* asparaginase, derived from cultures of *Erwinia carotovora,* has been used in these patients without cross-sensitivity.
- Don't use as sole agent to induce remission unless combination therapy is inappropriate. Not recommended for maintenance therapy.
- Risk of hypersensitivity increases with repeated dosages. Patients may be desensitized, but this doesn't rule out risk of allergic reactions. Routine administration of 2 IU I.V. test dose may identify high-risk patients.
- Because of vomiting, patients may need parenteral fluids for 24 hours or until oral fluids are tolerated.
- Monitor CBC and bone marrow function tests. Bone marrow regeneration may take 5 to 6 weeks.
- Obtain frequent serum amylase level determinations to check pancreatic status. If elevated, asparaginase should be discontinued.
- Tumor lysis can result in uric acid nephropathy. Prevent occurrence by increasing fluid intake. Allopurinol should be started before therapy begins.
- Warn patients to watch for signs of infection (fever, sore throat, fatigue) and bleeding (easy bruising, nosebleeds, bleeding gums, melena). Take temperature daily.
- Monitor blood and urine glucose before and during therapy. Watch for signs of hyperglycemia, such as glycosuria and polyuria.
- Preparation and administration of parenteral form of this drug is associated with carcinogenic, mutagenic, and teratogenic risks for personnel. Follow institutional policy to reduce risks.
- **I.V. use:** Give I.V. injection over 30 minutes through a running infusion of sodium chloride injection or 5% dextrose injection.
- For I.M. injection, limit dose at single injection site to 2 ml.
- Reconstitute with 2 to 5 ml of either sterile water for injection or sodium chloride injection.
- Don't shake vial; may cause loss of potency. Don't use cloudy solutions.
- Refrigerate unopened dry powder. Reconstituted solution is stable for 8 hours if refrigerated.

bacillus Calmette-Guérin (BCG), live intravesical

ImmuCyst†, TheraCys, TICE BCG

Pregnancy Risk Category: C

HOW SUPPLIED

TheraCys

Suspension (freeze-dried) for bladder instillation: 27 mg/vial

TICE BCG

Suspension (freeze-dried) for bladder instillation: approximately 50 mg/ampule

ACTION

Mechanism: Exact mechanism unknown. Instillation of the live bacterial suspension causes a local inflammatory response. Local infiltration of histiocytes and leukocytes is followed by a decrease in superficial tumors within the bladder.

Duration: median duration of response, about 4 years.

INDICATIONS & DOSAGE

In situ carcinoma of the urinary bladder (primary and relapsed) –

Adults: administer 3 reconstituted and diluted vials intravesically once weekly for 6 weeks (induction), followed by additional treatments at 3, 6, 12, 18, and 24 months (TheraCys); or, 1 bladder instillation (1 ampule suspended in 50 ml of sterile, preservative-free sodium chloride solution) once weekly for 6 weeks, and then once monthly for 6 to 12 months (TICE BCG).

ADVERSE REACTIONS

GI: nausea, vomiting, anorexia, diarrhea, mild abdominal pain.

GU: *dysuria, urinary frequency, hematuria,* cystitis, urinary urgency, urinary incontinence, urinary tract infection, cramps, pain, decreased bladder capacity, tissue in urine, local infection, renal toxicity, genital pain.

Hematologic: anemia, leukopenia, thrombocytopenia.

Hepatic: elevated liver enzymem levels.

Other: hypersensitivity reaction, malaise, *fever above 101° F (38.3° C),* chills, myalgia, arthralgia, ***disseminated mycobacterial infection.***

INTERACTIONS

Antibiotics: may attenuate the response to BCG intravesical. Avoid concomitant use.

Bone marrow suppressants, immunosuppressants, and radiation therapy: may impair the response to BCG intravesical by decreasing the immune response; may also increase the risk of osteomyelitis or disseminated BCG infection. Avoid concomitant use.

CONTRAINDICATIONS

- Contraindicated in immunocompromised patients, in those receiving immunosuppressive therapy (because of the risk of bacterial infection), and in those with urinary tract infection (because of the risk of increased bladder irritation or disseminated BCG infection). Also contraindicated in patients with fever of unknown origin. If fever is caused by an infection, the drug should be withheld until the patient has recovered.

NURSING CONSIDERATIONS

- Do not use as an immunizing agent for the prevention of cancer. Do not use to prevent tuberculosis; the drug should not be confused with BCG vaccine.
- This drug should not be handled or administered by a caregiver with a known immunologic deficiency.
- Do not administer BCG intravesical within 7 to 14 days of transurethral resection or biopsy. Fatal disseminated BCG infection has occurred after traumatic catheterization.
- Carefully monitor patient's urinary status because the drug causes an inflammatory response in the bladder.
- Closely monitor patients for evidence of systemic BCG infection. BCG infections are rarely detected by positive cultures. Withhold therapy if systemic infection is suspected (short-

term high fever above 103° F [39.4° C], or persistent fever above 101° F [38.3° C] over 2 days, or with severe malaise). Contact an infectious disease specialist for initiation of fast-acting antituberculosis therapy.

• Patients with a small bladder capacity may experience increased local irritation with the usual dose of BCG intravesical.

• Has the potential to cause hypersensitivity. Manage symptomatically.

• Tuberculin sensitivity may be rendered positive by BCG intravesical treatment. Determine patients' reactivity to tuberculin before therapy.

• To administer TheraCys, reconstitute only with 1 ml of the provided diluent per vial, just before use. Do not remove the rubber stopper to prepare the solution. Use immediately. Add the contents of the three reconstituted vials to 50 ml of sterile, preservative-free sodium chloride solution (final volume, 53 ml). Instill a urethral catheter into the bladder under aseptic conditions, drain the bladder, and then infuse 53 ml of the prepared solution by gravity feed. Remove the catheter and properly dispose of any unused drug.

• To administer TICE BCG, use thermosetting plastic or sterile glass containers and syringes. Draw 1 ml of sterile, preservative-free sodium chloride solution into a 3-ml syringe. Add to one ampule of the drug; gently expel back into the ampule three times to ensure thorough mixing. Use immediately. Dispense the cloudy suspension into the top end of a catheter-tipped syringe that contains 49 ml of sodium chloride solution. Gently rotate the syringe. Properly dispose of any unused drug.

• Handle drug and all material used for instillation of the drug as infectious material because it contains live attenuated mycobacteria. Dispose of all associated materials (syringes, catheters, and containers) as biohazardous waste.

• Use strict aseptic technique to administer the drug to minimize trauma to the GU tract and to prevent introducing other contaminants to the area.

• If there is evidence of traumatic catheterization, do not administer the drug. Subsequent treatment may resume after 1 week as if no interruption of the schedule occurred.

• Bladder irritation can be treated symptomatically with phenazopyridine, acetaminophen, and propantheline. Systemic hypersensitivity can be treated with diphenhydramine. In order to minimize the risk of systemic infection, some clinicians give isoniazid for 3 days starting on the first day of treatment.

• Tell patients to retain the drug in the bladder for 2 hours after instillation (if possible). For the first hour, have patients lie 15 minutes prone, 15 minutes supine, and 15 minutes on each side; the second hour may be spent in the sitting position.

• Instruct patients to sit when voiding.

• Instruct patients to disinfect any urine for 6 hours after instillation of the drug. To disinfect urine, add undiluted household bleach (5% sodium hypochlorite solution) in equal volume to voided urine to the toilet; allow to stand for 15 minutes before flushing.

• Tell patients to call if symptoms worsen or if any of the following symptoms develops: blood in the urine, fever and chills, frequent urge to urinate, painful urination, nausea, vomiting, joint pain, or rash.

• Caution patients that a cough that develops after therapy could indicate a life-threatening BCG infection and to report it to their doctor immediately.

etoposide (VP-16)

VePesid

Pregnancy Risk Category: D

HOW SUPPLIED
Capsules: 50 mg
Injection: 100 mg/5 ml

ACTION
Mechanism: A semisynthetic derivative of podophyllotoxin that arrests cell mitosis.
Duration: terminal elimination half-life, 4 to 11 hours.

INDICATIONS & DOSAGE
Testicular cancer –
Adults: 50 to 100 mg/m² P.O. or I.V. on 5 consecutive days q 3 to 4 weeks; or 100 mg/m² on days 1, 3, and 5 q 3 to 4 weeks.
Small-cell carcinoma of the lung, acute nonlymphocytic leukemia, Hodgkin's disease, non-Hodgkin's lymphoma, Ewing's sarcoma –
Adults: 35 mg/m² I.V. or P.O. daily for 4 consecutive days or 50 mg/m² I.V. or P.O. daily for 5 consecutive days q 3 or 4 weeks.
Kaposi's sarcoma –
Adults: 150 mg/m² P.O. or I.V. daily for 3 consecutive days q 4 weeks.

ADVERSE REACTIONS
CNS: occasional headache and fever, peripheral neuropathy.
CV: hypotension from rapid infusion.
GI: nausea and vomiting, anorexia, abdominal pain, *stomatitis.*
Hematologic: *anemia, **myelosuppression*** (dose-limiting), ***leukopenia, thrombocytopenia.***
Other: *reversible alopecia,* ***anaphylaxis*** (rare), phlebitis at injection site (infrequent).

INTERACTIONS
Warfarin: may further prolong PT.

CONTRAINDICATIONS
- Contraindicated in patients hypersensitive to the drug.
- Use cautiously in patients who have had previous cytotoxic or radiation therapy, and in those with impaired renal or hepatic function or recent infection.

NURSING CONSIDERATIONS
- Oral dosage is calculated according to body surface area; dose is rounded to the nearest 50 mg.
- Store capsules in refrigerator.
- Monitor blood pressure before infusion and at 30-minute intervals during infusion. If systolic blood pressure falls below 90 mm Hg, stop infusion and notify the doctor.
- Have diphenhydramine, hydrocortisone, epinephrine, and necessary emergency equipment available to establish an airway in case of anaphylaxis.
- Monitor CBC. Observe patients for signs of bone marrow suppression.
- Observe oral cavity for signs of ulceration.
- Etoposide has produced complete remissions in small-cell lung cancer and testicular cancer.
- Preparation and administration of parenteral form of this drug is associated with carcinogenic, mutagenic, and teratogenic risks for personnel. Follow institutional policy to reduce risks.
- **I.V. use:** Give drug by slow I.V. infusion (over at least 30 minutes) to prevent severe hypotension.
- The drug may be diluted for infusion in either D_5W or 0.9% sodium chloride solution to a concentration of 0.2 or 0.4 mg/ml. Higher concentrations may crystallize.
- Do not administer through membrane-type in-line filters because the diluent may dissolve the filter.
- Solutions diluted to 0.2 mg/ml are stable for 96 hours at room temperature in plastic or glass unprotected

from light; solutions diluted to 0.4 mg/ml are stable for 48 hours under the same conditions.

mitoxantrone hydrochloride

Novantrone

Pregnancy Risk Category: D

HOW SUPPLIED

Injection: 2 mg/ml in 10-ml, 12.5-ml, 15-ml vials

ACTION

Mechanism: Not fully understood; probably cell cycle-nonspecific. Reacts with DNA, producing cytotoxic effect.

Duration: terminal elimination half-life, about 6 days.

INDICATIONS & DOSAGE

Combination initial therapy for acute nonlymphocytic leukemia –

Adults: induction begins with 12 mg/m^2 I.V. daily on days 1 through 3, in combination with 100 mg/m^2 daily of cytarabine on days 1 through 7. A second induction may be given if response is not adequate. Maintenance therapy: 12 mg/m^2 on days 1 and 2, in combination with cytarabine on days 1 through 5.

ADVERSE REACTIONS

CNS: ***seizures,*** headache.
CV: ***CHF, arrhythmias,*** tachycardia.
EENT: conjunctivitis.
GI: *bleeding, abdominal pain, diarrhea, nausea, mucositis, vomiting, stomatitis.*
GU: renal failure, uric acid nephropathy.
Hematologic: ***myelosuppression.***
Hepatic: jaundice.
Respiratory: dyspnea, cough.
Skin: petechiae, ecchymoses.
Other: alopecia, hyperuricemia.

INTERACTIONS

Heparin: physically incompatible. Do not mix together.

CONTRAINDICATIONS

- Contraindicated in patients hypersensitive to mitoxantrone.
- Use cautiously in patients with prior exposure to anthracyclines or other cardiotoxic drugs.
- Patients with significant myelosuppression should not receive mitoxantrone unless the benefits outweigh the risks.

NURSING CONSIDERATIONS

- Uric acid nephropathy can be avoided by adequately hydrating the patient before and during therapy. Be prepared to administer allopurinol as ordered.
- Closely monitor hematologic and laboratory chemistry parameters.
- Infections should be treated with antibiotics, as ordered. If severe nonhematologic toxicity occurs during the first course of therapy, the second course should be delayed until patients recover.
- Inform patients that urine may appear blue-green within 24 hours after administration and some bluish discoloration of the sclera may occur. These effects are not harmful.
- Monitor left ventricular ejection fraction during administration.
- Preparation and administration of parenteral form of this drug is associated with mutagenic, teratogenic, and carcinogenic risks to personnel. Follow institutional policy to minimize risks.
- **I.V. use:** Available as an aqueous solution of 2 mg/ml in volumes of 10, 12.5, and 15 ml. Dilute dose in at least 50 ml of 0.9% sodium chloride injection or D_5W injection. Administer by direct injection into a free-flowing I.V. line of 0.9% sodium chloride or D_5W injection over at least 3 min-

utes. Mixing with other drugs is not recommended.

- Mitoxantrone is not a vesicant; however, if drug extravasates, discontinue infusion immediately.
- Store undiluted solution at room temperature. Once diluted, the mixture is stable for 7 days at room temperature.

paclitaxel

Taxol

Pregnancy Risk Category: D

HOW SUPPLIED

Injection: 30 mg/5 ml

ACTION

Mechanism: Prevents depolymerization of cellular microtubules, thus inhibiting the normal reorganization of the microtubule network necessary for mitosis and other vital cellular functions.

Duration: terminal half-life, 5½ to 17½ hours.

INDICATIONS & DOSAGE

Metastatic ovarian cancer after failure of first-line or subsequent chemotherapy –

Adults: 135 mg/m² I.V. over 24 hours q 3 weeks. Subsequent courses shouldn't be repeated until neutrophil count is ≥ 1,500/mm³ and platelet count is ≥ 100,000/mm³.

ADVERSE REACTIONS

CNS: *peripheral neuropathy.*

CV: *bradycardia, hypotension, abnormal ECG.*

GI: *nausea, vomiting, diarrhea, mucositis.*

Hematologic: ***neutropenia, leukopenia, thrombocytopenia,*** *anemia, bleeding.*

Hepatic: elevated liver enzyme levels.

Other: hypersensitivity reactions ***(anaphylaxis),*** alopecia, *myalgia, arthralgia,* phlebitis, cellulitis at injection site.

INTERACTIONS

Cisplatin: possible additive myelosuppressive effects. Use together cautiously.

Ketoconazole: inhibited paclitaxel metabolism. Use together cautiously.

CONTRAINDICATIONS

- Contraindicated in patients hypersensitive to the drug or to polyoxyethylated castor oil, a vehicle used in drug solution, and in patients with baseline neutrophil counts below 1,500/mm³.
- Use cautiously in patients who have received prior radiation therapy because these patients may display more frequent or more severe myelosuppression. Also use cautiously in patients with hepatic impairment.

NURSING CONSIDERATIONS

- Severe hypersensitivity reactions have occurred in as many as 2% of patients treated in early clinical trials. To reduce the incidence or severity of these reactions, patients should be pretreated with corticosteroids, such as dexamethasone, and antihistamines. Both histamine$_1$-receptor antagonists, such as diphenhydramine, and histamine$_2$-receptor antagonists, such as cimetidine or ranitidine, may be used.
- Continuously monitor patients for 30 minutes after initiating the infusion. Continue close monitoring throughout the infusion.
- Bone marrow toxicity is the most frequent and dose-limiting toxicity. Frequent monitoring of blood counts is necessary during therapy. Packed RBC or platelet transfusions may be necessary in severe cases. Institute bleeding precautions as appropriate.
- If patients develop significant cardiac conduction abnormalities during treatment, appropriate therapy should

be administered and continuous cardiac monitoring should be performed during subsequent infusions.

• Warn patients that alopecia is common (up to 82% of patients).

• Teach patients the signs and symptoms of peripheral neuropathy, such as a tingling or burning sensation or numbness in the extremities, and advise them to report these symptoms immediately. Although mild symptoms are common, severe symptoms occur infrequently. Dosage reduction may be necessary.

• Preparation and administration of parenteral form of this drug is associated with carcinogenic, mutagenic, and teratogenic risks for personnel. Follow institutional protocol for the safe handling, preparation, and administration of chemotherapeutic drugs. Mark all waste materials with CHEMOTHERAPY HAZARD labels.

• **I.V. use:** Concentrate must be diluted before infusion. Compatible solutions include 0.9% sodium chloride injection, D_5W, 5% dextrose in 0.9% sodium chloride injection, and 5% dextrose in Ringer's lactate injection. Dilute to a final concentration of 0.3 to 1.2 mg/ml. Diluted solutions are stable for 27 hours at room temperature.

• Prepare and store infusion solutions in glass containers. The undiluted concentrate shouldn't come in contact with polyvinylchloride I.V. bags or tubing. Store diluted solution in glass or polypropylene bottles, or use polypropylene or polyolefin bags. Administer through polyethylene-lined administration sets, and use an in-line 0.22-micron filter.

• Take care to avoid extravasation.

pentostatin (2′-deoxycoformycin; DCF)

Nipent

Pregnancy Risk Category: D

HOW SUPPLIED

Powder for injection: 10 mg/vial

ACTION

Mechanism: Inhibits the enzyme adenosine deaminase (ADA), causing an increase in intracellular levels of deoxyadenosine triphosphate. This leads to cell damage and death. Because the greatest activity of ADA is in cells of the lymphoid system (especially malignant T cells), pentostatin is useful in treating leukemias.

Duration: average terminal elimination half-life, 5 to 7 hours.

INDICATIONS & DOSAGE

Alpha-interferon-refractory hairy-cell leukemia –

Adults: 4 mg/m^2 every other week.

ADVERSE REACTIONS

CNS: *headache, neurologic symptoms, anxiety, confusion, depression, dizziness, insomnia, nervousness, paresthesia, somnolence, abnormal thinking, fatigue,* ***seizures.***

CV: ***arrhythmias,*** *abnormal ECG, thrombophlebitis, peripheral edema,* ***hemorrhage.***

EENT: abnormal vision, conjunctivitis, ear pain, eye pain, epistaxis, pharyngitis, rhinitis, sinusitis.

GI: *nausea, vomiting, anorexia, diarrhea, constipation, flatulence, stomatitis.*

GU: *hematuria, dysuria, increased BUN and creatinine levels.*

Hematologic: ***myelosuppression, leukopenia, anemia, thrombocytopenia, lymphadenopathy.***

Hepatic: *elevated liver enzyme levels.*

Respiratory: *cough, bronchitis, dyspnea, lung edema, pneumonia.*

Skin: photosensitivity, contact dermatitis, *ecchymosis, petechiae, rash, eczema, dry skin, herpes simplex or zoster, maculopapular rash, vesiculobullous rash, pruritus, seborrhea, discoloration, diaphoresis,* ***exfoliative dermatitis.***

Other: *fever, infection, pain,* ***hypersensitivity reactions,*** *chills, sepsis, chest pain, abdominal pain, back pain, flulike syndrome, asthenia, malaise, myalgia, arthralgia, weight loss, increased lactate dehydrogenase level.*

INTERACTIONS

Fludarabine: risk of severe or fatal pulmonary toxicity. Don't use together.
Vidarabine: increased incidence or severity of adverse effects associated with either drug. Avoid concomitant use.

CONTRAINDICATIONS

- Contraindicated in patients hypersensitive to the drug.
- Use cautiously and only under the supervision of a doctor qualified and experienced in the use of chemotherapeutic agents. Adverse reactions after pentostatin therapy are common.

NURSING CONSIDERATIONS

- Withhold or discontinue drug in patients with evidence of CNS toxicity, a severe rash, or an active infection. Drug may be resumed when the infection clears. Also avoid use in patients with renal damage (creatinine clearance of 60 ml/minute or less).
- Temporarily withhold drug if the absolute neutrophil count falls below 200/mm^3 and the pretreatment level was over 500/mm^3. No recommendations exist regarding dosage adjustments in patients with anemia, neutropenia, or thrombocytopenia.
- Drug should be used only in patients who have hairy-cell leukemia refractory to alpha-interferon. This is defined as disease that progresses after a minimum of 3 months of treatment with alpha-interferon or disease that does not exhibit a response after 6 months of therapy.
- Make sure patients are adequately hydrated before therapy. Administer 500 to 1,000 ml of D_5W in 0.45% sodium chloride injection. Give an additional 500 ml of D_5W after drug is administered.
- The optimal duration of therapy is unknown. Current recommendations suggest two additional courses of therapy after a complete response. If a partial response is not evident after 6 months of therapy, drug will be discontinued. If a partial response is evident, drug will be continued for another 6 months or for two courses of therapy after a complete response.
- Preparation and administration of parenteral form of this drug is associated with mutagenic, teratogenic, and carcinogenic risks to personnel. Follow institutional policy to reduce risks.
- Treat all spills and waste products with 5% sodium hypochlorite (household bleach).
- **I.V. use:** Add 5 ml of sterile water for injection to the vial containing pentostatin powder for injection. Mix thoroughly to make a solution of 5 mg/ml. Drug may be administered by I.V. bolus injection or diluted further in 25 or 50 ml of D_5W or 0.9% sodium chloride injection and infused over 20 to 30 minutes.
- Reconstituted solution contains no preservatives; use within 8 hours.

teniposide (VM-26)

Vumon

Pregnancy Risk Category: C

HOW SUPPLIED

Injection: 10 mg/ml

ACTION

Mechanism: A semisynthetic derivative of podophyllotoxin that arrests cell mitosis and causes breaks in DNA.
Duration: average terminal elimination half-life, 5 hours.

INDICATIONS & DOSAGE
Refractory childhood acute lymphoblastic leukemia –
Children: optimum dosage hasn't been established. In clinical trials, dosages ranged from 165 to 250 mg/m^2 I.V. once or twice weekly for 4 to 6 weeks. Usually used in combination with other agents.

ADVERSE REACTIONS
CV: hypotension from rapid infusion.
GI: nausea and vomiting, mucositis.
Hematologic: ***myelosuppression*** (dose-limiting), ***leukopenia, neutropenia, thrombocytopenia, anemia***.
Other: alopecia (rare), ***anaphylaxis*** (rare), hypersensitivity reactions (chills, fever, urticaria, tachycardia, ***bronchospasm,*** dyspnea, hypotension, flushing); mucositis; *phlebitis at injection site with extravasation.*

INTERACTIONS
Heparin: physically incompatible. Don't mix together.

CONTRAINDICATIONS
- Contraindicated in patients hypersensitive to the drug or to polyoxyethylated castor oil, an injection vehicle.
- Use cautiously in patients with a history of mild to moderate sensitivity to the drug. Also use cautiously and in lower doses in patients with Down syndrome because these patients may be particularly sensitive to myelosuppressive chemotherapy.

NURSING CONSIDERATIONS
- Some clinicians may decide to use this drug despite a patient's history of hypersensitivity because the therapeutic benefits may outweigh its risks. Such patients should be treated with antihistamines and corticosteroids before the infusion begins and should be closely watched during drug administration.
- Monitor baseline and periodic blood counts and renal and hepatic function tests.
- Monitor blood pressure before and at 30-minute intervals during infusion. If systolic blood pressure falls below 90 mm Hg, stop infusion and notify the doctor.
- Have on hand diphenhydramine, hydrocortisone, epinephrine, and appropriate emergency equipment to establish an airway in case of anaphylaxis.
- Drug may be given by local bladder instillation for bladder cancer.
- Preparation and administration of parenteral form of this drug is associated with carcinogenic, mutagenic, and teratogenic risks for personnel. Follow institutional policy to reduce risks.
- **I.V. use:** Dilute drug in either D_5W or 0.9% sodium chloride injection to a final concentration of 0.1, 0.2, 0.4, or 1 mg/ml. Don't agitate vigorously; precipitation of drug may occur. Discard cloudy solutions. Prepare and store the drug in glass containers. Infuse over 45 to 90 minutes to prevent hypotension.
- Don't mix with other drugs or solutions.
- Ensure careful placement of the I.V. catheter. Extravasation of the drug can result in local tissue necrosis or sloughing.
- Don't administer through a membrane-type in-line filter because the diluent may dissolve the filter.
- Solutions containing 0.5 to 1 mg/ml are stable for 4 hours; those containing 0.1 to 0.2 mg/ml are stable for 6 hours at room temperature.

vinblastine sulfate (VLB)
Alkaban-AQ, Velban, Velbe†‡

Pregnancy Risk Category: D

HOW SUPPLIED
Injection: 10-mg vials (lyophilized powder), 1 mg/ml in 10-ml vials

†Available in Canada only. ‡Available in Australia only. ◇Available OTC.

ACTION

Mechanism: Arrests mitosis in metaphase, blocking cell division.
Duration: terminal half-life, about 25 hours.

INDICATIONS & DOSAGE

Breast or testicular cancer, Hodgkin's and non-Hodgkin's lymphoma, choriocarcinoma, lymphosarcoma, neuroblastoma, mycosis fungoides, Kaposi's sarcoma, histiocytosis –
Adults: 0.1 mg/kg or 3.7 mg/m² I.V. weekly or q 2 weeks. May be increased to maximum dosage of 0.5 mg/kg or 18.5 mg/m² I.V. weekly according to response. Dosage should not be repeated if WBC count is less than 4,000/mm³.
Children: initial dose, 2.5 mg/m² I.V. Increase dose by 1.25 mg/m² until WBC count is below 3,000/mm³ or tumor response is seen. Maximum dosage is 12.5 mg/m² I.V. weekly.

ADVERSE REACTIONS

CNS: depression, *paresthesia, peripheral neuropathy and neuritis, numbness, loss of deep tendon reflexes, muscle pain and weakness,* ***seizures,*** headache.
CV: hypertension.
EENT: pharyngitis.
GI: *nausea, vomiting,* ulcer, bleeding, *constipation, ileus, anorexia, weight loss,* abdominal pain, *stomatitis.*
GU: oligospermia, aspermia, urine retention.
Hematologic: ***anemia, leukopenia*** (nadir, days 4 to 10; lasts another 7 to 14 days), ***thrombocytopenia.***
Respiratory: ***acute bronchospasm,*** shortness of breath.
Skin: dermatitis, vesiculation.
Other: reversible alopecia in 5% to 10% of patients, *pain in tumor site,* low-grade fever, hyperuricemia; *irritation, phlebitis,* cellulitis, necrosis with extravasation.

INTERACTIONS

Mitomycin: increased risk of bronchospasm and shortness of breath.
Phenytoin: decreased plasma phenytoin levels.

CONTRAINDICATIONS

- Contraindicated in patients with severe leukopenia or bacterial infection.
- Use cautiously in patients with jaundice or hepatic dysfunction.

NURSING CONSIDERATIONS

- Do not administer into a limb with compromised circulation.
- Decrease dose by 50% if bilirubin levels are greater than 3 mg/100 ml.
- After administering, monitor for development of life-threatening acute bronchospasm. If this occurs, notify the doctor immediately. Reaction is most likely to occur in patients who are also receiving mitomycin.
- To reduce nausea, give antiemetic before administering drug.
- Drug should be stopped if stomatitis occurs.
- Assess bowel activity. Give laxatives as needed. May use stool softeners prophylactically.
- Don't repeat dosage more frequently than every 7 days or severe leukopenia will develop.
- Less neurotoxic than vincristine.
- Assess for numbness and tingling in hands and feet. Assess gait for early evidence of footdrop.
- Warn patients that alopecia may occur, but that it's usually reversible.
- An adequate trial is 12 weeks. Reassure patients that therapeutic response isn't immediate.
- Take care to avoid confusing vinblastine with vincristine or the investigational agent vindesine.
- Preparation and administration of parenteral form of this drug is associated with carcinogenic, mutagenic, and teratogenic risks for personnel. Follow institutional policy to reduce risks.

• **I.V. use:** Inject directly into vein or tubing of running I.V. line over 1 minute. May also be given in 50 ml of D_5W or 0.9% sodium chloride solution infused over 15 minutes. If extravasation occurs, stop infusion immediately. The manufacturer recommends that moderate heat be applied to the area of leakage. Local injection of hyaluronidase may help disperse the drug. Some clinicians prefer to apply ice packs on and off every 2 hours for 24 hours, with local injection of hydrocortisone or 0.9% sodium chloride.
• Reconstitute 10-mg vial with 10 ml of sodium chloride injection or sterile water. This yields 1 mg/ml. Refrigerate reconstituted solution. Discard after 30 days.

vincristine sulfate

Oncovin, Vincasar PFS

Pregnancy Risk Category: D

HOW SUPPLIED

Injection: 1 mg/ml in 1-ml, 2-ml, 5-ml multiple-dose vials; 1 mg/ml in 1-ml, 2-ml preservative-free vials

ACTION

Mechanism: Arrests mitosis in metaphase, blocking cell division.
Duration: average terminal elimination half-life, 85 hours.

INDICATIONS & DOSAGE

Acute lymphoblastic and other leukemias, Hodgkin's disease, non-Hodgkin's lymphoma, lymphosarcoma, reticulum cell sarcoma, neuroblastoma, rhabdomyosarcoma, Wilms' tumor, Ewing's sarcoma, osteogenic and other sarcomas, lung and breast cancers –
Adults: 0.4 to 1.4 mg/m² I.V. weekly.
Children over 10 kg: 1.5 to 2 mg/m² I.V. weekly.
Children 10 kg and under: initially, 0.05 mg/kg I.V. weekly.
Maximum single dose (adults and children) is 2 mg.

ADVERSE REACTIONS

CNS: *peripheral neuropathy,* sensory loss, *loss of deep tendon reflexes, paresthesia, wristdrop and footdrop,* ataxia, cranial nerve palsies (headache, *jaw pain,* hoarseness, vocal cord paralysis, visual disturbances), *muscle weakness and cramps,* depression, agitation, insomnia; some neurotoxicities may be permanent.
CV: hypotension.
EENT: diplopia, optic and extraocular neuropathy, ptosis.
GI: diarrhea, *constipation, cramps,* ileus that mimics surgical abdomen, *nausea, vomiting,* anorexia, weight loss, dysphagia, ***intestinal necrosis,*** *stomatitis.*
GU: urine retention, SIADH, dysuria, polyuria.
Hematologic: rapidly reversible mild anemia and leukopenia.
Respiratory: ***acute bronchospasm.***
Other: *reversible alopecia* (up to 71% of patients), fever, severe local reaction with extravasation, *phlebitis,* cellulitis at injection site, hyperuricemia.

INTERACTIONS

Asparaginase: decreased hepatic clearance of vincristine.
Calcium channel blockers: enhanced vincristine accumulation in cells.
Digoxin: decreased digoxin effects. Monitor serum digoxin level.
Mitomycin: possibly increased frequency of bronchospasm and acute pulmonary reactions.

CONTRAINDICATIONS

• Contraindicated in patients hypersensitive to the drug. Do not administer to patients who are concurrently receiving radiation therapy through ports that include the liver.
• Use cautiously in patients with jaundice or hepatic dysfunction, neuromuscular disease, or infection, and

in those receiving other neurotoxic drugs. Dose may be reduced by 50% if bilirubin is above 3 mg/dl.

NURSING CONSIDERATIONS

- After administering, monitor for development of life-threatening acute bronchospasm. If this occurs, notify the doctor immediately. This reaction is most likely to occur in patients who are also receiving mitomycin.
- Monitor for hyperuricemia, especially in patients with leukemia or lymphoma. Maintain good hydration and administer allopurinol as ordered to prevent uric acid nephropathy.
- Monitor fluid intake and output. Fluid restriction may be necessary if SIADH develops.
- Because of the risk of neurotoxicity, don't give drug more than once a week. Children are more resistant to neurotoxicity than adults. Neurotoxicity is dose-related and usually reversible.
- Check for depression of Achilles tendon reflex, numbness, tingling, footdrop or wristdrop, difficulty in walking, ataxia, and slapping gait. Also check ability to walk on heels. Support patients when walking.
- Monitor bowel function. Give stool softener, laxative, or water before dosing. Constipation may be an early sign of neurotoxicity.
- Warn patients that alopecia may occur, but that it's usually reversible.
- Take care to avoid confusing vincristine with vinblastine or the investigational agent vindesine.
- Preparation and administration of parenteral form of this drug is associated with carcinogenic, mutagenic, and teratogenic risks for personnel. Follow institutional policy to reduce risks.
- **I.V. use:** Inject directly into vein or tubing of running I.V. line slowly over 1 minute. May also be given in 50 ml of D_5W or 0.9% sodium chloride solution infused over 15 minutes. If drug extravasates, stop infusion immediately. Apply ice packs on and off every 2 hours for 24 hours.
- The 5-mg vials are for multiple-dose use only. Don't administer entire vial to one patient as a single dose.
- All vials (1-mg, 2-mg, 5-mg) contain 1 mg/ml solution and should be refrigerated.

Immunosuppressants

azathioprine
cyclosporine
levamisole hydrochloride
lymphocyte immune globulin
muromonab-CD3

COMBINATION PRODUCTS
None.

azathioprine

Imuran, Thioprine‡

Pregnancy Risk Category: D

HOW SUPPLIED
Tablets: 50 mg
Injection: 100 mg

ACTION
Mechanism: Inhibits purine synthesis.
Peak: Levels peak in 1 to 2 hours.
Duration: rapidly cleared; not detectable in urine after 8 hours.

INDICATIONS & DOSAGE
Immunosuppression in kidney transplantation –
Adults and children: initially, 3 to 5 mg/kg P.O. or I.V. daily usually beginning on the day of transplantation. Maintain at 1 to 3 mg/kg daily (dosage varies considerably according to patient response).
Severe, refractory rheumatoid arthritis –
Adults: initially, 1 mg/kg P.O. as a single dose or as two doses. If patient response is not satisfactory after 6 to 8 weeks, dosage may be increased by 0.5 mg/kg daily (up to a maximum of 2.5 mg/kg daily) at 4-week intervals.

ADVERSE REACTIONS
EENT: mouth ulceration.
GI: nausea, vomiting, anorexia, ***pancreatitis,*** steatorrhea, esophagitis.
Hematologic: ***leukopenia, bone marrow suppression,*** anemia, ***pancytopenia, thrombocytopenia.***
Hepatic: ***hepatotoxicity,*** jaundice.
Skin: rash, pruritus.
Other: *immunosuppression* (possibly profound), arthralgia, muscle wasting, alopecia.

INTERACTIONS
Allopurinol: impaired inactivation of azathioprine. Decrease azathioprine dose to ¼ or ⅓ normal dose.
Nondepolarizing neuromuscular blocking agents: azathioprine may reverse the neuromuscular blockade.
Vaccines: decreased immune response. Postpone routine immunization.

CONTRAINDICATIONS
- Contraindicated in patients hypersensitive to the drug.
- Use cautiously in patients with hepatic or renal dysfunction.

NURSING CONSIDERATIONS
- Watch for early signs of hepatotoxicity: clay-colored stools, dark urine, pruritus, and yellow skin and sclera; and for increased alkaline phosphatase, bilirubin, AST, and ALT levels.
- In renal homotransplants, start drug 1 to 5 days before surgery.
- Monitor hemoglobin and WBC and platelet counts at least once monthly, more often at beginning of treatment. Drug should be stopped immediately when WBC count is less than 3,000/mm³ to prevent irreversible bone marrow suppression.
- Drug is a potent immunosuppres-

sant. Warn patients to report even mild infections (colds, fever, sore throat, and malaise).

- Instruct patients to avoid conception during therapy and for 4 months after stopping therapy.
- Warn patients that some thinning of hair is possible.
- To prevent bleeding, avoid all I.M. injections when platelet count is below 100,000/mm³.
- Therapeutic response usually occurs within 8 weeks. Patients taking this drug for refractory rheumatoid arthritis should know that it may take up to 12 weeks to be effective.
- **I.V. use:** Only for patients unable to tolerate oral medications. Reconstitute 100-mg vial with 10 ml of sterile water for injection. Visually inspect for particles before giving. Drug may be administered by direct I.V. injection or further diluted in 0.9% sodium chloride injection or D_5W and infused over 30 to 60 minutes.

cyclosporine (cyclosporin)

Sandimmun‡, Sandimmune

Pregnancy Risk Category: C

HOW SUPPLIED

Oral solution: 100 mg/ml
Injection: 50 mg/ml

ACTION

Mechanism: Inhibits the proliferation of T lymphocytes.
Peak: Plasma levels peak within 3½ hours after oral dose. **Duration:** terminal elimination half-life, about 19 hours.

INDICATIONS & DOSAGE

Prophylaxis of organ rejection in kidney, liver, bone marrow, or heart transplantation –
Adults and children: 15 mg/kg P.O. (oral solution) 4 to 12 hours before transplantation. Continue this daily dosage postoperatively for 1 to 2 weeks. Then gradually reduce dosage by 5% each week to maintenance level of 5 to 10 mg/kg/day. Alternatively, 4 to 5 mg/kg I.V. concentrate 4 to 12 hours before transplantation. Postoperatively, repeat this dosage daily until patients can tolerate oral solution.

ADVERSE REACTIONS

CNS: *tremor,* headache.
CV: hypertension.
EENT: *gum hyperplasia,* oral thrush.
GI: nausea, vomiting, diarrhea.
GU: ***nephrotoxicity.***
Hematologic: anemia, ***leukopenia, thrombocytopenia.***
Hepatic: ***hepatotoxicity.***
Skin: acne.
Other: sinusitis, flushing, increased low-density lipoprotein levels, ***infections, hirsutism.***

INTERACTIONS

Aminoglycosides, amphotericin B, co-trimoxazole, NSAIDs: increased risk of nephrotoxicity.
Amphotericin B, cimetidine, diltiazem, erythromycin, imipenem-cilastatin, ketoconazole, metoclopramide, prednisolone: may increase blood levels of cyclosporine. Monitor for increased toxicity.
Azathioprine, corticosteroids, cyclophosphamide, verapamil: increased immunosuppression.
Carbamazepine, isoniazid, phenobarbital, phenytoin, rifampin: possible decreased immunosuppressant effect. May need to increase cyclosporine dosage.
Vaccines: decreased immune response. Postpone routine immunization.

CONTRAINDICATIONS

- Contraindicated in patients hypersensitive to the drug. The injectable form contains polyoxylethylated castor oil (Cremophor EL), which may provoke hypersensitivity reactions in certain persons. Closely monitor patients receiving I.V. infusion of the drug.

NURSING CONSIDERATIONS

- Cyclosporine may cause nephrotoxicity. Monitor BUN and serum creatinine levels. Nephrotoxicity may develop 2 to 3 months after transplant surgery, possibly requiring dosage reduction. Promptly report to the doctor any signs or symptoms that suggest the development of nephrotoxicity.
- Differentiation between transplanted kidney rejection and cyclosporine-induced nephrotoxicity must be made.
- Monitor liver function tests for hepatotoxicity, which usually occurs during first month after transplant.
- Cyclosporine should always be given concomitantly with adrenal corticosteroids.
- Absorption of cyclosporine oral solution can be erratic. Monitor cyclosporine blood levels at regular intervals. In a recent study, absorption in children after liver transplant was enhanced by administering with water-soluble vitamin E.
- Measure oral doses carefully in an oral syringe. To increase palatability, mix with whole milk, chocolate milk, or fruit juice. Use a glass container to minimize adherence to container walls.
- Give dosage once daily in the morning. Encourage patients to take drug at the same time each day.
- Patients may take with meals if drug causes nausea. Anorexia, nausea, and vomiting are usually transient and most frequently occur at the start of therapy.
- Stress to patients that therapy should not be stopped without the doctor's approval.
- To prevent thrush, patients should swish and swallow nystatin four times daily.
- Cyclosporine has also been used to treat a variety of conditions, including psoriatic arthritis and ulcerative colitis.
- **I.V. use:** Usually reserved for patients who cannot tolerate oral medications. Cyclosporine I.V. concentrate is administered at one-third the oral dose and must be diluted before use. Dilute each milliliter of the concentrate in 20 to 100 ml of D_5W or 0.9% sodium chloride injection. Dilute immediately before administration; infuse over 2 to 6 hours.

levamisole hydrochloride

Ergamisol

Pregnancy Risk Category: C

HOW SUPPLIED

Tablets: 50 mg (base)

ACTION

Mechanism: Unknown. The effects of the drug on the immune system are complex. It appears to restore depressed immune function and may potentiate the actions of monocytes and macrophages and enhance T-cell responses.
Peak: Plasma levels peak in 1½ to 2 hours. **Duration:** elimination half-life, 3 to 4 hours; of active metabolite, 16 hours.

INDICATIONS & DOSAGE

Adjuvant treatment of Dukes' stage C colon cancer (with fluorouracil) after surgical resection –
Adults: 50 mg P.O. q 8 hours for 3 days. Therapy should begin no sooner than 7 days and no later than 30 days after surgery, provided that the patient is out of the hospital, ambulating, and maintaining normal oral nutrition; has well-healed wounds; and has recovered from any postoperative complications. Fluorouracil (450 mg/m²/day I.V.) is given for 5 days starting 21 to 34 days after surgery.

Maintenance dosage is 50 mg P.O. q 8 hours for 3 days q 2 weeks for 1 year. Given in conjunction with fluorouracil maintenance therapy (450 mg/m²/day by rapid I.V. push, once a week beginning 28 days after the initial 5-day course) for 1 year.

ADVERSE REACTIONS

CNS: *dizziness, headache, paresthesia, somnolence, depression, nervousness, insomnia, anxiety, fatigue, fever.*
CV: chest pain, edema.
EENT: blurred vision, conjunctivitis, *stomatitis, dysgeusia, altered sense of smell.*
GI: *nausea, diarrhea, vomiting, anorexia, abdominal pain, constipation, flatulence, dyspepsia.*
Hematologic: ***agranulocytosis, leukopenia, thrombocytopenia.***
Skin: *dermatitis,* ***exfoliative dermatitis,*** *pruritus, urticaria.*
Other: hyperbilirubinemia, rigors, *alopecia, infection, arthralgia, myalgia.*

INTERACTIONS

Ethanol: may precipitate a disulfiram-like reaction. Avoid concomitant use.
Phenytoin: plasma levels may be elevated when administered with levamisole and fluorouracil. Monitor phenytoin plasma levels.

CONTRAINDICATIONS

- Contraindicated in patients hypersensitive to the drug.
- Use cautiously and with close hematologic monitoring because agranulocytosis, which is sometimes fatal, may occur. Neutropenia is usually reversible when therapy is discontinued.
- Do not exceed recommended doses. Higher doses are associated with greater incidence of agranulocytosis.

NURSING CONSIDERATIONS

- If levamisole therapy begins 7 to 20 days after surgery, fluorouracil should be started with the second course of levamisole therapy. It should begin no sooner than 21 days and no later than 35 days after surgery. If levamisole is deferred until 21 to 30 days after surgery, fluorouracil therapy should begin with the first course of levamisole.
- Tell patients to promptly report the development of stomatitis or diarrhea. If either of these reactions occur during the initial course of fluorouracil therapy, discontinue drug and then begin weekly fluorouracil therapy 28 days after the start of the initial course. If stomatitis or diarrhea develops during the weekly doses of fluorouracil, defer fluorouracil therapy until these symptoms subside. Then restart fluorouracil therapy at reduced dosages (decrease dose by 20%).
- Dosage modifications are based on hematologic parameters. If WBC count is 2,500/mm³ to 3,500/mm³, don't administer fluorouracil until WBC count is above 3,500/mm³. When fluorouracil is restarted, reduce dosage by 20%. If WBC count stays below 2,500/mm³ for over 10 days after fluorouracil is withdrawn, discontinue levamisole.
- If platelet count is below 100,000/mm³, discontinue therapy with both fluorouracil and levamisole.
- Baseline CBC with differential, platelet count, and electrolyte levels, and liver function studies are necessary immediately before starting therapy. Then a CBC with differential and platelet count should be performed at weekly intervals before treatment with fluorouracil. Electrolyte levels and liver function studies should be repeated every 3 months for 1 year.
- Advise patients to immediately report any flulike symptoms, such as fever and chills.

lymphocyte immune globulin (antithymocyte globulin [equine], ATG)

Atgam

Pregnancy Risk Category: C

HOW SUPPLIED

Injection: 50 mg of equine IgG/ml in 5-ml ampules

ACTION

Mechanism: Inhibits cell-mediated immune responses by either altering T-cell function or eliminating antigen-reactive T cells.

Peak: Plasma levels peak after 5 days of therapy. **Duration:** elimination half-life, about 6 days.

INDICATIONS & DOSAGE

Prevention of acute renal allograft rejection –

Adults and children: 15 mg/kg I.V. daily for 14 days followed by alternate-day dosing for 14 days; the first dose should be given within 24 hours of transplantation.

Treatment of acute renal allograft rejection –

Adults and children: 10 to 15 mg/kg I.V. daily for 14 days followed by alternate-day dosing for 14 days. Therapy should be initiated when rejection is diagnosed.

ADVERSE REACTIONS

CNS: malaise, ***seizures,*** headache.

CV: ***hypotension,*** *chest pain,* thrombophlebitis, tachycardia, edema, iliac vein obstruction, renal artery stenosis.

EENT: ***laryngospasm.***

GI: *nausea, vomiting,* diarrhea, hiccups, epigastric pain, abdominal distention, stomatitis.

Hematologic: ***leukopenia, thrombocytopenia, hemolysis.***

Hepatic: elevated liver enzyme level.

Respiratory: *dyspnea,* ***pulmonary edema.***

Other: febrile reactions, serum sickness, ***anaphylaxis,*** rash, infections, arthralgia, night sweats, lymphadenopathy, hyperglycemia.

INTERACTIONS

Muromonab-CD3: increased risk of infection. Monitor closely.

CONTRAINDICATIONS

- Contraindicated in patients hypersensitive to the drug. An intradermal skin test is recommended at least 1 hour before the first dose. Marked local swelling or erythema larger than 10 mm indicates an increased potential for severe systemic reaction such as anaphylaxis. Severe reactions to the skin test, such as hypotension, tachycardia, dyspnea, generalized rash, or anaphylaxis, usually preclude further administration of the drug.
- Use cautiously in patients receiving additional immunosuppressive therapy (such as corticosteroids or azathioprine) because of the increased potential for infection. Do not dilute ATG concentrate with dextrose solutions or solutions with a low salt concentration because a precipitate may form. The proteins in ATG can be denatured by air. ATG is unstable in acidic solutions.

NURSING CONSIDERATIONS

- Monitor patients for signs of infection.
- ATG solutions must be filtered during administration; filters with pore sizes of 0.2 to 5 microns have been used.
- **I.V. use:** Concentrated drug for injection must be diluted before administration. Dilute the required dose in 250 to 1,000 ml of 0.45% or 0.9% sodium chloride injection. The final concentration of drug should not exceed 1 mg/ml. When adding ATG to the infusion solution, make sure the container is inverted so that the drug does not contact air inside the con-

tainer. Gently rotate or swirl the container to mix contents; do not shake because this may cause excessive foaming or denature the drug protein. Infuse with an in-line filter with a pore size of 0.2 to 1 micron, over no less than 4 hours (most institutions infuse over 4 to 8 hours).

- ATG concentrate is heat-sensitive; refrigerate at 35° to 47° F (2° to 8° C). Do not freeze.
- Do not use solutions that are more than 12 hours old, including actual infusion time.

muromonab-CD3

Orthoclone OKT3

Pregnancy Risk Category: C

HOW SUPPLIED

Injection: 1 mg/1 ml in 5-ml ampules

ACTION

Mechanism: Muromonab-CD3 is an IgG antibody that reacts in the T-lymphocyte membrane with a molecule (CD3) needed for antigen recognition. This drug depletes the blood of CD3-positive T cells, which leads to restoration of allograft function and reversal of rejection.

Onset: 10 to 15 minutes. **Duration:** elimination half-life, about 18 hours.

INDICATIONS & DOSAGE

Acute allograft rejection in renal transplant patients –

Adults: 5 mg I.V. bolus once daily for 10 to 14 days.

Children: 2.5 mg I.V. bolus once daily for 10 to 14 days.

ADVERSE REACTIONS

CNS: *tremors.*

CV: *chest pain.*

GI: *nausea, vomiting,* diarrhea.

Respiratory: ***severe pulmonary edema,*** *dyspnea.*

Other: *fever, chills, tremors,* ***infection.***

INTERACTIONS

Immunosuppressants: increased risk of infection. Monitor closely.

Live-virus vaccines: may potentiate replication and increase effects of virus vaccine.

CONTRAINDICATIONS

- Contraindicated in patients with fluid overload, as evidenced by chest X-ray or a weight gain greater than 3% within the week before treatment.

NURSING CONSIDERATIONS

- Muromonab-CD3 is a monoclonal antibody preparation. Patients develop antibodies to this preparation that can lead to loss of effectiveness and more severe adverse reactions if a second course of therapy is attempted. Therefore, experts believe that this drug should be used for only a single course of treatment.
- Most adverse reactions develop within ½ to 6 hours after the first dose.
- Treatment should begin in a facility that is equipped and staffed for cardiopulmonary resuscitation and where patients can be monitored closely.
- Assess patients for signs of fluid overload before treatment.
- Chest X-ray must be taken within 24 hours before starting drug treatment.
- Inform patients of expected adverse reactions, and reassure them that these will be less severe as treatment progresses.
- Administering an antipyretic before giving the drug may help lower incidence of expected pyrexia and chills. Corticosteroids may also be administered before first injection to help decrease the incidence of adverse reactions. Methylprednisolone sodium succinate (1 mg/kg) preinjection, followed by hydrocortisone sodium succinate (100 mg) 30 minutes postinjection, have been recommended to alleviate the severity of the first-dose reaction.

75
Vaccines and toxoids

BCG vaccine
cholera vaccine
diphtheria and tetanus toxoids, adsorbed
diphtheria and tetanus toxoids and pertussis vaccine
diphtheria and tetanus toxoids and acellular pertussis vaccine
***Haemophilus* b conjugate vaccines**
hepatitis B vaccine, recombinant
influenza virus vaccine, 1994-1995 trivalent types A & B (purified surface antigen)
influenza virus vaccine, 1994-1995 trivalent types A & B (subvirion or split virion)
influenza virus vaccine, 1994-1995 trivalent types A & B (whole virion)
Japanese encephalitis virus vaccine, inactivated
measles, mumps, and rubella virus vaccine, live
measles (rubeola) and rubella virus vaccine, live attenuated
measles (rubeola) virus vaccine, live attenuated
meningitis vaccine
mumps virus vaccine, live
plague vaccine
pneumococcal vaccine, polyvalent
poliovirus vaccine, live, oral, trivalent
poliovirus vaccine, inactivated
rabies vaccine, human diploid cell
rubella and mumps virus vaccine, live
rubella virus vaccine, live attenuated
tetanus toxoid, adsorbed
tetanus toxoid, fluid
typhoid vaccine
typhoid vaccine, oral
yellow fever vaccine

COMBINATION PRODUCTS
TETRAMUNE: 10 mcg purified Haemophilus b saccharide and approximately 25 mcg CRM_{197} protein, 12.5 Lf (limit flocculation) units inactivated diphtheria, 5 Lf units inactivated tetanus, and 4 protective units pertussis/0.5 ml.

BCG vaccine
Pregnancy Risk Category: C

HOW SUPPLIED
Intradermal vaccine: 3 to 26 million colony-forming units (CFU)/ml (Glaxo strain)
Percutaneous vaccine: 1 to 8×10^8 CFU/vial (Tice strain)

ACTION
Mechanism: A live, attenuated bacterial vaccine prepared from *Mycobacterium bovis* that promotes active immunity to tuberculosis.
Onset: 8 to 14 weeks.

INDICATIONS & DOSAGE
Tuberculosis exposure, cancer immunotherapy —
Adults and children 3 months and over: 0.1 ml (intradermal vaccine) or 0.2 to 0.3 ml (percutaneous vaccine) applied to cleaned skin followed by application of multiple-puncture disk.
Children under 3 months: 0.05 ml (intradermal vaccine).

ADVERSE REACTIONS
Systemic: lymphangitis, urticaria of trunk and limbs, lupus-like syndrome, lymphadenitis, osteomyelitis, flulike syndrome (fever, shivers, chills, nausea, vomiting), ***anaphylaxis***.

Other: lymph node and skin abscess, ulceration (2 to 3 weeks after injection) at injection site.

INTERACTIONS

Immunosuppressive therapy: may reduce response to BCG vaccine. Avoid if possible.
Isoniazid, rifampin, streptomycin: inhibited multiplication of BCG. Avoid using together.
Theophylline: may impair theophylline elimination.

CONTRAINDICATIONS

- Contraindicated in patients with hypogammaglobulinemia, in the presence of a positive tuberculin reaction (when meant for use as immunoprophylactic after exposure to tuberculosis), in immunosuppressed patients, in those with fresh smallpox vaccinations, in those who have suffered burns, and in patients receiving corticosteroid therapy. Patients should avoid this vaccine during pregnancy.
- Use cautiously in patients with chronic skin disease. Inject in area of healthy skin only.

NURSING CONSIDERATIONS

- Obtain history of allergies and reaction to immunization.
- Vaccine is of no value as immunoprophylactic in patients with positive tuberculin test.
- Keep epinephrine 1:1,000 available to treat anaphylaxis.
- Recommended injection site is over insertion of deltoid muscle.
- Do not shake vial after reconstitution. Use within 8 hours.
- Expected lesion forms in 7 to 14 days. Papules reach a maximum diameter of 3 mm, then start to fade.
- Allow at least 3 weeks between BCG and rubella vaccination.
- Don't administer to febrile children.
- Live vaccine; destroy by autoclaving or formaldehyde solution before disposal.
- Patients should have tuberculin skin test 2 to 3 months after BCG vaccination to determine success of vaccine.
- Use of BCG has shown some value in treating various cancers, such as leukemia, some lung cancers, malignant melanoma, multiple myeloma, and some breast tumors.

cholera vaccine

Pregnancy Risk Category: C

HOW SUPPLIED

Injection: suspension of killed *Vibrio cholerae* (each milliliter contains 8 units of Inaba and Ogawa serotypes) in 1-ml, 1.5-ml, and 20-ml vials

ACTION

Mechanism: Promotes active immunity to cholera.
Onset: within 2 weeks after second dose. **Duration:** 3 to 6 months.

INDICATIONS & DOSAGE

Primary immunization –
Adults and children over 10 years: two doses of 0.5 ml I.M. or 1 ml S.C., 1 week to 1 month apart, before traveling in cholera area. Booster is 0.5 ml q 6 months as long as protection is needed.
Children 6 months to 4 years: 0.2 ml I.M. or S.C. Boosters of same dose should be given q 6 months as long as protection is needed.
Children 5 to 10 years: 0.3 ml I.M. or S.C.

ADVERSE REACTIONS

Systemic: tachycardia, hypotension, diarrhea, urticaria, malaise, fever, flushing, headache, ***anaphylaxis***.
Other: *erythema, swelling, pain, induration at injection site.*

INTERACTIONS

Plague, typhoid, or other vaccines with systemic adverse reactions: enhanced toxicity. Don't use together.

*Liquid form contains alcohol.
**May contain tartrazine.

Common reactions are in italics; ***life-threatening,*** in bold italics.

Yellow fever vaccine: simultaneous administration may interfere with immune response to cholera vaccine and yellow fever vaccine. Administer 3 weeks apart.

CONTRAINDICATIONS

- Contraindicated in immunosuppressed patients or those on corticosteroid therapy. Not recommended for children under 6 months. Defer vaccination in patients with acute illness.

NURSING CONSIDERATIONS

- Obtain history of allergies and reaction to immunization.
- Vaccine is about 50% effective in reducing clinical illness incidence for 3 to 6 months.
- Keep epinephrine 1:1,000 available to treat anaphylaxis.
- Administer I.M. in deltoid muscle in adults and children over 3 years.
- I.M. and S.C. routes give higher levels of protection. May be given intradermally to adults and children over 5 years, but the volume of injection is limited to 0.2 ml.
- Advise patients that pain, induration, and swelling are common at the injection site for 24 to 48 hours.

diphtheria and tetanus toxoids, adsorbed

Pregnancy Risk Category: C

HOW SUPPLIED

Available in pediatric (DT) and adult (Td) strengths
Injection (for pediatric use): diphtheria toxoid 6.6 Lf (limit flocculation) units and tetanus toxoid 5 Lf units per 0.5 ml; diphtheria toxoid 10 Lf units and tetanus toxoid 5 Lf units per 0.5 ml; diphtheria toxoid 12.5 Lf units and tetanus toxoid 5 Lf units per 0.5 ml; diphtheria toxoid 15 Lf units and tetanus toxoid 10 Lf units per 0.5 ml
Injection (for adult use): diphtheria toxoid 1.5 Lf units and tetanus toxoid 5 Lf units per 0.5 ml; diphtheria toxoid 2 Lf units and tetanus toxoid 5 Lf units per 0.5 ml; diphtheria toxoid 2 Lf units and tetanus toxoid 10 Lf units per 0.5 ml

ACTION

Mechanism: Promotes immunity to diphtheria and tetanus by inducing production of antitoxins.
Onset: after third dose. **Duration:** 4 to 6 years.

INDICATIONS & DOSAGE

Primary immunization –
Adults and children over 7 years: use adult strength; 0.5 ml I.M. 4 to 6 weeks apart for two doses and a third dose 1 year later. Booster is 0.5 ml I.M. q 10 years.
Infants 6 weeks to 1 year: use pediatric strength; 0.5 ml I.M. at least 4 weeks apart for three doses. Give booster dose 6 to 12 months after third injection.
Children 1 to 6 years: use pediatric strength; 0.5 ml I.M. at least 4 weeks apart for two doses. Give booster dosage 6 to 12 months after the second injection. If the final immunizing dose is given after the seventh birthday, use the adult strength.

ADVERSE REACTIONS

Systemic: ***anaphylaxis,*** chills, fever, malaise.
Other: stinging, edema, erythema, pain, induration at injection site.

INTERACTIONS

None significant.

CONTRAINDICATIONS

- Contraindicated in immunosuppressed patients and in those receiving radiation or corticosteroid therapy. Defer vaccination in patients with respiratory illness and during polio outbreaks; also defer vaccinating those with acute illness except during emergency. When polio is a risk, use single antigen. In children under 6 years, use only when diphtheria, tetanus, and pertussis combination is contraindicated because of pertussis component.

NURSING CONSIDERATIONS
- Obtain history of allergies and reaction to immunization.
- Before injection, verify strength (pediatric or adult) of toxoid used.
- Keep epinephrine 1:1,000 available to treat anaphylaxis.
- Give in site not recently used for vaccines or toxoids.

diphtheria and tetanus toxoids and pertussis vaccine (DTP, DPT)
Tri-Immunol

diphtheria and tetanus toxoids and acellular pertussis vaccine
Acel-Imune

HOW SUPPLIED
whole-cell vaccine
Injection: 6.7 Lf (limit flocculation) units inactivated diphtheria, 5 Lf units inactivated tetanus, and 4 protective units pertussis per 0.5 ml, in 7.5-ml vials; 12.5 Lf units inactivated diphtheria, 5 Lf units inactivated tetanus, and 4 protective units pertussis per 0.5 ml, in 7.5-ml vials (Tri-Immunol)
acellular vaccine
Injection: 7.5 Lf units inactivated diphtheria, 5 Lf units inactivated tetanus, and 300 hemagglutinating units of acellular pertussis vaccine per 0.5 ml

ACTION
Mechanism: Promotes active immunity to diphtheria, tetanus, and pertussis by inducing production of antitoxins and antibodies.
Onset: after third dose. **Duration:** 4 to 6 years.

INDICATIONS & DOSAGE
Primary immunization –
Children 6 weeks to 6 years: 0.5 ml I.M. 2 months apart for three doses and a fourth dose 1 year later. Booster is 0.5 ml I.M. when starting school.

Not advised for adults or children over 6 years.

The acellular vaccine may be used only for the fourth or fifth dose in children 17 months to 7 years who have previously been immunized with three or four doses of the whole-cell vaccine.

ADVERSE REACTIONS
Systemic: ***seizures, encephalopathy.*** anorexia, vomiting, slight fever, chills, malaise, ***anaphylaxis, sudden infant death syndrome.***
Other: *soreness, redness,* expected nodule remaining several weeks at injection site.

INTERACTIONS
Immunosuppressive therapy: may reduce response to DPT vaccine. Avoid if possible.

CONTRAINDICATIONS
- Contraindicated in immunosuppressed patients, in those on corticosteroid therapy, and in those with a history of seizures. Defer vaccination in patients with acute febrile illness.
- Children with preexisting neurologic disorders should not receive pertussis component. Also, children who exhibit neurologic signs after DPT injection shouldn't receive pertussis component in any succeeding injections. Diphtheria and tetanus toxoids (DT) should be given instead.

NURSING CONSIDERATIONS
- Obtain history of allergies and reaction to immunization.
- Acellular vaccine may be associated

with a lower incidence of local pain and fever.
- DPT injection may be given at same time as trivalent oral polio vaccine.
- Keep epinephrine 1:1,000 available to treat anaphylaxis.
- Do not use for active infection.
- Administer only by deep I.M. injection, preferably in thigh or deltoid muscle. Don't give S.C.
- Shake before using. Refrigerate.
- An information booklet is available that describes the risks and benefits of this vaccine. Make sure parents read and understand the information before vaccine is administered.

Haemophilus b conjugate vaccines

Haemophilus b conjugate vaccine, diphtheria CRM_{197} protein conjugate (HbOC)
HibTITER

Haemophilus b conjugate vaccine, diphtheria toxoid conjugate (PRP-D)
ProHIBiT

Haemophilus b conjugate vaccine, meningococcal protein conjugate (PRP-OMP)
PedvaxHIB

HOW SUPPLIED

conjugate vaccine, diphtheria CRM_{197} protein conjugate
Injection: 10 mcg purified *Haemophilus* b saccharide and approximately 25 mcg CRM_{197} protein per 0.5 ml
conjugate vaccine, diphtheria toxoid conjugate
Injection: 25 mcg of *Haemophilus influenzae* type B (HIB) capsular polysaccharide and 18 mcg of diphtheria toxoid protein per 0.5 ml
conjugate vaccine, meningococcal protein conjugate
Powder for injection: 15 mcg *Haemophilus* b PRP, 250 mcg *Neisseria meningitidis* OMPC per dose

ACTION

Mechanism: Promotes active immunity to HIB; is a polymer of ribose, ribitol, and phosphate (PRP) and is covalently linked to highly antigenic substances, enabling the vaccine to promote an immune response in infants.
Onset: about 1 week. **Duration:** 1½ to 3 years.

INDICATIONS & DOSAGE

Immunization against HIB infection – conjugate vaccine, diphtheria CRM_{197} protein conjugate
Infants: 0.5 ml I.M. at age 2 months. Repeat at 4 months and 6 months.
A booster dose is required at age 15 months.
Previously unvaccinated infants 2 to 6 months: 0.5 ml I.M. Repeat in 2 months and again in 4 months for a total of three doses. Give a booster dose at age 15 months.
Previously unvaccinated infants 7 to 11 months: 0.5 ml I.M. Repeat in 2 months, for a total of two doses. Give a booster dose at age 15 months (but no sooner than 2 months after the last vaccination).
Previously unvaccinated infants 12 to 14 months: 0.5 ml I.M. Give a booster dose at age 15 months (but no sooner than 2 months after the first vaccination).
Previously unvaccinated children 15 months to 5 years: 0.5 ml I.M.
A booster dose is not required.
conjugate vaccine, diphtheria toxoid conjugate
Previously unvaccinated children 15 months to 5 years: 0.5 ml I.M.
A booster dose is not required. Not recommended for use in children under age 15 months.
conjugate vaccine, meningococcal protein conjugate
Infants: 0.5 ml I.M. at age 2 months.

Repeat at age 4 months. A booster dose is required at age 12 months.
Previously unvaccinated infants 2 to 6 months: 0.5 ml I.M. Repeat in 2 months. Give a booster dose at age 12 months.
Previously unvaccinated infants 7 to 11 months: 0.5 ml I.M. Repeat in 2 months. Give a booster dose at age 15 months (but no sooner than 2 months after the last vaccination).
Previously unvaccinated infants 12 to 14 months: 0.5 ml I.M. Give a booster dose at age 15 months (but no sooner than 2 months after the first vaccination).
Previously unvaccinated children 15 months to 5 years: 0.5 ml I.M. A booster dose is not required.

ADVERSE REACTIONS

Systemic: ***anaphylaxis,*** fever.
Other: *erythema, pain at injection site.*

INTERACTIONS

Immunosuppressive agents: may suppress antibody response to HIB vaccine.

CONTRAINDICATIONS

- Contraindicated in immunosuppressed patients. Defer immunization in patients with acute illness.

NURSING CONSIDERATIONS

- HIB is an important cause of meningitis in infants and preschool children.
- This vaccine protects against HIB only and will not protect children against any other microorganisms that cause meningitis.
- Diphtheria toxoid conjugate vaccine (ProHIBiT) is not recommended in children under 15 months.
- This vaccine and DPT may be given simultaneously. A combination product is commercially available.
- Don't administer to febrile children.
- Not routinely given to adults or children over 5 years unless they are at high risk for infection (including patients with chronic conditions such as functional asplenia, splenectomy, Hodgkin's disease, or sickle cell anemia).
- Children vaccinated with nonconjugated vaccine (no longer available in the United States) need not be routinely revaccinated if the primary immunization occurred at 24 months. However, if the first vaccination occurred at 18 to 23 months, revaccinate the child with conjugate vaccine, provided at least 2 months has elapsed.
- Keep epinephrine 1:1,000 available in case of anaphylaxis.
- Don't administer intradermally or I.V. Must administer I.M.
- Administer into anterolateral aspect of the upper thigh in small children. Injections may be made into the deltoid muscle of larger children if sufficient muscle mass is present.

hepatitis B vaccine, recombinant

Engerix-B, Recombivax HB

Pregnancy Risk Category: C

HOW SUPPLIED

Injection: 5 mcg HB_sAg/0.5 ml (Recombivax HB, pediatric injection); 10 mcg HB_sAg/0.5 ml (Engerix-B, pediatric injection); 10 mcg HB_sAg/ml (Recombivax HB); 20 mcg HB_sAg/ml (Engerix-B); 40 mcg HB_sAg/ml (Recombivax HB Dialysis Formulation)

ACTION

Mechanism: Promotes active immunity to hepatitis B.
Onset: 70% to 80% of recipients protected after second dose; >99% after third dose. **Duration:** at least 5 years for neonates; at least 7 years for adults.

INDICATIONS & DOSAGE

Immunization against infection from all known subtypes of hepatitis B; primary preexposure prophylaxis against hepatitis B; or postexposure prophylaxis (when given with hepatitis B immune globulin)–

Engerix-B

Adults and children over 10 years: initially, give 20 mcg (1-ml adult formulation) I.M., followed by a second dose of 20 mcg I.M. 30 days later. Give a third dose of 20 mcg I.M. 6 months after the initial dose.

Neonates and children up to 10 years: initially, give 10 mcg (0.5-ml pediatric formulation) I.M., followed by a second dose of 10 mcg I.M. 30 days later. Give a third dose of 10 mcg I.M. 6 months after the initial dose.

Adults undergoing dialysis or receiving immunosuppressants: initially, give 40 mcg I.M. (divided into two 20-mcg doses and administered at different sites). Follow with a second dose of 40 mcg I.M. in 30 days, and a final dose of 40 mcg I.M. 6 months after the initial dose.

Note: Certain populations (neonates born to infected mothers, persons recently exposed to the virus, and travelers to high-risk areas) may receive the vaccine on an abbreviated schedule, with the initial dose followed by a second dose in 1 month, and the third dose after 2 months. For prolonged maintenance of protective antibody titers, a booster dose is recommended 12 months after the initial dose.

Recombivax HB

Adults: initially, give 10 mcg (1-ml adult formulation) I.M., followed by a second dose of 10 mcg I.M. 30 days later. Give a third dose of 10 mcg I.M. 6 months after the initial dose.

Neonates and children up to 11 years: initially, give 2.5 mcg (0.25-ml pediatric formulation) I.M., followed by a second dose of 2.5 mcg I.M. 30 days later. Give a third dose of 2.5 mcg I.M. 6 months after the initial dose.

Children 11 to 19 years: initially, give 5 mcg (0.5-ml pediatric formulation) I.M., followed by a second dose of 5 mcg I.M. 30 days later. Give a third dose of 5 mcg I.M. 6 months after the initial dose.

Adults undergoing dialysis or receiving immunosuppressants: initially, give 40 mcg I.M. (use dialysis formulation, which contains 40 mcg/ml). Follow with a second dose of 40 mcg I.M. in 30 days, and give a final dose of 40 mcg I.M. 6 months after the initial dose.

ADVERSE REACTIONS

Systemic: headache, dizziness, nausea, vomiting, slight fever, transient malaise, flulike symptoms, myalgia.

Other: discomfort and local inflammation at injection site.

INTERACTIONS

None significant.

CONTRAINDICATIONS

- Contraindicated in patients hypersensitive to yeast; recombinant vaccines are derived from yeast cultures.
- Use cautiously in patients with any serious, active infections; compromised cardiac or pulmonary status; and in those for whom a febrile or systemic reaction could pose a serious risk.

NURSING CONSIDERATIONS

- Recombinant hepatitis B vaccine is not made with any human plasma products.
- Certain health care personnel (especially those working with dialysis patients, in blood banks, and in emergency medicine); selected patients

and patient contacts; populations in which the infection is endemic (Inuit [Alaskan], Indo-Chinese, and Haitian refugees); certain military personnel; morticians and embalmers; sexually active homosexual men; prostitutes; prisoners; and users of illicit injectable drugs are at increased risk of infection and should be considered for the vaccine.

- The American Academy of Pediatrics recommends hepatitis B vaccination for all neonates and encourages immunization for adolescents when resources allow.
- Give adults the vaccine in the deltoid muscle; give infants and young children the vaccine in the anterolateral aspect of the thigh. Never administer I.V.
- May be administered S.C. in persons at risk for hemorrhage, such as hemophiliacs. Otherwise, do not use this route; it may lead to an increased incidence or severity of local reactions.
- Although anaphylaxis has not been reported, always keep epinephrine available when administering this vaccine to counteract any possible reaction.
- Thoroughly agitate vial just before administration to restore suspension.
- Refrigerate both opened and unopened vials. Don't freeze.

influenza virus vaccine, 1994-1995 trivalent types A & B (purified surface antigen)

Flu-Imune

influenza virus vaccine, 1994-1995 trivalent types A & B (subvirion or split virion)

Fluogen Split, Fluzone Split, Flu-Shield

influenza virus vaccine, 1994-1995 trivalent types A & B (whole virion)

Fluzone (Whole)

Pregnancy Risk Category: C

HOW SUPPLIED

Injection: 15 mcg A/Texas/36/91-like (H1N1), 15 mcg A/Shadong (H3N2), and 15 mcg B/Panama/45/90 per 0.5 ml

ACTION

Mechanism: Promotes immunity to influenza by inducing production of antibodies.

Onset: 2 to 4 weeks. **Duration:** immunity declines gradually over 1 year.

INDICATIONS & DOSAGE

Influenza prophylaxis –

Adults and children over 12 years: 0.5 ml whole or split virus I.M. Only one dose is required.

Children 6 to 35 months: 0.25 ml split virus I.M. Repeat dose in 4 weeks unless child has been previously vaccinated.

Children 3 to 8 years: 0.5 ml split virus I.M. Repeat dose in 4 weeks unless child has been previously vaccinated.

Children 9 to 12 years: 0.5 ml split virus I.M. Only one dose is required.

ADVERSE REACTIONS

Systemic: ***anaphylaxis,*** fever, malaise, myalgia.

Other: erythema, induration, and soreness at injection site.

Fever and malaise reactions occur most often in children and in others not exposed to influenza viruses. Severe reactions in adults are rare.

INTERACTIONS

Theophylline, warfarin: clearance may be impaired.

CONTRAINDICATIONS

- Contraindicated in patients with hypersensitivity to eggs. Defer vaccination in patients with acute respiratory or other active infection.
- Use cautiously in patients with a history of sulfite allergy.

NURSING CONSIDERATIONS

- Obtain history of allergies, especially to eggs, and reaction to immunization.
- This vaccine is considered safe in pregnant patients. Vaccination shouldn't be postponed, regardless of the stage of pregnancy, in patients who have high-risk conditions and who will be in the first trimester of pregnancy when the flu season begins.
- Immunodeficient patients may receive two doses 1 month apart; however, little evidence suggests that booster doses improve the immunogenic response to the vaccine. Chemoprophylaxis with amantadine may be helpful.
- Ideally, perform vaccinations in November because outbreaks of influenza generally don't occur until December. Avoid administering the vaccine too early in the season because antibody titers may begin to decline before the flu season.
- Ensure that patients understand that annual vaccination using the current vaccine is necessary because immunity to influenza decreases in the year after the injection.
- Note that the combination of antigens used to create influenza vaccine changes annually even though some antigens may be the same as previous years. Do not use leftover supplies of 1993-1994 vaccine to immunize patients for the 1994-1995 flu season.
- Give children 12 years and under their second dose in December, if possible.
- Vaccines may be given to both children and adults throughout the flu season, even as late as April.
- Strongly recommended for anyone over 6 months; for patients with chronic disease, metabolic disorders, or medical conditions that put them at risk for complications from influenza; for health care workers, especially doctors, nurses, employees of nursing homes, volunteer workers, and other personnel in both hospital and outpatient settings; and for household members who may contact persons at high risk for medical complications of influenza. Also recommended for anyone who wishes to reduce the chance of infection.
- Influenza vaccine available as whole virus, split virus, and purified surface antigen preparations. Split virus and purified surface antigen vaccines cause somewhat fewer adverse reactions than whole virus in children.
- Fever, malaise, and myalgia may begin 6 to 12 hours after vaccination and persist 1 to 2 days. These systemic reactions are not common. Ensure that patients understand that the vaccine cannot cause influenza.
- Allergic reactions, which usually occur immediately, are extremely rare.
- Paralysis associated with Guillain-Barré syndrome is rare, and has only been associated with the 1976 vaccine.
- Advise patients about the risks of vaccination as compared with risk of influenza and its complications.
- Do not give children pertussis vaccine within 3 days of influenza virus vaccine. However, they may receive Haemophilus b vaccine; oral polio vaccine; measles, mumps, and rubella vaccine; or pneumococcal vaccine at the same time. Make injections at different sites.
- Although there is little information regarding influenza in persons with HIV, it is recommended that these pa-

tients receive the vaccine. Patients with advanced disease may exhibit a low response; there is no evidence that a booster dose will improve the immune response.

- Keep epinephrine 1:1,000 available to treat anaphylaxis.
- Thoroughly agitate vial just before administration to restore suspension.
- Give injections for adults and older children in deltoid muscle; for infants and children under 3 years, give in anterolateral aspect of thigh.

Japanese encephalitis virus vaccine, inactivated

Je-Vax

Pregnancy Risk Category: C

HOW SUPPLIED

Injection: 1-ml, 10-ml vials

ACTION

Mechanism: Provides active immunity against Japanese encephalitis (JE), a mosquito-borne arboviral flavivirus infection that's the leading cause of viral encephalitis in Asia.
Onset: after two doses in adults, or three doses in persons over age 60.
Duration: immunity endures less than 6 months if only two doses given; about 2 years if full primary immunization administered.

INDICATIONS & DOSAGE

Active immunization against JE–
Primary immunization schedule
Adults and children 3 years and over: 1 ml S.C. on days 0, 7, and 30.
Children 1 to 3 years: 0.5 ml S.C. on days 0, 7, and 30.
Booster doses
Adults and children 3 years and over: 1 ml S.C. q 2 years.
Children 1 to 3 years: 0.5 ml S.C. q 2 years.

ADVERSE REACTIONS

Systemic: *headache, dizziness,* hypotension, *nausea, vomiting, abdominal pain,* ***respiratory distress, anaphylaxis,*** *rash,* generalized urticaria, *fever, malaise, chills, myalgia or* angioedema of the face, oropharynx, extremities, or lips.
Other: *local tenderness and swelling at injection site.*

INTERACTIONS

None significant.

CONTRAINDICATIONS

- Contraindicated in patients hypersensitive to the drug or to thimerosal, a preservative, and in patients who exhibited severe adverse reactions, such as generalized urticaria or angioedema, to a prior dose of the vaccine. Because the vaccine is derived from mouse brain, its use is contraindicated in patients hypersensitive to substances of murine or neural origin.
- Use cautiously in pregnant or breast-feeding patients, elderly patients, and those with a history of urticaria after vaccines, drugs, or insect stings. Advanced age may be a risk factor for developing symptomatic illness after JE infection. JE acquired during pregnancy can cause intrauterine infection and fetal death.
- Before using the vaccine, the clinician must weigh the risks of adverse effects against the risks of exposure and illness as well as the availability, acceptability, and efficacy of repellents and other alternative protective measures.

NURSING CONSIDERATIONS

- The vaccine has been associated with a moderate incidence of local and mild systemic adverse effects. Local tenderness and swelling have been reported in up to 20% of those receiving the vaccine; systemic effects, such as fever, headache, malaise, or rash, in up to 10%. Serious reactions, such as generalized urticaria or angioedema, are uncommon (1% or less of those vaccinated).

• Generalized urticaria or angioedema may occur within minutes of vaccination. Most reactions occur within the first 10 days, with the majority occurring within 48 hours. However, adverse reactions that may be related to the vaccine have occurred as late as 17 days after the injection. Monitor patients closely for 30 minutes after injection. Warn them about the possibility of delayed generalized urticaria or delayed angioedema of the extremities, face, oropharynx or (especially) the lips.

• Reactions to the first dose have occurred a median of 12 hours after injection (88% happened within 3 days). The delay between the second dose and adverse effects was usually longer, with a median of 3 days and some effects not seen for 2 weeks. Some patients exhibited adverse reactions to the second or third dose, even when the first or second dose was well tolerated.

• Because of the possibility of delayed reactions, warn patients to remain in areas where medical care is available for 10 days after injection. Caution against international travel during this time. Advise patients to seek medical assistance as soon as any reaction appears.

• Encourage patients and parents to report adverse effects after vaccination. Health care providers should report these adverse effects to the U.S. Department of Health and Human Services Vaccine Adverse Event Reporting System (VAERS). Contact VAERS at (800) 822-7967 for information about the system and reporting forms.

• Use vaccine to provide protection against JE in persons planning to travel or reside in areas where the virus is endemic. It's not indicated for all persons traveling to or residing in Asia. For most travelers to Asia, the risk for acquiring JE is extremely low. Contact the Centers for Disease Control and Prevention at (404) 332-4555 for current travel advisories.

• Teach patients personal precautions that may avoid exposure to mosquito bites, such as using insect repellents and wearing protective clothing. Avoiding outdoor activities, especially during twilight periods and in the evening, will further reduce risk.

• Ensure that patients follow the recommended three-dose schedule for best results. When time constraints prohibit the use of this schedule, an abbreviated schedule with injections on days 0, 7, and 14 may be used.

• When it isn't possible to follow these schedules, a two-dose regimen with injections on days 0 and 7 may be used. Antibodies will be induced in about 80% of patients with this schedule. Don't use a two-dose regimen unless circumstances are unusual.

• Keep epinephrine 1:1,000 and other resuscitation equipment and drugs available to treat anaphylaxis and other adverse reactions.

• To prepare vaccine for injection, use supplied diluent (sterile water for injection). Add 1.3 ml of diluent to the single-dose vial and 11 ml of diluent to the 10-dose vial. Shake vial thoroughly to ensure dissolution of vaccine. After reconstitution, refrigerate vaccine (36° to 46° F [2° to 8° C]) for up to 8 hours.

measles, mumps, and rubella virus vaccine, live

M-M-RII

Pregnancy Risk Category: X

HOW SUPPLIED

Injection: single-dose vial containing not less than 1,000 $TCID_{50}$ (tissue culture infective doses) of attenuated measles virus derived from Enders' attenuated Edmonston strain (grown in chick embryo culture), 5,000 $TCID_{50}$ of the Jeryl Lynn (B level) mumps strain (grown in chick embryo culture), and the Wistar RA 27/3 strain of rubella virus (propagated in human diploid cell culture)

ACTION

Mechanism: Promotes immunity to measles, mumps, and rubella virus by inducing production of antibodies.
Onset: 2 to 6 weeks. **Duration:** at least 10 years; probably lifelong.

INDICATIONS & DOSAGE

Routine vaccination –
Children: administer 1 vial S.C. A two-dose schedule is recommended, with the first dose given at 15 months (12 months in high-risk areas) and the second dose given at the entry of school (kindergarten or first grade).
Measles outbreak control –
Children: if cases are occurring in children under 1 year, vaccinate children as young as 6 months. All students and their siblings should be revaccinated if they are without documentation of measles immunity.
Adults: school workers born in or after 1957 should be revaccinated if they are without proof of measles immunity. If the outbreak is in a medical facility, all workers born in or after 1957 should be revaccinated if they are without proof of immunity. Revaccination should be considered for persons born before 1957 as well.

ADVERSE REACTIONS

Systemic: urticaria, rash, fever, regional lymphadenopathy, ***anaphylaxis***.
Other: erythema at injection site.

INTERACTIONS

Immune serum globulin, plasma, whole blood: antibodies in serum may interfere with immune response. Don't use vaccine within 3 months of transfusion.

CONTRAINDICATIONS

- Contraindicated in immunosuppressed patients; in those with cancer, blood dyscrasia, gamma globulin disorders, fever, or active untreated tuberculosis; in those receiving corticosteroid or radiation therapy; and in pregnant patients.
- Use cautiously in patients hypersensitive to neomycin, chickens, ducks, eggs, or feathers. Defer immunization in patients with acute illness.

NURSING CONSIDERATIONS

- Obtain history of allergies, especially to antibiotics, chickens, ducks, eggs, feathers, or reaction to immunization.
- Incidence of adverse effects is low (0.5 to 4%).
- Presence of maternal antibodies may prevent response in children under 12 months.
- Treat fever with antipyretics, such as acetaminophen.
- The Immunization Practices Advisory Committee recommends that colleges and other post-high school educational institutions, as well as medical institutions employing health care providers, obtain documentation of the receipt of two doses of vaccine after age 1 (or other proof of immunity, such as infection, documented by a doctor). Combined measles, mumps, and rubella (MMR) vaccine is preferred.
- The Centers for Disease Control and Prevention recommends that, during a measles outbreak in a health care facility, susceptible personnel exposed to the measles virus (whether or not they received measles vaccine or immunoglobulin) avoid patient contact for days 5 through 21 after such exposure. If they become ill, they should avoid patient contact for at least 7 days after developing rash.

• Clinical trials indicate that vitamin A supplementation reduces morbidity and mortality in children with measles. In these studies, 100,000 to 400,000 IU daily have been used.
• Keep epinephrine 1:1,000 available to treat anaphylaxis.
• Inject in outer aspect of upper arm. Don't give I.V.
• Refrigerate; protect from light. Solution may be used if red, pink, or yellow, but must be clear.
• Use only diluent supplied. Discard 8 hours after reconstituting.

measles (rubeola) and rubella virus vaccine, live attenuated

M-R-Vax II

Pregnancy Risk Category: X

HOW SUPPLIED

Injection: single-dose vial containing not less than 1,000 $TCID_{50}$ (tissue culture infective doses) per 0.5 ml of attenuated measles virus derived from Enders' attenuated Edmonston strain (grown in chick embryo culture); 1,000 $TCID_{50}$ of the Wistar RA 27/3 strain of rubella virus

ACTION

Mechanism: Promotes immunity to measles and rubella virus by inducing production of antibodies.
Onset: 2 to 6 weeks. **Duration:** at least 10 years; probably lifelong.

INDICATIONS & DOSAGE

Immunization–
Children 15 months to puberty: 1 vial (1,000 units) S.C.

ADVERSE REACTIONS

Systemic: rash, fever, lymphadenopathy, ***anaphylaxis.***

INTERACTIONS

Immune serum globulin, plasma, whole blood: antibodies in serum may interfere with immune response. Don't use vaccine within 3 months of transfusion.
Tuberculin skin test: may temporarily decrease response to test. Defer skin testing.

CONTRAINDICATIONS

• Contraindicated in immunosuppressed patients; in those with cancer, blood dyscrasia, gamma globulin disorders, fever, or active untreated tuberculosis; in those receiving corticosteroid or radiation therapy; and in pregnant patients.
• Use cautiously in patients hypersensitive to neomycin, chickens, ducks, eggs, or feathers; when there is a history of febrile seizures; or in patients with head injury. Defer immunization in patients with acute illness.

NURSING CONSIDERATIONS

• Obtain history of allergies, especially to antibiotics, chickens, ducks, eggs, or feathers.
• Do not give within 1 month of other live virus vaccines, except oral poliovirus vaccine.
• Allow at least 3 weeks between BCG and rubella vaccines.
• Keep epinephrine 1:1,000 available to treat anaphylaxis.
• Inject in outer upper arm. Don't inject I.V.
• Use only diluent supplied. Discard 8 hours after reconstituting.
• Store in refrigerator and protect from light. Solution may be used if red, pink, or yellow, but must be clear (with no precipitation).

measles (rubeola) virus vaccine, live attenuated

Attenuvax

Pregnancy Risk Category: X

HOW SUPPLIED

Injection: single-dose vial containing not less than 1,000 $TCID_{50}$ (tissue culture infective doses) of attenuated measles virus derived from Enders' attenuated Edmonston strain (grown in chick embryo culture)

ACTION

Mechanism: Promotes immunity to measles virus by inducing production of antibodies.
Onset: 2 to 6 weeks. **Duration:** at least 13 years; probably lifelong.

INDICATIONS & DOSAGE

Immunization –
Adults and children age 15 months or over: 0.5 ml (1,000 units) S.C. A two-dose schedule is recommended, with the first dose given at age 15 months (age 12 months in high-risk areas) and the second dose given at the entry of school (kindergarten or first grade).
Measles outbreak control –
Children: if cases occur in children under age 1, vaccinate children as young as age 6 months. All students and their siblings should be revaccinated if they are without documentation of measles immunity.
Adults: school personnel born in or after 1957 should be revaccinated if they are without proof of measles immunity. If the outbreak is in a medical facility, all workers born in or after 1957 should be revaccinated if they are without proof of immunity. Revaccination should be considered for persons born before 1957 as well.

ADVERSE REACTIONS

Systemic: febrile seizures in susceptible children, anorexia, leukopenia, fever, rash, lymphadenopathy, ***anaphylaxis***.
Other: erythema, swelling, and tenderness at injection site.

INTERACTIONS

Immune serum globulin, plasma, whole blood: antibodies in serum may interfere with immune response. Don't use vaccine within 3 months of transfusion.
Tuberculin skin test: may temporarily decrease response to test. Defer skin testing.

CONTRAINDICATIONS

- Contraindicated in immunosuppressed patients; in those with cancer, blood dyscrasia, gamma globulin disorders, fever, or active untreated tuberculosis; in those receiving corticosteroid or radiation therapy; and in pregnant patients.
- Use cautiously in patients hypersensitive to neomycin, chickens, eggs, or feathers. Defer immunization in patients with acute illness or after administration of blood or plasma.

NURSING CONSIDERATIONS

- Obtain history of allergies, especially to antibiotics, chickens, eggs, or feathers, and reaction to immunization.
- Stress the importance of avoiding pregnancy for 3 months after vaccination. Offer to provide contraception information.
- May be given with oral poliovirus vaccine.
- The Immunization Practices Advisory Committee recommends that colleges and other post-high school educational institutions, as well as medical institutions employing health care providers, obtain documentation of the receipt of two doses of vaccine after age 1 (or other proof of immunity, such as infection, documented by a doctor). Combined measles, mumps, and rubella (MMR) vaccine is preferred.
- The Centers for Disease Control and Prevention recommends that, during a measles outbreak in a health care facility, susceptible personnel exposed to the measles virus (whether or not they received measles vaccine or immune globulin) avoid patient contact for days 5 through 21 after

such exposure. If they become ill, they should avoid patient contact for at least 7 days after developing rash.
• If attenuated measles vaccine is administered immediately after exposure to the disease, some protection may be provided. This level of protection is significantly increased if the vaccine is administered even a few days before exposure.
• Keep epinephrine 1:1,000 available to treat anaphylaxis.
• Do not give I.V.
• Use only diluent supplied. Discard 8 hours after reconstituting.
• Refrigerate and protect from light. Solution may be used if red, pink, or yellow, but must be clear (with no precipitation).

meningitis vaccine

Menomune-A/C, Menomune-A/C/Y/W-135

Pregnancy Risk Category: C

HOW SUPPLIED

Injection: 10-dose and 50-dose vials with vial of diluent

ACTION

Mechanism: Promotes active immunity to meningitis.
Onset: 10 to 14 days. **Duration:** antibody titers decline within 3 years.

INDICATIONS & DOSAGE

Meningococcal meningitis prophylaxis –
Adults and children over 2 years: 0.5 ml S.C.

ADVERSE REACTIONS

Systemic headache, malaise, chills, fever, muscle cramps, ***anaphylaxis***.
Other: *pain, erythema, and induration at injection site.*

INTERACTIONS

None significant.

CONTRAINDICATIONS

• Contraindicated in immunosuppressed and pregnant patients. Defer vaccination in patients with acute illness.

NURSING CONSIDERATIONS

• Obtain history of allergies and reaction to immunization.
• Stress to patients the importance of avoiding pregnancy for 3 months after vaccination. Offer to provide contraception information.
• Vaccine may be given with other immunizations.
• Some clinicians will revaccinate children if they are at high risk and previously received vaccine before age 4 years.
• Keep epinephrine 1:1,000 available to treat anaphylaxis.
• Do not give I.V.

mumps virus vaccine, live

Mumpsvax

Pregnancy Risk Category: X

HOW SUPPLIED

Injection: single-dose vial containing not less than 5,000 $TCID_{50}$ (tissue culture infective doses) of attenuated mumps virus derived from Jeryl Lynn mumps strain (grown in chick embryo culture) and vial of diluent

ACTION

Mechanism: Promotes active immunity to mumps.
Onset: 2 to 3 weeks. **Duration:** at least 15 years; probably lifelong.

INDICATIONS & DOSAGE

Immunization –
Adults and children over 1 year: 1 vial (5,000 units) S.C.

ADVERSE REACTIONS

CNS: febrile seizures (rare).
Other: *slight fever,* rash, malaise, mild allergic reactions.

INTERACTIONS
Immune serum globulin, plasma, whole blood: antibodies in serum may interfere with immune response. Don't use vaccine within 3 months of transfusion.
Tuberculin skin test: may temporarily decrease response to test. Defer skin testing.

CONTRAINDICATIONS
• Contraindicated in immunosuppressed patients; in those with cancer, blood dyscrasia, gamma globulin disorders, fever, or untreated active tuberculosis; in those receiving corticosteroid or radiation therapy; and in pregnant patients.
• Use cautiously in patients hypersensitive to neomycin, chickens, ducks, eggs, or feathers. Defer in patients with acute or febrile illness and for 3 months after transfusions or treatment with immune serum globulin.

NURSING CONSIDERATIONS
• Obtain history of allergies, especially to antibiotics, and reaction to immunization.
• Stress to patients the importance of avoiding pregnancy for 3 months after vaccination. Offer to provide contraception information.
• This vaccine should not be given less than 1 month before or after immunization with other live-virus vaccines; however, Attenuvax, Meruvax, or monovalent or trivalent live, oral poliovirus vaccine may be administered simultaneously.
• Not recommended for infants under 12 months because retained maternal mumps antibodies may interfere with the immune response.
• Treat fever with antipyretics.
• Keep epinephrine 1:1,000 available to treat anaphylaxis.
• Do not give I.V.
• Use only diluent supplied. Discard 8 hours after reconstituting.
• Refrigerate and protect from light. Solution may be used if red, pink, or yellow, but must be clear.

plague vaccine

Pregnancy Risk Category: C

HOW SUPPLIED
Injection: 2 billion killed plague bacilli (*Yersinia pestis*)/ml in 20-ml vials

ACTION
Mechanism: Promotes active immunity to plague.
Onset: over 90% of persons immune after the second dose. **Duration:** 6 to 12 months.

INDICATIONS & DOSAGE
Primary immunization and booster–
Adults and children over 10 years: 1 ml I.M. followed by 0.2 ml in 4 weeks, then 0.2 ml 6 months after the first dose. Booster is 0.1 to 0.2 ml q 6 months while in plague area.
Children under 1 year: ⅕ adult primary or booster dose.
Children 1 to 4 years: ⅖ adult primary or booster dose.
Children 5 to 10 years: ⅗ adult primary or booster dose.

ADVERSE REACTIONS
Systemic: headache, malaise, slight fever, lymphadenopathy, ***anaphylaxis.***
Other: swelling, *induration, and erythema* at injection site.

INTERACTIONS
Cholera, typhoid vaccine: increased risk of adverse effects. Don't give at the same time.

CONTRAINDICATIONS
• Contraindicated in immunosuppressed patients, pregnant patients, and in those hypersensitive to beef, soy, casein, or phenol. Defer in patients with respiratory infection.

NURSING CONSIDERATIONS
- Obtain history of allergies and reaction to immunization.
- Recommended for all laboratory and field personnel working with *Yersinia pestis.*
- Keep epinephrine 1:1,000 available to treat anaphylaxis.
- Deltoid area is the preferred injection site.

pneumococcal vaccine, polyvalent

Pneumovax 23, Pnu-Imune 23

Pregnancy Risk Category: C

HOW SUPPLIED

Injection: 25 mcg each of 23 polysaccharide isolates/0.5 ml

ACTION

Mechanism: Promotes active immunity to infections caused by *Streptococcus pneumoniae.*

Onset: 2 to 3 weeks. **Duration:** 5 to 10 years.

INDICATIONS & DOSAGE

Pneumococcal immunization –

Adults and children over 2 years: 0.5 ml I.M. or S.C.

Not recommended for children under 2 years.

ADVERSE REACTIONS

Systemic: ***anaphylaxis, slight fever.***

Other: soreness at injection site; severe local reaction can occur when revaccination takes place within 3 years.

INTERACTIONS

None significant.

CONTRAINDICATIONS
- Contraindicated in patients hypersensitive to the drug.

NURSING CONSIDERATIONS
- Check immunization history carefully to avoid revaccination within 3 years.
- Obtain history of allergies and reaction to immunization. Eggs and egg protein are not used during the manufacture of the vaccine; contains phenol as a preservative.
- Treat fever with mild antipyretics.
- Protects against 23 pneumococcal types, accounting for 90% of pneumococcal disease.
- May be administered to children to prevent pneumococcal otitis media.
- Recommended for all adults over 65 years.
- Simultaneous administration with influenza virus vaccine is safe and effective.
- When splenectomy is being considered, give vaccine at least 2 weeks before procedure to ensure adequate antibody response. This vaccine may be less effective in splenectomized patients.
- Keep epinephrine 1:1,000 available to treat anaphylaxis.
- Inject in deltoid or midlateral thigh. Don't inject I.V.
- Keep refrigerated. Reconstitution or dilution not necessary.

poliovirus vaccine, live, oral, trivalent (TOPV)

Orimune

poliovirus vaccine, inactivated (IPV)

IPOL, Polivax

Pregnancy Risk Category: C

HOW SUPPLIED

Oral vaccine: mixture of three live viruses (types 1, 2, and 3), grown in monkey kidney tissue culture, in 0.5-ml single-dose Dispettes

Inactivated virus vaccine injection: mixture of three types of poliovirus (types 1, 2, and 3) grown in tissue culture. IPOL employs monkey kidney cultures; Polivax employs human diploid cell cultures.

ACTION

Mechanism: Promotes immunity to poliomyelitis by inducing humoral antibodies and antibodies in the lymphatic tissue.
Onset: 1 to 2 weeks. **Duration:** many years; probably lifelong.

INDICATIONS & DOSAGE

Poliovirus immunization –
Children and nonimmunized adults: 0.5 ml P.O. (TOPV), followed by a second dose of 0.5 ml in 6 to 8 weeks. Give third 0.5-ml dose 6 to 12 months after second dose. A reinforcing dose of 0.5 ml should be given before entry to school.
Infants: administer 0.5 ml P.O. at 2 months, 4 months, and 18 months. Optional dose may be given at 6 months.
Poliovirus immunization in persons who cannot receive TOPV –
Adults: 0.5 ml S.C., followed by a second dose in 4 to 8 weeks. Administer a third dose in 6 to 12 months.
Children: 0.5 ml S.C. at 2 months and 4 months. Administer a third dose at 15 to 18 months. A reinforcing dose of 0.5 ml S.C. should be given before entry into school.

ADVERSE REACTIONS

Systemic: ***poliomyelitis.***

INTERACTIONS

Immune serum globulin, plasma, whole blood: antibodies in serum may interfere with immune response. Don't use vaccine within 3 months of transfusion.
Tuberculin skin test: may suppress response to skin test. Don't test for 6 weeks.

CONTRAINDICATIONS

• Oral vaccine is contraindicated in immunosuppressed patients; in those with cancer or immunoglobulin abnormalities; and in those receiving radiation, antimetabolite, alkylating agent, or corticosteroid therapy. These patients should receive IPV. Injectable vaccine is contraindicated in patients hypersensitive to neomycin or streptomycin.
• Defer oral vaccine in patients with vomiting or diarrhea. Defer both forms of vaccine in patients with acute illness.
• Immunodeficient patients or those with altered immune status may be at risk for developing the disease if live-virus vaccine is administered. These patients should receive parenteral form.
• Use with caution in siblings of child with known immunodeficiency syndrome. IPV is preferred.
• Should not be administered to neonates under 6 weeks.

NURSING CONSIDERATIONS

• Obtain history of allergies and reaction to immunization.
• The highest risk of poliovirus infection occurs after the first dose of the oral vaccine.
• Adults at high risk for exposure who have completed a primary course may receive another dose.
• Vaccine is not effective in modifying or preventing existing or incubating poliomyelitis.
• Oral vaccine is not for parenteral use.
• Keep frozen until used. Once thawed, if unopened, may refrigerate up to 30 days; if opened, up to 7 days. Thaw before administration.
• Color change from pink to yellow has no effect on efficacy of the vaccine. Yellow color results from vaccine being stored at low temperatures.
• Check the parents' immunization history when they bring in child for

vaccine; this is an excellent time for parents to receive booster immunizations.

• An information booklet is available that describes the risks and benefits of this vaccine. Make sure parents read and understand this information before vaccine is administered.

rabies vaccine, human diploid cell (HDCV)

Imovax

Pregnancy Risk Category: C

HOW SUPPLIED

Intradermal injection: 0.25 IU rabies antigen/dose
I.M. injection: 2.5 IU of rabies antigen/ml, in single-dose vial with diluent

ACTION

Mechanism: Promotes active immunity to rabies.
Onset: within 1 week. **Peak:** Antibody levels peak after 1 to 2 months.
Duration: about 1 year.

INDICATIONS & DOSAGE

Postexposure antirabies immunization –
Adults and children: five 1-ml doses of HDCV I.M. (for example, in the deltoid region). Give first dose as soon as possible after exposure; give an additional dose on each of days 3, 7, 14, and 28 after first dose. If lack of antibody response after this primary series exists, a booster dose is recommended.
Preexposure prophylaxis immunization for persons in high-risk groups –
Adults and children: three 1-ml injections administered I.M. Give first dose on day 0 (the first day of therapy), second dose on day 7, and third dose on either day 21 or 28. Alternatively, give 0.1 ml intradermally on the same dosage schedule.

ADVERSE REACTIONS

Systemic: headache, dizziness, nausea, abdominal pain, diarrhea, muscle aches, fever, ***anaphylaxis, serum sickness.***
Other: *pain, erythema, swelling, or itching at injection site.*

INTERACTIONS

Antimalarial drugs, corticosteroids, immunosuppressive agents: decreased response to rabies vaccine. Avoid concomitant use.

CONTRAINDICATIONS

• Use cautiously in patients with a history of hypersensitivity.
• When postexposure immunization is indicated, pregnancy is not a contraindication.

NURSING CONSIDERATIONS

• Corticosteroid therapy should be stopped during immunizing period unless therapy is essential for the treatment of other conditions.
• Some patients who receive booster doses experience serum sickness-like hypersensitivity reactions. These reactions usually respond to antihistamines.
• The Centers for Disease Control and Prevention recommends a booster dose with Imovax for all persons who have been potentially exposed to rabies since October 15, 1984, and who have received postexposure prophylaxis with Wyvac unless acceptable titers were proven.
• The alternative regimen of 0.1-ml doses is only for preexposure prophylaxis. For postexposure prophylaxis, only use the 1-ml doses.
• Keep epinephrine 1:1,000 available to treat anaphylaxis.
• Do not use intradermal route for postexposure rabies vaccination.

rubella and mumps virus vaccine, live

Biavax II

Pregnancy Risk Category: X

HOW SUPPLIED

Injection: single-dose vial containing not less than 1,000 $TCID_{50}$ (tissue culture infective doses) of the Wistar RA 27/3 rubella virus (propagated in human diploid cell culture) and not less than 5,000 $TCID_{50}$ of the Jeryl Lynn mumps strain (grown in chick embryo cell culture)

ACTION

Mechanism: Promotes immunity to rubella and mumps by inducing antibody production.
Onset: 2 to 6 weeks. **Duration:** 10 years or longer.

INDICATIONS & DOSAGE

Measles and mumps immunization–
Adults and children over 1 year: 1 vial (1,000 units) S.C.

ADVERSE REACTIONS

Systemic: polyneuritis, rash, thrombocytopenic purpura, urticaria, fever, arthritis, arthralgia, ***anaphylaxis,*** lymphadenopathy.
Other: pain, erythema, and induration at injection site.

INTERACTIONS

Immune serum globulin, plasma, whole blood: antibodies in serum may interfere with immune response. Don't give vaccine within 3 months of transfusion.
Tuberculin skin test: may temporarily decrease response to test. Defer skin testing.

CONTRAINDICATIONS

- Contraindicated in immunosuppressed patients; in those with cancer, blood dyscrasia, gamma globulin disorders, fever, or active untreated tuberculosis; and in those receiving corticosteroid or radiation therapy.
- Use cautiously in patients hypersensitive to neomycin, chickens, ducks, eggs, or feathers. Defer in patients with acute illness and after administration of immune serum globulin, blood, or plasma.
- Pregnancy should be avoided for 3 months after vaccination.

NURSING CONSIDERATIONS

- Obtain history of allergies, especially to antibiotics, chickens, ducks, eggs, or feathers, and reaction to immunization.
- Stress to patients the importance of avoiding pregnancy for 3 months after vaccination. Offer to provide contraception information.
- Allow an interval of at least 3 weeks between BCG and rubella vaccines.
- Keep epinephrine 1:1,000 available to treat anaphylaxis.
- Inject into outer upper arm. Don't inject I.V.
- Use only diluent supplied. Discard 8 hours after reconstituting.
- Refrigerate and protect from light. Solution may be used if red, pink, or yellow, but must be clear.

rubella virus vaccine, live attenuated (RA 27/3)

Meruvax II

Pregnancy Risk Category: X

HOW SUPPLIED

Injection: single-dose vial containing not less than 1,000 $TCID_{50}$ (tissue culture infective doses) of the Wistar RA 27/3 strain of rubella virus (propagated in human diploid cell culture)

ACTION

Mechanism: Promotes immunity to rubella by inducing production of antibodies.

Onset: 2 to 6 weeks. **Duration:** 10 years or longer.

INDICATIONS & DOSAGE
Measles immunization –
Adults and children over 1 year: 1 vial (1,000 units) S.C.

ADVERSE REACTIONS
Systemic: polyneuritis, rash, thrombocytopenic purpura, urticaria, *joint pain,* fever, arthritis, ***anaphylaxis,*** lymphadenopathy.
Other: pain, erythema, and induration at injection site.

INTERACTIONS
Immune serum globulin, plasma, whole blood: antibodies in serum may interfere with immune response. Don't use vaccine within 3 months of transfusion. Immune serum globulin may be given 2 weeks before vaccine.
Tuberculin skin test: may temporarily decrease response to test. Defer skin testing.

CONTRAINDICATIONS
- Contraindicated in immunosuppressed patients; in those with cancer, blood dyscrasia, gamma globulin disorders, fever, or active untreated tuberculosis; and in those receiving corticosteroid or radiation therapy.
- Use cautiously in patients hypersensitive to neomycin, chickens, ducks, eggs, or feathers. Defer immunization in patients with acute illness and after administration of human immune serum globulin, blood, or plasma.
- Pregnancy should be avoided for 3 months after vaccination.

NURSING CONSIDERATIONS
- Obtain history of allergies, especially to antibiotics, chickens, ducks, eggs, or feathers, and reaction to immunization.
- Stress to patients the importance of avoiding pregnancy for 3 months after vaccination. Offer to provide contraception information.
- Allow at least 3 weeks between BCG and rubella vaccines.
- Keep epinephrine 1:1,000 available to treat anaphylaxis.
- Inject into outer upper arm. Don't inject I.V.
- Refrigerate and protect from light. Solution may be used if red, pink, or yellow, but must be clear.
- Use only diluent supplied. Discard 8 hours after reconstituting.

tetanus toxoid, adsorbed

tetanus toxoid, fluid

Pregnancy Risk Category: C

HOW SUPPLIED
adsorbed
Injection: 5 to 10 Lf (limit flocculation) units of inactivated tetanus/0.5-ml dose, in 0.5-ml syringes and 5-ml vials
fluid
Injection: 4 to 5 Lf units of inactivated tetanus/0.5-ml dose, in 0.5-ml syringes and 7.5-ml vials

ACTION
Mechanism: Promotes immunity to tetanus by inducing antitoxin production.
Onset: after second dose. **Duration:** about 10 years.

INDICATIONS & DOSAGE
Primary immunization –
Adults and children over 6 years: 0.5 ml (adsorbed) I.M. 4 to 6 weeks apart for two doses; then third dose 6 to 12 months after the second. Alternatively, give 0.5 ml (fluid) I.M. or S.C. 4 to 8 weeks apart for three doses; then fourth dose of 0.5 ml 6 to 12 months after third dose.
Children 6 weeks to 6 years: 0.5 ml (adsorbed) I.M. at age 2, 4, and 6 months. Give a fourth dose at age 15

to 18 months. Give a fifth dose at age 4 to 6 years, just before entry into school.
Booster doses –
Adults: 0.5 ml I.M. at 10-year intervals.

ADVERSE REACTIONS
Systemic: tachycardia, hypotension, urticaria, pruritus, slight fever, chills, malaise, aches and pains, flushing, ***anaphylaxis***.
Other: erythema, induration, and nodule at injection site.

INTERACTIONS
Chloramphenicol: may interfere with response to tetanus toxoid.

CONTRAINDICATIONS
- Contraindicated in immunosuppressed patients and in those with immunoglobulin abnormalities. Defer vaccination in patients with acute illness and during polio outbreaks, except in emergencies.

NURSING CONSIDERATIONS
- Obtain history of allergies and reaction to immunization.
- Determine date of last tetanus immunization.
- Use for prevention, not treatment, of tetanus infections.
- Advise patients to avoid use of hot or cold compresses at injection site; these may increase severity of local reaction.
- Adsorbed form produces longer duration of immunity. Fluid form provides quicker booster effect in patients actively immunized previously.
- Do not confuse this drug with tetanus immune globulin, human.
- Keep epinephrine 1:1,000 available to treat anaphylaxis.

typhoid vaccine

typhoid vaccine, oral
Vivotif Berna Vaccine
Pregnancy Risk Category: C

HOW SUPPLIED
Injection: suspension of killed Ty-2 strain of *Salmonella typhi;* 8 units/ml in 5-ml, 10-ml, and 20-ml vials
Capsules (enteric-coated): 2 to 6 × 10^9 colony-forming units of viable *Salmonella typhi* $Ty^{21}a$ and 5 to 50 × 10^9 bacterial cells of nonviable $Ty^{21}a^2$

ACTION
Mechanism: Provides active immunity to typhoid fever.
Onset: immunity, at end of primary immunization. **Duration:** injection, 3 years; oral vaccine, 5 years.

INDICATIONS & DOSAGE
Primary immunization –
Adults and children over 10 years: 0.5 ml S.C. (injection); repeat in 4 weeks. Repeat protocol as booster q 3 years.
Adults: 1 capsule (oral vaccine) on alternate days taken 1 hour before meals for four doses. Repeat protocol as booster q 5 years.
Children 6 months to 10 years: 0.25 ml S.C. (injection); repeat in 4 weeks. Repeat protocol as booster q 3 years.

ADVERSE REACTIONS
CNS: headache.
GI: nausea.
Other: *fever,* malaise, ***anaphylaxis;*** swelling, pain, and inflammation at injection site.

INTERACTIONS
Sulfonamides, other antibiotics: may impair antibody response. Don't use together.

CONTRAINDICATIONS
• Contraindicated in immunosuppressed patients. Defer vaccination in patients with acute illness.

NURSING CONSIDERATIONS
• Obtain history of allergies and reaction to immunization.
• Treat fever with antipyretics.
• Keep epinephrine 1:1,000 available to treat anaphylaxis.
• When administering oral vaccine, ensure that patients understand the importance of taking all four doses. It is imperative to follow the alternate-day regimen.
• Tell patients to take oral vaccine with cold or lukewarm water and not to chew or crush enteric-coated capsules.
• Refrigerate oral vaccine at 35.5° to 50° F (2° to 10° C).
• Do not give parenteral form intradermally.
• Shake thoroughly before withdrawing from vial.

yellow fever vaccine
YF-Vax

Pregnancy Risk Category: D

HOW SUPPLIED
Injection: live, attenuated 17D yellow fever virus in 1- and 5-dose vials, with diluent; supplied only to designated yellow fever vaccination centers authorized to issue yellow fever vaccination certificates

ACTION
Mechanism: Provides active immunity to yellow fever.
Onset: 7 to 10 days. **Duration:** at least 30 to 35 years; probably lifelong.

INDICATIONS & DOSAGE
Primary vaccination –
Adults and children over 6 months: 0.5 ml deep S.C.; booster is 0.5 ml S.C. q 10 years.

ADVERSE REACTIONS
Systemic: ***anaphylaxis,*** fever, malaise.
Other: mild swelling, pain at injection site.

INTERACTIONS
Cholera vaccine: concurrent administration may interfere with immune response to both yellow fever vaccine and cholera vaccine. Administer 3 weeks apart.

CONTRAINDICATIONS
• Contraindicated in immunosuppressed patients; in those with cancer, gamma globulin deficiency, or hypersensitivity to chickens or eggs; or in those receiving corticosteroid or radiation therapy. Also contraindicated during pregnancy and in infants under 9 months, except in high-risk areas. Information regarding these areas can be obtained from the Centers for Disease Control and Prevention, Division of Vector-Borne Infectious Diseases, at (303) 221-6400.

NURSING CONSIDERATIONS
• Obtain history of allergies, especially to chicken or eggs, and reaction to immunization.
• Don't give yellow fever vaccine within 1 month of other live-virus vaccines; may be given concurrently with hepatitis B vaccine.
• Keep epinephrine 1:1,000 available to treat anaphylaxis.
• Reconstitute with sodium chloride injection that contains no preservatives (preservatives decrease potency).
• Keep frozen. Don't use unless shipping case contains some dry ice on arrival. Avoid vigorous shaking; carefully swirl mixture until suspension is uniform. Use within 1 hour after reconstituting. Discard remainder.

76

Antitoxins and antivenins

black widow spider antivenin
botulism antitoxin, bivalent equine
crotaline antivenin, polyvalent
diphtheria antitoxin, equine
***Micrurus fulvius* antivenin**

COMBINATION PRODUCTS
None.

black widow spider antivenin

Antivenin *(Latrodectus mactans)*

Pregnancy Risk Category: C

HOW SUPPLIED
Injection: combination package – 1 vial of antivenin (6,000 units/vial), one 2.5-ml vial of diluent (sterile water for injection), and one 1-ml vial of normal equine (horse) serum (1:10 dilution) for sensitivity testing

ACTION
Mechanism: Neutralizes and binds venom.
Peak: Serum levels peak 2 to 3 days after I.M. injection. **Duration:** elimination half-life, less than 15 days.

INDICATIONS & DOSAGE
Black widow spider bite –
Adults and children: 2.5 ml I.M. in deltoid. Second dose may be needed. In severe cases, antivenin may be given I.V.

ADVERSE REACTIONS
Systemic: hypersensitivity reactions, ***anaphylaxis, neurotoxicity.***

INTERACTIONS
None significant.

CONTRAINDICATIONS
- Contraindicated in patients hypersensitive to the drug.

NURSING CONSIDERATIONS
- Immobilize the patient; splint the bitten limb to prevent spread of venom.
- Test for sensitivity before giving the drug. Use 0.2 ml of a 1:10 dilution in 0.9% sodium chloride solution.
- Obtain accurate patient history of allergies, especially to horses, and reaction to immunization. Make sure epinephrine 1:1,000 is available in case of anaphylaxis.
- Venom is neurotoxic and may cause respiratory paralysis and seizures. Watch the patient carefully for 2 to 3 days.
- For best results, administer antivenin as soon as possible.
- **I.V. use:** Dilute antivenin in 10 to 50 ml of 0.9% sodium chloride solution and infuse over 15 minutes.

botulism antitoxin, bivalent equine

Pregnancy Risk Category: D

HOW SUPPLIED
Available through your state health department or the state epidemiologist's office.

ACTION
Mechanism: Neutralizes and binds toxin.
Duration: half-life, less than 15 days.

INDICATIONS & DOSAGE
Botulism –
Adults and children: 1 vial I.V. stat and q 4 hours, p.r.n., until the patient's condition improves.

*Liquid form contains alcohol.
**May contain tartrazine.

Common reactions are in italics; ***life-threatening,*** in bold italics.

ADVERSE REACTIONS
Systemic: hypersensitivity reactions, ***anaphylaxis,*** serum sickness (urticaria, pruritus, fever, malaise, arthralgia) may occur in 5 to 13 days.

INTERACTIONS
None significant.

CONTRAINDICATIONS
- Contraindicated in patients hypersensitive to the drug.

NURSING CONSIDERATIONS
- Test for sensitivity before giving the drug.
- Obtain accurate patient history of allergies, especially to horses, and reaction to immunization. Make sure epinephrine 1:1,000 is available in case of hypersensitivity reaction.
- For best results, administer antitoxin as soon as possible.
- **I.V. use:** Dilute antitoxin 1:10 in D_5W, $D_{10}W$, or 0.9% sodium chloride solution before giving. Give first 10 ml of dilution over 5 minutes; after 15 minutes, rate may be increased.
- Bivalent antitoxin contains antibodies against types A and B *Clostridium botulinum.* Antitoxins against all other types are available only from Centers for Disease Control and Prevention in Atlanta: Monday to Friday, 8 a.m. to 4:30 p.m. (E.S.T.) (404) 639-3670; nights, weekends, and holidays (emergencies only) (404) 639-2888.

crotaline antivenin, polyvalent
Pregnancy Risk Category: D

HOW SUPPLIED
Injection: combination package – one vial of lyophilized serum, one vial of diluent (10 ml bacteriostatic water for injection), and one 1-ml vial of normal horse serum (diluted 1:10) for sensitivity testing

ACTION
Mechanism: Neutralizes and binds venom of snakes of the species crotalids (pit vipers), including rattle snakes, water moccasins, and copperheads.
Duration: elimination half-life, less than 15 days.

INDICATIONS & DOSAGE
Crotalid (rattlesnake) bites –
Adults and children: initially, 10 to 50 ml I.V., depending on severity of bite and patient response. If large amount of venom, 70 to 100 ml I.V. directly into superficial vein. Subsequent doses based on patient's response; may give 10 ml q ½ to 2 hours, p.r.n. If bite is in extremity, inject part of initial dose at various sites around limb above swelling; don't inject in finger or toe. The smaller the patient, the larger the initial dose.

ADVERSE REACTIONS
Systemic: *hypersensitivity reactions,* ***anaphylaxis, neurotoxicity,*** *serum sickness.*

INTERACTIONS
Antihistamines: enhanced toxicity of crotaline venoms. Don't use together.

CONTRAINDICATIONS
- Contraindicated in patients hypersensitive to the drug.
- Use cautiously. Studies indicate that 60% of patients treated with this antivenin develop hypersensitivity.

NURSING CONSIDERATIONS
- Immobilize the patient immediately. Splint the bitten extremity.
- Test for sensitivity before giving drug. Give 0.02 to 0.03 ml of a 1:10 dilution in 0.9% sodium chloride solution intradermally. Read results after 5 to 10 minutes. Watch patients carefully for delayed allergic reaction or relapse.
- Obtain accurate patient history of

allergies, especially to horses, and reaction to immunization. Make sure epinephrine 1:1,000 is available in case of hypersensitivity reaction.
- Type and crossmatch blood as soon as possible because hemolysis from venom prevents accurate crossmatching.
- For best results, administer antivenin as soon as possible.
- Children, who have less resistance and less body fluid to dilute venom, may need twice the adult dose.
- Discard unused portion.
- If a large number of vials are administered, serum sickness may result. Administer corticosteroids as prescribed.

diphtheria antitoxin, equine

Pregnancy Risk Category: D

HOW SUPPLIED

Injection: not less than 500 units/ml in 10,000-unit and 20,000-unit vials

ACTION

Mechanism: Neutralizes and binds toxin.
Duration: elimination half-life, less than 15 days.

INDICATIONS & DOSAGE

Diphtheria prevention –
Adults and children: 1,000 to 5,000 units I.M.
Diphtheria treatment –
Adults and children: 20,000 to 80,000 units or more slow I.V. Additional doses may be given in 24 hours. I.M. route may be used in mild cases.

ADVERSE REACTIONS

Systemic: hypersensitivity reactions, ***anaphylaxis,*** serum sickness (urticaria, pruritus, fever, malaise, arthralgia) may occur in 7 to 12 days.

INTERACTIONS

None significant.

CONTRAINDICATIONS

- Contraindicated in patients hypersensitive to the drug.

NURSING CONSIDERATIONS

- Test for sensitivity before giving the drug.
- Obtain accurate patient history of allergies, especially to horses, and reaction to immunization. Make sure epinephrine 1:1,000 is available in case of hypersensitivity reaction.
- If patient has symptoms of diphtheria (sore throat, fever, tonsillar membrane), begin therapy immediately, without waiting for culture reports.
- For storage, refrigerate antitoxin at 35.6° to 50° F (2° to 10° C). Before administering, warm to 90° to 95° F (32.2° to 35° C), never higher.

Micrurus fulvius antivenin

Pregnancy Risk Category: D

HOW SUPPLIED

Injection: combination package with 10 ml diluent

ACTION

Mechanism: Neutralizes and binds coral snake venom.
Duration: elimination half-life, less than 15 days.

INDICATIONS & DOSAGE

Eastern and Texas coral snake bite –
Adults and children: 3 to 5 vials slow I.V. through running I.V. of 0.9% sodium chloride solution. Give first 1 to 2 ml over 3 to 5 minutes, and watch for signs of allergic reaction. If no signs develop, continue injection. Up to 10 vials may be needed.

Not effective for Sonoran or Arizona coral snake bites.

ADVERSE REACTIONS

Systemic: hypersensitivity reactions, ***anaphylaxis.***

*Liquid form contains alcohol.
**May contain tartrazine.

Common reactions are in italics; ***life-threatening,*** in bold italics.

INTERACTIONS
None significant.

CONTRAINDICATIONS
- Contraindicated in patients hypersensitive to the drug.

NURSING CONSIDERATIONS
- Test for sensitivity before giving the drug.
- Obtain accurate patient history of allergies, especially to horses, and reaction to immunization. Make sure epinephrine 1:1,000 is available in case of hypersensitivity reaction.
- Immobilize the patient and splint bitten limb to prevent spread of venom.
- For best results, administer antivenin as soon as possible (before onset of neurotoxic signs); treat asymptomatic patients because systemic signs usually develop late.
- Watch the patient carefully for 24 hours. Venom is neurotoxic and may cause respiratory paralysis.

77

Immune serums

cytomegalovirus immune globulin, intravenous
hepatitis B immune globulin, human
immune globulin intramuscular
immune globulin intravenous
rabies immune globulin, human
Rh_o(D) immune globulin, human
tetanus immune globulin, human
varicella-zoster immune globulin

COMBINATION PRODUCTS
None.

cytomegalovirus immune globulin, intravenous (CMV-IGIV)

CytoGam

Pregnancy Risk Category: C

HOW SUPPLIED
Powder for injection: 2.5 g with 50 ml sterile water diluent

ACTION
Mechanism: Provides passive immunity by supplying a relatively high concentration of immunoglobulin G (IgG) antibodies against CMV. Increasing these antibody levels in CMV-exposed patients may attenuate or reduce the incidence of serious CMV disease.
Duration: elimination half-life, 21 days or less.

INDICATIONS & DOSAGE
To attenuate primary CMV disease in seronegative kidney transplant recipients who receive a kidney from a CMV seropositive donor –
Adults: administer according to the following schedule.

– within 72 hours of transplantation: 150 mg/kg
– 2 weeks after transplantation: 100 mg/kg
– 4 weeks after transplantation: 100 mg/kg
– 6 weeks after transplantation: 100 mg/kg
– 8 weeks after transplantation: 100 mg/kg
– 12 weeks after transplantation: 50 mg/kg
– 16 weeks after transplantation: 50 mg/kg.

Administer initial dose at 15 mg/kg/hour. Increase to 30 mg/kg/hour after 30 minutes if no untoward reactions occur, then increase to 60 mg/kg/hour after another 30 minutes if no untoward reactions occur. Volume should not exceed 75 ml/hour. Subsequent doses may be administered at 15 mg/kg/hour for 15 minutes, increasing at 15-minute intervals in a stepwise fashion to 60 mg/kg/hour.

ADVERSE REACTIONS
Systemic: hypotension, nausea, vomiting, wheezing, ***anaphylaxis.***
Other: flushing, chills, muscle cramps, back pain, fever.

INTERACTIONS
Live-virus vaccines: may interfere with the immune response to live-virus vaccines. Vaccination should be deferred for at least 3 months.

CONTRAINDICATIONS
• Contraindicated in patients with history of sensitivity to other human Ig preparations and in patients with selective IgA deficiency.

NURSING CONSIDERATIONS
• Monitor the patient's vital signs closely preinfusion, midinfusion,

postinfusion, and before any increase in infusion rate.
- If anaphylaxis or drop in blood pressure occurs, discontinue infusion and administer CPR and drugs such as diphenhydramine and epinephrine.
- Drug has also been used for liver transplantation and allogeneic bone marrow transplantation.
- **I.V. use:** Reconstitute as follows: Remove tab portion of vial cap and clean rubber stopper with 70% alcohol or equivalent. Add 50 ml of sterile water for injection. *To avoid foaming, do not shake vial.* After adding water, release residual vacuum in vial to hasten dissolution. Rotate vial gently to wet all undissolved powder. Allow powder to dissolve for 30 minutes before administration. Inspect vial for clarity and particles.
- If possible, administer through a separate I.V. line using a constant infusion pump. Filters are unnecessary. If unable to administer through separate line, piggyback into preexisting line of sodium chloride injection or one of the following dextrose solutions with or without sodium chloride: dextrose 2.5% in water, D_5W, $D_{10}W$, or $D_{20}W$. Do not dilute more than 1:2 with any of the above solutions.
- Begin infusion within 6 hours of reconstitution and finish within 12 hours.
- Refrigerate powder for injection at 36° to 46° F (2° to 8° C). Do not store reconstituted drug.

hepatitis B immune globulin, human

H-BIG, Hep-B-Gammagee, HyperHep

Pregnancy Risk Category: C

HOW SUPPLIED
Injection: 1-ml, 4-ml, 5-ml vials

ACTION
Mechanism: Provides passive immunity to hepatitis B.
Onset: 1 to 6 days. **Peak:** Peak levels occur 3 to 11 days after I.M. administration. **Duration:** protective for 2 months or more; elimination half-life, 17 to 25 days.

INDICATIONS & DOSAGE
Hepatitis B exposure in high-risk patients –
Adults and children: 0.06 ml/kg I.M. within 7 days after exposure. Repeat 28 days after exposure.
Neonates born to patients who test positive for hepatitis B surface antigen (HB_sAg): 0.5 ml within 12 hours of birth. Repeat dose at 3 months and 6 months.

ADVERSE REACTIONS
Systemic: ***anaphylaxis.***

INTERACTIONS
Live-virus vaccines: may interfere with response to live-virus vaccines. Defer routine immunization for 3 months.

CONTRAINDICATIONS
- Contraindicated in patients with a history of anaphylactic reactions to immune serum.

NURSING CONSIDERATIONS
- Obtain history of allergies and reaction to immunizations. Make sure epinephrine 1:1,000 is available in case of anaphylaxis.
- Inject into anterolateral aspect of thigh or deltoid muscle areas in older children and adults; inject into anterolateral aspect of thigh for neonates and children under 3 years.
- For postexposure prophylaxis (for example, needle stick, direct contact), drug is usually given with hepatitis B vaccine.

immune globulin intramuscular (IGIM, IG, gamma globulin)
Gamastan, Gammar

immune globulin intravenous (IGIV)
Gamimune N, Gammagard S/D, Gammar-IV, Sandoglobulin, Venoglobulin-I

Pregnancy Risk Category: C

HOW SUPPLIED
intramuscular
Injection: 2-ml, 10-ml vials
intravenous
Injection: 5% in 10-ml, 50-ml, 100-ml vials (Gamimune N)
Powder for injection: 50 mg protein/ml in 0.5-g, 2.5-g, 5-g, 10-g vials (Gammagard); 2.5-g vials (Gammar-IV); 500-mg and 1-g vials; 1-g, 3-g, 6-g vials (Sandoglobulin); 2.5-g, 5-g vials (Venoglobulin-I)

ACTION
Mechanism: Provides passive immunity by increasing antibody titer. The primary component is IgG.
Peak: Serum levels peak 2 to 5 days after I.M. injection. **Duration:** serum half-life, 15 to 23 days.

INDICATIONS & DOSAGE
Agammaglobulinemia or hypogammaglobulinemia –
Adults: 30 to 50 ml I.M. monthly. Alternatively, administer 100 mg/kg I.V. (Gamimune N) monthly. Infuse at 0.01 to 0.02 ml/kg/minute for 30 minutes. For Sandoglobulin, administer 200 mg/kg I.V. monthly. Infuse at 0.5 to 1 ml/minute. After 15 to 30 minutes, increase infusion rate to 1.5 to 2.5 ml/minute.
Children: 20 to 40 ml I.M. monthly.
Hepatitis A exposure –
Adults and children: 0.02 to 0.04 ml/kg I.M. as soon as possible after exposure. Up to 0.1 ml/kg may be given after prolonged or intense exposure.
Posttransfusion hepatitis B –
Adults and children: 10 ml I.M. within 1 week after transfusion and 10 ml I.M. 1 month later.
Measles exposure –
Adults and children: 0.02 ml/kg I.M. within 6 days after exposure.
Modification of measles –
Adults and children: 0.04 ml/kg I.M. within 6 days after exposure.
Measles vaccine complications –
Adults and children: 0.02 to 0.04 ml/kg I.M.
Poliomyelitis exposure –
Adults and children: 0.3 to 0.4 ml/kg I.M. within 7 days after exposure.
Chicken pox exposure –
Adults and children: 0.2 to 1.3 ml/kg I.M. as soon as exposed.
Rubella exposure in first trimester of pregnancy –
Women: 0.2 to 0.4 ml/kg I.M. as soon as exposed.
Prophylaxis in primary immunodeficiencies –
Adults and children: 100 mg/kg by I.V. infusion monthly (Gamimune only). Infusion rate is 0.01 to 0.02 ml/kg/minute for 30 minutes. Rate can then be increased to 0.04 ml/minute for remainder of infusion.
Idiopathic thrombocytopenic purpura –
Adults: 0.4 g/kg Gamimune N or Sandoglobulin I.V. for 5 consecutive days or 1,000 mg/kg Gammagard. Additional doses may be given based on response. Give up to three doses (every other day) if necessary. Or, give Venoglobulin-I 500 mg/kg daily for 2 to 7 days.

ADVERSE REACTIONS
Systemic: angioedema, headache, urticaria, malaise, fever, nephrotic syndrome, ***anaphylaxis.***
Other: pain, erythema, muscle stiffness at injection site.

INTERACTIONS
Live-virus vaccines: Don't give within 3 months after administration of immune globulin.

CONTRAINDICATIONS
• Contraindicated in patients hypersensitive to the drug.

NURSING CONSIDERATIONS
• Obtain history of allergies and reaction to immunizations. Make sure epinephrine 1:1,000 is available in case of anaphylaxis.
• Do not give for prophylaxis against hepatitis A if 6 weeks or more have elapsed since exposure or after onset of clinical illness.
• **I.V. use:** I.V. products are not interchangeable. Gamimune-N, Sandoglobulin, and Venoglobulin-I do not require an in-line filter. Gammagard does require a filter, which is supplied by the manufacturer.
• Most adverse effects are related to a rapid infusion rate.
• When giving I.M., use anterolateral aspect of thigh or deltoid muscle for adults and anterolateral aspect of thigh for neonates and children under 3 years. Do not inject more than 3 ml at one injection site.

rabies immune globulin, human

Hyperab, Imogam

Pregnancy Risk Category: C

HOW SUPPLIED
Injection: 150 IU/ml in 2-ml, 10-ml vials

ACTION
Mechanism: Provides passive immunity to rabies.
Onset: within 24 hours. **Peak:** Peak levels occur in 2 to 13 days. **Duration:** elimination half-life, about 24 days.

INDICATIONS & DOSAGE
Rabies exposure –
Adults and children: 20 IU/kg I.M. at time of first dose of rabies vaccine. Use half of dose to infiltrate wound area. Give remainder I.M.

ADVERSE REACTIONS
Systemic: slight fever, ***anaphylaxis, angioedema.***
Other: pain, redness, induration at injection site.

INTERACTIONS
Corticosteroids and immunosuppressive agents: interferes with response. Avoid during postexposure immunization period.
Live-virus vaccines (measles, mumps, rubella, or polio): interferes with response to vaccine. Delay immunization if possible.

CONTRAINDICATIONS
• Contraindicated in patients hypersensitive to the drug.
• Repeated doses contraindicated after rabies vaccine is started.

NURSING CONSIDERATIONS
• Use only with rabies vaccine and immediate local treatment of wound. Don't give rabies vaccine and rabies immune globulin in same syringe or at same site. Give regardless of interval between exposure and initiation of therapy.
• Obtain history of animal bites, allergies, and reaction to immunizations. Have epinephrine 1:1,000 available to treat anaphylaxis.
• Don't administer live-virus vaccines within 3 months of rabies immune globulin.
• Don't administer more than 5 ml I.M. at one injection site; divide I.M. doses greater than 5 ml, and administer at different sites.
• This immune serum provides passive immunity. Do not confuse this drug with rabies vaccine, which is a

suspension of attenuated or killed microorganisms used to confer active immunity. The two drugs are often given together prophylactically after exposure to known or suspected rabid animals.

- Ask patients when last tetanus immunization was received; many doctors order a booster at this time.

Rh_o(D) immune globulin, human

Gamulin Rh, HypRho-D, MICRhoGAM, Mini-Gamulin Rh, Rhesonativ, RhoGAM

Pregnancy Risk Category: C

HOW SUPPLIED

Injection: 300 mcg of Rh_o(D) immune globulin/vial (standard dose); 50 mcg of Rh_o(D) immune globulin/vial (microdose)

ACTION

Mechanism: Suppresses the active antibody response and formation of anti-Rh_o(D) in Rh_o(D)-negative, D^u-negative individuals, exposed to Rh-positive blood.

Duration: elimination half-life, about 24 days.

INDICATIONS & DOSAGE

Rh exposure –

Adults (postabortion, postmiscarriage, ectopic pregnancy, or postpartum): transfusion unit or blood bank determines fetal packed RBC volume entering patient's blood; then gives one vial I.M. if fetal packed RBC volume is less than 15 ml. More than one vial I.M. may be required if large fetomaternal hemorrhage occurs. Must be given within 72 hours after delivery or miscarriage.

Transfusion accidents –

Adults and children: consult blood bank or transfusion unit at once. Must be given within 72 hours.

Postabortion or postmiscarriage to prevent Rh antibody formation –

Adults: consult transfusion unit or blood bank. One microdose vial will suppress immune reaction to 2.5 ml Rh_o(D)-positive RBCs. Ideally should be given within 3 hours, but may be given up to 72 hours after abortion or miscarriage.

ADVERSE REACTIONS

Systemic: slight fever, ***anaphylaxis.***
Others: discomfort at injection site.

INTERACTIONS

Live-virus vaccines: may interfere with response. Delay immunization if possible.

CONTRAINDICATIONS

- Contraindicated in Rh_o(D)-positive or D^u-positive patients and those previously immunized to Rh_o(D) blood factor.

NURSING CONSIDERATIONS

- Immediately after delivery, send a sample of neonate's cord blood to laboratory for typing and cross matching. Confirm if mother is Rh_o(D)-negative and D^u-negative. Administer to mother only if infant is Rh_o(D)-positive or D^u-positive.
- Obtain history of allergies and reaction to immunization. Be sure epinephrine 1:1,000 is available in case of anaphylaxis.
- MICRhoGAM is recommended for every patient undergoing abortion or miscarriage up to 12 weeks' gestation unless she is Rh_o(D)-positive or D^u-positive or has Rh antibodies, or the father or fetus is Rh-negative.
- Refrigerate at 36° to 46° F (2° to 8° C).
- This immune serum provides passive immunity to the patient exposed to Rh_o-positive fetal blood during pregnancy. Prevents formation of maternal antibodies (active immunity),

which would endanger future Rh_o-positive pregnancies.
• Defer vaccination with live-virus vaccines for 3 months after administration of Rh_o(D) immune globulin.
• Explain to patients how drug protects future Rh_o-positive fetuses.

tetanus immune globulin, human

Homo-Tet, Hu-Tet, Hyper-Tet†

Pregnancy Risk Category: C

HOW SUPPLIED
Injection: 250 units per vial or syringe

ACTION
Mechanism: Provides passive immunity to tetanus.
Peak: Peak levels occur 2 to 3 days after I.M. injection. **Duration:** half-life, 3½ to 4½ weeks; protection lasts about 4 weeks.

INDICATIONS & DOSAGE
Tetanus exposure –
Adults and children: 250 to 500 units I.M.
Tetanus treatment –
Adults and children: single doses of 3,000 to 6,000 units I.M. have been used. Optimal dosage schedules have not been established.

ADVERSE REACTIONS
Systemic: slight fever, hypersensitivity reactions, ***anaphylaxis.***
Other: pain, stiffness, erythema at injection site.

INTERACTIONS
None significant.

CONTRAINDICATIONS
• Use tetanus immune globulin only if wound is more than 24 hours old or patient has had fewer than two tetanus toxoid injections.

NURSING CONSIDERATIONS
• Obtain history of injury, tetanus immunizations, last tetanus toxoid injection, allergies, and reaction to immunizations. Have epinephrine 1:1,000 available to treat hypersensitivity reaction.
• Thoroughly clean wound and remove all foreign matter.
• Antibodies remain at effective levels for about 4 weeks, which is several times the duration of antitoxin-induced antibodies. Protects patients for the incubation period of most tetanus cases.
• Do not confuse this drug with tetanus toxoid. Tetanus immune globulin is not a substitute for tetanus toxoid, which should be given at the same time to produce active immunization. Don't give at same site as toxoid.
• Inject into the deltoid muscle for adults and children 3 years and older and into the anterolateral aspect of the thigh in neonates and children under 3 years.

varicella-zoster immune globulin (VZIG)

Pregnancy Risk Category: C

HOW SUPPLIED
Injection: 10% to 18% solution of the globulin fraction of human plasma containing 125 units of varicella-zoster virus antibody (volume is about 1.25 ml)

ACTION
Mechanism: Provides passive immunity to varicella-zoster virus.
Duration: mean elimination half-life, 21 days.

INDICATIONS & DOSAGE
Passive immunization of susceptible immunodeficient patients after exposure to varicella (chicken pox or herpes zoster) –
Children to 10 kg: 125 units I.M.

Children 10.1 to 20 kg: 250 units I.M.
Children 20.1 to 30 kg: 375 units I.M.
Children 30.1 to 40 kg: 500 units I.M.
Adults and children over 40 kg: 625 units I.M.

ADVERSE REACTIONS

Systemic: GI distress, malaise, headache, respiratory distress, ***anaphylaxis.***
Other: discomfort at injection site, rash.

INTERACTIONS

Live-virus vaccines: may interfere with response. Defer vaccination for 3 months after administration of VZIG.

CONTRAINDICATIONS

- Contraindicated in patients with a history of severe reaction to human immune serum globulin or thrombocytopenia.

NURSING CONSIDERATIONS

- For maximum benefit, administer as soon as possible after presumed exposure. May be of benefit when given as late as 96 hours after exposure.
- Obtain accurate patient history of allergies and reaction to immunization. Make sure epinephrine 1:1,000 is available in case of anaphylaxis.
- VZIG is not recommended for nonimmunosuppressed patients.
- Although usually restricted to children under 15 years, VZIG may be administered to adolescents and adults if necessary.
- Not commercially distributed. Available only from 20 regional U.S. distribution centers. These centers will distribute to Canada and overseas. Call the Centers for Disease Control and Prevention for details Monday to Friday, 8 a.m. to 4:30 p.m. (EST), (404) 639-3670; all other times, (404) 639-2888.
- Administer only by deep I.M. injection. Never administer I.V.
- Refrigerate vial.

Biological response modifiers

aldesleukin
epoetin alfa
filgrastim
interferon alfa-2a, recombinant
interferon alfa-2b, recombinant
interferon alfa-n3
interferon beta-1b, recombinant
interferon gamma-1b
sargramostim

COMBINATION PRODUCTS
None.

aldesleukin (interleukin-2, IL-2)

Proleukin

Pregnancy Risk Category: C

HOW SUPPLIED
Powder for injection: 22 million IU/vial

ACTION
Mechanism: Highly purified immunoregulatory protein known as lymphokine synthesized using genetically engineered *Escherichia coli.* The drug produced is similar to human interleukin-2 (IL-2): it enhances lymphocyte mitogenesis, stimulates long-term growth of IL-2-dependent cell lines, enhances lymphocyte cytotoxicity, induces both lymphokine-activated and natural killer cell activity, and induces the production of interferon gamma.
Onset: tumor regression, within 4 weeks. **Duration:** up to 12 months.

INDICATIONS & DOSAGE
Metastatic renal cell carcinoma –
Adults: 600,000 IU/kg (0.037 mg/kg) I.V. q 8 hours for 5 days (total of 14 doses). After a 9-day rest, repeat the sequence for another 14 doses. Repeat courses may be administered after a rest period of at least 7 weeks from hospital discharge.

ADVERSE REACTIONS
CNS: headache, *mental status changes, dizziness, sensory dysfunction, special senses disorders, syncope, motor dysfunction,* ***coma.***
CV: *hypotension, sinus tachycardia, arrhythmias, bradycardia,* ***PVCs,*** *premature atrial contractions, myocardial ischemia,* ***MI, CHF, cardiac arrest,*** myocarditis, endocarditis, *CVA,* pericardial effusion, thrombosis, ***capillary leak syndrome (CLS).***
GI: *nausea, vomiting, diarrhea, stomatitis, anorexia, bleeding, dyspepsia, constipation.*
GU: *oliguria,* ***anuria,*** *proteinuria, hematuria, dysuria,* urine retention, urinary frequency.
Hematologic: *anemia, thrombocytopenia, leukopenia,* coagulation disorders, leukocytosis, eosinophilia.
Hepatic: *jaundice;* ascites; hepatomegaly; *elevated bilirubin, serum transaminase, alkaline phosphatase levels.*
Respiratory: ***pulmonary congestion,*** *dyspnea,* ***pulmonary edema, respiratory failure, pleural effusion, apnea, pneumothorax,*** tachypnea.
Skin: *pruritus, erythema, rash, dryness,* ***exfoliative dermatitis,*** purpura, alopecia, petechiae.
Other: *elevated BUN and serum creatinine levels; hypomagnesemia; acidosis; hypocalcemia; hypophosphatemia; hypokalemia; hyperuricemia; hypoalbuminemia;* hypoproteinemia; hyponatremia; hyperkalemia; arthralgia; myalgia; *fever; chills;* abdominal, chest, or back pain; fatigue; weakness; malaise; edema; infections of the catheter tip, urinary tract, or in-

jection site; phlebitis; ***sepsis;*** weight gain; weight loss; conjunctivitis.

INTERACTIONS

Antihypertensives: increased risk of hypotension. Monitor closely.
Cardiotoxic, hepatotoxic, myelotoxic, or nephrotoxic drugs: enhanced toxicity. Avoid concomitant use.
Corticosteroids: decreased antitumor effectiveness of aldesleukin. Avoid concomitant use.
Psychotropic agents: unpredictable interaction. Because aldesleukin can alter CNS function, use together cautiously.

CONTRAINDICATIONS

- Contraindicated in patients hypersensitive to the drug or any component of the formulation and in patients with abnormal cardiac (thallium) stress test or pulmonary function tests.
- Retreatment is contraindicated in patients who experience any of the following adverse effects: pericardial tamponade; disturbances in cardiac rhythm that were uncontrolled or unresponsive to intervention; sustained ventricular tachycardia (five beats or more); chest pain accompanied by ECG changes, indicating MI or angina pectoris; renal dysfunction requiring dialysis for 72 hours or more; coma or toxic psychosis lasting 48 hours or more; seizures that were repetitive or difficult to control; ischemia or perforation of the bowel; GI bleeding requiring surgery.
- Do not use this drug unless the patient has had definitive tests documenting normal cardiac and pulmonary function. Use with extreme caution in patients with normal test results if they have a history of cardiac or pulmonary disease and in patients with a history of seizure disorders because the drug may cause seizures.
- Use cautiously and with close clinical monitoring because severe adverse effects usually accompany therapy at the recommended dosage.
- Use cautiously in patients who require large volumes of fluid (such as patients with hypercalcemia).

NURSING CONSIDERATIONS

- Monitor hematologic tests, including CBC, differential, and platelet counts; serum electrolyte levels; and renal and liver function tests, and obtain chest X-ray before therapy. Repeat daily during therapy.
- Administer only in a hospital under the direction of a doctor experienced in the use of chemotherapeutic agents. An intensive care facility and intensive care or cardiopulmonary specialists must be readily available.
- This drug has been associated with CLS, a condition that results from the loss of vascular tone, in which plasma proteins and fluids escape into the extravascular space. Mean arterial blood pressure begins to drop within 2 to 12 hours of treatment; edema and effusions may be severe, and death can result from hypoperfusion of major organs. Other conditions that accompany CLS include arrhythmias, MI, angina, mental status changes, renal insufficiency, respiratory distress or failure, and GI bleeding or infarction.
- Treat CLS with careful monitoring of fluid status, pulse, mental status, urine output, and organ perfusion. Central venous pressure monitoring is necessary.
- Fluid management or administration of pressor agents may be essential to treat CLS.
- Therapy is associated with impaired neutrophil function, which can lead to disseminated infection. Many studies employed prophylactic antibiotic therapy with oxacillin, nafcillin, ciprofloxacin, or vancomycin; check protocol and administer antibiotics as ordered. Monitor for infection. Treat

patients with bacterial infections before therapy.
- Withhold dose and notify doctor if patient develops moderate to severe lethargy or somnolence; continued administration can result in coma.
- Patients should be neurologically stable with a negative computed tomography scan for CNS metastases. Drug may exacerbate symptoms in patients with unrecognized or undiagnosed CNS metastases.
- Renal and hepatic impairment occurs during treatment; be prepared to adjust dosage of other drugs to compensate. Modify dosage by withholding a dose or interrupting therapy rather than by reducing the dose.
- Severe anemia or thrombocytopenia may occur. Administer packed RBCs or platelets, as ordered.
- **I.V. use:** To avoid altering the pharmacologic properties of the drug, reconstitute and dilute carefully, and follow manufacturer's recommendations. Do not mix with other drugs or albumin.
- Reconstitute the vial containing 22 million IU (1.3 mg) with 1.2 ml of sterile water for injection. Do not use bacteriostatic water or 0.9% sodium chloride injection; these diluents increase aggregation of drug. Direct the stream at the sides of the vial and gently swirl to reconstitute. Do not shake. The reconstituted solution will have a concentration of 18 million IU (1.1 mg)/ml. It should be particle-free and colorless to slightly yellow.
- Add the ordered dose of reconstituted drug to 50 ml of D_5W and infuse over 15 minutes. Do not use an in-line filter. Plastic infusion bags are preferred because they provide consistent drug delivery.
- Vials are for single-dose use and contain no preservatives. Discard unused portion.
- Refrigerate powder for injection or reconstituted solutions. Return drug to room temperature before administering to patients. After reconstitution and dilution, administer within 48 hours.
- IL-2 has been investigated for several cancers, including Kaposi's sarcoma, metastatic melanoma, colorectal cancer, and non-Hodgkin's lymphoma.

epoetin alfa (erythropoietin)

Epogen, Procrit

Pregnancy Risk Category: C

HOW SUPPLIED

Injection: 2,000 units/ml, 3,000 units/ml, 4,000 units/ml, 6,000 units/ml

ACTION

Mechanism: Mimics the effects of erythropoietin, a naturally occurring hormone produced by the kidneys. Epoetin alfa is one of the factors controlling the rate of red cell production. It acts on the erythroid tissues in the bone marrow, stimulating the mitotic activity of erythroid progenitor cells and early precursor cells. It functions as a growth factor and as a differentiating factor, enhancing the rate of RBC production.
Peak: Serum levels peak immediately after I.V. infusion or within 4 to 24 hours after S.C. administration.
Duration: elimination half-life, 4 to 16 hours.

INDICATIONS & DOSAGE

Anemia due to reduced production of endogenous erythropoietin, end-stage renal disease –
Adults: dosage is individualized. Starting dose is 50 to 100 units/kg I.V. three times weekly. (Nondialysis patients with chronic renal failure or patients receiving continuous peritoneal dialysis may receive the drug by S.C. injection or I.V.) Reduce dosage when target hematocrit is reached or if the hematocrit rises more than 4 points in

any 2-week period. Increase dosage if hematocrit does not increase by 5 to 6 points after 8 weeks of therapy. Maintenance dosage is usually 25 units/kg three times weekly.

Adjunctive treatment of HIV-infected patients with anemia secondary to zidovudine therapy–

Adults: 100 units/kg I.V. or S.C. three times weekly for 8 weeks or until target hemoglobin is reached.

ADVERSE REACTIONS

CNS: headache, ***seizures.***
CV: *hypertension,* decreased plasma volume.
GI: nausea, vomiting, diarrhea.
Hematologic: iron deficiency, elevated platelet count.
Skin: rash.
Other: increased clotting of arteriovenous grafts.

INTERACTIONS

None significant.

CONTRAINDICATIONS

- Contraindicated in patients with uncontrolled hypertension.

NURSING CONSIDERATIONS

- Monitor blood count. Hematocrit may rise and cause excessive clotting.
- When used in HIV-infected patients, individualize dosage based on response. Dosage recommendations are for patients with endogenous erythropoetin levels of 500 units/L or less and cumulative zidovudine doses of 4.2 g/week or less.
- Monitor blood pressure before initiating therapy. Up to 80% of patients with chronic renal failure have hypertension. Blood pressure may rise, especially when the hematocrit is increasing in the early part of therapy. Diet restrictions or drug therapy may be required to control blood pressure. Reduce dosage in patients who exhibit a rapid rise in hematocrit (more than 4 points in any 2-week period) because of the risk of hypertension.
- Advise patients to avoid hazardous activities, such as driving or operating heavy machinery, during initiation of therapy. A relationship between excessively rapid hematocrit rise and seizures may exist.
- Patients treated with epoetin alfa may require additional heparin to prevent clotting during dialysis treatments.
- After injection (usually within 2 hours), some patients complain of pain or discomfort in their limbs (long bones) and pelvis and of coldness and sweating. Symptoms may persist up to 12 hours and then disappear.
- Patients with end-stage renal disease may experience an improved appetite and enhanced well-being as a result of increased hematocrit.
- Epoetin alfa has also been used to correct the hemostatic defect associated with uremia.
- Advise patients that blood specimens will be drawn weekly for blood counts and that dosage adjustments may be made based on the results.
- The patient's response to epoetin alfa is dependent on amount of endogenous erythropoietin in the plasma. Patients with levels of 500 units/L or more usually have transfusion-dependent anemia and will probably not respond to the drug. Those with levels below 500 units/L usually respond well.
- **I.V. use:** Give by direct injection without dilution. Solution contains no preservatives. Discard unused portion. Do not mix with other drugs.

filgrastim (granulocyte colony-stimulating factor; G-CSF)

Neupogen

Pregnancy Risk Category: C

HOW SUPPLIED
Injection: 300 mcg/ml

ACTION
Mechanism: A glycoprotein that stimulates proliferation and differentiation of hematopoietic cells. Filgrastim is specific for neutrophils.
Onset: within 4 hours. **Peak:** Serum levels peak 4 to 5 hours after S.C. injection. **Duration:** terminal elimination half-life, 2 to 7 hours.

INDICATIONS & DOSAGE
To decrease the incidence of infection in patients with nonmyeloid malignancies receiving myelosuppressive antineoplastic agents –
Adults and children: 5 mcg/kg/day I.V. or S.C. as a single dose. Doses may be increased in increments of 5 mcg/kg for each chemotherapy cycle depending on the duration and severity of the nadir of the absolute neutrophil count (ANC).

ADVERSE REACTIONS
GU: hematuria, proteinuria.
Hematologic: ***thrombocytopenia.***
Skin: alopecia, exacerbation of preexisting conditions (such as psoriasis).
Other: *skeletal pain,* fever, splenomegaly, osteoporosis.

INTERACTIONS
Chemotherapeutic agents: rapidly dividing myeloid cells are potentially sensitive to cytotoxic agents. Do not use filgrastim concomitantly with chemotherapy.

CONTRAINDICATIONS
• Contraindicated in patients hypersensitive to proteins derived from *Escherichia coli.* Although the drug is a growth factor for neutrophils only, the potential exists for stimulation of myeloid tumor growth.
• Do not give the drug within 24 hours of cytotoxic chemotherapy.

NURSING CONSIDERATIONS
• A transiently increased neutrophil count is common 1 or 2 days after initiation of therapy. Give daily for up to 2 weeks or until the ANC has returned to 10,000/mm^3 after the expected chemotherapy-induced neutrophil nadir.
• Obtain CBC and platelet count before therapy and monitor twice weekly during therapy. Patients who receive this drug may potentially receive high doses of chemotherapy, which may increase the risk of chemotherapy-induced toxicities.
• Refrigerate at 36° to 46° F (2° to 8° C). Do not freeze; avoid shaking. Store at room temperature for a maximum of 6 hours; discard after 6 hours.
• Vials are for single-dose use and contain no preservatives. Once a dose is withdrawn, do not reenter vial. Discard unused portion.
• If patients will be self-administering the drug, teach them how to administer it and how to dispose of used needles, syringes, drug containers, and unused medicine. Give them a copy of the "information for patients" included with the product and ensure that they understand the information.
• **I.V. use:** Dilute in 50 to 100 ml of D_5W and give by intermittent infusion over 15 to 60 minutes or continuous infusion over 24 hours. If the final concentration of the drug is going to be 2 to 15 mcg/ml, add albumin at a concentration of 2 mg/ml (0.2%) to minimize binding of the drug to plastic containers or tubing.

interferon alfa-2a, recombinant (rIFN-A)
Roferon-A

Pregnancy Risk Category: C

HOW SUPPLIED
Injection: 3 million IU/vial; 18 million IU/multiple-dose vial

ACTION

Mechanism: Interferon alfa-2a is a sterile protein product produced by recombinant DNA techniques. Its exact mechanism of action is unknown, but appears to involve direct antiproliferative action against tumor cells or viral cells to inhibit replication, and modulation of host immune response by enhancing the phagocytic activity of macrophages and by augmenting specific cytotoxicity of lymphocytes for target cells.
Peak: Peak levels occur 15 to 60 minutes after I.V. administration, 1 to 8 hours after I.M. administration, or 6 to 8 hours after S.C. administration.
Duration: elimination half-life, about 5 hours.

INDICATIONS & DOSAGE

Hairy-cell leukemia –
Adults: for induction, give 3 million units S.C. or I.M. daily for 16 to 24 weeks. For maintenance, 3 million units S.C. or I.M. three times a week.
AIDS-related Kaposi's sarcoma –
Adults: for induction, give 36 million units S.C. or I.M. daily for 10 to 12 weeks. For maintenance, give 36 million units S.C. or I.M. three times a week.
Chronic hepatitis B –
Adults: 9 million units S.C. three times a week. Optimum duration of treatment is not known; studies have observed treatment for up to 48 weeks.

ADVERSE REACTIONS

CNS: *dizziness,* confusion, paresthesia, numbness, lethargy, depression, nervousness, difficulty in thinking or concentrating, insomnia, sedation, apathy, anxiety, irritability, fatigue, vertigo, gait disturbances, poor coordination.
CV: hypotension, chest pain, arrhythmias, palpitations, syncope, ***CHF,*** hypertension, edema.
EENT: visual disturbances, dryness or inflammation of the oropharynx, rhinorrhea, sinusitis, conjunctivitis, earache, eye irritation, rhinitis.
GI: *anorexia, nausea, diarrhea,* vomiting, abdominal fullness, abdominal pain, flatulence, constipation, hypermotility, gastric distress, dysgeusia.
GU: transient impotence.
Hematologic: ***leukopenia,*** mild thrombocytopenia.
Hepatic: ***hepatitis.***
Respiratory: ***bronchospasm,*** coughing, dyspnea, tachypnea.
Skin: *rash,* dryness, *pruritus,* partial alopecia, urticaria, flushing.
Other: inflammation at injection site (rare), flulike syndrome (fever, fatigue, myalgia, headache, chills, arthralgia), diaphoresis, hot flashes, excessive salivation, cyanosis.

INTERACTIONS

Aminophylline, theophylline: may reduce theophylline clearance. Monitor serum levels.
CNS depressants: enhanced CNS effects. Avoid concomitant use.
Live-virus vaccine: increased risk of adverse reactions and decreased antibody response. Don't use together.

CONTRAINDICATIONS

- Contraindicated in patients hypersensitive to the drug.
- Use cautiously in patients with severe hepatic or renal function impairment, seizure disorders, compromised CNS function, cardiac disease, or myelosuppression.
- Use with blood dyscrasia-causing medications, bone marrow suppressant, or radiation therapy may increase bone marrow suppressant effects. Dosage reduction may be required.

NURSING CONSIDERATIONS

- Neurotoxicity and cardiotoxicity are more common in elderly patients, especially those with underlying CNS or cardiac impairment.

• Obtain allergy history. Drug contains phenol as a preservative and serum albumin as a stabilizer.
• Use S.C. administration route in patients whose platelet count is below 50,000/mm³.
• Different brands of interferon may not be equivalent and may require different dosage.
• At the beginning of therapy, most patients experience flulike symptoms, which tend to diminish with continued therapy. Premedicate with acetaminophen to minimize symptoms.
• Make sure patients are well hydrated, especially during initial stages of treatment.
• Administer h.s. to minimize daytime drowsiness.
• Severe adverse reactions may require dosage reduction to one-half or discontinuation of therapy until reactions subside.
• Advise patients that laboratory tests will be performed before and periodically during therapy. Tests include a CBC with differential, platelet count, blood chemistry and electrolyte studies, liver function tests, and, if the patient has a preexisting cardiac disorder or advanced stages of cancer, ECGs.
• Interferons may decrease hemoglobin, hematocrit, WBC count, platelet count, and neutrophil count; increase PT and PTT; and increase serum levels of AST, ALT, lactate dehydrogenase, alkaline phosphatase, calcium, phosphorus, and fasting glucose, which are dose-related and reversible. Recovery occurs within several days or weeks after withdrawal of interferon.
• Periodically monitor for CNS adverse reactions, such as decreased mental status and dizziness, during therapy.
• Special precautions are required for patients who develop thrombocytopenia: exercise extreme care in performing invasive procedures; inspect injection site and skin frequently for signs of bruising; limit frequency of I.M. injections; test urine, emesis fluid, stool, and secretions for occult blood.
• Instruct patients in proper oral hygiene during treatment, because the bone marrow suppressant effects of interferon may lead to microbial infection, delayed healing, and gingival bleeding. Interferon may also decrease salivary flow.
• Advise patients to check with the doctor for instructions after missing a dose.
• If patients will be self-administering drug, teach them how to prepare and administer it and how to dispose of used needles, syringes, containers, and unused medication. Give them a copy of the "information for patients" included with the product and ensure that they understand the information. Also provide information on drug stability.
• Refrigerate the drug.
• Emphasize need to follow the doctor's instructions about taking and recording temperature, and how and when to take acetaminophen.
• Concurrent use with a live-virus vaccine may potentiate replication of vaccine virus, increase adverse reactions, and decrease patient's antibody response. Warn patients not to have any immunization without the doctor's approval and to avoid contact with persons who have taken oral polio vaccine. Patients are at increased risk for infection during therapy.
• Tell patients that drug may cause temporary loss of some hair, which should return when drug is withdrawn.

interferon alfa-2b, recombinant (IFN-alpha 2)

Intron A

Pregnancy Risk Category: C

HOW SUPPLIED

Injection: 3 million IU/vial with diluent, 5 million IU/vial with diluent, 10 million IU/vial with diluent, 25 million IU/vial with diluent, 50 million IU/vial with diluent

ACTION

Mechanism: A sterile protein product produced by recombinant DNA techniques. Its exact mechanism of action is unknown, but appears to involve direct antiproliferative action against tumor cells or viral cells to inhibit replication, and modulation of host immune response by enhancing the phagocytic activity of macrophages and by augmenting specific cytotoxicity of lymphocytes for target cells.
Peak: Peak levels occur 1 to 8 hours after I.M. administration, or 6 to 8 hours after S.C. administration.
Duration: elimination half-life, about 5 hours.

INDICATIONS & DOSAGE

Hairy-cell leukemia –
Adults: 2 million units/m² I.M. or S.C. three times a week.
Condylomata acuminata (genital or venereal warts) –
Adults: 1 million units/lesion intralesionally three times a week for 3 weeks.
AIDS-related Kaposi's sarcoma –
Adults: 30 million units/m² S.C. or I.M. three times a week.
Chronic hepatitis B –
Adults: 5 million units S.C. daily for up to 4 months.

ADVERSE REACTIONS

CNS: dizziness, confusion, paresthesia, lethargy, depression, difficulty in thinking or concentrating, insomnia, sedation, anxiety, *fatigue,* hypoesthesia, amnesia, agitation, weakness.
CV: hypotension, chest pain.
EENT: visual disturbances, hearing disorders, stye, pharyngitis, nasal congestion, sinusitis, rhinitis.
GI: *anorexia, nausea,* diarrhea, vomiting, abdominal pain, dyspepsia, constipation, loose stools, eructation, dry mouth, dysgeusia, stomatitis, gingivitis.
GU: transient impotence, gynecomastia.
Hematologic: ***leukopenia,*** mild thrombocytopenia.
Respiratory: dyspnea, coughing.
Skin: rash, dryness, pruritus, partial alopecia, urticaria, moniliasis, flushing, dermatitis.
Other: *flulike symptoms (fever, fatigue, headache, chills, muscle aches), arthralgia,* asthenia, rigors, leg cramps, arthrosis, bone disorders, back pain, increased diaphoresis, decreased libido, hypertonia, migraine, thirst.

INTERACTIONS

CNS depressants: enhanced CNS effects. Avoid concomitant use.
Live-virus vaccines: risk of enhanced adverse reactions to vaccine or decreased antibody response. Postpone immunization.

CONTRAINDICATIONS

- Contraindicated in patients hypersensitive to the drug.
- Use cautiously in patients with a history of cardiovascular disease, pulmonary disease, diabetes mellitus, coagulation disorders, and severe myelosuppression.
- Use with blood dyscrasia-causing medications, bone marrow suppressants, or radiation therapy may increase bone marrow suppressant effects. Dosage reduction may be required.

NURSING CONSIDERATIONS

- Periodically monitor for adverse CNS reactions, such as decreased mental status and dizziness, during therapy.

- Neurotoxicity and cardiotoxicity are more common in elderly patients, especially those with underlying CNS or cardiac impairment.
- Advise patients to avoid contact with persons with viral illness and those who have recently taken oral polio vaccine. Patients are at increased risk for infection during therapy.
- Use S.C. administration route in patients whose platelet count is below 50,000/mm³.
- Different brands of interferon may not be equivalent and may require different dosages.
- At the beginning of treatment, most patients experience flulike symptoms, which tend to diminish with continued therapy. Premedicate with acetaminophen to minimize flulike symptoms.
- Make sure patients are well hydrated, especially during initial treatment.
- Administer h.s. to minimize daytime drowsiness.
- Severe adverse reactions may require dosage reduction to one-half or discontinuation of therapy until reactions subside.
- Advise patients that laboratory tests will be performed before and periodically during therapy. Tests include a CBC with differential, platelet count, blood chemistry and electrolyte studies, liver function tests, and, if the patient has a preexisting cardiac disorder or advanced stages of cancer, ECGs.
- When administering interferon for condylomata acuminata, use only 10-million-IU vial because dilution of other strengths required for intralesional use results in a hypertonic solution. Do not reconstitute 10-million-IU vial with more than 1 ml of diluent. Use tuberculin or similar syringe and 25G to 30G needle. Do not inject too deeply beneath lesion or too superficially. As many as five lesions can be treated at one time. To ease discomfort, administer in evening with acetaminophen.
- Maximum response usually occurs 4 to 8 weeks after initiation of therapy. If results are not satisfactory after 12 to 16 weeks, a second course may be instituted. Patients with 6 to 10 condylomata may receive a second course of treatment; patients with more than 10 condylomata may receive additional courses.
- Interferons may decrease hemoglobin, hematocrit, WBC count, platelet count, and neutrophil count; increase PT and PTT; and increase serum levels of AST, ALT, lactate dehydrogenase, alkaline phosphatase, calcium, phosphorus, and fasting glucose, which are dose-related and reversible. Recovery occurs within several days or weeks after interferon withdrawal.
- Special precautions are required for patients who develop thrombocytopenia: exercise extreme care in performing invasive procedures; inspect injection site and skin frequently for signs of bruising; limit frequency of I.M. injections; test urine, emesis fluid, stool, and secretions for occult blood.
- Instruct patients in proper oral hygiene during treatment because the bone marrow suppressant effects of interferon may lead to microbial infection, delayed healing, and gingival bleeding. Interferon may also decrease salivary flow.
- Advise patients to check with the doctor for instructions after missing a dose.
- If patients will be self-administering drug, teach them how to prepare the injection and how to use a disposable syringe. Give information on drug stability.
- Refrigerate the drug.
- Emphasize need to follow the doctor's instructions about taking and recording temperature, and how and when to take acetaminophen.
- Tell patients drug may cause tempo-

rary loss of some hair, which should return when drug is withdrawn.

interferon alfa-n3

Alferon N

Pregnancy Risk Category: C

HOW SUPPLIED

Injection: 5 million units/ml in 1-ml vials

ACTION

Mechanism: A naturally occurring antiviral agent derived from human leukocytes. It attaches to membrane receptors and causes cellular changes, including increased protein synthesis.
Peak: Peak levels occur 6 to 8 hours after S.C. administration. **Duration:** elimination half-life, about 5 hours.

INDICATIONS & DOSAGE

Condylomata acuminata (genital or venereal warts) –
Adults: 0.05 ml/wart by intralesional injection. Treatment usually continues twice weekly for 8 weeks. Dosage should not exceed 0.5 ml (2.5 million units) per session.

ADVERSE REACTIONS

CNS: dizziness, light-headedness.
GI: dyspepsia, heartburn, vomiting, nausea.
Other: *acute hypersensitivity reactions with mild to moderate flulike syndrome (myalgia, fever, headache), arthralgia, back pain, malaise.*

INTERACTIONS

None reported.

CONTRAINDICATIONS

- Contraindicated in patients hypersensitive to interferon alfa and in those with a history of anaphylactic reactions to murine immunoglobulin, egg protein, or neomycin.
- Use cautiously in patients with debilitating illnesses (uncontrolled CHF, unstable angina, severe pulmonary disease, coagulation disorders, seizure disorders, severe myelosuppression, or diabetes mellitus with ketoacidosis) because of the association of interferon with a flulike syndrome.

NURSING CONSIDERATIONS

- Although anaphylaxis hasn't been reported, be prepared to treat acute hypersensitivity reactions. Teach patients how to recognize symptoms of hypersensitivity: hives or urticaria, tightness of the chest, wheezing, shortness of breath. Tell patients to report such symptoms immediately.
- Flulike symptoms may be relieved with acetaminophen.
- Explain to patients that warts will continue to disappear after completion of 8 weeks of therapy and discontinuation of drug.
- Inject each lesion at the base of the wart using a 30G needle.

interferon beta-1b, recombinant

Betaseron

Pregnancy Risk Category: C

HOW SUPPLIED

Powder for injection: 9.6 million IU (0.25 mg)

ACTION

Mechanism: A naturally occurring antiviral and immunoregulatory agent derived from human fibroblasts. It attaches to membrane receptors and causes cellular changes, including increased protein synthesis.
Peak: Serum levels are undetectable after the recommended dose; after higher doses, serum levels peak within 1 to 8 hours after S.C. administration. **Duration:** elimination half-life, 8 minutes to 4 hours.

INDICATIONS & DOSAGE
To reduce the frequency of exacerbations in patients with relapsing-remitting multiple sclerosis –
Adults: 8 million IU (0.25 mg) S.C. every other day.

ADVERSE REACTIONS
CNS: depression, anxiety, emotional lability, depersonalization, ***suicidal tendencies,*** confusion, somnolence, headache, dizziness.
EENT: laryngitis.
GI: diarrhea, constipation.
GU: *menstrual disorders (bleeding or spotting, early or delayed menses, decreased days of menstrual flow, menorrhagia).*
Hematologic: *decreased WBC and absolute neutrophil counts.*
Respiratory: dyspnea.
Other: *flulike symptoms (fever, chills, malaise, myalgia, diaphoresis),* elevated ALT levels, elevated bilirubin levels, breast pain, *pelvic pain; inflammation, pain, and necrosis at injection site, lymphadenopathy.*

INTERACTIONS
None significant.

CONTRAINDICATIONS
- Contraindicated in patients hypersensitive to interferon beta or human albumin.
- Use cautiously in women of childbearing age. Inconclusive evidence exists about the drug's teratogenic effects, but it may be an abortifacient.

NURSING CONSIDERATIONS
- Teach the patient how to self-administer S.C. injections, including solution preparation, use of aseptic technique, rotation of injection sites, and equipment disposal. Periodically reevaluate the patient's technique.
- Rotate injection sites to minimize local reactions.
- Warn patients of childbearing age about dangers to the fetus. If a patient becomes pregnant during therapy, tell her to notify the doctor and stop taking the drug.
- Taking interferon beta at bedtime may minimize the mild flulike symptoms that commonly occur.
- To reconstitute, inject 1.2 ml of the supplied diluent (0.54% sodium chloride injection) into the vial and gently swirl to dissolve drug. Do not shake. Reconstituted solution will contain 8 million IU (0.25 mg)/ml. Discard vials that contain particulate material or discolored solution.
- Inject immediately after preparation.
- Refrigerate the drug or reconstituted product (up to 3 hours) at 36° to 46° F (2° to 8° C). Do not freeze.

interferon gamma-1b
Actimmune

Pregnancy Risk Category: C

HOW SUPPLIED
Injection: 100 mcg (3 million units)/vial

ACTION
Mechanism: Acts as an interleukin-type lymphokine. It has potent phagocyte-activating properties and enhances the oxidative metabolism of tissue macrophages.
Peak: Peak levels occur within 4 hours after I.M. dose, 7 hours after S.C. use. **Duration:** half-life, about 3 hours after I.M. dose, about 6 hours after S.C.

INDICATIONS & DOSAGE
Chronic granulomatous disease –
Adults with a body surface area > 0.5 m²: 50 mcg/m² (1.5 million units/m²) I.M. three times weekly, preferably h.s. The preferred injection site is the deltoid or anterior thigh.
Adults with a body surface area

≤ 0.5 m²: 1.5 mcg/kg/dose three times weekly.

ADVERSE REACTIONS

CNS: fatigue, decreased mental status, gait disturbance.
GI: nausea, vomiting, diarrhea.
Hematologic: *myelosuppression* (at high doses).
Metabolic: elevated liver enzyme levels (at high doses).
Skin: rash.
Other: erythema or tenderness at the injection site, *flulike syndrome* (headache, fever, chills, myalgia, arthralgia).

INTERACTIONS

Myelosuppressive agents: possible additive myelosuppression. Monitor closely.
Zidovudine: increased plasma levels of zidovudine. Dosage adjustments are necessary when used at same time.

CONTRAINDICATIONS

- Contraindicated in patients hypersensitive to the drug or to genetically engineered products derived from *Escherichia coli.*
- Use cautiously in patients with cardiac disease, including arrhythmias, ischemia, or CHF. The flulike syndrome commonly seen at high doses of the drug can exacerbate these conditions.
- Use cautiously in patients with compromised CNS function or seizure disorders. CNS adverse reactions that may occur at high doses of the drug can exacerbate these conditions.
- Use myelosuppressive agents together with caution.

NURSING CONSIDERATIONS

- If patients will be self-administering drug, teach them how to administer it and how to dispose of used needles, syringes, containers, and unused medication. Give them a copy of the "information for patients" included with the product and ensure that they understand the information.
- At the beginning of therapy, most patients experience flulike symptoms, which tend to diminish with continued therapy. Premedicate with acetaminophen to minimize symptoms.
- Refrigerate drug immediately. Vials must be stored at 36° to 46° F (2° to 8° C); do not freeze. Do not shake the vial; avoid excessive agitation. Discard vials that have been left at room temperature for more than 12 hours.
- Each vial is for single-dose use only and does not contain a preservative. Discard unused portion.

---

sargramostim (granulocyte-macrophage colony-stimulating factor, GM-CSF)

Leukine

Pregnancy Risk Category: C

HOW SUPPLIED

Powder for injection: 250 mcg, 500 mcg

ACTION

Mechanism: A glycoprotein containing 127 amino acids manufactured by recombinant DNA technology in a yeast expression system. It differs from the natural human granulocyte-macrophage colony stimulating factor by substitution of leucine for arginine at position 23. The carbohydrate moiety may also be different. Sargramostim induces cellular responses by binding to specific receptors on cell surfaces of target cells.
Onset: 1 to 2 days. **Duration:** 3 to 7 days.

INDICATIONS & DOSAGE

Acceleration of hematopoietic reconstitution after autologous bone marrow transplantation in patients with non-Hodgkin's lymphoma or acute lymphoblastic leukemia or during autologous bone marrow transplantation in patients with Hodgkin's disease – **Adults:** 250 mcg/m² daily for 21 consecutive days given as a 2-hour I.V. infusion beginning 2 to 4 hours after bone marrow transplantation.

ADVERSE REACTIONS
CNS: malaise, CNS disorder.
CV: *blood dyscrasias,* hemorrhage.
GI: nausea, vomiting, diarrhea, anorexia, hemorrhage, GI disorder, stomatitis.
GU: urinary tract disorder, abnormal kidney function.
Hepatic: liver damage.
Respiratory: dyspnea, lung disorder.
Skin: alopecia, rash.
Other: fever, mucous membrane disorder, asthenia, edema, peripheral edema, ***sepsis.***

INTERACTIONS
Corticosteroids, lithium: may potentiate myeloproliferative effects of sargramostim. Use cautiously.

CONTRAINDICATIONS
• Contraindicated in patients with excessive leukemic myeloid blasts in bone marrow or peripheral blood and in those with hypersensitivity to the drug or any of its components or to yeast-derived products.
• Use cautiously in patients with preexisting cardiac disease, hypoxia, preexisting fluid retention, pulmonary infiltrates, CHF, or impaired renal or hepatic function because these conditions may be exacerbated.

NURSING CONSIDERATIONS
• Do not administer within 24 hours of last dose of chemotherapy or within 12 hours of last dose of radiotherapy because rapidly dividing progenitor cells may be sensitive to these cytotoxic therapies and drug would be ineffective.
• Reduce dose by half or temporarily discontinue if severe adverse reactions occur. Therapy may be resumed when reactions abate. Transient rashes and local reactions at the injection site may occur; no serious allergic or anaphylactic reactions have been reported.
• The effect of sargramostim may be limited in patients who have received extensive radiotherapy to hematopoietic sites for treatment of primary disease in the abdomen or chest or who have been exposed to multiple agents (alkylating, anthracycline antibiotics, antimetabolites) before autologous bone marrow transplantation.
• Stimulation of marrow precursors may result in rapid rise of WBC count; monitor CBC with differential, including examination for presence of blast cells biweekly, as prescribed. If blast cells appear or increase to 10% or more of the WBC count or if progression of the underlying disease occurs, discontinue therapy. If the absolute neutrophil count is above 20,000/mm³ or if platelet count is above 50,000/mm³, temporarily discontinue therapy or reduce dose by half.
• Blood counts return to normal or baseline levels within 3 to 7 days after stopping treatment.
• Sargramostim is effective in accelerating myeloid recovery in patients receiving bone marrow purged from monoclonal antibodies.
• The drug can act as a growth factor for any tumor type, particularly myeloid malignancies.
• **I.V. use:** Reconstitute with 1 ml of sterile water for injection. Direct stream of sterile water against side of vial and *gently swirl* contents to minimize foaming. Avoid excessive or vigorous agitation or shaking. Dilute in 0.9% sodium chloride solution. If final concentration is below 10 mcg/ml, add human albumin at a final concentration of 0.1% to the sodium chloride solution *before* adding sargramostim to prevent adsorption to components

of the delivery system. For a final concentration of 0.1% human albumin, add 1 mg human albumin/1 ml sodium chloride. Administer as soon as possible after mixing and no later than 6 hours after reconstituting.

- Vials are for single-dose use and contain no preservatives. Do not reenter the vial. Discard any unused portion.
- Refrigerate the sterile powder, reconstituted solution, and diluted solution for injection. Don't freeze or shake. Don't use after expiration date.
- Don't add other medications to infusion solution because no data exist regarding solution compatibility and stability.
- Sargramostim has been used to increase WBC counts in patients with myelodysplastic syndromes and in AIDS patients on zidovudine; to decrease nadir of leukopenia secondary to myelosuppressive chemotherapy; to decrease myelosuppression in preleukemic patients; to correct neutropenia in aplastic anemia; and to decrease transplant-associated organ system damage, particularly of liver and kidneys.

79
Ophthalmic anti-infectives

bacitracin
boric acid
chloramphenicol
ciprofloxacin hydrochloride
erythromycin
gentamicin
gentamicin sulfate
idoxuridine
natamycin
norfloxacin
polymyxin B sulfate
silver nitrate 1%
sulfacetamide sodium 10%
sulfacetamide sodium 15%
sulfacetamide sodium 30%
tetracycline hydrochloride
tobramycin
trifluridine
vidarabine

COMBINATION PRODUCTS

BLEPHAMIDE S.O.P. STERILE OPHTHALMIC OINTMENT: sulfacetamide sodium 10% and prednisolone acetate 0.2%.

CETAPRED OINTMENT: sulfacetamide sodium 10% and prednisolone acetate 0.25%.

CHLOROMYCETIN-HYDROCORTISONE OPHTHALMIC: chloramphenicol 0.25% and hydrocortisone acetate 0.5% (as the prepared solution).

CORTISPORIN OPHTHALMIC OINTMENT: polymyxin B sulfate 10,000 units, bacitracin zinc 400 units, neomycin sulfate 0.35%, and hydrocortisone 1%.

CORTISPORIN OPHTHALMIC SUSPENSION: polymyxin B sulfate 10,000 units, neomycin sulfate 0.35%, and hydrocortisone 1%.

ISOPTO CETAPRED: sulfacetamide sodium 10% and prednisolone acetate 0.25%.

MAXITROL OINTMENT/OPHTHALMIC SUSPENSION: dexamethasone 0.1%, neomycin sulfate 0.35%, and polymyxin B sulfate 10,000 units.

METIMYD OPHTHALMIC OINTMENT/SUSPENSION: sulfacetamide sodium 10% and prednisolone acetate 0.5%.

MYCITRACIN OPHTHALMIC OINTMENT: polymyxin B sulfate 5,000 units, neomycin sulfate 3.5 mg, and bacitracin 500 units.

NEODECADRON OPHTHALMIC OINTMENT: dexamethasone phosphate 0.1% and neomycin sulfate 0.35%.

NEOSPORIN OPHTHALMIC: polymyxin B sulfate 10,000 units, neomycin sulfate 1.75 mg, and gramicidin 0.025 mg.

NEOSPORIN OPHTHALMIC OINTMENT: polymyxin B sulfate 10,000 units, neomycin sulfate 3.5 mg, and bacitracin zinc 400 units/g.

NEOTAL: polymyxin B sulfate 5,000 units, neomycin sulfate 5 mg, and bacitracin zinc 400 units.

OPHTHA P/S OPHTHALMIC SUSPENSION: prednisolone acetate 0.5% and sulfacetamide sodium 10%.

OPHTHOCORT: chloramphenicol 1.0%, polymyxin B sulfate 10,000 units, and hydrocortisone acetate 0.5%.

OPTIMYD: prednisolone phosphate 0.5% and sulfacetamide sodium 10%.

POLYSPORIN OPHTHALMIC OINTMENT: polymyxin B sulfate 10,000 units and bacitracin zinc 500 units.

POLYTRIM OPHTHALMIC: trimethoprim sulfate 1 mg and polymyxin B sulfate 10,000 units/ml.

PRED G: prednisolone acetate 0.6%, gentamicin sulfate equivalent to gentamicin base 0.3%, chlorobutanol 0.5%, petrolatum, white petrolatum, mineral oil, and lanolin alcohol.

STATROL: neomycin sulfate 3.5 mg and polymyxin B sulfate 10,000 units.
SULFAPRED: sulfacetamide sodium 10%, prednisolone acetate 0.25%, and phenylephrine hydrochloride 0.125%.
TOBRADEX: dexamethasone 0.1%, tobramycin 0.3%, chlorobutanol 0.5%, mineral oil, and white petrolatum.
VASOCIDIN OPHTHALMIC OINTMENT: sulfacetamide sodium 10%, prednisolone acetate 0.5%, and phenylephrine hydrochloride 0.125%.
VASOCIDIN OPHTHALMIC SOLUTION: sulfacetamide sodium 10% and prednisolone phosphate 0.25%.
VASOSULF: sulfacetamide sodium 15% and phenylephrine hydrochloride 0.125%.

bacitracin

Pregnancy Risk Category: C

HOW SUPPLIED

Ophthalmic ointment: 500 units/g

ACTION

Mechanism: Inhibits protein synthesis. Bactericidal or bacteriostatic, depending on concentration and infection.
Peak: Systemic absorption is negligible.

INDICATIONS & DOSAGE

Ocular infections –
Adults and children: apply small amount of ointment into conjunctival sac several times daily or p.r.n. until favorable response is observed.

ADVERSE REACTIONS

EENT: slowed corneal wound healing, temporary visual haze.
Other: overgrowth of nonsusceptible organisms.

INTERACTIONS

Heavy metals (for example, silver nitrate): inactivation of bacitracin. Don't use together.

CONTRAINDICATIONS

- Contraindicated in patients hypersensitive to the drug.
- Use cautiously in patients with hereditary predisposition to antibiotic hypersensitivity.

NURSING CONSIDERATIONS

- Advise patients to watch for signs of sensitivity, such as itching lids, swelling, or constant burning. Tell patients who develop such signs to stop drug and notify doctor immediately.
- Teach patients how to apply; tell them only a small amount of ointment is needed and that it may cause blurred vision. Advise patients to wash hands before and after administering and not to touch tip of tube or dropper to eye or surrounding tissue. Tell patients to clean eye area of excessive exudate before application. Stress importance of compliance with recommended therapy.
- Ophthalmic solution not commercially available but may be prepared by pharmacy. Refrigerate up to 3 weeks in tightly closed, light-resistant container. Ophthalmic ointment may be stored at room temperature.
- Tell patients not to share eye medications, washcloths, or towels with family members. If anyone develops the same symptoms, the doctor should be notified.

boric acid

Blinx◇, Collyrium◇, Neo-Flo◇

Pregnancy Risk Category: C

HOW SUPPLIED

Ophthalmic ointment: 5%◇, 10%◇
Ophthalmic solution: 30 ml◇, 120 ml◇, 180 ml◇

*Liquid form contains alcohol.
**May contain tartrazine.

Common reactions are in italics; ***life-threatening,*** in bold italics.

ACTION

Mechanism: Unknown. However, drug has fungistatic and bacteriostatic properties.

Peak: Systemic absorption is negligible.

INDICATIONS & DOSAGE

For irrigation after tonometry, gonioscopy, foreign body removal, or use of fluorescein; to soothe and clean the eye –

Adults: apply eyewash p.r.n. Or apply 1 to 2 eyedrops into affected eye up to q.i.d. Or apply 5% or 10% ointment, p.r.n.

ADVERSE REACTIONS

Systemic: toxic if absorbed from abraded skin areas, granulating wounds, or ingestion.

INTERACTIONS

Idoxuridine, polyvinyl alcohol (Liquifilm): may form insoluble complex. Check with pharmacy on contents of other eye drugs and contact lens wetting solutions.

CONTRAINDICATIONS

- Contraindicated in patients with eye lacerations.

NURSING CONSIDERATIONS

- Don't apply to abraded cornea.
- Teach patients proper way to use eyewash: Fill eyecup half full. Apply the cup tightly to the affected eye and tilt head backward. Open the eye wide and rotate eyeball to thoroughly wash the eye. Always wash hands before and after instilling solution or ointment.
- Tell patients not to use with soft contact lenses.
- Tell patients not to share eye solution with family members.
- Avoid contaminating solution container. Don't use cloudy or discolored solutions.

chloramphenicol

AK-Chlor, Chloromycetin Ophthalmic, Chloroptic, Chloroptic S.O.P., Chlorsig‡, Fenicol†, Isopto Fenicol†, Ophthoclor Ophthalmic, Pentamycetin†

Pregnancy Risk Category: C

HOW SUPPLIED

Ophthalmic ointment: 1%
Ophthalmic solution: 0.5%
Powder for ophthalmic solution: 25 mg

ACTION

Mechanism: Inhibits protein synthesis. Bacteriostatic or bactericidal, depending on concentration.

Peak: Systemic absorption occurs, but has not been characterized; higher levels occur with ophthalmic ointment.

INDICATIONS & DOSAGE

Surface bacterial infection involving conjunctiva or cornea –

Adults and children: instill 1 drop of solution in eye q 1 to 4 hours around the clock until condition improves, or instill q.i.d., depending on severity of infection. Apply small amount of ointment to lower conjunctival sac h.s. as supplement to drops. May use ointment alone by applying a small amount of ointment to lower conjunctival sac q 3 to 6 hours or more frequently, if necessary. Continue until condition improves.

ADVERSE REACTIONS

EENT: optic atrophy in children, stinging or burning of eye after instillation, blurred vision (with ointment).

Hematologic: ***bone marrow hypoplasia with prolonged use, aplastic anemia.***

Other: overgrowth of nonsusceptible organisms; hypersensitivity reactions, including itching and burning eye, dermatitis, angioedema.

INTERACTIONS
None significant.

CONTRAINDICATIONS
- Contraindicated in minor infections. Do not use chloramphenicol when less potentially dangerous drugs are available.

NURSING CONSIDERATIONS
- Not for long-term use. Notify the doctor if no improvement occurs in 3 days.
- If patients have more than a superficial infection, use systemic therapy as well.
- Tell patients to watch for signs of sensitivity, such as itching lids, swelling, or constant burning. Patients who develop such signs should stop drug and notify the doctor immediately.
- Teach patients how to instill drops or apply ointment. Advise them to wash hands before and after administering ointment or solution, and warn them not to touch tip of applicator to eye or surrounding tissue. Tell them to clean eye area of excessive exudate before application and to apply light finger pressure on lacrimal sac for 1 minute after drops are instilled. Stress importance of compliance with recommended therapy.
- If chloramphenicol drops are to be given every hour, then tapered, follow order closely to ensure adequate anterior chamber levels.
- Store in tightly closed, light-resistant container.
- Tell patients not to share eye medications, washcloths, or towels with family members. If anyone develops the same symptoms, the doctor should be notified.
- Reconstitute powder for ophthalmic solution with supplied diluent. Use 5 ml of diluent to make a 0.5% solution, 10 ml of diluent to make a 0.25% solution, or 15 ml to make a 0.16% solution.

ciprofloxacin hydrochloride
Ciloxan

Pregnancy Risk Category: C

HOW SUPPLIED
Ophthalmic solution: 0.3% (base) in 2.5- and 5-ml containers

ACTION
Mechanism: Inhibits bacterial DNA gyrase, an enzyme necessary for bacterial replication. Bacteriostatic or bactericidal, depending on concentration.
Peak: Systemic absorption is negligible.

INDICATIONS & DOSAGE
Corneal ulcers caused by Pseudomonas aeruginosa, Staphylococcus aureus, S. epidermidis, Streptococcus pneumoniae, *and possibly* Serratia marcescens *and* Streptococcus viridans –
Adults and children over 12 years: 2 drops in the affected eye q 15 minutes for the first 6 hours; then 2 drops q 30 minutes for the remainder of the first day. On day 2, administer 2 drops hourly. On days 3 to 14, administer 2 drops q 4 hours.
Bacterial conjunctivitis caused by Staphylococcus aureus *and* S. epidermidis *and possibly* Streptococcus pneumoniae –
Adults and children over 12 years: 1 or 2 drops into the conjunctival sac of the affected eye q 2 hours while awake, for the first 2 days. Then 1 or 2 drops q 4 hours while awake, for the next 5 days.

ADVERSE REACTIONS
EENT: *local burning or discomfort, white crystalline precipitate* (in the superficial portion of the corneal defect in patients with corneal ulcers), *margin crusting, crystals or scales, foreign body sensation, itching, conjunctival hyperemia.*

Other: bad taste.

INTERACTIONS
None significant.

CONTRAINDICATIONS
• Contraindicated in patients with a history of hypersensitive to ciprofloxacin or other quinolone antibiotics. Don't inject this drug into the eye.
• Safety and efficacy in children under 12 years haven't been established. Because systemic ciprofloxacin has been shown to cause arthropathy in young animals, don't use this drug in children.
• It's unknown if drug is excreted in breast milk after application to the eye; however, systemically administered ciprofloxacin has been detected in human milk. Use caution.

NURSING CONSIDERATIONS
• Serious hypersensitivity reactions, including anaphylaxis, have occurred in patients receiving systemic quinolone therapy. Discontinue drug at the first sign of hypersensitivity reactions, such as skin rash.
• Prolonged use may result in overgrowth of nonsusceptible organisms, including fungi. Institute appropriate therapy if superinfection occurs.
• If corneal epithelium is still compromised after 14 days of treatment, continue therapy.
• Teach patients how to instill drops. Advise them to wash hands before and after administering solution and not to touch tip of dropper to eye or surrounding tissues. Tell patients to clean eye area of excessive exudate before instilling and to apply light finger pressure on lacrimal sac for 1 minute after drops are instilled. Stress importance of compliance with recommended therapy.
• Tell patients not to share eye medications, washcloths, or towels with family members. If anyone develops the same symptoms, the doctor should be notified.

erythromycin
Ilotycin Ophthalmic
Pregnancy Risk Category: C

HOW SUPPLIED
Ophthalmic ointment: 0.5%

ACTION
Mechanism: Inhibits protein synthesis. Bacteriostatic, but may be bactericidal in high concentrations or against highly susceptible organisms.
Peak: Systemic absorption is negligible.

INDICATIONS & DOSAGE
Acute and chronic conjunctivitis, trachoma, other eye infections –
Adults and children: apply 0.5% ointment 1 or more times daily, depending on severity of infection.
Prophylaxis of ophthalmia neonatorum –
Neonates: apply a ribbon of ointment approximately 0.5 to 2 cm long in the lower conjunctival sac of each eye shortly after birth.

ADVERSE REACTIONS
Eye: slowed corneal wound healing, blurred vision.
Other: overgrowth of nonsusceptible organisms with long-term use; hypersensitivity reactions, including itching and burning eyes, urticaria, dermatitis, ***angioedema***.

INTERACTIONS
None significant.

CONTRAINDICATIONS
• Contraindicated in patients hypersensitive to the drug.
• Has a limited antibacterial spectrum. Use only when sensitivity studies show it is effective against infect-

ing organisms. Don't use in infections of unknown etiology.

NURSING CONSIDERATIONS

- For prophylaxis of ophthalmia neonatorum, apply ointment no later than 1 hour after birth. Use in neonates born either by vaginal delivery or by cesarean section. Gently massage the eyelids for 1 minute to spread the ointment.
- Advise patients to watch for signs of sensitivity, such as itching lids, swelling, or constant burning. Tell patients who develop such signs to stop drug and notify the doctor immediately.
- Teach patients how to apply. Advise them to wash hands before and after administering ointment, and warn them not to touch tip of applicator to eye or surrounding tissue. Tell patients to clean eye area of excessive exudate before application and to apply light finger pressure on lacrimal sac for 1 minute after administering. Stress importance of compliance with recommended therapy.
- Warn patients that ointment may cause blurred vision.
- Store at room temperature in tightly closed, light-resistant container.
- Tell patients not to share eye medications, washcloths, or towels with family members. If anyone develops the same symptoms, the doctor should be notified.

gentamicin
Gentacidin

gentamicin sulfate
Garamycin Ophthalmic, Genoptic, Gentacidin, Gentak, Ocu-Gent

Pregnancy Risk Category: C

HOW SUPPLIED

gentamicin
Ophthalmic ointment: 0.3%
gentamicin sulfate
Ophthalmic ointment: 0.3% (base)
Ophthalmic solution: 0.3% (base)

ACTION

Mechanism: Inhibits protein synthesis.
Peak: Only small amounts of the drug are absorbed systemically.

INDICATIONS & DOSAGE

External ocular infections (conjunctivitis, keratoconjunctivitis, corneal ulcers, blepharitis, blepharoconjunctivitis, meibomianitis, and dacryocystitis) caused by susceptible organisms, especially Pseudomonas aeruginosa, Proteus, Klebsiella pneumoniae, Escherichia coli, *and other gram-negative organisms –*
Adults and children: instill 1 to 2 drops in eye q 4 hours. In severe infections, may use up to 2 drops q 1 hour. Apply ointment to lower conjunctival sac b.i.d. or t.i.d.

ADVERSE REACTIONS

EENT: burning, stinging, or blurred vision (with ointment), transient irritation (from solution).
Other: hypersensitivity reactions; overgrowth of nonsusceptible organisms with long-term use.

Systemic absorption from excessive use may cause systemic toxicities.

INTERACTIONS

None significant.

CONTRAINDICATIONS

- Contraindicated in patients hypersensitive to aminoglycosides.
- Use cautiously in patients with impaired renal function.
- Solution is not for injection in conjunctiva or anterior chamber of the eye.

NURSING CONSIDERATIONS

- Have culture taken before giving drug. Therapy may begin before culture results are known.
- If ophthalmic gentamicin is admin-

istered concomitantly with systemic gentamicin, carefully monitor serum gentamicin levels.

- Stress importance of following recommended therapy. *Pseudomonas* infections can cause complete vision loss within 24 hours if infection is not controlled.
- Tell patients to watch for signs of sensitivity, such as itching lids, swelling, or constant burning. Tell patients who develop such signs to stop drug and notify the doctor immediately.
- Teach patients how to instill drops or apply ointment. Advise them to wash hands before and after administering ointment or solution and not to touch tip of dropper to eye or surrounding tissues. Tell patients to clean eye area of excessive exudate before instilling and to apply light finger pressure on lacrimal sac for 1 minute after drops are instilled.
- Store away from heat.
- Tell patients not to share eye medications, washcloths, or towels with family members. If anyone develops the same symptoms, the doctor should be notified.

idoxuridine (IDU)

Herplex, Stoxil

Pregnancy Risk Category: C

HOW SUPPLIED

Ophthalmic ointment: 0.5%
Ophthalmic solution: 0.1%

ACTION

Mechanism: Interferes with DNA synthesis.
Onset: 5 to 8 days. **Peak:** Systemic absorption is unlikely; idoxuridine does not penetrate the cornea sufficiently to treat deep stromal infections or iritis.

INDICATIONS & DOSAGE

Herpes simplex keratitis –
Adults and children: instill 1 drop of solution into conjunctival sac q 1 hour during day and q 2 hours at night, or apply ointment to conjunctival sac q 4 hours or 5 times daily, with last dose h.s. A response should occur in 7 days; if not, discontinue and begin alternative therapy. Therapy should not be continued longer than 21 days.

ADVERSE REACTIONS

EENT: temporary visual haze; blurred vision (with ointment); irritation, pain, burning, or inflammation of eye; mild edema of eyelid or cornea; photophobia; small punctate defects in corneal epithelium; corneal ulceration; slowed corneal wound healing (with ointment).
Other: hypersensitivity reactions.

INTERACTIONS

Boric acid: precipitate formation; increased risk of ocular toxicity. Avoid concomitant use.

CONTRAINDICATIONS

- Contraindicated in patients with deep corneal ulceration.

NURSING CONSIDERATIONS

- Not for long-term use.
- Do not mix idoxuridine with other topical eye medications.
- Don't use old solution; causes ocular burning and has no antiviral activity.
- Advise patients to watch for signs of sensitivity, such as itching lids, swelling, or constant burning. Tell patients who develop such signs to stop drug and notify the doctor immediately.
- Teach patients how to instill drops or apply ointment. Advise them to wash hands before and after administering, and warn them not to touch dropper or tip to eye or surrounding tissue. Tell them to clean eye area of excessive exudate before application and to apply light finger pressure on lacrimal sac for 1 minute after drops are instilled. Stress importance of compliance with recommended therapy.

• Refrigerate idoxuridine 0.1% solution in a tightly closed, light-resistant container.
• Tell patients not to share eye medications, washcloths, or towels with family members. If anyone develops the same symptoms, the doctor should be notified.
• Tell patients to minimize photophobia by wearing sunglasses and avoiding prolonged exposure to sunlight.

natamycin

Natacyn

Pregnancy Risk Category: C

HOW SUPPLIED

Ophthalmic suspension: 5%

ACTION

Mechanism: increases fungal cell-membrane permeability.
Onset: 2 days. **Peak:** 2 to 4 weeks.

INDICATIONS & DOSAGE

Fungal keratitis –
Adults: initially, 1 drop instilled in conjunctival sac q 1 to 2 hours. After 3 to 4 days, reduce dosage to 1 drop six to eight times daily.
Blepharitis or fungal conjunctivitis –
Adults: instill 1 drop q 4 to 6 hours.

ADVERSE REACTIONS

EENT: ocular edema, hyperemia.

INTERACTIONS

None significant.

CONTRAINDICATIONS

• Contraindicated in patients hypersensitive to the drug.

NURSING CONSIDERATIONS

• Only antifungal available as ophthalmic preparation. Treatment of choice for fungal keratitis. May also be used to treat fungal blepharitis and conjunctivitis.
• Continue therapy for 14 to 21 days, or until active disease subsides. Reduce dosage gradually at 4- to 7-day intervals to ensure that organism has been eliminated. If infection does not improve within 7 to 10 days of therapy, clinical and laboratory reevaluation is recommended.
• Teach patients how to instill drops. Advise them to wash hands before and after administering solution and not to touch tip of dropper to eye or surrounding tissues. Tell them to clean eye area of excessive exudate before instilling and to apply light finger pressure on lacrimal sac for 1 minute after drops are instilled. Stress importance of compliance with recommended therapy.
• Tell patients not to share eye medications, washcloths, or towels with family members. If anyone develops the same symptoms, the doctor should be notified.
• Shake well before use. Refrigerate or store at room temperature.

norfloxacin

Chibroxin

Pregnancy Risk Category: C

HOW SUPPLIED

Ophthalmic solution: 0.3% in 5-ml containers

ACTION

Mechanism: Inhibits bacterial DNA gyrase, an enzyme necessary for bacterial replication. Bacteriostatic or bactericidal, depending on concentration.
Peak: Systemic absorption is negligible.

INDICATIONS & DOSAGE

Conjunctivitis caused by susceptible strains of bacteria –
Adults and children 1 year and over: 1 or 2 drops in the affected eye q.i.d. for up to 7 days. If condition warrants, 2 drops may be applied q 2

hours during the waking hours of the first day of treatment.

ADVERSE REACTIONS
EENT: local burning or discomfort, itching, chemosis, photophobia, conjunctival hyperemia.
Other: bad taste in mouth.

INTERACTIONS
Caffeine, cyclosporine, theophylline: impaired metabolism of these drugs with systemic norfloxacin. It's unknown if ophthalmic norfloxacin will have this effect. Monitor closely.
Oral anticoagulants: enhanced activity with systemic norfloxacin. It's unknown if ophthalmic norfloxacin will have this effect. Monitor closely.

CONTRAINDICATIONS
- Contraindicated in patients with a history of hypersensitivity to norfloxacin or other quinolone antibiotics. Drug shouldn't be injected into the eye.
- Use cautiously in breast-feeding patients. It's unknown if drug is excreted in breast milk.

NURSING CONSIDERATIONS
- Serious hypersensitivity reactions, including anaphylaxis, have occurred in patients receiving systemic quinolone therapy. Discontinue drug at the first sign of hypersensitivity, such as skin rash.
- Drug is indicated for treating conjunctivitis when caused by susceptible bacteria. Known susceptible strains include *Acinetobacter calcoaceticus, Aeromonas hydrophila, Haemophilus influenzae, Proteus mirabilis, Serratia marcescens, Staphylococcus aureus, S. epidermidis, S. warnerii,* and *Streptococcus pneumoniae.*
- Prolonged use may result in overgrowth of nonsusceptible organisms, including fungi. Institute appropriate therapy if superinfection occurs.
- Teach patients how to instill drops. Advise them to wash hands before and after administering and not to touch the tip of the tube or dropper to eye or surrounding tissue. Tell patients to clean eye area of excessive exudate before instilling. Stress the importance of compliance with recommended therapy.
- Tell patients not to share eye medications, washcloths, or towels with family members. If anyone develops the same symptoms, the doctor should be notified.
- Although systemically administered quinolones have been shown to cause arthropathy in young animals, ophthalmic norfloxacin has not produced this adverse effect.

polymyxin B sulfate

Pregnancy Risk Category: B

HOW SUPPLIED
Ophthalmic sterile powder for solution: 500,000-unit vials to be reconstituted to 20 to 50 ml

ACTION
Mechanism: Inhibits protein synthesis.
Peak: Systemic absorption is negligible.

INDICATIONS & DOSAGE
Used alone or in combination with other agents to treat corneal ulcers resulting from infection with Pseudomonas *or other gram-negative organism –*
Adults and children: instill 1 to 3 drops of 0.1% to 0.25% (10,000 to 25,000 units/ml) q 1 hour. Increase interval according to patient response; or up to 10,000 units subconjunctivally daily by the doctor. Do not exceed 2 million units daily.

ADVERSE REACTIONS
EENT: eye irritation, conjunctivitis.
Other: overgrowth of nonsusceptible

organisms, hypersensitivity reactions (local burning, itching).

INTERACTIONS
None significant.

CONTRAINDICATIONS
• Contraindicated in patients hypersensitive to the drug.

NURSING CONSIDERATIONS
• One of the most effective antibiotics against gram-negative organisms, especially *Pseudomonas.*
• Often used in combination with neomycin sulfate.
• In severe, life-threatening *Pseudomonas* infections, polymyxin B may be used as an ocular irrigant.
• Advise patients to watch for signs of sensitivity, such as itching lids, swelling, or constant burning. Tell patients who develop such signs to stop drug and notify the doctor immediately.
• Teach patients how to instill drops. Advise them to wash hands before and after administering solution, and warn them not to touch tip of dropper to eye or surrounding tissue. Tell patients to clean eye area of excessive exudate before application and to apply light finger pressure on lacrimal sac for 1 minute after drops are instilled. Stress importance of compliance with recommended therapy.
• Reconstitute carefully to ensure correct drug concentration in solution.
• Tell patients not to share eye medications, washcloths, or towels with family members. If anyone develops the same symptoms, the doctor should be notified.

silver nitrate 1%

Pregnancy Risk Category: C

HOW SUPPLIED
Ophthalmic solution: 1%

ACTION
Mechanism: Causes protein denaturation, which prevents gonorrheal ophthalmia neonatorum. Bacteriostatic, germicidal, and astringent.
Peak: Systemic absorption is negligible.

INDICATIONS & DOSAGE
Prevention of gonorrheal ophthalmia neonatorum –
Neonates: clean lids thoroughly; instill 2 drops of 1% solution into the lower conjunctival sac of each eye at the angle of the nasal bridge and eyes, no later than 1 hour after delivery.

ADVERSE REACTIONS
EENT: periorbital edema, temporary staining of lids and surrounding tissue, *conjunctivitis.*

INTERACTIONS
Bacitracin: inactivation of silver nitrate. Don't use together.

CONTRAINDICATIONS
• Contraindicated in patients hypersensitive to the drug.

NURSING CONSIDERATIONS
• Prophylaxis against gonococcal ophthalmia neonatorum is legally required for neonates in most states. Because of a high incidence of conjunctivitis (> 90%), many clinicians prefer antibiotic ointments such as erythromycin as an alternative.
• Never use concentrations greater than 1% in the eye.
• Apply within 1 hour of birth. Use in neonates born either by vaginal delivery or by cesarean section.
• Don't use repeatedly.
• If a concentrated solution is accidentally used in eye, prompt irrigation with 0.9% sodium chloride solution is advised to prevent severe eye irritation or blindness.
• Solution may stain skin and utensils. Handle carefully.

• May delay instillation slightly to allow neonate to bond with mother.
• Always wash hands before instilling solution.
• Store wax ampules away from light and heat.
• Don't irrigate eyes after instillation.

sulfacetamide sodium 10%

Bleph-10 Liquifilm Ophthalmic, Cetamide Ophthalmic, Sodium Sulamyd 10% Ophthalmic, Sulf-10 Ophthalmic

sulfacetamide sodium 15%

Isopto Cetamide Ophthalmic, Sulfacel-15 Ophthalmic

sulfacetamide sodium 30%

Sodium Sulamyd 30% Ophthalmic

Pregnancy Risk Category: C

HOW SUPPLIED

Ophthalmic ointment: 10%
Ophthalmic solution: 10%, 15%, 30%

ACTION

Mechanism: Prevents uptake of PABA, a metabolite of bacterial folic acid synthesis.
Onset: rapid. **Peak:** Systemic absorption is negligible. **Duration:** 1 to 4 hours for solution.

INDICATIONS & DOSAGE

Inclusion conjunctivitis, corneal ulcers, trachoma, chlamydial infection–
Adults and children: instill 1 to 2 drops of 10% solution into lower conjunctival sac q 2 to 3 hours during day, less often at night; or instill 1 to 2 drops of 15% solution into lower conjunctival sac q 1 to 2 hours initially, increasing interval as condition responds; or instill 1 drop of 30% solution into lower conjunctival sac q 2 hours. Instill ½" to 1" of 10% ointment into conjunctival sac q.i.d. and h.s. May use ointment at night along with drops during the day.

ADVERSE REACTIONS

EENT: slowed corneal wound healing (ointment), *pain on instilling eyedrop,* headache or brow pain, photophobia.
Other: hypersensitivity reactions (including itching or burning), overgrowth of nonsusceptible organisms, ***Stevens-Johnson syndrome.***

INTERACTIONS

Gentamicin (ophthalmic): in vitro *antagonism. Avoid using together.*
Local anesthetics (procaine, tetracaine), PABA derivatives: decreased sulfacetamide sodium action. Wait ½ to 1 hour after instilling anesthetic or PABA derivative before instilling sulfacetamide.
Silver preparations: precipitate formation. Avoid using together.

CONTRAINDICATIONS

• Contraindicated in patients hypersensitive to sulfonamides.
• Not recommended for children under 2 months.

NURSING CONSIDERATIONS

• Often used with oral tetracycline in treating trachoma and inclusion conjunctivitis.
• Replaced by other antibiotics in treating major ocular infections; still used in minor ocular infections.
• Warn patients that eyedrops burn slightly.
• Tell patients not to share eye medications, washcloths, or towels with family members. If anyone develops the same symptoms, the doctor should be notified.
• Advise patients to watch for signs of sensitivity, such as itching lids, swelling, or constant burning. Tell patients who develop such signs to stop drug and notify the doctor immediately.
• Teach patients how to instill drops

or apply ointment. Advise them to wash hands before and after administering ointment or solution and not to touch tip of dropper to eye or surrounding tissues. Tell them to clean eye area of excessive exudate before instilling and to apply light finger pressure on lacrimal sac for 1 minute after drops are instilled. Stress importance of compliance with recommended therapy.
- Wait at least 5 minutes before administering other eyedrops.
- Warn patients that solution may stain clothing.
- Store in tightly closed, light-resistant container away from heat.
- Don't use discolored solution.
- Tell patients to minimize photophobia by wearing sunglasses and avoiding prolonged exposure to sunlight.

tetracycline hydrochloride

Achromycin Ophthalmic

Pregnancy Risk Category: D

HOW SUPPLIED

Ophthalmic suspension: 1%
Ophthalmic ointment: 1%

ACTION

Mechanism: Inhibits protein synthesis. Bactericidal or bacteriostatic, depending upon concentration.
Peak: Systemic absorption is negligible.

INDICATIONS & DOSAGE

Superficial ocular infections and inclusion conjunctivitis –
Adults and children: apply a small amount of the ointment or instill 1 to 2 drops in eye b.i.d., q.i.d., or more often, depending on severity of infection.
Trachoma –
Adults and children: instill 2 drops in each eye b.i.d., t.i.d., or q.i.d. Continue for 1 to 2 months or longer, or apply a small amount of the ointment t.i.d. or q.i.d. for 30 days.
Prophylaxis of ophthalmia neonatorum –
Neonates: instill 1 to 2 drops of the suspension or apply ½″ to 1″ of the ointment into the lower conjunctival sac of each eye shortly after delivery.

ADVERSE REACTIONS

EENT: itching, blurred vision (with ointment).
Other: hypersensitivity reactions (eye itching and dermatitis); overgrowth of nonsusceptible organisms with long-term use.

INTERACTIONS

None significant.

CONTRAINDICATIONS

- Contraindicated in patients hypersensitive to the drug.
- Although unlikely, drug can cause permanent staining of teeth if used in children under age 8.

NURSING CONSIDERATIONS

- Tell patients or family that trachoma therapy should continue for 1 to 2 months or longer. Trachoma may cause blindness if left untreated or if not treated properly.
- Tell patients that gnats and flies are vectors of *Chlamydia trachomatis.* Warn patients with trachoma not to let gnats or flies settle around eye area. Also explain that infection is spread by direct contact, so handwashing is essential to prevent spread. Severe trachoma may require oral therapy as well.
- For prophylaxis of ophthalmia neonatorum, apply ointment no later than 1 hour after birth. Use in neonates born by either vaginal delivery or cesarean section.
- Tell patients to watch for signs of sensitivity, such as itching lids, swelling, or constant burning. Tell patients

who develop such signs to stop drug and notify the doctor immediately.

- Teach patients how to instill drops or apply ointment. Advise them to wash hands before and after administering ointment or solution and not to touch tip of dropper to eye or surrounding tissue. Tell patients to clean eye area of excessive exudate before applications and to apply light finger pressure on lacrimal sac for 1 minute after drops are instilled. Stress importance of compliance with recommended therapy.
- Store in tightly closed, light-resistant container.
- Remind patients to shake suspension well before use.
- Tell patients not to share eye medications, washcloths, or towels with family members. If anyone develops the same symptoms, the doctor should be notified.
- Ophthalmic ointment may be used with suspension to provide prolonged drug contact with affected area at night.

tobramycin

Tobrex

Pregnancy Risk Category: B

HOW SUPPLIED

Ophthalmic ointment: 0.3%
Ophthalmic solution: 0.3%

ACTION

Mechanism: Inhibits protein synthesis.
Peak: Systemic absorption is negligible.

INDICATIONS & DOSAGE

External ocular infections caused by susceptible gram-negative bacteria – **Adults and children:** in mild to moderate infections, instill 1 or 2 drops into the affected eye q 4 hours or apply a thin strip of ointment q 8 to 12 hours. In severe infections, instill 2 drops into the infected eye hourly until condition improves; then reduce frequency. Or, apply a thin strip of ointment q 3 to 4 hours until improvement; then reduce frequency.

ADVERSE REACTIONS

EENT: burning or stinging on instillation, lid itching, lid swelling, blurred vision (with ointment).
Other: hypersensitivity reactions.

INTERACTIONS

Tetracycline-containing eye preparations: incompatible with tyloxapol, an ingredient in Tobrex. Don't use together.

CONTRAINDICATIONS

- Contraindicated in patients hypersensitive to the drug.

NURSING CONSIDERATIONS

- Prolonged use may result in overgrowth of nonsusceptible organisms, including fungi.
- If topical ocular tobramycin is administered concomitantly with systemic tobramycin, carefully monitor serum levels.
- Clinical symptoms of tobramycin overdose include keratitis, erythema, increased lacrimation, edema, and lid itching. Stop drug and notify the doctor if any of these occurs.
- Tell patients not to share eye medications, washcloths, or towels with family members. If anyone develops the same symptoms, the doctor should be notified.
- Advise patients to watch for signs of sensitivity, such as itching lids, swelling, or constant burning. Tell patients who develop them to discontinue drug and notify the doctor immediately.
- Teach patients how to instill drops or apply ointment. Advise them to wash hands before and after administering ointment or solution and to avoid touching tip of dropper to eye or surrounding tissue. Tell them to clean eye area of excessive exudate before

application and to apply light finger pressure on lacrimal sac for 1 minute after drops are instilled. Stress importance of compliance with recommended therapy.
• Often used to combat gram-negative organisms that are resistant to gentamicin.
• When two different ophthalmic solutions are used, allow at least 5 minutes before instillation.

trifluridine

Viroptic Ophthalmic Solution 1%

Pregnancy Risk Category: C

HOW SUPPLIED
Ophthalmic solution: 1%

ACTION
Mechanism: Interferes with DNA synthesis.
Onset: 7 to 14 days. **Peak:** Systemic absorption is negligible.

INDICATIONS & DOSAGE
Primary keratoconjunctivitis and recurrent epithelial keratitis caused by herpes simplex virus, types I and II–
Adults: 1 drop of solution into the affected eye q 2 hours while patient is awake, to a maximum of 9 drops daily until corneal ulcer reepithelialization occurs; then 1 drop q 4 hours (minimum 5 drops daily) for an additional 7 days.

ADVERSE REACTIONS
Eye: *stinging on instillation,* edema of eyelids, increased intraocular pressure.
Other: hypersensitivity reactions.

INTERACTIONS
None significant.

CONTRAINDICATIONS
• Contraindicated in patients hypersensitive to the drug.

NURSING CONSIDERATIONS
• Prescribed only for those patients with clinical diagnosis of herpetic keratitis.
• Consider another form of therapy if improvement doesn't occur after 7 days' treatment or complete reepithelialization after 14 days' treatment. Don't use trifluridine more than 21 days continuously due to potential ocular toxicity.
• Watch for signs of increased intraocular pressure.
• Reassure patients that mild local irritation of the conjunctiva and cornea that occurs when solution is instilled is usually temporary.
• More effective than vidarabine or idoxuridine with fewer adverse reactions.
• Teach patients how to instill drops. Advise them to wash hands before and after administering solution and warn them not to touch tip of dropper to eye or surrounding tissue. Tell patients to clean eye area of excessive exudate before application and apply light finger pressure on lacrimal sac for 1 minute after drops are instilled. Stress importance of complying with recommended therapy.
• Tell patients not to share eye medications, washcloths, or towels with family members. If anyone develops the same symptoms, the doctor should be notified.
• Continue trifluridine for several days after steroid therapy.
• Keep refrigerated. Do not use if past the expiration date.

vidarabine

Vira-A Ophthalmic

Pregnancy Risk Category: C

HOW SUPPLIED
Ophthalmic ointment: 3% in 3.5-g tube (equivalent to 2.8% vidarabine)

ACTION
Mechanism: Interferes with DNA synthesis.
Peak: Systemic absorption is negligible.

INDICATIONS & DOSAGE
Acute keratoconjunctivitis, superficial keratitis, and recurrent epithelial keratitis resulting from herpes simplex types I and II –
Adults and children: instill ½" ointment into lower conjunctival sac five times daily at 3-hour intervals.

ADVERSE REACTIONS
EENT: temporary burning, itching, mild irritation, pain, lacrimation, foreign body sensation, conjunctival injection, superficial punctate keratitis, photophobia.
Other: hypersensitivity reactions.

INTERACTIONS
None significant.

CONTRAINDICATIONS
- Contraindicated in patients hypersensitive to the drug.
- Use cautiously and with close monitoring with steroids. Continue vidarabine for several days after steroid therapy.

NURSING CONSIDERATIONS
- Not for long-term use. Treatment should not exceed 21 days, or 3 to 5 days after healing. Warn patients not to exceed recommended frequency or duration of dosage.
- Not effective against RNA virus, adenoviral ocular infections, or bacterial, fungal, or chlamydial infections.
- Advise patients to watch for signs of sensitivity, such as itching lids, swelling, or constant burning. Tell patients who develop such signs to stop drug and notify the doctor immediately.
- Teach patients how to apply. Advise them to wash hands before and after administering ointment and to avoid touching tip of tube to eye or surrounding tissue. Tell patients to clean eye area of excessive exudate before application and to apply light finger pressure on lacrimal sac for 1 minute after drops are instilled.
- Store in tightly closed, light-resistant container.
- Tell patients not to share eye medications, washcloths, or towels with family members. If anyone develops the same symptoms, the doctor should be notified.
- Explain to patients that the ointment may produce a temporary visual haze.
- Tell patients to minimize photophobia by wearing sunglasses and avoiding prolonged exposure to sunlight.

80

Ophthalmic anti-inflammatory agents

dexamethasone
dexamethasone sodium phosphate
fluorometholone
flurbiprofen sodium
ketorolac tromethamine
medrysone
prednisolone acetate (suspension)
prednisolone sodium phosphate (solution)
suprofen

COMBINATION PRODUCTS
Corticosteroids for ophthalmic use are commonly combined with antibiotics and sulfonamides. See Chapter 78, OPHTHALMIC ANTI-INFECTIVES.

dexamethasone
Maxidex Ophthalmic Suspension

dexamethasone sodium phosphate
Decadron Phosphate Ophthalmic, Maxidex Ophthalmic

Pregnancy Risk Category: C

HOW SUPPLIED
dexamethasone
Ophthalmic suspension: 0.1%
dexamethasone sodium phosphate
Ophthalmic ointment: 0.05%
Ophthalmic solution: 0.1%

ACTION
Mechanism: Decreases the infiltration of WBCs at the site of inflammation.
Peak: Although systemic absorption occurs, plasma levels are very low and systemic effects are negligible.

INDICATIONS & DOSAGE
Uveitis; iridocyclitis; inflammatory conditions of eyelids, conjunctiva, cornea, anterior segment of globe; corneal injury from chemical or thermal burns, or penetration of foreign bodies; allergic conjunctivitis –
Adults and children: instill 1 to 2 drops of suspension or solution or apply ½″ to 1″ of ointment into conjunctival sac. In severe disease, drops may be used hourly, tapering to discontinuation as condition improves. In mild conditions, drops may be used up to four to six times daily or ointment applied t.i.d. or q.i.d. As condition improves, taper dosage to b.i.d. then once daily. Treatment may extend from a few days to several weeks.

ADVERSE REACTIONS
EENT: increased intraocular pressure; thinning of cornea, interference with corneal wound healing, increased susceptibility to viral or fungal corneal infection, corneal ulceration; with excessive or long-term use, glaucoma exacerbations, cataracts, defects in visual acuity and visual field, optic nerve damage; mild blurred vision; burning, stinging, or redness of eyes; watery eyes.
Other: systemic effects and adrenal suppression with excessive or long-term use.

INTERACTIONS
None significant.

CONTRAINDICATIONS
• Contraindicated in patients with acute superficial herpes simplex (dendritic keratitis), vaccinia, varicella, or other fungal or viral diseases of cornea and conjunctiva; ocular tubercu-

losis; or any acute, purulent, untreated infection of the eye.
• Use cautiously in patients with corneal abrasions that may be infected (especially with herpes).
• Use cautiously in patients with glaucoma (any form), because intraocular pressure may increase. Glaucoma medications may need to be increased to compensate.

NURSING CONSIDERATIONS
• Corneal viral and fungal infections may be exacerbated by steroid application.
• Warn patients to call the doctor immediately and to stop drug if visual acuity changes or visual field diminishes.
• Not for long-term use.
• Shake suspension well before use.
• May use eye pad with ointment.
• Teach patients how to instill drops or apply ointment. Advise them to wash hands before and after administering ointment or solution, and warn them not to touch dropper or tip to eye or surrounding tissue. Tell them to apply light finger pressure on lacrimal sac for 1 minute after instillation. Stress the importance of compliance with recommended therapy.
• Watch for corneal ulceration; may require stopping drug.
• Warn patients not to use leftover medication for a new eye inflammation; may cause serious problems.
• Tell patients not to share eye medications, washcloths, or towels with family members. If anyone develops similar symptoms, the doctor should be notified.

fluorometholone
FML Liquifilm Ophthalmic, FML S.O.P.

Pregnancy Risk Category: C

HOW SUPPLIED
Ophthalmic ointment: 0.1%
Ophthalmic suspension: 0.1%, 0.25%

ACTION
Mechanism: Decreases the infiltration of WBCs at inflammation site.
Peak: Although systemic absorption occurs, plasma levels are very low, and systemic effects are negligible.

INDICATIONS & DOSAGE
Inflammatory and allergic conditions of cornea, conjunctiva, sclera, anterior uvea –
Adults and children: instill 1 to 2 drops in conjunctival sac b.i.d. to q.i.d. May use q hour during first 1 to 2 days if needed. Alternatively, apply ½" ribbon of ointment to conjunctival sac q 4 hours, decreasing to one to three times a day as inflammation subsides.

ADVERSE REACTIONS
EENT: increased intraocular pressure, thinning of cornea, interference with corneal wound healing, corneal ulceration, increased susceptibility to viral or fungal corneal infections; with excessive or long-term use, glaucoma exacerbations, cataracts, decreased visual acuity, diminished visual field, optic nerve damage.
Other: systemic effects and adrenal suppression in excessive or long-term use.

INTERACTIONS
None significant.

CONTRAINDICATIONS
• Contraindicated in patients with vaccinia, varicella, acute superficial herpes simplex (dendritic keratitis), or other fungal or viral eye diseases; ocular tuberculosis; or any acute, purulent, untreated eye infection.
• Use cautiously in patients with corneal abrasions that may be contaminated (especially with herpes).

- Safety and efficacy in children under age 2 have not been established.

NURSING CONSIDERATIONS

- Not for long-term use.
- Shake well before using.
- Less likely to cause increased intraocular pressure with long-term use than other ophthalmic anti-inflammatory drugs (except medrysone).
- Store in tightly covered, light-resistant container.
- Advise patients to call the doctor immediately and to stop drug if visual acuity decreases or visual field diminishes.
- Teach patients how to instill drops or apply ointment. Advise them to wash hands before and after administering ointment or solution, and warn them not to touch dropper or tip to eye or surrounding tissue. Advise patients to apply light finger pressure on lacrimal sac for 1 minute after instillation.
- Warn patients not to use leftover medication for a new eye inflammation; may cause serious problems.
- Tell patients not to share eye medications, washcloths, or towels with family members. If anyone develops similar symptoms, the doctor should be notified.

flurbiprofen sodium

Ocufen Liquifilm

Pregnancy Risk Category: C

HOW SUPPLIED

Ophthalmic solution: 0.03%

ACTION

Mechanism: Blocks the synthesis of prostaglandins. Constricts the iris sphincter, inhibiting miosis by a mechanism independent of cholinergic action.

Peak: Peak levels in ocular tissues occurs within 30 to 60 minutes. **Duration:** elimination half-life, about 1½ hours.

INDICATIONS & DOSAGE

Inhibition of intraoperative miosis –

Adults: instill 1 drop into the eye undergoing surgery approximately every ½ hour, beginning 2 hours before surgery. Give a total of 4 drops.

ADVERSE REACTIONS

EENT: transient burning and stinging on instillation, ocular irritation.

INTERACTIONS

Acetylcholine, carbachol: may be rendered ineffective. Avoid concomitant use.

Anticoagulants: increased risk of bleeding if significant systemic absorption occurs. Monitor closely.

Epinephrine, other antiglaucoma agents: reduced ability to lower intraocular pressure. Don't use together.

CONTRAINDICATIONS

- Contraindicated in patients with epithelial herpes simplex keratitis.
- Use cautiously in patients who may be allergic to aspirin and other NSAIDs.
- Use cautiously in patients with bleeding tendencies and those who are receiving medications that may prolong clotting times.

NURSING CONSIDERATIONS

- Wound healing may be delayed.
- Advise patients to call the doctor immediately if visual acuity decreases or visual field diminishes.

ketorolac tromethamine

Acular

Pregnancy Risk Category:

HOW SUPPLIED

Ophthalmic solution: 0.5%

ACTION

Mechanism: An NSAID that inhibits the action of cyclooxygenase, an enzyme responsible for prostaglandin

synthesis. Prostaglandins mediate the inflammatory response and also cause miosis.
Peak: Systemic absorption is negligible.

INDICATIONS & DOSAGE
Relief of ocular itching caused by seasonal allergic conjunctivitis –
Adults: instill 1 drop into the conjunctival sac of each eye q.i.d.

ADVERSE REACTIONS
EENT: *transient stinging and burning on instillation,* superficial keratitis, superficial ocular infections.
Other: allergic reactions.

INTERACTIONS
None reported.

CONTRAINDICATIONS
- Contraindicated in patients hypersensitive to any component of the formulation.
- Because of the risk of serious adverse effects in the infant, don't administer to breast-feeding patients.
- Use cautiously in patients hypersensitive to other NSAIDs or aspirin and in patients with bleeding disorders.

NURSING CONSIDERATIONS
- Remind patients to store drug away from heat in a dark, tightly closed container and to protect drug from freezing.
- Teach patients how to instill drops. Advise them to wash hands before and after instilling solution, and warn them not to touch dropper or tip to eye or surrounding tissue. Advise patients to apply light finger pressure on lacrimal sac for 1 minute after instillation. Stress the importance of compliance with recommended therapy.
- Remind patients to discard drug when it's no longer needed.

medrysone
HMS Liquifilm Ophthalmic

Pregnancy Risk Category: C

HOW SUPPLIED
Ophthalmic suspension: 1%

ACTION
Mechanism: Decreases the infiltration of WBCs at the site of inflammation.
Peak: Although systemic absorption occurs, plasma levels are very low and systemic effects are negligible.

INDICATIONS & DOSAGE
Allergic conjunctivitis, vernal conjunctivitis, episcleritis, ophthalmic epinephrine sensitivity reaction –
Adults and children: instill 1 drop in conjunctival sac b.i.d. to q.i.d. May use q hour during first 1 to 2 days if needed.

ADVERSE REACTIONS
EENT: thinning of cornea, interference with corneal wound healing, increased susceptibility to viral or fungal corneal infection, corneal ulceration; with excessive or long-term use, glaucoma exacerbations, cataracts, visual acuity and visual field defects, optic nerve damage.
Other: systemic effects and adrenal suppression with excessive or long-term use.

INTERACTIONS
None significant.

CONTRAINDICATIONS
- Contraindicated in patients with vaccinia, varicella, acute superficial herpes simplex (dendritic keratitis), viral diseases of conjunctiva and cornea, ocular tuberculosis, fungal or viral eye diseases, iritis, uveitis, or any acute, purulent, untreated eye infection.
- Use cautiously in patients with cor-

neal abrasions that may be contaminated (especially with herpes).

NURSING CONSIDERATIONS
- Shake well before using. Don't freeze.
- Teach patients how to instill drops. Advise them to wash hands before and after instilling solution, and warn them not to touch dropper or tip to eye or surrounding tissue. Advise patients to apply light finger pressure on lacrimal sac for 1 minute after instillation. Stress the importance of compliance with recommended therapy.
- Warn patients not to use leftover medication for a new eye inflammation; may cause serious problems.
- Tell patients not to share eye medications, washcloths, or towels with family members. If anyone develops similar symptoms, the doctor should be notified.

prednisolone acetate (suspension)

Econopred Ophthalmic, Econopred Plus Ophthalmic, Pred-Forte, Pred Mild Ophthalmic

prednisolone sodium phosphate (solution)

AK-Pred, Hydeltrasol Ophthalmic, Inflamase Forte, Inflamase Ophthalmic, Ocu-Pred, Predsol Eye Drops‡

Pregnancy Risk Category: C

HOW SUPPLIED
acetate
Ophthalmic suspension: 0.12%, 0.125%, 1%
sodium phosphate
Ophthalmic solution: 0.125%, 1%

ACTION
Mechanism: Decreases the infiltration of WBCs at the site of inflammation.
Peak: Although systemic absorption occurs, plasma levels are very low and systemic effects are negligible.

INDICATIONS & DOSAGE
Inflammation of palpebral and bulbar conjunctiva, cornea, and anterior segment of globe –
Adults and children: instill 1 to 2 drops in eye of 0.12% to 1% suspension (acetate) or 0.125% to 1% solution (phosphate). In severe conditions, may be used hourly, tapering to discontinuation as inflammation subsides. In mild conditions, may be used up to four to six times daily.

ADVERSE REACTIONS
EENT: increased intraocular pressure; thinning of cornea, interference with corneal wound healing, increased susceptibility to viral or fungal corneal infection, corneal ulceration; with excessive or long-term use, glaucoma exacerbations, cataracts, visual acuity and visual field defects, optic nerve damage.
Other: systemic effects and adrenal suppression with excessive or long-term use.

INTERACTIONS
None significant.

CONTRAINDICATIONS
- Contraindicated in patients with acute, untreated, purulent, ocular infections; acute superficial herpes simplex (dendritic keratitis); vaccinia, varicella, or other viral or fungal eye diseases; or ocular tuberculosis.
- Use cautiously in patients with corneal abrasions that may be contaminated (especially with herpes).

NURSING CONSIDERATIONS
- Tell patients on long-term therapy to have frequent tonometric examinations.
- Shake suspension and check dosage before administering to ensure using

the correct strength. Store in tightly covered container.

- Teach patients how to instill drops. Advise them to wash hands before and after applying, and warn them not to touch dropper or tip to eye or surrounding area. Advise patients to apply light finger-pressure on lacrimal sac for 1 minute after instillation. Stress the importance of compliance with recommended therapy.
- Warn patients not to use leftover medication for a new eye inflammation; may cause serious problems.
- Tell patients not to share eye medications, washcloths, or towels with family members. If anyone develops similar symptoms, the doctor should be notified.

suprofen

Profenal

Pregnancy Risk Category: C

HOW SUPPLIED

Ophthalmic solution: 1%

ACTION

Mechanism: An NSAID that inhibits the action of cyclooxygenase, an enzyme responsible for the synthesis of prostaglandins. Prostaglandins mediate the inflammatory response and also cause miosis.

Peak: Systemic absorption is negligible.

INDICATIONS & DOSAGE

Inhibition of intraoperative miosis –

Adults: instill 2 drops into the conjunctival sac q 4 hours the day before surgery. On the day of surgery, instill 2 drops 3 hours, 2 hours, and 1 hour before surgery.

ADVERSE REACTIONS

EENT: *transient stinging and burning on instillation,* discomfort, itching, redness, iritis, pain, chemosis, photophobia, irritation, punctate epithelial staining.

Other: hypersensitivity reaction.

INTERACTIONS

Acetylcholine, carbachol: may be ineffective in patients treated with suprofen.

CONTRAINDICATIONS

- Contraindicated in patients hypersensitive to any component of the formulation and in patients with epithelial herpes simplex keratitis.
- Don't administer to breast-feeding patients because of the risk of serious adverse reactions in the infant.
- Use cautiously in patients hypersensitive to other NSAIDs or aspirin.
- Use cautiously in patients with bleeding disorders.

NURSING CONSIDERATIONS

- Advise patients to store drug away from heat in a dark, tightly closed container and to protect drug from freezing.
- Teach patients how to instill drops. Advise them to wash hands before and after administering solution and not to touch tip of dropper to eye or surrounding tissues. Tell patients to apply light finger pressure on lacrimal sac for 1 minute after drops are instilled. Stress importance of compliance with recommended therapy.
- Remind patients to discard drug when it's no longer needed.

81

Miotics

acetylcholine chloride
carbachol (intraocular)
carbachol (topical)
demecarium bromide
echothiophate iodide
isoflurophate
physostigmine salicylate
physostigmine sulfate
pilocarpine
pilocarpine hydrochloride
pilocarpine nitrate

COMBINATION PRODUCTS

E-PILO: epinephrine bitartrate 1% and pilocarpine hydrochloride 1%, 2%, 3%, 4%, or 6%.
ISOPTO P-ES: pilocarpine hydrochloride 2% and physostigmine salicylate 0.25%.
P_1E_1, P_2E_1, P_3E_1, P_4E_1, P_6E_1: epinephrine bitartrate 1% and pilocarpine hydrochloride 1%, 2%, 3%, 4%, or 6%.

acetylcholine chloride

Miochol

Pregnancy Risk Category: C

HOW SUPPLIED

Ophthalmic injection: 1%

ACTION

Mechanism: A cholinergic that causes contraction of the sphincter muscles of the iris, resulting in miosis, and that produces ciliary spasm, deepening of the anterior chamber, and vasodilation of conjunctival vessels of the outflow tract.
Onset: within seconds. **Duration:** about 10 minutes.

INDICATIONS & DOSAGE

Anterior segment surgery –
Adults and children: before or after securing sutures, the doctor gently instills 0.5 to 2 ml into anterior chamber.

ADVERSE REACTIONS

CV: bradycardia, hypotension.
EENT: corneal edema, clouding, or decompensation.
Respiratory: breathing difficulties.
Other: flushing, diaphoresis.

INTERACTIONS

None significant.

CONTRAINDICATIONS

- Contraindicated in patients hypersensitive to the drug or any of its components.

NURSING CONSIDERATIONS

- Reconstitute immediately before using, shaking vial gently until clear solution is obtained.
- Discard any unused solution.
- Don't gas-sterilize vial. Ethylene oxide may produce formic acid.

carbachol (intraocular)

Miostat

carbachol (topical)

Carbacel, Isopto Carbachol

Pregnancy Risk Category: C

HOW SUPPLIED

Topical ophthalmic solution: 0.75%, 1.5%, 2.25%, 3%
Intraocular injection: 0.01%

ACTION

Mechanism: A cholinergic that causes contraction of the sphincter muscles of the iris, resulting in miosis, and that produces ciliary spasm, deepening of the anterior

chamber, and vasodilation of conjunctival vessels of the outflow tract.
Onset: 10 to 20 minutes. **Peak:** Peak effect occurs 4 hours after topical application, 2 to 5 minutes after intraocular injection. **Duration:** about 8 hours after topical application, 24 hours after intraocular injection.

INDICATIONS & DOSAGE
To produce pupillary miosis in ocular surgery –
Adults: before or after securing sutures, the doctor gently instills 0.5 ml (intraocular form) into anterior chamber.
Open-angle glaucoma –
Adults: instill 1 to 2 drops (topical form) q 4 to 8 hours.

ADVERSE REACTIONS
CNS: headache.
EENT: spasm of eye accommodation, blurred vision, conjunctival vasodilation, eye and brow pain.
GI: abdominal cramps, diarrhea.
Respiratory: asthma.
Other: diaphoresis, flushing.

INTERACTIONS
Pilocarpine: additive effect. Use together cautiously.

CONTRAINDICATIONS
- Contraindicated in patients with acute iritis and corneal abrasion.
- Use cautiously in patients with acute heart failure, bronchial asthma, peptic ulceration, hyperthyroidism, GI spasm, Parkinson's disease, and urinary tract obstruction.

NURSING CONSIDERATIONS
- Used in open-angle glaucoma, especially when patients are resistant or allergic to pilocarpine hydrochloride or nitrate.
- Tell glaucoma patients that long-term use may be necessary. Stress compliance. Tell them to remain under medical supervision for periodic tonometric readings.
- In case of toxicity, give atropine parenterally.
- Teach patients how to instill. Advise them to wash hands before and after and to apply light finger-pressure on lacrimal sac for 1 minute after drops are instilled. Warn them not to exceed recommended dosage.
- Warn patients to avoid hazardous activities such as operating machinery or driving until temporary blurring subsides. Reassure patients that blurred vision usually diminishes with prolonged use.
- Patients with dark eyes (hazel or brown irises) may require stronger solutions or more frequent instillation because eye pigment may absorb the drug.
- If tolerance to the drug develops, the doctor may switch to another miotic for a short time.

demecarium bromide
Humorsol

Pregnancy Risk Category: X

HOW SUPPLIED
Ophthalmic solution: 0.125%, 0.25%

ACTION
Mechanism: An anticholinesterase drug that inhibits the enzymatic destruction of acetylcholine by inactivating cholinesterase, leaving acetylcholine free to act on the effector cells of the iridic sphincter and ciliary muscles, causing pupillary constriction and spasm of accommodation.
Onset: 15 to 60 minutes. **Peak:** Miotic effect peaks within 2 hours; intraocular pressure (IOP) reduction occurs within 24 hours. **Duration:** miosis, 3 to 10 days; IOP reduction, about 9 days.

INDICATIONS & DOSAGE

Acute angle-closure glaucoma after iridectomy, primary open-angle glaucoma –

Adults: instill 1 drop once or twice/day.

Convergent strabismus (uncomplicated) –

Adults: instill 1 drop daily for 2 to 3 weeks, then reduce to 1 drop q 2 days for 3 to 4 weeks. After reevaluation, instill 1 drop once or twice/week to once q 2 days as determined by the patient's condition. Reevaluate q 4 to 12 weeks, adjusting dosage as needed. Discontinue after 4 months if dosage required is 1 drop q 2 days.

Diagnostic use –

Adults: instill 1 drop daily for 2 weeks, then 1 drop q 2 days for 2 to 3 weeks.

ADVERSE REACTIONS

CNS: browache, unusual fatigue or weakness, headache.

CV: bradycardia, palpitations.

EENT: retinal detachment, iris cysts, conjunctival thickening, lens opacities, paradoxical increase in IOP, *lacrimation,* obstruction of nasolacrimal canals; eye pain, burning, redness, stinging and irritation; twitching eyelids; *blurred vision;* visual disturbances.

GI: nausea, vomiting, diarrhea, abdominal cramps or pain.

GU: loss of bladder control.

INTERACTIONS

Anticholinergics, antimyasthenics, other cholinesterase inhibitors: potential for additive toxicity. Monitor closely.

Carbamate or organophosphate-type insecticides (parathion, malathion): increased risk of systemic effects through respiratory tract or skin. Warn patients to protect themselves.

Cocaine: increased risk of cocaine toxicity; anticholinesterase effects may last weeks or months. Avoid concomitant use.

Epinephrine: additive effect, resulting in better control and lower dosages of both drugs.

Local anesthetics, ophthalmic tetracaine: increased risk of systemic toxicity and prolonged ocular anesthetic effect. Monitor closely.

Ophthalmic adrenocorticoids: increased IOP and decreased antiglaucoma effectiveness. Avoid concomitant use.

Ophthalmic belladonna alkaloids, cyclopentolate: may antagonize miotic effects. Avoid concomitant use.

Succinylcholine: enhanced neuromuscular blockade, possible CV collapse and prolonged respiratory depression or apnea may occur for several weeks or months after demecarium is discontinued. Advise the anesthesiologist that the patient has received demecarium.

CONTRAINDICATIONS

- Contraindicated in patients with bronchial asthma, pronounced bradycardia and hypotension, Down syndrome, seizure disorder, spastic GI disturbances, acute angle-closure glaucoma before iridectomy, Parkinson's disease, uveitis, marked vagotonia, MI, or history of retinal detachment.

NURSING CONSIDERATIONS

- Toxicity is cumulative; toxic systemic symptoms may not appear for weeks or months after start of therapy. Atropine sulfate S.C., I.M., or I.V. is antidote of choice.
- Administer phenylephrine concurrently, as ordered, to reduce incidence of iris cyst formation.
- Tell patients that regular medical supervision is required to check ocular pressure.
- Advise patients to carry medical identification card at all times during therapy.

• Teach patients how to instill demecarium. Advise them to wash hands before and after instilling drug, to avoid touching applicator tip to any surface, and to remove excess solution around eyes with clean tissue and without touching eye. Warn them not to exceed recommended dosage.
• If dose is missed, patients do not double dose. If schedule is every other day, instill as soon as possible if remembered same day; if remembered later, do not instill until next day, then skip a day and resume regular schedule. If schedule is once a day, instill as soon as possible. If not remembered until next day, skip missed dose and resume schedule. If schedule is more than once daily, instill as soon as possible. If close to time for next dose, skip missed dose and resume regular schedule.
• If tolerance to the drug develops after prolonged use, the doctor may switch to another miotic for a short time.

echothiophate iodide (ecothiopate iodide)

Phospholine Iodide

Pregnancy Risk Category: C

HOW SUPPLIED

Ophthalmic powder for solution: for reconstitution to make 0.03%, 0.06%, 0.125%, and 0.25% solutions

ACTION

Mechanism: An anticholinesterase drug that inhibits the enzymatic destruction of acetylcholine by inactivating cholinesterase, leaving acetylcholine free to act on the effector cells of the iridic sphincter and ciliary muscles, causing pupillary constriction and spasm of accommodation.
Onset: miosis, 10 to 30 minutes; intraocular pressure (IOP) reduction, 4 to 8 hours. **Peak:** Miotic effect peaks within 30 minutes; IOP reduction occurs within 24 hours. **Duration:** several days to 4 weeks.

INDICATIONS & DOSAGE

Primary open-angle glaucoma, conditions obstructing aqueous outflow –
Adults and children: instill 1 drop of 0.03% to 0.125% solution into conjunctival sac daily. Maximum dosage is 1 drop b.i.d. Use lowest possible dosage for continuous control of IOP.
Diagnosis of convergent strabismus –
Adults: instill 1 drop of 0.125% solution daily h.s. for 2 to 3 weeks.
Treatment of convergent strabismus –
Adults: instill 1 drop of 0.03% to 0.125% solution daily or every other day h.s.

ADVERSE REACTIONS

CNS: fatigue, muscle weakness, paresthesia, headache.
CV: bradycardia, hypotension.
EENT: ciliary spasm or spasm of eye accommodation, ciliary or circumcorneal injection, nonreversible cataract formation (time- and dose-related), reversible iris cysts, pupillary block, blurred or dimmed vision, eye or brow pain, twitching of eyelids, hyperemia, photophobia, lens opacities, lacrimation, retinal detachment.
GI: diarrhea, nausea, vomiting, abdominal pain, intestinal cramps, salivation.
GU: frequent urination.
Other: diaphoresis, flushing, ***bronchoconstriction.***

INTERACTIONS

Anticholinergics, ophthalmic belladonna alkaloids (such as atropine), cyclopentolate: antagonized miotic effects. Avoid concomitant use.
Cocaine: increased risk of cocaine toxicity. Avoid concomitant use.
Local anesthetics, ophthalmic tetracaine: increased rate of systemic toxicity and prolonged ocular anesthesia. Monitor closely.
Ophthalmic adrenocorticoids: in-

creased intraocular pressure and decreased antiglaucoma effectiveness. Avoid concomitant use.
Other cholinesterase inhibitors, organophosphate insecticides (parathion, malathion): possible additive effect causing systemic effects. Warn patients exposed to insecticides to protect themselves.
Succinylcholine: respiratory and CV collapse. Don't use together.
Systemic anticholinesterase agents for myasthenia gravis, pilocarpine: effects may be additive. Monitor patients for signs of toxicity.

CONTRAINDICATIONS

- Contraindicated in patients with acute angle-closure glaucoma, seizure disorders, vasomotor instability, parkinsonism, iodide hypersensitivity, active uveal inflammation, bronchial asthma, spastic GI conditions, urinary tract obstruction, peptic ulceration, severe bradycardia or hypotension, vascular hypertension, MI, or history of retinal detachment.
- Use cautiously in patients routinely exposed to organophosphate insecticides. May cause nausea, vomiting, and diarrhea, progressing to muscle weakness and respiratory difficulty.
- Also use cautiously in patients with myasthenia gravis receiving anticholinesterase therapy.

NURSING CONSIDERATIONS

- Toxicity is cumulative; toxic systemic symptoms may not appear for weeks or months after start of therapy. Atropine sulfate S.C., I.M., or I.V. is antidote of choice.
- A potent, long-acting, irreversible drug. Advise patients to carry medical identification card at all times during therapy.
- Tell patients to remain under constant medical supervision and not to exceed recommended dosage.
- Warn patients to report salivation, diarrhea, profuse diaphoresis, urinary incontinence, or muscle weakness to the doctor.
- Tell patients to instill drug at bedtime because it causes transient blurred vision. Warn patients that transient brow pain or dimmed or blurred vision is common at first but usually disappears within 5 to 10 days.
- Stop drug at least 2 weeks preoperatively if succinylcholine is to be used in surgery.
- Reconstitute powder using only diluent provided to avoid contamination. Discard refrigerated, reconstituted solution after 6 months; solution stored at room temperature, after 1 month.
- Teach patients how to instill drug. Advise them to wash hands before and after instilling drug, to avoid touching applicator tip to any surface and to apply light finger-pressure on lacrimal sac for 1 minute after instillation.

isoflurophate

Floropryl

Pregnancy Risk Category: X

HOW SUPPLIED

Ophthalmic ointment: 0.025%

ACTION

Mechanism: An anticholinesterase drug that inhibits the enzymatic destruction of acetylcholine by inactivating cholinesterase, leaving acetylcholine free to act on the effector cells of the iridic sphincter and ciliary muscles, causing pupillary constriction and spasm of accommodation.
Onset: miosis, within 10 minutes.
Peak: Miotic effect peaks within 20 minutes; intraocular pressure (IOP) reduction occurs within 24 hours.
Duration: miosis, 1 to 4 weeks; IOP reduction, up to 1 week.

INDICATIONS & DOSAGE
Glaucoma –
Adults: apply ¼" (0.5 cm) ribbon of ointment to conjunctiva q 8 to 72 hours.
Diagnosis of convergent strabismus (uncomplicated) –
Adults: apply ¼" ribbon of ointment to conjunctiva h.s. for 2 weeks.
Treatment of convergent strabismus –
Adults: apply ¼" ribbon of ointment to each eye h.s. for 2 weeks then once daily 2 to 7 days, depending on the patient's condition, for 2 months. If the patient cannot be maintained on every-2-day dosage, discontinue drug.

ADVERSE REACTIONS
CNS: headache, browache, unusual fatigue or weakness.
CV: slow or irregular heartbeat.
EENT: retinal detachment, iris cysts, conjunctival thickening, lens opacities, obstruction of nasolacrimal canals, paradoxical increase in IOP; *eye burning,* redness, pain, stinging or irritation; twitching of eyelids; *blurred vision;* visual disturbances.
GI: nausea, vomiting, diarrhea, abdominal cramps or pain.
GU: loss of bladder control.
Other: diaphoresis, flushing.

INTERACTIONS
Anticholinergics, antimyasthenics, other cholinesterase inhibitors: potential for additive toxicity. Monitor closely.
Carbamate or organophosphate-type insecticides (parathion, malathion): increased risk of systemic effects through respiratory tract or skin. Warn patients to protect themselves.
Cocaine: increased risk of cocaine toxicity; anticholinesterase effects may last weeks or months. Avoid concomitant use.
Epinephrine: additive effect, resulting in better control and lower dosages of both drugs.
Local anesthetics, ophthalmic tetracaine: increased risk of systemic toxicity, prolonged ocular anesthesia. Monitor closely.
Ophthalmic adrenocorticoids: increased IOP and decreased antiglaucoma effectiveness. Avoid concomitant use.
Ophthalmic belladonna alkaloids, cyclopentolate: may antagonize miotic effects. Avoid concomitant use.
Ophthalmic physostigmine: may shorten duration of action. Avoid concomitant use.
Succinylcholine: enhanced neuromuscular blockade, possible CV collapse, prolonged respiratory depression, or apnea may occur for several weeks or months after demecarium is discontinued. Advise the anesthesiologist that the patient has received demecarium.

CONTRAINDICATIONS
- Contraindicated in patients with bronchial asthma, pronounced bradycardia and hypotension, Down syndrome, seizure disorder, spastic GI disturbances, acute angle-closure glaucoma before iridectomy, Parkinson's disease, uveitis, marked vagotonia, MI, or history of retinal detachment.

NURSING CONSIDERATIONS
- Toxicity is cumulative; toxic systemic symptoms may not appear for weeks or months after therapy is discontinued. Atropine sulfate S.C., I.M., or I.V. is antidote of choice.
- Administer phenylephrine concurrently, as ordered, to reduce incidence of iris cyst formation.
- Tell patients that regular medical supervision is required to check ocular pressure.
- Advise patients to carry medical identification card at all times during therapy.
- Teach patients how to apply drug. Advise them to wash hands before and after application, to avoid touching

applicator tip to any surface and to wipe tip with clean tissue. Warn them not to exceed recommended dosage.
• If dose is missed, do not double dose. If schedule is every other day, apply as soon as possible if remembered same day; if remembered later, do not apply until next day, then skip a day and resume regular schedule. If schedule is once a day, apply as soon as possible. If not remembered until next day, skip missed dose and resume schedule. If schedule is more than once daily, apply as soon as possible. If close to time for next dose, skip missed dose and resume regular schedule.
• If tolerance to the drug develops after prolonged use, the doctor may switch to another miotic for a short time.

physostigmine salicylate
Isopto-Eserine

physostigmine sulfate
Eserine Sulfate

Pregnancy Risk Category: C

HOW SUPPLIED
salicylate
Ophthalmic solution: 0.25%, 0.5%
sulfate
Ophthalmic ointment: 0.25%

ACTION
Mechanism: Causes contraction of iris sphincter muscles resulting in miosis, and contraction of ciliary muscle, increasing outflow of aqueous humor and decreasing intraocular pressure.
Onset: within 30 minutes. **Duration:** 12 to 48 hours.

INDICATIONS & DOSAGE
Open-angle glaucoma –
Adults and children: instill 1 drop of solution b.i.d. to t.i.d. or apply a thin strip of ointment once daily to t.i.d.

ADVERSE REACTIONS
CNS: headache, weakness.
CV: slow or irregular heartbeat.
EENT: blurred vision, eye pain, burning, redness, stinging, eye irritation, twitching of eyelids, watering of eyes.
GI: nausea, vomiting, diarrhea.
GU: loss of bladder control.
Other: diaphoresis, muscle weakness, shortness of breath.

INTERACTIONS
Echothiophate, isoflurophate: duration of action may be shortened. Monitor closely.
Ophthalmic belladonna alkaloids: may antagonize miotic actions. Avoid concomitant use.

CONTRAINDICATIONS
• Contraindicated in patients with intolerance to physostigmine, active uveitis, or corneal injury.

NURSING CONSIDERATIONS
• Teach patients how to instill drug. Advise them to wash hands before and after instilling and to avoid touching applicator tip to any surface. Warn them not to exceed recommended dosage.
• Ointment may be used at night because of its longer duration of action.
• If tolerance to the drug develops, the doctor may switch to another miotic for a short time.

pilocarpine
Ocusert Pilo

pilocarpine hydrochloride
Adsorbocarpine, Isopto Carpine, Miocarpine†, Ocusert Pilo, Pilocar, Pilocel, Pilomiotin, Pilopine HS, Pilopt‡

*Liquid form contains alcohol.
**May contain tartrazine.
Common reactions are in italics; ***life-threatening,*** in bold italics.

pilocarpine nitrate

P.V. Carpine Liquifilm, Ocusert Pilo

Pregnancy Risk Category: C

HOW SUPPLIED

pilocarpine
Extended-release insert: 20 mcg/hour, 40 mcg/hour for 7 days
pilocarpine hydrochloride
Ophthalmic solution: 0.25%, 0.5%, 1%, 2%, 3%, 4%, 5%, 6%, 8%, 10%
Ophthalmic gel: 4%
pilocarpine nitrate
Ophthalmic solution: 1%, 2%, 4%

ACTION

Mechanism: A cholinergic that causes contraction of iris sphincter muscles, resulting in miosis, and that produces ciliary spasm, deepening of the anterior chamber, and vasodilation of conjunctival vessels of the outflow tract.
Onset: miosis, within 30 minutes; intraocular pressure (IOP) reduction, within 60 minutes. **Peak:** Miotic effect peaks within 30 minutes; IOP reduction occurs within 75 minutes.
Duration: miosis, up to 8 hours; IOP reduction, 4 to 14 hours with topical solution, up to 24 hours with gel.

INDICATIONS & DOSAGE

Primary open-angle glaucoma –
Adults and children: instill 1 to 2 drops once daily to q.i.d., as directed by the doctor, or apply ½″ (1cm) ribbon of 4% gel (Pilopine HS) h.s.

Alternatively, apply one Ocusert Pilo system (20 or 40 mcg/hour) q 7 days.

Emergency treatment of acute angle-closure glaucoma –
Adults and children: instill 1 drop of 2% solution q 5 minutes for three to six doses, followed by 1 drop q 1 to 3 hours until pressure is controlled.

ADVERSE REACTIONS

EENT: suborbital headache, *myopia,* ciliary spasm, *blurred vision,* conjunctival irritation, lacrimation, changes in visual field, *brow pain.*
GI: nausea, vomiting, abdominal cramps, diarrhea, salivation.
Respiratory: ***bronchoconstriction, pulmonary edema.***
Other: hypersensitivity reactions.

INTERACTIONS

Carbachol, echothiophate: additive effect. Don't use together.
Ophthalmic belladonna alkaloids (such as atropine and scopolamine), cyclopentolate: decreased pilocarpine antiglaucoma effectiveness and blocked mydriatic effects of these agents. Avoid concomitant use.
Phenylephrine: decreased dilation by phenylephrine. Don't use together.

CONTRAINDICATIONS

- Contraindicated in patients with acute iritis, acute inflammatory disease of anterior segment of eye or secondary glaucoma.
- Use cautiously in patients with bronchial asthma and hypertension.

NURSING CONSIDERATIONS

- Widely used drug to treat primary open-angle glaucoma. Also used to counteract effects of mydriatics and cycloplegics after surgery or ophthalmoscopic examination.
- May be used alternately with atropine to break adhesions or alone or with mannitol, urea, glycerol, or acetazolamide in acute angle-closure glaucoma before surgery.
- Instruct patients to apply gel at bedtime because it will blur vision. Warn patients to avoid hazardous activities such as operating machinery or driving until temporary blurring subsides.
- Warn patients that transient brow pain and myopia are common at first but usually disappear within 10 to 14 days.
- Teach patients how to instill pilocarpine. Advise them to wash hands before and after instilling drug and to

apply light finger-pressure on lacrimal sac for 1 minute after drops are instilled. Warn patients not to touch dropper or applicator tip to eye or surrounding tissue.

- If the Ocusert Pilo system falls out of the eye during sleep, patients should wash hands, rinse the insert in cool tap water, and reposition it in the eye. Also tell patients not to use a deformed insert.

82
Mydriatics

atropine sulfate
cyclopentolate hydrochloride
epinephrine hydrochloride
epinephryl borate
homatropine hydrobromide
phenylephrine hydrochloride
scopolamine hydrobromide
tropicamide

COMBINATION PRODUCTS
CYCLOMYDRIL OPHTHALMIC: cyclopentolate hydrochloride 0.2% and phenylephrine hydrochloride 1%.
MUROCOLL-2: scopolamine hydrobromide 0.3% and phenylephrine hydrochloride 10%.

atropine sulfate

Atropisol, Atropt‡, BufOpto Atropine, Isopto Atropine

Pregnancy Risk Category: C

HOW SUPPLIED
Ophthalmic ointment: 0.5%, 1%
Ophthalmic solution: 0.5%, 1%, 2%, 3%

ACTION
Mechanism: A potent mydriatic and cycloplegic whose anticholinergic action leaves the pupil under unopposed adrenergic influence, causing it to dilate.
Peak: Mydriatic effect peaks within 30 to 40 minutes; cycloplegic, within several hours. **Duration:** mydriasis, 7 to 12 days; cycloplegia, 14 days or more, especially in persons with heavily pigmented eyes.

INDICATIONS & DOSAGE
Acute iritis; uveitis –
Adults and children: instill 1 drop of 1% solution or ½″ (1cm) ribbon of ointment daily to b.i.d.
Cycloplegic refraction –
Adults: instill 1 to 2 drops of 1% solution 1 hour before refraction.
Children: instill 1 to 2 drops of 0.5% to 1% solution in each eye b.i.d. for 1 to 3 days before eye examination and 1 hour before refraction, or instill ½″ ribbon of ointment into conjunctival sac daily to t.i.d. 2 to 3 days before examination.

ADVERSE REACTIONS
CNS: irritability, confusion, somnolence, ataxia.
CV: tachycardia.
EENT: ocular congestion with long-term use, conjunctivitis, contact dermatitis of eye, ocular edema, *blurred vision,* eye dryness, *photophobia.*
GI: dry mouth, abdominal distention in infants.
Skin: dryness.
Other: flushing, fever.

INTERACTIONS
None significant.

CONTRAINDICATIONS
- Contraindicated in patients with acute angle-closure glaucoma.
- Use cautiously in infants, children, and elderly or debilitated patients. Also use cautiously in children with blond hair and blue eyes and in patients with Down syndrome or brain damage because they may be more susceptible to atropine or experience higher incidence of adverse reactions.

NURSING CONSIDERATIONS
- Not for internal use. Treat drops and ointment as poison; signs of poisoning are disorientation and confusion. Antidote of choice is physostigmine salicylate I.V. or I.M.
- Watch for signs of glaucoma: in-

creased intraocular pressure, ocular pain, headache, progressive blurring of vision.
- Teach patients how to instill atropine. Advise them to wash hands before and after instilling drug and to apply light finger-pressure on lacrimal sac for 1 minute after instillation. Warn patients not to touch dropper or tip of tube to eye or surrounding tissue.
- Warn patients to avoid hazardous activities such as operating machinery or driving until temporary blurring subsides.
- Advise patients to ease photophobia by wearing dark glasses.
- Tell patients to use sugarless hard candy or gum for dry mouth.

cyclopentolate hydrochloride

AK-Pentolate, Cyclogyl

Pregnancy Risk Category: C

HOW SUPPLIED

Ophthalmic solution: 0.5%, 1%, 2%

ACTION

Mechanism: A potent mydriatic and cycloplegic whose anticholinergic action leaves the pupil under unopposed adrenergic influence, causing it to dilate.

Onset: rapid. **Peak:** Peak effect occurs within 15 to 60 minutes. **Duration:** about 24 hours.

INDICATIONS & DOSAGE

Diagnostic procedures requiring mydriasis and cycloplegia –

Adults: instill 1 drop of 1% solution followed by 1 drop in 5 minutes. Use 2% solution in heavily pigmented irises.

Children: instill 1 drop of 0.5%, 1%, or 2% solution in each eye, followed in 5 minutes with 1 drop 0.5% or 1% solution, if necessary.

ADVERSE REACTIONS

CNS: irritability, confusion, somnolence, hallucinations, ataxia, ***seizures,*** behavioral disturbances in children.

CV: tachycardia.

EENT: eye burning on instillation, blurred vision, eye dryness, *photophobia,* ocular congestion, contact dermatitis in eye, conjunctivitis.

GU: urine retention.

Skin: dryness.

Other: flushing, fever.

INTERACTIONS

Carbachol, pilocarpine: may counteract mydriatic effect. Avoid concomitant use.

Long-acting cholinergic antiglaucoma agents: miotic actions may be inhibited. Avoid concomitant use.

CONTRAINDICATIONS

- Contraindicated in patients with acute angle-closure glaucoma.
- Use cautiously in elderly patients and in children with spastic paralysis.

NURSING CONSIDERATIONS

- Drug is superior to homatropine hydrobromide, and has a shorter duration of action. Physostigmine is antidote of choice.
- Teach patients how to instill drug. Advise them to wash hands before and after instilling drug and to apply light finger-pressure on lacrimal sac for 1 minute after drops are instilled. Warn patients not to touch tip of dropper to eye or surrounding tissue and that drug will burn when instilled.
- Warn patients to avoid hazardous activities, such as operating machinery or driving until temporary blurring subsides.
- Advise patients to ease photophobia by wearing dark glasses.

epinephrine hydrochloride
Epifrin, Glaucon

epinephryl borate
Epinal, Eppy/N

Pregnancy Risk Category: C

HOW SUPPLIED
epinephrine hydrochloride
Ophthalmic solution: 0.1%, 0.25%, 0.5%, 1%, 2%
epinephryl borate
Ophthalmic solution: 0.5%, 1%, 2%

ACTION
Mechanism: An adrenergic that dilates the pupil by contracting the dilator muscle.
Onset: mydriasis, within in a few minutes; intraocular pressure (IOP) reduction, within 1 hour. **Peak:** IOP reduction peaks within 4 to 8 hours.
Duration: mydriasis, several hours; IOP reduction, 12 to 24 hours.

INDICATIONS & DOSAGE
Open-angle glaucoma –
Adults: instill 1 drop of 0.5%, 1%, or 2% hydrochloride solution (or 0.5% or 1% epinephryl borate solution) b.i.d. Adjust dosage according to tonometric readings.
During surgery –
Adults: instill 1 or more drops of 0.1% hydrochloride solution up to three times.

ADVERSE REACTIONS
CNS: browache.
CV: palpitations, tachycardia.
EENT: corneal or conjunctival pigmentation or corneal edema in long-term use; follicular hypertrophy; chemosis; conjunctivitis; iritis; hyperemic conjunctiva; maculopapular rash; severe eye stinging, burning, and tearing on instillation.

INTERACTIONS
Cyclopropane, halogenated hydrocarbons: arrhythmias, tachycardia. Use together cautiously, if at all.
Digitalis glycosides: increased risk of arrhythmias. Monitor closely.
Local or systemic sympathomimetics: additive toxic effects. Avoid concomitant use.
MAO inhibitors: exaggerated adrenergic effects. Adjust dose of epinephrine carefully.
Topical miotics, beta-adrenergic blockers, osmotic agents, systemic carbonic anhydrase inhibitors: additive lowering of IOP. Use together cautiously.
Tricyclic antidepressants, antihistamines (diphenhydramine, dexchlorpheniramine): potentiated cardiac effects of epinephrine. Monitor closely.

CONTRAINDICATIONS
- Contraindicated in patients with shallow anterior chamber or acute angle-closure glaucoma.
- Use cautiously in elderly patients, pregnant patients, and those with diabetes mellitus, hypertension, Parkinson's disease, hyperthyroidism, aphakia (eye without lens), cardiac disease, or cerebral arteriosclerosis.

NURSING CONSIDERATIONS
- Don't substitute one salt if another one is ordered; epinephrine salts are not interchangeable.
- Also can be injected into anterior chamber to produce rapid mydriasis during cataract removal or can be used to control local bleeding during surgery.
- Monitor blood pressure and other vital signs.
- May stain soft contact lenses.
- Don't use darkened solution.
- Teach patients how to instill drug. Advise them to wash hands before and after instilling drug and to apply light finger-pressure on lacrimal sac for 1 minute after drops are instilled. Warn

patients not to touch tip of dropper to eye or surrounding tissue.

homatropine hydrobromide

Homatrine, Homatropine, Isopto Homatropine

Pregnancy Risk Category: C

HOW SUPPLIED

Ophthalmic solution: 2%, 5%

ACTION

Mechanism: Anticholinergic action leaves the pupil under unopposed adrenergic influence, causing it to dilate.

Onset: rapid. **Peak:** Mydriatic effect peaks within 10 to 30 minutes; cycloplegic effect, within 30 to 90 minutes. **Duration:** mydriasis, 6 hours to 4 days; cycloplegia, 10 hours to 2 days.

INDICATIONS & DOSAGE

Cycloplegic refraction –

Adults and children: instill 1 to 2 drops of 2% or 1 drop of 5% solution; if needed repeat in 5 to 10 minutes, for two or three doses.

Uveitis –

Adults and children: instill 1 to 2 drops of 2% or 1 drop of 5% solution up to q 3 to 4 hours.

ADVERSE REACTIONS

CNS: irritability, confusion, somnolence, ataxia.

CV: tachycardia.

EENT: eye irritation, *blurred vision, photophobia.*

GI: dry mouth.

Skin: dryness.

Other: flushing, fever.

INTERACTIONS

None significant.

CONTRAINDICATIONS

• Contraindicated in patients hypersensitive to the drug or to other belladonna alkaloids such as atropine and in those with acute angle-closure glaucoma.

• Use cautiously in infants and elderly or debilitated patients, children with blond hair and blue eyes, patients with cardiac disease, or those with increased intraocular pressure.

NURSING CONSIDERATIONS

• Homatropine is similar to atropine but weaker, with a shorter duration of action. May produce symptoms of atropine poisoning, such as severe dryness of mouth or tachycardia.

• Teach patients how to instill drug. Advise them to wash hands before and after instilling drug and to apply light finger-pressure on lacrimal sac for 1 minute after drops are instilled. Warn patients not to touch tip of dropper to eye or surrounding tissue.

• Warn patients to avoid hazardous activities such as operating machinery or driving until temporary blurring subsides.

• Advise patients to ease photophobia by wearing dark glasses.

• Tell patients to use sugarless hard candy or gum for dry mouth.

phenylephrine hydrochloride

AK-Dilate, AK-Nefrin Ophthalmic◊, I-Phrine 2.5%, Isopto Frin◊, Mydfrin, Neo-Synephrine, Prefrin Liquifilm

Pregnancy Risk Category: C

HOW SUPPLIED

Ophthalmic solution: 0.12%◊, 2.5%, 10%

ACTION

Mechanism: An adrenergic that dilates the pupil by contracting the dilator muscle.

Onset: rapid. **Peak:** Mydriatic effect peaks within 15 to 60 minutes after using the 2.5% solution; 10 to 90 minutes after using the 10% solution.

*Liquid form contains alcohol.
**May contain tartrazine.

Common reactions are in italics; ***life-threatening,*** in bold italics.

Duration: 2.5% solution, about 3 hours. 10% solution, 3 to 7 hours.

INDICATIONS & DOSAGE

Mydriasis without cycloplegia –

Adults and children: instill 1 drop of 2.5% or 10% solution before examination.

Mydriasis and vasoconstriction –

Adults and adolescents: instill 1 drop of 2.5% or 10% solution; repeat in 1 hour if needed.

Children: instill 1 drop of 2.5% solution; repeat in 1 hour if needed.

To relieve eye redness –

Adults: instill 1 to 2 drops of 0.12% solution daily up to q.i.d.

Chronic mydriasis –

Adults and adolescents: instill 1 drop of 2.5% or 10% solution b.i.d. or t.i.d.

Children: instill 1 drop of 2.5% solution b.i.d. or t.i.d.

Posterior synechia (adhesion of iris) –

Adults and children: instill 1 drop of 10% solution.

Do not use 10% concentration in infants.

ADVERSE REACTIONS

CNS: browache, headache.

CV: *hypertension* (with 10% solution), tachycardia, palpitations, ***PVCs.***

EENT: transient eye burning or stinging on instillation, blurred vision, reactive hyperemia of eye, allergic conjunctivitis, iris floaters, acute angle-closure glaucoma, rebound miosis.

Other: pallor, trembling, diaphoresis, dermatitis.

INTERACTIONS

Guanethidine: increased mydriatic and pressor effects of phenylephrine. Use together cautiously.

Levodopa (systemic): reduced mydriatic effect of phenylephrine. Use together cautiously.

MAO inhibitors, beta blockers: may cause arrhythmias because of increased pressor effect. Use together cautiously.

Topically applied atropine, cyclopentolate, homatropine, scopolamine: may increase dilation of pupil. Use together cautiously.

Tricyclic antidepressants: potentiated cardiac effects of epinephrine. Use together cautiously.

CONTRAINDICATIONS

• Contraindicated in patients with idiopathic orthostatic hypotension or acute angle-closure glaucoma and in those wearing soft contact lens.

• Systemic adverse reactions are less likely with 2.5% solution; adverse reactions and toxicity are much more likely with 10% solution.

• Avoid 10% solution and use cautiously in patients with marked hypertension or cardiac disorders, in children of low body weight, and in elderly patients.

NURSING CONSIDERATIONS

• Do not use brown solutions or solutions that contain precipitate.

• Teach patients how to instill drug. Advise them to wash hands before and after instilling drug and to apply light finger-pressure on lacrimal sac for 1 minute after drops are instilled. Warn patients not to touch tip of dropper to eye or surrounding tissue.

• Warn patients not to exceed recommended dosage because systemic effects can result. Monitor blood pressure and pulse rate.

• Advise patients to contact the doctor if condition persists longer than 12 hours after discontinuation of the drug.

• Warn patients to avoid hazardous activities such as operating machinery or driving until temporary blurring subsides.

• Advise patients to ease photophobia by wearing dark glasses.

scopolamine hydrobromide

Isopto Hyoscine

Pregnancy Risk Category: C

HOW SUPPLIED

Ophthalmic solution: 0.25%

ACTION

Mechanism: Anticholinergic action leaves the pupil under unopposed adrenergic influence, causing it to dilate.

Onset: rapid. **Peak:** Mydriatic effect peaks within 15 to 30 minutes; cycloplegic effect, within 30 to 45 minutes.
Duration: up to 1 week.

INDICATIONS & DOSAGE

Cycloplegic refraction –
Adults: instill 1 to 2 drops of 0.25% solution 1 hour before refraction.
Children: instill 1 drop of 0.25% solution b.i.d. for 2 days before refraction.
Iritis, uveitis –
Adults: instill 1 to 2 drops of 0.25% solution daily b.i.d. or t.i.d.
Children: instill 1 drop once daily to t.i.d.

ADVERSE REACTIONS

CNS: ataxia, irritability, confusion, delirium, somnolence, acute psychotic reactions, hallucinations.
CV: tachycardia.
EENT: ocular congestion with prolonged use, conjunctivitis, *blurred vision,* eye dryness, increased intraocular pressure (IOP), *photophobia.*
GI: dry mouth.
Skin: dryness, contact dermatitis.
Other: flushing, fever.

INTERACTIONS

None significant.

CONTRAINDICATIONS

- Contraindicated in patients with shallow anterior chamber and acute angle-closure glaucoma.
- Use with extreme caution (if at all) in infants and small children.
- Use cautiously in patients with cardiac disease or increased IOP and in elderly patients.

NURSING CONSIDERATIONS

- Scopolamine may be used in patients sensitive to atropine because it's faster acting and has a shorter duration of action and fewer adverse reactions.
- Observe patients closely for adverse CNS effects (such as disorientation and delirium).
- Teach patients how to instill drug. Advise them to wash hands before and after instilling drug and to apply light finger-pressure on lacrimal sac for 1 minute after drops are instilled. Warn patients to avoid touching tip of dropper to eye or surrounding tissue.
- Warn patients to avoid hazardous activities such as operating machinery or driving until temporary blurring subsides.
- Advise patients to ease photophobia by wearing dark glasses.

tropicamide

Mydriacyl, Tropicacyl

Pregnancy Risk Category: C

HOW SUPPLIED

Ophthalmic solution: 0.5%, 1%

ACTION

Mechanism: The shortest-acting cycloplegic available, whose anticholinergic action leaves the pupil under unopposed adrenergic influence, causing it to dilate.

Onset: rapid. **Peak:** Mydriatic effect peaks within 20 to 40 minutes; cycloplegic effect, within 20 to 35 minutes.
Duration: up to 7 hours.

INDICATIONS & DOSAGE

Cycloplegic refraction –
Adults: instill 1 drop of 1% solution;

repeat in 5 minutes. If needed, instill additional drop in 20 to 30 minutes.
Children: instill 1 drop of 0.5% or 1% solution; repeat in 5 minutes, if needed.
Fundus examinations –
Adults and children: instill 1 to 2 drops of 0.5% solution in each eye 15 to 20 minutes before examination.

ADVERSE REACTIONS
CNS: ataxia, irritability, confusion, somnolence, hallucinations, behavioral disturbances in children.
EENT: *transient eye stinging on instillation,* increased intraocular pressure, *blurred vision, photophobia; dry throat.*
GI: dry mouth.
Skin: dryness.
Other: flushing, fever.

INTERACTIONS
None significant.

CONTRAINDICATIONS
- Contraindicated in patients with shallow anterior chamber and acute angle-closure glaucoma.
- Use cautiously in elderly patients.

NURSING CONSIDERATIONS
- Tropicamide's mydriatic effect is greater than its cycloplegic effect.
- Teach patients how to instill drug. Advise them to wash hands before and after instilling drug and to apply light finger-pressure on lacrimal sac for 1 minute after drops are instilled. Warn patients not to touch tip of dropper to eye or surrounding tissue.
- Warn patients that drug causes transient stinging.
- Warn patients to avoid hazardous activities such as operating machinery or driving until temporary blurring subsides.
- Advise patients to ease photophobia by wearing dark glasses.

83

Ophthalmic vasoconstrictors

naphazoline hydrochloride
tetrahydrozoline hydrochloride
zinc sulfate

COMBINATION PRODUCTS

ALBALON-A LIQUIFILM: naphazoline hydrochloride 0.05% and antazoline phosphate 0.5%.
BLEPHAMIDE LIQUIFILM SUSPENSION: phenylephrine hydrochloride 0.12%, sulfacetamide sodium 10%, and prednisolone acetate 0.2%.
EDTA: 1.4% polyvinyl alcohol, polysorbate 80, sodium thiosulfate, and benzalkonium chloride.
PHENYLZIN◇: zinc sulfate 0.25% and phenylephrine hydrochloride 0.12%.
PREFRIN-A: phenylephrine hydrochloride 0.12%, pyrilamine maleate 0.1%, and antipyrine 0.1%.
VASOCIDIN OPHTHALMIC OINTMENT: phenylephrine hydrochloride 0.125%, sulfacetamide sodium 10%, and prednisolone acetate 0.5%.
VASOCIDIN OPHTHALMIC SOLUTION: phenylephrine hydrochloride 0.125%, sulfacetamide sodium 10%, and prednisolone sodium phosphate 0.25%.
VASOCON-A OPHTHALMIC SOLUTION: naphazoline hydrochloride 0.05% and antazoline phosphate 0.5%.
ZINCFRIN◇: phenylephrine hydrochloride 0.12% and zinc sulfate 0.25%.

naphazoline hydrochloride

AK-Con, Albalon Liquifilm, Allerest◇, Clear Eyes◇, Degest 2◇, Estivin II, Naphcon◇, Naphcon Forte, Optazine‡, Vasoclear◇, Vasocon Regular

Pregnancy Risk Category: C

HOW SUPPLIED

Ophthalmic solution: 0.012%◇, 0.02%, 0.03%, 0.1%

ACTION

Mechanism: Causes vasoconstriction by local adrenergic action on the blood vessels of the conjunctiva.
Onset: 10 minutes. **Duration:** 2 to 6 hours.

INDICATIONS & DOSAGE

Ocular congestion, irritation, itching –
Adults: instill 1 to 3 drops of 0.1% solution q 3 to 4 hours or 1 to 2 drops of 0.012% to 0.03% solution up to q.i.d.

ADVERSE REACTIONS

CNS: headache, dizziness, nervousness, weakness.
EENT: transient eye stinging, pupillary dilation, eye irritation, photophobia, blurred vision, increased intraocular pressure.
GI: nausea.
Other: diaphoresis.

INTERACTIONS

Tricyclic antidepressants, MAO inhibitors: hypertensive crisis if naphazoline is systemically absorbed. Use together cautiously.

CONTRAINDICATIONS

- Contraindicated in patients hypersensitive to any of drug's ingredients, in patients with acute angle-closure glaucoma, and in children.
- Use cautiously in patients with hyperthyroidism, cardiac disease, hypertension, or diabetes mellitus and in elderly patients.

NURSING CONSIDERATIONS

- Most widely used ocular decongestant.
- Not recommended for use in infants and children; can produce marked sedation and coma if ingested.
- Teach patients how to instill drug. Advise them to wash hands before and after instilling drug and to apply light finger-pressure on lacrimal sac for 1 minute after drops are instilled. Warn them not to touch tip of dropper to eye or surrounding tissue.
- Warn patients not to exceed recommended dosage. Rebound congestion and conjunctivitis may occur with frequent or prolonged use.
- Tell patients to notify the doctor if photophobia, blurred vision, pain, or lid edema develops.
- Store in tightly closed container.

tetrahydrozoline hydrochloride

Murine Plus◇, Optigene◇, Soothe◇, Tetrasine◇, Visine◇

Pregnancy Risk Category: C

HOW SUPPLIED

Ophthalmic solution: 0.05%◇

ACTION

Mechanism: Causes vasoconstriction by local adrenergic action on the blood vessels of the conjunctiva.
Onset: within a few minutes. **Duration:** 4 to 8 hours.

INDICATIONS & DOSAGE

Ocular congestion, irritation, and allergic conditions –
Adults and children over 2 years: instill 1 to 2 drops of 0.05% solution b.i.d. or t.i.d. or as directed by the doctor.

ADVERSE REACTIONS

CNS: depression, headache, drowsiness, insomnia, dizziness, tremor.
CV: ***cardiac arrhythmias.***
EENT: transient eye stinging, pupillary dilation, increased intraocular pressure, eye irritation, iris floaters in elderly patients.

INTERACTIONS

Guanethidine, MAO inhibitors, tricyclic antidepressants: hypertensive crisis if tetrahydrozoline is systemically absorbed. Don't use together.

CONTRAINDICATIONS

- Contraindicated in patients hypersensitive to the drug or any of its components, in patients receiving MAO inhibitors, and in those with acute angle-closure glaucoma.
- Use cautiously in patients with hyperthyroidism, heart disease, hypertension, or diabetes mellitus and in elderly patients.

NURSING CONSIDERATIONS

- Teach patients how to instill drug. Advise them to wash hands before and after instilling drug and to apply light finger-pressure on lacrimal sac for 1 minute after drops are instilled. Warn them not to touch tip of dropper to eye or surrounding tissue.
- Caution patients not to share eye medications with others.
- Warn patients not to exceed recommended dosage. Rebound congestion may occur with frequent or prolonged use.
- Tell patients to stop drug and notify the doctor if redness or irritation persists or increases or if no relief occurs within 2 days.

zinc sulfate

Bufopto Zinc Sulfate◇, Eye-Sed Ophthalmic◇, Op-Thal-Zin◇

Pregnancy Risk Category: C

HOW SUPPLIED

Ophthalmic solution: 0.217%◇

ACTION

Mechanism: A decongestant astringent that causes astringent and weak antiseptic action on the conjunctiva.

Duration: 6 to 12 hours.

INDICATIONS & DOSAGE

Ocular congestion, irritation –

Adults and children: instill 1 to 2 drops of 0.217% solution b.i.d. or t.i.d.

ADVERSE REACTIONS

EENT: eye irritation.

INTERACTIONS

None significant.

CONTRAINDICATIONS

- Use cautiously in patients with shallow anterior chamber or predisposition to acute angle-closure glaucoma.

NURSING CONSIDERATIONS

- Teach patients how to instill drug. Advise them to wash hands before and after instilling drug and to apply light finger-pressure on lacrimal sac for 1 minute after drops are instilled. Warn them not to touch tip of dropper to eye or surrounding tissue.
- Tell patients to stop drug and notify the doctor if redness or irritation persists or increases or if no relief occurs within 3 days.
- Store in tightly closed container.

84

Miscellaneous ophthalmics

apraclonidine hydrochloride
artificial tears
betaxolol hydrochloride
botulinum toxin type A
dapiprazole hydrochloride
dipivefrin
eye irrigation solutions
fluorescein sodium
glycerin, anhydrous
isosorbide
levobunolol hydrochloride
levocabastine hydrochloride
lodoxamide tromethamine
metipranolol hydrochloride
sodium chloride, hypertonic
timolol maleate

COMBINATION PRODUCTS
FLURESS: fluorescein sodium 0.25% and benoxinate hydrochloride 0.4%.

apraclonidine hydrochloride
Iopidine

Pregnancy Risk Category: C

HOW SUPPLIED
Ophthalmic solution: 1%

ACTION
Mechanism: An alpha-adrenergic agonist that reduces intraocular pressure (IOP), possibly by decreasing production of aqueous humor.
Onset: within 1 hour. **Peak:** Peak effect occurs within 3 to 5 hours. **Duration:** at least 12 hours.

INDICATIONS & DOSAGE
Prevention or control of IOP elevation after argon laser trabeculoplasty or iridotomy –
Adults: instill 1 drop of 1% solution 1 hour before initiation of laser surgery on the anterior segment, followed by 1 drop immediately after surgery.

ADVERSE REACTIONS
CNS: insomnia, irritability, dream disturbances, headache.
CV: bradycardia, vasovagal attack, palpitations, hypotension, orthostatic hypotension.
EENT: upper eyelid elevation, conjunctival blanching and microhemorrhage, mydriasis, eye burning or discomfort, foreign body sensation in eye, eye dryness and itching, blurred vision, nasal burning or dryness, or increased pharyngeal secretions.
GI: abdominal pain, discomfort, diarrhea, vomiting, taste disturbances, dry mouth.
Skin: pruritus not associated with rash.
Other: sweaty palms, body heat sensation, decreased libido, extremity pain or numbness, allergic response.

INTERACTIONS
Topical pilocarpine or beta-adrenergic blockers: additive effects in lowering IOP. Use together cautiously.

CONTRAINDICATIONS
• Contraindicated in patients hypersensitive to apraclonidine or clonidine.

NURSING CONSIDERATIONS
• Closely monitor patients who tend to develop exaggerated decreases in IOP after drug therapy.
• Drug's systemic effects (altered heart rate and blood pressure) are uncommon after usual dose, but closely monitor patients with severe systemic disease, including hypertension.
• Observe patients closely for vasovagal attack during laser surgery.

artificial tears

Adsorbotear◇, Hypotears◇, Isopto Alkaline◇, Isopto Plain◇, Isopto Tears◇, Lacril◇, Lacrisert, Liquifilm Forte◇, Liquifilm Tears◇, Lyteers◇, Methulose◇, Moisture Drops◇, Neo-Tears◇, Refresh◇, Tearisol◇, Tears Naturale◇, Tears Plus◇, Ultra Tears◇, Visculose◇

Pregnancy Risk Category: C

HOW SUPPLIED

Ophthalmic solution: 2 ml◇, 15 ml◇, 30 ml◇
Ocular insert: 5 mg (hydroxypropyl cellulose)

ACTION

Mechanism: Augments insufficient tear production.
Onset: immediate.

INDICATIONS & DOSAGE

Insufficient tear production –
Adults and children: instill 1 to 2 drops of solution in eye t.i.d., q.i.d., or p.r.n.
Moderate to severe dry eye syndromes, including keratoconjunctivitis sicca –
Adults: insert 1 Lacrisert rod daily into inferior cul-de-sac. Some patients may require twice-daily use.

ADVERSE REACTIONS

EENT: eye discomfort; eye burning or pain on instillation; blurred vision (especially with Lacrisert); crust formation on eyelids and eyelashes in products with high viscosity, such as Adsorbotear, Isopto Tears, and Tearisol.

INTERACTIONS

Borate external irrigation solutions: may form gummy deposits on the lid when used with artificial tear products containing polyvinyl alcohol (Liquifilm Forte, Liquifilm Tears). Keep the patient's eyelids clean.

CONTRAINDICATIONS

- Contraindicated in patients hypersensitive to the drug or any of its components.
- Do not administer with contact lens in place unless product is designated for this use.

NURSING CONSIDERATIONS

- Teach patients how to instill product. Advise them to wash hands before and after instilling and to avoid touching tip of dropper or container to eye, surrounding tissue, or other surface.
- Instruct patients that product should be used by only one person to prevent the spread of infection.
- Lacrisert rod should be inserted with special applicator that is included in the package. Familiarize patient with included illustrated instructions.
- Tell patients to discontinue use and contact the doctor if condition worsens or does not improve.

betaxolol hydrochloride

Betoptic

Pregnancy Risk Category: C

HOW SUPPLIED

Ophthalmic solution: 0.5%
Ophthalmic suspension: 0.25%

ACTION

Mechanism: A cardioselective beta blocker that reduces formation and possibly increases outflow of aqueous humor.
Onset: ½ to 1 hour. **Peak:** Intraocular pressure (IOP) reduction peaks after a single dose within about 2 hours; with repeated use, within about 2 weeks. **Duration:** 12 or more hours.

INDICATIONS & DOSAGE

Chronic open-angle glaucoma and ocular hypertension –
Adults: instill 1 drop of 0.5% solu-

tion or 1 to 2 drops of 0.25% suspension b.i.d.

ADVERSE REACTIONS

CNS: insomnia, confusion.
EENT: *eye stinging upon instillation,* occasional tearing, photophobia.

INTERACTIONS

Calcium channel blockers: AV conduction disturbances, ventricular failure, and hypotension if significant systemic absorption occurs. Monitor closely.
Cocaine: may inhibit betaxolol's effects. Avoid concomitant use.
Digitalis glycosides: excessive bradycardia; patients may require ECG monitoring if significant systemic absorption occurs.
Inhalation hydrocarbon anesthetics: prolonged severe hypotension if significant systemic absorption occurs. Tell the anesthesiologist that the patient is receiving ophthalmic betaxolol.
Ophthalmic epinephrine, dipivefrin: may produce mydriasis. Use together cautiously.
Oral antidiabetic agents, insulin: risk of hypoglycemia or hyperglycemia if significant systemic absorption occurs. Dosage adjustments or hypoglycemic medication may be necessary.
Phenothiazines: additive hypotensive effects; increased risk of adverse effects if significant systemic absorption occurs. Monitor closely.
Reserpine: excessive beta blockade. Monitor closely.
Systemic beta blockers: additive effects. Monitor closely.

CONTRAINDICATIONS

- Contraindicated in patients with sinus bradycardia, greater-than-first-degree AV block, cardiogenic shock, or overt heart failure.
- Use cautiously in patients with restricted pulmonary function, diabetes mellitus, or a history of heart failure.

NURSING CONSIDERATIONS

- Encourage patients to comply with twice-daily dosage regimen.
- Some patients may need a few weeks' treatment to stabilize IOP-lowering response. Determine IOP after 4 weeks of treatment.
- Teach patients how to instill drug. Advise them to wash hands before and after instilling drug and to apply light finger-pressure on lacrimal sac for 1 minute after instillation. Warn patients not to touch tip of dropper to eye or surrounding tissue. Be sure to shake suspension well before instilling.
- Advise patients to ease photophobia by wearing dark glasses.

botulinum toxin type A

Botox

Pregnancy Risk Category: C

HOW SUPPLIED

Powder for injection: 100 units/vial

ACTION

Mechanism: A protein that produces a neuromuscular paralysis by binding to acetylcholine receptors on the motor end-plate and that may inhibit the release of acetylcholine from presynaptic nerve endings.
Onset: 1 or 2 days after injection.
Peak: Peak effect occurs within 1 to 2 weeks after a single injection. **Duration:** 2 to 6 weeks.

INDICATIONS & DOSAGE

Strabismus –
Adults and children 12 years and over: injections should be made only by doctors familiar with the technique, which involves surgical exposure of the region as well as electromyographic guidance of the injection needle.

Dosage varies with the degree of deviation (lower doses are used for small deviations). For vertical muscles and for horizontal strabismus of < 20 prism diopters, the usual dosage is 1.25 to 2.5 units injected into any one muscle. For horizontal strabismus of 20 to 50 prism diopters, dosage is 2.5 to 5 units into any one muscle. For persistent (greater than 1 month's duration) palsy of the sixth cranial nerve, dosage is 1.25 to 2.5 units into the medial rectus muscle.

Subsequent injections for recurrent or residual strabismus should not be made until 7 to 14 days after the initial dose and unless substantial function has returned to the injected and adjacent muscles. Dosage may be increased up to twice the initial dose for patients experiencing incomplete paralysis; subsequent doses in patients with adequate response should not be increased. The maximum single dose for any one muscle is 25 units.

Blepharospasm –
Adults: initially, 1.25 to 2.5 units injected into the medial and lateral pretarsal orbicularis oculi of the upper lid and into the lateral pretarsal orbicularis oculi of the lower lid. Effects should be apparent within 3 days and peak within 1 to 2 weeks. Dosage may be doubled if inadequate paralysis is achieved; however, exceeding 5 units/site produces no apparent benefit. Each treatment lasts about 3 months and can be repeated indefinitely.

Cumulative dosage should not exceed 200 units/month.

ADVERSE REACTIONS

EENT: double or blurred vision, spacial disorientation, *ptosis, vertical deviation* (after treatment of strabismus), *eye irritation* (after treatment of blepharospasm), *swelling of eyelid.*
Skin: diffuse rash, ecchymosis.

INTERACTIONS

None significant.

CONTRAINDICATIONS

- Contraindicated in patients hypersensitive to the drug or any of its components.

NURSING CONSIDERATIONS

- Have epinephrine readily available in case of an anaphylactic reaction.
- Reconstitute the drug with preservative-free 0.9% sodium chloride solution. The vacuum in the vial should be noticeable when reconstituting. Inject the diluent into the vial gently because severe agitation can denature the protein.
- Reconstituting with 1 ml of 0.9% sodium chloride solution produces a concentration of 10 units/0.1 ml; adding 2 ml yields 5 units/0.1 ml. Adding more diluent (such as 4 ml to produce 2.5 units/0.1 ml or 8 ml to yield 1.25 units/0.1 ml) or using different injection volumes may also be used to adjust dosage.
- Reconstituted drug should be clear, colorless, and free of particulate matter. Record the date and time of reconstitution. Keep reconstituted drug in the refrigerator until use. Administer within 4 hours of removal from the freezer.
- Several drops of an ocular decongestant and a topical anesthetic may be applied before treating strabismus.
- Prepare the injection by drawing slightly more volume than needed into a sterile 1-ml syringe. Expel air bubbles in the barrel of the syringe and attach an electromyographic injection needle (if treating strabismus), such as a 1.5-inch, 27G needle. Expel excess drug into an appropriate waste container while checking for leakage around the needle. Be sure to use a new needle and syringe for each injection.
- Freeze at or below 23° F (−5° C).
- Has been used investigationally to treat torticollis and some other spastic muscle disorders.

dapiprazole hydrochloride

Rēv-Eyes

Pregnancy Risk Category: B

HOW SUPPLIED

Ophthalmic powder: 25 mg/vial with 5 ml diluent and dropper supplied

ACTION

Mechanism: Blocks alpha-adrenergic receptors in smooth muscle, producing miosis through an effect on the dilator muscle of the iris.

Onset: rapid.

INDICATIONS & DOSAGE

Mydriasis –

Adults: instill 2 drops, followed in 5 minutes by another 2 drops.

ADVERSE REACTIONS

CNS: headache, browache.

EENT: *circumcorneal injection lasting 20 minutes,* eye burning on instillation, ptosis, lid erythema, lid edema, chemosis, eye itching or dryness, punctate keratitis, corneal edema, photophobia, tearing, blurry vision.

INTERACTIONS

None significant.

CONTRAINDICATIONS

- Contraindicated in patients hypersensitive to the drug or any of its components; when pupil constriction is undesirable, as in acute iritis; to reduce intraocular pressure (IOP); and to treat open-angle glaucoma.

NURSING CONSIDERATIONS

- Dapiprazole has no significant activity on ciliary muscle contraction, nor does it significantly alter IOP in normotensive eyes or in eyes with increased IOP. Eye color can affect the rate of pupillary constriction, but not the final pupil size.
- Do not use in same patient more than once per week.
- To prepare, remove and discard aluminum seals and rubber stoppers from both drug and diluent vials. Pour diluent into drug vial and attach dropper assembly. Shake vial to ensure mixing.
- To avoid contamination, do not touch dropper to any surface.
- Store at room temperature for 21 days. Discard any discolored solution.

dipivefrin

Propine

Pregnancy Risk Category: B

HOW SUPPLIED

Ophthalmic solution: 0.1%

ACTION

Mechanism: A prodrug of epinephrine, dipivefrin is converted to epinephrine in the eye. The liberated epinephrine appears to decrease aqueous production and increase aqueous outflow.

Onset: within 30 minutes. **Peak:** Peak effect occurs within 1 hour.

Duration: 12 hours or more.

INDICATIONS & DOSAGE

Intraocular pressure (IOP) reduction in chronic open-angle glaucoma –

Adults: for initial glaucoma therapy, instill 1 drop of 0.1% solution q 12 hours.

ADVERSE REACTIONS

CV: tachycardia, hypertension.

EENT: eye burning or stinging.

INTERACTIONS

Digitalis glycosides, inhalation hydrocarbon anesthetics, tricyclic antidepressants: increased risk of adverse cardiac effects if significant systemic absorption occurs. Monitor closely.

Ophthalmic beta blockers, osmotic agents, systemically administered car-

bonic anhydrase inhibitors: additive lowering of IOP. Use together cautiously. Monitor for potential adverse effects.
Systemic sympathomimetics: possible additive effects if significant systemic absorption occurs. Monitor closely.

CONTRAINDICATIONS
- Contraindicated in patients with acute angle-closure glaucoma.
- Use cautiously in patients with aphakia.

NURSING CONSIDERATIONS
- May have fewer adverse reactions than conventional epinephrine therapy.
- Often used concomitantly with other antiglaucoma drugs.
- Teach patients how to instill dipivefrin. Advise them to wash hands before and after instilling drug and to avoid touching tip of dropper to eye or surrounding tissue.

eye irrigation solutions

Blinx◇, Collyrium◇, Dacriose◇, Eye-Stream◇, I-Lite Eye Drops◇, Lauro Eye Wash◇, Lavoptik Eye Wash◇, Murine Eye Drops◇, Neo-Flo◇, Sterile 0.9% sodium chloride◇

HOW SUPPLIED
Ophthalmic solution: 15 ml◇, 30 ml◇, 120 ml◇, 180 ml◇

ACTION
Mechanism: Cleans the eye.
Onset: immediate.

INDICATIONS & DOSAGE
Eye irrigation –
Adults and children: flush eye with 1 to 2 drops t.i.d., q.i.d., or p.r.n.

ADVERSE REACTIONS
None reported.

INTERACTIONS
Products containing polyvinyl alcohol: may form gel and gummy deposits on the eye. Keep the patient's eyelids clean.

CONTRAINDICATIONS
- Contraindicated in patients hypersensitive to the drug or any of its components.

NURSING CONSIDERATIONS
- Instruct patients that product should be used by only one person to prevent the spread of infection.
- Teach patients how to instill solution. Advise them to wash hands before and after instilling solution and to avoid touching tip of container to eye, surrounding tissue, or other surface. Teach patients to turn their head to side, irrigating from inner to outer canthus.
- Store in tightly closed, light-resistant container. Check expiration date.

fluorescein sodium

Fluorescite, Fluor-I-Strip, Fluor-I-Strip A.T., Ful-Glo, Funduscein Injections

Pregnancy Risk Category: C

HOW SUPPLIED
Ophthalmic solution: 2%
Ophthalmic strips: 0.6 mg, 1 mg, 9 mg
Parenteral injection: 10%, 25%

ACTION
Mechanism: A water-soluble dye that produces an intense green fluorescence in alkaline solution (pH 5.0 or less) or a bright yellow if viewed under cobalt blue illumination.
Onset: immediate.

INDICATIONS & DOSAGE
Diagnostic in corneal abrasions and foreign bodies; fitting hard contact

lenses; lacrimal patency; fundus photography; applanation tonometry – **Adults and children:** instill 1 drop of 2% solution followed by irrigation; or moisten strip with sterile water, touch conjunctiva or fornix with moistened tip, and flush eye with irrigating solution. Patient should blink several times after application.
Retinal angiography –
Adults: 5 ml of 10% solution (500 mg) or 3 ml of 25% solution (750 mg) rapidly injected into antecubital vein.
Children: 0.077 ml of 10% solution (7.7 mg/kg body weight) or 0.044 ml of 25% solution (11 mg/kg body weight) rapidly injected into antecubital vein.

ADVERSE REACTIONS
Topical use:
EENT: eye stinging or burning, yellow tears.
Intravenous use:
CNS: headache persisting for 24 to 36 hours, dizziness, syncope, ***seizures.***
CV: hypotension, ***shock, cardiac arrest, thrombophlebitis.***
GI: nausea, vomiting.
GU: bright yellow urine (persists for 24 to 36 hours).
Skin: yellow skin discoloration (fades in 6 to 12 hours).
Other: hypersensitivity reactions, including urticaria and ***anaphylaxis;*** extravasation at injection site.

INTERACTIONS
None significant.

CONTRAINDICATIONS
- Use cautiously in patients with history of allergy or bronchial asthma.

NURSING CONSIDERATIONS
- Always use aseptic technique. Easily contaminated by *Pseudomonas aeruginosa.*
- Defects appear green under normal light or bright yellow under cobalt blue illumination. Foreign bodies are surrounded by a green ring. Similar lesions of the conjunctiva are delineated in orange-yellow.
- **I.V. use:** Keep an antihistamine, epinephrine, and oxygen available when giving parenterally.
- Warn patients that urine will be bright yellow after injection and that routine urinalysis will be abnormal within 1 hour after injection.
- Never instill dye while patients are wearing soft contact lenses; fluorescein will ruin them.
- Use topical anesthetic before instilling to relieve burning and irritation.
- Don't freeze; store below 80° F (26.7° C).

glycerin, anhydrous
Ophthalgan

Pregnancy Risk Category: C

HOW SUPPLIED
Ophthalmic solution: 7.5-ml containers

ACTION
Mechanism: Removes excess fluid from the cornea.
Onset: immediate.

INDICATIONS & DOSAGE
Corneal edema before ophthalmoscopy or gonioscopy in acute open-angle glaucoma and bullous keratitis –
Adults and children: instill 1 to 2 drops after instilling a local anesthetic.

ADVERSE REACTIONS
EENT: pain if instilled without topical anesthetic.

INTERACTIONS
None significant.

CONTRAINDICATIONS
- Contraindicated in patients hypersensitive to the drug.

NURSING CONSIDERATIONS

- Anhydrous glycerin is used to temporarily restore corneal transparency when cornea is too edematous to permit diagnosis.
- Use topical tetracaine or proparacaine before instilling to prevent discomfort.
- Don't touch tip of dropper to eye, surrounding tissue, or tear-film; anhydrous glycerin will absorb moisture.

isosorbide

Ismotic

Pregnancy Risk Category: C

HOW SUPPLIED

Oral solution: 45% (100 g/225 ml) in 220-ml containers

ACTION

Mechanism: Acts as an osmotic agent by promoting redistribution of water and thereby producing diuresis.
Onset: within 4 hours.

INDICATIONS & DOSAGE

Short-term reduction of intraocular pressure (IOP) caused by glaucoma –
Adults: initially, 1.5 g/kg P.O. Usual dosage range is 1 to 3 g/kg.

ADVERSE REACTIONS

CNS: vertigo, light-headedness, lethargy, headache, confusion.
GI: gastric discomfort, diarrhea, anorexia, nausea, vomiting.
Other: hypernatremia, hyperosmolality, thirst.

INTERACTIONS

None significant.

CONTRAINDICATIONS

- Contraindicated in patients with anuria caused by severe renal disease, severe dehydration, acute pulmonary edema, and hemorrhagic glaucoma.
- Give additional doses cautiously, especially in patients with diseases associated with sodium retention, such as CHF.

NURSING CONSIDERATIONS

- Isosorbide is especially useful for rapid reduction of IOP. May be used to interrupt acute attack of glaucoma before laser surgery.
- To improve palatability, pour medication over cracked ice and tell patients to sip it.
- Monitor patients closely for 5 to 10 minutes after administration.
- Tell patients that this drug may induce thirst. In patients with diseases associated with sodium retention, carefully monitor fluid and electrolyte balance.

levobunolol hydrochloride

Betagan

Pregnancy Risk Category: C

HOW SUPPLIED

Ophthalmic solution: 0.25%, 0.5%

ACTION

Mechanism: A nonselective beta blocker that reduces formation and possibly increases outflow of aqueous humor.
Onset: within 1 hour. **Peak:** Intraocular pressure (IOP) reduction peaks within 2 to 6 hours after a single dose; within 2 to 3 weeks after repeated use. **Duration:** up to 24 hours.

INDICATIONS & DOSAGE

Chronic open-angle glaucoma and ocular hypertension –
Adults: instill 1 to 2 drops once daily or b.i.d.

ADVERSE REACTIONS

CNS: headache, dizziness, depression.
CV: slight reduction in resting heart rate.
EENT: *transient eye stinging and*

burning; decreased corneal sensitivity with long-term use.
GI: nausea.
Skin: urticaria.
Other: evidence of beta blockade and systemic absorption *(hypotension, bradycardia, syncope, **asthmatic attacks in patients with a history of asthma,** and CHF).*

INTERACTIONS
Propranolol, metoprolol, and other oral beta-adrenergic blockers: increased ocular and systemic effect. Use together cautiously.
Reserpine and other catecholamine-depleting drugs: enhanced hypotensive and bradycardiac effects. Monitor closely.
Topical miotics, dipivefrin, epinephrine; systemically administered carbonic anhydrase inhibitors: additive lowered IOP. Use together cautiously.

CONTRAINDICATIONS
- Contraindicated in patients with bronchial asthma, a history of bronchial asthma or severe COPD; sinus bradycardia; second- or third-degree AV block; cardiac failure; and cardiogenic shock.
- Use cautiously in patients with chronic bronchitis and emphysema, diabetes mellitus, and hyperthyroidism.

NURSING CONSIDERATIONS
- Teach patients how to instill levobunolol. Advise them to wash hands before and after instilling drug and to apply light finger-pressure on lacrimal sac for 1 minute after drops are instilled. Warn patients not to touch dropper to eye or surrounding tissue.

levocabastine hydrochloride
Livostin
Pregnancy Risk Category: C

HOW SUPPLIED
Ophthalmic suspension: 0.5%

ACTION
Mechanism: Selectively blocks ophthalmic histamine H_1 receptors.
Duration: at least 2 hours.

INDICATIONS & DOSAGE
Temporary relief of seasonal allergic conjunctivitis –
Adults: instill 1 drop in each affected eye q.i.d. for up to 2 weeks.

ADVERSE REACTIONS
CNS: headache, fatigue, somnolence.
EENT: transient eye discomfort upon instillation (burning, stinging), eye discharge, dryness, pain, or redness; lacrimation; eyelid edema; visual disturbances; pharyngitis.
GI: dry mouth, nausea.
Respiratory: cough, dyspnea.
Skin: rash.

INTERACTIONS
None significant.

CONTRAINDICATIONS
- Contraindicated in patients hypersensitive to the drug or any of its components.
- Use cautiously in breast-feeding patients.

NURSING CONSIDERATIONS
- Teach patients how to instill levocabastine. Advise them to wash hands before and after instilling drug and to avoid touching tip of dropper to eye or surrounding tissue. Be sure to shake suspension well before instilling.
- Patients may experience transient discomfort or burning upon instillation. Tell them to contact the doctor if pain persists.
- Advise patients not to wear soft contact lenses during therapy.
- Store drug at room temperature; avoid freezing. Do not use if solution is discolored.

lodoxamide tromethamine

Alomide

Pregnancy Risk Category: B

HOW SUPPLIED

Ophthalmic solution: 0.1%

ACTION

Mechanism: Stabilizes mast cells and prevents the release of inflammation mediators.
Duration: elimination half-life, 8.5 hours.

INDICATIONS & DOSAGE

Vernal conjunctivitis, vernal keratoconjunctivitis, vernal keratitis –
Adults and children over 2 months: instill 1 to 2 drops in each affected eye q.i.d. for up to 3 months.

ADVERSE REACTIONS

CNS: headache, dizziness, somnolence.
EENT: transient eye discomfort upon instillation (burning, stinging); anterior chamber cells; blepharitis; blurred vision; chemosis; corneal erosion, ulcer, or abrasion; crystalline deposits; epitheliopathy; sensation of foreign body, stickiness, or warmth; hyperemia; keratitis; keratopathy; ocular edema, discharge, swelling, fatigue, itching, or allergy; pruritus; scales on eyelids or eyelash; tearing; dry nose.
GI: nausea, stomach discomfort.
Skin: rash.

INTERACTIONS

None significant.

CONTRAINDICATIONS

- Contraindicated in patients hypersensitive to the drug or any of its components.
- Use cautiously in breast-feeding patients.

NURSING CONSIDERATIONS

- Teach patients how to instill lodoxamide. Advise them to wash hands before and after instilling drug and to avoid touching tip of dropper to eye or surrounding tissue.
- Tell patients to contact the doctor if discomfort or burning persists upon instillation.
- Advise patients not to wear soft contact lenses during therapy.

metipranolol hydrochloride

OptiPranolol

Pregnancy Risk Category: C

HOW SUPPLIED

Ophthalmic solution: 0.3% in 5- or 10-ml dropper bottles

ACTION

Mechanism: A noncardioselective beta-adrenergic blocker. Exact ocular antihypertensive effect is unknown, but appears to reduce aqueous production and to reduce elevated and normal intraocular pressure (IOP) with or without glaucoma with little or no effect on pupil size or accommodation. IOP above 24 mm Hg is reduced an average of 20% to 26%.
Onset: 30 minutes. **Peak:** Peak effect occurs within about 2 hours. **Duration:** about 24 hours.

INDICATIONS & DOSAGE

IOP reduction in ocular conditions, including ocular hypertension and chronic open-angle glaucoma –
Adults: instill 1 drop into affected eye b.i.d. If IOP is not at a satisfactory level, concomitant therapy to lower it may be instituted.

ADVERSE REACTIONS

CNS: headache, anxiety, dizziness, depression, somnolence, nervousness, asthenia, browache.
CV: hypertension, ***MI,*** atrial fibrillation, angina, palpitation, bradycardia.

EENT: transient local eye discomfort, tearing, conjunctivitis, eyelid dermatitis, blurred vision, blepharitis, abnormal vision, photophobia, eye edema, rhinitis, epistaxis.
GI: nausea.
Respiratory: dyspnea, bronchitis, cough.
Skin: rash.
Other: hypersensitivity reactions, myalgia.

INTERACTIONS
Antithyroid agents, antihypertensives: increased risk of systemic metipranolol toxicity. Monitor closely.

CONTRAINDICATIONS
• Contraindicated in patients hypersensitive to the drug or any of its components and in patients with bronchial asthma, history of bronchial asthma or severe COPD, second- or third-degree AV block, cardiac failure, and cardiogenic shock.
• Use cautiously in patients with nonallergic bronchospasm, chronic bronchitis, emphysema, diabetes mellitus (especially in those subject to spontaneous hypoglycemia), hyperthyroidism, or cerebrovascular insufficiency.

NURSING CONSIDERATIONS
• A slight increase in outflow facility has been demonstrated with metipranolol. Like other noncardioselective beta-adrenergic blockers, metipranolol does not have significant local anesthetic (membrane-stabilizing) actions or intrinsic sympathomimetic activity.
• The efficacy of using more than one drop twice daily has not been proven. The normal eye can retain about 10 microliters of fluid, and the average dropper delivers 25 to 50 microliters/drop. If multiple drops are needed, the best interval between drops is 5 minutes.
• Pilocarpine, other miotics, or systemic carbonic anhydrase inhibitors may be administered concomitantly if IOP is not adequately controlled.
• Check expiration date on bottle before use. Do not use if eyedrops have changed color.
• Teach patients how to instill metapranolol. Instruct them to first wash hands thoroughly and then tilt back or lie down and gaze upward. Tell them to gently grasp lower eyelid below eyelashes and pull eyelid away from eye to form a pouch. Then have them place dropper directly over eye, avoiding contact with eye or any surface; look up just before applying drop; and look down for several seconds after instillation and slowly release eyelid. Tell patients to close eyes gently for 1 to 2 minutes and to apply gentle pressure to inside corner of eye at bridge of nose to retard draining of solution from intended area. Warm them not to rub eye or rinse dropper.

sodium chloride, hypertonic

Adsorbonac Ophthalmic Solution, Muro-128 Ointment, Sodium Chloride Ointment 5%

Pregnancy Risk Category: C

HOW SUPPLIED
Ophthalmic ointment: 5%
Ophthalmic solution: 2%, 5%

ACTION
Mechanism: An osmotic agent that removes excess fluid from the cornea.
Onset: immediate.

INDICATIONS & DOSAGE
Postoperative corneal edema after cataract extraction or corneal transplantation; trauma or bullous keratopathy –
Adults and children: instill 1 to 2 drops q 3 to 4 hours, or apply ointment h.s.

ADVERSE REACTIONS
EENT: slight eye stinging.
Other: hypersensitivity reactions.

INTERACTIONS
None significant.

CONTRAINDICATIONS
• Contraindicated in patients hypersensitive to the drug or any of its components.

NURSING CONSIDERATIONS
• If patients experience severe headache, pain, rapid change in vision, acute redness of eyes, sudden appearance of floating spots, pain on exposure to light, or double vision, drug should be discontinued.
• Tell patients to prevent caking on dropper bottle tip by putting a few drops of sterile irrigation solution inside bottle cap.
• Warn patients that ointment may cause blurred vision.
• Teach patients how to instill drug. Advise them to wash hands before and after instilling drug and to apply light finger-pressure on lacrimal sac for 1 minute after drops are instilled. Warn patients not to touch dropper to eye or surrounding tissue.
• Store in tightly closed container.

timolol maleate
Timoptic Solution
Pregnancy Risk Category: C

HOW SUPPLIED
Ophthalmic solution: 0.25%, 0.5%

ACTION
Mechanism: A beta blocker that reduces aqueous formation and possibly increases aqueous outflow.
Onset: within 30 minutes. **Peak:** Peak effect occurs within 1 to 5 hours. **Duration:** about 24 hours.

INDICATIONS & DOSAGE
Chronic open-angle, secondary, and aphakic glaucomas; ocular hypertension–
Adults: initially, instill 1 drop of 0.25% solution in each affected eye b.i.d.; maintenance dosage is 1 drop daily. If no response, instill 1 drop of 0.5% solution in each affected eye b.i.d. If intraocular pressure (IOP) is controlled, reduce dosage to 1 drop daily.

ADVERSE REACTIONS
CNS: headache, depression, fatigue.
CV: slight reduction in resting heart rate.
Eye: minor eye irritation, decreased corneal sensitivity with long-term use.
GI: anorexia.
Other: apnea in infants, *evidence of beta blockade and systemic absorption (hypotension, bradycardia, syncope,* ***asthmatic attacks in patients with a history of asthma,*** and *CHF).*

INTERACTIONS
Calcium channel blockers, digitalis glycosides, quinidine: increased risk of adverse cardiac effects if significant amounts of timolol are systemically absorbed. Use together cautiously.
Fentanyl, general anesthetics: excessive hypotension. Monitor closely.
Metoprolol tartrate, propranolol, other oral beta-adrenergic blockers: increased ocular and systemic effects. Use together cautiously.
Reserpine and other catecholamine-depleting drugs: enhanced hypotensive and bradycardiac effects. Avoid concurrent use.

CONTRAINDICATIONS
• Contraindicated in patients hypersensitive to the drug.
• Use cautiously in patients with bronchial asthma, sinus bradycardia, second- or third-degree heart block,

cardiogenic shock, right ventricular failure resulting from pulmonary hypertension, CHF, severe cardiac disease, and in infants with congenital glaucoma.

NURSING CONSIDERATIONS

- Some patients may need a few weeks' treatment to stabilize pressure-lowering response. Determine IOP after 4 weeks of treatment.
- Can be used safely in patients with glaucoma who wear conventional hard contact lenses.
- Systemic beta-blocking effects can mask some signs of hypoglycemia in diabetic patients. Monitor these patients carefully.
- Teach patients how to instill timolol. Advise them to wash hands before and after instilling drug and to apply light finger-pressure on lacrimal sac for 1 minute after drops are instilled. Warn patients not to touch dropper to eye or surrounding tissue.

85
Otics

acetic acid
boric acid
carbamide peroxide
chloramphenicol
triethanolamine polypeptide oleate-condensate

COMBINATION PRODUCTS
BOROFAIR OTIC: acetic acid 2% and aluminum acetate 2%.
COLY-MYCIN S OTIC: each ml contains neomycin SO_4 3.3 mg, colistin SO_4 3 mg, hydrocortisone acetate 10 mg, and thonzonium bromide 0.05%.
CORTISPORIN OTIC: each ml contains neomycin SO_4 5 mg, polymyxin B 10,000 units, and hydrocortisone 1%.
TRI-OTIC: each ml contains chloroxylenol 1 mg, pramoxine hydrochloride 10 mg, and hydrocortisone 10 mg.
OTOCORT: polymyxin B sulfate equal to 10,000 units of polymyxin B; hydrocortisone 1% 10 mg; neomycin sulfate equal to 3.5 mg of neomycin base.

acetic acid
Domeboro Otic, VoSol Otic

Pregnancy Risk Category: C

HOW SUPPLIED
Otic solution: 2% acetic acid in aluminum acetate solution (Domeboro Otic), 2% acetic acid with 3% propylene glycol diacetate (VoSol Otic)

ACTION
Mechanism: Inhibits or destroys bacteria in the ear canal.
Onset: 15 to 30 minutes.

INDICATIONS & DOSAGE
External ear canal infection –
Adults and children: instill 4 to 6 drops into ear canal t.i.d. or q.i.d.; or insert saturated wick for first 24 hours, then continue with instillations.
Prophylaxis of swimmer's ear –
Adults and children: 2 drops in each ear b.i.d.

ADVERSE REACTIONS
EENT: ear irritation, and itching.
Skin: urticaria.
Other: overgrowth of nonsusceptible organisms.

INTERACTIONS
None significant.

CONTRAINDICATIONS
• Use cautiously in patients with perforated eardrum.

NURSING CONSIDERATIONS
• Has anti-infective, anti-inflammatory, and antipruritic effects. *Pseudomonas aeruginosa* is particularly sensitive to this drug.
• Reculture any persistent drainage.
• Warn patients to avoid touching ear with dropper to prevent reinfection.

boric acid
Aurocaine 2◇, Auro-Dri◇, Dri/Ear◇, Ear-Dry◇

Pregnancy Risk Category: C

HOW SUPPLIED
Otic solution: 2.75% boric acid in isopropyl alcohol

ACTION
Mechanism: Weak bacteriostatic that inhibits or destroys bacteria in the ear canal; also is a fungistatic agent.
Onset: 15 to 30 minutes.

INDICATIONS & DOSAGE
External ear canal infection –
Adults and children: 3 to 6 drops into ear canal; plug with cotton. Repeat t.i.d. or q.i.d.

ADVERSE REACTIONS
EENT: ear irritation or ear itching.
Skin: urticaria.
Other: overgrowth of nonsusceptible organisms.

INTERACTIONS
None significant.

CONTRAINDICATIONS
- Contraindicated in patients with a perforated eardrum or excoriated membranes in ear.

NURSING CONSIDERATIONS
- Watch for signs of superinfection (continual pain, inflammation, fever).
- Tell patients using cotton plug to always moisten with medication.
- Warn patients to avoid touching ear with dropper to prevent reinfection.

carbamide peroxide
Debrox◇

Pregnancy Risk Category: C

HOW SUPPLIED
Otic solution: 6.5% carbamide in glycerin or glycerin and propylene glycol

ACTION
Mechanism: A ceruminolytic that emulsifies and disperses accumulated cerumen.
Onset: 15 to 30 minutes.

INDICATIONS & DOSAGE
Impacted cerumen –
Adults and children: 5 to 10 drops into ear canal b.i.d. Allow solution to remain in ear canal for 15 to 30 minutes; remove with warm water.

ADVERSE REACTIONS
None reported.

INTERACTIONS
None significant.

CONTRAINDICATIONS
- Contraindicated in patients with a perforated eardrum.
- Use in children under 12 years only under a doctor's direction.

NURSING CONSIDERATIONS
- Tell patients to call the doctor if redness, pain, or swelling persists.
- Warn patients to avoid touching ear with dropper to prevent reinfection.
- Tell patients to flush ear gently with warm water, using a rubber bulb syringe.

chloramphenicol
Chloromycetin Otic, Sopamycetin†

Pregnancy Risk Category: C

HOW SUPPLIED
Otic solution: 0.5%

ACTION
Mechanism: Inhibits or destroys bacteria in the ear canal.
Onset: 15 to 30 minutes.

INDICATIONS & DOSAGE
External ear canal infection –
Adults and children: 2 to 3 drops into ear canal t.i.d.

ADVERSE REACTIONS
EENT: ear itching or burning, sore throat.
Skin: pruritus, urticaria, vesicular or maculopapular dermatitis, angioedema.
Other: overgrowth of nonsusceptible organisms, burning.

INTERACTIONS
None significant.

CONTRAINDICATIONS
• Contraindicated in patients with a perforated eardrum.

NURSING CONSIDERATIONS
• Obtain history of use and reaction to drug.
• Watch for signs of superinfection (continued pain, inflammation, fever). Avoid prolonged use.
• Reculture any persistent drainage.
• Watch for signs of sore throat (early sign of toxicity).
• Warn patients to avoid touching ear with dropper to avoid reinfection.

triethanolamine polypeptide oleate-condensate
Cerumenex

Pregnancy Risk Category: C

HOW SUPPLIED
Otic solution: 10% in 6-ml, 12-ml bottles with droppers

ACTION
Mechanism: A ceruminolytic that emulsifies and disperses accumulated cerumen.
Onset: 15 to 30 minutes.

INDICATIONS & DOSAGE
Impacted cerumen –
Adults and children: fill ear canal with solution and insert cotton plug. After 15 to 30 minutes, flush ear with warm water.

ADVERSE REACTIONS
EENT: ear erythema or pruritus.
Skin: severe eczema.

INTERACTIONS
None significant.

CONTRAINDICATIONS
• Contraindicated in perforated eardrum, otitis media, and otitis externa.

NURSING CONSIDERATIONS
• If you suspect hypersensitivity, do patch test by placing 1 drop of drug on inner forearm; cover with small bandage. Read results in 24 hours. If any reaction (redness, swelling) occurs, don't use drug.
• Advise patients to discontinue the drug if adverse reactions occur and to contact the doctor immediately.
• Warn patients that this medication is for use only in the ears.
• Tell patients not to use drops more often than prescribed.
• Teach patients how to apply the drug. Moisten cotton plug with medication before insertion. Leave cotton in place for a maximum of 30 minutes. Flush ear gently with warm water, using a rubber bulb syringe.
• Keep container tightly closed and away from moisture.

Nasal agents

beclomethasone dipropionate
budesonide
dexamethasone sodium phosphate
ephedrine sulfate
epinephrine hydrochloride
flunisolide
naphazoline hydrochloride
oxymetazoline hydrochloride
phenylephrine hydrochloride
tetrahydrozoline hydrochloride
xylometazoline hydrochloride

COMBINATION PRODUCTS
4-WAY NASAL SPRAY◊: phenylephrine hydrochloride 0.5%, naphazoline hydrochloride 0.05%, and pyrilamine maleate 0.2%.

beclomethasone dipropionate

Aldecin Aqueous Nasal Spray, Beconase AQ Nasal Spray, Beconase Nasal Inhaler, Vancenase AQ Nasal Spray, Vancenase Nasal Inhaler

Pregnancy Risk Category: C

HOW SUPPLIED
Nasal aerosol: 42 mcg/metered spray, 50 mcg/metered spray‡
Nasal spray: 0.042%, 50 mcg/metered spray‡

ACTION
Mechanism: A corticosteroid that decreases nasal inflammation, mainly by stabilizing leukocyte lysosomal membranes.
Duration: 6 to 12 hours.

INDICATIONS & DOSAGE
Relief of symptoms of seasonal or perennial rhinitis; prevention of recurrence of nasal polyps after surgical removal–
Adults and children over 12 years: usual dosage is 1 spray (42 mcg) in each nostril b.i.d. to q.i.d. (total dosage 168 to 336 mcg daily). Most patients require 1 spray in each nostril t.i.d. (252 mcg daily).

ADVERSE REACTIONS
CNS: headache.
EENT: *mild transient nasal burning and stinging,* nasal congestion, sneezing, epistaxis, watery eyes, nasopharyngeal fungal infections.
GI: nausea, vomiting.

INTERACTIONS
None significant.

CONTRAINDICATIONS
- Contraindicated in patients hypersensitive to the drug.
- Use cautiously, if at all, in patients with active or quiescent respiratory tract tubercular infections or untreated fungal, bacterial, or systemic viral or ocular herpes simplex infections. Also use cautiously in patients who have recently had nasal septal ulcers, nasal surgery, or trauma.

NURSING CONSIDERATIONS
- Warn the patient not to exceed recommended dosages because doing so will not suppress hypothalamic-pituitary-adrenal function.
- Beclomethasone is not effective for acute exacerbations. Decongestants or antihistamines may be needed.
- Advise the patient to use drug regularly as prescribed because its effectiveness depends on regular use.
- Explain that the drug's therapeutic effects, unlike those of decongestants, are not immediate. Most patients

achieve benefit within a few days, but some may require 2 to 3 weeks.
• Tell the patient to notify the doctor if symptoms don't improve within 3 weeks or if nasal irritation persists.
• Observe the patient for fungal infections.
• Teach the patient good nasal and oral hygiene.
• To instill, instruct the patient to shake the container before using; to blow nose to clear nasal passages; and to tilt head slightly forward and insert nozzle into nostril, pointing away from septum. Tell him to hold the other nostril closed and then to inspire gently and spray. Next, have him shake the container again and repeat in the other nostril.
• The nasal spray pump should be pumped three or four times before the first use, and once or twice before first use each day. The cap and nosepiece of the activator should be cleaned in warm water every day, then allowed to air dry.

budesonide

Rhinocort

Pregnancy Risk Category: C

HOW SUPPLIED

Nasal spray: 32 mcg/metered spray (7-g canister)

ACTION

Mechanism: A corticosteroid that decreases nasal inflammation, mainly by inhibiting the activities of specific cells and the mediators involved in the allergic response.
Duration: 12 to 24 hours.

INDICATIONS & DOSAGE

Symptoms of seasonal or perennial allergic rhinitis –
Adults and children over 6 years: 2 sprays in each nostril in the morning and evening or 4 sprays in each nostril in the morning. Maintenance dosage should be the fewest number of sprays needed to control symptoms.

ADVERSE REACTIONS

CNS: nervousness.
EENT: *nasal irritation, epistaxis, pharyngitis,* reduced sense of smell, nasal pain, hoarseness.
GI: bad taste, dry mouth, dyspepsia, nausea.
Respiratory: *cough,* moniliasis, wheezing, dyspnea.
Skin: facial edema, rash, pruritus, contact dermatitis.
Other: myalgia, hypersensitivity reactions.

INTERACTIONS

None significant.

CONTRAINDICATIONS

• Contraindicated in patients hypersensitive to the drug or any of its components and in those who have had recent septal ulcers, nasal surgery, or nasal trauma until total healing has occurred.
• Use cautiously in patients with tuberculous infections; untreated fungal, bacterial, or systemic viral infections; or ocular herpes simplex.

NURSING CONSIDERATIONS

• Tell the patient to contact the doctor if symptoms do not improve in 3 weeks or if condition worsens.
• Warn the patient not to exceed prescribed dosage or use for long periods of time because of the risk of hypothalamic-pituitary-adrenal axis suppression.
• To instill, instruct the patient to shake the container before using; to blow nose to clear nasal passages; and to tilt head slightly forward and insert nozzle into nostril, pointing away from septum. Tell him to hold the other nostril closed and then to inspire gently and spray. Next, have him shake container again and repeat in the other nostril.

• Teach the patient good nasal and oral hygiene.
• Instruct the patient that the product should be used by one person only to prevent the spread of infection.
• Advise the patient not to break, incinerate, or store canister in extreme heat; contents under pressure.

dexamethasone sodium phosphate

Decadron Phosphate Turbinaire

Pregnancy Risk Category: C

HOW SUPPLIED

Nasal aerosol: 100 mcg/metered spray, 170 doses/canister

ACTION

Mechanism: Decreases nasal inflammation, mainly by stabilizing leukocyte lysosomal membranes.
Duration: 6 to 8 hours.

INDICATIONS & DOSAGE

Allergic or inflammatory conditions, nasal polyps –
Adults: 2 sprays in each nostril b.i.d. or t.i.d. Maximum dosage is 12 sprays daily.
Children 6 to 12 years: 1 or 2 sprays in each nostril b.i.d. Maximum 8 sprays daily.

Each spray delivers 0.1 mg dexamethasone sodium phosphate equal to 0.084 mg dexamethasone.

ADVERSE REACTIONS

EENT: nasal irritation, dryness, rebound nasal congestion.
Other: hypersensitivity reactions, systemic effects with prolonged use (pituitary-adrenal suppression, sodium retention, ***CHF,*** hypertension, hypokalemia, headaches, ***seizures,*** peptic ulceration, ecchymoses, petechiae, masking of infection).

INTERACTIONS

None significant.

CONTRAINDICATIONS

• Contraindicated in breast-feeding patients (systemic absorption can occur) and in cutaneous tuberculosis and fungal and herpetic lesions.
• Use cautiously in patients with diabetes mellitus, peptic ulceration, or tuberculosis.

NURSING CONSIDERATIONS

• Underlying bacterial infection should be controlled with anti-infectives. Notify the doctor if you suspect an infection.
• Irritation or sensitivity may require stopping drug.
• Fluid retention can occur from systemic absorption.
• Don't break, incinerate, or store canister in extreme heat; contents under pressure.
• To instill, instruct the patient to shake the container before using; to blow nose to clear nasal passages; and to tilt head slightly forward and insert nozzle into nostril, pointing away from septum. Tell him to hold the other nostril closed and then to inspire gently and spray. Next, have him shake container again and repeat in the other nostril.
• Teach the patient good nasal and oral hygiene.
• Warn the patient that product should be used by only one person to prevent spread of infection.
• Hypertension and hypokalemia can occur with systemic absorption. Frequently monitor blood pressure and serum potassium level. Advise the patient to contact the doctor if he experiences fever, joint or muscle aches, or extreme tiredness.
• Gradually reduce dosage as nasal condition improves.
• Warn the patient to avoid prolonged use because of the risk of hypothalamic-pituitary-adrenal-axis suppression.

ephedrine sulfate

Vicks Vatronol Nose Drops◊

Pregnancy Risk Category: C

HOW SUPPLIED

Nasal solution: 0.5%◊

ACTION

Mechanism: Causes local vasoconstriction of dilated arterioles, reducing blood flow and nasal congestion.
Duration: up to 6 hours.

INDICATIONS & DOSAGE

Nasal congestion –
Adults and children: Instill 3 to 4 drops of 0.5% solution into each nostril. Use no more frequently than q 4 hours.

ADVERSE REACTIONS

CNS: nervousness, excitation.
CV: *tachycardia.*
EENT: rebound nasal congestion with long-term or excessive use.
Other: mucosal irritation.

INTERACTIONS

MAO inhibitors: hypertensive crisis if ephedrine is absorbed. Don't use together.

CONTRAINDICATIONS

- Use cautiously in patients with hyperthyroidism, coronary artery disease, hypertension, or diabetes mellitus.

NURSING CONSIDERATIONS

- Tell patients not to exceed recommended dosage and use only when needed.
- Teach patients how to instill nosedrops.
- Instruct patients that product should be used by only one person to prevent spread of infection.

epinephrine hydrochloride

Adrenalin Chloride

Pregnancy Risk Category: C

HOW SUPPLIED

Nasal solution: 0.1%

ACTION

Mechanism: Causes local vasoconstriction of dilated arterioles, reducing blood flow and nasal congestion.
Onset: within 5 minutes. **Duration:** 1 hour or less.

INDICATIONS & DOSAGE

Nasal congestion, local superficial bleeding –
Adults and children: instill 1 or 2 drops of solution.

ADVERSE REACTIONS

CNS: nervousness, excitation.
CV: *tachycardia.*
EENT: rebound nasal congestion, slight sting upon application.

INTERACTIONS

None significant.

CONTRAINDICATIONS

- Use cautiously in patients with hyperthyroidism, coronary artery disease, hypertension, or diabetes mellitus.

NURSING CONSIDERATIONS

- Tell patients not to exceed recommended dosage and to use only when needed.
- Teach patients how to instill nosedrops.
- Instruct patients that product should be used by only one person to prevent spread of infection.

flunisolide

Nasalide, Rhinalar Nasal Mist‡

Pregnancy Risk Category: C

HOW SUPPLIED
Nasal inhalant: 25 mcg/metered spray, 200 doses/bottle‡
Nasal solution: 0.25 mg/ml in pump spray bottle

ACTION
Mechanism: Decreases nasal inflammation, mainly by stabilizing leukocyte lysosomal membranes.
Duration: about 12 hours.

INDICATIONS & DOSAGE
Symptoms of seasonal or perennial rhinitis –
Adults: starting dose is 2 sprays (50 mcg) in each nostril b.i.d. Total daily dosage is 200 mcg. If necessary, dosage may be increased to 2 sprays in each nostril t.i.d. Maximum total daily dosage is 8 sprays in each nostril (400 mcg daily).
Children 6 to 14 years: starting dose is 1 spray (25 mcg) in each nostril t.i.d. or 2 sprays (50 mcg) in each nostril b.i.d. Total daily dosage is 150 to 200 mcg. Maximum total daily dosage is 4 sprays in each nostril (200 mcg daily).

ADVERSE REACTIONS
CNS: headache.
EENT: *mild, transient nasal burning and stinging,* nasal congestion, nasopharyngeal fungal infection, sneezing, epistaxis, watery eyes.
GI: nausea, vomiting.

INTERACTIONS
None significant.

CONTRAINDICATIONS
- Contraindicated in patients hypersensitive to the drug.
- Use cautiously, if at all, in patients with active or quiescent respiratory tract tubercular infections or in untreated fungal, bacterial, or systemic viral or ocular herpes simplex infections. Also use cautiously in patients who have recently had nasal septal ulcers, nasal surgery, or nasal trauma.

NURSING CONSIDERATIONS
- Advise patients to use drug regularly, as prescribed, because its effectiveness depends on regular use.
- Explain that the drug's therapeutic effects, unlike those of decongestants, are not immediate. Most patients achieve benefit within a few days, but some may require 2 to 3 weeks.
- Warn patients not to exceed recommended dosage to avoid suppression of hypothalamic-pituitary-adrenal function. Warn patients not to exceed this dosage.
- Flunisolide is not effective for acute exacerbations. Decongestants or antihistamines may be needed.
- Patients with dryness and crusting of the nasal mucosa may prefer the liquid spray of flunisolide to the aerosolized powder of beclomethasone.
- Tell patients to stop drug and notify the doctor if symptoms don't improve within 3 weeks or if nasal irritation persists.
- To instill, instruct patients to shake the container before using; to blow nose to clear nasal passages; and to tilt head slightly forward and insert nozzle into nostril, pointing away from septum. Tell them to hold the other nostril closed, and then to inspire gently and spray. Next, have them shake container again and repeat in the other nostril. Tell patients to clean nosepiece with warm water if it becomes clogged.

naphazoline hydrochloride
Privine◇

Pregnancy Risk Category: C

HOW SUPPLIED
Nasal drops: 0.05% solution
Nasal spray: 0.05% solution

ACTION
Mechanism: Causes local vasoconstriction of dilated arterioles, reducing blood flow and nasal congestion.
Onset: within 10 minutes. **Duration:** 2 to 6 hours.

INDICATIONS & DOSAGE
Nasal congestion –
Adults: apply 2 drops or sprays of 0.05% solution to nasal mucosa q 3 to 4 hours.
Children 6 to 12 years: apply 1 to 2 drops or sprays; repeat q 3 to 6 hours, p.r.n. Use no longer than 3 to 5 days.

ADVERSE REACTIONS
EENT: rebound nasal congestion with excessive or long-term use, sneezing, stinging, dryness of mucosa.
Other: systemic effects in children after excessive or long-term use, marked sedation.

INTERACTIONS
None significant.

CONTRAINDICATIONS
- Contraindicated in patients with acute angle-closure glaucoma.
- Use cautiously in patients with hyperthyroidism, heart disease, hypertension, or diabetes mellitus.

NURSING CONSIDERATIONS
- Warn patients not to exceed recommended dosage.
- Teach patients how to apply. For nasal drops, instruct patients to tilt head back as far as possible, instill drops, then lean head forward while inhaling and to repeat procedure for other nostril. For nasal spray, instruct patients to hold spray container and head upright. Tell patients not to shake the container.
- Instruct patients that product should be used by only one person to prevent spread of infection.
- Tell patients to contact the doctor if nasal congestion persists after 5 days.

oxymetazoline hydrochloride

Afrin◇, Afrin Children's Strength Nose Drops◇, Allerest 12-Hour Nasal◇, Chlorphed-LA◇, Coricidin Nasal Mist◇, Dristan Long Lasting◇, Drixine Nasal‡, Duramist Plus◇, Duration◇, 4-Way Long-Acting Nasal, Genasal Spray◇, Neo-Synephrine 12 Hour◇, Nostrilla◇, NTZ Long Acting Nasal◇, Sinarest 12-Hour◇, Sinex Long-Acting◇, Twice-A-Day Nasal◇

Pregnancy Risk Category: C

HOW SUPPLIED
Nasal solution: 0.025%◇, 0.05%◇

ACTION
Mechanism: Causes local vasoconstriction of dilated arterioles, reducing blood flow and nasal congestion.
Onset: 5 to 10 minutes. **Peak:** Peak effect occurs within 6 hours. **Duration:** less than 12 hours.

INDICATIONS & DOSAGE
Nasal congestion –
Adults and children over 6 years: apply 2 to 4 drops or sprays of 0.05% solution to nasal mucosa b.i.d.
Children 2 to 6 years: apply 2 to 3 drops of 0.025% solution to nasal mucosa b.i.d. Use no longer than 3 to 5 days. Dosage for younger children has not been established.

ADVERSE REACTIONS
CNS: headache, drowsiness, dizziness, insomnia, possible sedation.
CV: palpitations, ***CV collapse,*** hypertension.
EENT: rebound nasal congestion or irritation with excessive or long-term use, dryness of nose and throat, in-

creased nasal discharge, stinging, sneezing.
Other: systemic effects in children with excessive or long-term use.

INTERACTIONS
None significant.

CONTRAINDICATIONS
- Use cautiously in patients with hyperthyroidism, cardiac disease, hypertension, or diabetes mellitus.

NURSING CONSIDERATIONS
- Tell patients not to exceed recommended dosage and to use only when needed.
- Warn patients that excessive use may cause bradycardia, hypotension, dizziness, and weakness.
- Teach patients how to apply oxymetazoline. Tell them to hold head upright to minimize swallowing of medication, then sniff spray briskly.
- Instruct patients that product should be used by only one person to prevent spread of infection.

phenylephrine hydrochloride
Alconefrin 12◇, Alconefrin 25◇, Alconefrin 50◇, Doktors◇, Duration◇, Neo-Synephrine◇, Nostril◇, Rhinall◇, Rhinall-10◇, Sinex◇, St. Joseph Measured Dose Nasal Decongestant◇

Pregnancy Risk Category: C

HOW SUPPLIED
Nasal jelly: 0.5%
Nasal solution: 0.125%, 0.16%, 0.2%, 0.25%, 0.5%, 1%

ACTION
Mechanism: Causes local vasoconstriction of dilated arterioles, reducing blood flow and nasal congestion.
Onset: rapid. **Duration:** ½ to 4 hours.

INDICATIONS & DOSAGE
Nasal congestion –
Adults: apply 1 to 2 drops or sprays of 0.125% to 1% solution or small amount of jelly to nasal mucosa q 4 hours, p.r.n.
Children under 6 years: apply 2 to 3 drops or sprays of 0.125% solution q 4 hours, p.r.n.
Children 6 to 12 years: apply 1 to 2 drops or sprays of 0.25% solution q 4 hours, p.r.n.

ADVERSE REACTIONS
CNS: headache, tremor, dizziness, nervousness.
CV: *palpitations, tachycardia, PVCs,* hypertension, pallor.
EENT: transient burning or stinging, dryness of nasal mucosa, rebound nasal congestion with continued use.
GI: nausea.

INTERACTIONS
None significant.

CONTRAINDICATIONS
- Contraindicated in patients with acute angle-closure glaucoma.
- Use cautiously in patients with hyperthyroidism, hypertension, diabetes mellitus, or ischemic cardiac disease.

NURSING CONSIDERATIONS
- Tell patients not to exceed recommended dosage and to use only when needed.
- Advise patients to contact the doctor if symptoms persist beyond 3 days.
- Teach patients how to apply phenylephrine. Tell them to hold head upright to minimize swallowing of medication, then sniff spray briskly.
- Instruct patients that product should be used by only one person to prevent spread of infection.

tetrahydrozoline hydrochloride

Tyzine Drops, Tyzine Pediatric Drops

Pregnancy Risk Category: C

HOW SUPPLIED

Nasal solution: 0.05%, 0.1%

ACTION

Mechanism: Causes local vasoconstriction of dilated arterioles, reducing blood flow and nasal congestion.
Onset: within a few minutes. **Duration:** 4 to 8 hours.

INDICATIONS & DOSAGE

Nasal congestion –
Adults and children over 6 years: apply 2 to 4 drops of 0.1% solution or spray to nasal mucosa q 4 to 6 hours, p.r.n.
Children 2 to 6 years: apply 2 to 3 drops of 0.05% solution to nasal mucosa q 4 to 6 hours, p.r.n.

ADVERSE REACTIONS

EENT: transient burning, stinging; sneezing, rebound nasal congestion in excessive or long-term use.

INTERACTIONS

None significant.

CONTRAINDICATIONS

- Contraindicated in children under 2 years and in patients with acute angle-closure glaucoma. The 0.1% solution is contraindicated in children under 6 years.
- Use cautiously in patients with hyperthyroidism, hypertension, and diabetes mellitus.

NURSING CONSIDERATIONS

- Tell patients not to exceed recommended dosage and to use only as needed for 3 to 5 days.
- Teach patients how to apply tetrahydrozoline. Tell them to hold head upright to minimize swallowing of medication, then sniff spray briskly.
- Instruct patients that product should be used by only one person to prevent spread of infection.

xylometazoline hydrochloride

4-Way Long Acting, Neo-Synephrine II, Otrivin, Sine-Off Nasal Spray, Sinex-L.A.

Pregnancy Risk Category: C

HOW SUPPLIED

Nasal solution: 0.05%, 0.1%

ACTION

Mechanism: Causes local vasoconstriction of dilated arterioles, reducing blood flow and nasal congestion.
Onset: 5 to 10 minutes. **Duration:** 5 to 6 hours.

INDICATIONS & DOSAGE

Nasal congestion –
Adults and children over 12 years: apply 2 to 3 drops or 1 to 2 sprays of 0.1% solution to nasal mucosa q 8 to 10 hours.
Children 6 months to 12 years: apply 2 to 3 drops or 1 spray of 0.05% solution to nasal mucosa q 8 to 10 hours.
Infants under 6 months: instill 1 drop of 0.05% solution into each nostril q 6 hours p.r.n.

ADVERSE REACTIONS

EENT: transient burning, stinging; dryness or ulceration of nasal mucosa; sneezing; rebound nasal congestion or irritation with excessive or long-term use.

INTERACTIONS

None significant.

CONTRAINDICATIONS

- Contraindicated in patients with acute angle-closure glaucoma.

• Use cautiously in patients with hyperthyroidism, cardiac disease, hypertension, diabetes mellitus, and advanced arteriosclerosis.

NURSING CONSIDERATIONS

• Tell patients not to exceed recommended dose and to use only as needed for 3 to 5 days.
• Teach patients how to apply xylometazoline. Have patients hold head upright to minimize swallowing of medication, then sniff spray briskly.
• Instruct patients that product should be used by only one person to prevent spread of infection.

87

Local anti-infectives

acyclovir
amphotericin B
bacitracin
butoconazole nitrate
carbol-fuchsin solution
chloramphenicol
chlortetracycline hydrochloride
ciclopirox olamine
clindamycin phosphate
clotrimazole
econazole nitrate
erythromycin
gentamicin sulfate
gentian violet
haloprogin
iodochlorhydroxyquin
ketoconazole
mafenide acetate
metronidazole (topical)
miconazole nitrate
mupirocin
naftifine
neomycin sulfate
nitrofurazone
nystatin
oxiconazole nitrate
podofilox
silver sulfadiazine
sulconazole nitrate
terbinafine hydrochloride
terconazole
tetracycline hydrochloride
tioconazole
tolnaftate
undecylenic acid and zinc undecylenate

COMBINATION PRODUCTS

BENZAMYCIN GEL: erythromycin 3% and benzoyl peroxide 5%.
CORDRAN-N CREAM, OINTMENT: flurandrenolide 0.05% and neomycin sulfate 0.5%.
LANABIOTIC◇: polymyxin B sulfate 5,000 units, neomycin sulfate 5 mg, bacitracin 500 units, and lidocaine 40 mg/g.
LOTRISONE CREAM: clotrimazole 1% and betamethasone dipropionate 0.05%.
MYCITRACIN OINTMENT◇: polymyxin B sulfate 5,000 units, bacitracin 500 units, and neomycin sulfate 3.5 mg/g.
MYCOLOG II CREAM, OINTMENT: triamcinolone acetonide 0.1% and nystatin 100,000 units/g.
NEO-CORTEF OINTMENT: hydrocortisone acetate 1% and neomycin sulfate 0.5%.
NEODECADRON CREAM: dexamethasone phosphate 0.1% and neomycin sulfate 0.5%.
NEO-POLYCIN OINTMENT◇: polymyxin B sulfate 5,000 units, neomycin sulfate 5 mg, and zinc bacitracin 400 units/g.
NEOSPORIN CREAM†◇: polymyxin B sulfate 10,000 units and neomycin sulfate 5 mg.
NEOSPORIN OINTMENT◇: polymyxin B sulfate 5,000 units, bacitracin zinc 400 units, and neomycin sulfate 5 mg/g.
POLYSPORIN OINTMENT◇: polymyxin B sulfate 10,000 units and zinc bacitracin 500 units/g.
SULFACET-R LOTION: sulfacetamide sodium 10% and sulfur 5%.
VIOFORM-HYDROCORTISONE MILD CREAM, RACET CREAM: iodochlorhydroxyquin 3% and hydrocortisone 0.5%.
VYTONE CREAM: hydrocortisone 1% and iodoquinol 1%.

acyclovir

Zovirax

Pregnancy Risk Category: C

HOW SUPPLIED
Ointment: 5%

ACTION
Mechanism: Inhibits herpes simplex and varicella-zoster viral DNA synthesis by interfering with viral DNA polymerase action.
Duration: terminal elimination half-life, about 3½ hours.

INDICATIONS & DOSAGE
Initial herpes genitalis; limited, non-life-threatening mucocutaneous herpes simplex virus infections in immunocompromised patients –
Adults and children: thoroughly cover all lesions q 3 hours six times daily for 7 days. Although dosage will vary depending on the total lesion area, use approximately a ½″ ribbon of ointment on each 4″ square of surface area.

ADVERSE REACTIONS
Skin: transient burning and stinging, rash, pruritus.

INTERACTIONS
None significant.

CONTRAINDICATIONS
- Contraindicated in patients hypersensitive to the drug.

NURSING CONSIDERATIONS
- For cutaneous use only; don't apply to the eye.
- Apply with a finger cot or rubber glove to prevent autoinoculation of other body sites and transmission of infection to other persons.
- As ordered, initiate therapy as early as possible after onset of signs and symptoms of herpes.
- Most studies show that topically applied acyclovir is not effective when used to treat recurrent genital herpes.
- Emphasize importance of compliance for successful therapy.
- Teach the patient that virus transmission can occur during treatment.

amphotericin B
Fungizone

Pregnancy Risk Category: B

HOW SUPPLIED
Cream: 3%
Lotion: 3%
Ointment: 3%

ACTION
Mechanism: Usually fungistatic; binds to sterols in the fungal cell membrane.
Onset: variable.

INDICATIONS & DOSAGE
Cutaneous or mucocutaneous candidal infections –
Adults and children: apply liberally b.i.d. to q.i.d. for 1 to 3 weeks; treat interdigital lesions, paronychias, and onychomycoses for several months because relapses are common.

ADVERSE REACTIONS
Skin: possible drying, contact sensitivity, erythema, burning, pruritus.

INTERACTIONS
None significant.

CONTRAINDICATIONS
- Contraindicated in patients hypersensitive to the drug.

NURSING CONSIDERATIONS
- Clean area before applying.
- Cream or lotion is preferred for such areas as groin folds, armpit, and neck creases.
- Watch for and report signs of local irritation. Cream may dry the skin; ointment may irritate if applied to moist hairy areas.
- Avoid occlusive dressings.
- Store at room temperature; avoid freezing.

• Well tolerated, even by infants, for long periods.
• Tell the patient to continue using medication for full length of time prescribed, even if condition has improved.
• Cream discolors skin slightly when rubbed in; lotion or ointment may stain nail lesions but not skin if thoroughly rubbed in.
• Tell the patient that discoloration of fabric caused by cream or lotion can usually be removed by washing; discoloration by ointment, with cleaning fluid.
• Discontinue drug if irritation or hypersensitivity occurs, and notify the doctor.

bacitracin

Baciguent◇, Bacitin†

Pregnancy Risk Category: C

HOW SUPPLIED

Ointment: 500 units/g

ACTION

Mechanism: Bactericidal or bacteriostatic, depending on organism and concentration of drug; inhibits bacterial cell-wall synthesis. Effective mainly against gram-positive organisms, such as staphylococci and streptococci.
Peak: Effects peak in 1 to 2 hours.
Duration: 6 to 8 hours.

INDICATIONS & DOSAGE

Topical infections, impetigo, abrasions, cuts, and minor burns or wounds –
Adults and children: apply thin film b.i.d., t.i.d., or p.r.n., depending on severity of condition.

ADVERSE REACTIONS

Skin: stinging, rashes, other allergic reactions; pruritus, burning, or swelling of lips or face.
Systemic: *possible systemic adverse reactions when used over large areas for prolonged periods, including potential nephrotoxicity and ototoxicity; hypersensitivity reactions;* tightness in chest, hypotension.

INTERACTIONS

None significant.

CONTRAINDICATIONS

• Contraindicated in patients hypersensitive to the drug and for application in the external ear canal if the eardrum is perforated.
• Use cautiously in patients allergic to neomycin; possible cross-sensitivity.

NURSING CONSIDERATIONS

• Clean area before applying, especially areas with crusted or suppurative lesions.
• Consider alternative treatment for burns that cover more than 20% of body surface, especially if the patient suffers impaired renal function.
• If no improvement occurs or condition worsens, tell the patient to stop using and notify the doctor.
• Prolonged use may result in overgrowth of nonsusceptible organisms, particularly *Candida* species.

butoconazole nitrate

Femstat

Pregnancy Risk Category: C

HOW SUPPLIED

Vaginal cream: 2% supplied with applicators

ACTION

Mechanism: Controls or destroys fungus by disrupting cell-membrane permeability, causing osmotic instability.
Onset: 3 days.

INDICATIONS & DOSAGE

Vulvovaginal mycotic infections caused by Candida *species –*

*Liquid form contains alcohol. *Common* reactions are in italics; ***life-threatening,*** in bold italics.
**May contain tartrazine.

Adults: 1 applicatorful intravaginally h.s. for 3 days. If necessary, treatment can be extended for another 3 days.

ADVERSE REACTIONS
GU: vulvovaginal itching, soreness, and swelling.
Skin: finger itching.

INTERACTIONS
None significant.

CONTRAINDICATIONS
- Contraindicated in patients hypersensitive to the drug and during the first trimester of pregnancy.

NURSING CONSIDERATIONS
- Butoconazole may be used with oral contraceptive and antibiotic therapy.
- May be used during second and third trimester of pregnancy only.
- Diagnosis of *Candida* vulvovaginal infection should be confirmed by smears or cultures.
- Symptom resolution comparable to 7-day miconazole cream therapy.
- Teach the patient how to apply, and tell her not to use tampons during treatment.
- Tell the patient's sexual partner to wear a condom during intercourse until treatment is complete. He should consult the doctor if he experiences penile itching, redness, or discomfort.
- Advise the patient to keep affected area cool and dry, wear loose-fitting cotton clothing, avoid feminine hygiene sprays, wash daily with unscented soap, dry thoroughly with a clean towel, and maintain proper hygiene by wiping perineum from front to back to prevent reinfection.

carbol-fuchsin solution (Castellani's paint, Magenta paint)
Castaderm

Pregnancy Risk Category: C

HOW SUPPLIED
Topical solution: 0.3% basic fuchsin, 4.5% phenol, 10% resorcinol, 5% acetone, and 10% alcohol

ACTION
Mechanism: A fungicidal and bactericidal agent that disrupts protein synthesis.
Onset: on contact.

INDICATIONS & DOSAGE
Tinea, dermatophytoses, skin infections –
Adults and children: apply liberally once daily or b.i.d.

ADVERSE REACTIONS
Hematologic: possible bone marrow hypoplasia with prolonged use or at frequent intervals.
Skin: *contact dermatitis.*

INTERACTIONS
None significant.

CONTRAINDICATIONS
- Contraindicated in patients hypersensitive to the drug.

NURSING CONSIDERATIONS
- Clean skin with soap and water before application. Don't apply to eroded skin or over extensive areas.
- Warn the patient to expect a stinging sensation, usually followed by the drug's local anesthetic effect.
- Apply over a small area in an initial test; if contact dermatitis or sensitivity occurs, discontinue.
- Discontinue after 1 week if no improvement shown; consult the doctor. Toxicities may develop in long-term use.
- Solution is poisonous; warn the patient against swallowing drug. Store in tight, light-resistant container.
- Instruct the patient to continue using for full treatment period prescribed, even if condition has improved.

- Useful in treating moist eczematous dermatitis, especially in hairy areas.
- Will stain clothing.

chloramphenicol

Chloromycetin

Pregnancy Risk Category: C

HOW SUPPLIED

Cream: 1%

ACTION

Mechanism: Inhibits bacterial protein synthesis; effective against most gram-positive and gram-negative bacteria, and *Chlamydia, Mycoplasma,* and *Rickettsia.*

Onset: variable.

INDICATIONS & DOSAGE

Superficial skin infections caused by susceptible bacteria –

Adults and children: after thoroughly cleaning the skin, apply t.i.d. or q.i.d.

ADVERSE REACTIONS

Skin: possible contact sensitivity; burning, urticaria, pruritus, angioedema in hypersensitive patients.

INTERACTIONS

None significant.

CONTRAINDICATIONS

- Contraindicated in patients hypersensitive to the drug or any components of the formulation.

NURSING CONSIDERATIONS

- If no improvement occurs or if condition worsens, stop using and report to the doctor.
- Prolonged use may result in overgrowth of fungi or other nonsusceptible organisms.
- Systemically administered chloramphenicol has been linked to serious adverse reactions and toxicity; tell the patient to avoid prolonged or frequent intermittent use.
- Topical use of this drug should be supplemented by appropriate systemic medication for all but very superficial infections.
- Discontinue if hypersensitivity reactions develop, and notify the doctor.
- Tell the patient to continue using for full treatment period prescribed, even if condition has improved.

chlortetracycline hydrochloride

Aureomycin 3%◊

Pregnancy Risk Category: D

HOW SUPPLIED

Ointment: 3%

ACTION

Mechanism: Usually bacteriostatic; disrupts protein synthesis in susceptible organisms, including *Rickettsia, Chlamydia, Mycoplasma,* spirochetes, and other gram-positive and gram-negative organisms.

Onset: variable; minimal systemic absorption.

INDICATIONS & DOSAGE

Superficial skin infections caused by susceptible bacteria –

Adults and children: rub into affected area b.i.d. or t.i.d.

ADVERSE REACTIONS

Skin: *dermatitis,* drying.

INTERACTIONS

Abrasive or medicated soaps or cleansers; acne preparations or other preparations containing peeling agents (benzoyl peroxide, resorcinol, salicylic acid, sulfur, tretinoin); alcohol-containing products (after-shave, cosmetics, perfumed toiletries, shaving creams or lotions); astringent soaps or cosmetics; isotretinoin; medicated cosmetics or cover-ups: may cause cumulative drying or irritation, resulting in excessive skin irritation. Use together cautiously.

CONTRAINDICATIONS
• Contraindicated in patients hypersensitive to the drug.

NURSING CONSIDERATIONS
• Drug has lanolin base; don't use in patients allergic to wool.
• Prolonged use may result in overgrowth of nonsusceptible organisms.
• If no improvement occurs or if condition worsens, stop using and report to the doctor.
• Treated skin fluoresces under ultraviolet light.

ciclopirox olamine

Loprox

Pregnancy Risk Category: B

HOW SUPPLIED
Cream: 1%
Lotion: 1%

ACTION
Mechanism: Depletes essential fungal intracellular substrates by blocking amino acid transport and alters cell-membrane integrity.
Duration: elimination half-life, about 1½ hours; most of absorbed drug excreted within 8 hours.

INDICATIONS & DOSAGE
Tinea pedis, cruris, corporis, and versicolor; cutaneous candidiasis –
Adults and children over 10 years: massage gently into the affected and surrounding areas b.i.d., in the morning and evening.

ADVERSE REACTIONS
Skin: pruritus, burning.

INTERACTIONS
None significant.

CONTRAINDICATIONS
• Contraindicated in patients hypersensitive to the drug.

NURSING CONSIDERATIONS
• If hypersensitivity reaction occurs, discontinue treatment, and notify the doctor.
• Tell patient to continue using drug for the full treatment period even though symptoms may have improved, usually 1 week after clearing. Tell the patient to notify the doctor if no improvement occurs after 4 weeks.
• Don't use occlusive dressings.
• Hypopigmentation from tinea versicolor will resolve gradually.

clindamycin phosphate

Cleocin T Gel, Lotion, Solution; Cleocin Vaginal Cream

Pregnancy Risk Category: B

HOW SUPPLIED
Gel: 1%
Lotion: 1%
Topical solution: 1%
Vaginal cream: 2%

ACTION
Mechanism: Bacteriostatic or bactericidal, depending on concentration of drug and susceptibility of organism; suppresses growth of susceptible organisms in sebaceous glands by blocking protein synthesis. Also active against most aerobic gram-positive cocci.
Onset: variable; minimal systemic absorption. **Peak:** Effects peak in 8 to 24 hours for intravaginal use. **Duration:** maximum benefits, 8 to 12 weeks with topical use.

INDICATIONS & DOSAGE
Inflammatory acne vulgaris, grades II and III –
Adults and adolescents: apply to skin b.i.d., morning and evening; solution may be used up to q.i.d.

Bacterial vaginosis –
Adults: 1 applicatorful intravaginally h.s. for 7 consecutive days.

ADVERSE REACTIONS

GI: upset, diarrhea, bloody diarrhea, abdominal pain, colitis (including pseudomembranous colitis).
GU: *cervicitis or vaginitis,* Candida albicans overgrowth, *vulvar irritation.*
Skin: *dryness,* rash, redness, pruritus, swelling, irritation, contact dermatitis.

INTERACTIONS

Abrasive or medicated soaps or cleansers; acne preparations or other preparations containing peeling agents (benzoyl peroxide, resorcinol, salicylic acid, sulfur, tretinoin); alcohol-containing products (after-shave, cosmetics, perfumed toiletries, shaving creams or lotions); astringent soaps or cosmetics; isotretinoin; medicated cosmetics or cover-ups: potential cumulative drying or irritation, resulting in excessive skin irritation. Use cautiously.

CONTRAINDICATIONS

- Contraindicated in patients hypersensitive to the drug and those with a history of ulcerative colitis, regional enteritis, or antibiotic-associated colitis.

NURSING CONSIDERATIONS

- Instruct the patient to wash area with warm water and soap, rinse, and pat dry before application and to wait 30 minutes after washing or shaving to apply. Warn the patient to avoid too frequent washing of area. Tell him to cover entire affected area, but to avoid contact with eyes, nose, mouth, and other mucous membranes.
- When used intravaginally, ensure that the patient understands how to use the applicators that come with the drug.
- For treating acne, drug may be used concurrently with tretinoin or benzoyl peroxide as well as systemic antibiotics. Caution the patient to notify the doctor if skin becomes excessively dry.
- Warn the patient not to smoke while applying topical solution.
- Tell the patient to use only as prescribed.
- If diarrhea occurs, tell the patient to check with the doctor or pharmacist before using antidiarrheal medication because it may worsen the condition.
- Tell the patient to dab, not roll, applicator-tipped bottle. If tip becomes dry, the patient should invert bottle and depress tip several times to moisten.

clotrimazole

Canesten†, Gyne-Lotrimin◇, Lotrimin, Mycelex, Mycelex-G, Mycelex-OTC◇, Mycelex-7◇

Pregnancy Risk Category: B

HOW SUPPLIED

Lozenges: 1%
Cream: 1%
Topical lotion: 1%
Topical solution: 1%
Vaginal cream: 1%◇
Vaginal tablets: 100 mg◇, 500 mg
Combination pack: vaginal inserts 100 mg and vulvar cream 1%◇

ACTION

Mechanism: Alters fungal cell-wall permeability and produces osmotic instability.
Onset: variable; minimal systemic absorption. **Duration:** up to 3 hours for lozenge; 72 hours for vaginal cream or tablets.

INDICATIONS & DOSAGE

Superficial fungal infections (tinea pedis, tinea cruris, tinea corporis, or tinea versicolor; candidiasis) –

Adults and children: apply thinly and massage into affected and surrounding area, morning and evening, for 2 to 8 weeks.
Vulvovaginal candidiasis –
Adults: insert two 100-mg vaginal tablets daily h.s. for 3 consecutive days, or one 500-mg vaginal tablet daily h.s. for 3 days; or 1 applicatorful vaginal cream daily h.s. for 3 days.
Oropharyngeal candidiasis –
Adults and children: dissolve lozenge over 15 to 30 minutes in mouth five times daily for 14 consecutive days.

ADVERSE REACTIONS
GI: nausea and vomiting (with lozenges).
GU: *mild vaginal burning or irritation with vaginal use.*
Hepatic: elevated AST levels (from lozenges).
Skin: blistering, *erythema,* edema, pruritus, burning, stinging, peeling, urticaria, skin fissures, general irritation.

INTERACTIONS
None significant.

CONTRAINDICATIONS
• Contraindicated in patients hypersensitive to the drug.
• Also contraindicated for ophthalmic use.

NURSING CONSIDERATIONS
• Clean area before applying.
• Warn the patient not to use occlusive wrappings or dressings.
• Watch for and report irritation or sensitivity; discontinue if irritation occurs.
• Improvement usually demonstrated within a week; if no improvement occurs in 4 weeks, diagnosis should be reviewed.
• Emphasize the need to continue treatment for full course even if symptoms have improved.
• Ensure that the patient understands that frequent or persistent yeast infections may be a symptom of a more serious medical problem, such as immunodeficiency or AIDS.
• When compliance is a problem, mild to moderate vaginal candidiasis may be treated with a single 500-mg tablet.
• Hypopigmentation from tinea versicolor will resolve gradually.
• Topical preparation may stain clothing.

econazole nitrate
Ecostatin, Spectazole

Pregnancy Risk Category: C

HOW SUPPLIED
Cream: 1%

ACTION
Mechanism: Alters fungal cell-wall permeability and promotes osmotic instability.
Onset: rapid.

INDICATIONS & DOSAGE
Tinea pedis, tinea cruris, and tinea corporis; cutaneous candidiasis –
Adults and children: rub into affected areas once daily for at least 2 weeks.
Cutaneous candidiasis –
Adults and children: rub into affected areas b.i.d.

ADVERSE REACTIONS
Skin: burning, pruritus, stinging, erythema.

INTERACTIONS
Topical corticosteroids: may inhibit antifungal effect.

CONTRAINDICATIONS
• Contraindicated in patients hypersensitive to the drug.

NURSING CONSIDERATIONS

- Clean affected area before applying.
- If condition persists or worsens or if irritation (burning, pruritus, stinging, redness) occurs, discontinue use and report this to doctor.
- Tell the patient to use medication for entire treatment period, even though symptoms may have improved. Notify the doctor if no improvement occurs after 2 weeks (tinea cruris, tinea corporis, and tinea versicolor) or 4 weeks (tinea pedis).
- Don't use occlusive dressings.
- Hypopigmentation from tinea versicolor will resolve gradually.
- May stain clothing.

erythromycin

Akne-mycin, A/T/S, Del-Mycin, Erycette, EryDerm, EryGel, Ery-Sol†, ETS†, Sans-Acne†, T-Stat†, Staticin

Pregnancy Risk Category: B

HOW SUPPLIED

Ointment: 2%
Topical gel: 2%
Topical solution: 1.5%*, 2%*
Pledgets: 2%

ACTION

Mechanism: Usually bacteriostatic; disrupts protein synthesis in susceptible bacteria. Effective against most aerobic and anaerobic gram-positive bacteria, *Rickettsia, Chlamydia, Mycoplasma,* and a few gram-negative bacteria.
Onset: variable.

INDICATIONS & DOSAGE

Superficial skin infections due to susceptible organisms, inflammatory acne vulgaris –
Adults and children: apply to affected area b.i.d.

ADVERSE REACTIONS

Skin: sensitivity reactions, erythema, burning, *dryness, pruritus.*

INTERACTIONS

Abrasive or medicated soaps or cleansers; acne preparations or other preparations containing peeling agents (benzoyl peroxide, resorcinol, salicylic acid, sulfur, tretinoin); alcohol-containing products (after-shave, cosmetics, perfumed toiletries, shaving creams or lotions); astringent soaps or cosmetics; isotretinoin; medicated cosmetics or cover-ups: may cause cumulative drying or irritation, resulting in excessive skin irritation. Use cautiously.

CONTRAINDICATIONS

- Contraindicated in patients hypersensitive to the drug.

NURSING CONSIDERATIONS

- Wash, rinse, and dry affected areas before application.
- Prolonged use may be necessary when treating acne vulgaris; such use may result in overgrowth of nonsusceptible organisms.
- If no improvement occurs or if condition worsens, stop using and notify the doctor.
- Don't use near eyes, nose, mouth, or other mucous membranes.

gentamicin sulfate

Garamycin, G-Myticin

Pregnancy Risk Category: C

HOW SUPPLIED

Cream: 0.1%
Ointment: 0.1%

ACTION

Mechanism: A bactericidal agent that disrupts bacterial protein synthesis by binding to ribosomes.
Onset: variable.

*Liquid form contains alcohol.
**May contain tartrazine.

INDICATIONS & DOSAGE

Primary and secondary bacterial infections, superficial burns, skin ulcers, infected insect bites and stings, infected lacerations and abrasions, wounds from minor surgery –
Adults and children over 1 year: rub in small amount gently t.i.d. or q.i.d., with or without gauze dressing.

ADVERSE REACTIONS

Skin: minor skin irritation, possible photosensitivity, allergic contact dermatitis.

INTERACTIONS

None significant.

CONTRAINDICATIONS

- Contraindicated in patients hypersensitive to the drug. May exhibit cross-sensitivity with other aminoglycosides, such as neomycin.

NURSING CONSIDERATIONS

- Clean affected area before applying.
- If no improvement occurs or if condition worsens, stop using and notify the doctor.
- Use only in selected patients; widespread use may lead to resistant organisms.
- Avoid use on large skin lesions or over a wide area because of possible systemic toxic effects.
- Prolonged use may result in overgrowth of nonsusceptible organisms.
- May be used to treat bacterial infections that have not responded to other antibacterial agents.
- Store in cool place.
- Remove crusts before application of gentamicin in impetigo contagiosa to enhance absorption.

gentian violet (methylrosaniline chloride, crystal violet)

Genapax

Pregnancy Risk Category: C

HOW SUPPLIED

Topical solution: 1%◇, 2%◇
Tampons: 5 mg

ACTION

Mechanism: Unknown, although drug has fungistatic and antibacterial activity.
Onset: variable.

INDICATIONS & DOSAGE

Superficial skin infections; lesions, particularly those caused by Candida albicans –
Adults and children: apply with swab b.i.d. or t.i.d. for 3 days.
Vaginal fungal infections –
Adults: insert 1 tampon for 3 to 4 hours daily or b.i.d. for 12 days. For resistant infections, insert an additional tampon h.s.

ADVERSE REACTIONS

Skin: *permanent discoloration if applied to granulation tissue;* irritation or ulceration of mucous membranes.

INTERACTIONS

None significant.

CONTRAINDICATIONS

- Contraindicated in patients hypersensitive to the drug.

NURSING CONSIDERATIONS

- Keep affected area clean, dry, and exposed to air to prevent spread of infection.
- Do not use on ulcerative facial lesions.
- Apply carefully to avoid undue staining. Will stain skin and clothing.
- Do not use occlusive dressings.

• Tattooing of the skin may occur if applied to granulation tissue.
• Toxicity has occurred after ingestion or with excessive use.

haloprogin

Halotex

Pregnancy Risk Category: B

HOW SUPPLIED
Cream: 1%
Topical solution: 1%

ACTION
Mechanism: Unknown, although drug has fungistatic and fungicidal activity.
Onset: variable.

INDICATIONS & DOSAGE
Superficial fungal infections (tinea pedis, tinea cruris, tinea corporis, tinea manuum, and tinea versicolor) –
Adults: apply liberally b.i.d. for 2 to 3 weeks. Intertriginous lesions may require 4 weeks of therapy.

ADVERSE REACTIONS
Skin: burning sensation, irritation, vesicle formation, increased maceration, *pruritus, or exacerbation of preexisting lesions.*

INTERACTIONS
None significant.

CONTRAINDICATIONS
• Contraindicated in patients hypersensitive to the drug.

NURSING CONSIDERATIONS
• Diagnosis should be reconsidered if no improvement occurs after 4 weeks of therapy.
• Tell the patient to continue using for full treatment period prescribed, even if condition has improved.
• Tell the patient to notify the doctor if increased irritation occurs.
• Don't allow drug to come in contact with the eyes.

iodochlorhydroxyquin (clioquinol)

Ala-Quin, Corque, Cortin, Torofor◊, Vioform◊

Pregnancy Risk Category: C

HOW SUPPLIED
Cream: 3%
Ointment: 3%
Lotion: 3%

ACTION
Mechanism: Unknown, although drug has fungistatic and fungicidal activity.
Onset: variable; minimal systemic absorption.

INDICATIONS & DOSAGE
Inflamed skin conditions, including eczema, tinea pedis, tinea cruris, and tinea corporis –
Adults and children over 2 years: apply a thin layer b.i.d. or t.i.d. Continue for 1 week after cessation of symptoms. Treat tinea pedis or tinea corporis for 4 weeks, tinea cruris for 2 weeks.

ADVERSE REACTIONS
CNS: neurotoxicity (with systemic absorption).
Skin: *possible burning, pruritus, acneiform eruptions,* allergic contact dermatitis.
Other: altered protein-bound iodine levels (with systemic absorption).

INTERACTIONS
Systemic corticosteroids: possible increased absorption. Use together cautiously.

CONTRAINDICATIONS
• Contraindicated in patients hypersensitive to the drug, iodine, or iodine-containing preparations; in chil-

dren under age 2; or in patients with tuberculosis, vaccinia, or varicella.

NURSING CONSIDERATIONS
- Don't use to treat diaper rash. Drug is also not effective in the treatment of fungal infections of the scalp or nails.
- Note all adverse reactions and precautions related to each component of combination antifungal products.
- Presence of drug in urine may cause false-positive result for phenylketonuria or inaccurate thyroid function tests; discontinue drug at least 1 month before such tests.
- Drug will stain fabric and hair.

ketoconazole
Nizoral

Pregnancy Risk Category: C

HOW SUPPLIED
Cream: 2%
Shampoo: 2%

ACTION
Mechanism: An imidazole that inhibits yeast growth by altering the permeability of the cell membrane.
Onset: variable; minimal systemic absorption.

INDICATIONS & DOSAGE
Tinea corporis, tinea pedis, tinea cruris, and tinea versicolor caused by susceptible organisms; seborrheic dermatitis; cutaneous candidiasis – **Adults:** cover the affected and immediate surrounding area once daily for at least 2 weeks. Treat seborrheic dermatitis for 4 weeks. When using shampoo, wet hair, lather, and massage for 1 minute. Rinse and repeat, but leave drug on scalp for 3 minutes before rinsing. Shampoo twice weekly for 4 weeks, with at least 3 days between shampooing.

ADVERSE REACTIONS
Skin: severe irritation, pruritus, stinging.
Other: swelling, inflammation.

INTERACTIONS
None significant.

CONTRAINDICATIONS
- Contraindicated in patients hypersensitive to the drug.

NURSING CONSIDERATIONS
- Discontinue if hypersensitivity reaction occurs, and notify the doctor.
- Most patients show improvement soon after treatment begins. However, treatment of tinea cruris or tinea corporis should continue for at least 2 weeks, or tinea pedis for 4 to 8 weeks, to reduce the possibility of recurrence.
- Check with the doctor if condition worsens; drug may have to be discontinued and diagnosis redetermined.

mafenide acetate
Sulfamylon

Pregnancy Risk Category: C

HOW SUPPLIED
Cream: 8.5%

ACTION
Mechanism: Unknown, although it interferes with bacterial cellular metabolism.
Onset: variable; minimal systemic absorption.

INDICATIONS & DOSAGE
Adjunctive treatment of second- and third-degree burns to prevent infection caused by susceptible organisms (especially Pseudomonas aeruginosa*)* – **Adults and children:** apply 1/16" thickness of cream daily or b.i.d. to clean, debrided wounds. Reapply p.r.n. to keep burned area covered.

ADVERSE REACTIONS
Hematologic: eosinophilia.
Skin: pain, *burning sensation,* rash, pruritus, swelling, hives, blisters, erythema.
Other: *metabolic acidosis,* facial edema.

INTERACTIONS
None significant.

CONTRAINDICATIONS
• Contraindicated in patients hypersensitive to the drug.
• Use cautiously in patients with acute renal failure and in those with known hypersensitivity to sulfonamides.

NURSING CONSIDERATIONS
• Clean area before applying, bathing patient daily, if possible.
• Use reverse isolation technique with sterile gloves and instruments when applying cream to minimize risk of further wound contamination.
• Closely monitor acid-base balance, especially in patients with pulmonary and renal dysfunction. If acidosis occurs, discontinue use for 24 to 48 hours.
• Mafenide can cause pain and burning at application site; if either occurs, notify the doctor. Severe and prolonged pain may indicate allergy; if these or other allergic reactions occur, treatment may have to be temporarily discontinued.
• Sometimes difficult to distinguish between adverse reactions and effects of severe burn.
• Keep burn areas medicated at all times.

metronidazole (topical)
MetroGel, MetroGel-Vaginal
Pregnancy Risk Category: B

HOW SUPPLIED
Topical gel: 0.75%
Vaginal gel: 0.75%

ACTION
Mechanism: Unknown; may cause bactericidal effect by interacting with bacterial DNA. Active against many anaerobic gram-negative bacilli, anaerobic gram-positive cocci, *Gardnerella vaginalis,* and *Campylobacter fetus.*
Onset: variable; minimal systemic absorption from intact skin. **Peak:** Effects peak 6 to 12 hours after intravaginal use.

INDICATIONS & DOSAGE
Acne rosacea –
Adults: apply a thin film to affected area b.i.d., morning and evening. Significant results should appear within 3 weeks and continue for 9 weeks. Adjust frequency and duration of therapy after response is seen.
Bacterial vaginosis –
Adults: 1 applicatorful b.i.d., morning and evening, for 5 days.

ADVERSE REACTIONS
Topical gel
EENT: lacrimation (if drug applied around the eyes).
Vaginal form
CNS: dizziness, light-headedness, headache.
GI: cramps, pain, nausea, diarrhea, constipation, metallic or bad taste in mouth.
GU: *cervicitis, vaginitis.*
Skin: rash, *transient redness, dryness, mild burning, stinging.*
Other: overgrowth of nonsusceptible organisms, decreased appetite.

INTERACTIONS
Oral anticoagulants: may potentiate anticoagulant effect. Monitor the patient for potential adverse reactions.

CONTRAINDICATIONS
- Contraindicated in patients hypersensitive to metronidazole or its ingredients (such as parabens).
- Use cautiously in patients with history or evidence of blood dyscrasia; chemically related compounds are associated with blood dyscrasia.
- Use vaginal gel cautiously in patients with CNS diseases; a theoretical risk of seizures, and peripheral neuropathy exist because these adverse reactions are associated with the oral form. However, plasma levels after typical doses of vaginal gel are usually less than 5% of those seen after a 500-mg oral dose.

NURSING CONSIDERATIONS
- Instruct the patient using topical gel to avoid use of drug around the eyes. Also advise the patient to clean area thoroughly before use, but wait 15 to 20 minutes after cleaning the skin before applying drug to minimize risk of local irritation. Cosmetics may be used after applying drug.
- If local reactions occur, advise the patient to apply less frequently or to discontinue and contact the doctor.
- Topical metronidazole therapy has not been associated with the adverse effects observed with parenteral or oral metronidazole therapy (including disulfiram-like reactions after alcohol ingestion). However, some of the drug can be absorbed after topical use.

---

miconazole nitrate

Micatin◇, Monistat-Derm Cream and Lotion, Monistat 3 Vaginal Suppository, Monistat 7 Vaginal Cream◇, Monistat 7 Vaginal Suppository◇

Pregnancy Risk Category: C

HOW SUPPLIED
Cream: 2%◇
Lotion: 2%◇
Powder: 2%◇
Spray: 2%◇
Vaginal cream: 2%◇
Vaginal suppositories: 100 mg◇, 200 mg

ACTION
Mechanism: A fungicidal imidazole that disrupts fungal cell-membrane permeability.
Peak: Effects peak within 6 days.

INDICATIONS & DOSAGE
Tinea pedis, tinea cruris, tinea corporis, and tinea versicolor; cutaneous candidiasis (moniliasis); common dermatophyte infections –
Adults and children: apply or spray sparingly b.i.d. for 2 to 4 weeks.
Vulvovaginal candidiasis –
Adults: 1 applicatorful or 100 mg suppository (Monistat 7) inserted intravaginally h.s. for 7 days; repeat course if necessary. Alternatively, insert 200 mg suppository (Monistat 3) intravaginally h.s. for 3 days.

ADVERSE REACTIONS
GU: vulvovaginal burning, pruritus, or irritation with vaginal cream.
Skin: irritation, burning, maceration.

INTERACTIONS
None significant.

CONTRAINDICATIONS
- Contraindicated in patients hypersensitive to the drug.

NURSING CONSIDERATIONS
- For perineal or intravaginal use only. Keep out of eyes.
- Discontinue if sensitivity or chemical irritation occurs.
- Tell the patient to continue using for full treatment period prescribed, even if condition has improved.
- Ensure that the patient understands that frequent or persistent yeast infections may be a symptom of a more serious medical problem, such as immunodeficiency or AIDS.

• Do not use occlusive dressings.
• Tell the patient to cautiously insert intravaginal forms high into the vagina with applicator provided.
• May stain clothing.
• Concurrent use of intravaginal forms and certain latex products, such as vaginal contraceptive diaphragms, are not recommended because of possible interaction.

mupirocin
Bactroban
Pregnancy Risk Category: C

HOW SUPPLIED
Ointment: 2%

ACTION
Mechanism: Inhibits bacterial protein and RNA synthesis; active against *Staphylococcus aureus* (including methicillin-resistant and beta-lactamase producing strains), *S. saprophyticus,* and *Streptococcus pyogenes.*
Onset: variable; minimal systemic absorption from intact skin.

INDICATIONS & DOSAGE
Common bacterial skin infections caused by susceptible bacteria, impetigo –
Adults and children: apply to affected areas t.i.d. for 1 to 2 weeks.

ADVERSE REACTIONS
Skin: burning, pruritus, stinging, rash.

INTERACTIONS
None significant.

CONTRAINDICATIONS
• Contraindicated in patients hypersensitive to the drug.

NURSING CONSIDERATIONS
• Local reactions appear to be caused by the polyethylene glycol vehicle.
• If no improvement occurs in 3 to 5 days or condition worsens, notify the doctor immediately.
• Prolonged use may cause overgrowth of nonsusceptible bacteria and fungi.
• Do not use to treat eye infections or burns.

naftifine
Naftin
Pregnancy Risk Category: B

HOW SUPPLIED
Cream: 1%
Gel: 1%

ACTION
Mechanism: A broad-spectrum fungicidal agent; inhibits sterol biosynthesis in susceptible fungi by blocking the enzyme squalene 2,3 epoxidase.
Onset: variable; minimal absorption from intact skin.

INDICATIONS & DOSAGE
Tinea corporis, tinea pedis, or tinea cruris –
Adults: apply to affected area once daily with the cream, or b.i.d. in the morning and evening with the gel.

ADVERSE REACTIONS
Skin: *burning, stinging,* dryness, pruritus, local irritation.

INTERACTIONS
None significant.

CONTRAINDICATIONS
• Contraindicated in patients hypersensitive to the drug.

NURSING CONSIDERATIONS
• Not for ophthalmic use. Instruct the patient to keep cream away from mucous membranes (eyes, nose, and mouth).
• Don't use occlusive dressings unless directed otherwise by the doctor.

- Instruct the patient to wash hands after application.
- Therapy should be reevaluated if no improvement occurs after 4 weeks.
- Instruct the patient to discontinue therapy and notify the doctor if irritation or sensitivity develops.
- Cultures should be done to confirm diagnosis before therapy.

neomycin sulfate

Mycifradin†, Myciguent◇, Neo-Rx

Pregnancy Risk Category: C

HOW SUPPLIED

Cream: 0.5%◇
Ointment: 0.5%◇

ACTION

Mechanism: Disrupts bacterial protein synthesis by binding to bacterial ribosomes.
Onset: variable.

INDICATIONS & DOSAGE

Prevention or treatment of topical bacterial infections, minor burns, wounds, skin grafts, following surgical procedures, primary pyodermas, pruritus, trophic ulcerations, otitis externa –
Adults and children: rub into affected area 1 to 3 times a day.

ADVERSE REACTIONS

Skin: *rashes, contact dermatitis,* urticaria.
Systemic: *possible nephrotoxicity, ototoxicity, and* ***neuromuscular blockade.***

INTERACTIONS

None significant.

CONTRAINDICATIONS

- Contraindicated in patients hypersensitive to the drug.

NURSING CONSIDERATIONS

- If no improvement occurs or if condition worsens, stop using and report to the doctor.
- Don't use on more than 20% of the body surface or on patients with impaired renal function unless risk-to-benefit ratio has been assessed.
- Prolonged use may result in overgrowth of nonsusceptible organisms.
- In combination products containing corticosteroids, use of occlusive dressings increases corticosteroid absorption and the likelihood of systemic effects.
- Enhanced systemic absorption occurs on denuded or abraded areas.
- Watch for signs of hypersensitivity and contact dermatitis.
- Evaluate patients for signs of ototoxicity with prolonged or extended use.

nitrofurazone

Furacin

Pregnancy Risk Category: C

HOW SUPPLIED

Cream: 0.2%
Ointment: 0.2% (soluble dressing)
Topical solution: 0.2%

ACTION

Mechanism: Broad-spectrum antibiotic that inhibits bacterial enzymes involved in carbohydrate metabolism.
Onset: variable; minimal systemic absorption.

INDICATIONS & DOSAGE

Adjunctive treatment of second- and third-degree burns (especially when resistance to other antibiotics and sulfonamides occurs); prevention of skin allograft rejection –
Adults and children: apply directly to lesion daily or every few days, depending on severity of burn. May also be applied to dressings used to cover affected area.

ADVERSE REACTIONS
GU: possible renal toxicity.
Skin: *erythema, pruritus,* burning, edema, severe reactions (vesiculation, denudation, ulceration), *allergic contact dermatitis.*

INTERACTIONS
None significant.

CONTRAINDICATIONS
- Contraindicated in patients hypersensitive to the drug.
- Use cautiously in patients with known or suspected renal impairment. Monitor serum creatinine levels regularly.

NURSING CONSIDERATIONS
- Clean wound as indicated by the doctor before reapplying dressings.
- If irritation, sensitization, or infection occurs, discontinue use.
- When using wet dressing, protect skin around wound with zinc oxide ointment.
- Store solution in tight, light-resistant containers (brown bottles). Avoid exposure to direct light, prolonged heat, and alkaline materials.
- Drug may discolor in light but still retains its potency.
- Discard cloudy solutions if warming to 55° to 60° C (131° to 140° F) does not restore clarity.
- Use reverse isolation or sterile application technique to prevent further wound contamination.

nystatin
Mycostatin, Nadostine†, Nilstat
Pregnancy Risk Category: B

HOW SUPPLIED
Cream: 100,000 units/g
Ointment: 100,000 units/g
Powder: 100,000 units/g
Vaginal tablets: 100,000 units

ACTION
Mechanism: disrupts integrity of fungal cell wall, promoting osmotic instability.
Onset: 24 to 72 hours.

INDICATIONS & DOSAGE
Cutaneous and mucocutaneous infections caused by Candida albicans, *such as oral thrush, diaper rash, and vulvovaginal candidiasis –*
Adults and children: apply to affected area once daily or b.i.d. for 2 weeks.
Vulvovaginal candidiasis –
Adults: 1 vaginal tablet daily or b.i.d. for 14 days.

ADVERSE REACTIONS
Skin: occasional contact dermatitis from preservatives in some formulations.

INTERACTIONS
None significant.

CONTRAINDICATIONS
- Contraindicated in patients hypersensitive to the drug.

NURSING CONSIDERATIONS
- Generally well tolerated by all age groups, including debilitated infants.
- Preparation does not stain skin or mucous membranes.
- Cream is recommended for intertriginous areas; powder, for very moist areas; ointment, for dry areas.
- Tell the female patient to continue using drug during her menstrual period.
- Tell the patient to use drug for the full prescribed period, even if condition has improved. Immunosuppressed patients may use the drug chronically.
- Do not use occlusive dressings.
- Refrigerate vaginal tablets.

oxiconazole nitrate

Oxistat

Pregnancy Risk Category: B

HOW SUPPLIED

Cream: 1%
Lotion: 1%

ACTION

Mechanism: Inhibits ergosterol synthesis in fungal cell walls, causing osmotic instability and cell lysis.
Onset: variable. **Peak:** Effects peak in 2 to 4 weeks.

INDICATIONS & DOSAGE

Cutaneous candidiasis; tinea pedis, cruris, tinea versicolor, and tinea corporis caused by Trichophyton rubrum, T. mentagrophytes, *and* Epidermophyton floccosum –
Adults: apply to affected area once daily or b.i.d. Treat tinea cruris and tinea corporis for 2 weeks, tinea pedis for 1 month to minimize risk of recurrence.

ADVERSE REACTIONS

Skin: pruritus, burning, stinging, contact dermatitis, irritation, scaling, tingling, pain.

INTERACTIONS

None significant.

CONTRAINDICATIONS

- Contraindicated in patients hypersensitive to the drug or any component of the formulation.
- Use cautiously in breast-feeding patients; oxiconazole is excreted in breast milk.

NURSING CONSIDERATIONS

- Tell the patient to discontinue drug and contact the doctor if local irritation occurs.
- Ensure that the patient understands that drug is for external use only.

Drug shouldn't touch the eyes or vagina.

podofilox

Condylox*

Pregnancy Risk Category: C

HOW SUPPLIED

Topical solution: 0.5%*

ACTION

Mechanism: Unknown; a keratolytic agent that causes local necrosis of wart tissue.
Onset: variable; minimal absorption.

INDICATIONS & DOSAGE

External genital warts (condylomata acuminata) –
Adults: apply to affected areas q 12 hours for 3 consecutive days; then withhold for 4 consecutive days. Repeat as needed up to 4 weeks until warts disappear.

ADVERSE REACTIONS

CNS: insomnia, dizziness.
GI: vomiting.
GU: foreskin retraction, dyspareunia, hematuria.
Skin: burning, pain, inflammation, erosion, pruritus, tingling, *tenderness,* chafing, scarring, vesicle formation, crusting edema, dryness and peeling.

INTERACTIONS

None significant.

CONTRAINDICATIONS

- Contraindicated in patients hypersensitive to or intolerant of any component of the medication (contains 95% alcohol).
- Do not use to treat genital warts in the perianal area or on mucous membranes of the genital area, including the urethra, rectum, and vagina.

NURSING CONSIDERATIONS

- If no response occurs after 4 weeks of therapy, alternative therapy should be considered.
- Tell the patient that the drug is for external use only. Systemic administration has caused hematologic toxicity, hematuria, seizures, and GI disturbances.
- Tell the patient that additional applications will not improve efficacy but can increase adverse reactions and the risk of systemic absorption, which is associated with substantial toxicity.
- Teach the patient how to apply the drug:
  - Dampen the supplied cotton-tipped applicator with drug and touch it to the wart.
  - Apply least amount needed to cover the lesion; 0.5 ml or less, and covering less than 10 cm² (4″) of wart tissue.
  - Allow the area to dry before allowing skin to retract.
  - Dispose of used applicator properly and wash hands thoroughly afterward.
- Tell the patient to avoid contact with eyes. If eye contact occurs, the patient should flush the area with plenty of water and contact the doctor immediately.

silver sulfadiazine

Flamazine†, Flint SSD, Silvadene, SSD-AF, Thermazene

Pregnancy Risk Category: C

HOW SUPPLIED

Cream: 1%

ACTION

Mechanism: Broad-spectrum sulfonamide that acts on cell membrane and cell wall; bactericidal for many gram-positive and gram-negative organisms.

Onset: on contact. **Duration:** elimination half-life of absorbed sulfadiazine, about 24 hours.

INDICATIONS & DOSAGE

Prevention and treatment of wound infection, especially in second- and third-degree burns –

Adults and children: apply 1/16″ thickness to clean debrided burn wound daily or b.i.d.

ADVERSE REACTIONS

Hematologic: ***neutropenia*** (in 3% to 5% of those receiving extensive applications).

Skin: pain, burning, rashes, itching.

INTERACTIONS

Topical proteolytic enzymes: inactivation of enzymes. Do not use together.

CONTRAINDICATIONS

- Contraindicated in premature and full-term neonates during first month of life. Drug may increase possibility of kernicterus.
- Use with caution in patients hypersensitive to sulfonamides.

NURSING CONSIDERATIONS

- Use reverse isolation or sterile application technique to prevent wound contamination.
- If hepatic or renal dysfunction occurs, consider discontinuing drug.
- Inspect the patient's skin daily, and note any changes. Notify the doctor if burning or excessive pain develops.
- Use only on affected areas. Keep these areas medicated at all times.
- Monitor serum sulfadiazine concentrations and renal function, and check urine for sulfa crystals in patients with extensive burns.
- Bathe the patient daily, if possible.
- Discard darkened cream, which indicates drug is ineffective.

sulconazole nitrate

Exelderm

Pregnancy Risk Category: C

HOW SUPPLIED

Topical solution: 1%
Cream: 1%

ACTION

Mechanism: Unknown; an imidazole derivative that inhibits the growth of both fungi and yeast.
Onset: variable; minimal absorption.
Peak: Effects peak in 3 to 4 weeks.

INDICATIONS & DOSAGE

Tinea cruris, tinea corporis, tinea pedis, or tinea versicolor –
Adults: massage a small amount of drug into affected area daily to b.i.d. for 3 weeks. Treat tinea pedis with cream b.i.d. daily for 4 weeks.

ADVERSE REACTIONS

Skin: pruritus, burning, stinging.

INTERACTIONS

None significant.

CONTRAINDICATIONS

- Contraindicated in patients hypersensitive to any component of the formulation.

NURSING CONSIDERATIONS

- If irritation develops during treatment, tell the patient to discontinue drug and contact the doctor. If no improvement occurs after 4 weeks, diagnosis should be reconsidered.
- Clinical improvement is usually apparent within 1 week, with symptomatic relief in just a few days. Explain to the patient the necessity of completing the full course of therapy, even after symptoms subside, to prevent recurrence.
- Efficacy against tinea pedis (athlete's foot) has not been proven with the topical solution; use only the cream.
- Tell the patient to avoid touching the eyes with the drug and to wash hands thoroughly after applying.

terbinafine hydrochloride

Lamisil

Pregnancy Risk Category: B

HOW SUPPLIED

Cream: 1%

ACTION

Mechanism: Fungicidal; selectively inhibits an early step in synthesis of sterols used by fungi for cell-wall synthesis.
Onset: variable.

INDICATIONS & DOSAGE

Interdigital tinea pedis, tinea cruris, and tinea corporis –
Adults: cover affected area and immediate surrounding area b.i.d. for at least 1 week.

ADVERSE REACTIONS

Skin: irritation, burning, pruritus, dryness.

INTERACTIONS

None significant.

CONTRAINDICATIONS

- Contraindicated in patients hypersensitive to the drug.

NURSING CONSIDERATIONS

- Tell the patient to discontinue drug and contact the doctor if irritation or sensitivity develops.
- Therapy shouldn't exceed 4 weeks.
- Teach the patient proper use of drug. Tell the patient to use only as directed for the full recommended course, even if symptoms disappear; and not to apply near the eyes, mouth, or mucous membranes or use occlusive dressings unless so directed.

• Observe patients for 2 to 4 weeks after therapy is complete to determine if treatment was successful; review the diagnosis if the condition persists beyond this observation period.

terconazole

Terazol 3 Vaginal Suppositories, Terazol 7 Vaginal Cream

Pregnancy Risk Category: C

HOW SUPPLIED

Vaginal cream: 0.4%, 0.8%
Vaginal suppositories: 80 mg

ACTION

Mechanism: Unknown; may increase fungal cell-membrane permeability (*Candida* species only).
Onset: variable; minimal systemic absorption.

INDICATIONS & DOSAGE

Vulvovaginal candidiasis –
Adults: insert 1 applicatorful of cream or 1 suppository into vagina h.s. Use 0.4% cream for 7 consecutive days; 0.8% cream or 80 mg suppository for 3 consecutive days. Repeat course if necessary after reconfirmation by smear or culture.

ADVERSE REACTIONS

CNS: headache.
Skin: vulvovaginal burning, irritation, *pruritus.*
Other: fever, chills, body aches.

INTERACTIONS

None significant.

CONTRAINDICATIONS

• Contraindicated in patients with known sensitivity to terconazole or any inactive ingredients in formulation.

NURSING CONSIDERATIONS

• Discontinue if the patient develops fever, chills, other flulike symptoms, or sensitivity.
• Some photosensitivity reactions were observed after dermal use; none with vaginal use.
• Continue treatment during the menstrual period; therapeutic effect of terconazole is unaffected by menstruation. However, tell the patient not to use tampons.
• Tell the patient to use for full treatment period prescribed. Explain how to prevent reinfection.
• Vaginal burning or pruritus is reportedly less frequent with terconazole than with miconazole or clotrimazole.

tetracycline hydrochloride

Achromycin, Topicycline

Pregnancy Risk Category: D

HOW SUPPLIED

Ointment: 3%
Topical solution: 2.2 mg/ml

ACTION

Mechanism: A broad-spectrum antibiotic that disrupts bacterial protein synthesis; usually bacteriostatic.
Onset: variable; minimal systemic absorption.

INDICATIONS & DOSAGE

Acne vulgaris –
Adults and children over 12 years: rub generously into affected areas b.i.d. until skin is thoroughly covered.
Prevention or treatment of superficial skin infections caused by susceptible bacteria –
Adults: apply to affected area b.i.d. in morning and evening or t.i.d.

ADVERSE REACTIONS

Skin: temporary stinging or burning on application; slight yellowing of treated skin, especially in patients with light complexions; severe dermatitis.

INTERACTIONS

Abrasive or medicated soaps or cleansers; acne preparations or other preparations containing peeling agents (benzoyl peroxide, resorcinol, salicylic acid, sulfur, tretinoin); alcohol-containing products (after-shave, cosmetics, perfumed toiletries, shaving creams or lotions); astringent soaps or cosmetics; isotretinoin; medicated cosmetics or cover-ups: may cause cumulative drying or irritation, resulting in excessive skin irritation. Use cautiously.

CONTRAINDICATIONS

- Contraindicated in patients hypersensitive to the drug.

NURSING CONSIDERATIONS

- Wash area before applying.
- If no improvement occurs or if condition worsens, stop using and notify the doctor.
- Prolonged use may result in overgrowth of nonsusceptible organisms.
- Tell the patient that she may continue normal use of cosmetics.
- Store at room temperature, away from excessive heat.
- Tell the patient not to share medication with family members.
- Advise the patient to use or discard the drug within 2 months.
- Explain that floating plug in bottle of Topicycline – an inert and harmless result of proper reconstitution of the preparation – shouldn't be removed.
- Significant systemic effects are unlikely because serum levels with topical tetracycline hydrochloride are much lower than those for orally administered drug.
- Increase or decrease applicator pressure against the skin to control flow rate of solution.

tioconazole

Vagistat

Pregnancy Risk Category: C

HOW SUPPLIED

Vaginal ointment: 6.5%

ACTION

Mechanism: A fungicidal imidazole that alters cell-wall permeability.

Onset: hours to days.

INDICATIONS & DOSAGE

Vulvovaginal candidiasis –

Adults: insert 1 applicatorful (about 4.6 g) intravaginally h.s.

ADVERSE REACTIONS

GU: *burning, pruritus,* discharge, vulvar edema and swelling, irritation.

INTERACTIONS

None significant.

CONTRAINDICATIONS

- Contraindicated in patients hypersensitive to the drug or other imidazole antifungal agents (miconazole, ketoconazole).

NURSING CONSIDERATIONS

- To avoid contamination of the ointment, open the applicator just before using it.
- Review proper use of the drug with the patient. Written instructions for the patient are available with the product. Tell the patient to insert drug high into the vagina.
- If irritation or sensitivity occurs, tell the patient to discontinue drug and report adverse reaction to the doctor.
- Emphasize the need to complete the full course of therapy, even after symptoms have improved. The patient should continue using the drug, even during her menstrual period.
- Tell the patient to use a sanitary napkin to avoid staining her clothing.

• Advise the patient to avoid sexual intercourse during therapy, or advise partner to use a condom to prevent reinfection.

tolnaftate

Aftate for Athlete's Foot◇, Aftate for Jock Itch◇, Dr. Scholl's Athlete's Foot Powder◇, Dr. Scholl's Athlete's Foot Spray◇, Footwork◇, Fungatin◇, Genaspor◇, NP-27◇, Tinactin◇, Ting◇, Zeasorb-AF◇

Pregnancy Risk Category: C

HOW SUPPLIED

Aerosol liquid: 1% (36% alcohol)◇
Aerosol powder: 1% (14% alcohol)◇
Cream: 1%◇
Gel: 1%◇
Powder: 1%◇
Pump spray liquid: 1% (36% alcohol)◇
Topical solution: 1%◇

ACTION

Mechanism: Fungistatic and fungicidal activity. Mechanism is unknown.
Onset: variable.

INDICATIONS & DOSAGE

Superficial fungal infections of the skin; infections due to common pathogenic fungi; tinea pedis, tinea cruris, tinea corporis, and tinea versicolor–
Adults and children: apply ¼" to ½" ribbon of cream or 3 drops of lotion to cover area about the size of one hand; same amount of cream or 3 drops of lotion to cover toes and interdigital webs of one foot; or gel, powder, or spray to cover affected area. Apply and massage gently into skin b.i.d. for 2 to 6 weeks.

ADVERSE REACTIONS

Skin: possible irritation.

INTERACTIONS

None significant.

CONTRAINDICATIONS

• Contraindicated in patients hypersensitive to the drug.

NURSING CONSIDERATIONS

• Discontinue if condition worsens. Check with the doctor.
• Odorless, greaseless; won't stain or discolor skin, hair, nails, or clothing.
• Use only a small quantity of cream or lotion; treated area should not be wet with solution.
• Commonly used to treat tinea pedis (athlete's foot). If no improvement occurs after 10 days, consult the doctor.
• Tell the patient to continue using for full treatment period prescribed, even if condition has improved. Treatment should continue for at least 2 weeks after symptoms have resolved to prevent reinfection.
• Don't use to treat fungal infections of the hair or nails; tolnaftate is ineffective against these fungi.
• Powder or aerosol may be used inside socks and shoes of persons susceptible to tinea infections.

undecylenic acid and zinc undecylenate

Cruex◇, Desenex◇, Desenex Aerosol◇, Quinsana Plus◇

Pregnancy Risk Category: C

HOW SUPPLIED

Cream: 15 g
Ointment: 15 g, 30 g
Powder: 2% undecylenic acid and 20% zinc undecylenate◇

ACTION

Mechanism: Unknown, although drug has fungistatic and fungicidal activity.
Onset: variable; minimal systemic absorption.

INDICATIONS & DOSAGE
Tinea pedis, tinea cruris, and tinea corporis (except nails and hairy areas) –
Adults and children: apply b.i.d. to thoroughly clean area. Treat tinea cruris for 2 weeks, tinea pedis or tinea corporis for 4 weeks.

ADVERSE REACTIONS
Skin: possible irritation.

INTERACTIONS
None significant.

CONTRAINDICATIONS
- Contraindicated in patients hypersensitive to the drug.

NURSING CONSIDERATIONS
- Tell the patient to continue using for full treatment period prescribed, even if condition has improved.
- Apply for at least 2 weeks to minimize risk of relapse.
- Liquids are preferable for hairy areas; powders in moist areas such as skin folds. Ointment or cream should be used at night, but the powder may be used during the day.

Scabicides and pediculicides

benzyl benzoate lotion
crotamiton
lindane
permethrin
pyrethrins

COMBINATION PRODUCTS
None.

benzyl benzoate lotion

Scabanca†

Pregnancy Risk Category: C

HOW SUPPLIED
Lotion: 14% (with benzocaine 2%)
Emulsion: 50%

ACTION
Mechanism: Unknown.
Onset: on contact with parasite.

INDICATIONS & DOSAGE
Parasitic infestation (scabies, Phthirus pubis, Pediculus humanus capitis) –
Adults and children: scrub entire body with soap and water. Remove scales or crusts. Then apply the lotion undiluted over entire body, except the face and scalp, while still damp. Be sure to apply around nails. Let dry. Apply second coat on the most involved areas. Bathe after 24 hours.

ADVERSE REACTIONS
Skin: *irritation, pruritus; contact dermatitis with repeated applications.*

INTERACTIONS
None significant.

CONTRAINDICATIONS
- Contraindicated when skin is raw or inflamed.

NURSING CONSIDERATIONS
- Retreatment may be indicated if mites reappear or new lesions form, which occurs in 7 to 10 days.
- Preferred over lindane for treatment of infants, young children, and pregnant or breast-feeding patients.
- Do not apply to face, eyes, mucous membranes, or urethral meatus. If accidental contact with eyes occurs, flush with water and notify the doctor.
- Notify the doctor immediately if skin irritation or hypersensitivity develops; tell the patient to discontinue drug and to wash it off skin.
- Instruct the patient to change and sterilize (boil, launder, dry clean, or apply very hot iron) all clothing and bed linen after drug is washed off.
- Reassure the patient that although itching may continue for several weeks, it will cease; continued itching does not indicate that therapy is ineffective.
- Apply topical corticosteroids as prescribed if dermatitis develops from scratching.
- After application for lice infestation, use a fine-tooth comb dipped in white vinegar to remove nits from hairy areas.
- Instruct the patient to reapply drug if it is washed off during treatment time.
- Do not apply to infants' or small children's hands because they put hands in their mouths.
- Make sure hospitalized patients are placed in isolation, with linen-handling precautions until treatment is completed.
- Tell the patient to warn other family members and sexual contacts about infestation. Sexual contacts should be treated simultaneously.

• Store drug in light-resistant container; avoid exposure to excessive heat.

crotamiton

Eurax

Pregnancy Risk Category: C

HOW SUPPLIED

Cream: 10%

ACTION

Mechanism: Unknown.

Onset: on contact with parasite.

INDICATIONS & DOSAGE

Parasitic infestation (scabies) –
Adults and children: scrub entire body with soap and water. Remove scales or crusts. Then apply a thin layer of cream over entire body, from chin down (with special attention to folds, creases, interdigital spaces, and genital area). Apply second coat in 24 hours. Wait additional 48 hours, then wash off.

Itching –
Adults and children: apply locally b.i.d. or t.i.d.

ADVERSE REACTIONS

Skin: *irritation.*

INTERACTIONS

None significant.

CONTRAINDICATIONS

• Contraindicated when skin is raw or inflamed.

NURSING CONSIDERATIONS

• Do not apply to face, eyes, mucous membranes, or urethral meatus. If accidental contact with eyes occurs, flush with water and notify the doctor.
• Notify the doctor immediately if skin irritation or hypersensitivity develops; tell the patient to discontinue drug and to wash it off skin.
• Instruct the patient to change and sterilize (boil, launder, dry clean, or apply very hot iron) all clothing and bed linen after drug is washed off.
• After application for lice infestation, use a fine-tooth comb dipped in white vinegar to remove nits from hairy areas.
• Apply topical corticosteroids as prescribed if dermatitis develops from scratching.
• Estimate amount of cream needed per application; most patients have a tendency to overuse scabicides. For most adults, a single tube of cream provides a sufficient amount for two applications.
• Tell the patient to warn other family members and sexual contacts about infestation. Sexual contacts should be treated simultaneously.
• Instruct the patient to reapply drug if it is washed off during treatment time.
• Make sure hospitalized patients are placed in isolation, with special linen-handling precautions until treatment is completed.
• Repeat treatment as prescribed if mites reappear or new lesions form, which may occur after 7 to 10 days.
• Monthly maintenance treatments may be necessary in long-term care facilities, where infestation is a problem.

lindane

Gamma Benzene, gBh†, Kildane, Kwell, Kwellada†, Scabene

Pregnancy Risk Category: C

HOW SUPPLIED

Cream: 1%
Lotion: 1%
Shampoo: 1%

ACTION

Mechanism: Appears to inhibit neuronal membrane function in arthropods, causing neuronal hyperactivity,

seizures, and death after penetrating the parasites' exoskeleton.
Onset: about 3 hours.

INDICATIONS & DOSAGE
Parasitic infestation (scabies, pediculosis)—
Adults and children: scrub entire body with soap and water; let skin dry thoroughly before using.

Apply thin layer of cream or lotion over entire skin surface (with special attention to folds, creases, interdigital spaces, and genital area) for scabies, or to hairy areas for pediculosis. After 8 to 12 hours, wash off drug. Repeat process in 1 week if mites appear or new lesions develop.

Apply shampoo undiluted to affected area and work into lather for 4 to 5 minutes; small amounts of water may enhance formation of lather. Apply 30 ml of shampoo for short hair, 45 ml for medium length hair, or 60 ml for long hair. Rinse thoroughly and rub dry with towel.

ADVERSE REACTIONS
CNS: *dizziness,* ***seizures.***
Skin: *irritation with repeated use.*

INTERACTIONS
None significant.

CONTRAINDICATIONS
- Contraindicated in patients hypersensitive to the drug and those with seizure disorders and when skin is raw or inflamed.
- Contraindicated in premature neonates.
- Use cautiously in infants and young children; there is a greater risk for CNS toxicity in this group.

NURSING CONSIDERATIONS
- Do not apply to open areas, acutely inflamed skin, or to face, eyes, mucous membranes, or urethral meatus. If accidental contact with eyes occurs, flush with water and notify the doctor. Avoid inhaling vapors.
- Notify the doctor immediately if skin irritation or hypersensitivity develops; tell patient to discontinue drug and to wash it off skin.
- Discourage repeated use, which can lead to skin irritation, systemic toxicity, or seizures. Repeat use only if live lice or nits are found after 1 week.
- Warn the patient that itching may continue for several weeks after effective treatment, especially in scabies.
- Apply topical corticosteroids or administer oral antihistamines as prescribed for pruritus.
- Instruct the patient to change and sterilize (boil, launder, dry clean, or apply very hot iron) all clothing and bed linen after drug is washed off.
- After application for lice infestation, use a fine-tooth comb dipped in white vinegar to remove nits from hairy areas.
- Use shampoo to clean combs or brushes; wash them thoroughly afterward. Warn the patient not to use routinely.
- Instruct the patient to reapply drug if it is washed off during treatment time.
- Make sure that hospitalized patients are placed in isolation, with special linen-handling precautions until treatment is completed.
- Tell patients to warn other family members and sexual contacts about infestation. Sexual contacts should be treated simultaneously.
- Modest amounts (6% to 13%) are absorbed through intact skin. Absorption is increased if used with creams, oils, or lotions or if applied to face, scalp, axillae, neck, scrotum, or irritated or broken skin.

permethrin
Elimite, Nix
Pregnancy Risk Category: B

HOW SUPPLIED

Topical liquid (cream-rinse): 1%

ACTION

Mechanism: Acts on the parasites' nerve cells to disrupt the sodium channel current, causing paralysis of the parasite.

Onset: 10 to 15 minutes. **Duration:** residual activity persists about 10 days.

INDICATIONS & DOSAGE

Infestation with Pediculus humanus capitis *(head lice) and its nits –*

Adults and children: use after hair has been washed with shampoo, rinsed with water, and towel-dried. Apply 25 to 50 ml of liquid to saturate the hair and scalp. Allow to remain on hair for 10 minutes before rinsing off with water.

ADVERSE REACTIONS

Skin: pruritus, burning, stinging, tingling, numbness or scalp discomfort, mild erythema, scalp rash.

INTERACTIONS

None significant.

CONTRAINDICATIONS

- Contraindicated in patients hypersensitive to pyrethrins or chrysanthemums.
- Do not use on children under 2 months.

NURSING CONSIDERATIONS

- A single treatment is usually all that is necessary. Combing of nits is not required for effectiveness but drug package supplies a fine-tooth comb for cosmetic use as desired.
- Retreat as prescribed if lice are observed 7 days after the initial application.
- Explain to the patient that treatment with permethrin may temporarily worsen the symptoms of head lice infestation, such as pruritus, erythema, and edema.
- Tell the patient that headgear, scarfs, coats, and bed linens should be disinfected by machine washing using hot water and machine drying for at least 20 minutes, using the hot cycle. Dry-clean nonwashable items and seal in a plastic bag for 2 weeks, or spray with a product designed to eliminate lice and their nits.
- Tell the patient to warn other family members and sexual contacts about infestation. Sexual contacts should be treated simultaneously.

pyrethrins

A-200 Pyrinate◇, Barc◇, Blue Gel, R&C, Pronto, Pyrinyl◇, RID◇, TISIT◇, Triple X◇

Pregnancy Risk Category: C

HOW SUPPLIED

Shampoo: pyrethrins 0.17% and piperonyl butoxide 2%; pyrethrins 0.3% and piperonyl butoxide 3%

Topical gel: pyrethrins 0.18% and piperonyl butoxide 2.2%; pyrethrins 0.33% and piperonyl butoxide 3%; pyrethrins 0.3% and piperonyl butoxide 4%

Topical solution: pyrethrins 0.18% and piperonyl butoxide 2%; pyrethrins 0.2%, piperonyl butoxide 2%, and deodorized kerosene 0.8%; pyrethrins 0.3% and piperonyl butoxide 3%

ACTION

Mechanism: Acts as contact poison that disrupts parasite's nervous system, causing parasite paralysis and death.

Onset: about 10 to 20 minutes.

INDICATIONS & DOSAGE

Infestations of head, body, and pubic (crab) lice and their eggs –

Adults and children: apply to hair, scalp, or other infested areas until entirely wet. Allow to remain for 10 minutes but no longer. Wash thoroughly with warm water and soap or shampoo. Remove dead lice and eggs with fine-tooth comb. Repeat treatment, if necessary, in 7 to 10 days to kill newly hatched lice. Do not exceed two applications within 24 hours.

ADVERSE REACTIONS

Skin: *irritation with repeated use.*

INTERACTIONS

None significant.

CONTRAINDICATIONS

- Contraindicated in patients hypersensitive to the drug or when skin is raw or inflamed.
- Contraindicated in patients allergic to ragweed.
- Use cautiously in infants and small children.

NURSING CONSIDERATIONS

- Do not apply to open areas or acutely inflamed skin or to face, eyes, mucous membranes, or urethral meatus. If accidental contact with eyes occurs, flush with water and notify the doctor.
- Discourage repeated use, which can lead to skin irritation and possible systemic toxicity.
- All preparations contain petroleum distillates. Notify the doctor immediately if skin irritation develops; tell the patient to discontinue drug and to wash it off skin.
- Apply topical corticosteroids or oral antihistamines as prescribed if dermatitis develops from scratching.
- Instruct the patient to change and sterilize (boil, launder, dry clean, or apply very hot iron) all clothing and bed linen after drug is washed off.
- Pyrethrins and lindane may be equally effective for lice infestation, but pyrethrins may be less hazardous.
- Teach the patient to remove dead parasites with a fine-tooth comb.
- Not effective against scabies.
- Tell the patient to warn other family members and sexual contacts about infestation. Sexual contacts should be treated simultaneously.

89
Topical corticosteroids

alclometasone dipropionate
amcinonide
betamethasone benzoate
betamethasone dipropionate
betamethasone valerate
clobetasol propionate
clocortolone pivalate
desonide
desoximetasone
dexamethasone
dexamethasone sodium phosphate
diflorasone diacetate
fluocinolone acetonide
fluocinonide
flurandrenolide
fluticasone propionate
halcinonide
halobetasol propionate
hydrocortisone
hydrocortisone acetate
hydrocortisone butyrate
hydrocortisone valerate
mometasone furoate
triamcinolone acetonide

COMBINATION PRODUCTS
Corticosteroids for topical use are commonly combined with antibiotics and antifungals. (See Chapter 87, LOCAL ANTI-INFECTIVES.)

alclometasone dipropionate
Alclovate, Logoderm‡

Pregnancy Risk Category: C

HOW SUPPLIED
Cream: 0.05%
Ointment: 0.05%

ACTION
Mechanism: Diffuses across cell membranes to form complexes with specific cytoplasmic receptors. Exhibits anti-inflammatory, antipruritic, vasoconstrictive, and antiproliferative activity. Considered a group IV (low-potency) agent, according to vasoconstrictive properties.
Peak: Plasma levels are highest when applied to inflamed or damaged skin, eyelids, or scrotal area; lowest when applied to intact normal skin, palms of hands, or soles of feet.

INDICATIONS & DOSAGE
Inflammation associated with corticosteroid-responsive dermatoses –
Adults: apply a thin film to affected areas b.i.d. or t.i.d. Gently massage until the medication disappears.

ADVERSE REACTIONS
Skin: burning, pruritus, irritation, dryness, erythema, folliculitis, striae, acneiform eruptions, perioral dermatitis, hypopigmentation, hypertrichosis, allergic contact dermatitis; *secondary infection, maceration, atrophy, striae, miliaria* (with occlusive dressings).
Systemic: ***hypothalamic-pituitary-adrenal (HPA) axis suppression,*** Cushing's syndrome, hyperglycemia, glucosuria.

INTERACTIONS
None significant.

CONTRAINDICATIONS
- Contraindicated in patients hypersensitive to the drug.
- Use cautiously in patients with viral skin diseases such as varicella, vaccinia, or herpes simplex and in patients with fungal infections or bacterial skin infections.

NURSING CONSIDERATIONS

• Warn the patient not to use for more than 14 consecutive days; potential for systemic absorption and HPA axis suppression exists.

• Avoid application near eyes or mucous membranes. Do not apply to face, armpits, groin, or under breasts unless specifically ordered.

• Systemic absorption likely with use of occlusive dressings, prolonged treatment, or application to extensive body surface. Monitor the patient for systemic adverse reactions.

• Children may absorb larger amounts of drug and be more prone to systemic toxicity.

• Stop drug and notify the doctor if the patient develops signs of systemic absorption, skin irritation or ulceration, hypersensitivity, or infection.

• If antifungal agents or antibiotics are used concomitantly, corticosteroids should be discontinued until infection is controlled.

• Gently wash skin before applying. To prevent skin damage, rub medication in gently, leaving a thin coat. When treating hairy sites, part hair and apply directly to lesions.

• If an occlusive dressing is ordered, do not leave it in place longer than 16 hours each day or use it on infected or exudative lesions.

• Notify the doctor and remove occlusive dressing if fever develops.

• Change dressings as ordered by the doctor. Discontinue drug and notify the doctor if skin infection, striae, or atrophy occurs.

• To prevent recurrence, continue treatment for a few days after lesions clear.

• Repeated application can result in diminished effectiveness.

amcinonide

Cyclocort

Pregnancy Risk Category: C

HOW SUPPLIED

Cream: 0.1%
Lotion: 0.1%
Ointment: 0.1%

ACTION

Mechanism: Diffuses across cell membranes to form complexes with specific cytoplasmic receptors. Exhibits anti-inflammatory, antipruritic, vasoconstrictive, and antiproliferative activity. Considered a group II (high-potency) agent according to vasoconstrictive properties.

Peak: Plasma levels are highest when applied to inflamed or damaged skin, eyelids, or scrotal area; lowest when applied to intact normal skin, palms of hands, or soles of feet.

INDICATIONS & DOSAGE

Inflammation associated with corticosteroid-responsive dermatoses –

Adults and children: apply a light film to affected areas b.i.d. or t.i.d. Rub cream in gently and thoroughly until it disappears.

ADVERSE REACTIONS

Skin: burning, pruritus, irritation, dryness, erythema, folliculitis, striae, acneiform eruptions, perioral dermatitis, hypopigmentation, hypertrichosis, allergic contact dermatitis; *secondary infection, maceration, atrophy, striae, miliaria* (with occlusive dressings).

Systemic: ***hypothalamic-pituitary-adrenal (HPA) axis suppression,*** Cushing's syndrome, hyperglycemia, glucosuria.

INTERACTIONS

None significant.

CONTRAINDICATIONS

• Contraindicated in patients hypersensitive to the drug.

• Use cautiously in patients with viral diseases of skin such as varicella, vaccinia, or herpes simplex and in patients with fungal infections or bacterial skin infections.

NURSING CONSIDERATIONS

- Avoid application near eyes or mucous membranes. Do not use on face, armpits, groin, in ear canal, or under breasts unless specifically ordered.
- Systemic absorption likely with use of occlusive dressings, prolonged treatment, or extensive body-surface treatment. Monitor patients for systemic adverse reactions.
- Children may absorb larger amounts of drug and be more prone to systemic toxicity. Avoid using plastic pants or tight-fitting diapers on treated areas in young children.
- Stop drug and notify the doctor if the patient develops signs of systemic absorption, skin irritation or ulceration, hypersensitivity, or infection.
- If antifungal agents or antibiotics are being used concomitantly, corticosteroids should be stopped until infection is controlled.
- Gently wash skin before applying. To prevent skin damage, rub medication in gently, leaving a thin coat. Part hair and apply directly to lesion when treating hairy sites.
- If an occlusive dressing is ordered, do not leave it in place longer than 16 hours each day or use it on infected or exudative lesions.
- For patients with eczematous dermatitis whose skin may be irritated by adhesive material, hold dressing in place with gauze, elastic bandages, stockings, or stockinette.
- Notify the doctor and remove occlusive dressing if fever develops.
- Change dressings as ordered. Discontinue drug and notify the doctor if skin infection, striae, or atrophy occurs.
- To prevent recurrence, continue treatment for a few days after lesions clear.

betamethasone benzoate

Benisone, Uticort

betamethasone dipropionate

Alphatrex, Diprolene, Diprolene AF, Diprosone, Maxivate, Psorion

betamethasone valerate

Betatrex, Beta-Val, Betnovate†‡, Valisone

Pregnancy Risk Category: C

HOW SUPPLIED

benzoate

Cream: 0.025%
Gel: 0.025%
Lotion: 0.025%
Ointment: 0.025%

dipropionate

Aerosol: 0.1%
Cream: 0.05%
Lotion: 0.05%
Ointment: 0.05%

valerate

Aerosol: 0.1%
Cream: 0.01%, 0.1%
Lotion: 0.1%
Ointment: 0.1%

ACTION

Mechanism: Diffuses across cell membranes to form complexes with specific cytoplasmic receptors. Exhibits anti-inflammatory, antipruritic, vasoconstrictive, and antiproliferative activity. Considered a group III (medium-potency) agent according to vasoconstrictive properties.

Peak: Plasma levels are highest when applied to inflamed or damaged skin, eyelids, or scrotal area; lowest when applied to intact normal skin, palms of hands, or soles of feet.

INDICATIONS & DOSAGE

Inflammation associated with corticosteroid-responsive dermatoses –

Adults and children: clean area; apply cream, ointment, lotion, aerosol spray, or gel sparingly daily to q.i.d.

ADVERSE REACTIONS

Skin: burning, pruritus, irritation, dryness, erythema, folliculitis, striae, acneiform eruptions, perioral dermatitis, hypopigmentation, hypertrichosis, allergic contact dermatitis; *secondary infection, maceration, atrophy, striae, miliaria* (with occlusive dressings).

Systemic: ***hypothalamic-pituitary-adrenal (HPA) axis suppression,*** Cushing's syndrome, hyperglycemia, and glucosuria (with betamethasone dipropionate).

INTERACTIONS

None significant.

CONTRAINDICATIONS

- Contraindicated in patients hypersensitive to the drug.
- Use cautiously in patients with viral diseases of skin such as varicella, vaccinia, or herpes simplex and in patients with fungal infections or bacterial skin infections.

NURSING CONSIDERATIONS

- Avoid application near eyes, mucous membranes, or in ear canal.
- Because of alcohol content of vehicle, gel preparations may cause mild, transient stinging, especially if used on or near excoriated skin.
- Systemic absorption likely with use of occlusive dressings, prolonged treatment, or extensive body-surface treatment. Monitor the patient for systemic adverse reactions.
- Children may absorb larger amounts of drug and be more prone to systemic toxicity. Avoid the use of plastic pants or tight-fitting diapers on treated areas when used in young children.
- Stop drug and notify the doctor if the patient develops signs of systemic absorption, skin irritation or ulceration, hypersensitivity, or infection.
- If antifungal agents or antibiotics are used concomitantly, corticosteroids should be stopped until infection is controlled.
- Gently wash skin before applying. To prevent skin damage, rub medication in gently, leaving a thin coat. When treating hairy sites, part hair and apply directly to lesions.
- If an occlusive dressing is ordered, do not leave it in place longer than 16 hours each day. Do not use occlusive dressings on infected or exudative lesions.
- For patients with eczematous dermatitis whose skin may be irritated by adhesive material, hold dressing in place with gauze, elastic bandages, stockings, or stockinette.
- Notify the doctor and remove occlusive dressing if fever develops.
- Change dressings as ordered. Discontinue drug and notify the doctor if infection, striae, or atrophy occurs.
- To prevent recurrence, treatment should be continued for a few days after lesions clear.
- Note that Diprolene and Diprolene AF may not be substituted generically because other products have different potencies.

clobetasol propionate

Dermovate†, Temovate

Pregnancy Risk Category: C

HOW SUPPLIED

Cream: 0.05%
Lotion: 0.05%
Ointment: 0.05%

ACTION

Mechanism: Diffuses across cell membranes to form complexes with specific cytoplasmic receptors. Exhibits anti-inflammatory, antipruritic, vasoconstrictive, and antiproliferative activity. Considered a group I (very

high-potency) agent according to vasoconstrictive properties.
Peak: Plasma levels are highest when applied to inflamed or damaged skin, eyelids, or scrotal area; lowest when applied to intact normal skin, palms of hands, or soles of feet.

INDICATIONS & DOSAGE
Inflammation associated with corticosteroid-responsive dermatoses –
Adults: apply a thin layer to affected skin areas b.i.d., in the morning and evening for a maximum of 14 days. Total dosage should not exceed 50 g weekly.

ADVERSE REACTIONS
Skin: burning, pruritus, irritation, dryness, erythema, folliculitis, perioral dermatitis, allergic contact dermatitis, hypopigmentation, hypertrichosis, acneiform eruptions.
Systemic: ***hypothalamic-pituitary-adrenal (HPA) axis suppression,*** Cushing's syndrome, hyperglycemia, glucosuria.

INTERACTIONS
None significant.

CONTRAINDICATIONS
- Contraindicated in patients hypersensitive to the drug.
- Use cautiously in patients with viral skin diseases such as varicella, vaccinia, or herpes simplex and in patients with fungal infections or bacterial skin infections.
- Not recommended for use in children under 12 years.

NURSING CONSIDERATIONS
- Warn the patient not to use for longer than 14 consecutive days; risk of systemic absorption and HPA axis suppression.
- Avoid application near eyes, mucous membranes, or in ear canal.
- Don't use occlusive dressings or bandage, cover, or wrap treated areas.
- Stop drug and notify the doctor if the patient develops signs of systemic absorption, skin irritation or ulceration, hypersensitivity, or infection.
- If antifungal agents or antibiotics are used concomitantly, corticosteroids should be stopped until infection is controlled.
- Gently wash skin before applying. To prevent skin damage, rub medication in gently, leaving a thin coat. When treating hairy sites, part hair and apply directly to lesions.
- Discontinue drug and notify the doctor if skin infection, striae, or atrophy occurs.
- Repeated application can result in diminished effectiveness.
- Do not refrigerate.

clocortolone pivalate
Cloderm
Pregnancy Risk Category: C

HOW SUPPLIED
Cream: 0.1%

ACTION
Mechanism: Diffuses across cell membranes to form complexes with specific cytoplasmic receptors. Exhibits anti-inflammatory, antipruritic, vasoconstrictive, and antiproliferative activity. Considered a group III (medium-potency) agent according to vasoconstrictive properties.
Peak: Plasma levels are highest when applied to inflamed or damaged skin, eyelids, or scrotal area; lowest when applied to intact normal skin, palms of hands, or soles of feet.

INDICATIONS & DOSAGE
Inflammation associated with corticosteroid-responsive dermatoses –
Adults and children: apply cream sparingly to affected areas once daily to q.i.d. and rub in gently.

ADVERSE REACTIONS

Skin: burning, pruritus, irritation, dryness, erythema, folliculitis, striae, acneiform eruptions, perioral dermatitis, hypertrichosis, hypopigmentation, allergic contact dermatitis; *secondary infection, maceration, atrophy, striae, miliaria* (with occlusive dressings).
Systemic: ***hypothalamic-pituitary-adrenal (HPA) axis suppression,*** Cushing's syndrome, hyperglycemia, glucosuria.

INTERACTIONS

None significant.

CONTRAINDICATIONS

- Contraindicated in patients hypersensitive to the drug.
- Use cautiously in patients with viral diseases of skin such as varicella, vaccinia, or herpes simplex and in patients with fungal infections or bacterial skin infections.

NURSING CONSIDERATIONS

- Avoid application near eyes or mucous membranes.
- Systemic absorption likely with use of occlusive dressings, prolonged treatment, or extensive body-surface treatment. Monitor the patient for systemic adverse reactions.
- Children may absorb larger amounts of drug and be more prone to systemic toxicity. Avoid using plastic pants or tight-fitting diapers on treated areas in young children.
- Stop drug and notify the doctor if the patient develops signs of systemic absorption, skin irritation or ulceration, hypersensitivity, or infection.
- If antifungal agents or antibiotics are being used concomitantly, corticosteroids should be stopped until infection is controlled.
- Gently wash skin before applying. To prevent skin damage, rub medication in gently, leaving a thin coat. When treating hairy sites, part hair and apply directly to lesions.
- If an occlusive dressing is ordered, don't leave it in place longer than 16 hours each day; don't use occlusive dressings on infected or exudative lesions.
- For patients with eczematous dermatitis whose skin may be irritated by adhesive material, hold dressing in place with gauze, elastic bandages, or stockinette.
- Notify the doctor and remove occlusive dressing if fever develops.
- Change dressings as ordered. Discontinue drug and notify the doctor if skin infection, striae, or atrophy occurs.
- To prevent recurrence, continue treatment for a few days after lesions clear.

---

desonide

DesOwen, Tridesilon

Pregnancy Risk Category: C

HOW SUPPLIED

Cream: 0.05%
Ointment: 0.05%

ACTION

Mechanism: Diffuses across cell membranes to form complexes with specific cytoplasmic receptors. Exhibits anti-inflammatory, antipruritic, vasoconstrictive, and antiproliferative activity. Considered a group IV (low-potency) agent according to vasoconstrictive properties.
Peak: Plasma levels are highest when applied to inflamed or damaged skin, eyelids, or scrotal area; lowest when applied to intact normal skin, palms of hands, or soles of feet.

INDICATIONS & DOSAGE

Inflammation associated with corticosteroid-responsive dermatoses –
Adults and children: clean area; ap-

ply cream or ointment sparingly b.i.d. to q.i.d.

ADVERSE REACTIONS

Skin: burning, pruritus, irritation, dryness, erythema, folliculitis, perioral dermatitis, allergic contact dermatitis, hypertrichosis, hypopigmentation, acneiform eruptions; *maceration of skin, secondary infection, atrophy, striae, miliaria* (with occlusive dressings).

Systemic: ***hypothalamic-pituitary-adrenal (HPA) axis suppression,*** Cushing's syndrome, hyperglycemia, glucosuria.

INTERACTIONS

None significant.

CONTRAINDICATIONS

- Contraindicated in patients hypersensitive to the drug.
- Use cautiously in patients with viral diseases of skin such as varicella, vaccinia, or herpes simplex and in patients with fungal infections or bacterial skin infections.

NURSING CONSIDERATIONS

- Avoid application near eyes, mucous membranes, or in ear canal.
- Systemic absorption likely with use of occlusive dressings, prolonged treatment, or extensive body-surface treatment. Monitor the patient for systemic adverse reactions.
- Children may absorb larger amounts of drug and be more prone to systemic toxicity. Avoid using plastic pants or tight-fitting diapers on treated areas in young children.
- Stop drug and notify the doctor if patient develops signs of systemic absorption, skin irritation or ulceration, hypersensitivity, or infection.
- If antifungal agents or antibiotics are used concomitantly, corticosteroids should be stopped until infection is controlled.
- Gently wash skin before applying. To prevent skin damage, rub medication in gently, leaving a thin coat. When treating hairy sites, part hair and apply directly to lesions.
- If an occlusive dressing is ordered, don't leave dressing in place longer than 16 hours each day; don't use occlusive dressings on infected or exudative lesions.
- For patients with eczematous dermatitis whose skin may be irritated by adhesive material, hold dressing in place with gauze, elastic bandages, stockings, or stockinette.
- Notify the doctor and remove occlusive dressing if fever develops.
- Change dressing as ordered. Discontinue drug and notify doctor if skin infection, striae, or atrophy occurs.
- To prevent recurrence, continue treatment for a few days after lesions clear.

desoximetasone

Topicort

Pregnancy Risk Category: C

HOW SUPPLIED

Cream: 0.05%, 0.25%
Gel: 0.05%
Ointment: 0.25%

ACTION

Mechanism: Diffuses across cell membranes to form complexes with specific cytoplasmic receptors. Exhibits anti-inflammatory, antipruritic, vasoconstrictive, and antiproliferative activity. Considered a group III (medium-potency) agent according to vasoconstrictive properties.

Peak: Plasma levels are highest when applied to inflamed or damaged skin, eyelids, or scrotal area; lowest when applied to intact, normal skin, palms of hands, or soles of feet.

INDICATIONS & DOSAGE
Inflammation associated with corticosteroid-responsive dermatoses –
Adults and children: clean area; apply cream, gel, or ointment sparingly once daily to b.i.d.

ADVERSE REACTIONS
Skin: burning, pruritus, irritation, dryness, erythema, folliculitis, hypertrichosis, acneiform eruptions, perioral dermatitis, hypopigmentation, allergic contact dermatitis; *maceration, secondary infection, atrophy, striae, miliaria* (with occlusive dressings).
Systemic: ***hypothalamic-pituitary-adrenal (HPA) axis suppression,*** Cushing's syndrome, hyperglycemia, glucosuria.

INTERACTIONS
None significant.

CONTRAINDICATIONS
• Contraindicated in patients hypersensitive to the drug.
• Use cautiously in patients with viral diseases of skin such as varicella, vaccinia, or herpes simplex and in patients with fungal infections or bacterial skin infections.

NURSING CONSIDERATIONS
• Avoid application near eyes, mucous membranes, or in ear canal.
• Systemic absorption likely with use of occlusive dressings, prolonged treatment, or extensive body-surface treatment. Monitor patients for systemic adverse reactions.
• Children may absorb larger amounts of drug and be more prone to systemic toxicity. Avoid using plastic pants or tight-fitting diapers on treated areas in young children.
• Stop drug and notify the doctor if the patient develops signs of systemic absorption, skin irritation or ulceration, hypersensitivity, or infection.
• If antifungal agents or antibiotics are used concomitantly, corticosteroids should be stopped until infection is controlled.
• Gently wash skin before applying. To prevent skin damage, rub medication in gently, leaving a thin coat. When treating hairy sites, part hair and apply directly to lesions.
• If an occlusive dressing is ordered, don't leave dressing in place longer than 16 hours each day; don't use occlusive dressings on infected or exudative lesions.
• For patients with eczematous dermatitis whose skin may be irritated by adhesive material, hold dressing in place with gauze, elastic bandages, stockings, or stockinette.
• Notify the doctor and remove occlusive dressing if fever develops.
• Change dressing as ordered. Discontinue drug and notify doctor if skin infection, stiae, or atrophy occurs.
• To prevent recurrence, continue treatment for a few days after lesions clear.
• Gel contains alcohol and may cause burning or irritation in open lesions.
• Store in tightly sealed containers.

dexamethasone
Aeroseb-Dex, Decaderm, Decaspray

dexamethasone sodium phosphate
Decadron Phosphate

Pregnancy Risk Category: C

HOW SUPPLIED
dexamethasone
Aerosol: 0.01%, 0.04%
Gel: 0.1%
dexamethasone sodium phosphate
Cream: 0.1%

ACTION
Mechanism: Diffuses across cell membranes to form complexes with specific cytoplasmic receptors. Ex-

hibits anti-inflammatory, antipruritic, vasoconstrictive, and antiproliferative activity. Considered a group IV (low-potency) agent according to vasoconstrictive properties.
Peak: Plasma levels are highest when applied to inflamed or damaged skin, eyelids, or scrotal area; lowest when applied to intact normal skin, palms of hands, or soles of feet.

INDICATIONS & DOSAGE

Inflammation associated with corticosteroid-responsive dermatoses –
Adults and children: clean area; apply cream, gel, or aerosol sparingly b.i.d. to q.i.d.

For aerosol use on scalp, shake can well and apply to dry scalp after shampooing. Hold can upright. Slide applicator tube under hair so that it touches scalp. Spray while moving tube to all affected areas, keeping tube under hair and in contact with scalp throughout spraying, which should take about 2 seconds. Spot spray inadequately covered areas by sliding applicator tube through hair to touch scalp, then pressing and immediately releasing spray button. Don't massage medication into scalp or spray forehead or near eyes.

ADVERSE REACTIONS

Skin: burning, pruritus, irritation, dryness, erythema, folliculitis, hypertrichosis, acneiform eruptions, perioral dermatitis, hypopigmentation, allergic contact dermatitis; *maceration, secondary infection, atrophy, striae, miliaria* (with occlusive dressings).
Systemic: ***hypothalamic-pituitary-adrenal (HPA) axis suppression,*** Cushing's syndrome, hyperglycemia, glucosuria.

INTERACTIONS

None significant.

CONTRAINDICATIONS

- Contraindicated in patients hypersensitive to the drug.
- Use cautiously in patients with viral diseases of skin such as varicella, vaccinia, or herpes simplex and in patients with fungal infections or bacterial skin infections.

NURSING CONSIDERATIONS

- Avoid application near eyes, mucous membranes, or in ear canal.
- Systemic absorption likely with use of occlusive dressings, prolonged treatment, or extensive body-surface treatment. Monitor the patient for systemic adverse reactions.
- Children may absorb larger amounts of drug and be more prone to systemic toxicity. Avoid using plastic pants or tight-fitting diapers on treated areas in young children.
- Stop drug and notify the doctor if the patient develops signs of systemic absorption, skin irritation or ulceration, hypersensitivity, or infection.
- If antifungal agents or antibiotics are used concomitantly, corticosteroids should be stopped until infection is controlled.
- Gently wash skin before applying. To prevent skin damage, rub medication in gently, leaving a thin coat. When treating hairy sites, part hair and apply directly to lesions.
- If an occlusive dressing is ordered, don't leave it in place longer than 16 hours each day; don't use occlusive dressings on infected or exudative lesions.
- For patients with eczematous dermatitis whose skin may be irritated by adhesive material, hold dressing in place with gauze, elastic bandages, stockings, or stockinette.
- Notify the doctor and remove occlusive dressing if fever develops.
- Change dressing as ordered. Discontinue drug and notify doctor if skin infection, striae, or atrophy occurs.

• Aerosol preparation contains alcohol and may produce irritation or burning in open lesions. When using around the face, cover the patient's eyes and warn against inhalation of the spray. To avoid freezing tissues, do not spray longer than 3 seconds or closer than 6″ (15 cm).
• To prevent recurrence, continue treatment for a few days after lesions clear.

diflorasone diacetate

Florone, Flutone, Maxiflor, Psorcon

Pregnancy Risk Category: C

HOW SUPPLIED

Cream: 0.05%
Ointment: 0.05%

ACTION

Mechanism: Diffuses across cell membranes to form complexes with specific cytoplasmic receptors. Exhibits anti-inflammatory, antipruritic, vasoconstrictive, and antiproliferative activity. Considered a group II (high-potency) agent according to vasoconstrictive properties.
Peak: Plasma levels are highest when applied to inflamed or damaged skin, eyelids, or scrotal area; lowest when applied to intact normal skin, palms of hands, or soles of feet.

INDICATIONS & DOSAGE

Inflammation associated with corticosteroid-responsive dermatoses –
Adults and children: clean area; apply sparingly in a thin film. Apply cream b.i.d. to q.i.d.; apply ointment daily to t.i.d. because it is more potent.

ADVERSE REACTIONS

Skin: burning, pruritus, irritation, dryness, erythema, folliculitis, perioral dermatitis, hypertrichosis, hypopigmentation, acneiform eruptions; *maceration, secondary infection, atrophy, striae, miliaria* (with occlusive dressings).
Systemic: ***hypothalamic-pituitary-adrenal (HPA) axis suppression***, Cushing's syndrome, hyperglycemia, glucosuria.

INTERACTIONS

None significant.

CONTRAINDICATIONS

• Contraindicated in patients hypersensitive to the drug.
• Use cautiously in patients with viral diseases of skin such as varicella, vaccinia, or herpes simplex and in patients with fungal infections or bacterial skin infections.
• Use very cautiously in young children. This is a high-potency corticosteroid.

NURSING CONSIDERATIONS

• Avoid application near eyes, mucous membranes, or in ear canal.
• Systemic absorption likely with use of occlusive dressings, prolonged treatment, or extensive body-surface treatment. Monitor the patient for systemic adverse reactions.
• Children may absorb larger amounts of drug and be more prone to systemic toxicity. Avoid using plastic pants or tight-fitting diapers on treated areas in young children.
• Stop drug and notify the doctor if the patient develops signs of systemic absorption, skin irritation or ulceration, hypersensitivity, or infection.
• If antifungal agents or antibiotics are used concomitantly, corticosteroids should be stopped until infection is controlled.
• Before applying, gently wash skin. To prevent skin damage, rub medication in gently, leaving a thin coat. When treating hairy sites, part hair and apply directly to lesions.
• If an occlusive dressing is ordered, don't leave it in place longer than 16 hours each day; don't use occlusive

dressings on infected or exudative lesions on in combination with Psorcon.

- For patients with eczematous dermatitis whose skin may be irritated by adhesive material, hold dressing in place with gauze, elastic bandages, stockings, or stockinette.
- Notify the doctor and remove occlusive dressing if fever develops.
- Change dressing as ordered. Discontinue drug and notify the doctor if skin infection, striae, or atrophy occurs.
- Diflorasone is often effective with once-daily application.

fluocinolone acetonide

Fluocet, Fluonid, Flurosyn, Synalar, Synemol

Pregnancy Risk Category: C

HOW SUPPLIED
Cream: 0.01%, 0.025%, 0.2%
Ointment: 0.025%
Topical solution: 0.01%

ACTION
Mechanism: Diffuses across cell membranes to form complexes with specific cytoplasmic receptors. Exhibits anti-inflammatory, antipruritic, vasoconstrictive, and antiproliferative activity. Considered a group III (medium-potency) agent according to vasoconstrictive properties.
Peak: Plasma levels are highest when applied to inflamed or damaged skin, eyelids, or scrotal area; lowest when applied to intact normal skin, palms of hands, or soles of feet.

INDICATIONS & DOSAGE
Inflammation associated with corticosteroid-responsive dermatoses –
Adults and children: clean area; apply cream, ointment, or topical solution sparingly b.i.d. to q.i.d. Treat multiple or extensive lesions sequentially, applying to only small areas at any one time.

ADVERSE REACTIONS
Skin: burning, pruritus, irritation, dryness, erythema, folliculitis, hypertrichosis, hypopigmentation, acneiform eruptions, perioral dermatitis, allergic contact dermatitis; *maceration, secondary infection, atrophy, striae, miliaria* (with occlusive dressings).
Systemic: ***hypothalamic-pituitary-adrenal (HPA) axis suppression,*** Cushing's syndrome, hyperglycemia, glucosuria.

INTERACTIONS
None significant.

CONTRAINDICATIONS
- Contraindicated in patients hypersensitive to the drug.
- Use cautiously in patients with viral diseases of skin such as varicella, vaccinia, or herpes simplex and in patients with fungal infections or bacterial skin infections.

NURSING CONSIDERATIONS
- Avoid application near eyes, mucous membranes, or in ear canal.
- Systemic absorption likely with use of occlusive dressings, prolonged treatment, or extensive body-surface treatment. Monitor the patient for systemic adverse reactions.
- Children may absorb larger amounts of drug and be more prone to systemic toxicity. In young children, avoid using plastic pants or tight-fitting diapers on treated areas.
- Stop drug and notify the doctor if the patient develops signs of systemic absorption, skin irritation or ulceration, hypersensitivity, or infection.
- If antifungal agents or antibiotics are used concomitantly, corticosteroids should be stopped until infection is controlled.
- Gently wash skin before applying. To prevent skin damage, rub medication in gently, leaving a thin coat.

When treating hairy sites, part hair and apply directly to lesions.
- If an occlusive dressing is ordered, don't leave it in place longer than 16 hours each day; don't use occlusive dressings on infected or exudative lesions.
- For patients with eczematous dermatitis whose skin may be irritated by adhesive material, hold dressing in place with gauze, elastic bandages, stockings, or stockinette.
- Notify the doctor and remove occlusive dressing if fever develops.
- Change dressing as ordered. Discontinue drug and notify the doctor if skin infection, striae, or atrophy occurs.
- Fluonid solution on dry lesions may increase dryness, scaling, or pruritus; on denuded or fissured areas, may produce burning or stinging. If burning or stinging persists and dermatitis has not improved, discontinue use of solution.

fluocinonide

Lidemol†, Lidex, Lidex-E, Topsyn

Pregnancy Risk Category: C

HOW SUPPLIED

Cream: 0.05%
Gel: 0.05%
Ointment: 0.05%
Topical solution: 0.05%

ACTION

Mechanism: Diffuses across cell membranes to form complexes with specific cytoplasmic receptors. Exhibits anti-inflammatory, antipruritic, vasoconstrictive, and antiproliferative activity. Considered a group II (high-potency) agent according to vasoconstrictive properties.
Peak: Plasma levels are highest when applied to inflamed or damaged skin, eyelids, or scrotal area; lowest when applied to intact, normal skin, palms of hands, or soles of feet.

INDICATIONS & DOSAGE

Inflammation associated with corticosteroid-responsive dermatoses –
Adults and children: clean area; apply cream, gel, ointment, or topical solution sparingly t.i.d. or q.i.d.

ADVERSE REACTIONS

Skin: burning, pruritus, irritation, dryness, erythema, folliculitis, hypertrichosis, hypopigmentation, acneiform eruptions, perioral dermatitis, allergic contact dermatitis; *maceration, secondary infection, atrophy, striae, miliaria* (with occlusive dressings).
Systemic: ***hypothalamic-pituitary-adrenal (HPA) axis suppression,*** Cushing's syndrome, hyperglycemia, glucosuria.

INTERACTIONS

None significant.

CONTRAINDICATIONS

- Contraindicated in patients hypersensitive to the drug.
- Use cautiously in patients with viral diseases of skin such as varicella, vaccinia, or herpes simplex and in patients with fungal infections or bacterial skin infections.

NURSING CONSIDERATIONS

- Avoid application near eyes, mucous membranes, or in ear canal.
- Systemic absorption likely with use of occlusive dressings, prolonged treatment, or extensive body-surface treatment. Monitor the patient for systemic adverse reactions.
- Children may absorb larger amounts of drug and be more prone to systemic toxicity. In young children, avoid using plastic pants or tight-fitting diapers on treated areas.
- Stop drug and notify the doctor if patient develops signs of systemic absorption, skin irritation or ulceration, hypersensitivity, or infection.
- If antifungal agents or antibiotics

are used concomitantly, corticosteroids should be stopped until infection is controlled.
- Gently wash skin before applying. To prevent skin damage, rub medication in gently, leaving a thin coat. When treating hairy sites, part hair and apply directly to lesion.
- If an occlusive dressing is ordered, don't leave it in place longer than 16 hours each day; don't use occlusive dressings on infected or exudative lesions.
- For patients with eczematous dermatitis whose skin may be irritated by adhesive material, hold dressing in place with gauze, elastic bandages, stockings, or stockinette.
- Notify the doctor and remove occlusive dressing if fever develops.
- Change dressing as ordered. Discontinue drug and notify the doctor if skin infection, striae, or atrophy occurs.
- To prevent recurrence, continue treatment for a few days after lesions clear.

flurandrenolide

Cordran, Cordran SP, Cordran Tape, Drenison†, Drenison ¼†, Drenison Tape†

Pregnancy Risk Category: C

HOW SUPPLIED

Cream: 0.025%, 0.05%
Lotion: 0.05%
Ointment: 0.025%, 0.05%
Tape: 4 mcg/cm^2

ACTION

Mechanism: Diffuses across cell membranes to form complexes with specific cytoplasmic receptors. Exhibits anti-inflammatory, antipruritic, vasoconstrictive, and antiproliferative activity. Considered a group III (medium-potency) agent according to vasoconstrictive properties.
Peak: Plasma levels are highest when applied to inflamed or damaged skin, eyelids, or scrotal area; lowest when applied to intact normal skin, palms of hands, or soles of feet.

INDICATIONS & DOSAGE

Inflammation associated with corticosteroid-responsive dermatoses –
Adults and children: clean area; apply cream, lotion, or ointment sparingly b.i.d. or t.i.d.

Apply Cordran tape q 12 to 24 hours. Before applying tape, clean skin carefully, removing scales, crust, and dried exudate. Allow skin to dry for 1 hour before applying new tape. Shave or clip hair to allow good contact with skin and comfortable removal. If tape ends loosen prematurely, trim off and replace with fresh tape.

ADVERSE REACTIONS

Skin: burning, pruritus, irritation, dryness, erythema, folliculitis, hypertrichosis, hypopigmentation, acneiform eruptions, allergic contact dermatitis; *maceration, secondary infection, atrophy, striae, miliaria* (with occlusive dressings); purpura, stripping of epidermis, furunculosis (with tape).
Systemic: ***hypothalamic-pituitary-adrenal (HPA) axis suppression,*** Cushing's syndrome, hyperglycemia, glucosuria.

INTERACTIONS

None significant.

CONTRAINDICATIONS

- Contraindicated in patients hypersensitive to the drug.
- Use cautiously in patients with viral diseases of skin such as varicella, vaccinia, or herpes simplex and in patients with fungal infections or bacterial skin infections.

NURSING CONSIDERATIONS

• Tape not advised for exudative lesions or lesions in intertriginous areas.
• Replace tape every 12 hours or, if well tolerated and adherence is satisfactory, every 24 hours. Do not tear Cordran tape; cut it with scissors.
• Avoid application near eyes, mucous membranes, or in ear canal.
• Systemic absorption likely with use of occlusive dressings, prolonged treatment, or extensive body-surface treatment. Monitor the patient for systemic adverse reactions.
• Children may absorb larger amounts of drug and be more prone to systemic toxicity. Avoid using plastic pants or tight-fitting diapers on treated areas in young children.
• Stop drug and notify the doctor if the patient develops signs of systemic absorption, skin irritation or ulceration, hypersensitivity, or infection.
• If antifungal agents or antibiotics are used concomitantly, corticosteroids should be stopped until infection is controlled.
• Gently wash skin before applying. To prevent skin damage, rub medication in gently, leaving a thin coat. When treating hairy sites, part hair and apply directly to lesions.
• If an occlusive dressing is ordered, don't leave it in place longer than 16 hours each day; don't use occlusive dressings on infected or exudative lesions.
• For patients with eczematous dermatitis whose skin may be irritated by adhesive material, hold dressing in place with gauze, elastic bandages, stockings, or stockinette.
• Notify the doctor and remove occlusive dressing if fever develops.
• Discontinue drug and notify the doctor if skin infection, striae, or atrophy occurs.
• To prevent recurrence, continue treatment for a few days after lesions clear.

fluticasone propionate

Cutivate

Pregnancy Risk Category: C

HOW SUPPLIED

Cream: 0.05%
Ointment: 0.005%

ACTION

Mechanism: Diffuses across cell membranes to form complexes with specific cytoplasmic receptors. Exhibits anti-inflammatory, antipruritic, vasoconstrictive, and antiproliferative activity. Considered a group III (medium-potency) agent according to vasoconstrictive properties.
Peak: Plasma levels are highest when applied to inflamed or damaged skin, eyelids, or scrotal area; lowest when applied to intact normal skin, palms of hands, or soles of feet.

INDICATIONS & DOSAGE

Inflammation associated with corticosteroid-responsive dermatoses –
Adults and children: apply cream or ointment sparingly to affected area b.i.d. and rub in gently and completely. Treatment beyond 2 consecutive weeks is not recommended; total dosage should not exceed 50 g weekly in adults, 15 g weekly in children.

ADVERSE REACTIONS

Skin: stinging, burning, pruritus, irritation, dryness, erythema, folliculitis, skin atrophy, leukoderma, vesicles, rash, hypertrichosis, acneiform eruptions, hypopigmentation, perioral dermatitis, allergic contact dermatitis, secondary infection, striae, miliaria.
Significant systemic absorption can produce the following reactions:
CNS: euphoria, insomnia, headache, psychotic behavior, pseudotumor cerebri, mental changes, nervousness, restlessness.
CV: ***CHF,*** hypertension, edema.
EENT: cataracts, glaucoma, thrush.

GI: peptic ulceration, irritation, increased appetite.
Other: immunosuppression, increased susceptibility to infection, hypokalemia, sodium retention, fluid retention, weight gain, ***hypothalamic-pituitary-adrenal (HPA) axis suppression,*** Cushing's syndrome, hyperglycemia, glucosuria, osteoporosis, muscle atrophy, growth suppression in children, withdrawal syndrome.

INTERACTIONS
None significant.

CONTRAINDICATIONS
- Contraindicated in patients hypersensitive to the drug or any of its components and in patients with viral, fungal, herpetic, or tubercular skin lesions.
- Use cautiously in pediatric patients. Children may be more susceptible to topical steroid-induced HPA axis suppression because they may absorb proportionally larger amounts of the drug.
- Use cautiously in breast-feeding patients because systemically administered corticosteroids are known to appear in breast milk and may suppress growth.
- Do not use to treat rosacea, perioral dermatitis, or acne.

NURSING CONSIDERATIONS
- Do not mix drug with other bases or vehicles; this may affect potency.
- Consider changing to a less potent agent if adverse reactions occur.
- One-time coverage of the adult body requires 12 to 26 g. Use of more than 50 g weekly is not recommended.
- Discontinue drug if local irritation or systemic infection, absorption, or hypersensitivity occur.
- Tell the patient to notify the doctor if the condition persists or worsens or if burning or irritation develops.
- Tell the patient to avoid prolonged use and contact with eyes; warn the patient not to apply around eyes, genitals, or rectum, on face and in skin creases.

halcinonide
Halciderm, Halog

Pregnancy Risk Category: C

HOW SUPPLIED
Cream: 0.025%, 0.1%
Ointment: 0.1%
Topical solution: 0.1%

ACTION
Mechanism: Diffuses across cell membranes to form complexes with specific cytoplasmic receptors. Exhibits anti-inflammatory, antipruritic, vasoconstrictive, and antiproliferative activity. Considered a group II (high-potency) agent according to vasoconstrictive properties.
Peak: Plasma levels are highest when applied to inflamed or damaged skin, eyelids, or scrotal area; lowest when applied to intact normal skin, palms of hands, or soles of feet.

INDICATIONS & DOSAGE
Inflammation associated with corticosteroid-responsive dermatoses –
Adults and children: clean area; apply cream, ointment, or topical solution sparingly b.i.d. or t.i.d.

ADVERSE REACTIONS
Skin: burning, pruritus, irritation, dryness, erythema, folliculitis, hypertrichosis, hypopigmentation, acneiform eruptions, allergic contact dermatitis; *maceration, secondary infection, atrophy, striae, miliaria* (with occlusive dressings).
Systemic: ***hypothalamic-pituitary-adrenal (HPA) axis suppression,*** Cushing's syndrome, hyperglycemia, glucosuria.

INTERACTIONS
None significant.

CONTRAINDICATIONS
• Contraindicated in patients hypersensitive to the drug.
• Use cautiously in patients with viral diseases of skin such as varicella, vaccinia, or herpes simplex and in patients with fungal infections or bacterial skin infections.

NURSING CONSIDERATIONS
• Avoid application near eyes, mucous membranes, or in ear canal.
• Systemic absorption especially likely with use of occlusive dressings, prolonged treatment, or extensive body-surface treatment. Monitor the patient for systemic adverse reactions.
• Children may absorb larger amounts of drug and be more prone to systemic toxicity. Avoid using plastic pants or tight-fitting diapers on treated areas in young children.
• Stop drug and notify the doctor if the patient develops signs of systemic absorption, skin irritation or ulceration, hypersensitivity, or infection.
• If antifungal agents or antibiotics are used concomitantly, corticosteroids should be stopped until infection is controlled.
• Gently wash skin before applying. To prevent skin damage, rub medication in gently, leaving a thin coat. When treating hairy sites, part hair and apply directly to lesions.
• Gently rub small amount of cream into lesion until it disappears. Reapply, leaving a thin coating on lesion, and cover with occlusive dressing, if ordered. Apply ointment to lesion and cover with occlusive dressing, if ordered. Do not leave dressing in place longer than 16 hours each day.
• Don't use occlusive dressings on infected or exudative lesions.
• Good results have been obtained by applying occlusive dressings in evening and removing them in morning providing 12-hour occlusion. Medication should then be reapplied in the morning, without use of occlusive dressings during the day.
• For patients with eczematous dermatitis whose skin may be irritated by adhesive material, hold dressing in place with gauze, elastic bandages, stockings, or stockinette.
• Notify the doctor and remove occlusive dressing if fever develops.
• Change dressing as ordered. Discontinue drug and notify doctor if skin infection, striae, or atrophy occurs.
• To prevent recurrence, continue treatment for a few days after lesions clear.

halobetasol propionate
Ultravate
Pregnancy Risk Category: C

HOW SUPPLIED
Cream: 0.05%
Ointment: 0.05%

ACTION
Mechanism: Diffuses across cell membranes to form complexes with specific cytoplasmic receptors. Exhibits anti-inflammatory, antipruritic, vasoconstrictive, and antiproliferative activity. Considered a group I (very high-potency) agent according to vasoconstrictive properties.
Peak: Plasma levels are highest when applied to inflamed or damaged skin, eyelids, or scrotal area; lowest when applied to intact normal skin, palms of hands, or soles of feet.

INDICATIONS & DOSAGE
Inflammation associated with corticosteroid-responsive dermatoses –
Adults: apply cream or ointment sparingly to affected area b.i.d. and rub in gently and completely. Treatment beyond 2 consecutive weeks is

not recommended. Total dosage should not exceed 50 g weekly.

ADVERSE REACTIONS
Skin: stinging, burning, pruritus, irritation, dryness, erythema, folliculitis, skin atrophy, leukoderma, vesicles, rash, hypertrichosis, acneiform eruptions, hypopigmentation, perioral dermatitis, allergic contact dermatitis, secondary infection, striae, miliaria.
Significant systemic absorption can produce the following reactions:
CNS: euphoria, insomnia, headache, mental changes, nervousness, psychotic behavior, restlessness, pseudotumor cerebri, fatigue, dizziness, syncope.
CV: ***CHF,*** *hypertension, hypotension.*
EENT: cataracts, glaucoma, thrush.
GI: peptic ulceration, GI irritation, increased appetite, nausea, anorexia.
Other: edema, hypokalemia, weight gain, ***hypothalamic-pituitary-adrenal (HPA) axis suppression,*** Cushing's syndrome, hyperglycemia, glucosuria, fluid retention, osteoporosis, muscle atrophy, myalgia, arthralgia, fever, growth suppression in children.

INTERACTIONS
None significant.

CONTRAINDICATIONS
- Contraindicated in patients hypersensitive to the drug or any of its components and in patients with viral, fungal, herpetic, or tubercular skin lesions.
- Also contraindicated in pediatric patients because their higher ratio of skin surface to body mass increases susceptibility to systemic absorption and toxicity.
- Use cautiously in breast-feeding patients because systemically administered corticosteroids are known to appear in breast milk and may suppress growth.
- Do not use drug to treat rosacea or perioral dermatitis.

NURSING CONSIDERATIONS
- Some systemic absorption usually occurs and may cause HPA axis suppression, Cushing's syndrome, hyperglycemia, and glucosuria, which are reversible after discontinuation of therapy.
- Corticotropin stimulation, morning plasma cortisol, and urinary cortisol tests are useful in determining the extent of HPA axis suppression.
- If HPA axis suppression occurs, discontinue drug, reduce frequency of application, or substitute a less potent corticosteroid, as prescribed.
- Do not use occlusive dressings with this drug.
- Discontinue if infection occurs and notify the doctor.
- Avoid use on face, groin, or axilla.
- Tell the patient that drug is for external use only, as directed by the doctor. Tell him to avoid contact with eyes and not to cover, bandage, or wrap treated area unless directed by the doctor. Tell the patient not to use more often or for any condition other than prescribed.
- Tell the patient to notify the doctor of any signs of stinging, burning, or irritation.

hydrocortisone

Acticort, Aeroseb-HC, Bactine HC◇, CaldeCort, Carmol HC, Cetacort, Cort-Dome, Cortef◇, Cortenema, Cortinal, Cortizone 5◇, Cortril, Cremesone, Delacort, DermaCort◇, Dermolate◇, Dermtex HC, Durel-Cort, Ecosone, HC Cream, HI-Cor-2.5, Hycortole, Hydrocortex, HydroTex, Hytone, Ivocort, Maso-Cort, Microcort, Nutracort, Orabase HCA, Penecort, Proctocort, Rhus Tox HC, Rocort, Squibb-HC‡, Synacort, T/Scalp, Unicort

hydrocortisone acetate
CortaGel, Cortaid◇, Cortamed†, Cortef, Corticaine, Corticreme†, Cortifoam, Dermacort‡, Dermacort Ointment‡, Epifoam, Gynecort, Hydrocortisone Acetate, Lanacort, MyCort Lotion, Proctofoam-HC

hydrocortisone butyrate
Locoid

hydrocortisone valerate
Westcort Cream

Pregnancy Risk Category: C

HOW SUPPLIED
hydrocortisone
Aerosol: 0.5%
Cream: 0.25%◇, 0.5%◇, 1%◇, 2.5%
Gel: 1%
Lotion: 0.125%, 0.25%, 0.5%◇, 1%, 2%, 2.5%
Ointment: 0.5%◇, 1%◇, 2.5%
Topical solution: 1%
hydrocortisone acetate
Cream: 0.5%◇
Lotion: 0.5%◇
Ointment: 0.5%◇, 1%
Rectal foam: 90 mg/application
hydrocortisone butyrate
Cream: 0.1%
Ointment: 0.1%
hydrocortisone valerate
Cream: 0.2%
Ointment: 0.2%

ACTION
Mechanism: Diffuses across cell membranes to form complexes with specific cytoplasmic receptors. Exhibits anti-inflammatory, antipruritic, vasoconstrictive, and antiproliferative activity. Considered a group IV (low-potency) agent according to vasoconstrictive properties.
Peak: Plasma levels are highest when applied to inflamed or damaged skin, eyelids, or scrotal area; lowest when applied to intact normal skin, palms of hands, or soles of feet.

INDICATIONS & DOSAGE
Inflammation associated with corticosteroid-responsive dermatoses; adjunctive topical management of seborrheic dermatitis of scalp –
Adults and children: clean area; apply cream, gel, lotion, ointment, or topical solution sparingly daily to q.i.d. Spray aerosol onto affected area daily to q.i.d. until acute phase is controlled; then reduce dosage to one to three times weekly as needed.
Inflammation associated with proctitis –
Adults: 1 applicatorful of rectal foam P.R. daily or b.i.d. for 2 to 3 weeks, then every other day as necessary.

ADVERSE REACTIONS
Skin: burning, pruritus, irritation, dryness, erythema, folliculitis, hypertrichosis, hypopigmentation, acneiform eruptions, allergic contact dermatitis; *maceration, secondary infection, atrophy, striae, miliaria* (with occlusive dressings).
Systemic: ***hypothalamic-pituitary-adrenal (HPA) axis suppression,*** Cushing's syndrome, hyperglycemia, glucosuria.

INTERACTIONS
None significant.

CONTRAINDICATIONS
- Contraindicated in patients hypersensitive to the drug.
- Use cautiously in patients with viral diseases of skin such as varicella, vaccinia, or herpes simplex and in patients with fungal infections or bacterial skin infections.

NURSING CONSIDERATIONS
- Avoid application near eyes, mucous membranes, or in ear canal; may be safely used on face, groin, armpits, and under breasts.
- Systemic absorption likely with use of occlusive dressings, prolonged treatment, or extensive body-surface

treatment. Monitor the patient for systemic adverse reactions.
• Children may absorb larger amounts of drug and be more prone to systemic toxicity. Avoid using plastic pants or tight-fitting diapers on treated areas in young children.
• Stop drug and notify the doctor if the patient develops signs of systemic absorption, skin irritation or ulceration, hypersensitivity, or infection.
• If antifungal agents or antibiotics are used concomitantly, corticosteroids should be stopped until infection is controlled.
• Gently wash skin before applying. To prevent skin damage, rub medication in gently, leaving a thin coat. When treating hairy sites, part hair and apply directly to lesions.
• If an occlusive dressing is ordered, don't leave it in place longer than 16 hours each day; don't use occlusive dressings on infected or exudative lesions.
• For patients with eczematous dermatitis whose skin may be irritated by adhesive material, hold dressing in place with gauze, elastic bandages, stockings, or stockinette.
• Notify the doctor and remove occlusive dressing if fever develops.
• Change dressing as ordered. Discontinue drug and notify doctor if skin infection, striae, or atrophy occurs.
• Aerosol preparation contains alcohol and may produce irritation or burning in open lesions. When using around the face, cover the patient's eyes and warn against inhalation of the spray. Do not spray longer than 3 seconds or closer than 6″ (15 cm) to avoid freezing of tissues. Apply to dry scalp after shampooing; no need to massage medication into scalp after spraying.
• To prevent recurrence, continue treatment for a few days after lesions clear.

mometasone furoate
Elocon

Pregnancy Risk Category: C

HOW SUPPLIED
Cream: 0.1%
Ointment: 0.1%

ACTION
Mechanism: Diffuses across cell membranes to form complexes with specific cytoplasmic receptors. Exhibits anti-inflammatory, antipruritic, vasoconstrictive, and antiproliferative activity. Considered a group III (medium-potency) agent according to vasoconstrictive properties.
Peak: Plasma levels are highest when applied to inflamed or damaged skin, eyelids, or scrotal area; lowest when applied to intact normal skin, palms of hands, or soles of feet.

INDICATIONS & DOSAGE
Inflammation associated with corticosteroid-responsive dermatoses –
Adults: apply cream or ointment to affected areas once daily.

ADVERSE REACTIONS
Skin: burning, erythema, pruritus, atrophy, irritation, acneiform eruptions, hypopigmentation, allergic contact dermatitis.
Systemic: ***hypothalamic-pituitary-adrenal (HPA) axis suppression,*** Cushing's syndrome, hyperglycemia, glucosuria.

INTERACTIONS
None significant.

CONTRAINDICATIONS
• Contraindicated in patients hypersensitive to the drug.
• Use cautiously in patients with viral diseases of skin such as varicella, vaccinia, or herpes simplex and in patients with fungal infections or bacterial skin infections.

• Use cautiously in young children.

NURSING CONSIDERATIONS
• Avoid application near eyes, mucous membranes, or in ear canal.
• Systemic absorption likely with use of occlusive dressings, prolonged treatment, or extensive body-surface treatment. Monitor the patient for systemic adverse reactions.
• Do not use occlusive dressings with this drug.
• Children may absorb larger amounts of drug and be more prone to systemic toxicity.
• Stop drug and notify the doctor if the patient develops signs of systemic absorption, skin irritation or ulceration, hypersensitivity, or infection.
• If antimicrobial agents are used concomitantly, corticosteroids should be stopped until infection is controlled.
• Gently wash skin before applying. To prevent skin damage, rub medication in gently, leaving a thin coat. When treating hairy sites, part hair and apply directly to lesions.

triamcinolone acetonide

Aristocort, Flutex, Kenalog, Kenalone‡, Triacet

Pregnancy Risk Category: C

HOW SUPPLIED
Aerosol: 0.2 mg/2-second spray
Cream: 0.02%‡, 0.025%, 0.1%, 0.5%
Lotion: 0.025%, 0.1%
Ointment: 0.02%‡, 0.025%, 0.1%, 0.5%
Paste: 0.1%

ACTION
Mechanism: Diffuses across cell membranes to form complexes with specific cytoplasmic receptors. Exhibits anti-inflammatory, antipruritic, vasoconstrictive, and antiproliferative activity. Considered a group III (medium-potency) agent according to vasoconstrictive properties.
Peak: Plasma levels are highest when applied to inflamed or damaged skin, eyelids, or scrotal area; low levels result when applied to intact, normal skin, palms of hands, or soles of feet.

INDICATIONS & DOSAGE
Inflammation associated with corticosteroid-responsive dermatoses –
Adults and children: clean area; apply aerosol, cream, lotion, or ointment sparingly b.i.d. to q.i.d.
Inflammation associated with oral lesions –
Adults and children: apply paste t.i.d. and h.s. Apply a small amount without rubbing and press to lesion in mouth until a thin film develops.

ADVERSE REACTIONS
Skin: burning, pruritus, irritation, dryness, erythema, folliculitis, hypertrichosis, hypopigmentation, acneiform eruptions, perioral dermatitis, allergic contact dermatitis; *maceration, secondary infection, atrophy, striae, miliaria* (with occlusive dressings).
Systemic: ***hypothalmic-pituitary-adrenal (HPA) axis suppression,*** Cushing's syndrome, hyperglycemia, glucosuria.

INTERACTIONS
None significant.

CONTRAINDICATIONS
• Contraindicated in patients hypersensitive to the drug.
• Use cautiously in patients with viral diseases of skin such as varicella, vaccinia, or herpes simplex and in patients with fungal infections or bacterial skin infections.

NURSING CONSIDERATIONS
• Avoid application near eyes or in ear canal.
• Systemic absorption likely with use

of occlusive dressings, prolonged treatment, or extensive body-surface treatment. Monitor the patient for systemic adverse reactions.

- Children may absorb larger amounts of drug and be more prone to systemic toxicity. Avoid using plastic pants or tight-fitting diapers on treated areas in young children.
- Stop drug and notify the doctor if the patient develops signs of systemic absorption, skin irritation or ulceration, hypersensitivity, or infection.
- If antifungal agents or antibiotics are used concomitantly, corticosteroids should be stopped until infection is controlled.
- Gently wash skin before applying. To avoid skin damage, rub medication in gently, leaving a thin coat. When treating hairy sites, part hair and apply directly to lesions.
- Aerosol preparation contains alcohol and may produce irritation or burning in open lesions. When using about the face, cover the patient's eyes and warn against inhalation of the spray. Do not spray longer than 3 seconds or closer than 6″ (15 cm) to avoid freezing of tissues.
- If an occlusive dressing is ordered, don't leave it in place longer than 16 hours each day; don't use occlusive dressings on infected or exudative lesions.
- Change dressing as ordered. Discontinue drug and notify the doctor if skin infection, striae, or atrophy occurs.

90

Vitamins and minerals

vitamin A

vitamin B complex
cyanocobalamin
hydroxocobalamin
folic acid
leucovorin calcium
niacin
niacinamide
pyridoxine hydrochloride
riboflavin
thiamine hydrochloride

vitamin C
vitamin D
cholecalciferol
ergocalciferol
vitamin E

vitamin K analogues
menadione/menadiol sodium diphosphate
phytonadione

sodium fluoride
sodium fluoride, topical

trace elements
chromium
copper
iodine
manganese
selenium
zinc

COMBINATION PRODUCTS

M.T.E.-4: zinc sulfate 1 mg, copper sulfate 0.4 mg, manganese sulfate 0.1 mg, and chromium chloride 4 mcg per ml.

M.T.E.-4 CONCENTRATED: zinc sulfate 5 mg, copper sulfate 1 mg, manganese sulfate 0.5 mg, and chromium chloride 10 mcg per ml.

M.T.E.-5: zinc sulfate 1 mg, copper sulfate 0.4 mg, manganese sulfate 0.1 mg, chromium chloride 4 mcg, and selenium (as selenious acid) 20 mcg per ml.

M.T.E.-5 CONCENTRATED: zinc sulfate 5 mg, copper sulfate 1 mg, manganese sulfate 0.5 mg, chromium chloride 10 mcg, and selenium (as selenious acid) 60 mcg per ml.

M.T.E.-6: zinc sulfate 1 mg, copper sulfate 0.4 mg, manganese sulfate 0.1 mg, chromium chloride 4 mcg, selenium (as selenious acid) 20 mcg, and sodium iodide 25 mcg per ml.

M.T.E.-6 CONCENTRATED: zinc sulfate 5 mg, copper sulfate 1 mg, manganese sulfate 0.5 mg, chromium chloride 10 mcg, selenium (as selenious acid) 60 mcg, and sodium iodide 75 mcg per ml.

M.T.E.-7: zinc sulfate 1 mg, copper sulfate 0.4 mg, manganese sulfate 0.1 mg, chromium chloride 4 mcg, selenium (as selenious acid) 20 mcg, and sodium iodide 25 mcg per ml.

MULTIPLE TRACE ELEMENT: zinc sulfate 1 mg, copper sulfate 0.4 mg, manganese sulfate 0.1 mg, and chromium chloride 4 mcg per ml.

MULTIPLE TRACE ELEMENT CONCENTRATED: zinc sulfate 5 mg, copper sulfate 1 mg, manganese sulfate 0.5 mg, and chromium chloride 10 mcg per ml.

MULTITRACE: zinc chloride 1 mg, copper chloride 0.4 mg, manganese chloride 0.1 mg, and chromium chloride 4 mcg per ml.

MULTITRACE 5: zinc sulfate 1 mg, copper sulfate 0.4 mg, manganese sulfate 0.1 mg, chromium chloride 4 mcg, and selenium (as selenious acid) 20 mcg per ml.

MULTITRACE CONCENTRATE: zinc chloride 5 mg, copper chloride 1 mg, manganese chloride 0.5 mg, and chromium chloride 10 mcg per ml.

MULTITRACE PEDIATRIC: zinc sulfate 1 mg, copper sulfate 0.1 mg, manganese sulfate 0.025 mg, and chromium chloride 1 mcg per ml.
NEOTRACE-4: zinc sulfate 1.5 mg, copper sulfate 0.1 mg, manganese sulfate 0.025 mg, and chromium chloride 0.85 mcg per ml.
PEDIATRIC MULTIPLE TRACE ELEMENT: zinc sulfate 0.5 mg, copper sulfate 0.1 mg, manganese sulfate 0.03 mg, and chromium chloride 1 mcg per ml.
PEDTRACE-4: zinc sulfate 0.5 mg, copper sulfate 0.1 mg, manganese sulfate 0.025 mg, and chromium chloride 0.85 mcg per ml.
P.T.E.-4: zinc sulfate 1 mg, copper sulfate 0.1 mg, manganese sulfate 0.025 mg, and chromium chloride 1 mcg per ml.
P.T.E.-5: zinc sulfate 1 mg, copper sulfate 0.1 mg, manganese sulfate 0.025 mg, chromium chloride 1 mcg, and selenium (as selenious acid) 15 mcg per ml.
T.E.C.: zinc sulfate 1 mg, copper sulfate 0.4 mg, manganese sulfate 0.1 mg, and chromium chloride 4 mcg per ml.
TRACE METALS ADDITIVE: zinc chloride 0.8 mg, copper chloride 0.2 mg, manganese chloride 0.16 mg, and chromium chloride 2 mcg per ml.
B complex vitamins◇
B complex vitamins with iron◇
B complex with vitamin C◇
B vitamin combinations◇
Calcium and vitamin products◇
Fluoride with vitamins◇
Geriatric supplements with multivitamins and minerals◇
Miscellaneous vitamins and minerals◇
Multivitamins◇
Multivitamins and minerals with hormones◇
Multivitamins with B_{12}◇
Vitamin A and D combinations◇

vitamin A (retinol)

Acon, Aquasol A, Del-Vi-A

Pregnancy Risk Category: A (X if > RDA)

HOW SUPPLIED

Tablets: 10,000 IU
Capsules: 10,000 IU◇, 25,000 IU, 50,000 IU
Drops: 30 ml with dropper (5,000 IU/0.1 ml)
Injection: 2-ml vials (5,000 IU/ml with 0.5% chlorobutanol, polysorbate 80, butylated hydroxyanisol, and butylated hydroxytoluene)

ACTION

Mechanism: Coenzyme that stimulates retinal function, bone growth, and differentiation of epithelial tissues.
Peak: Normal serum levels peak at 300 to 700 ng/ml in adults and children, 200 to 500 ng/ml in infants.

INDICATIONS & DOSAGE

Recommended daily allowance (RDA) –
Note: RDAs have been converted to retinol equivalents (RE). One RE has the activity of 0.3 mcg all-*trans* retinol, 6 mcg beta carotene, or 12 mcg carotenoid provitamins.
Neonates and infants to 1 year: 375 mcg RE or 1,875 IU.
Children 1 to 3 years: 400 mcg RE or 2,000 IU.
Children 4 to 6 years: 500 mcg RE or 2,500 IU.
Children 7 to 10 years: 700 mcg RE or 3,500 IU.
Males over 11 years: 1,000 mcg RE or 5,000 IU.
Females over 11 years: 800 mcg RE or 4,000 IU.
Pregnant women: 800 mcg RE or 4,000 IU.
Lactating women (first 6 months): 1,300 mcg RE or 6,500 IU.

†Available in Canada only. ‡Available in Australia only. ◇Available OTC.

Lactating women (second 6 months): 1,200 mcg RE or 6,000 IU.
Severe vitamin A deficiency –
Adults and children over 8 years: 50,000 to 100,000 IU I.M. or 100,000 to 500,000 IU P.O. for 3 days, followed by 50,000 IU I.M. or P.O. for 2 weeks; then 10,000 to 20,000 IU P.O. for 2 months. Follow with adequate dietary nutrition and RDA vitamin A supplements.
Infants under 1 year: 7,500 to 15,000 IU I.M. daily for 10 days.
Children 1 to 8 years: 17,500 to 35,000 IU I.M. daily for 10 days.
Maintenance dosage to prevent recurrence of vitamin A deficiency –
Children under 4 years: 10,000 IU I.M. daily for 2 months, then adequate dietary nutrition and RDA vitamin A supplements.
Children 4 to 8 years: 15,000 IU I.M. daily for 2 months, then adequate dietary nutrition and RDA vitamin A supplements.

ADVERSE REACTIONS

Adverse reactions are usually seen only with toxicity.
CNS: irritability, headache, ***increased intracranial pressure,*** fatigue, lethargy, malaise, vertigo, visual disturbances.
EENT: miosis, papilledema, exophthalmos.
GI: anorexia, epigastric pain, diarrhea, nausea, vomiting.
GU: hypomenorrhea.
Hematologic: hypoplastic anemia, leukocytosis, thrombocytopenia.
Hepatic: jaundice, hepatomegaly, ***cirrhosis,*** elevated liver enzymes.
Skin: alopecia; drying, cracking, scaling of skin; pruritus; lip fissures; massive desquamation; increased pigmentation; night sweating; brittle nails.
Other: skeletal – slow growth, decalcification of bone, hypercalcemia, hypercalciuria, fractures, hyperostosis, periostitis, premature closure of epiphyses, migratory arthralgia, cortical thickening over the radius and tibia, bulging fontanelles; splenomegaly.

INTERACTIONS

Cholestyramine resin, mineral oil: reduced GI absorption of fat-soluble vitamins. If needed, give mineral oil at bedtime.
Isotretinoin, multivitamins containing vitamin A: increased risk of toxicity. Avoid concomitant use.
Warfarin: increased risk of bleeding. Monitor PT closely.

CONTRAINDICATIONS

- Contraindicated for oral administration in patients with malabsorption syndrome; if malabsorption is from inadequate bile secretion, oral route may be used with concurrent administration of bile salts (dehydrocholic acid). Also contraindicated in hypervitaminosis A.
- I.V. administration contraindicated except for special water-miscible forms intended for infusion with large parenteral volumes. I.V. push of vitamin A of any type is also contraindicated (anaphylaxis or anaphylactoid reactions and death have resulted).
- Use cautiously in pregnant patients, avoiding doses exceeding RDA.

NURSING CONSIDERATIONS

- Evaluate the patient's vitamin A intake from fortified foods, dietary supplements, self-administered drugs, and prescription drug sources.
- To avoid toxicity, advise the patient against self-administration of megadoses of vitamins without specific indications. Also stress that the patient should not share prescribed vitamins with family members or others.
- Monitor for adverse reactions if dosage is high.
- Acute toxicity has resulted from single doses of 25,000 IU/kg of body weight; 350,000 IU in infants and

over 2 million IU in adults have also proved acutely toxic. Doses that do not exceed the RDA are usually nontoxic.

- Chronic toxicity in infants (3 to 6 months) has resulted from doses of 18,500 IU daily for 1 to 3 months. In adults, chronic toxicity has resulted from doses of 50,000 IU daily for over 8 months; 500,000 IU daily for 2 months, and 1 million IU daily for 3 days.
- Monitor the patient closely for skin disorders; high dosages may induce chronic toxicity.
- Liquid preparations available if nasogastric administration is necessary. May be mixed with cereal or fruit juice.
- Record dietary and bowel habits, and report abnormalities to doctor.
- Adequate vitamin A absorption requires suitable protein, vitamin E, and zinc intake and bile secretion; give supplemental salts if necessary. Zinc supplements may be necessary in patients receiving long-term total parenteral nutrition.
- Absorption is fastest and most complete with water-miscible preparations, intermediate with emulsions, and slowest with oil suspensions.
- Protect from light and heat.

cyanocobalamin (vitamin B_{12})

Anacobin†, Bedoce, Bedoz†, Bioglan B_{12} Plus‡, Crysti-12, Crystamine, Cyanabin†, Cyanocobalamin, Cyano-Gel, Cyanoject, Cyomin, Dodex, Ener-B◇, Kaybovite, Poyamin, Rubesol-1000, Rubion†, Rubramin, Sigamine

hydroxocobalamin (vitamin B_{12a})

Alpha-Ruvite, Codroxomin, Droxomin, Hydrobexan, Hydro-Cobex, Hydro-Crysti-12, LA-12, Rubesol-L.A.

Pregnancy Risk Category: A (C if > RDA)

HOW SUPPLIED

cyanocobalamin
Tablets: 25 mcg◇, 50 mcg◇, 100 mcg◇, 250 mcg◇
Injection: 30 mcg/ml, 100 mcg/ml, 1,000 mcg/ml
hydroxocobalamin
Injection: 30 mcg/ml, 100 mcg/ml, 120 mcg/ml, 1,000 mcg/ml

ACTION

Mechanism: Coenzyme that stimulates metabolic functions. Necessary for cell replication and hematopoiesis.
Onset: normoblastic erythroid progenitor cells appear 8 hours after I.M. injection; CNS symptoms of deficiency subside in 24 hours; platelet and granulocyte effects occur in 10 to 14 days. **Peak:** Plasma levels peak ½ to 2 hours after S.C. or I.M. injection. **Duration:** about 48 hours.

INDICATIONS & DOSAGE

Recommended daily allowance (RDA) for cyanocobalamin –
Neonates and infants to 6 months: 0.3 mcg.
Infants 6 months to 1 year: 0.5 mcg.
Children over 1 year to 3 years: 0.7 mcg.
Children 4 to 6 years: 1 mcg.
Children 7 to 10 years: 1.4 mcg.
Adults and children 11 years and over: 2 mcg.
Pregnant women: 2.2 mcg.
Lactating women: 2.6 mcg.
Vitamin B_{12} deficiency caused by inadequate diet, subtotal gastrectomy, or any other condition, disorder, or disease except malabsorption related to

†Available in Canada only. ‡Available in Australia only. ◇Available OTC.

pernicious anemia or other GI disease –
Adults: 30 to 100 mcg hydroxocobalamin S.C. or I.M. daily for 5 to 10 days, depending on severity of deficiency. Maintenance dosage is 100 to 200 mcg I.M. once monthly. For subsequent prophylaxis, advise adequate nutrition and daily RDA vitamin B_{12} supplements.
Children: 30 to 100 mcg hydroxocobalamin S.C. or I.M. daily for 5 to 10 days, depending on severity of deficiency. Maintenance dosage is at least 60 mcg/month I.M. or S.C. For subsequent prophylaxis, advise adequate nutrition and daily RDA vitamin B_{12} supplements.
Pernicious anemia or vitamin B_{12} malabsorption –
Adults: initially, 100 mcg hydroxocobalamin I.M. daily for 5 days, then 100 to 200 mcg I.M. once monthly until remission occurs. Then 100 mcg I.M. once monthly for life. If neurologic complications are present, follow initial therapy with 100 to 1,000 mcg I.M. once q 2 weeks before starting monthly regimen.
Children: 1,000 to 5,000 mcg hydroxocobalamin I.M. or S.C. over 2 or more weeks in 100-mcg increments; then 60 mcg I.M. or S.C. monthly for life.
Methylmalonic aciduria –
Neonates: 1,000 mcg hydroxocobalamin I.M. daily for 11 days with a protein-restricted diet.
Schilling test flushing dose –
Adults and children: 1,000 mcg hydroxocobalamin I.M. in a single dose.

ADVERSE REACTIONS

CV: peripheral vascular thrombosis.
GI: transient diarrhea.
Skin: itching, transitory exanthema, urticaria.
Other: ***anaphylaxis, anaphylactoid reactions with parenteral administration***, pain or burning at S.C. or I.M. injection sites.

INTERACTIONS

Aminoglycosides, chloramphenicol, colchicine, para-aminosalicylic acid and salts: malabsorption of vitamin B_{12}. Don't use concomitantly.

CONTRAINDICATIONS

- Contraindicated for parenteral administration in patients hypersensitive to vitamin B_{12} or cobalt.
- Therapeutic dosage contraindicated before proper diagnosis; vitamin B_{12} therapy may mask folate deficiency.
- Use cautiously in anemic patients with coexisting cardiac, pulmonary, or hypertensive disease; in early Leber's disease; in patients with severe vitamin B_{12}-dependent deficiencies, especially those receiving cardiotonic glycosides (monitor closely the first 2 to 3 days for hypokalemia, fluid overload, pulmonary edema, CHF, and hypertension); and in gout (monitor serum uric acid for hyperuricemia).

NURSING CONSIDERATIONS

- Vitamin B_{12} is usually nontoxic.
- Infection, tumors, or renal, hepatic, and other debilitating diseases may reduce therapeutic response.
- Deficiencies are more common in strict vegetarians and their breast-fed infants.
- Stress need for patients with pernicious anemia to return for monthly injections. Although total body stores may last 3 to 6 years, anemia will recur if not treated monthly.
- May cause false-positive intrinsic factor antibody test.
- Closely monitor serum potassium levels for first 48 hours. Give potassium supplement if necessary.
- Don't mix parenteral liquids in same syringe with other medications.
- Protect from light and heat. Do not refrigerate or freeze.
- Hydroxocobalamin is approved for I.M. use only. Its only advantage over cyanocobalamin is its longer duration.
- Physically incompatible with dex-

trose solutions, alkaline or strongly acidic solutions, oxidizing or reducing agents, heavy metals, chlorpromazine, phytonadione, prochlorperazine, and many other drugs.

- Large oral doses of vitamin B_{12} should not be given routinely; such doses increase risk of hypersensitivity reactions.

folic acid (vitamin B_9)

Folvite, Novofolacid†

Pregnancy Risk Category: A (C if > RDA)

HOW SUPPLIED

Tablets: 0.1 mg, 0.4 mg, 0.8 mg, 1 mg

Injection: 10-ml vials (5 mg/ml with 1.5% benzyl alcohol or 10 mg/ml with 1.5% benzyl alcohol and 0.2% EDTA)

ACTION

Mechanism: Stimulates normal erythropoiesis and nucleoprotein synthesis.

Peak: Levels peak 60 to 90 minutes after I.M. injection, 8 to 12 hours after oral administration. **Duration:** plasma half-life, 6 days; half-life of folate stored in the liver, 400 days.

INDICATIONS & DOSAGE

Recommended daily allowance (RDA) –

Neonates and infants to 6 months: 25 mcg.

Infants 6 months to 1 year: 35 mcg.

Children over 1 year to 3 years: 50 mcg.

Children 4 to 6 years: 75 mcg.

Children 7 to 11 years: 100 mcg.

Children 11 to 14 years: 150 mcg.

Males 15 years and over: 200 mcg.

Females 15 years and over: 180 mcg.

Pregnant women: 400 mcg.

Lactating women (first 6 months): 280 mcg.

Lactating women (second 6 months): 260 mcg.

Megaloblastic or macrocytic anemia secondary to folic acid or other nutritional deficiency, hepatic disease, alcoholism, intestinal obstruction, excessive hemolysis –

Adults and children over 4 years: 1 mg P.O., S.C., or I.M. daily for 4 to 5 days. After anemia secondary to folic acid deficiency is corrected, proper diet and RDA supplements are necessary to prevent recurrence.

Children under 4 years: up to 0.3 mg P.O., S.C., or I.M. daily.

Pregnant and lactating women: 0.8 mg P.O., S.C., or I.M. daily.

Prevention of megaloblastic anemia in pregnancy and fetal damage –

Adults: 1 mg P.O., S.C., or I.M. daily throughout pregnancy.

Nutritional supplement –

Adults: 0.1 mg P.O., S.C., or I.M. daily.

Children: 0.05 mg P.O. daily.

To test folic acid deficiency in patients with megaloblastic anemia without masking pernicious anemia –

Adults and children: 0.1 to 0.2 mg P.O. or I.M. for 10 days while maintaining a diet low in folate and vitamin B_{12}.

Tropical sprue –

Adults: 3 to 15 mg P.O. daily.

ADVERSE REACTIONS

Respiratory: ***bronchospasm.***

Skin: allergic reactions (rash, pruritus, erythema).

Other: general malaise.

INTERACTIONS

Anticonvulsants such as phenobarbital and phenytoin: increased anticonvulsant metabolism and decreased blood levels. Monitor closely.

Chloramphenicol: antagonism of folic acid. Monitor for decreased folic acid effect. Use together cautiously.

CONTRAINDICATIONS

• Contraindicated in normocytic, refractory, or aplastic anemias; as sole agent in treating pernicious anemia because it may mask neurologic effects; in treating patients with methotrexate, pyrimethamine, or trimethoprim overdose; and in undiagnosed anemia because it may mask pernicious anemia patients.

NURSING CONSIDERATIONS

• Patients with small-bowel resections and intestinal malabsorption may require parenteral administration routes.
• Don't mix with other medications in same syringe for I.M. injections.
• Protect from light and heat; store at room temperature.
• May use concurrent folic acid and vitamin B_{12} therapy if supported by diagnosis.
• Reticulosis, reversion to normoblastic hematopoiesis, and return to normal hemoglobin indicate folic acid deficiency.
• Proper nutrition is necessary to prevent recurrence of anemia.
• Patients with pernicious anemia should avoid multivitamins containing folic acid.
• Carefully monitor hematologic response to folic acid in patients receiving chloramphenicol concurrently with folic acid.

leucovorin calcium (citrovorum factor, folinic acid)

Wellcovorin

Pregnancy Risk Category: C

HOW SUPPLIED

Tablets: 5 mg, 10 mg, 15 mg, 25 mg
Injection: 1-ml ampule (3 mg/ml with 0.9% benzyl alcohol or 5 mg/ml, with methyl and propyl parabens)
Powder for injection: 50 mg/vial, 100 mg/vial, 350 mg/vial

ACTION

Mechanism: A reduced form of folic acid that is readily converted to other folic acid derivatives.
Onset: 5 minutes after I.V. administration, 10 to 20 minutes after I.M. administration, 20 to 30 minutes after oral administration. **Peak:** Levels peak within 10 minutes after I.V. administration, less than 1 hour after I.M. administration, or 2 to 3 hours after oral administration. **Duration:** 3 to 6 hours.

INDICATIONS & DOSAGE

Overdose of folic acid antagonist –
Adults and children: P.O., I.M., or I.V. dose equivalent to weight of antagonist given.
Leucovorin rescue after high methotrexate dose in treatment of malignancy –
Adults and children: 10 mg/m² P.O., I.M., or I.V. q 6 hours until methotrexate levels fall below 5 x 10-8 M.
Hematologic toxicity caused by pyrimethamine therapy –
Adults and children: 5 mg P.O. or I.M. daily.
Hematologic toxicity caused by trimethoprim therapy –
Adults and children: 400 mcg to 5 mg P.O. or I.M. daily.
Megaloblastic anemia caused by congenital enzyme deficiency –
Adults and children: 3 to 6 mg I.M., then 1 mg P.O. or I.M. daily for life.
Folate-deficient megaloblastic anemia –
Adults and children: up to 1 mg of leucovorin I.M daily. Duration of treatment depends on hematologic response.
Palliative treatment of advanced colorectal carcinoma –
Adults: 20 mg/m² I.V., followed by fluorouracil 425 mg/m² I.V. daily for 5 consecutive days. Repeat at 4-week intervals for two additional courses; then at intervals of 4 to 5 weeks if tolerated.

ADVERSE REACTIONS
Respiratory: ***bronchospasm.***
Skin: hypersensitivity reactions (rash, pruritus, erythema).

INTERACTIONS
Fluorouracil: may enhance fluorouracil toxicity. Avoid concomitant use.

CONTRAINDICATIONS
- Contraindicated in patients hypersensitive to the drug or folic acid (possible cross-sensitivity).
- Contraindicated in treating undiagnosed anemia, because it may mask pernicious anemia.
- Use cautiously in patients with pernicious anemia; hemolytic remission may occur while neurologic manifestations remain progressive.

NURSING CONSIDERATIONS
- Do not confuse leucovorin (folinic acid) with folic acid.
- Follow leucovorin rescue schedule and protocol closely to maximize therapeutic response.
- Do not administer leucovorin simultaneously with systemic methotrexate. Time intervals have ranged from 0 to 72 hours after methotrexate.
- Protect from light and heat, especially reconstituted parenteral preparations.
- **I.V. use:** When using powder for injection, reconstitute 50-mg vial with 5 ml, 100-mg vial with 10 ml, or 350-mg vial with 17 ml of sterile water or bacteriostatic water for injection. When doses are greater than 10 mg/m^2, don't use diluents containing benzyl alcohol.
- Don't exceed 160 mg/minute when giving by direct injection.

niacin (vitamin B_3, nicotinic acid)
Niac, Niacor, Nico-400, Nicobid◇, Nicolar**, Nicotinex

niacinamide (nicotinamide)◇
Pregnancy Risk Category: A (C if > RDA)

HOW SUPPLIED
niacin
Tablets: 25 mg◇, 50 mg◇, 100 mg◇, 250 mg◇, 500 mg
Tablets (timed-release): 150 mg◇, 250 mg◇, 500 mg◇, 750 mg◇
Capsules (timed-release): 125 mg◇, 250 mg◇, 300 mg◇, 400 mg◇, 500 mg
Elixir: 50 mg/5 ml◇
Injection: 100 mg/ml in 30-ml vials
niacinamide
Tablets: 50 mg◇, 100 mg◇, 500 mg◇
Tablets (timed-release): 1,000 mg◇
Injection: 100 mg/ml

ACTION
Mechanism: Niacin and nicotinic acid stimulate lipid metabolism, tissue respiration, and glycogenolysis; niacin decreases synthesis of low-density lipoproteins and inhibits lipolysis in adipose tissue.
Onset: triglyceride levels begin to decrease within several hours; cholesterol levels within several days. **Peak:** Serum levels peak 45 minutes after oral administration.

INDICATIONS & DOSAGE
Recommended daily allowance (RDA) –
Neonates and infants to 6 months: 5 mg.
Infants 6 months to 1 year: 6 mg.
Children 1 to 3 years: 9 mg.
Children 4 to 6 years: 12 mg.
Children 7 to 10 years: 13 mg.
Males 11 to 14 years: 17 mg.
Males 15 to 18 years: 20 mg.
Males 19 to 50 years: 19 mg.
Males 51 years and over: 15 mg.
Females 11 to 50 years: 15 mg.
Females 51 years and over: 13 mg.
Pregnant women: 17 mg.
Lactating women: 20 mg.

Pellagra –
Adults: 10 to 20 mg P.O., S.C., I.M., or I.V. daily, depending on severity of niacin deficiency. Maximum daily recommended dosage is 500 mg, divided into ten 50-mg doses.
Children: up to 300 mg P.O. or 100 mg I.V. daily, depending on severity of niacin deficiency.

After symptoms subside, advise adequate nutrition and RDA supplements to prevent recurrence.

Peripheral vascular disease and circulatory disorders –
Adults: 250 to 800 mg P.O. daily in divided doses.

Hyperlipidemias, especially with hypercholesterolemia –
Adults: 1.5 to 3 g P.O. daily in two to four divided doses with or after meals, increased at intervals to 6 g daily.

ADVERSE REACTIONS

Most adverse reactions are dose-dependent.
CNS: dizziness, transient headache.
CV: *excessive peripheral vasodilation (especially niacin).*
GI: *nausea, vomiting, diarrhea,* possible activation of peptic ulceration, epigastric or substernal pain.
Hepatic: ***hepatic dysfunction.***
Skin: *flushing,* pruritus, dryness.
Other: hyperglycemia, hyperuricemia.

INTERACTIONS

Antihypertensive drugs (sympathetic or ganglionic blockers): potential additive vasodilating effect, causing postural hypotension. Use together cautiously; also warn the patient about postural hypotension.

CONTRAINDICATIONS

- Contraindicated in patients with hepatic dysfunction, active peptic ulcers, severe hypotension, or arterial hemorrhage.
- Use cautiously in patients with gallbladder disease, diabetes mellitus, and gout.

NURSING CONSIDERATIONS

- Monitor hepatic function and blood glucose early in therapy.
- To minimize GI side effects, give with meals.
- Timed-release niacin or niacinamide may prevent excessive flushing that occurs with large doses. However, timed-release niacin has been associated with hepatic dysfunction, even at doses as low as 1 g/day.
- Aspirin (80 to 325 mg P.O. 30 minutes before niacin dose) may reduce the flushing response to niacin.
- Stress that this substance is a potent medication, not just a vitamin, and may cause serious adverse effects. Explain importance of adhering to therapeutic regimen.
- Advise patient against self-medicating for hyperlipidemia.
- **I.V. use:** Give slow I.V. (no faster than 2 mg/minute). Explain harmlessness of flushing syndrome to ease anxiety.

---

pyridoxine hydrochloride (vitamin B_6)

Beesix, Hexa-Betalin, Hexacrest, Nestrex◇, Rodex

Pregnancy Risk Category: A (C if > RDA)

HOW SUPPLIED

Tablets: 10 mg◇, 25 mg◇, 50 mg◇, 100 mg◇, 200 mg◇, 250 mg◇, 500 mg◇
Tablets (timed-release): 500 mg
Injection: 100 mg/ml

ACTION

Mechanism: Acts as a coenzyme that stimulates various metabolic functions, including amino acid metabolism.
Duration: half-life, 15 to 20 days.

*Liquid form contains alcohol.
**May contain tartrazine.

Common reactions are in italics; ***life-threatening,*** in bold italics.

INDICATIONS & DOSAGE
Recommended daily allowance (RDA) –
Neonates and infants to 6 months: 0.3 mg.
Infants 6 months to 1 year: 0.6 mg.
Children 1 year to 3 years: 1 mg.
Children 4 to 6 years: 1.1 mg.
Children 7 to 10 years: 1.4 mg.
Males 11 to 14 years: 1.7 mg.
Males 15 years and over: 2 mg.
Females 11 to 14 years: 1.4 mg.
Females 15 to 18 years: 1.5 mg.
Females 19 years and over: 1.6 mg.
Pregnant women: 2.2 mg.
Lactating women: 2.1 mg.
Dietary vitamin B_6 deficiency –
Adults: 10 to 20 mg P.O., I.M., or I.V. daily for 3 weeks, then 2 to 5 mg daily as a supplement to a proper diet.
Children: 100 mg P.O., I.M., or I.V. to correct deficiency, then an adequate diet with supplementary RDA doses to prevent recurrence.
Seizures related to vitamin B_6 deficiency or dependency –
Adults and children: 100 mg I.M. or I.V. in single dose.
Vitamin B_6-responsive anemias or dependency syndrome (inborn errors of metabolism) –
Adults: up to 600 mg P.O., I.M., or I.V. daily until symptoms subside, then 50 mg daily for life.
Children: 100 mg I.M. or I.V., then 2 to 10 mg I.M. or 10 to 100 mg P.O. daily.
Prevention of vitamin B_6 deficiency during drug therapy –
Adults and children: 10 to 50 mg P.O. daily for penicillamine, or 100 to 300 mg P.O. daily for cycloserine, hydralazine, or isoniazid.
Drug-induced vitamin B_6 deficiency –
Adults and children: 50 to 200 mg P.O., I.M., or I.V. daily for 3 weeks, followed by 25 to 100 mg P.O., I.M., or I.V. daily to prevent relapse.
Antidote for cycloserine poisoning –
Adults: 100 to 300 mg P.O., I.M., or I.V. daily in divided doses.
Antidote for isoniazid poisoning –
Adults: 1 to 4 g I.V., followed by 1 g I.M. q 30 minutes until the amount of pyridoxine administered equals the amount of isoniazid ingested.

ADVERSE REACTIONS
CNS: drowsiness, paresthesia.

INTERACTIONS
Levodopa: decreased levodopa effect. Avoid concomitant use.
Phenobarbital, phenytoin: decreased anticonvulsant serum levels, increasing risk of seizures. Avoid concomitant use.

CONTRAINDICATIONS
• Contraindicated in patients hypersensitive to pyridoxine.

NURSING CONSIDERATIONS
• Excessive protein intake increases daily pyridoxine requirements; carefully monitor the patient's diet and snacking habits.
• Stress importance of compliance and of good nutrition if prescribed for maintenance therapy to prevent recurrence of deficiency. Explain that pyridoxine in combination therapy with isoniazid has a specific therapeutic purpose and is not just a vitamin. Explain importance of adhering to therapeutic regimen.
• Patients taking high doses (2 to 6 g/day) may experience difficulty walking because of diminished proprioceptive and sensory function.
• When used to treat isoniazid toxicity, expect to also administer anticonvulsants.
• Advise patients taking levodopa alone to avoid multivitamins containing pyridoxine because of decreased levodopa effect.
• **I.V. use:** Inject undiluted drug into I.V. line containing a free-flowing compatible solution. Alternatively, infuse diluted drug over prescribed du-

ration for intermittent infusions. Do not use for continuous infusion.
• Protect from light. Do not use solution if it contains a precipitate, although slight darkening is acceptable.
• If sodium bicarbonate is required to control acidosis in isoniazid toxicity, do not mix in same syringe with pyridoxine.

riboflavin (vitamin B_2)◊

Pregnancy Risk Category: A (C if > RDA)

HOW SUPPLIED

Tablets: 10 mg◊, 25 mg◊, 50 mg◊, 100 mg◊
Tablets (sugar-free): 50 mg◊, 100 mg◊

ACTION

Mechanism: Converts to two other coenzymes that are necessary for normal tissue respiration.
Duration: half-life, 1 to 1½ hours.

INDICATIONS & DOSAGE

Recommended daily allowance (RDA) –
Neonates and infants to 6 months: 0.4 mg.
Infants 6 months to 1 year: 0.5 mg.
Children 1 year to 3 years: 0.8 mg.
Children 4 to 6 years: 1.1 mg.
Children 7 to 10 years: 1.2 mg.
Males 11 to 14 years: 1.5 mg.
Males 15 to 18 years: 1.8 mg.
Males 19 to 50 years: 1.7 mg.
Males 51 years and over: 1.4 mg.
Females 11 to 50 years: 1.3 mg.
Females 51 years and over: 1.2 mg.
Pregnant women: 1.6 mg.
Lactating women (first 6 months): 1.8 mg.
Lactating women (second 6 months): 1.7 mg.
Riboflavin deficiency or adjunct to thiamine treatment for polyneuritis or cheilosis secondary to pellagra –
Adults and children over 12 years: 5 to 50 mg P.O. daily, depending on severity.
Children under 12 years: 2 to 10 mg P.O. daily, depending on severity.
For maintenance, increase nutritional intake and supplement with vitamin B complex.

ADVERSE REACTIONS

GU: bright yellow urine (with high doses).

INTERACTIONS

Propantheline, other anticholinergics: decreased rate and extent of absorption. Avoid concomitant use.

CONTRAINDICATIONS

None reported.

NURSING CONSIDERATIONS

• Stress proper nutritional habits to prevent recurrence of deficiency.
• Riboflavin deficiency usually accompanies other vitamin B complex deficiencies and may require multivitamin therapy.
• Encourage patient to take riboflavin with meals because food increases its absorption.
• May be given I.M. or I.V. as a component of multiple vitamins.
• Protect from air and light.

thiamine hydrochloride (vitamin B_1)

Apatate Drops, Betamin‡, Beta-Sol‡, Biamine, Thia

Pregnancy Risk Category: A (C if > RDA)

HOW SUPPLIED

Tablets: 5 mg◊, 10 mg◊, 25 mg◊, 50 mg◊, 100 mg◊, 250 mg◊, 500 mg◊
Elixir: 2.25 mg/5 ml (with alcohol 10%)◊
Injection: 100 mg/ml

ACTION

Mechanism: Combines with adenosine triphosphate to form a coenzyme necessary for carbohydrate metabolism.

Peak: Levels peak in several days.

INDICATIONS & DOSAGE

Recommended daily allowance (RDA) –

Neonates and infants to 6 months: 0.3 mg.

Infants 6 months to 1 year: 0.4 mg.

Children over 1 year to 3 years: 0.7 mg.

Children 4 to 6 years: 0.9 mg.

Children 7 to 10 years: 1 mg.

Males 11 to 14 years: 1.3 mg.

Males 15 to 50 years: 1.5 mg.

Males 51 years and over: 1.2 mg.

Females 11 to 50 years: 1.1 mg.

Females 51 years and over: 1 mg.

Pregnant women: 1.5 mg.

Lactating women: 1.6 mg.

Beriberi –

Adults: depending on severity, 10 to 500 mg I.M. t.i.d. for 2 weeks, followed by dietary correction and multivitamin supplement containing 5 to 100 mg thiamine daily for 1 month.

Children: depending on severity, 10 to 50 mg I.M. daily for several weeks with adequate diet.

Anemia secondary to thiamine deficiency; polyneuritis secondary to alcoholism, pregnancy, or pellagra –

Adults: 100 mg P.O. daily.

Children: 10 to 50 mg P.O. daily in divided doses.

Wernicke's encephalopathy –

Adults: 500 mg to 1 g I.V. for crisis therapy, followed by 100 mg b.i.d. for maintenance; or 50 mg I.V. bolus followed by 50 mg I.M. daily until symptoms improve.

Wet beriberi with myocardial failure –

Adults and children: 100 to 500 mg I.V. for emergency treatment.

ADVERSE REACTIONS

CNS: restlessness.

CV: ***hypotension after rapid I.V. injection, angioedema,*** cyanosis.

EENT: tightness of throat (allergic reaction).

GI: nausea, hemorrhage, diarrhea.

Respiratory: pulmonary edema.

Skin: feeling of warmth, pruritus, urticaria, sweating.

Other: ***anaphylactoid reactions,*** weakness.

INTERACTIONS

Neuromuscular blockers: enhanced neuromuscular blockade. Clinical significance unknown.

CONTRAINDICATIONS

- Contraindicated in patients hypersensitive to thiamine products.
- I.V. push is contraindicated, except when treating life-threatening myocardial failure in wet beriberi.

NURSING CONSIDERATIONS

- Thiamine malabsorption is most likely in alcoholism, cirrhosis, or GI disease.
- Clinically significant deficiency can occur in approximately 3 weeks of totally thiamine-free diet. Thiamine deficiency usually requires concurrent treatment for multiple deficiencies.
- Doses larger than 30 mg t.i.d. may not be fully utilized. After tissue saturation with thiamine, it is excreted in urine as pyrimidine.
- If beriberi occurs in a breast-fed infant, both mother and child should be treated with thiamine.
- **I.V. use:** Dilute before administration.
- Administer large I.V. doses cautiously; give the patient skin test before therapy if he has a history of hypersensitivity reactions. Have epinephrine on hand to treat anaphylaxis should it occur.
- Use parenteral administration only when P.O. route is not feasible.

• Unstable in alkaline solutions; do not use with materials that yield alkaline solutions.

vitamin C (ascorbic acid)

Ascorbicap◊, Cebid Timecelles◊, Cecon◊, Cee-1000 T.D.◊, Cenolate◊, Cevalin◊, Cevi-Bid, Ce-Vi-Sol*, Cevita◊, C-Span◊, Dull-C◊, Flavettes‡, Redoxon†, Solucap C, Vita C Crystals◊

Pregnancy Risk Category: A (C if > RDA)

HOW SUPPLIED

Tablets: 25 mg◊, 50 mg◊, 100 mg◊, 250 mg◊, 500 mg◊, 1,000 mg◊
Tablets (chewable): 100 mg◊, 250 mg◊, 500 mg◊, 1,000 mg◊
Tablets (effervescent): 1,000 mg sugar-free◊
Tablets (timed-release): 500 mg◊, 750 mg◊, 1,000 mg◊, 1,500 mg
Capsules (timed-release): 500 mg◊
Crystals: 100 g (4 g/tsp)◊, 500 g (4 g/tsp)◊
Lozenges: 60 mg◊
Oral liquid: 50 ml (35 mg/0.6 ml)*◊
Oral solution: 60 mg/ml◊, 100 mg/ml◊
Powder: 100 g (4 g/tsp)◊, 500 g (4 g/tsp)◊
Syrup: 20 mg/ml in 120 ml, 480 ml◊; 500 mg/5 ml in 5 ml◊, 10 ml◊, 120 ml◊, 473 ml◊
Injection: 100 mg/ml in 2-ml, 10-ml ampules; 250 mg/ml in 10-ml ampules and 10-ml, 30-ml, 50-ml vials; 500 mg/ml in 2-ml, 5-ml ampules and 50-ml vials; 500 mg/ml (with monothioglycerol) in 1-ml ampules

ACTION

Mechanism: Stimulates collagen formation and tissue repair; involved in oxidation-reduction reactions throughout the body.
Peak: Levels peak within 3 hours after an oral dose.

INDICATIONS & DOSAGE

Recommended daily allowance (RDA) –
Neonates and infants to 6 months: 30 mg.
Infants 6 months to 1 year: 35 mg.
Children 1 to 3 years: 40 mg.
Children 4 to 10 years: 45 mg.
Children 11 to 14 years: 50 mg.
Children 15 years and over, adults: 60 mg.
Pregnant women: 70 mg.
Lactating women (first 6 months): 95 mg.
Lactating women (second 6 months): 90 mg.
Frank and subclinical scurvy –
Adults: depending on severity, 100 mg to 2 g P.O., S.C., I.M., or I.V. daily, then at least 50 mg daily for maintenance.
Children: depending on severity, 100 to 300 mg P.O., S.C., I.M., or I.V. daily, then at least 35 mg daily for maintenance.
Infants: 50 to 100 mg P.O., I.M., I.V., or S.C. daily.
Extensive burns, delayed fracture or wound healing, postoperative wound healing, severe febrile or chronic disease states –
Adults: 200 to 500 mg S.C., I.M., or I.V. daily.
Children: 100 to 200 mg P.O., S.C., I.M., or I.V. daily.
Prevention of vitamin C deficiency in patients with poor nutritional habits or increased requirements –
Adults: 45 to 60 mg P.O., S.C., I.M., or I.V. daily.
Pregnant and lactating women: at least 60 mg P.O., S.C., I.M., or I.V. daily.
Children: at least 40 mg P.O., S.C., I.M., or I.V. daily.
Infants: at least 35 mg P.O., S.C., I.M., or I.V. daily.
Potentiation of methenamine in urine acidification –
Adults: 4 to 12 g P.O. daily in divided doses.

*Liquid form contains alcohol.
**May contain tartrazine.

Common reactions are in italics; ***life-threatening,*** in bold italics.

ADVERSE REACTIONS

CNS: faintness or dizziness with fast I.V. administration.
GI: nausea, vomiting, diarrhea, epigastric burning, esophagitis, intestinal obstruction.
GU: acid urine, oxaluria, renal calculi, ***renal failure.***
Hematologic: hemolysis.
Other: discomfort at injection site.

INTERACTIONS

Aspirin (high doses): increased risk of ascorbic acid deficiency. Monitor the patient closely.
Oral iron supplements: increased iron absorption (a beneficial drug interaction).
Warfarin: decreased anticoagulant effect. Avoid concomitant use.

CONTRAINDICATIONS

- Use cautiously in patients with G6PD deficiency.

NURSING CONSIDERATIONS

- When administering for urine acidification, check urine pH to ensure efficacy.
- **I.V. use:** Administer I.V. infusion cautiously in patients with renal insufficiency.
- Avoid rapid I.V. administration.
- Protect solution from light, and refrigerate ampules.

---

vitamin D

cholecalciferol (vitamin D_3)

Delta-D◊, Vitamin D_3◊

ergocalciferol (vitamin D_2)

Calciferol, Drisdol, Radiostol†, Radiostol Forte†, Vitamin D

Pregnancy Risk Category: A (D if > RDA)

HOW SUPPLIED

Tablets: 1.25 mg (50,000 IU)
Capsules: 0.625 mg (25,000 IU), 1.25 mg (50,000 IU)
Oral liquid: 8,000 IU/ml in 60-ml dropper bottle◊
Injection: 12.5 mg (500,000 IU)/ml

ACTION

Mechanism: Promotes absorption and utilization of calcium and phosphate, helping to regulate calcium homeostasis.
Onset: about 30 days. **Peak:** Serum levels peak 4 to 8 hours after an oral dose. **Duration:** half-life of circulating vitamin D, about 19 days.

INDICATIONS & DOSAGE

Recommended daily allowance (RDA) for cholecalciferol –
Neonates and infants to 6 months: 300 IU.
Infants 6 months to adults 24 years: 400 IU.
Adults 25 years and over: 200 IU.
Pregnant or lactating women: 400 IU.
Rickets and other vitamin D deficiency diseases; renal osteodystrophy –
Adults: initially, 12,000 IU P.O. or I.M. daily, usually increased as indicated by response up to 500,000 IU daily or up to 800,000 IU daily for vitamin D-resistant rickets.
Children: 1,500 to 5,000 IU P.O. or I.M. daily for 2 to 4 weeks, repeated after 2 weeks, if necessary. Alternatively, give single dose of 600,000 IU.

Monitor serum calcium levels daily to guide dosage. After correction of deficiency, maintenance includes adequate diet and RDA supplements.
Hypoparathyroidism –
Adults and children: 50,000 to 200,000 IU P.O. or I.M. daily, with 4-g calcium supplement.

ADVERSE REACTIONS

Adverse reactions listed are usually seen only in vitamin D toxicity.

CNS: headache, dizziness, ataxia, weakness, somnolence, decreased libido, overt psychosis, ***seizures.***
CV: ***calcifications of soft tissues, including the heart.***
EENT: rhinorrhea, conjunctivitis (calcific), photophobia, tinnitus.
GI: anorexia, nausea, vomiting, constipation, diarrhea, dry mouth, metallic taste.
GU: polyuria, albuminuria, hypercalciuria, nocturia, ***impaired renal function,*** renal calculi.
Skin: pruritus.
Other: bone and muscle pain, bone demineralization, weight loss, ***hypercalcemia,*** hyperphosphatemia.

INTERACTIONS

Cholestyramine resin, mineral oil: inhibited GI absorption of oral vitamin D. Space doses. Use together cautiously.
Corticosteroids: antagonized effect of vitamin D. Monitor vitamin D levels closely.
Digitalis glycosides: increased risk of arrhythmias. Monitor serum calcium levels.
Magnesium-containing antacids: possible hypermagnesemia, especially in patients with chronic renal failure. Monitor serum magnesium levels.
Phenobarbital, phenytoin: increased vitamin D metabolism and decreased effectiveness. Monitor closely.
Thiazide diuretics: may cause hypercalcemia in patients with hypoparathyroidism. Monitor closely.

CONTRAINDICATIONS

- Contraindicated in patients with hypercalcemia, hypervitaminosis A, or renal osteodystrophy with hyperphosphatemia.
- Use cautiously in cardiac patients, especially those receiving digitalis glycosides.

NURSING CONSIDERATIONS

- Monitor the patient's eating and bowel habits; dry mouth, nausea, vomiting, metallic taste, and constipation may be early signs and symptoms of toxicity.
- Patients with hyperphosphatemia require dietary phosphate restrictions and binding agents to avoid metastatic calcifications and renal calculi.
- Monitor serum and urine calcium, potassium, and urea levels frequently when high therapeutic dosages are used.
- Malabsorption from inadequate bile or hepatic dysfunction may require addition of exogenous bile salts to oral vitamin D.
- I.M. injection of vitamin D dispersed in oil is preferable in patients unable to absorb the oral form.
- This vitamin is fat-soluble. Warn the patient of the dangers of increasing dosage without consulting the doctor.
- Dosages of 60,000 IU/day can cause hypercalcemia.
- Tell patients taking vitamin D to restrict their intake of magnesium-containing antacids.

vitamin E (tocopherol)

Aquasol E◊, Eprolin◊, Pertropin◊, Solucap E◊, Tocopher◊

Pregnancy Risk Category: A (C if > RDA)

HOW SUPPLIED

Tablets: 100 IU◊, 200 IU◊, 400 IU◊, 500 IU◊, 600 IU◊, 1,000 IU◊
Tablets (chewable): 100 IU◊, 200 IU◊, 400 IU◊
Capsules: 50 IU◊, 100 IU◊, 200 IU◊, 400 IU◊, 600 IU◊, 1,000 IU◊
Oral solution: 50 IU/ml◊

ACTION

Mechanism: Acts as an antioxidant and protects RBC membranes against hemolysis.

Duration: half-life after I.M. use, 44 hours.

INDICATIONS & DOSAGE

Recommended daily allowance (RDA) –
Note: RDAs for vitamin E have been converted to alpha-tocopherol equivalents (α-TE). One α-TE equals 1 mg of D-alpha tocopherol or 1.49 IU.
Neonates and infants to 6 months: 3 α-TE or 4 IU.
Infants 6 months to 1 year: 4 α-TE or 6 IU.
Children over 1 year to 3 years: 6 α-TE or 9 IU.
Children 4 to 10 years: 7 α-TE or 10 IU.
Males 11 years and over: 10 α-TE or 15 IU.
Females 11 years and over: 8 α-TE or 12 IU.
Pregnant women: 10 α-TE or 15 IU.
Lactating women (first 6 months): 12 α-TE or 18 IU.
Lactating women (second 6 months): 11 α-TE or 16 IU.
Vitamin E deficiency in premature neonates and in patients with impaired fat absorption –
Adults: depending on severity, 60 to 75 IU P.O. daily.
Children: 1 IU/kg daily.

ADVERSE REACTIONS

None reported with recommended dosages.

INTERACTIONS

Cholestyramine resin, mineral oil: inhibited GI absorption of oral vitamin E. Space doses. Use together cautiously.
Vitamin K: antagonized effects of vitamin K possible with large doses of vitamin E. Avoid concurrent use.

CONTRAINDICATIONS

None reported.

NURSING CONSIDERATIONS

- Water-miscible forms more completely absorbed in GI tract.
- Tell the patient that tablets should not be crushed and capsules should not be opened. An oral solution and chewable tablets are commercially available.
- Monitor the patient with liver or gallbladder disease for response to therapy. Adequate bile is essential for vitamin E absorption.
- Requirements increase with rise in dietary polyunsaturated acids.
- May protect other vitamins against oxidation.
- This vitamin is fat-soluble. Discourage the patient from self-medication with megadoses, which can cause thrombophlebitis.

menadione/menadiol sodium diphosphate (vitamin K_3)

Synkavite†, Synkayvite

Pregnancy Risk Category: C (X near term)

HOW SUPPLIED

Tablets: 10 mg‡
Injection: 5 mg/ml, 10 mg/ml, 37.5 mg/ml

ACTION

Mechanism: An antihemorrhagic factor that promotes hepatic formation of active prothrombin.
Onset: 1 to 2 hours.

INDICATIONS & DOSAGE

Hypoprothrombinemia secondary to vitamin K malabsorption or drug therapy, or when oral administration is desired and bile secretion is inadequate –
Adults: 5 to 10 mg P.O., or 5 to 15 mg I.M. or I.V. daily to b.i.d., titrated to the patient's requirements.

ADVERSE REACTIONS
CNS: headache, ***kernicterus.***
GI: nausea, vomiting.
Skin: allergic rash, pruritus, urticaria.
Other: pain, hematoma at injection site.

INTERACTIONS
Cholestyramine resin, mineral oil: inhibited GI absorption of oral vitamin K. Space doses. Use together cautiously.
Oral anticoagulants: impaired effectiveness. Increase in oral anticoagulant dosage may be required.

CONTRAINDICATIONS
• Contraindicated in treatment of hereditary hypoprothrombinemia (because vitamin K_3 can paradoxically worsen the disorder); in patients with hepatocellular disease, unless it is caused by biliary obstruction; in treatment of heparin-induced bleeding; and during the last weeks of pregnancy to avoid toxic reactions in neonates.
• Contraindicated in neonates (especially premature neonates) because it can cause hemolytic anemia, hyperbilirubinemia, kernicterus, brain damage, and death.
• Use cautiously in patients with G6PD deficiency to avoid hemolysis. In severe bleeding, do not delay other measures, such as giving fresh frozen plasma or whole blood. Use large dosages cautiously in severe hepatic disease.

NURSING CONSIDERATIONS
• Do not use vitamin K_3 to treat hypoprothrombinemia induced by oral anticoagulants; phytonadione (vitamin K_1) is the drug of choice.
• Considered more toxic than vitamin K_1.
• Failure to respond to vitamin K_3 may indicate coagulation defects.
• Excessive use of vitamin K_3 may temporarily defeat oral anticoagulant therapy, requiring higher doses of oral anticoagulant or interim use of heparin.
• Monitor PT to determine dosage effectiveness.
• Observe for signs of adverse reactions and report them to the doctor.
• Use caution in handling bulk menadione powder; it irritates the skin and respiratory tract.
• This vitamin is fat-soluble.
• **I.V. use:** Infusion rate shouldn't exceed 1 mg/minute.
• Effects of I.V. injections are more rapid but shorter-lived than S.C. or I.M. injections.
• Protect parenteral products from light.

phytonadione (vitamin K_1)
AquaMEPHYTON, Konakion, Mephyton
Pregnancy Risk Category: C

HOW SUPPLIED
Tablets: 5 mg
Injection (aqueous colloidal solution): 2 mg/ml, 10 mg/ml
Injection (aqueous dispersion): 2 mg/ml, 10 mg/ml

ACTION
Mechanism: An antihemorrhagic factor that promotes hepatic formation of active prothrombin.
Onset: 24 to 48 hours. **Peak:** Plasma levels peak within 12 hours after oral dose.

INDICATIONS & DOSAGE
Recommended daily allowance (RDA) –
Neonates and infants to 6 months: 5 mcg.
Infants 6 months to 1 year: 10 mcg.
Children 1 year to 3 years: 15 mcg.
Children 4 to 6 years: 20 mcg.
Children 7 to 10 years: 30 mcg.

Children 11 to 14 years: 45 mcg.
Males 15 to 18 years: 65 mcg.
Males 19 to 24 years: 70 mcg.
Males 25 years and over: 80 mcg.
Females 15 to 18 years: 55 mcg.
Females 19 to 24 years: 60 mcg.
Females 25 years and over; pregnant or lactating women: 65 mcg.
Hypoprothrombinemia secondary to vitamin K malabsorption, drug therapy, or excessive vitamin A dosage –
Adults: depending on severity, 2.5 to 10 mg P.O., S.C., or I.M. repeated and increased up to 50 mg if necessary.
Infants: 2 mg P.O. or parenterally.
Children: 5 to 10 mg P.O. or parenterally.

I.V. injection rate for infants and children should not exceed 3 mg/m²/minute or a total of 5 mg.
Hypoprothrombinemia secondary to effect of oral anticoagulants –
Adults: 2.5 to 10 mg P.O., S.C., or I.M. based on PT, repeated if necessary within 12 to 48 hours after oral dose or within 6 to 8 hours after parenteral dose. In emergency, give 10 to 50 mg slow I.V., rate not to exceed 1 mg/minute, repeated q 4 hours, p.r.n.
Prevention of hemorrhagic disease –
Neonates: 0.5 to 1 mg S.C. or I.M. immediately after birth, repeated within 6 to 8 hours, if needed, especially if mother received oral anticoagulants or long-term anticonvulsant therapy during pregnancy.
To differentiate between hepatocellular disease or biliary obstruction as source of hypoprothrombinemia –
Adults and children: 10 mg I.M. or S.C.
Prevention of hypoprothrombinemia related to vitamin K deficiency in long-term parenteral nutrition –
Adults: 5 to 10 mg S.C. or I.M. weekly.
Children: 2 to 5 mg S.C. or I.M. weekly.
Prevention of hypoprothrombinemia in infants receiving less than 0.1 mg/liter vitamin K in breast milk or milk substitutes –
Infants: 1 mg S.C. or I.M. monthly.

ADVERSE REACTIONS

CNS: dizziness, seizurelike movements.
CV: transient hypotension after I.V. administration, rapid and weak pulse, cardiac irregularities.
GI: nausea, vomiting.
Respiratory: ***bronchospasm,*** dyspnea.
Skin: diaphoresis, flushing, erythema.
Other: cramp-like pain, ***anaphylaxis and anaphylactoid reactions*** (usually after rapid I.V. administration); pain, swelling, and hematoma at injection site.

INTERACTIONS

Cholestyramine resin, mineral oil: inhibited GI absorption of oral vitamin K. Space doses. Use together cautiously.

CONTRAINDICATIONS

- Contraindicated in patients with hereditary hypoprothrombinemia; bleeding secondary to heparin therapy or overdose; or hepatocellular disease, unless caused by biliary obstruction (vitamin K can paradoxically worsen the hypoprothrombinemia). Oral administration is contraindicated if bile secretion is inadequate, unless supplemented with bile salts.
- Use cautiously, if at all, during last weeks of pregnancy to avoid toxic reactions in neonates, and in patients with G6PD deficiency to avoid hemolysis. Use large dosages cautiously in patients with severe hepatic disease.

NURSING CONSIDERATIONS

- Failure to respond to vitamin K may indicate coagulation defects.
- If severe bleeding occurs, don't delay other measures, such as fresh frozen plasma or whole blood.

- Monitor PT to determine dosage effectiveness.
- Observe the patient closely for signs of flushing, weakness, tachycardia, and hypotension; may progress to shock.
- Phytonadione therapy for hemorrhagic disease in infants causes fewer adverse reactions than do other vitamin K analogues.
- Check brand name labels for administration route restrictions.
- This vitamin is fat-soluble.
- **I.V. use:** Dilute with 0.9% sodium chloride injection, D_5W, or D_5W in 0.9% sodium chloride injection. Administer I.V. by slow infusion over 2 to 3 hours. Infusion rate shouldn't exceed 1 mg/minute in adults or 3 mg/m^2/minute in children.
- Effects of I.V. injection are more rapid but shorter-lived than S.C. or I.M. injections.
- Protect parenteral products from light. Wrap infusion container with aluminum foil.
- Anticipate order of weekly addition of 5 to 10 mg of phytonadione to total parenteral nutrition solutions.

sodium fluoride

Fluor-A-Day†, Fluoritab,Fluorodex, Fluotic†, Flura, Flura-Drops, Flura-Loz, Karidium, Luride, Luride Lozi-Tabs, Luride-SF, Luride-SF Lozi-Tabs, Pediaflor, Pedi-Dent†, Pharmaflur, Pharmaflur df, Pharmaflur 1.1, Phos-Flur, Solu-Flur†

sodium fluoride, topical

ACT◊, Fluorigard◊, Fluorinse, Gel Kam, Gel-Tin◊, Karigel, Karigel-N, Listermint with Fluoride, Minute Gel, Point-Two, PreviDent, Stop◊, Thera-Flur, Thera-Flur-N

Pregnancy Risk Category: C

HOW SUPPLIED

sodium fluoride
Tablets: 1 mg
Tablets (chewable): 0.5 mg, 1 mg
Drops: 0.125 mg/drop, 0.25 mg/drop, 0.2 mg/ml, 0.5 mg/ml
Lozenges: 1 mg
sodium fluoride, topical
Gel: 0.1%, 0.5%, 1.23%
Gel drops: 0.5%
Rinse: 0.01%◊, 0.02%◊, 0.09%

ACTION

Mechanism: May catalyze bone remineralization. Mechanism is unknown.
Peak: Levels peak within 30 minutes after an oral dose. **Duration:** half-life, about 6 hours.

INDICATIONS & DOSAGE

Prevention of dental caries –
Adults and children over 12 years: 5 to 10 ml of rinse or thin ribbon of gel applied to teeth with toothbrush or mouth trays for at least 1 minute h.s.
Children under 3 years: 0.5 mg P.O. (tablet or drops) daily.
Children 3 to 6 years: 1 mg P.O. (tablet or lozenge) daily.
Children 6 to 12 years: 5 to 10 ml of rinse or thin ribbon of gel applied to teeth with toothbrush or mouth trays for at least 1 minute h.s.
Osteoporosis –
Adults: 20 to 60 mg P.O. daily.

ADVERSE REACTIONS

CNS: headache, weakness.
GI: gastric distress, nausea, vomiting, bad taste (salty, soapy).
Skin: hypersensitivity reactions, such as atopic dermatitis, eczema, and urticaria.
Other: staining of teeth.

INTERACTIONS

None significant.

CONTRAINDICATIONS
• Contraindicated when fluoride intake from drinking water exceeds 0.7 ppm.

NURSING CONSIDERATIONS
• Chronic toxicity (fluorosis) may result from prolonged use of higher-than-recommended doses.
• Advise the patient to notify the dentist if tooth mottling occurs.
• Tablets may be dissolved in mouth, chewed, or swallowed whole.
• Drops may be administered orally undiluted or mixed with fluids or food.
• Topical rinses and gels should not be swallowed by children under 3 years or if water supply is fluorinated. Most effective when used immediately after brushing teeth. Tell the patient to rinse around and between teeth for 1 minute, then spit out.
• Tell the patient to dilute drops or rinses in plastic rather than glass containers.
• Fluoride in prenatal vitamins has produced healthier teeth in infants.

trace elements

chromium (chromic chloride)
Chrometrace

copper (cupric chloride, cupric sulfate)
Coppertrace

iodine (sodium iodide)
Iodopen

manganese (manganese chloride, manganese sulfate)
Mangatrace

selenium (selenious acid)
Selenitrace

zinc (zinc chloride, zinc sulfate)
Zinctrace

Pregnancy Risk Category: C

HOW SUPPLIED
chromium
Injection: 4 mcg/ml
copper
Injection: 0.4 mg/ml
iodine
Injection: 100 mcg/ml
manganese
Injection: 0.1 mg/ml, 0.5 mg/ml
selenium
Injection: 40 mcg/ml, 50 mcg/ml
zinc
Injection: 1 mg/ml, 5 mg/ml

ACTION
Mechanism: Participates in synthesis and stabilization of proteins and nucleic acids in subcellular and membrane transport systems.
Peak: Levels peak immediately after an I.V. infusion.

INDICATIONS & DOSAGE
Prevention of individual trace element deficiencies in patients receiving long-term total parenteral nutrition –
Chromium –
Adults: 10 to 15 mcg I.V. daily.
Children: 0.14 to 0.20 mcg/kg I.V. daily.
Copper –
Adults: 0.5 to 1.5 mg I.V. daily.
Children: 20 mcg/kg I.V. daily.
Iodine –
Adults: 1 mcg/kg I.V. daily.
Manganese –
Adults: 0.15 to 0.8 mcg I.V. daily.
Children: 2 to 10 mcg/kg I.V. daily.
Selenium –
Adults: 40 to 120 mcg I.V. daily.
Children: 3 mcg/kg I.V. daily.
Zinc –
Adults: 2 to 4 mg I.V. daily.
Children: 0.05 to 0.1 mg/kg I.V. daily.

ADVERSE REACTIONS
None reported.

INTERACTIONS
None significant at recommended dosages.

CONTRAINDICATIONS
• Contraindicated in pregnant and lactating patients.

NURSING CONSIDERATIONS
• Check serum levels of trace elements in patients who have received total parenteral nutrition (TPN) for 2 months or longer. Give supplement if ordered. Call the doctor's attention to low serum levels of these elements.
• Normal serum levels are 0.85 ng/ml chromium; 0.07 to 0.15 mg/ml copper; 4 to 20 mcg/100 ml manganese; 0.1 to 0.19 mcg/ml selenium; and 0.05 to 0.15 mg/100 ml zinc.
• Solutions of trace elements are compounded by pharmacy for addition to TPN solutions according to various formulas. One common trace element solution is Shil's solution, which contains copper 1 mg/ml, iodide 0.06 mg/ml, manganese 0.4 mg/ml, and zinc 2 mg/ml.
• **I.V. use:** Cautiously infuse diluted solution through a patent I.V. line over the ordered duration. Direct injection and intermittent infusion are not recommended.

91
Calorics

amino acid infusions, crystalline
amino acid infusions in dextrose
amino acid infusions with electrolytes
amino acid infusions with electrolytes in dextrose
amino acid infusions for hepatic failure
amino acid infusions for high metabolic stress
amino acid infusions for renal failure
corn oil
dextrose
fat emulsions
fructose
invert sugar
medium-chain triglycerides

COMBINATION PRODUCTS
Various products contain dextrose, fructose, or invert sugar in combination with electrolytes.

amino acid infusions, crystalline
Aminosyn, Aminosyn II, Aminosyn-PF, FreAmine III, Novamine, Travasol, TrophAmine

amino acid infusions in dextrose
Aminosyn II with dextrose

amino acid infusions with electrolytes
Aminosyn with electrolytes, Aminosyn II with electrolytes, FreAmine III with electrolytes, ProcalAmine with electrolytes, Travasol with electrolytes

amino acid infusions with electrolytes in dextrose
Aminosyn II with electrolytes in dextrose

amino acid infusions for hepatic failure
HepatAmine

amino acid infusions for high metabolic stress
Aminosyn-HBC, BranchAmin, FreAmine HBC

amino acid infusions for renal failure
Aminess, Aminosyn-RF, NephrAmine, RenAmin

Pregnancy Risk Category: C

HOW SUPPLIED
Injection: 250 ml, 500 ml, 1,000 ml, 2,000 ml containing amino acids in varying concentrations
amino acid infusions, crystalline
Aminosyn: 3.5%, 5%, 7%, 8.5%, 10%
Aminosyn II: 3.5%, 5%, 7%, 8.5%, 10%
Aminosyn-PF: 7%, 10%
FreAmine III: 8.5%, 10%
Novamine: 11.4%, 15%
Travasol: 5.5%, 8.5%, 10%
TrophAmine: 6%, 10%
amino acid infusions in dextrose
Aminosyn II: 3.5% in 5% dextrose, 3.5% in 25% dextrose, 4.25% in 10% dextrose, 4.25% in 20% dextrose, 4.25% in 25% dextrose, 5% in 25% dextrose
amino acid infusions with electrolytes
Aminosyn: 3.5%, 7%, 8.5%
Aminosyn II: 3.5%, 7%, 8.5%, 10%
FreAmine III: 3%, 8.5%
ProcalAmine: 3%

Travasol: 3.5%, 5.5%, 8.5%
amino acid infusions with electrolytes in dextrose
Aminosyn II: 3.5% with electrolytes in 5% dextrose, 4.25% with electrolytes in 10% dextrose
amino acid infusions for hepatic failure
HepatAmine: 8%
amino acid infusions for high metabolic stress
Aminosyn-HBC: 7%
BranchAmin: 4%
FreAmine HBC: 6.9%
amino acid infusions for renal failure
Aminess: 5.2%
Aminosyn-RF: 5.2%
NephrAmine: 5.4%
RenAmin: 6.5%

ACTION

Mechanism: Provides a substrate for protein synthesis or enhances conservation of existing body protein. Formulations for hepatic failure and high metabolic stress contain essential and nonessential amino acids, with high concentrations of the branched chain amino acids isoleucine, leucine, and valine. Formulations for patients with renal failure contain histidine and minimal amounts of essential amino acids; nonessential amino acids are synthesized from excess ammonia in the blood of the uremic patient, thus lowering azotemia.
Peak: Serum levels peak immediately after an I.V. infusion.

INDICATIONS & DOSAGE

Total parenteral nutrition in patients who cannot or will not eat–
Adults: 1 to 1.5 g/kg I.V. daily.
Children under 10 kg: 2 to 4 g/kg I.V. daily.
Children over 10 kg: 20 to 25 g/kg I.V. daily for the first 10 kg, then 1 to 1.25 g/kg I.V. daily for each kg over 10 kg.
Nutritional support in patients with cirrhosis, hepatitis, and hepatic encephalopathy–
Adults: 80 to 120 g of amino acids (12 to 18 g of nitrogen) I.V. daily of the formulation for hepatic failure.
Nutritional support in patients with high metabolic stress–
Adults: 1.5 g/kg I.V. daily of the formulation for high metabolic stress.
Nutritional support in patients with renal failure–
Adults: 0.3 to 0.5 g/kg I.V. daily (up to total of 26 g daily). Patients on dialysis may require 1 to 1.2 g/kg daily.

ADVERSE REACTIONS

CNS: mental confusion, unconsciousness, headache, dizziness.
CV: hypervolemia, ***CHF*** (in susceptible patients), ***pulmonary edema,*** exacerbation of hypertension (in predisposed patients), thrombophlebitis.
GI: nausea, vomiting.
GU: glycosuria, osmotic diuresis.
Hepatic: fatty liver.
Skin: chills, flushing, feeling of warmth.
Other: hypersensitivity reactions, tissue sloughing at infusion site caused by extravasation, *catheter sepsis,* thrombosis, *rebound hypoglycemia* (when long-term infusions are abruptly stopped), hyperglycemia, metabolic acidosis, alkalosis, hypophosphatemia, ***hyperosmolar nonketotic syndrome,*** hyperammonemia, ***electrolyte imbalances,*** dehydration (if hyperosmolar solutions are used).

INTERACTIONS

None significant.

CONTRAINDICATIONS

- Contraindicated in patients with anuria and in patients with inborn errors of amino acid metabolism, such as maple syrup urine disease and isovaleric acidemia. Also contraindicated in patients with severe uncorrected electrolyte or acid-base imbalances, hyperammonemia, and decreased circulating blood volume.

- Use cautiously in patients with renal insufficiency or failure, cardiac disease, or hepatic impairment.
- Use extra caution in pediatric patients and in neonates, especially those with low birth weight.
- Administer cautiously to diabetic patients; insulin may be required to prevent hyperglycemia. Administer cautiously in cardiac insufficiency; may cause circulatory overload. Patients with fluid restriction may tolerate only 1 to 2 liters.

NURSING CONSIDERATIONS

- Safe and effective use of parenteral nutrition requires a knowledge of nutrition as well as clinical expertise in the recognition and treatment of potential complications. Frequent evaluation of the patient and laboratory determinations are necessary.
- Monitor serum electrolytes, glucose and BUN levels, and renal and hepatic function. Monitor serum calcium frequently.
- Individualize dosage to metabolic and clinical response as determined by nitrogen balance and body weight corrected for fluid balance.
- Add vitamins, electrolytes, and trace elements as ordered.
- Monitor for extraordinary electrolyte losses that may occur during nasogastric suction, vomiting, or drainage from GI fistula.
- **I.V. use:** Control infusion rate carefully with infusion pump. If infusion rate falls behind, notify the doctor; do not increase the rate to catch up.
- Limit peripheral infusions to 2.5% amino acids and dextrose 10%. Check infusion site frequently for erythema, inflammation, irritation, tissue sloughing, necrosis, and phlebitis. Change peripheral I.V. sites routinely to prevent irritation and infection. If a subclavian catheter is used, administer solution into the midsuperior vena cava.
- Protect bottles from light until use.
- Check fractional urine every 6 hours for glycosuria initially, then every 12 to 24 hours in stable patients. Abrupt onset of glycosuria may be an early sign of impending sepsis.
- Assess body temperature every 4 hours; elevation may indicate sepsis or infection.
- If the patient has chills, fever, or other signs of sepsis, replace I.V. tubing and bottle and send them to the laboratory to be cultured.

corn oil

Lipomul

Pregnancy Risk Category: C

HOW SUPPLIED

Liquid: 473-ml container with 10 g corn oil/15 ml (sugar-free)

ACTION

Mechanism: Source of calories and fatty acids.
Peak: Serum levels peak within 2 hours.

INDICATIONS & DOSAGE

To increase caloric intake –
Adults: 45 ml P.O. b.i.d. to q.i.d. after or between meals, alone or with proteins, milk, or other nutritional energy sources.
Children: 30 ml P.O. daily to q.i.d. after or between meals, alone or with proteins, milk, or other nutritional energy sources.

ADVERSE REACTIONS

GI: nausea, vomiting, diarrhea.

INTERACTIONS

Griseofulvin: increased GI absorption of griseofulvin. A beneficial interaction.

CONTRAINDICATIONS

- Contraindicated in patients with gallbladder calculi or complete GI obstruction.
- Use cautiously in patients with steatorrhea, partial GI obstruction, or enterostomies.

NURSING CONSIDERATIONS

- To minimize nausea, diarrhea, and vomiting, give more frequent, smaller doses with meals or mixed with milk.
- Dosage varies greatly with individual requirements; 30 ml of the emulsion provides 180 calories.

dextrose (D-glucose)

Pregnancy Risk Category: C

HOW SUPPLIED

Injection: 3-ml ampule (10%); 5-ml ampule (10%); 10 ml (25%); 50 ml (5% and 50% available in vial, ampule, and Bristoject); 70-ml pin-top vial (70% for additive use only); 100 ml (5%); 250 ml (5%, 10%); 400 ml (5%); 500 ml (5%, 10%, 20%, 30%, 40%, 50%, 60%, 70%); 650 ml (38.5%); 1,000 ml (2.5%, 5%, 10%, 20%, 30%, 40%, 50%, 60%, 70%)

ACTION

Mechanism: A simple water-soluble sugar that minimizes glyconeogenesis and promotes anabolism in patients who can't receive sufficient oral caloric intake.

Peak: Serum levels peak immediately after I.V. infusion.

INDICATIONS & DOSAGE

Fluid replacement and caloric supplementation in patients who can't maintain adequate oral intake or who are restricted from doing so –

Adults and children: dosage depends on fluid and caloric requirements. Use peripheral I.V. infusion of 2.5%, 5%, or 10% solution or central I.V. infusion of 20% solution for minimal fluid needs. Use 50% solution to treat insulin-induced hypoglycemia. Use 40% to 70% solutions diluted in admixtures, normally amino acid solutions, for total parenteral nutrition (TPN) given through a central vein.

ADVERSE REACTIONS

CNS: confusion, ***unconsciousness in hyperosmolar nonketotic syndrome.***

CV: with fluid overload – ***pulmonary edema, exacerbated hypertension, and CHF*** in susceptible patients. Prolonged or concentrated infusions may cause *phlebitis and venous sclerosis,* especially when administered peripherally.

GU: glycosuria, osmotic diuresis.

Skin: sloughing and tissue necrosis, if extravasation occurs with concentrated solutions.

Other: with rapid infusion of concentrated solution or prolonged infusion – hyperglycemia, hypervolemia, hyperosmolarity. Rapid termination of long-term infusions may cause hypoglycemia from rebound hyperinsulinemia.

INTERACTIONS

None significant.

CONTRAINDICATIONS

- Contraindicated in patients with hyperglycemia, diabetic coma, intracranial or intraspinal hemorrhage, or delirium tremens.
- Use cautiously in patients with cardiac or pulmonary disease, hypertension, renal insufficiency, urinary obstruction, or hypovolemia.

NURSING CONSIDERATIONS

- Monitor fluid intake and output and weight carefully, especially patients with renal function impairment.
- Check vital signs frequently. Report adverse effects promptly.
- **I.V. use:** Control infusion rate carefully; maximal rate is 0.5 g/kg/hour. Use infusion pump when infusing

with amino acids for TPN. Never infuse concentrated solutions rapidly; may cause hyperglycemia and fluid shift.

• Monitor serum glucose levels carefully. Prolonged therapy with D_5W can cause depletion of pancreatic insulin production and secretion. If blood glucose level exceeds 200 mg/dl for more than 3 days, discontinue infusion.

• Never stop hypertonic solutions abruptly. If necessary, have dextrose 10% in water solution available to treat hypoglycemia if rebound hyperinsulinemia occurs.

• Don't give dextrose solutions without sodium chloride solution in blood transfusions; may cause clumping of RBCs. Use central veins to infuse dextrose solutions with concentrations greater than 10%.

• Take care to prevent extravasation. Check injection site frequently to prevent irritation, tissue sloughing, necrosis, and phlebitis.

• Watch closely for signs of fluid overload, especially if fluid intake is restricted.

fat emulsions

Intralipid 10%, Intralipid 20%, Liposyn II 10%, Liposyn II 20%, Liposyn III 10%, Liposyn III 20%

Pregnancy Risk Category: C

HOW SUPPLIED

Injection: 50 ml (10%, 20%), 100 ml (10%, 20%), 200 ml (10%, 20%), 250 ml (10%, 20%), 500 ml (10%, 20%)

ACTION

Mechanism: Provides neutral triglycerides, predominantly unsaturated fatty acids; acts as a source of calories; and prevents fatty acid deficiency. When substituted for dextrose as a source of calories, fat emulsions decrease carbon dioxide production.

Peak: Serum levels peak immediately after I.V. infusion. **Duration:** elimination half-life, about 30 minutes; reversal of fatty acid deficiency, 2 weeks.

INDICATIONS & DOSAGE

Intralipid:

Source of calories as adjunct to total parenteral nutrition (TPN) –

Adults: 1 ml/minute I.V. for 15 to 30 minutes (10% emulsion); 0.5 ml/minute I.V. for 15 to 30 minutes (20% emulsion). If no adverse reactions occur, increase rate to deliver 500 ml over 4 to 8 hours; total daily dosage should not exceed 2.5 g/kg.

Children: 0.1 ml/minute for 10 to 15 minutes (10% emulsion), 0.05 ml/minute I.V. for 10 to 15 minutes (20% emulsion). If no adverse reactions occur, increase rate to deliver 1 g/kg over 4 hours; daily dosage should not exceed 4 g/kg. Equals 60% of daily caloric intake; protein-carbohydrate TPN should supply remaining 40%.

Fatty acid deficiency –

Adults and children: 8% to 10% of total caloric intake I.V.

Liposyn:

Prevention of fatty acid deficiency –

Adults: 500 ml (10% emulsion) I.V. twice weekly. Infuse initially at a rate of 1 ml/minute for 30 minutes. Rate may be increased but should not exceed 500 ml over 4 to 6 hours.

Children: 5 to 10 ml/kg (10% emulsion) I.V. daily. Infuse initially at a rate of 0.1 ml/minute for 30 minutes. Rate may be increased but should not exceed 100 ml/hour.

ADVERSE REACTIONS

Early reactions to fat overload:

CNS: headache, sleepiness, dizziness.

EENT: pressure over eyes.

GI: nausea, vomiting.

Hematologic: ***hypercoagulability, thrombocytopenia in neonates*** (rare).

Respiratory: dyspnea, cyanosis.

Skin: flushing, diaphoresis.
Other: hyperlipidemia, fever, chest and back pains, hypersensitivity reactions, irritation at infusion site.
Delayed reactions:
CNS: focal seizures.
CV: ***shock.***
Hematologic: thrombocytopenia, leukopenia, leukocytosis.
Hepatic: transient increases in liver function test values, hepatomegaly.
Other: fever, splenomegaly, ***fat accumulation in lungs.***

INTERACTIONS
None significant.

CONTRAINDICATIONS
• Contraindicated in hyperlipidemia, lipid nephrosis, or acute pancreatitis accompanied by hyperlipidemia.
• Use cautiously in patients with severe hepatic disease; pulmonary disease; anemia; or blood coagulation disorders, including thrombocytopenia; and in patients at risk for fat embolism.
• Also use cautiously in premature infants because they are susceptible to I.V. fat overload.

NURSING CONSIDERATIONS
• Monitor the patient for adverse reactions, especially during first ½ of infusion.
• **I.V. use:** Avoid rapid infusion, and use an infusion pump to regulate rate.
• Check platelet count frequently in neonates receiving fat emulsions I.V.
• Lipids support bacterial growth, so change all I.V. tubing before each infusion. Check injection site daily. Report signs of inflammation or infection promptly.
• Carefully monitor serum triglycerides and free fatty acids in infants.
• May be mixed with amino acid solution, dextrose, electrolytes, and vitamins in the same I.V. container. Check with the pharmacist for acceptable proportions and compatibility information.
• Manufacturers do not recommend using an in-line filter for administering fat emulsions because fat particles are larger than the pores of a standard 0.22-micron cellulose filter. However, an in-line filter with pores of 1.2 micron or larger is sometimes used to remove particulate matter.
• Do not use fat emulsion if it separates or becomes oily.
• Refrigeration is not necessary.
• Monitor serum lipid levels closely when the patient is receiving fat emulsion therapy. Lipemia must clear between dosing.
• Monitor hepatic function carefully in long-term use.
• Intralipid and Liposyn differ mainly by their fatty acid components.

fructose (levulose)

Pregnancy Risk Category: C

HOW SUPPLIED
Injection: 1,000 ml (10% or 100 g/liter)

ACTION
Mechanism: Minimizes glyconeogenesis and promotes anabolism in patients who can't receive sufficient oral caloric intake.
Peak: Serum levels peak immediately after I.V. infusion.

INDICATIONS & DOSAGE
Source of carbohydrate calories, primarily when fluid replacement is also indicated, and as a dextrose substitute for patients with diabetes –
Adults and children: dosage depends on caloric needs. I.V. infusion rate should not exceed 1 g/kg/hour. Single liter of 10% solution yields 375 calories.

ADVERSE REACTIONS

CV: increased pulse rate, precipitation or exacerbation of ***CHF*** in susceptible patients, thrombophlebitis.
Hepatic: hepatomegaly.
Respiratory: increased respiratory rate, ***pulmonary edema***.
Other: metabolic acidosis, hypervolemia, tissue sloughing from extravasation at infusion site.

INTERACTIONS

None significant.

CONTRAINDICATIONS

- Contraindicated in patients with hereditary fructose intolerance or gout or in patients receiving therapy for hypoglycemia.
- Use cautiously in patients with cardiac disease, hypertension, pulmonary disease, hypervolemia, renal insufficiency, or urinary tract obstructions.

NURSING CONSIDERATIONS

- Monitor the patient for signs of fluid overload, pulmonary edema, or CHF.
- **I.V. use:** Control infusion rate carefully. Direct injection or intermittent infusion is not recommended.
- Change infusion sites regularly to avoid irritation with prolonged therapy. Take care to avoid extravasation.
- Don't use unless the solution is clear and the seal is intact.

invert sugar

Travert

Pregnancy Risk Category: C

HOW SUPPLIED

Injection: 5%, 10%, 10% with electrolytes

ACTION

Mechanism: Composed of equal amounts of dextrose and fructose; minimizes glyconeogenesis and promotes anabolism in patients who can't receive sufficient oral caloric intake.
Peak: Serum levels peak immediately after I.V. infusion.

INDICATIONS & DOSAGE

Nonelectrolyte fluid replacement and caloric supplementation solution –
Adults and children: dosage depends on the patient's age, weight, and clinical need. I.V. infusion rate should not exceed 1 g/kg/hour. A single liter of 5% invert sugar yields 375 calories. Most patients receive 1 to 3 liters of 10% solution daily.

ADVERSE REACTIONS

CNS: confusion, unconsciousness in ***hyperosmolar nonketotic syndrome***.
CV: increased pulse rate, precipitation or exacerbation of ***CHF*** in susceptible patients, hypertension, thrombophlebitis.
GU: glycosuria, osmotic diuresis.
Respiratory: ***pulmonary edema.***
Other: hypervolemia, hyperglycemia, hyperosmolarity, sloughing with extravasation at infusion site.

INTERACTIONS

None significant.

CONTRAINDICATIONS

- Contraindicated in patients with hereditary fructose intolerance, hyperglycemia, diabetic coma, intracranial or intraspinal hemorrhage, or delirium tremens.
- Use cautiously in patients with cardiac disease, hypertension, pulmonary disease, hypervolemia, renal insufficiency, or urinary tract obstruction.

NURSING CONSIDERATIONS

- Monitor the patient for signs of fluid overload, pulmonary edema, or CHF. Monitor blood pressure frequently.
- Monitor serum glucose levels closely. Prolonged therapy can cause

decreased pancreatic insulin production and secretion. Rapid termination of long-term infusion may cause hypoglycemia from rebound hyperinsulinemia.
- Monitor fluid intake and output and weight closely, especially in patients with renal function impairment.
- Check vital signs frequently, notifying the doctor promptly if adverse reactions occur.
- **I.V. use:** Take care to avoid extravasation, and change infusion sites regularly to avoid irritation with prolonged therapy.

medium-chain triglycerides

M.C.T.◇

Pregnancy Risk Category: C

HOW SUPPLIED

Oil: 960 ml (115 calories/15 ml)◇

ACTION

Mechanism: Source of rapidly hydrolyzable lipid.
Peak: Serum levels peak within 4 hours.

INDICATIONS & DOSAGE

Inadequate digestion or absorption of food fats –
Adults: 15 ml P.O. t.i.d. or q.i.d. Maximum of 100 ml/day.

ADVERSE REACTIONS

CNS: reversible ***coma*** in susceptible patients (such as those with advanced hepatic cirrhosis).
GI: *nausea, vomiting, diarrhea, abdominal distention, cramps.*

INTERACTIONS

None significant.

CONTRAINDICATIONS

- Contraindicated in patients with advanced hepatic disease or abetalipoproteinemia.
- Use cautiously in patients with portacaval shunts.

NURSING CONSIDERATIONS

- To minimize GI adverse reactions, give smaller, more frequent doses with meals, mixed with salad dressing, or in chilled fruit juice.
- More easily absorbed than long-chain fats; not dependent on bile salts for emulsification.
- Rapid metabolism provides quick energy.
- May be useful in lowering cholesterol levels. Also used in patients with short-bowel syndrome.
- Provides 7.7 calories/ml. No essential fatty acids are provided.

92
Antigout agents

allopurinol
colchicine
probenecid
sulfinpyrazone

COMBINATION PRODUCTS
COLBENEMID, PROBEN-C, PROBENECID WITH COLCHICINE: probenecid 500 mg and colchicine 0.5 mg.

allopurinol
Alloremed‡, Capurate‡, Lopurin, Zyloprim

Pregnancy Risk Category: C

HOW SUPPLIED
Tablets (scored): 100 mg, 300 mg
Capsules: 100 mg‡, 300 mg‡

ACTION
Mechanism: Reduces uric acid production by inhibiting the biochemical reactions preceding its formation.
Onset: 24 to 48 hours. **Peak:** Allopurinol levels peak in 2 to 6 hours; oxypurinol (active metabolite) levels, in 3 to 4 hours. **Duration:** 1 to 2 weeks.

INDICATIONS & DOSAGE
Gout, primary or secondary to hyperuricemia; secondary to diseases such as acute or chronic leukemia, polycythemia vera, multiple myeloma, and psoriasis –
Dosage varies with severity of disease; can be given as single dose or divided, but doses larger than 300 mg should be divided.
Adults: mild gout, 200 to 300 mg P.O. daily; severe gout with large tophi, 400 to 600 mg P.O. daily. Same dosage for maintenance in secondary hyperuricemia.
Hyperuricemia secondary to malignancies –
Children under 6 years: 50 mg P.O. t.i.d.
Children 6 to 10 years: 300 mg P.O. daily or divided t.i.d.
Prevention of acute gouty attacks –
Adults: 100 mg P.O. daily; increase at weekly intervals by 100 mg without exceeding maximum dose (800 mg), until serum uric acid falls to 6 mg/100 ml or less.
Prevention of uric acid nephropathy during cancer chemotherapy –
Adults: 600 to 800 mg P.O. daily for 2 to 3 days, with high fluid intake.
Recurrent calcium oxalate calculi –
Adults: 200 to 300 mg P.O. daily in single or divided doses.

In impaired renal function in adults: 200 mg P.O. daily if creatinine clearance is 10 to 20 ml/minute; 100 mg P.O. daily if less than 10 ml/minute; 100 mg P.O. more than 24 hours apart if less than 3 ml/minute.

ADVERSE REACTIONS
CNS: drowsiness, headache.
EENT: cataracts, retinopathy.
GI: nausea, vomiting, diarrhea, abdominal pain.
Hematologic: ***agranulocytosis,*** anemia, ***aplastic anemia.***
Hepatic: altered liver function studies, ***hepatitis.***
Skin: *rash, usually maculopapular;* ***exfoliative,*** urticarial, and purpuric lesions; ***erythema multiforme;*** severe furunculosis of nose; ichthyosis, ***toxic epidermal necrolysis.***

INTERACTIONS
Amoxicillin, ampicillin, bacampicillin: increased possibility of skin rash. Avoid concomitant use.
Anticoagulants: potentiation of anti-

coagulant effect. Dosage adjustments may be necessary.
Antineoplastic agents: increased potential for bone marrow suppression. Monitor the patient carefully.
Chlorpropamide: possible increased hypoglycemic effect. Avoid concomitant use.
Diazoxide, diuretics, ethanol, mecamylamine, pyrazinamide: increased serum acid concentration. Adjust dosage of allopurinol.
Ethacrynic acid, thiazide diuretics: increased risk of allopurinol toxicity. Reduce dosage of allopurinol and closely monitor renal function.
Uricosuric agents: additive effect. May be used to therapeutic advantage.
Urine-acidifying agents (ammonium chloride, ascorbic acid, potassium or sodium phosphate): may increase the possibility of kidney stone formation. Monitor the patient carefully.
Xanthines: increased serum theophylline levels. Adjust dosage of theophyllines.

CONTRAINDICATIONS
- Contraindicated in patients with hypersensitivity to the drug and in those with idiopathic hemochromatosis.
- Use cautiously in patients with cataracts and hepatic or renal disease.

NURSING CONSIDERATIONS
- Discontinue at first sign of rash, which may precede severe hypersensitivity or other adverse reaction. Rash is more common in patients taking diuretics and in those with renal disorders. Tell the patient to report all adverse reactions immediately.
- Allopurinol may predispose the patient to amoxicillin- or ampicillin-induced rash; allopurinol may cause rash even weeks after discontinuation.
- Monitor fluid intake and output; daily urine output of at least 2 liters and maintenance of neutral or slightly alkaline urine are desirable. Encourage the patient to drink plenty of fluids while taking this drug unless otherwise contraindicated.
- If renal insufficiency occurs at any time during treatment, reduce allopurinol dosage.
- Periodically monitor CBC and hepatic and renal function, especially at start of therapy.
- If the patient is taking allopurinol for treatment of recurrent calcium oxalate stones, advise him to also reduce his dietary intake of animal protein, sodium, refined sugars, oxalate-rich foods, and calcium.
- Optimal benefits of therapy may require 2 to 6 weeks of therapy. Because acute gouty attacks may occur during this time, concurrent use of colchicine may be prescribed prophylactically.
- To minimize GI adverse reactions, administer with or immediately after meals.
- Evaluate drug's effectiveness using serum uric acid level.
- Because drug may cause drowsiness, advise the patient to refrain from driving car or performing hazardous tasks requiring mental alertness until CNS effects of the drug are known.

colchicine
Colchicine MR‡, Colgout‡, Colsalide, Novocolchicine†

Pregnancy Risk Category: D

HOW SUPPLIED
Tablets: 0.5 mg (1/120 grain), 0.6 mg (1/100 grain) as sugar-coated granules
Injection: 1 mg (1/60 grain)/2 ml

ACTION
Mechanism: As antigout agent, apparently decreases WBC motility, phagocytosis, and lactic acid production, decreasing urate crystal deposits and reducing inflammation. As antiosteolytic agent, apparently inhibits

mitosis of osteoprogenitor cells and decreases osteoclast activity.
Onset: 15 minutes after I.V. use, 30 minutes after oral use. **Peak:** Levels peak 45 minutes to 1 hour after oral use; however, serum levels don't correlate well with therapeutic action.
Duration: 12 hours.

INDICATIONS & DOSAGE

Prevention of acute gout attacks as prophylactic or maintenance therapy –
Adults: 0.5 or 0.6 mg P.O. daily. Patients who normally have one attack per year or less should receive the drug only 3 or 4 days per week; patients who have more than one attack per year should receive the drug daily. In severe cases, give 1 to 1.8 mg daily.
Prevention of gout attacks in patients undergoing surgery –
Adults: 0.5 to 0.6 mg P.O. t.i.d. 3 days before and 3 days after surgery.
Acute gout, acute gouty arthritis –
Adults: initially, 1 to 1.2 mg P.O., then 0.5 or 0.6 mg q hour, or 1 to 1.2 mg q 2 hours until pain is relieved; nausea, vomiting, or diarrhea ensues; or the maximum dosage of 10 mg is reached. Alternatively, give 2 mg I.V. followed by 0.5 mg I.V. q 6 hours if necessary. (Note that some clinicians prefer to give a single I.V. injection of 3 mg.) Total I.V. dosage over 24 hours (one course of treatment) should not exceed 4 mg.
Familial Mediterranean fever suppression –
Adults: acute attack – 0.6 mg P.O. hourly for four doses, then q 2 hours for four doses on the first day. Then, give 1.2 mg P.O. q 12 hours for 2 days. Maintenance dosage is 0.5 to 0.6 mg P.O. b.i.d. to t.i.d.

ADVERSE REACTIONS

CNS: peripheral neuritis.
GI: *nausea, vomiting, abdominal pain, diarrhea.*
Hematologic: ***aplastic anemia and agranulocytosis with prolonged use;*** nonthrombocytopenic purpura.
Skin: urticaria, dermatitis.
Other: alopecia, severe local irritation if extravasation occurs.

INTERACTIONS

Ethanol: may impair efficacy of colchicine prophylaxis. Don't use together.
Loop diuretics: may decrease efficacy of colchicine prophylaxis. Avoid concomitant use.
Phenylbutazone: may increase risk of leukopenia or thrombocytopenia. Avoid concomitant use.
Vitamin B_{12}: impaired absorption of vitamin B_{12}. Avoid concomitant use.

CONTRAINDICATIONS

- Use cautiously in patients with hepatic dysfunction, cardiac disease, blood dyscrasia, renal disease, or GI disorders, and in elderly or debilitated patients.

NURSING CONSIDERATIONS

- Colchicine is a toxic drug and fatalities have resulted from overdose. After a full course of I.V. colchicine (4 mg), don't give any more colchicine by any route for at least 7 days.
- First sign of acute overdosage may be GI symptoms, followed by vascular damage, muscle weakness, and ascending paralysis. Delirium and seizures may occur without the patient losing consciousness.
- Discontinue colchicine as soon as gout pain is relieved or at the first sign of GI symptoms.
- Colchicine has no effect on nongouty arthritis.
- **I.V. use:** Give by slow I.V. push over 2 to 5 minutes. Be sure to avoid extravasation because colchicine is very irritating to tissues. Don't dilute colchicine injection with dextrose 5% injection or any other fluid that might change pH of colchicine solution. If

lower concentration of colchicine injection is needed, dilute with 0.9% sodium chloride solution or sterile water for injection and administer over 2 to 5 minutes by direct injection. Preferably, inject into the tubing of a free-flowing I.V. solution. However, don't inject if diluted solution becomes turbid.

- Do not administer I.M. or S.C.; severe local irritation occurs.
- Give with meals to reduce GI effects as maintenance therapy. May be used with uricosuric agents.
- Baseline laboratory studies, including CBC, should precede therapy and be repeated periodically.
- Monitor fluid intake and output, and keep output at 2,000 ml daily.
- Store in tightly closed, light-resistant container.

probenecid

Benemid, Benn, Benuryl†, Probalan, Robenecid

Pregnancy Risk Category: B

HOW SUPPLIED

Tablets: 500 mg

ACTION

Mechanism: Blocks renal tubular reabsorption of uric acid, increasing excretion, and inhibits active renal tubular secretion of many weak organic acids, such as penicillins and cephalosporins.

Onset: 1 hour. **Peak:** Serum levels peak in 2 to 4 hours; peak effects occur in 3 hours. **Duration:** 8 to 10 hours.

INDICATIONS & DOSAGE

Adjunct to penicillin or cephalosporin therapy –

Adults and children over 50 kg: 500 mg P.O. q.i.d.

Children 2 to 14 years or under 50 kg: initially, 25 mg/kg P.O., then 40 mg/kg in divided doses q.i.d.

Gonorrhea –

Adults: 3.5 g ampicillin P.O. with 1 g probenecid P.O. given together; or 1 g probenecid P.O. 30 minutes before dose of 4.8 million units of aqueous penicillin G procaine I.M., injected at two different sites.

Hyperuricemia of gout, gouty arthritis –

Adults: 250 mg P.O., b.i.d. for first week, then 500 mg b.i.d., to maximum of 2 g daily. Maintenance dosage is 500 mg daily for 6 months.

ADVERSE REACTIONS

CNS: *headache,* dizziness.
CV: hypotension.
GI: anorexia, nausea, vomiting, sore gums, *gastric distress.*
GU: urinary frequency, renal colic.
Hematologic: ***hemolytic anemia.***
Skin: dermatitis, pruritus.
Other: flushing, fever, alopecia.

INTERACTIONS

Ethanol: increased urate levels. Avoid use.
Indomethacin: decreased indomethacin excretion. Lower indomethacin dosages may be required.
Methotrexate: decreased methotrexate excretion. Lower methotrexate dosage may be required. Serum levels should be determined.
Oral antidiabetic agents: enhanced hypoglycemic effect. Monitor blood glucose levels closely. Dosage adjustment may be required.
Salicylates: inhibited uricosuric effect of probenecid, causing urate retention. Do not use together.

CONTRAINDICATIONS

- Contraindicated in patients with blood dyscrasia; acute gout attack; penicillin therapy in known renal impairment; gouty nephropathy; urinary tract stones or obstruction; and azotemia or hyperuricemia secondary to cancer chemotherapy, radiation, or

myeloproliferative neoplastic diseases.
• Use cautiously in patients with peptic ulceration and renal impairment.

NURSING CONSIDERATIONS
• Typically preferred over sulfinpyrazone because probenecid produces fewer and less severe GI and hematologic adverse reactions.
• Contains no analgesic or anti-inflammatory agent, and is of no value during acute gout attacks. Don't initiate therapy until acute attack subsides.
• Patients with gout should avoid all medications that contain aspirin. which may precipitate gout. Acetaminophen may be used for pain.
• Suitable for long-term use; no cumulative effects or tolerance reported.
• Ineffective in patients with chronic renal insufficiency (glomerular filtration rate less than 30 ml/minute).
• Periodic BUN and renal function tests recommended in long-term therapy.
• May increase frequency, severity, and length of acute gout attacks during first 6 to 12 months of therapy. Prophylactic colchicine or another anti-inflammatory agent is given during first 3 to 6 months.
• Tell patient with gout to avoid alcohol; it increases urate level.
• Force fluids to maintain minimum daily output of 2 to 3 liters. Alkalinize urine with sodium bicarbonate or potassium citrate as ordered. These measures will prevent hematuria, renal colic, urate stone development, and costovertebral pain.
• To minimize GI distress, give with milk, food, or antacids. Continued disturbances might indicate need to lower dosage.
• Tell the patient with gout to limit intake of foods high in purine: anchovies, liver, sardines, kidneys, sweetbreads, peas, and lentils.
• Instruct the patient and his family that drug must be taken regularly as ordered or gout attacks may result. Tell him to visit the doctor regularly so uric acid can be monitored and dosage adjusted, if necessary. Lifelong therapy may be required in patients with hyperuricemia.
• May produce false-positive glucose tests with Benedict's solution or Clinitest, but not with glucose oxidase method (Clinistix, Diastix, Tes-Tape).
• Decreases urinary excretion of 17-ketosteroids, Bromsulphalein (BSP), aminohippuric acid, and iodine-related organic acids, interfering with laboratory procedures.

sulfinpyrazone
Anturan†, Anturane

Pregnancy Risk Category: C

HOW SUPPLIED
Tablets: 100 mg
Capsules: 200 mg

ACTION
Mechanism: Blocks renal tubular reabsorption of uric acid, increasing excretion, and inhibits platelet aggregation.
Peak: Serum levels peak 1 to 2 hours after administration. **Duration:** 4 to 6 hours.

INDICATIONS & DOSAGE
Inhibition of platelet aggregation, increase of platelet survival time in treatment of thromboembolic disorders, angina, MI, transient cerebral ischemic attacks, peripheral arterial atherosclerosis –
Adults: 200 mg P.O. q.i.d.
Maintenance therapy for common gout; reduction or prevention of joint changes and tophi formation –
Adults: 100 to 200 mg P.O. b.i.d. first week, then 200 to 400 mg P.O.

b.i.d. Maximum dosage is 800 mg daily.

ADVERSE REACTIONS

CNS: dizziness, vertigo, tinnitus.
GI: *nausea, dyspepsia,* epigastric pain, blood loss, reactivation of peptic ulcerations.
Hematologic: ***agranulocytosis, blood dyscrasia*** (rare).
Skin: rash.

INTERACTIONS

Oral anticoagulants: increased anticoagulant effect and risk of bleeding. Use together cautiously.
Oral antidiabetic agents: increased effects. Monitor closely.
Probenecid: inhibited renal excretion of sulfinpyrazone. Use together cautiously.
Salicylates: inhibited uricosuric effect of sulfinpyrazone. Do not use together.

CONTRAINDICATIONS

- Contraindicated in patients with hypersensitivity to pyrazole derivatives (including oxyphenbutazone and phenylbutazone); active peptic ulceration; gouty nephropathy; urolithiasis or urinary obstruction; bone marrow suppression; azotemia; hyperuricemia secondary to cancer chemotherapy, radiation, or myeloproliferative neoplastic diseases; or blood dyscrasia; and during or within 2 weeks after gout attack.
- Use cautiously in patients with diminished hepatic or renal function.

NURSING CONSIDERATIONS

- Recommended for patients unresponsive to probenecid. Suitable for long-term use; neither cumulative effects nor tolerance develops.
- Contains no analgesic or anti-inflammatory agent and is of no value during acute gout attacks.
- Warn patients with gout not to take any aspirin-containing medications because these may precipitate gout. Acetaminophen may be used for pain.
- Periodic BUN, CBC, and renal function studies advised during long-term use.
- May increase frequency, severity, and length of acute gout attacks during first 6 to 12 months of therapy. Prophylactic colchicine or another anti-inflammatory agent is given during first 3 to 6 months.
- Therapy, especially at start, may lead to renal colic and formation of uric acid stones. Until acid levels are normal (about 6 mg/dl), monitor fluid intake and output closely.
- Force fluids to maintain minimum daily output of 2 to 3 liters. Alkalinize urine with sodium bicarbonate or other agent as ordered.
- To minimize GI disturbances, give with milk, food, or antacids.
- Patients with gout should avoid foods high in purine: anchovies, liver, sardines, kidneys, sweetbreads, peas, and lentils.
- Instruct the patient and his family that drug must be taken regularly as ordered or gout attacks may result. Tell him to visit the doctor regularly so blood levels can be monitored and dosage adjusted if necessary.
- Lifelong therapy may be required in patients with hyperuricemia.
- Decreases urinary excretion of aminohippuric acid, interfering with laboratory test results.
- Alkalinizing agents are used therapeutically to increase sulfinpyrazone activity, preventing urolithiasis.
- Use in treating thromboembolic conditions is investigational and is most often directed at prevention of recurrent MI.

93
Enzymes

chymopapain
fibrinolysin and desoxyribonuclease
hyaluronidase

COMBINATION PRODUCTS
CHYMORAL-100: 100,000 units enzymatic activity; trypsin and chymotrypsin in ratio of 6:1.
GRANULEX AEROSOL: trypsin 0.1 mg, balsam Peru 72.5 mg, and castor oil 650 mg/0.82 ml.
ORENZYME BITABS ENTERIC-COATED TABLETS: 100,000 units trypsin and 8,000 units chymotrypsin.

chymopapain
Chymodiactin, Discase

Pregnancy Risk Category: C

HOW SUPPLIED
Powder for injection: 4,000 units/vial, 10,000 units/vial; each unit of chymopapain also known as 1 picoKatal (pKat)

ACTION
Mechanism: Hydrolyzes noncollagenous proteins in the chondromucoprotein of the nucleus pulposus.
Peak: 1 week.

INDICATIONS & DOSAGE
Herniated lumbar intervertebral disk –
Adults: 2,000 to 4,000 pKat units/disk injected intradiskally. Maximum dosage in patients with multiple disk herniation is 10,000 units.

ADVERSE REACTIONS
Systemic: ***anaphylaxis, anaphylactoid reaction; paraplegia, cerebral hemorrhage, acute transverse myelitis,*** nausea, headache, dizziness, leg weakness, paresthesia, numbness of legs and toes.
Other: *back pain, stiffness, back spasm.*

INTERACTIONS
None significant.

CONTRAINDICATIONS
• Contraindicated in patients with history of allergy to papaya or meat tenderizers; in patients who have previously received an injection of chymopapain; and in those with severe spondylolisthesis in addition to spinal stenosis, severe progressing paralysis, or evidence of spinal cord tumor or a cauda equina lesion. Most clinicians advocate pretreatment with antihistamine (both H_1 and H_2 blockers).

NURSING CONSIDERATIONS
• Should be used only by doctors qualified and experienced to perform laminectomy, diskectomy, or other spinal procedures, and who have received specialized training in chemonucleolysis. Drug shouldn't be injected in any region other than the lumbar spine. Chymopapain is extremely toxic if injected into the subarachnoid space.
• Monitor patients very closely for anaphylactoid reaction (0.5% of patients). Can be immediate or delayed up to 1 hour after injection and can last for minutes to several hours or longer. Watch for hypotension and bronchospasm, possibly leading to laryngeal edema, arrhythmias, cardiac arrest, coma, and death. Other signs of allergic response include erythema, pilomotor erection, rash, pruritic urticaria, conjunctivitis, vasomotor rhini-

tis, angioedema, or various GI disturbances.
- A ChymoFAST test can detect hypersensitivity to chymopapain.
- Keep an I.V. line open to rapidly manage anaphylaxis. Keep epinephrine and steroids readily available.
- Instruct the patient to anticipate delayed allergic reactions, such as rash, urticaria, or pruritus, which may occur as late as 15 days after injection. The patient should report these to the doctor immediately.
- The patient may experience back pain or involuntary muscle spasm in the lower back for several days after injection. Reassure the patient that this is common and will not be chronic.
- Use within 60 minutes after reconstitution. Discard unused drug.

fibrinolysin and desoxyribonuclease

Elase

Pregnancy Risk Category: C

HOW SUPPLIED

Powder for solution: 25 units fibrinolysin and 15,000 units desoxyribonuclease in 30-ml vial
Ointment: 30 units fibrinolysin and 20,000 units desoxyribonuclease in 30-g tube (with applicator)

ACTION

Mechanism: Fibrinolysin attacks fibrin of blood clots and fibrinous exudates; desoxyribonuclease attacks DNA. Combined enzymatic action debrides wound surfaces and promotes healing.
Onset: on administration. **Duration:** up to 24 hours.

INDICATIONS & DOSAGE

Debridement of inflammatory and infected lesions, including surgical wounds, ulcerative lesions, second- and third-degree burns, circumcision, episiotomy, abscesses, fistulas, and sinus tracts –
Adults and children: apply ointment to lesions daily to t.i.d. for as long as enzyme action is desired. Alternatively, apply solution prepared from powder topically as a liquid, spray, or wet dressing.

For wet-to-dry dressing, mix 1 vial of Elase powder with 10 to 50 ml of 0.9% sodium chloride solution; saturate strips of fine gauze with solution. Pack ulcerated area with Elase gauze. Allow gauze to dry in contact with ulcerated lesion for about 6 to 8 hours. Remove dried gauze and repeat t.i.d. or q.i.d.

Mild-to-moderate cervicitis or vaginitis –
Adults: insert 5 ml ointment using applicator supplied, once daily h.s. for 5 days or until tube is empty.

Irrigation of infected wounds, empyema cavities, abscesses, otorhinolaryngologic wounds, subcutaneous hematomas –
Adults and children: dilute prepared solution and irrigate wound p.r.n., depending on extent and severity of wound.

For solution as irrigating agent, drain cavity and replace Elase every 6 to 10 hours to reduce amount of by-product accumulation and to minimize loss of enzyme activity.

ADVERSE REACTIONS

Systemic: hyperemia with high doses, hypersensitivity reactions.

INTERACTIONS

None significant.

CONTRAINDICATIONS

- Contraindicated for parenteral use.

NURSING CONSIDERATIONS

- Dense, dry eschar must be removed surgically before enzymatic debridement. Enzyme must be in constant contact with substrate. Remove accu-

mulated necrotic debris periodically and replenish the enzyme at least once daily.
- Ensure that wound-dressing techniques are performed carefully under aseptic conditions and that antibiotic therapy is instituted as ordered.
- Clean wound with water, 0.9% sodium chloride solution, or hydrogen peroxide and dry gently; cover with thin layer of Elase. Cover with nonadherent dressing.
- Change dressing at least once and preferably two to three times daily. Flush away necrotic debris and reapply ointment. Frequency of application may be more important than the amount of drug used.
- Prepare solution just before use and discard after 24 hours.

hyaluronidase

Wydase

Pregnancy Risk Category: C

HOW SUPPLIED

Injection: 150 units/vial, 1,500 units/vial; 150 units/ml in 1-ml, 10-ml vials

ACTION

Mechanism: Hydrolyzes hyaluronic acid, promoting diffusion of fluids in tissues.

Onset: on administration.

INDICATIONS & DOSAGE

Adjunct to increase absorption and dispersion of other injected drugs –
Adults and children: 150 units added to solution containing other medication.

Hypodermoclysis –
Adults and children over 3 years: 150 units injected S.C. before clysis or injected into clysis tubing near needle for each 1,000 ml clysis solution.

Excretory urography when contrast medium is given S.C. –
Adults and children: with the patient in a prone position, give 75 units S.C. over each scapula, followed by injection of contrast medium at same sites.

ADVERSE REACTIONS

Skin: rash, urticaria, irritation.

INTERACTIONS

Local anesthetics: increased potential for toxic local reaction. Use together cautiously.

CONTRAINDICATIONS

- Use cautiously in patients with blood-clotting abnormalities, severe hepatic or renal disease.

NURSING CONSIDERATIONS

- Not recommended for I.V. use.
- Do not inject into acutely inflamed or cancerous areas.
- In patients with hypodermoclysis, adjust dosage, rate of injection, and type of solution according to the patient's response.
- Perform a skin test for sensitivity. Avoid injecting into diseased areas (may spread infection), and observe injection site for local reactions.
- Avoid getting solution in eyes; if solution does get in eyes, flush with water at once.
- Protect from heat. Do not use cloudy or discolored solution.
- For children, 15 units are added to each 100 ml of solution. The drip rate should not exceed 2 ml/minute.
- Hyaluronidase is incompatible with epinephrine and heparin. Don't add to any solutions containing these drugs.

94
Oxytocics

carboprost tromethamine
dinoprostone
ergonovine maleate
methylergonovine maleate
oxytocin, synthetic injection
oxytocin, synthetic nasal solution

COMBINATION PRODUCTS
None.

carboprost tromethamine
Hemabate
Pregnancy Risk Category: C

HOW SUPPLIED
Injection: 250 mcg/ml

ACTION
Mechanism: A prostaglandin that produces strong, prompt contractions of uterine smooth muscle, possibly mediated by calcium and cAMP.
Peak: Serum levels peak in 15 to 60 minutes. **Duration:** average time to abortion, 16 hours; elimination complete in 24 hours.

INDICATIONS & DOSAGE
To abort pregnancy between 13th and 20th weeks of gestation –
Adults: initially, administer 250 mcg deep I.M. Administer subsequent doses of 250 mcg at intervals of 1½ to 3½ hours, depending on uterine response. Dosage may be increased in increments to 500 mcg if contractility is inadequate after several 250-mcg doses. Total dosage should not exceed 12 mg.
Postpartum hemorrhage caused by uterine atony not managed by conventional methods –
Adults: 250 mcg by deep I.M. injection. Administer repeat doses at 15- to 90-minute intervals, as necessary. Maximum total dosage is 2 mg.

ADVERSE REACTIONS
GI: *vomiting, diarrhea,* nausea.
Other: *fever,* chills.

INTERACTIONS
None significant.

CONTRAINDICATIONS
- Contraindicated in patients with pelvic inflammatory disease or active cardiac, pulmonary, renal, or hepatic disease.
- Use cautiously in patients with history of asthma; hypertension; cardiovascular, renal, or hepatic disease; anemia; jaundice; diabetes; seizure disorders; or previous uterine surgery.

NURSING CONSIDERATIONS
- Unlike other prostaglandin abortifacients, carboprost is administered by I.M. injection. Injectable form avoids risk of expelling vaginal suppositories, which may occur in the presence of profuse vaginal bleeding.
- Carboprost should be used only by trained personnel in a hospital setting.

dinoprostone
Prostin E_2, Prepidil
Pregnancy Risk Category: C

HOW SUPPLIED
Vaginal suppositories: 20 mg
Endocervical gel: 0.5 mg per application (2.5-ml syringe)

ACTION
Mechanism: A prostaglandin that produces strong, prompt contractions of uterine smooth muscle, possibly mediated by calcium and cAMP.

Onset: 10 minutes for suppositories, 15 to 30 minutes for gel. **Duration:** 2 to 3 hours for suppositories, 6 to 12 hours for gel.

INDICATIONS & DOSAGE

To abort second-trimester pregnancy; to evacuate uterus in missed abortion, intrauterine fetal deaths up to 28 weeks of gestation, or benign hydatidiform mole –
Adults: insert 20-mg suppository high into posterior vaginal fornix. Repeat q 3 to 5 hours until abortion is complete.
Ripening of an unfavorable cervix in pregnant patients at or near term –
Adults: administer contents of one syringe; if cervix remains unfavorable after 6 hours, repeat dosage. Do not give more than 1.5 mg (three applications) per 24 hours.

ADVERSE REACTIONS

CNS: headache, *dizziness.*
CV: hypotension (in large doses).
GI: *nausea, vomiting, diarrhea.*
GU: vaginal pain, vaginitis.
Respiratory: ***bronchospasm.***
Other: *nocturnal leg cramps, fever, shivering, chills, joint inflammation.*

INTERACTIONS

Ethanol: inhibited effectiveness of dinoprostone with high doses. Avoid concomitant use.

CONTRAINDICATIONS

- Contraindicated in patients with pelvic inflammatory disease or history of pelvic surgery, incisions, uterine fibroids, or cervical stenosis.
- Use cautiously in patients with asthma, seizure disorders, anemia, diabetes, hypertension or hypotension, jaundice, and cardiovascular, renal, or hepatic disease.

NURSING CONSIDERATIONS

- Administer only when critical care facilities are readily available.
- When used as an abortifacient, the patient may be pretreated with an antiemetic and an antidiarrheal agent.
- Abortion should be complete within 30 hours.
- Just before use, warm dinoprostone suppositories in their wrapping to room temperature. After administration, patient should remain supine for 10 minutes.
- Freeze suppositories at – 20° C (– 4° F).
- Dinoprostone-induced fever is self-limiting and transient and occurs in approximately 50% of all patients. Treat with water or alcohol sponging and increased fluid intake, not with aspirin.
- Check vaginal discharge daily.
- When used for cervical ripening, have the patient lying on her back, with the cervix visualized using a speculum. Using aseptic technique, use the catheter provided with the drug to administer the gel into the cervical canal just below the level of the internal os.
- Use the contents of the syringe for one patient only. Discard the syringe, catheter, and any unused drug after administration; do not attempt to administer the small amount of drug remaining in the catheter.

ergonovine maleate (ergometrine maleate)

Ergotrate Maleate

HOW SUPPLIED

Injection: 0.2 mg/ml

ACTION

Mechanism: Increases motor activity of the uterus by direct stimulation; prolonged uterine contraction helps control hemorrhage.
Onset: 2 to 5 minutes after I.M. use; immediate after I.V. use. **Duration:** 3 hours after I.M. use; 45 minutes after I.V. use.

INDICATIONS & DOSAGE
Prevention or treatment of postpartum and postabortion hemorrhage from uterine atony or subinvolution –
Adults: 0.2 mg I.M. q 2 to 4 hours, for maximum of five doses; or 0.2 mg I.V. (for severe uterine bleeding or other life-threatening emergencies only) over 1 minute while blood pressure and uterine contractions are monitored. I.V. dose may be diluted to 5 ml with 0.9% sodium chloride solution. Decrease dosage if severe uterine cramping occurs.

ADVERSE REACTIONS
CNS: dizziness, headache.
CV: ***hypertension,*** chest pain.
EENT: tinnitus.
GI: nausea, vomiting.
GU: uterine cramping.
Other: diaphoresis, dyspnea, hypersensitivity reactions.

INTERACTIONS
Dopamine, I.V. oxytocin, regional anesthetics: excessive vasoconstriction. Use together cautiously.

CONTRAINDICATIONS
• Contraindicated for induction or augmentation of labor, before delivery of placenta, in threatened spontaneous abortion, and in patients with allergy or sensitivity to ergot preparations.
• Use cautiously in patients with hypertension, cardiac disease, venoatrial shunts, mitral valve stenosis, obliterative vascular disease, sepsis, and hepatic or renal impairment.

NURSING CONSIDERATIONS
• Administer only when the patient can be meticulously observed. Uterine hyperstimulation during labor may lead to uterine tetany, which may impair placental blood flow and cause amniotic fluid embolism.
• Monitor and record blood pressure, pulse rate, and uterine response. Report sudden changes in vital signs, frequent periods of uterine relaxation, and character and amount of vaginal bleeding.
• Hypocalcemia may decrease the patient's response. If the patient is not also taking digitalis glycosides, cautious administration of calcium gluconate I.V. may produce desired oxytocic action.
• Keep the patient warm.
• Store drug in tightly closed, light-resistant container. Discard if discolored.
• **I.V. use:** Store I.V. solutions below 8° C (46.4° F). Daily stock may be kept at cool room temperature for 60 days.
• I.V. ergonovine is also used to diagnose coronary artery spasm (Prinzmetal's angina).

methylergonovine maleate
Methergine

HOW SUPPLIED
Tablets: 0.2 mg
Injection: 0.2 mg/ml

ACTION
Mechanism: Increases motor activity of the uterus by direct stimulation.
Onset: 2 to 5 minutes after I.M. use, 5 to 15 minutes after oral use, immediate after I.V. use. **Peak:** Serum levels peak 30 minutes after oral use.
Duration: 45 minutes after I.M. use; 3 hours or more after oral use.

INDICATIONS & DOSAGE
Prevention and treatment of postpartum hemorrhage caused by uterine atony or subinvolution –
Adults: 0.2 mg I.M. q 2 to 5 hours for maximum of five doses; or 0.2 mg I.V. (excessive uterine bleeding or other emergencies) over 1 minute while blood pressure and uterine contractions are monitored. I.V. dose may be diluted to 5 ml with 0.9% sodium

chloride solution. After initial I.M. or I.V. dose, may give 0.2 to 0.4 mg P.O. q 6 to 12 hours for 2 to 7 days. Decrease dosage if severe cramping occurs.

ADVERSE REACTIONS
CNS: dizziness, headache, ***seizures, CVA*** with I.V. use.
CV: hypertension, ***MI,*** transient chest pain, palpitations, peripheral vasoconstriction, gangrene.
EENT: tinnitus.
GI: *nausea, vomiting.*
Respiratory: dyspnea.
Other: diaphoresis, hypersensitivity reactions, ***uterine tetany.***

INTERACTIONS
Dopamine, I.V. oxytocin, regional anesthetics, vasoconstrictors: excessive vasoconstriction. Use together cautiously.

CONTRAINDICATIONS
- Contraindicated for induction of labor; before delivery of placenta; in patients with hypertension, toxemia, or sensitivity to ergot preparations; and in threatened spontaneous abortion.
- Use cautiously in patients with sepsis; obliterative vascular disease; and hepatic, renal, or cardiac disease.

NURSING CONSIDERATIONS
- Monitor and record blood pressure, pulse rate, and uterine response; report any sudden change in vital signs, frequent periods of uterine relaxation, and character and amount of vaginal bleeding.
- Contractions may continue 3 hours or more after P.O. or I.M. administration.
- **I.V. use:** Drug should not be routinely administered I.V. because of the risk of severe hypertension and CVA. If it must be given by this route, administer slowly over 1 minute with careful blood pressure monitoring. Contractions begin immediately after I.V. use and continue for up to 45 minutes.
- Store in tightly closed, light-resistant containers. Discard if discolored.
- Store I.V. solutions below 8° C (46.4° F). Daily stock may be kept at room temperature for 60 to 90 days.

oxytocin, synthetic injection
Oxytocin, Pitocin, Syntocinon

Pregnancy Risk Category: B

HOW SUPPLIED
Injection: 10 units/ml ampule or vial

ACTION
Mechanism: Causes potent and selective stimulation of uterine and mammary gland smooth muscle.
Onset: 3 to 5 minutes after I.M. use, immediate after I.V. use. **Duration:** 1 hour after I.V. use, 2 to 3 hours after I.M. use; plasma half-life, 3 to 5 minutes.

INDICATIONS & DOSAGE
Induction or stimulation of labor –
Adults: initially, 1 ml (10 units) ampule in 1,000 ml of dextrose 5% injection or 0.9% sodium chloride solution I.V. infused at 1 to 2 milliunits/minute. Increase rate at 15- to 30-minute intervals until normal contraction pattern is established. Maximum infusion rate is 1 to 2 ml (20 milliunits)/minute. Decrease rate when labor is firmly established.
Reduction of postpartum bleeding after expulsion of placenta –
Adults: 10 to 40 units added to 1,000 ml of D_5W or 0.9% sodium chloride solution infused at rate necessary to control bleeding, usually 10 to 20 milliunits/minute. Also, 1 ml (10 units) can be given I.M. after delivery of the placenta.
Incomplete or inevitable abortion –
Adults: 10 units of oxytocin I.V. in

500 ml of 0.9% sodium chloride solution or dextrose 5% in 0.9% sodium chloride solution. Infuse at rate of 10 to 20 milliunits/minute.

ADVERSE REACTIONS

Maternal –
CNS: ***subarachnoid hemorrhage*** from hypertension; ***seizures or coma*** from water intoxication.
CV: ***hypertension;*** increased heart rate, systemic venous return, and cardiac output; ***arrhythmias.***
GI: nausea, vomiting.
Hematologic: afibrinogenemia; may be related to postpartum bleeding.
Other: hypersensitivity reactions ***(anaphylaxis),*** tetanic uterine contractions, ***abruptio placentae, impaired uterine blood flow,*** pelvic hematoma, ***increased uterine motility.***
Fetal –
CV: bradycardia, tachycardia, ***PVCs.***
Hematologic: hyperbilirubinemia.
Respiratory: ***anoxia, asphyxia.***

INTERACTIONS

Cyclopropane anesthetics: less pronounced bradycardia and hypotension. Use together cautiously.
Thiopental anesthetics: possible delayed induction. Use together cautiously.
Vasoconstrictors: severe hypertension if oxytocin is given within 3 to 4 hours of vasoconstrictor in patients receiving caudal block anesthetic. Avoid concomitant use.

CONTRAINDICATIONS

- Contraindicated when cephalopelvic disproportion is present or when delivery requires conversion, as in transverse lie; in fetal distress, when delivery isn't imminent; and in patients with severe toxemia, partial placenta previa, prematurity, and other obstetric emergencies.
- Use with extreme caution during first and second stages of labor because cervical laceration, uterine rupture, and maternal and fetal death have been reported.
- Use cautiously in patients with history of cervical or uterine surgery (including cesarean section), grand multiparity, uterine sepsis, traumatic delivery, or overdistended uterus and in primiparas over 35 years.

NURSING CONSIDERATIONS

- Used to induce or reinforce labor only when pelvis is known to be adequate, when vaginal delivery is indicated, when fetal maturity is assured, and when fetal position is favorable. Should be used only in hospital where critical care facilities and doctor are immediately available.
- Oxytocin should never be given simultaneously by more than one route.
- Monitor and record uterine contractions, heart rate, blood pressure, intrauterine pressure, fetal heart rate, and character of blood loss every 15 minutes.
- Antidiuretic effect may lead to fluid overload, seizures, and coma. Monitor fluid intake and output.
- If contractions occur less than 2 minutes apart and if contractions above 50 mm Hg are recorded, or if contractions last 90 seconds or longer, stop infusion, turn the patient on her side, and notify the doctor.
- Have magnesium sulfate (20% solution) available for relaxation of the myometrium.
- **I.V. use:** Don't give by I.V. bolus injection. Administer by infusion only; give by piggyback infusion so the drug may be discontinued without interrupting the I.V. line. Use an infusion pump.
- Not recommended for routine I.M. use. However, 10 units may be given I.M. after delivery of placenta to control postpartum uterine bleeding.

oxytocin, synthetic nasal solution

Syntocinon

HOW SUPPLIED

Nasal solution: 40 units/ml

ACTION

Mechanism: Stimulates impaired milk ejection.
Onset: 3 to 5 minutes. **Duration:** 1 to 3 hours.

INDICATIONS & DOSAGE

Promotion of initial milk ejection; possible relief of postpartum breast engorgement –
Adults: 1 spray into one or both nostrils 2 or 3 minutes before breastfeeding or pumping breasts.

ADVERSE REACTIONS

None reported.

INTERACTIONS

None significant.

CONTRAINDICATIONS

- Contraindicated in patients hypersensitive to the drug.

NURSING CONSIDERATIONS

- Instruct the patient to clear nasal passages first. With the patient's head in vertical position, hold squeeze bottle upright and eject solution into nostril.

95

Spasmolytics

flavoxate hydrochloride
oxybutynin chloride

COMBINATION PRODUCTS
None.

flavoxate hydrochloride

Urispas

Pregnancy Risk Category: C

HOW SUPPLIED

Tablets: 100 mg

ACTION

Mechanism: Produces direct spasmolytic effect on smooth muscles of the urinary tract and provides some local anesthesia and analgesia.
Peak: Levels peak within 2 hours.

INDICATIONS & DOSAGE

Symptomatic relief of dysuria, urinary frequency and urgency, nocturia, incontinence, and suprapubic pain associated with urologic disorders –
Adults and children over 12 years: 100 to 200 mg P.O. t.i.d. to q.i.d.

ADVERSE REACTIONS

CNS: *confusion* (especially in elderly patients), nervousness, dizziness, headache, drowsiness, difficulty concentrating.
CV: tachycardia, palpitations.
EENT: *dry throat, blurred vision,* disturbed eye accommodation.
GI: abdominal pain, constipation (with high doses), dry mouth, nausea, vomiting.
Skin: urticaria, dermatoses.
Other: fever.

INTERACTIONS

None significant.

CONTRAINDICATIONS

- Contraindicated in patients with pyloric or duodenal obstruction, obstructive intestinal lesions or ileus, achalasia, GI hemorrhage, or obstructive uropathies of lower urinary tract.
- Use cautiously in patients suspected of having glaucoma.

NURSING CONSIDERATIONS

- Check history for other drug use before giving drugs with anticholinergic adverse reactions. Such reactions may be intensified by flavoxate.
- Warn patients to avoid hazardous activities such as operating machinery or driving until the CNS effects of the drug are known.
- Tell patients to contact the doctor if they experience adverse reactions to the drug or if symptoms do not improve.

oxybutynin chloride

Ditropan

Pregnancy Risk Category: C

HOW SUPPLIED

Tablets: 5 mg
Syrup: 5 mg/5 ml

ACTION

Mechanism: Produces a direct spasmolytic effect and an antimuscarinic (atropine-like) effect on urinary tract smooth muscles, increasing urinary bladder capacity and providing some local anesthesia and mild analgesia.
Onset: 30 to 60 minutes. **Peak:** Levels peak within 3 to 4 hours. **Duration:** 6 to 10 hours.

INDICATIONS & DOSAGE

Antispasmodic for neurogenic bladder–

Adults: 5 mg P.O. b.i.d. to t.i.d., to maximum of 5 mg q.i.d.

Children over 5 years: 5 mg P.O. b.i.d., to maximum of 5 mg t.i.d.

ADVERSE REACTIONS

CNS: *drowsiness,* dizziness, insomnia. restlessness, impaired alertness.

CV: *palpitations, tachycardia.*

EENT: *transient blurred vision,* mydriasis, cycloplegia.

GI: nausea, vomiting, *constipation,* bloated feeling, *dry mouth.*

GU: impotence, *urinary hesitancy or urine retention.*

Skin: rash, urticaria, allergic reactions.

Other: decreased diaphoresis, fever, suppression of lactation, flushing.

INTERACTIONS

None significant.

CONTRAINDICATIONS

- Contraindicated in patients with myasthenia gravis, GI obstruction, glaucoma, adynamic ileus, megacolon, severe or ulcerative colitis, or obstructive uropathy, or in elderly or debilitated patients with intestinal atony.
- Use cautiously in elderly patients and in patients with autonomic neuropathy, reflux esophagitis, and hepatic or renal disease.
- May aggravate symptoms of hyperthyroidism, coronary artery disease, CHF, arrhythmias, tachycardia, hypertension, or prostatic hyperplasia.

NURSING CONSIDERATIONS

- To minimize tendency toward tolerance, stop therapy periodically to determine whether patients can get along without it.
- Before giving oxybutynin, confirm neurogenic bladder by cystometry and rule out partial intestinal obstruction in patients with diarrhea, especially those with colostomy or ileostomy. Periodically evaluate patient's response to therapy by cystometry.
- If urinary tract infection is present, patients should receive antibiotics concomitantly.
- Warn patients to avoid hazardous activities such as operating machinery or driving until CNS effects of the drug are known.
- Caution patients that using drug during very hot weather may precipitate fever or heatstroke because it suppresses diaphoresis.
- Advise patients to store the drug in tightly closed containers at 59° to 86° F (15° to 30° C).

96

Gold salts

auranofin
aurothioglucose
gold sodium thiomalate

COMBINATION PRODUCTS
None.

auranofin

Ridaura
Pregnancy Risk Category: C

HOW SUPPLIED
Capsules: 3 mg

ACTION
Mechanism: Unknown. Anti-inflammatory effects in rheumatoid arthritis are probably caused by inhibition of sulfhydryl systems, which alters cellular metabolism. Auranofin may also alter enzyme function and immune response and suppress phagocytic activity.
Onset: 1 to 3 months, possibly 6 months. **Peak:** Serum levels peak within 2 hours. **Duration:** may last for months after drug is discontinued.

INDICATIONS & DOSAGE
Rheumatoid arthritis –
Adults: 6 mg P.O. daily, either as 3 mg b.i.d. or 6 mg once daily. After 6 months, may be increased to 9 mg daily.

ADVERSE REACTIONS
GI: *diarrhea, abdominal pain, nausea, vomiting,* stomatitis, enterocolitis, anorexia, metallic taste, dyspepsia, flatulence.
GU: proteinuria, hematuria, nephrotic syndrome, glomerulonephritis.
Hematologic: ***thrombocytopenia*** (with or without purpura), ***aplastic anemia, agranulocytosis,*** leukopenia, eosinophilia.
Hepatic: jaundice, elevated liver enzymes.
Respiratory: interstitial pneumonitis.
Skin: *rash, pruritus, dermatitis,* ***exfoliative dermatitis.***

INTERACTIONS
Phenytoin: may increase phenytoin blood levels. Monitor for toxicity.

CONTRAINDICATIONS
- Contraindicated in patients with history of necrotizing enterocolitis, pulmonary fibrosis, exfoliative dermatitis, bone marrow aplasia, or severe hematologic disorders.
- Use cautiously with other drugs that cause blood dyscrasias. Also use cautiously in patients who have preexisting renal, hepatic, or inflammatory bowel disease or skin rash.

NURSING CONSIDERATIONS
- Remind patients to see their doctor for monthly platelet counts. Auranofin should be discontinued if platelet count falls below $100,000/mm^3$, if hemoglobin drops suddenly, if granulocytes are below $1,500/mm^3$, or if leukopenia (WBC count below $4,000/mm^3$) or eosinophilia (eosinophils > 75%) is present.
- Reassure patients that beneficial drug effect may be delayed as long as 3 months. However, if response is inadequate and maximum dose has been reached, expect the doctor to discontinue auranofin.
- Encourage patients to take drug as prescribed and not to alter dosage schedule.
- Diarrhea is the most common adverse reaction. Tell patients to continue taking drug if they experience

mild diarrhea, and to contact the doctor immediately if blood is noted in stool.

• Advise patients to report any rashes or other skin problems immediately. Pruritus in many instances precedes dermatitis; any pruritic skin eruption while patients are receiving auranofin should be considered a reaction to this drug until proven otherwise. Stop therapy until reaction subsides.

• Advise patients that stomatitis is preceded in many instances by a metallic taste, which should be reported to the doctor immediately. Promote careful oral hygiene during therapy.

• Tell patients to continue taking concomitant drug therapy, such as NSAIDs, if prescribed.

• Advise patients to have regular urinalysis. If proteinuria or hematuria is detected, discontinue drug because it can produce a nephrotic syndrome or glomerulonephritis.

• Auranofin, like injectable gold preparations, should be prescribed only for selected rheumatoid arthritis patients. Warn patients not to give the drug to others.

aurothioglucose

Gold-50‡, Solganal

gold sodium thiomalate

Myochrysine

Pregnancy Risk Category: C

HOW SUPPLIED

aurothioglucose

Injection (suspension): 50 mg/ml in sesame oil with aluminum monostearate 2% and propylparaben 0.1% in a 10-ml container

gold sodium thiomalate

Injection: 10 mg/ml, 50 mg/ml with benzyl alcohol

ACTION

Mechanism: Unknown. Anti-inflammatory effects in rheumatoid arthritis are probably caused by inhibition of sulfhydryl systems, which alters cellular metabolism. Gold salts may also alter enzyme function and immune response and suppress phagocytic activity.

Onset: weeks to months. **Peak:** Serum levels peak within 36 hours. **Duration:** may continue for several months after drug is discontinued.

INDICATIONS & DOSAGE

Rheumatoid arthritis –

aurothioglucose

Adults: initially, 10 mg I.M., followed by 25 mg for second and third doses at weekly intervals. Then, 50 mg weekly until 1 g has been given. If improvement occurs without toxicity, continue 25 to 50 mg at 3- to 4-week intervals indefinitely as maintenance therapy.

Children 6 to 12 years: ¼ usual adult dosage. Or 1 mg/kg I.M. once weekly for 20 weeks.

gold sodium thiomalate

Adults: initially, 10 mg I.M., followed by 25 mg in 1 week. Then, 50 mg weekly until 14 to 20 doses have been given. If improvement occurs without toxicity, continue 50 mg q 2 weeks for four doses; then, 50 mg q 3 weeks for four doses; then, 50 mg every month indefinitely as maintenance therapy. If relapse occurs during maintenance therapy, resume injections at weekly intervals.

Children: 1 mg/kg I.M. weekly for 20 weeks. If response is good, may be given q 3 to 4 weeks indefinitely.

ADVERSE REACTIONS

CNS: *dizziness,* syncope.

CV: bradycardia, hypotension.

EENT: corneal gold deposition, corneal ulcers.

GI: *metallic taste, stomatitis,* difficulty swallowing, nausea, vomiting.

GU: albuminuria, proteinuria, ***nephrotic syndrome,*** nephritis, acute tubular necrosis.

Hematologic: ***thrombocytopenia*** (with or without purpura), ***aplastic anemia, agranulocytosis,*** leukopenia, eosinophilia.
Hepatic: hepatitis, jaundice.
Skin: photosensitivity; *rash and dermatitis in 20% of patients* (may lead to fatal ***exfoliative dermatitis*** if drug is not stopped).
Other: ***anaphylaxis, angioedema,*** diaphoresis.

INTERACTIONS

None significant.

CONTRAINDICATIONS

- Contraindicated in patients hypersensitive to the drug and in patients with severe uncontrollable diabetes, renal disease, hepatic dysfunction, hypertension, heart failure, systemic lupus erythematosus, Sjögren's syndrome, and skin rash.
- Use cautiously with other drugs that cause blood dyscrasias.

NURSING CONSIDERATIONS

- Gold compounds are typically used only in active rheumatoid arthritis that has not responded adequately to salicylates, rest, and physical therapy. Some clinicians advocate earlier use before disease progression.
- Administer only under constant supervision of a doctor who is thoroughly familiar with drug's toxicities and benefits.
- Keep dimercaprol on hand to treat acute toxicity.
- Most adverse reactions are readily reversible if drug is stopped immediately.
- Advise patients to report any skin rashes or problems immediately. Pruritus precedes dermatitis in many instances; any pruritic skin eruption while patients are receiving gold therapy should be considered a reaction to therapy until proven otherwise. Stop therapy until reaction subsides.
- Advise patients that stomatitis is preceded in many instances by a metallic taste, which should be reported to the doctor immediately. Promote careful oral hygiene during therapy.
- If adverse reactions are mild, some rheumatologists resume gold therapy after 2 to 3 weeks' rest.
- Administer all gold salts I.M., preferably intragluteally. Drug is pale yellow; don't use if it darkens.
- Aurothioglucose is a suspension. Immerse vial in warm water and shake vigorously before injecting.
- Observe patients for 30 minutes after administration because of possible anaphylactoid reaction.
- When giving gold sodium thiomalate, have patients lie down and remain recumbent for 10 to 20 minutes after injection to minimize hypotension.
- Analyze urine for protein and sediment changes before each injection.
- Monitor CBC, including platelet count, before every second injection during therapy.
- Monitor platelet counts if patients develop purpura or ecchymoses.
- Gold therapy may alter liver function studies.
- Inform patients that benefits of therapy may not appear for 3 to 4 months or longer.
- Advise patients that increased joint pain may occur for 1 to 2 days after injection but usually subsides after a few injections.
- Tell patients to avoid sunlight and artificial ultraviolet light to minimize the risk of photosensitivity.
- Stress need for close medical follow-ups and frequent blood and urine tests during therapy.

97

Diagnostic skin tests

coccidioidin
histoplasmin
mumps skin test antigen
tuberculin purified protein derivative
tuberculosis multiple-puncture tests

COMBINATION PRODUCTS
None.

coccidioidin

Spherulin
Pregnancy Risk Category: C

HOW SUPPLIED
Injection: 1:100 dilution (1 ml), 1:10 dilution (0.5 ml)

ACTION
Mechanism: Causes a T-cell-mediated immune response.
Onset: 4 to 12 hours. **Peak:** Reaction peaks within 24 to 48 hours. **Duration:** 5 days or longer.

INDICATIONS & DOSAGE
Suspected coccidioidomycosis; to assess cell-mediated immunity –
Adults and children: 0.1 ml of 1:100 dilution intradermally into flexor surface of the forearm. Use tuberculin syringe with 26G or 27G ½″ needle. In persons nonreactive to this form, repeat test using 1:10 dilution.

ADVERSE REACTIONS
Systemic: hypersensitivity reactions (vesiculation, ulceration, necrosis), ***anaphylaxis,*** Arthus reaction.

INTERACTIONS
None significant.

CONTRAINDICATIONS
- Contraindicated in patients hypersensitive to thimerosal.

NURSING CONSIDERATIONS
- Give drug intradermally; S.C. injection invalidates test. If erythema without induration appears when the test should be read, injection was probably S.C. Repeat test.
- If coccidioidomycosis is suspected because of clinical manifestations or X-ray findings and the 1:100 dilution is negative, the 1:10 dilution may be used.
- Read test at 24 and 48 hours. Induration of 5 mm or more indicates a positive reaction (cell-mediated immune response). Erythema does not indicate a delayed hypersensitivity reaction or a positive reaction.
- Test HIV-positive and high-risk patients for anergy to verify a negative reaction.
- Reactivity to this test may be depressed or suppressed for as long as 4 to 6 weeks in individuals who have received concurrent or recent immunization with certain vaccines (for example, measles or influenza), in those receiving corticosteroids or immunosuppressants, in severely malnourished patients, in patients with HIV, and in those who have had viral infections (rubeola, influenza, mumps, and probably others).
- Obtain history of allergies and reactions to skin tests.
- If severe reaction occurs, use cold packs or topical corticosteroids to relieve pain or itching.
- Keep epinephrine 1:1,000 available in case of hypersensitivity reaction.
- Tell patients not to wash off circle marked on skin for serial skin tests because it aids in reading test results.

• It is not necessary to cover the area with a bandage.
• Obtain history of any recent residence in or travel to endemic areas – southern California, Arizona, New Mexico, and western Texas.

histoplasmin

Histolyn-CYL

Pregnancy Risk Category: C

HOW SUPPLIED

Injection: vials containing 10 doses of 0.1 ml

ACTION

Mechanism: Causes a T-cell-mediated immune response.
Onset: 8 to 12 hours. **Peak:** Response peaks within 24 to 48 hours. **Duration:** 5 days or longer.

INDICATIONS & DOSAGE

To differentiate histoplasmosis from coccidioidomycosis, tuberculosis, sarcoidosis, or other mycotic or bacterial infections; to assess T-cell-mediated immunity –
Adults and children: 0.1 ml intradermally into flexor surface of the forearm. Use tuberculin syringe with 26G or 27G ½" needle.

ADVERSE REACTIONS

Skin: urticaria, ulceration, or necrosis in highly sensitive patients.
Systemic: ***anaphylaxis.***

INTERACTIONS

None significant.

CONTRAINDICATIONS

• Contraindicated in patients known to be positive reactors.

NURSING CONSIDERATIONS

• Give drug intradermally; S.C. injection invalidates test. If erythema without induration appears when test should be read, injection was probably S.C. Repeat test.
• Read test within 24 to 48 hours. Induration of 5 mm or more indicates a positive reaction; erythema does not indicate a positive reaction. In some instances, maximum reactions may not be present until fourth day.
• Positive reaction may indicate past infection or mild subacute or chronic histoplasmosis or related fungal infection, such as coccidioidomycosis or blastomycosis.
• Test HIV-positive and high-risk patients for anergy to verify a negative reaction.
• Reactivity to this test may be depressed or suppressed for as long as 4 to 6 weeks in individuals who have received concurrent or recent immunization with certain virus vaccines (for example, measles or influenza), in those who are receiving corticosteroids or immunosuppressants, in severely malnourished patients, in patients with HIV, and in those who have had viral infections (rubeola, influenza, mumps, and probably others).
• Serologic titers are boosted in many instances by a previous skin test. Draw serologic sample before skin test or at least 96 hours after test administration.
• Give tuberculin skin test concurrently with histoplasmin test.
• Obtain history of allergies and reactions to skin tests.
• If severe reaction occurs, use cold packs or topical corticosteroids to relieve pain and itching.
• Obtain history of any recent residence in or travel to endemic areas – central (Ohio Valley) and eastern United States and Africa.

mumps skin test antigen

MSTA

Pregnancy Risk Category: C

HOW SUPPLIED
Injection (suspension): 20 complement-fixing units/ml

ACTION
Mechanism: Causes a T-cell-mediated immune response.
Onset: 6 to 12 hours. **Peak:** Effect peaks within 48 to 72 hours. **Duration:** 5 days or longer.

INDICATIONS & DOSAGE
To assess T-cell-mediated immunity – **Adults and children:** 0.1 ml intradermally into flexor surface of the forearm. Use tuberculin syringe with 26G or 27G ½″ needle.

ADVERSE REACTIONS
Systemic: hypersensitivity reactions (vesiculation, ulceration), ***anaphylaxis,*** Arthus reaction.

INTERACTIONS
None significant.

CONTRAINDICATIONS
- Contraindicated in patients allergic to thimerosal.
- Use cautiously in patients hypersensitive to eggs, feathers, or chicken.

NURSING CONSIDERATIONS
- Mumps skin test antigen is used to assess T-cell function for immunocompetence, not exposure to mumps.
- Read test at 48- and 72-hour intervals. Induration of 5 mm or more indicates a positive reaction (cell-mediated immune response). Erythema does not indicate a delayed hypersensitivity reaction.
- Reactivity to this test may be depressed or suppressed for as long as 4 to 6 weeks in individuals who have received concurrent or recent immunization with certain vaccines (for example, measles or influenza), in those receiving corticosteroids or immunosuppressants, in severely malnourished patients, in patients with HIV, and in those who have had viral infections (rubeola, influenza, mumps, and probably others).
- Keep epinephrine 1:1,000 available in case of hypersensitivity reaction.
- Obtain history of allergies and reactions to skin tests.
- If severe reaction occurs, use cold packs or topical corticosteroids to relieve pain or itching.
- Store vials in refrigerator.

tuberculin purified protein derivative (PPD)

Aplisol, PPD-stabilized Solution (Mantoux test), Tubersol

Pregnancy Risk Category: C

HOW SUPPLIED
Injection: 1 tuberculin unit (TU)/0.1 ml, 5 TU/0.1 ml, 250 TU/0.1 ml

ACTION
Mechanism: Causes a cell-mediated immune response.
Onset: 4 hours. **Peak:** Response peaks within 48 to 72 hours. **Duration:** 5 to 7 days.

INDICATIONS & DOSAGE
Diagnosis of tuberculosis (past, latent, or current infection) – **Adults and children:** initially, 1 TU (0.1 ml of appropriate solution) intradermally into flexor surface of the forearm. Use tuberculin syringe with 26G or 27G ½″ needle. Retest with 5 TU and, if negative, 250 TU. If still no response, the individual is nonreactive.

ADVERSE REACTIONS
Skin: pruritus, vesiculation.
Systemic: hypersensitivity reactions, ***anaphylaxis,*** Arthus reaction.
Other: pain, ulceration, necrosis.

INTERACTIONS
None significant.

CONTRAINDICATIONS
• Contraindicated in known tuberculin-positive reactors; severe reactions may occur.

NURSING CONSIDERATIONS
• Give drug intradermally; S.C. injection invalidates test results. Bleb (6 to 10 mm in diameter) must form on skin upon intradermal injection.
• Read test within 48 to 72 hours. Induration of 15 mm or more indicates a significant reaction (formerly called positive reaction). Significance of reaction is determined by its size and by circumstances. For example, a reaction of 5 mm or more may be considered significant in patients who have had close contact with persons with known tuberculosis, in patients with HIV or at risk for HIV, or patients with chest X-rays indicating old tuberculosis scars. A reaction of 10 mm or more may be considered significant in patients born in Asia, Africa, or Latin America; HIV-negative I.V. drug users; medically underserved low-income populations; residents of long-term care facilities; or high-risk patients, such as those with diabetes or renal failure, or those receiving immunosuppressants. Induration of 5 mm or less in persons not belonging to these groups implies that infection is unlikely. Amount of induration – not erythema – at the site determines the significance of the reaction.
• Patients immunized with BCG vaccine should react positively.
• If reaction is positive, test further to confirm diagnosis. Report all known cases of tuberculosis to the appropriate public health agency.
• Test HIV-positive and high-risk patients for anergy to verify a negative reaction.
• Reactivity to this test may be depressed or suppressed for as long as 4 to 6 weeks in individuals who have received concurrent or recent immunization with certain vaccines (for example, measles or influenza), in those receiving corticosteroids or immunosuppressants, in severely malnourished patients, in patients with HIV, and in those who have had viral infections (rubeola, influenza, mumps, and probably others).
• Obtain history of allergies and reactions to skin tests.
• If severe reaction occurs, use cold packs or topical corticosteroids to relieve pain and itching.
• Keep epinephrine 1:1,000 available in case of hypersensitivity reaction.
• Strongly positive tests can result in scarring at test site.
• Never give initial test with second test strength (250 TU). Use only when patients have a negative response to a 5-TU PPD but have the clinical signs and symptoms of tuberculosis.
• When retesting, know that the first test will not exert a booster phenomenon. Test may be repeated immediately at a different site at least 5 cm from first site.

tuberculosis multiple-puncture tests

Aplitest (dried purified protein derivative [PPD]), Mono-Vacc Test (liquid Old Tuberculin [OT]), Sclavo Test (dried PPD), Tine Test (dried OT, dried PPD)

Pregnancy Risk Category: C

HOW SUPPLIED
Test: 5 tuberculin units (TU)/device

ACTION
Mechanism: Causes a cell-mediated immune response.
Onset: 4 to 8 hours. **Peak:** Effect peaks within 48 to 72 hours. **Duration:** 5 days.

INDICATIONS & DOSAGE
Screening for tuberculosis –
Adults and children: clean skin thoroughly with alcohol; make skin taut on

flexor surface of forearm and press points firmly into selected site. Hold device at injection site for about 3 seconds to ensure depositing of the dried tuberculin B in tissue lymph.

ADVERSE REACTIONS
Systemic: hypersensitivity reactions (vesiculation, ulceration, necrosis), ***anaphylaxis***.

INTERACTIONS
Aminocaproic acid, corticosteroids: false-negative or insignificant reactions to tuberculosis multiple-puncture tests. Don't administer concomitantly.

CONTRAINDICATIONS
- Contraindicated in known tuberculin-positive reactors.

NURSING CONSIDERATIONS
- Read test within 48 to 72 hours. Verify questionable or positive reactions by the Mantoux test. Induration of 1 to 2 mm indicates a significant reaction. Induration – not erythema – at the site determines the significance of the reaction.
- False-positive reaction can occur in sensitive patients. False-negative reaction can occur from anergy or poor technique.
- Reactivity to this test may be depressed or suppressed for as long as 4 to 6 weeks in individuals who have received concurrent or recent immunization with certain vaccines (for example, measles or influenza), in those receiving corticosteroids or immunosuppressants, in severely malnourished patients, in patients with HIV, and in those who have had viral infections (rubeola, influenza, mumps, and probably others) or miliary tuberculosis.
- If vesiculation is present, test should be interpreted as positive.
- Rarely, minimal bleeding can occur at the puncture site. It does not interfere with interpretation of the test results.
- Report all cases of tuberculosis to the appropriate public health agency.
- Obtain history of allergies, especially to acacia (a stabilizer in the Tine Test), and reactions to skin tests.
- Keep epinephrine 1:1,000 available in case of hypersensitivity reaction.
- If severe reaction occurs, use cold packs or topical corticosteroids to relieve pain and itching.

98

Miscellaneous antagonists and antidotes

activated charcoal
aminocaproic acid
ammonia, aromatic spirits
deferoxamine mesylate
digoxin immune FAB (ovine)
dimercaprol
doxapram hydrochloride
D-penicillamine
edetate calcium disodium
edetate disodium
flumazenil
ipecac syrup
naloxone hydrochloride
naltrexone hydrochloride
pralidoxime chloride
protamine sulfate
sodium cellulose phosphate
sodium polystyrene sulfonate
succimer
trientine hydrochloride

(See also Chapter 37, ANTICHOLINERGICS.)
(See also Chapter 39, ADRENERGIC BLOCKERS [SYMPATHOLYTICS].)

COMBINATION PRODUCTS
None.

activated charcoal

Actidose-Aqua◇, Charcoaide◇, Charcocaps◇, Liqui-Char◇, Superchar◇

Pregnancy Risk Category: C

HOW SUPPLIED
Tablets: 200 mg‡◇, 300 mg‡◇, 325 mg◇, 650 mg◇
Capsules: 260 mg◇
Powder: 30 g◇, 50 g◇
Oral suspension: 0.625 g/5 ml◇, 0.83 g/5 ml◇, 1 g/5 ml◇, 1.25 g/5 ml◇

ACTION
Mechanism: An adsorbent that adheres to many drugs and chemicals, inhibiting their absorption from the GI tract.
Onset: immediate.

INDICATIONS & DOSAGE
Flatulence or dyspepsia –
Adults: 600 mg to 5 g P.O. t.i.d. or q.i.d.
Poisoning –
Adults: initially, 1 g/kg (30 to 100 g) P.O. or 5 to 10 times the amount of poison ingested as a suspension in 180 to 240 ml of water.
Children: 5 to 10 times estimated weight of drug or chemical ingested. Minimum dose is 30 g P.O. in 250 ml water to make a slurry. Give preferably within 30 minutes of poisoning. Larger dose is necessary if food is in the stomach.

For treating poisoning or overdosage with acetaminophen, amphetamines, antimony, arsenic, aspirin, atropine, barbiturates, camphor, cocaine, digitalis glycosides, glutethimide, ipecac, malathion, morphine, poisonous mushrooms, opium, oxalic acid, parathion, phenol, phenothiazines, potassium permanganate, propoxyphene, quinine, strychnine, sulfonamides, or tricyclic antidepressants.

ADVERSE REACTIONS
GI: black stools, nausea, constipation.

INTERACTIONS
Acetylcysteine, ipecac: render charcoal ineffective. Don't administer together, or lavage stomach until all charcoal is removed.

CONTRAINDICATIONS
- Contraindicated in semiconscious or unconscious patients unless airway

is protected, and then use cautiously. Can be given by nasogastric tube after lavage.

NURSING CONSIDERATIONS

- Because activated charcoal absorbs and inactivates syrup of ipecac, give after emesis is complete.
- Powder form is most effective. Mix with tap water to form consistency of thick syrup. Adding a small amount of fruit juice or flavoring will make mix more palatable.
- Preparations made with sorbitol have a laxative effect that lessens the risk of severe constipation or fecal impaction.
- Don't give in ice cream, milk, or sherbet, which reduce absorptive capacity.
- If patients vomit shortly after administration, dose may need to be repeated.
- Space doses at least 1 hour apart from other drugs if treatment is for any indication other than poisoning.
- Follow treatment with stool softener or laxative to prevent constipation.
- Warn patients that feces will be black.

aminocaproic acid

Amicar

Pregnancy Risk Category: C

HOW SUPPLIED

Tablets: 500 mg
Syrup: 250 mg/ml
Injection: 5 g/20 ml for dilution, 24 g/96 ml for infusion

ACTION

Mechanism: Inhibits plasminogen activator substances and, to a lesser degree, blocks antiplasmin activity by inhibiting fibrinolysis.
Onset: 1 hour to 3 days. **Peak:** Levels peak within 2 hours of oral dose.

INDICATIONS & DOSAGE

Excessive bleeding resulting from hyperfibrinolysis –
Adults: initially, 5 g P.O. or slow I.V. infusion, followed by 1 to 1.25 g hourly until bleeding is controlled. Maximum dosage is 30 g daily.
Prevention of hemorrhage after dental surgery in hemophiliacs –
Adults: initially, 6 g P.O. immediately after surgery, then 6 g P.O. q 6 hours for 9 to 10 days.

ADVERSE REACTIONS

CNS: dizziness, malaise, headache.
CV: hypotension, bradycardia, ***arrhythmias*** (with rapid I.V. infusion).
EENT: tinnitus, nasal stuffiness, conjunctival suffusion.
GI: nausea, cramps, diarrhea.
Hematologic: generalized thrombosis.
Skin: rash.
Other: malaise, myopathy.

INTERACTIONS

Estrogens, oral contraceptives: increased probability of hypercoagulability. Use together cautiously.

CONTRAINDICATIONS

- Contraindicated in patients with active intravascular clotting.
- Use cautiously in patients with thrombophlebitis or with cardiac, hepatic, or renal disease.

NURSING CONSIDERATIONS

- Monitor coagulation studies, heart rhythm, and blood pressure. Notify the doctor of any change immediately.
- **I.V. use:** Dilute solution with sterile water for injection, 0.9% sodium chloride injection, D_5W, or Ringer's injection. Infuse slowly. Don't give by direct or intermittent injection.
- Drug is sometimes helpful as an adjunct in treating hemophilia. Also used as an antidote for alteplase, anistreplase, streptokinase, or urokinase;

is not beneficial in treating thrombocytopenia.

ammonia, aromatic spirits◊

Pregnancy Risk Category: C

HOW SUPPLIED

Solution: 30 ml◊, 60 ml◊, 120 ml◊; pints◊; gallons◊
Inhalant: 0.33 ml◊, 0.4 ml◊

ACTION

Mechanism: Irritates the sensory receptors in the nasal membranes, producing reflex stimulation of the respiratory centers.
Onset: immediate.

INDICATIONS & DOSAGE

Fainting –
Adults and children: inhale as needed.

ADVERSE REACTIONS

EENT: irritation.

INTERACTIONS

None significant.

CONTRAINDICATIONS

None reported.

NURSING CONSIDERATIONS

• Avoid inhaling vapors when administering drug.

deferoxamine mesylate

Desferal
Pregnancy Risk Category: C

HOW SUPPLIED

Powder for injection: 500 mg

ACTION

Mechanism: Chelates iron by binding ferric ions.
Onset: immediate.

INDICATIONS & DOSAGE

Adjunctive treatment of acute iron intoxication –
Adults and children: 1 g I.M. or I.V. followed by 500 mg I.M. or I.V. for two doses, q 4 hours; then 500 mg I.M. or I.V. q 4 to 12 hours. I.V. infusion rate shouldn't exceed 15 mg/kg hourly. Maximum dosage is 6 g in 24 hours.
Chronic iron overload from multiple transfusions –
Adults and children: 500 mg to 1 g I.M. daily and 2 g slow I.V. infusion in separate solution along with each unit of blood transfused. I.V. infusion rate shouldn't exceed 15 mg/kg hourly. Maximum dosage is 6 g daily. Alternatively, 20 to 40 mg/kg via S.C. infusion pump over 8 to 24 hours.

ADVERSE REACTIONS

CV: tachycardia with long-term use.
EENT: blurred vision, cataracts, hearing loss.
GI: diarrhea and abdominal discomfort with long-term use.
GU: dysuria with long-term use.
Other: hypersensitivity reactions (cutaneous wheal formation, pruritus, rash, ***anaphylaxis***); pain and induration at injection site; leg cramps, fever; after rapid I.V. administration – *erythema, urticaria, hypotension,* ***shock.***

INTERACTIONS

Ascorbic acid: may enhance the effects of deferoxamine and increase tissue toxicity of iron. Use together with extreme caution and close monitoring.

CONTRAINDICATIONS

• Contraindicated in patients with severe renal disease or anuria.
• Use cautiously in patients with impaired renal function.

NURSING CONSIDERATIONS
- Monitor fluid intake and output carefully.
- I.M. route is preferred.
- **I.V. use:** Use I.V. only when patients have cardiovascular collapse or shock. Change to I.M. as soon as possible.
- To reconstitute, add 2 ml of sterile water for injection to each ampule. Make sure drug is completely dissolved. Reconstituted solution is good for 1 week at room temperature. Protect from light.
- After reconstitution, add to 0.9% sodium chloride solution, D_5W, or lactated Ringer's solution and infuse at a rate not exceeding 15 mg/kg hourly.
- Warn patients that urine may be red.
- Have epinephrine 1:1,000 readily available to treat hypersensitivity reaction.
- Recommend regular eye examinations during long-term therapy.
- Used investigationally to treat aluminum toxicity.

digoxin immune FAB (ovine)
Digibind

Pregnancy Risk Category: C

HOW SUPPLIED
Injection: 40-mg vial

ACTION
Mechanism: Binds molecules of digoxin and digitoxin, making them unavailable for binding at site of action on cells.
Onset: 30 minutes. **Duration:** 2 to 6 hours.

INDICATIONS & DOSAGE
Potentially life-threatening digoxin or digitoxin intoxication –
Adults and children: I.V. dosage varies according to the amount of digoxin or digitoxin to be neutralized. Each vial binds about 0.6 mg digoxin or digitoxin. Average dosage is 10 vials (400 mg). However, if the toxicity resulted from acute digoxin ingestion, and neither a serum digoxin level nor an estimated ingestion amount is known, 20 vials (800 mg) should be administered. See package insert for complete, specific dosage instructions.

ADVERSE REACTIONS
CV: ***CHF*** and rapid ventricular rate (both caused by reversal of the digitalis glycoside's therapeutic effects).
Other: hypersensitivity reactions, hypokalemia.

INTERACTIONS
None reported.

CONTRAINDICATIONS
- Use cautiously in patients known to be allergic to ovine proteins. In these high-risk patients, skin testing is recommended because digoxin immune FAB is derived from digoxin-specific antibody fragments obtained from immunized sheep.

NURSING CONSIDERATIONS
- Use only for life-threatening overdose in patients in shock or cardiac arrest; with ventricular arrhythmias, such as ventricular tachycardia or fibrillation; with progressive bradycardia, such as severe sinus bradycardia; or with second- or third-degree AV block not responsive to atropine.
- It's best to infuse the drug through a 0.22-micron membrane filter. However, give by bolus injection if cardiac arrest seems imminent.
- Monitor potassium level closely.
- In most patients, signs of digitalis toxicity disappear within a few hours.
- Because drug will interfere with digitalis immunoassay measurements, standard serum digoxin levels will be

misleading until drug is cleared from body (about 2 days).

- **I.V. use:** Reconstitute 40-mg vial with 4 ml of sterile water for injection. Gently roll vial to dissolve the powder. Reconstituted solution contains 10 mg/ml. Drug may be given by direct injection if cardiac arrest seems imminent. Alternatively, dilute with 0.9% sodium chloride injection to an appropriate volume and give by intermittent infusion.
- Refrigerate powder for injection. Reconstitute drug immediately before use. Reconstituted solutions may be refrigerated for 4 hours.

dimercaprol

BAL in Oil

Pregnancy Risk Category: D

HOW SUPPLIED
Injection: 100 mg/ml

ACTION
Mechanism: Forms complexes with heavy metals.
Peak: Level peaks within 30 to 60 minutes. **Duration:** 4 hours.

INDICATIONS & DOSAGE
Severe arsenic or gold poisoning –
Adults and children: 3 mg/kg deep I.M. q 4 hours for 2 days, then q.i.d. on third day, then b.i.d. for 10 days.
Mild arsenic or gold poisoning –
Adults and children: 2.5 mg/kg deep I.M. q.i.d. for 2 days, then b.i.d. on third day, then once daily for 10 days.
Mercury poisoning –
Adults and children: initially, 5 mg/kg deep I.M., then 2.5 mg/kg daily or b.i.d. for 10 days.
Acute lead encephalopathy or lead level greater than 100 mcg/ml –
Adults and children: 4 mg/kg deep I.M., then q 4 hours with edetate calcium disodium (12.5 mg/kg I.M.). Use separate sites. Maximum dosage is 5 mg/kg per dose.

ADVERSE REACTIONS
CNS: pain or tightness in throat, chest, or hands; headache; paresthesia; muscle pain or weakness.
CV: *transient increase in blood pressure* (returns to normal in 2 hours), *tachycardia.*
EENT: blepharospasm, conjunctivitis, lacrimation, rhinorrhea, excessive salivation.
GI: *halitosis; nausea; vomiting; burning sensation in lips, mouth, and throat; abdominal pain.*
GU: *dysuria;* renal damage if alkaline urine not maintained.
Other: *fever (especially in children),* diaphoresis, pain in teeth, sterile abscess, pain at injection site, decreased iodine uptake.

INTERACTIONS
Iron: toxic metal complex formed; concurrent therapy contraindicated. Wait 24 hours after last dimercaprol dose.
^{131}I uptake thyroid tests: decreased. Don't schedule patient for this test during course of dimercaprol therapy.

CONTRAINDICATIONS
- Contraindicated in pregnancy except to treat life-threatening poisoning and in patients with hepatic dysfunction (except postarsenical jaundice) or acute renal insufficiency.
- Also contraindicated for iron, cadmium, or selenium toxicity. The complex formed is highly toxic, even fatal.
- Use cautiously in patients with hypertension.

NURSING CONSIDERATIONS
- Drug is ineffective in arsine gas poisoning.
- Use ephedrine or antihistamine to prevent or relieve mild adverse reactions.
- Don't give I.V.; give by deep I.M. route only.
- Keep urine alkaline to prevent renal

damage. Oral sodium bicarbonate may be ordered.

- Drug has an unpleasant, garlic-like odor.
- Be careful not to let drug come in contact with skin, because it may cause a skin reaction.
- Solution with slight sediment is usable.

doxapram hydrochloride

Dopram

Pregnancy Risk Category: C

HOW SUPPLIED

Injection: 20 mg/ml (benzyl alcohol 0.9%)

ACTION

Mechanism: Acts either directly on the central respiratory centers in the medulla or indirectly on the chemoreceptors.
Onset: immediate. **Duration:** 6 to 8 hours.

INDICATIONS & DOSAGE

Postanesthesia respiratory stimulation, drug-induced CNS depression, chronic pulmonary disease associated with acute hypercapnia –
Adults: 0.5 to 1 mg/kg of body weight (up to 2 mg/kg in CNS depression) by I.V. injection or infusion. Maximum dosage is 4 mg/kg, up to 3 g/day. Infusion rate is 1 to 3 mg/minute. In postanesthesia use, initial dosage is 5 mg/minute.
COPD –
Adults: 1 to 2 mg/minute by I.V. infusion. Maximum dosage is 3 mg/minute for a maximum duration of 2 hours.

ADVERSE REACTIONS

CNS: ***seizures,*** *headache,* dizziness, apprehension, disorientation, pupillary dilation, bilateral Babinski's signs, paresthesia.
CV: *chest pain and tightness, variations in heart rate, hypertension,* lowered T waves.
EENT: sneezing, ***laryngospasm.***
GI: nausea, vomiting, diarrhea.
GU: urine retention, bladder stimulation with incontinence.
Respiratory: cough, ***bronchospasm.***
Skin: pruritus.
Other: hiccups, rebound hypoventilation, fever, muscle spasms, diaphoresis, flushing.

INTERACTIONS

MAO inhibitors, sympathomimetics: potentiate adverse cardiovascular effects. Use together cautiously.

CONTRAINDICATIONS

- Contraindicated in patients with seizure disorders; head injury; cardiovascular disorders; frank uncompensated heart failure; severe hypertension; CVA; respiratory failure or incompetence secondary to neuromuscular disorders, muscle paresis, flail chest, obstructed airway, pulmonary embolism, pneumothorax, restrictive respiratory disease, acute bronchial asthma, or extreme dyspnea; or hypoxia not associated with hypercapnia.
- Use cautiously in patients with bronchial asthma, severe tachycardia or arrhythmias, cerebral edema or increased CSF pressure, hyperthyroidism, pheochromocytoma, or metabolic disorders.

NURSING CONSIDERATIONS

- Most doctors strongly discourage use as an analeptic.
- Use only in surgical or emergency room situations.
- **I.V. use:** Administer slowly; rapid infusion may cause hemolysis. Doxapram is physically incompatible with strongly alkaline drugs such as thiopental sodium, aminophylline, or sodium bicarbonate.
- Establish adequate airway before administering drug. Prevent patients

from aspirating vomitus by placing them on their side.
• Monitor blood pressure, heart rate, deep tendon reflexes, and arterial blood gases before giving drug and every 30 minutes afterward.
• Be alert for signs of overdosage: hypertension, tachycardia, arrhythmias, skeletal muscle hyperactivity, and dyspnea. Discontinue drug if patients show signs of increased arterial carbon dioxide or oxygen tension, or if mechanical ventilation is started. May give I.V. injection of anticonvulsant.
• Avoid extravasation, which may lead to thrombophlebitis and local skin irritation.

D-penicillamine

Cuprimine, Depen, D-Penamine‡
Pregnancy Risk Category: D

HOW SUPPLIED
Tablets: 125 mg‡, 250 mg
Capsules: 125 mg, 250 mg

ACTION
Mechanism: Chelates heavy metals and may inhibit collagen formation.
Onset: immediate.

INDICATIONS & DOSAGE
Wilson's disease –
Adults: 250 mg P.O. q.i.d. 30 to 60 minutes before meals. Adjust dosage to achieve urinary copper excretion of 0.5 to 1 mg daily.
Children: 20 mg/kg P.O. daily divided q.i.d. before meals. Adjust dosage to achieve urinary copper excretion of 0.5 to 1 mg daily.
Cystinuria –
Adults: 250 mg to 1 g P.O. q.i.d. before meals. Adjust dosage to achieve urinary cystine excretion of less than 100 mg daily when renal calculi are present, or 100 to 200 mg daily when no calculi are present. Maximum dosage is 5 g daily.
Children: 30 mg/kg P.O. daily divided q.i.d. before meals. Adjust dosage to achieve urinary cystine excretion of less than 100 mg daily when renal calculi are present, or 100 to 200 mg daily when no calculi are present.
Rheumatoid arthritis –
Adults: initially, 125 to 250 mg P.O. daily, with increases of 250 mg q 2 to 3 months if necessary. Maximum dosage is 1.5 g daily.

ADVERSE REACTIONS
EENT: tinnitus.
GU: ***nephrotic syndrome, glomerulonephritis,*** proteinuria.
Hepatic: hepatotoxicity.
Hematologic: *leukopenia, eosinophilia, thrombocytopenia, monocytosis, granulocytopenia,* elevated sedimentation rate, lupus-like syndrome.
Skin: friability, especially at pressure spots; wrinkling; erythema; urticaria; ecchymoses.
Other: reversible taste impairment, especially of salts and sweets; hair loss; myasthenia gravis syndrome with long-term use; *decreased pyridoxine (may cause optic neuritis),* decreased zinc and mercury. About one-third of patients develop allergic reactions *(rash, pruritus, fever), arthralgia, lymphadenopathy, or pneumonitis.*

INTERACTIONS
Antacids, oral iron: decreased effectiveness of D-penicillamine. Give at least 2 hours apart.

CONTRAINDICATIONS
• Contraindicated in pregnant patients with cystinuria.
• Use cautiously in patients with penicillin allergy; cross-sensitivity may occur. However, most patients hypersensitive to penicillin can receive penicillamine.

*Liquid form contains alcohol.
**May contain tartrazine.

NURSING CONSIDERATIONS

• Give dose on empty stomach to facilitate absorption, preferably 1 hour before or 3 hours after meals.
• If patients have a skin reaction, give antihistamines as prescribed. Handle patients carefully to avoid skin damage.
• Monitor CBC and renal and hepatic function every 2 weeks for the first 6 months, then monthly.
• Monitor urinalysis regularly for protein loss.
• Rash and fever are important signs of toxicity; report them to the doctor immediately.
• Withhold drug and notify the doctor if WBC count falls below 3,500/mm^3 or platelet count falls below 100,000/mm^3. A progressive decline in platelet or WBC count in three successive blood tests may necessitate temporary cessation of therapy, even if such counts are within normal limits.
• Patients should receive supplemental pyridoxine daily.
• Advise patients to report early signs of granulocytopenia: fever, sore throat, chills, bruising, and prolonged bleeding time.
• Tell patients to maintain adequate fluid intake, especially at night.
• Tell patients that therapeutic effect may be delayed up to 3 months in treatment of rheumatoid arthritis.
• Reassure patients that taste impairment usually resolves in 6 weeks without changes in dosage.

edetate calcium disodium

Calcium Disodium Versenate, Calcium EDTA

Pregnancy Risk Category: C

HOW SUPPLIED

Injection: 200 mg/ml

ACTION

Mechanism: Forms stable, soluble complexes with metals, particularly lead.

Onset: 1 hour. **Peak:** Effect peaks after 24 to 48 hours. **Duration:** 4 to 5 days.

INDICATIONS & DOSAGE

Lead poisoning (blood levels greater than 50 mcg/dl) –
Adults and children: 1 g/m^2 I.V. or I.M. daily in divided doses at 12-hour intervals for 3 to 5 days.
Acute lead encephalopathy or blood lead levels above 100 mcg/dl –
Adults and children: 1.5 g/m^2 I.V. or I.M. daily in divided doses at 12-hours intervals for 3 to 5 days, usually in conjunction with dimercaprol. A second course may be administered in 4 days but preferably 2 to 3 weeks later.

ADVERSE REACTIONS

CNS: headache, paresthesia, numbness, fatigue (4 to 8 hours after infusion).
CV: ***arrhythmias,*** hypotension.
EENT: sneezing and nasal congestion (4 to 8 hours after infusion).
GI: anorexia, nausea, vomiting.
GU: proteinuria, hematuria; ***nephrotoxicity with renal tubular necrosis leading to fatal nephrosis.***
Other: arthralgia, myalgia, hypercalcemia; sudden fever, chills, and excessive thirst (4 to 8 hours after infusion).

INTERACTIONS

None significant.

CONTRAINDICATIONS

• Contraindicated in patients with severe renal disease or anuria.
• Because I.V. use may increase intracranial pressure, do not administer by that route to treat lead encephalopathy. Give by I.M. route instead.

NURSING CONSIDERATIONS

• Do not confuse with edetate disodium, which is used to treat hypercalcemia.
• **I.V. use:** Dilute with D_5W or 0.9%

sodium chloride injection to a concentration of 2 to 4 mg/ml. Infuse one-half of the daily dose over 1 hour in asymptomatic patients or 2 hours in symptomatic patients. Give the rest of the infusion at least 6 hours later. Alternatively, give by slow infusion over at least 8 hours.
• I.M. route preferred, especially for children and patients with lead encephalopathy.
• Procaine hydrochloride may be added to I.M. solution to minimize pain. Watch for local reactions.
• Force fluids to facilitate lead excretion, except in patients with lead encephalopathy.
• Monitor fluid intake and output, urinalysis, BUN, and ECGs daily.
• To avoid toxicity, use with dimercaprol.

edetate disodium

Disodium EDTA, Disotate, Endrate
Pregnancy Risk Category: C

HOW SUPPLIED
Injection: 150 mg/ml

ACTION
Mechanism: Chelates with metals, such as calcium, to form a stable, soluble complex.
Onset: immediate.

INDICATIONS & DOSAGE
Hypercalcemic crisis –
Adults: 50 mg/kg by slow I.V. infusion added to 500 ml of D_5W or 0.9% sodium chloride solution. Maximum dosage is 3 g/day.
Children: 40 to 70 mg/kg by slow I.V. infusion, diluted to a maximum concentration of 30 mg/ml in D_5W or 0.9% sodium chloride solution. Maximum dosage is 70 mg/kg/day.

ADVERSE REACTIONS
CNS: circumoral paresthesia, numbness, headache, malaise, fatigue, muscle pain or weakness.
CV: hypertension, thrombophlebitis, orthostatic hypotension.
EENT: erythema.
GI: nausea, vomiting, diarrhea, anorexia, abdominal cramps.
GU: in excessive doses – nephrotoxicity with urinary urgency, nocturia, dysuria, polyuria, proteinuria, renal insufficiency, ***renal failure, tubular necrosis.***
Skin: dermatitis.
Other: ***severe hypocalcemia,*** decreased magnesium, pain at site of infusion.

INTERACTIONS
None significant.

CONTRAINDICATIONS
• Contraindicated in patients with anuria, known or suspected hypocalcemia, significant renal disease, active or healed tubercular lesions, history of seizures or intracranial lesions, and generalized arteriosclerosis associated with aging.
• Use cautiously in patients with limited cardiac reserve, CHF, hypokalemia, or diabetes mellitus.

NURSING CONSIDERATIONS
• Other drug treatments for hypercalcemia are safer and more effective than edetate disodium.
• No scientific evidence exists that the drug is safe or effective for treatment of atherosclerosis and related disorders.
• Don't use to treat lead toxicity; use edetate calcium disodium instead.
• **I.V. use:** Dilute before use. Avoid rapid I.V. infusion; profound hypocalcemia may occur, leading to tetany, seizures, arrhythmias, and respiratory arrest. Not recommended for direct or intermittent injection. Avoid extravasation.

• Record I.V. site used, and avoid repeated use of the same site, which increases likelihood of thrombophlebitis.
• Monitor ECG and renal function tests frequently.
• Obtain serum calcium after each dose.
• Keep I.V. calcium available to treat hypocalcemia.
• Keep patients in bed for 15 minutes after infusion to avoid orthostatic hypotension. Monitor blood pressure closely.
• If generalized systemic reactions – fever, chills, back pain, emesis, muscle cramps, urinary urgency – occur 4 to 8 hours after infusion, report them to the doctor. Treatment is usually supportive. Symptoms generally subside within 12 hours.

flumazenil

Romazicon

Pregnancy Risk Category: C

HOW SUPPLIED

Injection: 0.1 mg/ml in 5- and 10-ml multiple-dose vials

ACTION

Mechanism: Benzodiazepine antagonist that competitively inhibits the actions of benzodiazepines on the gamma-aminobutyric acid-benzodiazepine receptor complex.
Onset: 1 to 2 minutes. **Duration:** 1 to 4 hours.

INDICATIONS & DOSAGE

Complete or partial reversal of sedative effects of benzodiazepines after anesthesia or short diagnostic procedures (conscious sedation) –
Adults: initially, 0.2 mg I.V. over 15 seconds. If patient does not reach the desired level of consciousness after 45 seconds, repeat dose. Repeat at 1-minute intervals until a cumulative dose of 1 mg has been given (initial dose plus four additional doses). Most patients respond after 0.6 to 1 mg of drug. In case of resedation, dosage may be repeated after 20 minutes; however, no more than 1 mg should be given at any one time, and no more than 3 mg/hour.
Suspected benzodiazepine overdose –
Adults: initially, 0.2 mg I.V. over 15 seconds. If patient does not reach the desired level of consciousness after 30 seconds, administer 0.3 mg over 30 seconds. If patient still does not respond adequately, give 0.5 mg over 30 seconds; repeat 0.5-mg doses at 1-minute intervals until a cumulative dose of 3 mg has been given. Most patients suffering from benzodiazepine overdose respond to cumulative doses between 1 and 3 mg; rarely, patients who respond partially after 3 mg may require additional doses. Do not give more than 5 mg over 5 minutes initially. Sedation that persists after this dosage is unlikely to be caused by benzodiazepines. In case of resedation, dosage may be repeated after 20 minutes; however, no more than 1 mg should be given at any one time, and no more than 3 mg/hour.

ADVERSE REACTIONS

CNS: *dizziness, abnormal or blurred vision, headache,* ***seizures,*** fatigue, agitation, emotional lability.
CV: ***arrhythmias,*** cutaneous vasodilation.
GI: nausea, vomiting.
Other: *diaphoresis, pain at injection site.*

INTERACTIONS

Antidepressants; drugs that can cause seizures or arrhythmias: seizures or arrhythmias can develop after effect of benzodiazepine overdose is removed. Use flumazenil with caution in cases of mixed overdose.

CONTRAINDICATIONS

- Contraindicated in patients hypersensitive to flumazenil or benzodiazepines; patients who show evidence of serious tricyclic or tetracyclic antidepressant overdose; those who received benzodiazepine to treat a potentially life-threatening condition (such as status epilepticus); and in benzodiazepine-dependent patients (flumazenil may precipitate seizures).
- Use cautiously in patients at high risk for developing seizures, including patients undergoing concurrent sedative-hypnotic drug withdrawal; patients who have recently received multiple doses of a parenteral benzodiazepine; patients displaying some signs of seizure activity; patients who may be at risk for unrecognized benzodiazepine dependence, such as intensive care unit patients; patients with head injury because of the risk of precipitating seizures; those who have received neuromuscular blockers; psychiatric patients because the drug has precipitated panic attacks in those with panic disorder; and alcohol-dependent patients.

NURSING CONSIDERATIONS

- Dosage adjustments don't appear necessary in elderly patients.
- Safety and efficacy in children have not been established.
- Drug can be administered by direct injection or diluted with a compatible solution. Discard unused drug that has been drawn into a syringe or diluted within 24 hours.
- **I.V. use:** Administer drug into an I.V. line in a large vein with a free-flowing I.V. solution to minimize pain at the injection site. Compatible solutions include D_5W, lactated Ringer's injection, or 0.9% sodium chloride.
- Monitor patients closely for resedation that may occur after reversal of benzodiazepine effects because flumazenil's duration of action is shorter than that of all benzodiazepines. Duration of monitoring period depends on specific drug being reversed. Monitor closely after long-acting benzodiazepines such as diazepam, or after high doses of short-acting benzodiazepines, such as 10 mg of midazolam. In most cases, severe resedation is unlikely in patients who fail to show signs of resedation 2 hours after a 1-mg dose of flumazenil.
- Warn patients not to perform hazardous activities, such as operating heavy equipment or driving, within 24 hours of procedure because of resedation risk.
- Do not expect patients to recall information told to them in the postprocedure period because drug does not reverse the amnesic effects of benzodiazepines. Tell family members important instructions or give patients written instructions.
- Tell patients to avoid alcohol, CNS depressants, and OTC drugs for 24 hours.

ipecac syrup*

Pregnancy Risk Category:C

HOW SUPPLIED

Syrup: 70 mg powdered ipecac/ml* ◇

ACTION

Mechanism: Induces vomiting by acting locally on the gastric mucosa and centrally on the chemoreceptor trigger zone.

Onset: 15 to 30 minutes. **Duration:** 20 to 25 minutes.

INDICATIONS & DOSAGE

To induce vomiting in poisoning –

Adults and children over 12 years: 30 ml P.O., followed by 200 to 300 ml of water.

Children under 1 year: 5 to 10 ml P.O., followed by 100 to 200 ml of water or milk. If necessary, repeat dose once after 20 minutes.

Children 1 year to 12 years: 15 ml

*Liquid form contains alcohol.
**May contain tartrazine.

P.O., followed by about 200 ml of water or milk.

ADVERSE REACTIONS
CNS: depression.
CV: ***arrhythmias,*** bradycardia, hypotension, atrial fibrillation, or ***fatal myocarditis*** after ingestion of excessive dose.
GI: diarrhea.

INTERACTIONS
Activated charcoal: neutralized emetic effect. Don't give together; may give activated charcoal after vomiting.

CONTRAINDICATIONS
- Contraindicated in semicomatose or unconscious patients, or those with severe inebriation, seizures, shock, or loss of gag reflex.
- Don't give after ingestion of petroleum distillates (for example, kerosene, gasoline) or volatile oils; retching and vomiting may cause aspiration and lead to bronchospasm, pulmonary edema, or aspiration pneumonitis. Vegetable oil will delay absorption of these substances. Don't give after ingestion of caustic substances, such as lye; additional injury to the esophagus and mediastinum can occur.

NURSING CONSIDERATIONS
- Clearly indicate ipecac *syrup,* not single word "ipecac," to avoid confusion with fluidextract, which is 14 times more concentrated and, if inadvertently used instead of syrup, may cause death. Fluidextract is no longer commercially available in the United States.
- No systemic toxicity occurs with doses of 30 ml or less.
- Ipecac syrup usually induces vomiting within 20 to 30 minutes.
- Stomach is usually emptied completely; vomitus also may contain some intestinal material.
- If two doses do not induce vomiting, gastric lavage is necessary.
- In antiemetic toxicity, ipecac syrup is usually effective if less than 1 hour has passed since ingestion of antiemetic.
- Recommend that 1 oz (30 ml) of syrup be readily available in the home when child becomes 1 year old for immediate use in case of emergency.
- Ipecac syrup is now commonly abused by bulimics who binge and then purge.

naloxone hydrochloride
Narcan

Pregnancy Risk Category: B

HOW SUPPLIED
Injection: 0.4 mg/ml, 1 mg/ml

ACTION
Mechanism: Displaces previously administered narcotic analgesics from their receptors (competitive antagonism). Has no pharmacologic activity of its own.
Onset: 1 to 2 minutes after I.V. use, 2 to 5 minutes after S.C. or I.M. use.
Duration: 45 minutes to 4 hours.

INDICATIONS & DOSAGE
Known or suspected narcotic-induced respiratory depression, including that caused by pentazocine and propoxyphene –
Adults: 0.4 to 2 mg I.V., S.C., or I.M. May repeat q 2 to 3 minutes, p.r.n. If no response is observed after 10 mg has been administered, the diagnosis of narcotic-induced toxicity should be questioned.
Postoperative narcotic depression –
Adults: 0.1 to 0.2 mg I.V. q 2 to 3 minutes, p.r.n. Adult concentration is 0.4 mg/ml.
Children: 0.01 mg/kg dose I.M., I.V., or S.C. May repeat q 2 to 3 minutes.
Note: If initial dose of 0.01 mg/kg does not result in clinical improvement,

up to 10 times this dose (0.1 mg/kg) may be needed.
Neonates (asphyxia neonatorum): 0.01 mg/kg I.V. into umbilical vein. May repeat q 2 to 3 minutes for three doses.

ADVERSE REACTIONS
CV: tachycardia and hypertension with higher-than-recommended doses.
GI: nausea and vomiting with higher-than-recommended doses.
Other: tremors and withdrawal symptoms in narcotic-dependent patients with higher-than-recommended doses.

INTERACTIONS
None significant.

CONTRAINDICATIONS
- Contraindicated in patients hypersensitive to the drug.
- Use cautiously in patients with cardiac irritability and opiate addiction. Abrupt reversal of opiate-induced CNS depression may result in nausea, vomiting, diaphoresis, tachycardia, CNS excitement, and increased blood pressure.

NURSING CONSIDERATIONS
- Drug is effective only in reversing respiratory depression caused by opiates, not against other drug-induced respiratory depression. Flumazenil should be used to treat respiratory depression caused by diazepam or other benzodiazepines. However, recent reports indicate that naloxone may reverse coma induced by ethanol intoxication.
- **I.V. use:** Continuous I.V. infusion is necessary in many instances to control adverse effects of epidurally administered morphine. Adult concentration (0.4 mg) may be diluted by mixing 0.5 ml with 9.5 ml of sterile water or sodium chloride solution for injection to make neonatal concentration (0.02 mg/ml).
- Duration of action of the narcotic may exceed that of naloxone and patients may relapse into respiratory depression.
- Monitor respiratory depth and rate. Be prepared to provide oxygen, ventilation, and other resuscitation measures.
- Respiratory rate increases within 1 to 2 minutes. Effect lasts 1 to 4 hours, but dosage may have to be repeated q 20 minutes.
- Be aware that patients who received naloxone to reverse opioid-induced respiratory depression may exhibit tachypnea.
- Used investigationally to treat the senile dementia of Alzheimer's disease, to improve circulation in refractory shock, and to relieve certain kinds of chronic constipation.

naltrexone hydrochloride
Trexan
Pregnancy Risk Category: C

HOW SUPPLIED
Tablets: 50 mg

ACTION
Mechanism: Reversibly blocks the subjective effects of intravenously administered opioids by occupying opiate receptors in the brain.
Onset: 15 to 30 minutes. **Peak:** Effects peak after 12 hours. **Duration:** about 24 hours.

INDICATIONS & DOSAGE
Adjunct for maintenance of opioid-free state in detoxified individuals –
Adults: initially, 25 mg P.O. If no withdrawal signs occur within 1 hour, give an additional 25 mg. Once patient has been started on 50 mg q 24 hours, flexible maintenance schedule may be used. From 50 to 150 mg may be given daily, depending on the schedule prescribed.

ADVERSE REACTIONS
CNS: *insomnia, anxiety, nervousness, headache,* depression.
GI: *nausea, vomiting,* anorexia, *abdominal pain.*
Hepatic: hepatotoxicity.
Other: *muscle and joint pain.*

INTERACTIONS
None significant.

CONTRAINDICATIONS
- Contraindicated in patients receiving opioid analgesics, opioid-dependent patients, patients in acute opioid withdrawal, and in those with positive urine screen for opioids or acute hepatitis or liver failure.
- Use cautiously in patients with mild liver disease or history of recent liver disease.

NURSING CONSIDERATIONS
- Naltrexone should be used only as part of a comprehensive rehabilitation program.
- Treatment shouldn't begin until patients receive naloxone challenge, a provocative test of opioid dependency. If signs of opioid withdrawal persist after naloxone challenge, don't administer naltrexone.
- Patients must be completely free of opioids before taking naltrexone or severe withdrawal symptoms may occur. Patients who have been addicted to short-acting opioids, such as heroin and meperidine, must wait at least 7 days after the last opioid dose before starting naltrexone. Patients who have been addicted to longer-acting opioids, such as methadone, should wait at least 10 days.
- In an emergency, patients receiving naltrexone may be given an opioid analgesic, but the dose must be higher than usual to surmount naltrexone's effect. Monitor for respiratory depression from the opioid; it may be longer and deeper.
- For patients expected to be poor compliers, try a flexible maintenance dosage regimen: 100 mg on Monday and Wednesday, 150 mg on Friday.
- Advise patients to carry a medical identification card. Warn them to tell medical personnel that they are taking naltrexone.
- Give patients names of nonopioid drugs that they can continue to take for pain, diarrhea, or cough.

pralidoxime chloride (pyridine-2-aldoxime methochloride; 2-PAM)
Protopam Chloride

Pregnancy Risk Category: C

HOW SUPPLIED
Injection: 1 g/20 ml in 20-ml vial without diluent or syringe; 1 g/20 ml in 20-ml vial with diluent, syringe, needle, and alcohol swab (emergency kit); 600 mg/2 ml auto-injector, parenteral

ACTION
Mechanism: Reactivates cholinesterase that has been inactivated by organophosphorus pesticides and related compounds, permiting degradation of accumulated acetylcholine and facilitating normal functioning of neuromuscular junctions.
Onset: 1 hour.

INDICATIONS & DOSAGE
Antidote for organophosphate poisoning –
Adults: 1 to 2 g in 100 ml of sodium chloride solution by I.V. infusion over 15 to 30 minutes. If pulmonary edema is present, give by slow I.V. push over 5 minutes. Repeat in 1 hour if muscle weakness persists. Additional doses may be given cautiously. Use I.M. or S.C. injection if I.V. is not feasible.
Children: 20 to 40 mg/kg I.V.

Cholinergic crisis in myasthenia gravis –
Adults: 1 to 2 g I.V., followed by increments of 250 mg I.V. q 5 minutes.

ADVERSE REACTIONS

CNS: dizziness, headache, drowsiness, excitement, manic behavior after recovery of consciousness.
CV: tachycardia.
EENT: blurred vision, diplopia, impaired accommodation, ***laryngospasm.***
GI: nausea.
Other: muscular weakness, muscle rigidity, hyperventilation.

INTERACTIONS

None significant.

CONTRAINDICATIONS

- Contraindicated in patients poisoned with Sevin, a carbamate insecticide, because it increases drug's toxicity.
- Use with extreme caution in patients with renal insufficiency or myasthenia gravis (overdosage may precipitate myasthenic crisis), and in patients with asthma or peptic ulceration.

NURSING CONSIDERATIONS

- Use in hospitalized patients only; have respiratory and other supportive measures available. If possible, obtain accurate medical history and chronology of poisoning. Give as soon as possible after poisoning; treatment is most effective if initiated within 24 hours after exposure.
- Initial measures should include removal of secretions, maintenance of patent airway, and artificial ventilation if needed. After dermal exposure to organophosphate, remove the patient's clothing and wash his skin and hair with sodium bicarbonate, soap, water, and alcohol as soon as possible. A second washing may be necessary. When washing the patient, wear protective gloves and clothes to avoid exposure.
- Draw blood for cholinesterase levels before giving pralidoxime.
- **I.V. use:** Give I.V. preparation slowly as diluted solution. Dilute with sterile water without preservatives.
- To ameliorate muscarinic effects and block accumulation of acetylcholine associated with organophosphate poisoning, atropine 2 to 4 mg I.V. may be given along with pralidoxine if cyanosis is not present. (If cyanosis is present, atropine should be given I.M.) Give atropine every 5 to 6 minutes until signs and symptoms of atropine toxicity (flushing, tachycardia, dry mouth, blurred vision, excitement, delirium, and hallucinations) appear; maintain atropinization for at least 48 hours.
- Drug relieves paralysis of respiratory muscles but is less effective in relieving depression of respiratory center.
- Drug is not effective against poisoning due to phosphorus, inorganic phosphates, or organophosphates with no anticholinesterase activity.
- It is difficult to distinguish between toxic effects produced by atropine or by organophosphate compounds and those resulting from pralidoxime. Observe patient for 48 to 72 hours if poison was ingested. Delayed absorption may occur from lower bowel.
- Observe the patient with myasthenia gravis treated for overdose of cholinergic drugs closely for signs of rapid weakening. This patient can pass quickly from a cholinergic crisis to a myasthenic crisis, and requires more cholinergic drugs to treat the myasthenia. Keep edrophonium (Tensilon) available in such situations for establishing differential diagnosis.
- Caution the patient treated for organophosphate poisoning to avoid contact with insecticides for several weeks.
- Although not approved, subconjunctival injection of pralidoxime has been used to reverse adverse ocular reactions

resulting from splashing into the eye or systemic overdose of organophosphates.

protamine sulfate

Pregnancy Risk Category: C

HOW SUPPLIED
Injection: 10 mg/ml

ACTION
Mechanism: A heparin antagonist that forms a physiologically inert complex with heparin sodium.
Onset: within 1 minute. **Duration:** 2 hours.

INDICATIONS & DOSAGE
Heparin overdose –
Adults: dosage based on venous blood coagulation studies, usually 1 mg for each 90 to 115 units of heparin. Give diluted to 1% (10 mg/ml) by slow I.V. injection over 1 to 3 minutes. Maximum dosage is 50 mg/10 minutes.

ADVERSE REACTIONS
CV: fall in blood pressure, bradycardia.
Respiratory: dyspnea.
Other: transitory flushing, feeling of warmth, ***anaphylaxis, anaphylactoid reactions.***

INTERACTIONS
None significant.

CONTRAINDICATIONS
- Use cautiously after cardiac surgery.

NURSING CONSIDERATIONS
- Calculate dosage carefully. One mg of protamine neutralizes 90 to 115 units of heparin depending on the salt (heparin calcium or heparin sodium) and the source of heparin (beef or pork).
- **I.V. use:** Administer slowly by direct I.V. injection. Have equipment available to treat shock.
- Monitor patients continually. Check vital signs frequently.
- Watch for spontaneous bleeding (heparin "rebound"), especially in patients undergoing dialysis and in those who have undergone cardiac surgery.
- Protamine sulfate may act as anticoagulant in very high doses.

sodium cellulose phosphate

Calcibind

Pregnancy Risk Category: C

HOW SUPPLIED
Powder: 2.5-g packets or 300-g bulk. Inorganic phosphate content approximately 34%; sodium content approximately 11%.

ACTION
Mechanism: Binds calcium in the GI tract and decreases the amount absorbed.
Onset: hours to days.

INDICATIONS & DOSAGE
Absorptive hypercalciuria type I with recurrent calcium oxalate or calcium phosphate renal stones –
Adults: 15 g/day P.O. (5 g with each meal) in patients with urine calcium greater than 300 mg/day. When urine calcium declines to less than 150 mg/day, reduce dosage to 10 g/day (5 g with dinner, 2.5 g with two remaining meals).

ADVERSE REACTIONS
CNS: drowsiness, mood or mental changes, ***seizures,*** trembling.
GI: anorexia, nausea, vomiting, discomfort, diarrhea, dyspepsia.
GU: hyperoxaluria, hypomagnesuria.
Other: acute arthralgia.

INTERACTIONS
Calcium-containing products, dairy products: worsened hypercalcemia. Avoid use.
Magnesium-containing products: may bind drug. Separate doses by at least 1 hour.
Vitamin C: risk of nephrolithiasis. Avoid excessive intake.

CONTRAINDICATIONS
• Contraindicated in patients with primary or secondary hyperparathyroidism, including renal hypercalciuria; hypomagnesemic states; bone disease; hypocalcemic states; normal or low intestinal absorption; renal excretion of calcium; or enteric hyperoxaluria.
• Use cautiously in patients with CHF or ascites.

NURSING CONSIDERATIONS
• Drug is recommended only for the type of absorptive hypercalciuria in which both intestinal calcium absorption and urine calcium remain abnormally high even with a calcium-restricted diet. When administered inappropriately it may cause hypocalciuria, which could stimulate parathyroid function and lead to parathyroid bone disease.
• Instruct patients to maintain a calcium-restricted diet and avoid all dairy products.
• Patients taking sodium cellulose phosphate may develop hyperoxaluria and hypomagnesuria, which predispose them to stone formation. Advise patients to restrict dietary intake of oxalates (found in spinach, rhubarb, chocolate, and tea).
• Tell patients to avoid vitamin C because it can increase urine oxalate.
• Encourage fluid intake. Urine output should be at least 2 liters/day.
• Advise patients to mix powder with 8 oz of fruit juice, water, or a soft drink and to take it with meals. Remind patients to refill glass, mix, and drink all of the fluid to get the full dose.
• Encourage a low-sodium diet because drug has 2 to 3 mEq of sodium/g. Tell patients to avoid salty foods and to avoid adding salt at the table.
• Because of the difficulty involved in managing sodium cellulose phosphate therapy, many doctors prefer to treat hypercalciuria with a low-calcium diet, high fluid intake, and thiazides, when necessary.

sodium polystyrene sulfonate
Kayexalate, Resonium A, SPS

Pregnancy Risk Category: C

HOW SUPPLIED
Powder: 1-lb jar (3.5 g/teaspoon)
Suspension: 60 ml*, 120 ml*, 200 ml*, 480 ml*, 500 ml*

ACTION
Mechanism: Potassium-removing resin exchanges sodium ions for potassium ions in the intestine: 1 g of sodium polystyrene sulfonate is exchanged for 0.5 to 1 mEq of potassium. The resin is then eliminated. Much of the exchange capacity is used for cations other than potassium (calcium and magnesium) and possibly for fats and proteins.
Onset: hours to days.

INDICATIONS & DOSAGE
Hyperkalemia –
Adults: 15 g P.O. daily to q.i.d. in water or sorbitol (3 to 4 ml/g of resin). Alternatively, mix powder with appropriate medium – aqueous suspension or diet appropriate for renal failure – and instill in nasogastric tube.

Or, give 30 to 50 g/100 ml of sorbitol q 6 hours as warm emulsion deep into sigmoid colon (20 cm). In persistent vomiting or paralytic ileus, high-retention enema of sodium polysty-

rene sulfonate (30 g) suspended in 200 ml of 10% methylcellulose, 10% dextrose, or 25% sorbitol solution.
Children: 1 g of resin P.O. or P.R. for each mEq of potassium to be removed.

Oral administration preferred because drug should remain in intestine for at least 6 hours; otherwise, consider nasogastric administration.

ADVERSE REACTIONS

GI: *constipation,* fecal impaction (in elderly patients), anorexia, gastric irritation, nausea, vomiting, *diarrhea* (with sorbitol emulsions).
Other: ***hypokalemia,*** hypocalcemia, hypomagnesemia, sodium retention.

INTERACTIONS

Antacids and laxatives (nonabsorbable cation-donating types, including magnesium hydroxide): systemic alkalosis and reduced potassium exchange capability. Don't use together.

CONTRAINDICATIONS

- Use cautiously in elderly patients, in patients on digitalis glycoside therapy, and in patients with hypokalemia, severe CHF, severe hypertension, or marked edema.

NURSING CONSIDERATIONS

- Treatment may result in potassium deficiency. Monitor serum potassium levels at least once daily. Treatment is usually stopped when potassium is reduced to 4 or 5 mEq/L.
- Watch for other signs of hypokalemia: irritability, confusion, arrhythmias, ECG changes, severe muscle weakness and sometimes paralysis, and digitalis toxicity in digitalized patients.
- If hyperkalemia is severe, do not depend solely on polystyrene resin to lower serum potassium. Dextrose 50% with regular insulin I.V. push may be given.
- Monitor for symptoms of other electrolyte deficiencies (magnesium, calcium) because drug is nonselective. Monitor serum calcium in patients receiving sodium polystyrene therapy for more than 3 days. Supplementary calcium may be needed.
- Drug contains about 100 mg sodium/g. Watch for sodium overload. About ⅓ of resin's sodium is retained.
- Premixed forms are available (SPS and others).
- Do not heat resin; this will impair the drug's effectiveness. Mix resin only with water or sorbitol for P.O. administration. Above all, *never* mix with orange juice (high potassium content) to disguise taste.
- Chill oral suspension for greater palatability.
- If sorbitol is given, it may be mixed with resin suspension.
- Consider solid form. Resin cookie and candy recipes are available; ask pharmacist or dietitian to supply.
- Watch for constipation in oral or nasogastric administration. Use sorbitol (10 to 20 ml of 70% syrup every 2 hours as needed) to produce one or two watery stools daily.
- If preparing manually, mix polystyrene resin only with water and sorbitol for rectal use. Do not use mineral oil for rectal administration to prevent impaction; ion exchange requires aqueous medium. Sorbitol content prevents impaction.
- Prevent fecal impaction in elderly patients by administering resin rectally. Give cleansing enema before rectal administration. Explain to patients the need to retain enema – for 6 to 10 hours is ideal, but 30 to 60 minutes is acceptable.
- Prepare rectal dose at room temperature. Stir emulsion gently during administration.
- Use #28 French rubber tube for rectal dose; insert 20 cm into sigmoid colon. Tape tube in place. Alternatively, consider a Foley catheter with a 30-ml balloon inflated distal to anal sphincter

to aid in retention. This is especially helpful for patients with poor sphincter control (for example, after CVA). Use gravity flow. Drain returns constantly through Y-tube connection. Place patient in knee-chest position or with hips on pillow for a while if back-leakage occurs.

• After rectal administration, flush tubing with 50 to 100 ml of nonsodium fluid to ensure delivery of all medication. Flush rectum to remove the resin.

succimer

Chemet

Pregnancy Risk Category: C

HOW SUPPLIED

Capsules: 100 mg

ACTION

Mechanism: A chelating agent that forms water-soluble complexes with lead and increases its excretion in urine.

Onset: several days.

INDICATIONS & DOSAGE

Lead poisoning in children with blood lead levels above 45 mcg/dl –

Children: initially, 10 mg/kg or 350 mg/m² q 8 hours for 5 days. Round dosage as appropriate to nearest 100 mg (see chart). Then, decrease frequency of administration to q 12 hours for an additional 2 weeks of therapy.

Weight (kg)	*Dose (mg)*
8 to 15	100
16 to 23	200
24 to 34	300
35 to 44	400
>45	500

ADVERSE REACTIONS

CNS: *drowsiness, dizziness, sensory motor neuropathy, sleepiness, paresthesia, headache.*

CV: arrhythmias.

EENT: plugged ears, cloudy film in eyes, otitis media, watery eyes, sore throat, rhinorrhea, nasal congestion.

GI: *nausea, vomiting, diarrhea, loss of appetite,* abdominal cramps, hemorrhoidal symptoms, *metallic taste in mouth.*

GU: decreased urination, difficult urination, proteinuria.

Hematologic: increased platelet count, intermittent eosinophilia.

Respiratory: cough, head cold.

Skin: papular rash, herpetic rash, mucocutaneous eruptions, pruritus.

Other: *leg, kneecap, back, stomach, rib, or flank pain; flulike symptoms;* moniliasis; *elevated serum AST, ALT, alkaline phosphatase, or cholesterol levels.*

INTERACTIONS

None reported.

CONTRAINDICATIONS

• Contraindicated in patients hypersensitive to the drug.

• Use cautiously in patients with compromised renal function.

NURSING CONSIDERATIONS

• Concurrent administration of succimer with other chelating agents is not recommended. Patients who have received edetate calcium disodium with or without dimercaprol may use succimer as subsequent therapy after a 4-week interval.

• Elevated blood lead levels and associated symptoms may return rapidly after drug is discontinued because of redistribution of lead from bone to soft tissues and blood. Monitor patients at least once weekly for rebound blood lead levels.

• Transient mild elevations of serum transaminases have been observed. Monitor serum transaminase before and at least weekly during therapy. Patients with history of liver disease should be monitored more closely.

• False-positive results for ketones in urine using nitroprusside reagents

(Ketostix) and falsely decreased levels of serum uric acid and CK have been reported.

- Tell parents of young children who cannot swallow capsules that capsule can be opened and its contents sprinkled on a small amount of soft food. Alternatively, medicated beads from capsule may be poured on a spoon; follow with flavored beverage, such as a fruit drink.
- Identifying and removing sources of lead in child's environment is critical to successful therapy. Chelation therapy is not a substitute for preventing further exposure and should not be used to permit continued exposure.
- Severity of lead intoxication should be used as a guide for more frequent blood lead monitoring. Measure severity by initial blood lead level and by rate and degree of rebound of blood lead level.
- Course of treatment lasts 19 days. Repeated courses may be necessary if indicated by weekly monitoring of blood lead levels.
- A minimum of 2 weeks between courses is recommended unless high blood lead levels indicate need for immediate therapy.
- Tell patients to consult the doctor if rash occurs. Consider possibility of allergic or other mucocutaneous reactions each time drug is used.

---

trientine hydrochloride
Cuprid

Pregnancy Risk Category: C

HOW SUPPLIED
Capsules: 250 mg

ACTION
Mechanism: Chelates copper and increases its urinary excretion.
Onset: hours to days.

INDICATIONS & DOSAGE
Wilson's disease in patients who cannot tolerate penicillamine –
Adults: 750 to 2,000 mg P.O. daily in two, three, or four divided doses.
Children: 500 to 1,500 mg P.O. daily in two, three, or four divided doses.

The optimal long-term maintenance dosage should be determined q 6 to 12 months, according to serum copper analysis.

ADVERSE REACTIONS
Hematologic: iron-deficiency anemia.
Other: hypersensitivity reactions (rash), fever.

INTERACTIONS
Mineral supplements, including iron: may block trientine absorption. Administer at least 2 hours apart.

CONTRAINDICATIONS
- Contraindicated in patients with known or suspected hypersensitivity to the drug.
- Not recommended for use in patients with rheumatoid arthritis, biliary cirrhosis, or cystinuria.
- Use cautiously in patients with or at risk for iron-deficiency anemia. Patients (especially women) should be closely monitored for evidence of iron-deficiency anemia throughout therapy.
- Also use cautiously in patients with idiopathic or penicillamine-induced systemic lupus erythematosus because drug may reactivate the disease.

NURSING CONSIDERATIONS
- Observe patients for signs of hypersensitivity reactions, such as skin rash.
- Tell patients to take trientine on an empty stomach at least 1 hour before or 2 hours after meals, and at least 1 hour apart from any other drug, food, or milk.
- Tell patients to swallow capsules

whole with water and not to open or chew them.

- Exposure to capsule contents may cause contact dermatitis. If capsule is accidentally opened and contents spilled on skin, tell patients to wash site thoroughly.
- Urge patients to faithfully follow trientine regimen and low-copper diet as prescribed.
- Tell patients to take their temperature every night and report any fevers or skin eruptions, especially during the first month of therapy.

99
Uncategorized drugs

acetohydroxamic acid
alglucerase
alprostadil
aprotinin
benzoyl peroxide cleansers
benzoyl peroxide creams
benzoyl peroxide gels
benzoyl peroxide lotions
calcipotriene
capsaicin
cisapride
clomiphene citrate
diazoxide, oral
etretinate
finasteride
gallium nitrate
isotretinoin
levocarnitine
levomethadyl acetate hydrochloride
masoprocol
mesalamine
mesna
methoxsalen
minoxidil (topical)
olsalazine sodium
pamidronate disodium
pentoxifylline
ritodrine hydrochloride
sodium benzoate and sodium phenylacetate
strontium 89 chloride
ticlopidine hydrochloride
tiopronin
tretinoin

COMBINATION PRODUCTS
None.

acetohydroxamic acid
Lithostat

Pregnancy Risk Category: X

HOW SUPPLIED
Tablets (scored): 250 mg

ACTION
Mechanism: Prevents formation of renal stones by inhibiting bacterial urease activity.
Peak: Serum levels peak within 15 to 60 minutes.

INDICATIONS & DOSAGE
Infection-related kidney stones—
Adults: 250 mg P.O. t.i.d. or q.i.d. at 6- to 8-hour intervals when the stomach is empty. Maximum daily dosage is 1.5 g.
Children: 10 mg/kg/day P.O. in two or three divided doses.

ADVERSE REACTIONS
CNS: *mild headache, depression, anxiety, nervousness.*
CV: phlebitis, palpitations.
GI: *nausea, vomiting, diarrhea, constipation, anorexia.*
Hematologic: ***hemolytic anemia.***
Skin: *nonpruritic, macular rash on arms and face.*
Other: alopecia, deep vein thrombosis, malaise.

INTERACTIONS
Methenamine: may produce synergistic effects.
Oral iron supplements: reduced absorption of acetohydroxamic acid. Check with the doctor, who may request that iron be administered I.M.

CONTRAINDICATIONS
- Contraindicated in patients whose physical state and disease are amenable to surgery and appropriate antibiotics, in patients whose urine is infected by nonurease-producing organisms, during pregnancy, and in patients with poor renal function.
- Use cautiously in patients predisposed to deep vein thrombosis.

NURSING CONSIDERATIONS

- A negative Coombs' test for hemolytic anemia has occurred in patients receiving acetohydroxamic acid.
- Monitor CBC, including reticulocyte count, after 2 weeks of therapy, then at 3-month intervals for duration of treatment. If laboratory findings indicate hemolytic anemia, discontinue drug.
- Reduced dosage may be necessary in renal impairment.
- Skin rash is more common during prolonged use and with concomitant use of alcoholic beverages. The rash appears 30 to 45 minutes after ingestion of alcoholic beverages and disappears spontaneously in 30 to 60 minutes. Although skin rash doesn't usually require treatment, advise patients to avoid alcohol.
- Patients may also be given methenamine to enhance response to acetohydroxamic acid.

alglucerase (glucocerebrosidase, glucosylceramidase, glucocerebrosidase-beta-glucosidase)

Ceredase

Pregnancy Risk Category: C

HOW SUPPLIED

Injection: 80 IU/ml in 5-ml bottles

ACTION

Mechanism: Appears to reduce glycolipid accumulation by acting as a catalyst for the hydrolysis of glucocerebroside to glucose and ceramide – part of the normal degradation pathway for lipids.

Onset: 3 to 6 months. **Duration:** 6 months after therapy.

INDICATIONS & DOSAGE

Long-term endogenous enzyme (glucosylceramidase) replacement therapy in confirmed Type I Gaucher's disease –

Adults and children: individualize dosage; initially, up to 60 units/kg I.V. may be used. Infusion should run over 1 to 2 hours and be given once q 2 weeks. Frequency of infusion may be adjusted based on severity of disease or patient convenience. Once response is established, reduce dosage for maintenance at 3- to 6-month intervals.

ADVERSE REACTIONS

GI: abdominal discomfort, nausea, vomiting.

Other: chills, slight fever, discomfort, burning, swelling at injection site.

INTERACTIONS

None significant.

CONTRAINDICATIONS

- Contraindicated in patients hypersensitive to the drug.

NURSING CONSIDERATIONS

- Alglucerase is purified from a large pool of human placental tissue collected from selected donors. Although the risk of viral contamination from slow-acting or latent viruses is believed to be remote, the risks and benefits of therapy must be carefully assessed before administration.
- Monitor response parameters to use lowest effective dose.
- Hemoglobin levels may normalize after 6 months of therapy. Improved mineralization may also occur after prolonged treatment.
- **I.V. use:** To prepare solution, dilute appropriate amount of alglucerase with 0.9% sodium chloride solution to a final volume not to exceed 100 ml. Use an in-line particulate filter during administration. Because alglucerase is preservative-free, use immediately.
- Do not shake bottle. Shaking may denature the glycoprotein and render it biologically inactive.

• Store at 39° F (4° C). Do not use solution that is discolored or that contains particles.

alprostadil

Prostin VR Pediatric

HOW SUPPLIED
Injection: 500 mcg/ml

ACTION
Mechanism: A prostaglandin derivative that relaxes the smooth muscle of the ductus arteriosus.
Onset: 30 minutes.

INDICATIONS & DOSAGE
Palliative therapy for temporary maintenance of patency of ductus arteriosus until surgery can be performed–
Infants: 0.05 to 0.1 mcg/kg/minute by I.V., intra-arterial, or intra-aortic infusion. When therapeutic response is achieved, reduce infusion rate to give lowest dosage that will maintain response. Maximum dosage is 0.4 mcg/kg/minute. Alternatively, administer through umbilical artery catheter placed at ductal opening.

ADVERSE REACTIONS
CNS: ***seizures.***
CV: bradycardia, hypotension, tachycardia.
GI: diarrhea.
Hematologic: ***disseminated intravascular coagulation.***
Other: ***apnea, flushing, fever, sepsis.***

INTERACTIONS
None significant.

CONTRAINDICATIONS
• Contraindicated in neonates with respiratory distress syndrome.
• Use cautiously in neonates with bleeding tendencies because drug inhibits platelet aggregation.

NURSING CONSIDERATIONS
• **I.V. use:** This drug is not recommended for direct injection or intermittent infusion. Administer by continuous infusion using a constant-rate pump. Infuse through a large peripheral or central vein or through an umbilical artery catheter placed at the level of the ductus arteriosus. If flushing occurs from peripheral vasodilation, reposition catheter.
• Reduce infusion rate if fever or significant hypotension occurs.
• Dilute drug before administering. Prepare fresh solution daily; discard solution after 24 hours.
• Do not use diluents that contain benzyl alcohol. Fatal toxic syndrome may occur.
• In infants with restricted pulmonary blood flow, measure drug's effectiveness by monitoring blood oxygenation. In infants with restricted systemic blood flow, measure drug's effectiveness by monitoring systemic blood pressure and blood pH.
• Monitor arterial pressure by umbilical artery catheter, auscultation, or Doppler transducer. Slow rate of infusion if arterial pressure falls significantly.
• Apnea and bradycardia may reflect drug overdose. If the signs occur, stop infusion immediately.
• CV and CNS adverse reactions are more frequent in infants weighing less than 2 kg and in those receiving infusions for longer than 48 hours.
• Keep respiratory support available.

aprotinin

Trasylol

Pregnancy Risk Category: B

HOW SUPPLIED
Injection: 10,000 KIU(kallikrein inactivator units)/ml (1.4 mg/ml) in 100-ml and 200-ml vials

ACTION

Mechanism: A naturally occurring protease inhibitor that acts as a systemic hemostatic agent, decreasing bleeding and turnover of coagulation factors. It inhibits fibrinolysis by affecting kallikrein and plasmin, prevents triggering of the contact phase of the coagulation pathway, and increases the resistance of platelets to damage from mechanical injury and high plasmin levels that occur during cardiopulmonary bypass.
Onset: immediate. **Peak:** Peak levels occur immediately after I.V. infusion.
Duration: plasma half-life, 2½ hours.

INDICATIONS & DOSAGE

To reduce blood loss or the need for transfusion in patients undergoing coronary artery bypass grafts –
Adults: start with a 1-ml test dose at least 10 minutes before the loading dose. If no allergic reaction is evident, anesthesia may be induced while the loading dose of 200 ml is given slowly over 20 to 30 minutes. When the loading dose is complete, sternotomy may be performed. Before bypass is initiated, prime the cardiopulmonary bypass circuit with 200 ml of drug by replacing an aliquot of the priming fluid with the drug. Give a continuous infusion at a rate of 50 ml/hour until the patient leaves the operating room.

ADVERSE REACTIONS

CV: ***cardiac arrest, CHF, MI, heart failure, ventricular tachycardia,*** atrial fibrillation, atrial flutter, hypotension, supraventricular tachycardia.
GU: nephrotoxicity
Respiratory: pneumonia, respiratory disorder, ***bronchospasm.***
Other: hypersensitivity reactions, ***anaphylaxis,*** fever.

INTERACTIONS

None significant.

CONTRAINDICATIONS

- Contraindicated in patients hypersensitive to beef because the drug is prepared from bovine lung.
- Use drug cautiously and monitor patients closely for hypersensitivity reaction. Patients may experience anaphylaxis after the full therapeutic dose even if they remained asymptomatic after the test dose. If symptoms of hypersensitivity occur (skin eruptions, itching, dyspnea, nausea, tachycardia), discontinue the infusion immediately and provide supportive treatment.

NURSING CONSIDERATIONS

- Patients with a history of allergies to drugs or other substances may be at higher risk of developing an allergic reaction to aprotinin.
- Test dose is particularly important in patients who have previously received the drug because they have a higher risk of anaphylaxis. In such patients, pretreatment with an antihistamine is recommended.
- Monitor patients for increased serum creatinine levels and other signs of nephrotoxicity. If nephrotoxicity occurs, it is usually mild and reversible.
- Aprotinin will increase levels for activated clotting time and PTT. It may increase CK and transaminase levels and may falsely prolong whole blood clotting times when determined by surface activation methods, such as the Hemachron method.
- **I.V. use:** Aprotinin is incompatible with amino acids, corticosteroids, fat emulsions, heparin, and tetracyclines. Don't add any drugs to the I.V. container and use a separate I.V. line.
- Administer all doses through a central line.
- To avoid hypotension, make sure patients are supine when the loading dose is given.
- Store between 2° and 25° C (36° and 77° F). Protect from freezing.

benzoyl peroxide cleansers

Benzac W Wash 5, Benzac W Wash 10, Desquam-X 5 Wash, Desquam-X 10 Wash, Fostex 10% BPO Cleansing◇, Fostex 10% BPO Wash◇, Oxy-10 Wash◇, PanOxyl 5◇, PanOxyl 10◇

benzoyl peroxide creams

Acne-Aid◇, Clearasil Maximum Strength◇, Cuticura Acne◇ Fostex 10% BPO Tinted◇, Oxy 10 Cover◇

benzoyl peroxide gels

5 Benzagel, 10 Benzagel, Benzac 5, Benzac W 5, Benzac W 10, Benzac W 2 ½, Ben-Aqua 5, Ben-Aqua 10, Buf-Oxal 10◇, Clear By Design◇, Del Aqua 5◇, Del Aqua 10◇, Desquam-E, Desquam-X 5, Desquam-X 10, Desquam-X 2.5, Fostex 5% BPO◇, Fostex 10% BPO◇, PanOxyl 5, PanOxyl 10, PanOxyl AQ 5, PanOxyl AQ 10, PanOxyl AQ 2 ½, Persa-Gel, Persa-Gel W 5%, Persa-Gel W 10%, Xerac BP5◇, Xerac BP10◇, Zeroxin-5, Zeroxin-10

benzoyl peroxide lotions

Acne-10◇, Ben-Aqua 5◇, Benoxyl 5◇, Benoxyl 10◇, Clearasil 10◇, Loroxide◇, Oxy 5◇, Oxy 10◇, Vanoxide◇

Pregnancy Risk Category: C

HOW SUPPLIED

Cream: 5%◇, 10%◇
Gel: 2.5%◇, 5%◇, 10%◇
Liquid cleanser: 5%, 10%◇
Lotion: 5%◇, 5.5%◇, 10%◇
Soap (bar): 5%◇, 10%◇

ACTION

Mechanism: Antimicrobial and comedolytic activity. Mechanism is unknown.
Onset: variable.

INDICATIONS & DOSAGE

Acne –
Adults and children: apply once daily to q.i.d., depending on tolerance and effect.

ADVERSE REACTIONS

Skin: stinging on application, warmth, painful irritation, pruritus, vesicles, allergic contact dermatitis.

INTERACTIONS

Abrasives, medical soaps and cleansers, acne preparations and preparations containing peeling agents, topical alcohol preparations (including cosmetics, after-shave, cologne): cumulative irritation of skin or excessive drying of skin. Use together cautiously.

CONTRAINDICATIONS

- Contraindicated in patients sensitive to the drug or any its components.

NURSING CONSIDERATIONS

- Initiate therapy with 2.5% or 5% preparation; change to 10% strength after 3 to 4 weeks or as tolerance develops.
- Patients with fair skin or patients living in very dry climates should begin with one application daily.
- Tell patients to wash face thoroughly 20 to 30 minutes before applying.
- Warn patients not to use near eyes, on mucous membranes, or on denuded or highly inflamed skin.
- Warn patients that drug may bleach hair or clothing.
- Dryness, redness, and peeling should occur 3 to 4 days after starting treatment. Tell patients to discontinue temporarily if these common reactions cause considerable discomfort.
- Advise patients to discontinue use if painful irritation or vesicles develop.

calcipotriene

Dovonex

Pregnancy Risk Category: C

HOW SUPPLIED

Ointment: 0.005%

ACTION

Mechanism: A synthetic vitamin D_3 analogue that regulates the development and production of skin cells.
Onset: within 2 weeks. **Peak:** Marked improvement noted after 8 weeks.

INDICATIONS & DOSAGE

Moderate plaque psoriasis –
Adults: apply a thin layer to the affected area b.i.d. Rub in gently and completely.

ADVERSE REACTIONS

Skin: *burning, pruritus, irritation,* atrophy, dermatitis, dry skin, erythema, folliculitis, hyperpigmentation, peeling, rash, worsening of psoriasis.
Other: hypercalcemia.

INTERACTIONS

None significant.

CONTRAINDICATIONS

- Contraindicated in patients hypersensitive to the drug or any components in the preparation. Also contraindicated in patients with hypercalcemia or evidence of vitamin D toxicity.
- Use cautiously in breastfeeding patients.
- Use cautiously in elderly patients; they may experience more severe adverse skin reactions.

NURSING CONSIDERATIONS

- Tell patients to discontinue the drug and call the doctor if the drug irritates lesions or surrounding uninvolved skin.
- Advise patients not to use the drug on the face, in the eyes, orally, or vaginally. Tell them to wash their hands after applying the ointment.
- Advise patients to apply only a thin layer of the ointment. Transient elevations of serum calcium have been reported, especially when excess dosage is applied.

capsaicin

Axsain◊, Zostrix◊

Pregnancy Risk Category: C

HOW SUPPLIED

Cream: 0.025%◊ (Zostrix◊), 0.075%◊ (Axsain◊)

ACTION

Mechanism: May deplete substance P, the principal neurotransmitter for pain, in peripheral type C sensory fibers. Exact mechanism unknown.
Onset: within minutes.

INDICATIONS & DOSAGE

Temporary relief of pain after herpes zoster infections –
Adults and children 2 years and over: 0.025% cream applied to affected areas not more than q.i.d.
Neuralgias, such as postsurgical pain and painful diabetic neuropathy; pain associated with osteoarthritis or rheumatoid arthritis –
Adults and children over 2 years: 0.075% cream applied to affected areas not more than q.i.d.

ADVERSE REACTIONS

Skin: redness, *stinging or burning on application.*

INTERACTIONS

None significant.

CONTRAINDICATIONS

- Contraindicated in patients hypersensitive to the drug.

NURSING CONSIDERATIONS

- Avoid getting drug in eyes or on broken skin.
- Transient burning or stinging with application is usually evident at initial therapy but will decrease with cautious use. However, this effect will persist in patients who use the drug less frequently than three times a day.
- Do not bandage area tightly after applying drug.
- Tell patients who are self-medicating with capsaicin to contact the doctor if symptoms persist beyond 2 to 4 weeks or resolve and shortly reappear.
- Tell patients to wash hands after applying drug.

cisapride

Propulsid

Pregnancy Risk Category: C

HOW SUPPLIED

Tablets: 10 mg

ACTION

Mechanism: Stimulates serotonin-4 (5-HT_4) receptors, enhancing the release of acetylcholine at the myenteric plexus and increasing GI motility.

Onset: 30 to 60 minutes. **Peak:** Plasma levels peak within 1 to 1½ hours. **Duration:** terminal half-life, 6 to 12 hours.

INDICATIONS & DOSAGE

Symptoms of nocturnal heartburn caused by gastroesophageal reflux disease –

Adults: initially, 10 mg P.O. q.i.d. 15 minutes before meals and h.s. If response is inadequate, increase to 20 mg q.i.d.

ADVERSE REACTIONS

CNS: *headache.*

CV: tachycardia.

GI: *diarrhea, abdominal pain,* nausea, constipation, flatulence, dyspepsia.

GU: frequency, urgency, vaginitis.

Respiratory: rhinitis, sinusitis, cough.

Skin: rash, pruritus.

Other: flulike symptoms, pain, fever.

INTERACTIONS

Anticholinergics: decreased effectiveness of cisapride. Avoid concomitant use.

Anticoagulants: may increase clotting times. Monitor closely.

Benzodiazepines, ethanol: enhanced sedation. Avoid concomitant use.

Cimetidine, ranitidine: increased absorption of these agents; cimetidine increases cisapride levels. Use together cautiously.

CONTRAINDICATIONS

- Contraindicated in patients hypersensitive to the drug. Also contraindicated in patients in whom increased GI motility may be harmful, such as those with mechanical obstruction, hemorrhage, or perforation of the GI tract.
- Use cautiously in breastfeeding patients because small amounts of the drug are excreted in breast milk.

NURSING CONSIDERATIONS

- Remind patients to avoid alcohol and sedatives while using this drug.
- Advise patients to immediately report any adverse effects to their doctor.

clomiphene citrate

Clomid

Pregnancy Risk Category: X

HOW SUPPLIED

Tablets: 50 mg

ACTION

Mechanism: Appears to stimulate release of pituitary gonadotropins, folli-

cle-stimulating hormone, and luteinizing hormone. This results in maturation of the ovarian follicle, ovulation, and development of the corpus luteum.
Onset: 4 days; however, may take several cycles before ovulation occurs.

INDICATIONS & DOSAGE
To induce ovulation –
Adults: 50 to 100 mg P.O. daily for 5 days, starting any time; or 50 to 100 mg P.O. daily starting on day 5 of menstrual cycle (first day of menstrual flow is day 1). Repeat until conception occurs or until three courses of therapy are completed.

ADVERSE REACTIONS
CNS: headache, restlessness, insomnia, dizziness, light-headedness, depression, fatigue, tension.
CV: hypertension.
EENT: blurred vision, diplopia, scotoma, photophobia.
GI: nausea, vomiting, bloating, distention, increased appetite, weight gain.
GU: urinary frequency and polyuria; ovarian enlargement and cyst formation, which regress spontaneously when drug is stopped.
Skin: urticaria, rash, dermatitis.
Other: *hot flashes,* reversible alopecia, *breast discomfort, hyperglycemia.*

INTERACTIONS
None significant.

CONTRAINDICATIONS
- Contraindicated in patients with undiagnosed abnormal genital bleeding, ovarian cyst, hepatic disease or dysfunction, or a history of thrombophlebitis or thromboembolism.
- Use cautiously in patients with hypertension, mental depression, migraines, seizures, diabetes mellitus, and gonadotropin sensitivity. Report development or worsening of these conditions to doctor; may require stopping drug.

NURSING CONSIDERATIONS
- Tell patients there is a possibility of multiple births with this drug. Risk increases with higher doses.
- Teach patients to take and chart basal body temperature to ascertain whether ovulation has occurred.
- Advise patients to stop drug and contact the doctor immediately if abdominal symptoms or pain occurs because these may indicate ovarian enlargement or ovarian cyst.
- Reassure patients that ovulation generally occurs after the first course of therapy. If pregnancy does not occur, course of therapy may be repeated twice.
- Advise patients to stop drug and contact the doctor immediately if pregnancy is suspected because the drug may have teratogenic effect.
- Tell patients to report signs of impending visual toxicity – blurred vision, diplopia, scotoma, or photophobia – to the doctor immediately.
- Drug may cause dizziness or visual disturbances. Warn patients to avoid hazardous activities such as driving or operating machinery until CNS effects are known.

diazoxide, oral
Proglycem
Pregnancy Risk Category: C

HOW SUPPLIED
Capsules: 50 mg
Oral suspension: 50 mg/ml in 30-ml bottle

ACTION
Mechanism: Inhibits release of insulin from the pancreas and decreases peripheral utilization of glucose.
Onset: 1 hour. **Duration:** 8 hours.

INDICATIONS & DOSAGE
Hypoglycemia from a variety of conditions resulting in hyperinsulinism –
Adults and children: 3 to 8 mg/kg P.O. daily, in three equally divided doses q 8 hours.
Infants and neonates: 8 to 15 mg/kg P.O. daily, in two or three equally divided doses q 8 to 12 hours.

ADVERSE REACTIONS
CV: arrhythmias.
EENT: diplopia.
GI: nausea, vomiting, anorexia, taste alteration.
Hematologic: leukopenia, thrombocytopenia.
Other: *severe hypertrichosis (hair growth) in 25% of adults and higher percentage of children; sodium and fluid retention, ketoacidosis and hyperosmolar nonketotic syndrome, hyperuricemia.*

INTERACTIONS
Alpha-adrenergic blockers: antagonism of diazoxide inhibition of insulin release. Avoid concomitant use.
Anticoagulants: increased anticoagulant effect. Adjust dosage of anticoagulant.
Antigout agents: increased serum uric acid. Adjust dosage of antigout agent.
Antihypertensive agents, peripheral vasodilators: additive hypotensive effects. Monitor blood pressure.
Beta-adrenergic blockers: increased hypotensive effect. Monitor blood pressure.
Hydantoin anticonvulsants: decreased anticonvulsant effects and decreased hyperglycemic effect of diazoxide. Don't use together.
Thiazide diuretics: may potentiate hyperglycemic, hyperuricemic, and hypotensive effects. Monitor appropriate laboratory values.

CONTRAINDICATIONS
- Contraindicated in patients hypersensitive to thiazides and in patients with functional hypoglycemia.

NURSING CONSIDERATIONS
- Oral diazoxide does not significantly lower blood pressure in the dosages used to treat hypoglycemia.
- Drug's most important use is to manage hypoglycemia from hyperinsulinism in infants and children.
- Monitor urine regularly for glucose and ketones; report any abnormalities to the doctor.
- If not effective after 2 or 3 weeks, drug should be stopped.
- Reassure patients that hair growth on arms and forehead is a common adverse reaction that subsides when drug treatment is completed.
- Explain importance of following dietary restrictions for successful therapy.
- Advise patients to report to the doctor any adverse reactions, including excessive thirst, fruity breath odor, or urinary frequency.

etretinate
Tegison
Pregnancy Risk Category: X

HOW SUPPLIED
Capsules: 10 mg, 25 mg

ACTION
Mechanism: Inhibits ornithine decarboxylase, an enzyme that regulates cell growth and differentiation. May also block neutrophil migration into the epidermis.
Onset: initial response, 8 to 16 weeks.

INDICATIONS & DOSAGE
Severe recalcitrant psoriasis, including erythrodermia and generalized pustular types in patients unresponsive to standard therapy (topical tar plus

UVB light, psoralens plus UVA light, systemic corticosteroids, and methotrexate) – **Adults:** initially, 0.75 to 1 mg/kg P.O. daily in divided doses. Maximum initial dosage is 1.5 mg/kg daily. After initial response, begin maintenance dosage of 0.5 to 0.75 mg/kg daily.

ADVERSE REACTIONS

CNS: *benign intracranial hypertension (pseudotumor cerebri), fatigue, headache,* dizziness, lethargy.
CV: thrombosis, edema.
EENT: *eye pain, blurred vision, dry eyes,* photosensitivity, decreased night vision.
GI: *appetite change, nausea, sore tongue, chapped lips, dry mouth.*
Hematologic: ***blood dyscrasia,*** anemia, altered PT.
Hepatic: ***hepatitis,*** elevated liver enzymes.
GU: *WBCs in urine,* proteinuria, hematuria.
Respiratory: dyspnea.
Skin: *peeling, pruritus.*
Other: *bone pain, hypokalemia or hyperkalemia, hyperlipidemia.*

INTERACTIONS

Ethanol: increased risk of hypertriglyceridemia. Avoid concomitant use.
Hepatotoxic medications (including methotrexate): increased risk of hepatotoxicity. Monitor closely.
Tetracyclines: increased risk of pseudotumor cerebri. Avoid concomitant use.
Vitamin A: additive toxic effects. Avoid concomitant use.

CONTRAINDICATIONS

- Contraindicated in patients who are pregnant, who intend to become pregnant, or who may not use reliable contraception during and after treatment (drug causes severe birth defects).

NURSING CONSIDERATIONS

- Women of childbearing age must not receive etretinate unless pregnancy is excluded by a pregnancy test within 2 weeks before initiating therapy. Therapy may begin on second or third day of next normal menstrual period.
- Warn patients to use effective contraception for 1 month before therapy begins, during treatment, and for an indefinite time after treatment is discontinued.
- Significant residual blood levels of etretinate have been reported as long as 2.9 years after discontinuation of treatment. Consequently, the period of time after treatment during which pregnancy must be avoided to prevent teratogenicity is unknown.
- Monitor liver function tests every 1 to 2 weeks for the first 1 to 2 months of therapy, and every 1 to 3 months thereafter. Suspected hepatotoxicity requires discontinuation of etretinate.
- Monitor blood lipids every 1 to 2 weeks during treatment.
- Advise patients to take drug with milk or fatty food to enhance absorption.
- Advise patients never to double the dose. Tell them to take a missed dose as soon as possible. If it's nearly time for the next dose, skip missed dose and resume schedule.
- Tell patients to report possible early signs of pseudotumor cerebri – headache, nausea and vomiting, and visual disturbances – to the doctor promptly. If these reactions are present, immediately check for papilledema. If present, discontinue drug immediately.
- Advise diabetic patients to monitor blood glucose closely. Adjustments of hypoglycemic medications may be necessary.
- Warn patients not to take vitamin A supplements, to avoid possible additive adverse reactions.
- Reassure patients that transient ex-

acerbation of psoriasis is common during beginning of therapy.

- Advise patients to expect dry skin and possible difficulty tolerating contact lenses during treatment.
- Tell patients to avoid excess bright sun and to use a sunblock to prevent photosensitivity reactions.
- Advise patients to report visual difficulties.
- Advise patients to use ice or sugarless hard candy or gum for dry mouth and to check with the dentist if this continues beyond 2 weeks.

finasteride

Proscar

Pregnancy Risk Category: X

HOW SUPPLIED

Tablets: 5 mg

ACTION

Mechanism: Competitively inhibits steroid 5α-reductase, an enzyme responsible for formation of the potent androgen 5α-dihydrotestosterone (DHT) from testosterone. Because DHT influences development of the prostate gland, decreasing levels of this hormone in adult males should relieve the symptoms associated with benign prostatic hyperplasia (BPH).

Peak: Serum levels peak within 2 to 6 hours.

INDICATIONS & DOSAGE

Symptomatic BPH –

Adults: 5 mg P.O. daily.

ADVERSE REACTIONS

GU: impotence, decreased volume of ejaculate.

Other: decreased libido.

INTERACTIONS

Theophylline: may increase theophylline clearance and decrease theophylline half-life. Monitor theophylline levels.

CONTRAINDICATIONS

- Contraindicated in patients hypersensitive to the drug, in pregnant and breastfeeding patients, and in children.
- Use cautiously in patients with hepatic dysfunction because drug is metabolized extensively in the liver. No dosage adjustments are necessary in patients with renal impairment; decreased urinary excretion of metabolites is associated with increased excretion of metabolites in the feces.

NURSING CONSIDERATIONS

- Although drug's elimination rate is decreased in elderly patients, dosage adjustments aren't necessary.
- Baseline and periodic digital rectal examinations are recommended. Drug will decrease serum prostate-specific antigen (PSA) levels, even in prostate cancer. However, in clinical trials, drug didn't appear to decrease the rate of prostate cancer detection.
- Before therapy, closely evaluate patients for conditions that might mimic BPH, including hypotonic bladder; prostate cancer, infection, or stricture; or relevant neurologic conditions.
- Carefully evaluate sustained increases in serum PSA levels, which could indicate noncompliance with therapy.
- Because it's impossible to identify which patients will respond to finasteride, a minimum of 6 months of therapy may be necessary.
- Carefully monitor patients who have a large residual urine volume or severely diminished urine flow; these patients may not be candidates for finasteride therapy.
- Long-term effects on the complications of BPH, including acute urinary obstruction, and incidence of surgery are unknown.
- Warn women who are or may become pregnant not to handle crushed

tablets because of risk of adverse effects on a male fetus.

- Caution patients whose sexual partner is or may become pregnant to discontinue drug or take precautions to avoid exposing her to his semen.
- Reassure patients that finasteride may decrease volume of ejaculate but doesn't appear to impair normal sexual function. However, impotence and decreased libido have occurred in less than 4% of patients.
- Drug's effectiveness as adjuvant therapy after radical prostatectomy, as adjuvant treatment of prostate cancer, and as treatment of male pattern baldness, acne, and hirsutism is currently under investigation.

gallium nitrate

Ganite

Pregnancy Risk Category: C

HOW SUPPLIED

Injection: 25 mg/ml

ACTION

Mechanism: Appears to reduce hypercalcemia by inhibiting resorption of bone and reducing bone turnover in patients with increased bone turnover. Exact mechanism unknown.
Onset: within 48 hours. **Duration:** 4 to 14 days.

INDICATIONS & DOSAGE

Symptomatic, unresponsive hypercalcemia caused by cancer –
Adults: 200 mg/m^2 as a continuous I.V. infusion daily for 5 consecutive days or until serum calcium is normal. Lower doses (100 mg/m^2) may be given to patients with mild hypercalcemia.

ADVERSE REACTIONS

CNS: lethargy, confusion.
CV: tachycardia, lower extremity edema, decreased mean systolic and diastolic blood pressures.
EENT: visual or hearing impairment, acute optic neuritis.
GI: nausea and vomiting, diarrhea, constipation.
GU: ***acute renal failure,*** *increased BUN and creatinine levels.*
Hematologic: anemia, leukopenia.
Respiratory: dyspnea, crackles and rhonchi, pulmonary infiltrates, pleural effusion.
Other: *hypophosphatemia, hypocalcemia, decreased serum bicarbonate.*

INTERACTIONS

Nephrotoxic drugs, such as aminoglycosides or amphotericin B: increased risk of nephrotoxicity. Avoid concomitant use.

CONTRAINDICATIONS

- Contraindicated in patients with severe renal impairment. Keep in mind association of hypercalcemia with decreased renal function in cancer patients. Drug should *not* be used in patients with asymptomatic hypercalcemia (generally, serum calcium levels of less than 12 mg/dl).

NURSING CONSIDERATIONS

- Make sure that patients are adequately hydrated, either with oral fluids or I.V. sodium chloride solution, before using drug and during infusion. Establish adequate urine flow (2 liters/day) before treatment. Diuretic therapy is not recommended before correction of hypovolemia. Avoid overhydration, especially in patients with decreased CV function.
- **I.V. use:** Dilute daily dose in 1 liter of 0.9% sodium chloride injection or D_5W. Discard unused portion (drug contains no preservatives).
- Rapid I.V. infusion or dosage over 200 mg/m^2 may increase risk of nephrotoxicity or cause nausea and vomiting.
- Monitor renal function, including fluid intake and output and BUN and serum creatinine levels, during ther-

apy. Discontinue drug if serum creatinine rises above 2.5 mg/dl.

- Monitor serum calcium levels, and assess patients for signs of hypocalcemia, including a positive Chvostek's sign. If hypocalcemia occurs, discontinue drug. Treatment of hypocalcemia may be required.
- Overdosage is usually treated with vigorous hydration, sometimes with diuretics, for 2 to 3 days. Carefully monitor fluid intake and output and renal function. Short-term therapy with I.V. calcium may also be needed.
- If patients require treatment with a potentially nephrotoxic drug, such as an aminoglycoside, discontinue gallium nitrate therapy and continue hydration for several days after administration of the nephrotoxic drug. Monitor renal function closely.
- Transient hypophosphatemia is common. Patients may require oral phosphorus supplements.
- Advise patients to report hearing or vision problems. In early clinical trials, a few patients experienced hearing loss and optic neuritis after high-dose gallium nitrate therapy when combined with investigational antineoplastic agents.

isotretinoin

Accutane, Roaccutane‡

Pregnancy Risk Category: X

HOW SUPPLIED

Capsules: 10 mg, 20 mg, 40 mg

ACTION

Mechanism: Normalizes keratinization, reversibly decreases size of sebaceous glands, and alters composition of sebum to a less viscous form that is less likely to cause follicular plugging.

Peak: Plasma levels peak in about 3 hours.

INDICATIONS & DOSAGE

Severe cystic acne unresponsive to conventional therapy –

Adults and adolescents: 0.5 to 2 mg/kg P.O. daily in two divided doses for 15 to 20 weeks.

ADVERSE REACTIONS

CNS: headache, fatigue, *pseudotumor cerebri* (benign intracranial hypertension).

EENT: *conjunctivitis,* corneal deposits, dry eyes, visual disturbances.

GI: nonspecific GI symptoms, gum bleeding and inflammation, nausea, vomiting.

Hematologic: anemia, elevated platelet count.

Hepatic: elevated AST, ALT, and alkaline phosphatase levels.

Skin: *cheilosis, rash, dry skin,* peeling of palms and toes, skin infection, photosensitivity.

Other: *hypertriglyceridemia, musculoskeletal pain (skeletal hyperostosis),* thinning of hair, hyperglycemia.

INTERACTIONS

Ethanol: increased risk of hypertriglyceridemia. Avoid concomitant use.

Tetracyclines: increased risk of pseudotumor cerebri. Avoid concomitant use.

Vitamin A, products containing vitamin A: increased toxic effects of isotretinoin. Don't use together without the doctor's permission.

CONTRAINDICATIONS

- Contraindicated in women of childbearing age unless patient has had a negative serum pregnancy test within 2 weeks before beginning therapy; will begin drug therapy on second or third day of next menstrual period; and will comply with stringent contraceptive measures for 1 month before therapy, during therapy, and for at least 1 month after therapy. *Severe fetal abnormalities may occur if used during pregnancy.*

• Also contraindicated in patients hypersensitive to parabens, which are used as preservatives.

NURSING CONSIDERATIONS

• Monitor serum lipid studies and liver function tests before therapy begins and then at regular intervals until response to drug is established, usually about 4 weeks.
• Monitor blood glucose regularly.
• Monitor CK levels in patients who participate in vigorous physical activity.
• Most adverse reactions appear to be dose-related, occurring at dosages greater than 1 mg/kg daily. They are generally reversible when therapy is discontinued or dosage is reduced.
• Patients who experience headache, nausea and vomiting, or visual disturbances should be screened for papilledema. Signs and symptoms of pseudotumor cerebri require immediate discontinuation of therapy and prompt neurologic intervention.
• A second course of therapy, if needed, shouldn't be started until at least 8 weeks after completion of first course because improvement may continue after withdrawal of drug.
• Warn patients that contact lenses may feel uncomfortable during isotretinoin therapy.
• Warn patients against using abrasives, medicated soaps and cleansers, acne preparations containing peeling agents, and topical alcohol preparations (including cosmetics, aftershave, cologne) because these agents cause cumulative irritation or excessive drying of skin.
• Drug may have additive effect if used with other agents that cause photosensitivity. Tell patients to avoid prolonged exposure to the sun and to use sunblock.
• Tell patients to immediately report any visual disturbances and bone, muscle, or joint pain.
• Advise patients to take drug with or shortly after meals to ensure adequate absorption.

levocarnitine (L-carnitine)

Carnitor, Vitacarn

Pregnancy Risk Category: B

HOW SUPPLIED

Tablets: 330 mg
Capsules: 250 mg
Oral liquid: 100 mg/ml

ACTION

Mechanism: Facilitates transport of fatty acids into cellular mitochondria. The fatty acids are then used to produce energy.
Peak: Plasma levels peak within 2 to 4 hours.

INDICATIONS & DOSAGE

Primary systemic carnitine deficiency –
Adults: 990 mg (three tablets) P.O. b.i.d. or t.i.d. Alternatively, 10 to 30 ml (1 to 3 g) of oral liquid daily.
Children: 50 to 100 mg/kg/day P.O. in divided doses of either the tablet, capsule, or oral liquid.

All dosages depend on the clinical response. Higher dosages may be given. However, for children, maximum dosage is 3 g/day.

ADVERSE REACTIONS

GI: *nausea, vomiting, cramps, diarrhea.*
Other: body odor.

INTERACTIONS

D,L-carnitine (sold as vitamin B_T): inhibition of levocarnitine and possible deficiency. Avoid concomitant use.
Valproic acid: increased requirement for carnitine. Adjust dosage as ordered.

CONTRAINDICATIONS

None reported.

NURSING CONSIDERATIONS

- Monitor patient's tolerance during first week of therapy and after increasing dosage.
- Monitor blood chemistries and plasma carnitine concentrations periodically, as well as vital signs and patient's overall clinical condition.
- Give enteral liquid alone or dissolved in drinks or liquid food.
- Space doses evenly every 3 to 4 hours and give drug with or after meals, if possible.
- Use entire or partial contents of containers of liquid immediately after opening; discard any unused contents.
- Do not refrigerate solution.
- Tell patients to consume oral liquid slowly to minimize GI distress. If GI intolerance persists, dosage may have to be reduced.
- Warn patients to avoid "vitamin B_T" in health food stores. This will interact with the drug and render it ineffective.
- Caution patients not to share drug with others. Some people have used it to improve athletic performance.

levomethadyl acetate hydrochloride

ORLAAM

Controlled Substance Schedule II

Pregnancy Risk Category: C

HOW SUPPLIED

Oral solution: 10 mg/ml

ACTION

Mechanism: A synthetic opiate agonist structurally similar to methadone that suppresses symptoms of withdrawal in opiate-tolerant individuals by cross-substituting for opiate agonists. Long-term administration may produce sufficient tolerance to block the euphoric effects of opiate agonists.

Onset: 2 to 4 hours. **Duration:** 48 to 72 hours.

INDICATIONS & DOSAGE

Opiate addiction –

Adults: dosage is highly individualized. Initially, 20 to 40 mg three times a week. Increase subsequent doses in increments of 5 to 10 mg until steady state is reached, usually within 1 week. Most patients are stable on 60 to 90 mg three times a week. Maximum dosage is 140 mg three times a week.

ADVERSE REACTIONS

CNS: drowsiness, sedation.

CV: bradycardia, edema, prolonged QT interval.

EENT: blurred vision, rhinitis.

GI: *abdominal pain, diarrhea, constipation, dry mouth, nausea, vomiting.*

GU: *impotence, difficulty with ejaculation.*

Respiratory: *cough.*

Skin: *rash, diaphoresis.*

Other: yawning, arthralgia, asthenia, back pain, chills, flulike syndrome, malaise, abstinence syndrome with sudden withdrawal.

INTERACTIONS

Carbamazepine, phenobarbital, phenytoin, rifampin: increased hepatic enzyme activity; may increase levomethadyl's peak activity or shorten its duration of action. Monitor closely.

Cimetidine, erythromycin, ketoconazole: decreased hepatic enzyme activity; may decrease levomethadyl's peak activity or prolong its duration of action. Monitor closely.

Naloxone; pentazocine or other opioid agonist-antagonists: may precipitate abstinence syndrome. Don't use together.

CONTRAINDICATIONS

- Contraindicated in patients hypersensitive to the drug.
- Use cautiously in patients with cardiac conduction defects or with hepatic or renal failure.

NURSING CONSIDERATIONS

- Levomethadyl is to be used only by certain licensed and approved clinics. There are no recognized clinical uses for the drug outside of addiction treatment programs. Levomethadyl may only be dispensed by treatment programs approved by the FDA, DEA, and designated state authority. By law, take-home doses of levomethadyl are forbidden.
- This drug should never be administered on a daily basis because of the risk of fatal overdose.
- If administering to women of childbearing age, monthly pregnancy tests are recommended. Patients should be switched to methadone if pregnancy occurs.
- When used to replace methadone, the suggested initial dose is 1.2 to 1.3 times the daily methadone dose three times a week, not to exceed 120 mg. Adjust dosage according to clinical response. The crossover to methadone should be done in a single dose rather than decreasing doses of methadone and increasing doses of levomethadyl.
- Most patients can tolerate the 72-hour interval between weekly regimens. If withdrawal is a problem during the 72-hour interval, increase the preceding dose or switch to an alternate-day schedule. Never give levomethadyl on 2 consecutive days; instead, give small supplemental doses of methadone. Consider the risk of drug diversion before giving patients take-home methadone.

masoprocol

Actinex

Pregnancy Risk Category: B

HOW SUPPLIED

Cream: 10%

ACTION

Mechanism: Antiproliferative activity against keratinocytes in vitro. Exact mechanism unknown.
Onset: several days.

INDICATIONS & DOSAGE

Actinic (solar) keratoses –
Adults: apply a sufficient amount of cream to cover area b.i.d., in morning and evening, for 28 days.

ADVERSE REACTIONS

EENT: eye irritation.
Skin: *erythema, flaking, dryness, pruritus, burning, soreness,* bleeding, crusting, blistering, oozing, rash, irritation, stinging, tightness, tingling.

INTERACTIONS

None significant.

CONTRAINDICATIONS

- Contraindicated in patients hypersensitive to the drug or any component of the formulation. Drug contains sulfites, which may cause allergic reactions in sensitive individuals.
- Use cautiously near the eyes because drug may cause pain and burning if it comes into contact with them. If such contact occurs, rinse with plenty of water.

NURSING CONSIDERATIONS

- Instruct patients to wash and dry the area, then gently massage in the cream (avoiding eyes and mucous membranes of nose and mouth) until evenly distributed; and to wash hands after applying drug with fingers. Tell them not to use occlusive dressings or to apply makeup or any other skin product without their doctor's approval.
- Local skin reactions are common but don't interfere with drug's effectiveness. Explain to patients that these reactions will clear within 2 weeks of discontinuing drug. However, if se-

vere reactions occur, such as oozing or blistering, patients should discontinue drug and contact their doctor immediately.

• Warn patients to avoid unnecessary exposure to sun to prevent actinic (solar) kercatoses. Advise patients to wear protective clothing and to use sunblock.

mesalamine

Rowasa, Pentasa

Pregnancy Risk Category: B

HOW SUPPLIED

Capsules: 250 mg
Rectal suspension: 4 g/60 ml
Suppositories: 500 mg

ACTION

Mechanism: an active metabolite of sulfasalazine; probably acts topically by inhibiting prostaglandin production in the colon. Exact mechanism unknown.
Onset: up to 3 weeks.

INDICATIONS & DOSAGE

Active mild to moderate distal ulcerative colitis, proctitis, or proctosigmoiditis –
Adults: 1 g P.O. q.i.d or 500 mg P.R. (suppository) b.i.d., or 4 g as a retention enema once daily (preferably h.s.). Rectal dosage form should be retained overnight (for about 8 hours). Usual course of therapy is 3 to 6 weeks.

ADVERSE REACTIONS

CNS: headache, dizziness, fatigue, malaise.
GI: abdominal pain, cramps, discomfort, flatulence, diarrhea, rectal pain, bloating, nausea, *pancolitis.*
Skin: itching, rash, urticaria, hair loss.
Other: wheezing, ***anaphylaxis*** (rare), fever.

INTERACTIONS

None significant.

CONTRAINDICATIONS

• Contraindicated in patients hypersensitive to the drug, its components, or salicylates.
• Use cautiously in patients with renal impairment. Problems have not been documented, but nephrotoxic potential from absorbed mesalamine exists.

NURSING CONSIDERATIONS

• Because it contains potassium metabisulfite, mesalamine may cause hypersensitivity reactions in patients sensitive to sulfites.
• Patients intolerant of sulfasalazine may also be hypersensitive to mesalamine; instruct patients to discontinue drug if they experience a fever or rash.
• Monitor periodic renal function studies in patients on long-term mesalamine therapy.
• Instruct patients to carefully follow instructions supplied with medication.

mesna

Mesnex

Pregnancy Risk Category: B

HOW SUPPLIED

Injection: 100 mg/ml

ACTION

Mechanism: Prevents ifosfamide-induced hemorrhagic cystitis by reacting with urotoxic ifosfamide metabolites.
Onset: immediate. **Peak:** Serum levels peak immediately.

INDICATIONS & DOSAGE

Prophylaxis of hemorrhagic cystitis in patients receiving ifosfamide –
Adults: dosage varies with amount of ifosfamide administered. Usual dosage is 240 mg/m² as an I.V. bolus w

administration of ifosfamide. Repeat dosage at 4 hours and 8 hours after administration of ifosfamide.

ADVERSE REACTIONS

GI: soft stools, nausea, vomiting, diarrhea, dysgeusia.

Note: Because mesna is used concomitantly with ifosfamide and other chemotherapeutic agents, it is difficult to determine adverse reactions attributable solely to mesna.

INTERACTIONS

None significant.

CONTRAINDICATIONS

- Contraindicated in patients hypersensitive to mesna or thiol-containing compounds.

NURSING CONSIDERATIONS

- Monitor urine samples daily in patients receiving mesna for hematuria.
- Up to 6% of patients may not respond to drug's protective effects.
- Mesna is not effective in preventing hematuria from other causes (such as thrombocytopenia).
- Although formulated to prevent hemorrhagic cystitis from ifosfamide, it will not protect against other toxicities associated with ifosfamide therapy.
- Mesna may interfere with diagnostic tests for urine ketones.
- **I.V. use:** Prepare I.V. solution by diluting commercially available ampules with D_5W solution, dextrose 5% and 0.9% sodium chloride injection, 0.9% sodium chloride injection, or lactated Ringer's solution.
- Mesna I.V. is incompatible with cisplatin.
- Diluted solutions are stable for 24 hours at room temperature; however, refrigerate after preparation and use within 6 hours. After opening ampule, discard any unused drug because it decomposes quickly into an inactive compound.

methoxsalen (topical)

Oxsoralen-Ultra

Pregnancy Risk Category: C

HOW SUPPLIED

Lotion: 1%

ACTION

Mechanism: May enhance melanogenesis, either directly or secondarily, to an inflammatory process.

Onset: 1 to 2 hours. **Duration:** 6 to 8 hours; effects may persist for 2 days.

INDICATIONS & DOSAGE

To induce repigmentation in vitiligo; psoriasis –

Adults and children over 12 years: apply lotion to small, well-defined vitiliginous lesions, allow to dry 1 to 2 minutes, and then reapply 2 to 2½ hours before measured periods of long-wave ultraviolet exposure. After exposure, wash lesions with soap and water and protect area with sunblock. Although manufacturer recommends weekly treatment, some doctors may treat q 3 to 5 days.

ADVERSE REACTIONS

Skin: edema, erythema, painful blistering, burning, peeling, pruritus.

INTERACTIONS

Photosensitizing agents: may increase methoxsalen toxicity. Don't use together.

CONTRAINDICATIONS

- Contraindicated in patients sensitive to psoralen compounds and in patients with porphyria, acute lupus erythematosus, xerodoma, melanoma, skin cancer, or hydromorphic and polymorphic light eruptions.
- Use cautiously in patients with familial history of sunlight allergy, GI diseases, or chronic infection.

NURSING CONSIDERATIONS

- Regulate therapy carefully. Overdosage or overexposure to light can cause serious burning or blistering. Tell patients to avoid excessive sunlight during therapy.
- Protect patient's eyes and lips during light exposure treatments.
- Monthly liver function tests should be done on patients with vitiligo (especially at beginning of therapy).

minoxidil (topical)

Rogaine

Pregnancy Risk Category: C

HOW SUPPLIED

Topical solution: 2%

ACTION

Mechanism: Stimulates hair growth, possibly by dilating arterial microcapillaries around hair follicles.

Onset: 4 months. **Duration:** up to a few months after discontinuing therapy.

INDICATIONS & DOSAGE

Male pattern baldness (alopecia androgenetica) of the vertex and scalp – **Adults:** apply 1 ml of 2% solution to affected area b.i.d. Maximum daily dosage is 2 ml.

ADVERSE REACTIONS

CNS: headache, dizziness, faintness, light-headedness.

CV: edema, chest pain, hypertension, hypotension, palpitations, increased or decreased pulse rate.

EENT: sinusitis.

GU: urinary tract infection, renal calculi, urethritis.

Respiratory: bronchitis, upper respiratory infection.

Skin: irritant dermatitis, allergic contact dermatitis, eczema, hypertrichosis, local erythema, pruritus, dry skin or scalp, flaking, alopecia, exacerbation of hair loss.

Other: back pain, tendinitis, edema, weight gain.

INTERACTIONS

Topical corticosteroids, petrolatum, topical retinoids, or other drugs that may enhance skin absorption: increased risk of systemic effects of minoxidil. Do not apply minoxidil with other drugs.

CONTRAINDICATIONS

- Contraindicated in patients hypersensitive to the drug or any component of the solution.

NURSING CONSIDERATIONS

- Patients need to have normal, healthy scalps before beginning therapy, because absorption of drug through irritated skin may cause adverse systemic effects.
- Treatment is most likely to succeed in patients with balding area smaller than 4″ (10 cm) that developed within the past 10 years.
- Advise patients with history of heart disease that drug may exacerbate their illness.
- Teach patients to monitor pulse rate and body weight.
- Advise patients of need for medical follow-ups 1 month after initiation of therapy and every 6 months thereafter.
- Teach patients how to apply topical minoxidil. Hair and scalp should be thoroughly dry before application, and drug should not be applied to any other body areas. Tell patients not to use drug on irritated or sunburned scalp, or with any other medication on scalp. Tell patients to thoroughly wash hands after application.
- Warn patients to avoid inhaling any spray or mist from drug. They should avoid spraying around eyes, because solution contains alcohol and may be irritating.
- Advise patients that therapy will be prolonged and will continue for at

least 4 months before clinical effects appear. About 40% of patients will see moderate to dense hair growth.

- Tell patients that discontinuing drug may result in loss of new hair growth. New hair growth is usually fine and may be colorless, but will resemble existing hair after continued treatment.

olsalazine sodium

Dipentum

Pregnancy Risk Category: C

HOW SUPPLIED

Capsules: 250 mg

ACTION

Mechanism: After oral administration, converts to 5-aminosalicylic acid (5-ASA or mesalamine) in the colon, where it has a local anti-inflammatory effect.
Peak: Serum levels peak in 30 to 90 minutes.

INDICATIONS & DOSAGE

Maintenance of remission of ulcerative colitis in patients intolerant of sulfasalazine –
Adults: 500 mg P.O. b.i.d. with meals.

ADVERSE REACTIONS

CNS: headache, depression, vertigo, dizziness.
GI: *diarrhea,* nausea, abdominal pain, heartburn.
Skin: rash, itching.
Other: arthralgia.

INTERACTIONS

None significant.

CONTRAINDICATIONS

- Contraindicated in patients hypersensitive to salicylates.
- Use cautiously in patients with preexisting renal disease. Although problems have not been reported with this drug, the possibility of renal tubular damage from absorbed mesalamine or its metabolites must be considered.

NURSING CONSIDERATIONS

- In clinical trials, 17% of all patients reported diarrhea during therapy. Although diarrhea appears dose-related, it is difficult to distinguish from worsening of disease symptoms. Exacerbation of disease has been noted with similar drugs.
- Regularly monitor BUN and creatinine levels and urinalysis in patients with preexisting renal disease.
- Teach patients to take drug in evenly divided doses and with food to minimize adverse GI reactions.

pamidronate disodium

Aredia

Pregnancy Risk Category: C

HOW SUPPLIED

Injection: 30 mg/vial

ACTION

Mechanism: An antihypercalcemic agent that inhibits resorption of bone. Adsorbs to hydroxyapatite crystals in bone and may directly block dissolution of calcium phosphate. Drug apparently doesn't inhibit bone formation or mineralization.
Onset: 1 to 2 days. **Duration:** 2 to 3 weeks.

INDICATIONS & DOSAGE

Moderate to severe hypercalcemia associated with cancer (with or without metastases) –
Adults: dosage depends on severity of hypercalcemia. Serum calcium levels should be corrected for serum albumin:

$$\text{Corrected serum calcium (CCa) (in mg/dl)} = \text{serum calcium (in mg/dl)} + 0.8\,(4 - \text{serum albumin (in g/dl)})$$

Patients with moderate hypercalcemia (CCa levels of 12 to 13.5 mg/dl) may receive 60 to 90 mg by I.V. infusion over 24 hours. Patients with severe hypercalcemia (CCa levels over 13.5 mg/dl) may receive 90 mg by I.V. infusion over 24 hours.

ADVERSE REACTIONS

CNS: ***seizures.***
CV: *fluid overload, hypertension.*
GI: *abdominal pain, anorexia, constipation, nausea, vomiting.*
GU: *urinary tract infection.*
Hematologic: *leukopenia, thrombocytopenia, anemia.*
Other: *hypophosphatemia, hypokalemia, hypomagnesemia, hypocalcemia, bone pain, fever, redness, swelling, pain.*

INTERACTIONS

None significant.

CONTRAINDICATIONS

- Contraindicated in patients hypersensitive to the drug or to other biphosphonates, such as etidronate.
- Use with extreme caution and consider the risks and benefits in patients with renal impairment.

NURSING CONSIDERATIONS

- Drug should be used only after patients have been vigorously hydrated with sodium chloride solution. In patients with mild to moderate hypercalcemia, hydration alone may be sufficient.
- Because drug can cause electrolyte disturbances, carefully monitor serum electrolytes, especially calcium, phosphate, and magnesium. Short-term administration of calcium may be necessary in patients with severe hypocalcemia. Also monitor creatinine level, CBC and differential, hematocrit, and hemoglobin.
- Carefully monitor patients with preexisting anemia, leukopenia, or thrombocytopenia during first 2 weeks of therapy.
- Monitor patient's temperature. In clinical trials, 27% of patients experienced an elevation of 1° C for 24 to 48 hours after therapy.
- **I.V. use:** Reconstitute vial with 10 ml of sterile water for injection. After drug is completely dissolved, add to 1,000 ml of 0.45% or 0.9% sodium chloride injection or D_5W. Do not mix with infusion solutions that contain calcium, such as Ringer's injection or lactated Ringer's injection. Visually inspect for precipitate before administering.
- Give only by I.V. infusion. Animal studies have shown evidence of nephropathy when drug is given as a bolus.
- Solution is stable for 24 hours at room temperature.

pentoxifylline

Trental

Pregnancy Risk Category: C

HOW SUPPLIED

Tablets (extended-release): 400 mg

ACTION

Mechanism: Improves capillary blood flow by increasing RBC flexibility and lowering blood viscosity.
Onset: 2 to 4 weeks; clinical effects, at least 8 weeks. **Peak:** Serum levels peak within 2 to 4 hours but are not related to drug effect.

INDICATIONS & DOSAGE

Intermittent claudication caused by chronic occlusive vascular disease –
Adults: 400 mg P.O. t.i.d. with meals.

ADVERSE REACTIONS

CNS: headache, dizziness.
GI: dyspepsia, nausea, vomiting.

INTERACTIONS
Anticoagulants: increased anticoagulant effect. Adjust anticoagulant dosage as ordered.
Antihypertensives: increased hypotensive effect. Dosage adjustments may be necessary.

CONTRAINDICATIONS
• Contraindicated in patients who are intolerant to methylxanthines such as caffeine, theophylline, and theobromine.

NURSING CONSIDERATIONS
• Drug is useful in patients who are not good surgical candidates.
• Elderly patients may be more sensitive to drug's effects.
• Tell patients not to discontinue drug during the first 8 weeks of therapy unless directed by their doctor.
• Instruct patients to swallow medication whole, without breaking, crushing, or chewing.
• Advise patients to take with meals to minimize GI upset.
• Tell patients to report any GI or CNS adverse reactions; the doctor may reduce the dosage.
• Advise patients to avoid smoking because nicotine causes vasoconstriction that can worsen their condition.

ritodrine hydrochloride
Yutopar

Pregnancy Risk Category: B

HOW SUPPLIED
Tablets: 10 mg
Injection: 10-mg in 5-ml vial or ampule, 15 mg/ml in 10-ml vial

ACTION
Mechanism: A beta-receptor agonist that stimulates the $beta_2$-adrenergic receptors in uterine smooth muscle, inhibiting contractility.
Onset: 30 to 60 minutes after oral administration, 5 minutes after I.V. administration.

INDICATIONS & DOSAGE
Preterm labor–
Adults: dilute 150 mg (3 ampules) in 500 ml of fluid, yielding a final concentration of 0.3 mg/ml. Usual initial dose is 0.1 mg/minute I.V., to be gradually increased by 0.05 mg/minute q 10 minutes until desired result is obtained. Effective dosage usually ranges from 0.15 to 0.35 mg/minute.

Note: I.V. infusion should be continued for 12 to 24 hours after contractions have stopped. Oral maintenance: 10 mg approximately 30 minutes before termination of I.V. therapy. Usual dosage for first 24 hours of maintenance is 10 mg P.O. q 2 hours. Thereafter, usual dosage is 10 to 20 mg P.O. q 4 to 6 hours. Total daily dosage should not exceed 120 mg.

ADVERSE REACTIONS
Intravenous:
CNS: nervousness, anxiety, headache.
CV: *dose-related alterations in blood pressure, palpitations,* ***pulmonary edema,*** *tachycardia,* ECG changes.
GI: nausea, vomiting.
Other: erythema, *hyperglycemia,* hypokalemia.
Oral:
CNS: tremors, nervousness.
CV: palpitations.
GI: nausea, vomiting.
Skin: rash.

INTERACTIONS
Beta-adrenergic blockers: may inhibit ritodrine's action. Avoid concurrent use.
Corticosteroids: may produce pulmonary edema in mother. Monitor patient closely.
Inhalation anesthetics: potentiated adverse cardiac effects, arrhythmias, and hypotension. Monitor patient closely.

Sympathomimetics: additive sympathomimetic effects. Use together cautiously.

CONTRAINDICATIONS

- Contraindicated in pregnant women before 20th week of pregnancy and in women with antepartum hemorrhage, eclampsia, intrauterine fetal death, chorioamnionitis, maternal cardiac disease, pulmonary hypertension, maternal hyperthyroidism, or uncontrolled maternal diabetes mellitus.

NURSING CONSIDERATIONS

- Monitor blood glucose concentrations during infusion, especially in diabetic mother.
- **I.V. use:** Because cardiovascular responses are common and more pronounced during I.V. administration, closely monitor cardiovascular effects – including maternal pulse rate and blood pressure, and fetal heart rate. Maternal tachycardia of over 140 beats/minute or persistent respiratory rate of over 20 breaths/minute may be a sign of impending pulmonary edema.
- Discontinue drug if pulmonary edema develops.
- Monitor amount of fluids administered I.V. to prevent circulatory overload.
- Don't use ritodrine I.V. if solution is discolored or contains a precipitate.

sodium benzoate and sodium phenylacetate

Ucephan

Pregnancy Risk Category: C

HOW SUPPLIED

Oral solution: 10 g sodium benzoate and 10 g sodium phenylacetate per 100 ml

ACTION

Mechanism: Activates metabolic pathways that are ineffective in patients with urea cycle enzymopathies, resulting in decreased ammonia formation.
Onset: variable.

INDICATIONS & DOSAGE

Prevention or treatment of hyperammonemia in patients with urea cycle enzymopathy –
Children: 2.5 ml/kg P.O. daily in three to six equally divided doses. Maximum daily dosage is 100 ml.

ADVERSE REACTIONS

GI: nausea and vomiting.

INTERACTIONS

Penicillin, probenecid: may impair renal excretion of conjugated metabolites. Monitor the patient for toxicity.

CONTRAINDICATIONS

- Contraindicated in patients hypersensitive to sodium benzoate or sodium phenylacetate.
- Use cautiously in neonates with hyperbilirubinemia.

NURSING CONSIDERATIONS

- Drug may compete with bilirubin for binding sites on serum albumin.
- Drug is not intended as sole therapy for patients with urea cycle enzymopathies. It is most effective when combined with a low-protein diet and amino acid supplementation.
- Dilute each dose in 4 to 8 oz of infant formula or milk and administer with meals. Inspect mixture for compatibility if other liquids are used. Drug may precipitate in some solutions, especially acidic solutions such as fruit juice, depending on concentration and pH.
- Carefully measure required dosage because stock solution is very concentrated.
- Avoid getting solution on skin or clothing; lingering odor of drug may be offensive.
- Drug is structurally similar to salic-

ylates. Watch for salicylate-associated adverse reactions, including mild respiratory alkalosis and exacerbation of peptic ulcerations.

strontium 89 (^{89}Sr) chloride

Metastron

Pregnancy Risk Category: D

HOW SUPPLIED

Injection: 4 millicuries (mCi)/10 ml

ACTION

Mechanism: Acts as a calcium analogue that is actively taken up by bone, particularly in areas of active osteogenesis such as metastatic bone tumors. The drug locally irradiates tissue with beta radiation.
Onset: rapidly taken up by bone within hours of injection. **Peak:** Pain relief typically takes 7 to 20 days.
Duration: physical half-life, 50½ days; strontium turnover, about 14 days in normal bone, and longer in metastatic lesions.

INDICATIONS & DOSAGE

Relief of bone pain in patients with painful metastatic lesions –
Adults: 4 mCi by slow I.V. injection over 1 to 2 minutes.

ADVERSE REACTIONS

CV: cutaneous flushing with rapid injection.
Hematologic: ***bone marrow suppression.***
Other: transient increase in pain ("flare" reaction).

INTERACTIONS

Calcium supplements: decreased strontium 89's effectiveness. Discontinue calcium supplements about 2 weeks before strontium-89 administration.
Cytotoxic agents: additive bone marrow suppression. Monitor closely.

CONTRAINDICATIONS

- Contraindicated in breast-feeding patients and in patients with severe bone marrow suppression.
- Use cautiously in patients with platelet counts below 60,000/mm^3 or WBC counts below 2,400/mm^3.
- Because the drug is a potential carcinogen, use should be restricted to patients with documented metastatic bone cancer.

NURSING CONSIDERATIONS

- Because of the delayed onset of pain relief, this drug should not be used in patients with a short life expectancy.
- Frequently assess the degree of pain relief after administration of the drug. During the first week, a transient increase in pain may necessitate a dosage increase in concomitantly administered analgesics. Pain relief from strontium 89 usually occurs after 2 to 3 weeks. In clinical trials, over 75% of patients received substantial pain relief, allowing a reduction or elimination of opiate analgesics.
- Advise women of childbearing age to avoid becoming pregnant while taking this drug.
- Follow institutional safety measures to minimize radiation exposure. Urinary excretion of radiation is greatest during the first 2 days after administration.
- Teach patients proper radiation precautions; tell them to flush the toilet twice, wipe any spilled urine with a tissue that is subsequently flushed, and immediately launder any linens soiled with blood or urine during the first few days after treatment. Make sure patients understand that the drug has a low level of radioactivity and that they will pose no risk to family members.
- Consider placing an indwelling urinary catheter in incontinent patients to minimize contaminating the environment with radiation.

ticlopidine hydrochloride

Ticlid

Pregnancy Risk Category: B

HOW SUPPLIED

Tablets: 250 mg

ACTION

Mechanism: An antiplatelet agent that blocks adenosine diphosphate-induced platelet-fibrinogen and platelet-platelet binding.

Onset: 6 hours. **Peak:** Effects peak after 3 to 5 days. **Duration:** 24 to 48 hours.

INDICATIONS & DOSAGE

To reduce risk of thrombotic stroke in patients with history of stroke or who have experienced stroke precursors –
Adults: 250 mg P.O. b.i.d. with meals.

ADVERSE REACTIONS

CNS: dizziness, anorexia.
CV: vasculitis.
EENT: epistaxis, conjunctival hemorrhage.
GI: *diarrhea, nausea, dyspepsia,* vomiting, flatulence, *pain,* bleeding, light-colored stools.
GU: hematuria, ***nephrotic syndrome,*** dark-colored urine.
Hematologic: neutropenia, ***pancytopenia, hemolytic anemia, immune thrombocytopenia.***
Hepatic: hepatitis, cholestatic jaundice.
Respiratory: *allergic pneumonitis.*
Skin: *rash,* purpura, pruritus, ecchymosis, maculopapular rash, urticaria, thrombocytopenic purpura, subcutaneous bleeding.
Other: hypersensitivity reactions, postoperative bleeding, systemic lupus erythematosus, ***serum sickness,*** arthropathy, myositis, ***hyponatremia,*** *increased serum cholesterol levels,* peripheral neuropathy.

INTERACTIONS

Antacids: decreased plasma ticlopidine levels. Separate administration times by at least 2 hours.
Aspirin: effects of aspirin on platelets potentiated. Avoid concomitant use.
Cimetidine: decreased clearance of ticlopidine and increased risk of toxicity. Avoid concomitant use.
Digoxin: slight decrease in serum digoxin levels. Monitor serum digoxin levels.
Theophylline: decreased theophylline clearance and risk of toxicity. Monitor closely and adjust theophylline dosage as ordered.

CONTRAINDICATIONS

• Contraindicated in patients hypersensitive to the drug; in patients with hematopoietic disorders, such as neutropenia, thrombocytopenia, or disorders of hemostasis; in patients with active pathologic bleeding, such as peptic ulceration or active intracranial bleeding; and in those with severe hepatic impairment.
• Use cautiously and with close monitoring of CBC and WBC differentials. Moderate to severe neutropenia and agranulocytosis have occurred in patients taking ticlopidine, usually within the first 3 weeks to 3 months of therapy.

NURSING CONSIDERATIONS

• Determine CBC and WBC differentials at the second week of therapy and repeat every 2 weeks until end of third month. Increase frequency of tests in patients showing signs of declining neutrophil count or if count is 30% less than baseline. After first 3 months of therapy, CBC and WBC differential determinations should be performed only in patients showing signs of infection.
• Thrombocytopenia has occurred rarely. Drug should be discontinued in patients having a platelet count of 80,000/mm³ or less. If necessary, give

methylprednisolone 20 mg I.V. to normalize bleeding time within 2 hours. Platelet transfusions may also be used.
- Monitor baseline liver function tests and repeat whenever liver dysfunction is suspected. Monitor closely, especially during first 4 months of treatment.
- If ticlopidine is being substituted for a fibrinolytic or anticoagulant, tell patients to discontinue those drugs before starting ticlopidine therapy.
- Advise patients to discontinue drug 10 to 14 days before undergoing elective surgery.
- Stress importance of regular blood tests. Because neutropenia can result in increased risk of infection, tell patients to immediately report any signs of infection, such as fever, chills, or sore throat.
- Also tell patients to immediately report yellow skin or sclera, severe or persistent diarrhea, skin rashes, subcutaneous bleeding, light-colored stools, or dark urine.
- Explain to patients that drug will prolong the bleeding time and that any unusual or prolonged bleeding should be reported. Advise patients to tell dentists and other doctors that they are taking ticlopidine.
- Tell patients to avoid aspirin and aspirin-containing products and to check with their doctor or pharmacist before taking any OTC medications.
- Tell patients to take drug with meals; this substantially increases bioavailability and improves GI tolerance.
- Used investigationally to treat intermittent claudication, chronic arterial occlusion, subarachnoid hemorrhage, primary glomerulonephritis, and sickle cell disease.
- When used preoperatively, ticlopidine may decrease incidence of graft occlusion in patients receiving coronary artery bypass grafts and reduce severity of drop in platelet count in patients receiving extracorporeal hemoperfusion during open heart surgery.

tiopronin
Thiola

Pregnancy Risk Category: C

HOW SUPPLIED
Tablets: 100 mg

ACTION
Mechanism: Forms a water-soluble chemical complex with cysteine in the urine, increasing cysteine solubility and preventing formation of urinary cysteine stones.
Onset: variable.

INDICATIONS & DOSAGE
Prevention of urinary cysteine stone formation in patients with severe homozygous cysteinuria (urinary cysteine excretion exceeding 500 mg/day) unresponsive to other therapies –
Adults: 800 mg P.O. daily, divided t.i.d.
Children: 15 mg/kg P.O. daily, divided t.i.d.

ADVERSE REACTIONS
GI: hypogeusia.
Skin: rash, pruritus, wrinkling, friability.
Other: drug fever, lupus erythematosus-like reaction.

INTERACTIONS
None significant.

CONTRAINDICATIONS
- Contraindicated in patients with a history of agranulocytosis, aplastic anemia, or thrombocytopenia.

NURSING CONSIDERATIONS
- The following conservative measures to treat cysteinuria should be attempted before tiopronin is administered. Patients should drink at least 3

*Liquid form contains alcohol.
**May contain tartrazine.

Common reactions are in italics; ***life-threatening,*** in bold italics.

liters of fluid daily, including at least two 8-oz glasses of water at each meal and at bedtime. Urine output should be at least 3 liters daily, and urine pH should be 6.5 to 7. Excessive alkalization of urine may precipitate calcium stones. Urine pH should not exceed 7.

- Dosage is usually adjusted to keep urine cysteine levels below 250 mg/L.
- Monitor CBC, platelet counts, hemoglobin, serum albumin, liver function tests, 24-hour urine protein, and routine urinalysis at 3- to 6-month intervals during treatment.
- Frequently monitor urine cysteine during first 6 months of treatment to identify optimal dosage level and then at least every 6 months.
- Drug fever may develop, especially during first month of therapy. Expect drug to be discontinued until fever subsides and to be reinstituted at lower dosages.
- Generalized rash with mild pruritus that develops in first few months of therapy may be controlled with antihistamines and will disappear after discontinuing the drug. A rash accompanied by intense pruritus may appear on the trunk after 6 months of therapy. This rash disappears slowly after discontinuing drug.
- Whenever possible, have patients take tiopronin at least 1 hour before or 2 hours after meals.
- Advise patients to have annual abdominal X-ray to assess for presence of stones.
- Tell patients to report any signs or symptoms of hematologic abnormalities, including fever, sore throat, bleeding or bruising, and chills. Blood dyscrasias have been reported in patients receiving other drugs for cysteinuria.
- Studies indicate that about two-thirds of patients who cannot tolerate penicillamine will tolerate tiopronin.

tretinoin (vitamin A acid, retinoic acid)

Retin-A, StieVAA†

Pregnancy Risk Category: B

HOW SUPPLIED

Cream: 0.025%, 0.05%, 0.1%
Gel: 0.025%, 0.01%
Solution: 0.05%

ACTION

Mechanism: Inhibits comedones by increasing epidermal cell mitosis and turnover.
Onset: beneficial effects, within 6 weeks.

INDICATIONS & DOSAGE

Acne vulgaris (especially grades I, II, and III), fine wrinkles from photodamaged skin –
Adults and children: clean affected area and lightly apply solution once daily h.s.

ADVERSE REACTIONS

Skin: *feeling of warmth, slight stinging, local erythema, peeling,* chapping, swelling, blistering, crusting, temporary hyperpigmentation or hypopigmentation.

INTERACTIONS

Topical preparations containing sulfur, resorcinol, or salicylic acid: increased risk of skin irritation. Don't use together.

CONTRAINDICATIONS

- Contraindicated in patients hypersensitive to any tretinoin component.
- Use cautiously in patients with eczema.

NURSING CONSIDERATIONS

- Patients should not discontinue the drug if it causes transient exacerbation of inflammatory lesions. If severe local irritation develops, discontinue temporarily and readjust dosage when application is resumed. Some redness and scaling are normal reactions.

- Relapses generally occur within 3 to 6 weeks after therapy is stopped.
- Instruct patients to clean area thoroughly before application and to avoid getting drug in eyes, mouth, or mucous membranes.
- Tell patients to wash face with mild soap no more than two or three times a day. Warn against using strong or medicated cosmetics, soaps, or other skin cleansers. Also advise patients to avoid topical products containing alcohol, astringents, spices, and lime because these may interfere with drug.
- Instruct patients to minimize exposure to sunlight or ultraviolet rays during treatment. If patients become sunburned, delay therapy until sunburn subsides. Tell patients who can't avoid exposure to sunlight to use SPF 15 sunblock and to wear protective clothing.
- Warn patients that they may experience increased sensitivity to wind or cold temperatures.

100
Investigational drugs

amsacrine
azacytidine
docetaxel
domperidone
famciclovir
flunarizine hydrochloride
fluvoxamine
halofantrine
hexoprenaline sulfate
ketotifen fumarate
metformin
mifepristone
perindopril
riluzole
semustine
stavudine
tolrestat
trimebutine maleate
varicella vaccine
vindesine sulfate

COMBINATION PRODUCTS
None.

amsacrine (m-AMSA)
Amsidyl†
Pregnancy Risk Category: C

HOW SUPPLIED
Injection: 50 mg/ml†

ACTION
Intercalates DNA and inhibits DNA synthesis, producing a cytotoxic effect.

INDICATIONS & DOSAGE
Ovarian cancer, lymphomas –
Adults: 30 to 50 mg/m²/day I.V. for 3 days, or 90 to 180 mg/m² as a single dose.
Acute myelogenous leukemia –
Adults: by 75 to 120 mg/m²/day for 5 days I.V. or by intra-arterial infusion.

ADVERSE REACTIONS
CNS: *seizures* at dosages as low as 40 mg/m²/day.
CV: *ventricular arrhythmias* (rare) and *cardiac arrest,* possibly caused by the diluent.
GI: infrequent and mild nausea and vomiting, stomatitis at higher doses.
Hematologic: *leukopenia* (usually dose-limiting), mild thrombocytopenia.
Hepatic: abnormal liver function tests.
Other: *local irritation and mild phlebitis.*

INTERACTIONS
None significant.

CONTRAINDICATIONS
- Contraindicated in patients hypersensitive to the drug.
- Use cautiously in patients with impaired hepatic function.

NURSING CONSIDERATIONS
- To prepare solution, add 1.5 ml of amsacrine from the ampule (50 mg/ml) to the vial containing 13.5 ml of lactic acid. The combined solution will contain 5 mg/ml of amsacrine and is stable for 48 hours at room temperature.
- Use glass syringes for combining the amsacrine and lactic acid. The diluent in the amsacrine may dissolve plastic syringes.
- The solution may be further diluted for infusion with D_5W to minimize vein irritation. Administer doses of less than 100 mg in at least 100 ml of D_5W, doses of 100 to 199 mg in 250 ml of D_5W, and doses of 200 mg or greater in a minimum of 500 ml of D_5W. Diluted solutions are stable for 48 hours at room temperature.

- Infuse solutions slowly over several hours to minimize vein irritation.
- Do not add amsacrine to 0.9% sodium chloride or other chloride-containing solutions or heparin. Precipitation may occur.
- Do not administer amsacrine through membrane-type in-line filters. The diluent may dissolve the filter.
- Inform the patient that the drug may turn the urine orange.
- Monitor CBC and liver function tests.
- Monitor patients closely for CNS and cardiac toxicity during administration.
- Avoid direct contact of amsacrine with skin to prevent possible sensitization.
- Preparation of parenteral form of the drug is associated with carcinogenic, mutagenic, and teratogenic risks for personnel. Follow institutional policy to reduce risks.

azacytidine (5-azacytidine)

HOW SUPPLIED

Injection: 100-mg vials

ACTION

Mechanism: An antimetabolite that disrupts the translation of nucleic acid sequences into protein.

INDICATIONS & DOSAGE

Acute lymphocytic and acute myelogenous leukemia –
Adults and children: 200 to 300 mg/m²/day I.V. for 5 to 10 days. Repeated at 2- to 3-week intervals.

ADVERSE REACTIONS

CNS: infrequent neurotoxicities, including generalized muscle pain and weakness.
CV: *hypotension* from rapid infusion.
GI: *severe nausea and vomiting, diarrhea.*
Hematologic: *leukopenia* (usually dose-limiting), *thrombocytopenia.*
Hepatic: hepatotoxicity (rare).
Other: drug fever.

INTERACTIONS

Myelosuppressants: additive myelosuppression. Monitor closely.

CONTRAINDICATIONS

- Contraindicated in patients hypersensitive to the drug and in those with liver disease.

NURSING CONSIDERATIONS

- Information is based on current literature and may change with further clinical experience.
- Instruct the patient to report any signs of neurotoxicity, such as muscle pain and weakness.
- Monitor temperature, CBC, and liver function tests.
- **I.V. use:** Reconstitute drug, using 19.9 ml of sterile water for injection. The final concentration will be 5 mg/ml. Dilute to a final concentration of 0.2 to 2 mg/ml using lactated Ringer's injection.
- After reconstitution, administer drug promptly.
- Give by slow I.V. infusion to prevent severe hypotension. Monitor blood pressure before infusion and at 30-minute intervals during infusion. If systolic blood pressure falls below 90 mm Hg, stop infusion and notify the doctor.
- Nausea and vomiting may be reduced with continuous infusions. Tolerance to nausea and vomiting develops during prolonged treatment.
- For stability reasons, azacytidine should be diluted only in lactated Ringer's solution.
- Drug may be given S.C. if necessary. Mix drug in a smaller quantity of diluent (3 to 5 ml for a 100-mg vial) for S.C. administration.

docetaxel

Taxotere

HOW SUPPLIED

Injection: 40 mg/ml in 50-ml vial

ACTION

Mechanism: Prevents depolymerization of cellular microtubules by inhibiting the normal reorganization of the microtubule network necessary for mitosis and other vital cellular functions.
Duration: elimination half-life, 12 to 18 hours.

INDICATIONS & DOSAGE

Ovarian cancer, small-cell and non-small-cell lung cancer, breast cancer –
Adults: 100 mg/m² I.V. once q 21 days.

ADVERSE REACTIONS

CNS: malaise, neuropathy.
CV: fluid retention, edema.
GI: *nausea, vomiting.*
Hematologic: ***neutropenia,*** *anemia, thrombocytopenia.*
Skin: macropapular eruptions, desquamation.
Other: mucositis, hypersensitivity reactions ***(anaphylaxis)*.**

INTERACTIONS

Myelosuppressants: possible additive toxicity. Use together cautiously.

CONTRAINDICATIONS

- Contraindicated in patients hypersensitive to the drug.

NURSING CONSIDERATIONS

- Information is based on current literature and may change with further clinical experience.
- Docetaxel is a semisynthetic derivative of paclitaxel. Docetaxel is made from the needles of the yew tree *Taxus baccata,* a readily renewable resource, while paclitaxel is extracted from the bark of *Taxus brevifolia.* Docetaxol is twice as potent as paclitaxel.
- Tell the patient to report signs of edema to the doctor.
- Pretreatment with diuretics is being studied to control fluid retention and edema.
- Docetaxol is being investigated to treat colon cancer and melanoma.
- **I.V. use:** Studies are underway to determine the most stable I.V. formulation of the drug. Check with the manufacturer for recommendations regarding dilution and admixture compatibility.
- Follow institutional protocol for the safe handling, preparation, and administration of chemotherapeutic drugs. Dispose of all waste materials properly.

domperidone

Motilium†‡

HOW SUPPLIED

Tablets: 10 mg†‡

ACTION

Mechanism: Blocks peripheral dopamine receptors, including those in the medullary chemoreceptor trigger zone (located outside the blood-brain barrier). In the GI tract, it enhances motility in the stomach and small intestine.

INDICATIONS & DOSAGE

Symptoms of upper GI motility disorders associated with gastritis and diabetic gastroparesis; prevention of nausea and vomiting caused by antiparkinsonian medications –
Adults: 10 mg P.O. t.i.d. to q.i.d. 30 minutes before meals and h.s. Maximum dosage is 20 mg P.O. q.i.d.

ADVERSE REACTIONS
CNS: headache.
GI: dry mouth.
Other: galactorrhea, gynecomastia, menstrual irregularities, hot flashes, rash.

INTERACTIONS
Antacids, histamine$_2$-antagonists: may impair absorption of domperidone. Separate administration times.
Anticholinergic agents: decreased domperidone effectiveness. Avoid concomitant use.
Orally administered drugs: altered GI motility, possibly impairing absorption of orally administered drugs. Dosage adjustments may be necessary.

CONTRAINDICATIONS
• Contraindicated in patients hypersensitive to the drug and in patients with mechanical obstruction of the GI tract or GI hemorrhage.

NURSING CONSIDERATIONS
• Information is based on current literature and may change with further clinical experience.
• Parenteral domperidone has also been tested as an antiemetic for patients receiving chemotherapy. Doses up to 1 mg/kg appear to be effective and well tolerated.

---

famciclovir
Famvir

Pregnancy Risk Category: B

HOW SUPPLIED
Tablets: 500 mg

ACTION
Mechanism: A guanosine nucleoside that is converted to penciclovir, which enters viral cells and inhibits DNA polymerase and viral DNA synthesis.
Peak: Plasma levels peak within 1 hour. **Duration:** plasma elimination half-life, 2 to 3 hours.

INDICATIONS & DOSAGE
Acute herpes zoster –
Adults: 500 mg P.O. q 8 hours.
In patients with reduced renal function: If creatinine clearance is greater than or equal to 60 ml/minute/1.73m^2, 500 mg P.O. q 8 hours; if 40-59 ml/minute/1.73m^2, 500 mg P.O. q 12 hours; if 20-39 ml/minute/1.73 m^2, 500 mg P.O. q 24 hours.

ADVERSE REACTIONS
CNS: *headache,* fatigue.
GI: diarrhea, *nausea.*

INTERACTIONS
Probenecid: may increase plasma concentrations of famciclovir. Monitor patient for increased adverse effects.

CONTRAINDICATIONS
• Contraindicated in patients hypersensitive to the drug.

NURSING CONSIDERATIONS
• Information is based on current literature and may change with further clinical experience.
• Famciclovir may be taken without regard to meals.
• Teach patients how to prevent spread of infection to others.
• Urge patients to recognize the early symptoms of herpes infection, such as tingling, itching, or pain. Treatment is more effective if therapy is started within 48 hours of rash onset.

---

flunarizine hydrochloride
Sibelium†

HOW SUPPLIED
Capsules: 5 mg†

ACTION
Mechanism: A calcium channel blocker that blocks the entry of calcium ions into specialized channels within the membrane of smooth muscle cells. Unlike many other calcium channel blockers, flunarizine doesn't affect the SA or AV node of the heart and doesn't cause peripheral vasodilation. Drug also has weak antihistamine activity.

INDICATIONS & DOSAGE
Prophylaxis of vascular headache –
Adults: 10 mg P.O. daily, in the evening.

ADVERSE REACTIONS
CNS: *drowsiness, sedation, fatigue,* depression, extrapyramidal symptoms, sleep disturbances, insomnia, anxiety, dizziness, vertigo.
GI: nausea, vomiting, heartburn, discomfort, dry mouth.
Other: *weight gain, increased appetite,* asthenia, muscle aches, rash.

INTERACTIONS
Mephenytoin, other anticonvulsants: lowered steady-state levels of mephenytoin and other anticonvulsants. Monitor anticonvulsant blood levels.
Oral contraceptives: possible galactorrhea. Monitor closely.

CONTRAINDICATIONS
- Contraindicated in patients hypersensitive to the drug and in those with Parkinson's disease, other preexisting extrapyramidal disorders, or a history of mental depression.
- Use cautiously in patients with hepatic failure. Elderly patients may require lower dosages.

NURSING CONSIDERATIONS
- Information is based on current literature and may change with further clinical experience.
- Drug is used to reduce the frequency of migraine attacks. To a lesser extent, it reduces the severity of the attack; it doesn't appear to change duration. Make sure patients understand that flunarizine isn't useful for treating acute attacks and that daily use is necessary for best drug effect.
- Sedation or drowsiness may occur, especially at the start of therapy. Tell patients to avoid hazardous activities that require alertness, such as driving, until CNS effects of the drug are known.
- Extrapyramidal symptoms may develop during therapy. Elderly patients are particularly at risk. Advise patients to report movement or coordination disturbances to the doctor.

fluvoxamine
Luvox

ACTION
Mechanism: Inhibits the CNS neuronal uptake of serotonin. Not a tricyclic derivative; considered an atypical antidepressant.
Peak: Plasma levels peak in 2 to 8 hours after an oral dose. **Duration:** elimination half-life, 15 hours.

INDICATIONS & DOSAGE
Depression –
Adults: 50 to 100 mg P.O. daily.

ADVERSE REACTIONS
CNS: *somnolence, headache, agitation, insomnia, tremor, hypokinesia, asthenia, anorexia, dizziness, syncope.*
GI: *nausea, vomiting, constipation, dry mouth.*

INTERACTIONS
Propranolol, warfarin: possible increased serum levels of these drugs. Monitor closely and adjust dosage as ordered.

CONTRAINDICATIONS
- Contraindicated in patients hypersensitive to the drug.
- Use cautiously in patients at high risk for suicide.

NURSING CONSIDERATIONS
- Information is based on current literature and may change with further clinical experience.
- Drug may also be effective in the treatment of obsessive-compulsive disorders and panic attacks, and in improving memory in patients with alcohol amnestic disorder (Korsakoff's syndrome).
- Like other antidepressants, maximum benefit may not be seen for 4 weeks or more after the initiation of therapy.

halofantrine
Halfan

ACTION
Mechanism: Halofantrine, a phenanthrenemethanol derivative structurally similar to mefloquine, is an antimalarial agent that is active against multidrug-resistant *Plasmodium falciparum.*

INDICATIONS & DOSAGE
P. falciparum *malaria –*
Adults and children over 40 kg: 500 mg P.O. q 6 hours for three doses. A second course of therapy may be recommended after 7 days.

ADVERSE REACTIONS
GI: *abdominal pain, vomiting, diarrhea.*
Skin: pruritus, rash.

INTERACTIONS
None significant.

CONTRAINDICATIONS
- Contraindicated in patients hypersensitive to the drug.

NURSING CONSIDERATIONS
- Information is based on current literature and may change with further clinical experience.
- Drug's effectiveness in treating *P. ovale, P. vivax,* or *P. malariae* infections hasn't been determined.
- Drug absorption after oral administration is erratic and variable. Diet, genetic factors, and racial factors may also influence bioavailability of the drug.

hexoprenaline sulfate
Delaprem

ACTION
Mechanism: A beta$_2$-selective adrenergic agonist that stimulates uterine beta$_2$ receptors, resulting in a decrease in the frequency or intensity of uterine muscle contractions.

INDICATIONS & DOSAGE
Tocolysis in preterm labor –
Adults: Individualize dosage. Some studies employed I.V. bolus injections of 7.5 mcg, resulting in decreased uterine activity within 13 minutes, lasting about 33 minutes. Other studies used continuous I.V. infusion of 0.38 mcg/minute for 20 minutes.

ADVERSE REACTIONS
CV: tachycardia (maternal and fetal), supraventricular or ventricular arrhythmias, ***MI,*** hypotension.
Respiratory: ***pulmonary edema.***
Other: tremor, hyperglycemia, hypokalemia.

CONTRAINDICATIONS
- Contraindicated in patients hypersensitive to the drug.

NURSING CONSIDERATIONS
- Information is based on current literature and may change with further clinical experience.
- Hexoprenaline appears to cause

fewer adverse effects than currently used tocolytic agents, such as ritodrine or terbutaline.
• Closely monitor maternal and fetal heart rates during therapy.
• Drug has also been used to treat fetal heart rate disturbances, a measure of fetal distress, during labor. Increases in fetal heart rate probably aren't caused by a direct action of the drug because animal studies have shown that less than 1% of a dose crosses the placenta.

ketotifen fumarate
Zaditen

HOW SUPPLIED
Tablets: 1 mg
Capsules: 1 mg
Elixir: 1 mg/5 ml*

ACTION
Mechanism: Like cromolyn, ketotifen stabilizes mast cells. However, it has a number of other pharmacologic effects that may contribute to its action, including antihistamine, phosphodiesterase-inhibiting, and calcium channel blocking effects and possible activity on $beta_2$-adrenergic receptors.

INDICATIONS & DOSAGE
Asthma prophylaxis; allergic rhinitis and conjunctivitis –
Adults: 1 mg P.O. b.i.d. with food. May be increased to 2 mg b.i.d.

ADVERSE REACTIONS
CNS: sedation, tiredness, dizziness, headache, drowsiness.
GI: dry mouth, nausea.
Respiratory: exacerbation of asthma, ***bronchospasm, status asthmaticus.***
Other: increased appetite and weight gain.

INTERACTIONS
Alcohol: may potentiate adverse reactions. Avoid concomitant use.
Oral antidiabetic agents: reversible fall in platelet count. Avoid concomitant use.

CONTRAINDICATIONS
• Contraindicated in patients hypersensitive to the drug.

NURSING CONSIDERATIONS
• Information is based on current literature and may change with further clinical experience. Ketotifen is currently available in Europe.
• Long-term therapy is necessary for asthma prophylaxis. Studies lasting less than 4 weeks have not shown consistent benefits, but patients taking the drug for 3 months or more consider the drug effective.
• Warn patients to avoid hazardous activities that require alertness, such as operating heavy machinery or driving, until CNS effects of the drug are known.

metformin
Glucophage†

HOW SUPPLIED
Tablets: 500 mg†

ACTION
Mechanism: A substituted biguanide that produces its antidiabetic effects only in the presence of insulin. It facilitates insulin's action on peripheral receptor sites and may increase the number of insulin receptors. It has no effect on pancreatic beta cells.

INDICATIONS & DOSAGE
To control diabetes in stable, mild, nonketosis-prone type II diabetic patients –
Adults: initially, 500 mg P.O. t.i.d., preferably with food. Adjust dosage upward as necessary, not to exceed 2.5 g daily.

ADVERSE REACTIONS
GI: epigastric discomfort, nausea, vomiting, diarrhea, anorexia, metallic taste.
Other: *lactic acidosis.*

INTERACTIONS
Anticoagulants: may increase the elimination of oral anticoagulants. Monitor PT carefully during changes in metformin dosage.
Corticosteroids, diuretics, nicotinic acid, oral contraceptives: may produce hyperglycemia and reduce effectiveness of metformin therapy. Dosage adjustment may be necessary.

CONTRAINDICATIONS
• Contraindicated in patients hypersensitive to the drug; in those with insulin-dependent diabetes, a history of ketoacidosis, liver disease, lactic acidosis or a history of lactic acidosis, or renal dysfunction; during acute stress (surgery, severe infections, or trauma); in pregnant patients; and in patients undergoing pyelography or angiography, which may precipitate temporary oliguria.

NURSING CONSIDERATIONS
• Information is based on current literature and may change with further clinical experience.
• Lactic acidosis is a potentially fatal complication of biguanide therapy. Phenformin (DBI), a similar compound, was withdrawn from the U.S. market in the mid-1970s after it was associated with this adverse reaction. If vomiting occurs, drug should be discontinued immediately and the patient assessed for lactic acidosis.
• Drug should be discontinued 2 days before elective surgery or angiographic exams. Renal function should be assessed before drug is restarted.
• Metformin will not prevent the development of complications from diabetes mellitus.
• Advise the patient of the importance of good dietary management to control his diabetes. Metformin therapy should not be used in place of good diet.
• Advise the patient to take metformin with food to minimize gastric irritation.
• Warn the patient to avoid alcohol consumption while taking metformin to prevent elevation of blood lactate levels.
• Impaired absorption of vitamin B_{12} and folic acid has been reported in some patients on long-term therapy. Serum levels of these cofactors should be measured every 1 or 2 years.
• The drug should be temporarily discontinued once or twice a year to assess the need for continued therapy.

mifepristone (RU 486)
Mifegyne

ACTION:
Mechanism: Blocks progesterone and glucocorticoid receptors, but doesn't block estrogen or mineralocorticoid receptors. Has weak antagonist activity at androgen receptors.

INDICATIONS & DOSAGE
Early termination of pregnancy –
Adults: 600 mg P.O.
Postcoital contraception –
Adults: 600 mg P.O. within 3 days of unprotected intercourse.
Cushing's syndrome –
Adults: 20 mg/kg P.O. daily.

ADVERSE REACTIONS
CNS: headache.
GI: *abdominal pain, nausea, vomiting, diarrhea.*
GU: *excessive bleeding.*

CONTRAINDICATIONS
• Contraindicated in patients hypersensitive to the drug.

NURSING CONSIDERATIONS

- Information is based on current literature and may change with further clinical experience.
- When used as an abortifacient, drug should be used within 60 days of first missed period. Usually administered with a prostaglandin analogue, which will increase uterine activity.
- Drug has been used investigationally for tamoxifen-resistant breast cancer with evidence of progesterone receptors, open-angle glaucoma, and induction of labor.

perindopril

Aceon

HOW SUPPLIED

Tablets: 2 mg, 4 mg, 8 mg

ACTION

Mechanism: An ACE inhibitor that blocks the conversion of angiotensin I to angiotensin II, a potent vasoconstrictor.

INDICATIONS & DOSAGE

Hypertension –

Adults: initially, 4 mg P.O. once daily. Titrate dosage to a maximum of 16 mg daily.

ADVERSE REACTIONS

CNS: headache, mood disturbances, sleep disorder, dizziness, light-headedness.
GI: nausea, abdominal pain, diarrhea.
GU: impotence.
Respiratory: *cough.*
Other: increased serum potassium levels, rash.

INTERACTIONS

Diuretics, other antihypertensives: additive antihypertensive effects. Monitor closely.
Potassium supplements, potassium-sparing diuretics: risk of hyperkalemia. Avoid concomitant use.

CONTRAINDICATIONS

- Contraindicated in patients hypersensitive to the drug.
- Also contraindicated during pregnancy because other ACE inhibitors have been shown to cause fetal harm during the second and third trimesters.

NURSING CONSIDERATIONS

- Information is based on current literature and may change with further clinical experience.
- Instruct the patient to take the drug on an empty stomach because absorption may be reduced by food.
- Remind the patient to check with the doctor or pharmacist before taking any other prescription or OTC medications.
- Monitor the patient for development of cough and notify the doctor if it occurs.

riluzole

HOW SUPPLIED

Tablets: 50 mg

ACTION

Mechanism: Modulates the effects of the excitatory neurotransmitter glutamate in the CNS.

INDICATIONS & DOSAGE

Amyotrophic lateral sclerosis (ALS) –

Adults: 50 mg P.O. b.i.d.

ADVERSE REACTIONS

CNS: asthenia, depression, incoordination.
CV: increased blood pressure.
EENT: rhinitis.
GI: constipation, nausea, abdominal pain, dysphagia.
Respiratory: *respiratory disorders.*

Other: stiffness, fasiculations, mild hepatotoxicity.

INTERACTIONS
None significant.

CONTRAINDICATIONS
- Contraindicated in patients hypersensitive to the drug.

NURSING CONSIDERATIONS
- Information is based on current literature and may change with further clinical experience.
- Early studies indicate that the drug improves survival in patients with ALS. However, survival effects depend on the site of onset. Patients with bulbar-onset disease have a more positive drug response than those with limb-onset disease.
- Encourage the patient to continue drug therapy despite the mild adverse reactions.

semustine (methyl CCNU)

ACTION
Mechanism: A nitrosourea compound that probably acts as an alkylating agent. The drug cross-links DNA and also inhibits several key enzymatic processes.

INDICATIONS & DOSAGE
Advanced GI tumors, brain tumors, Hodgkin's and non-Hodgkin's lymphomas –
Adults: 150 to 200 mg/m^2 P.O. q 6 to 8 weeks.

ADVERSE REACTIONS
GI: *acute nausea and vomiting 2 to 6 hours after administration, anorexia.*
GU: renal toxicity.
Hematologic: *delayed thrombocytopenia* (about 4 weeks) *and leukopenia* (about 6 weeks). *Myelosuppression* may be cumulative.
Hepatic: elevated liver enzyme levels.
Respiratory: ***pulmonary fibrosis*** with prolonged use.

CONTRAINDICATIONS
- Contraindicated in patients hypersensitive to the drug.
- Use cautiously with other nephrotoxic drugs.

NURSING CONSIDERATIONS
- Monitor renal and liver function tests.
- Capsules are usually refrigerated but are stable for 1 year at room temperature. Avoid high temperatures and excessive moisture.
- To ensure absorption, give drug on an empty stomach.
- Monitor CBC for delayed myelosuppression, up to 4 weeks for the onset of thrombocytopenia and 6 weeks for leukopenia.

stavudine (2,3 didehydro-3-deoxythymidine, d4T)

Zerit

Pregnancy Risk Category: C

HOW SUPPLIED
Capsules: 15 mg, 20 mg, 30 mg, 40 mg

ACTION
Mechanism: A primidine nucleoside analogue that prevents replication of HIV by inhibiting the enzyme reverse transcriptase.
Duration: plasma elimination half-life, 1 to 1½ hours.

INDICATIONS & DOSAGE
Patients with advanced HIV infection who are intolerant or unresponsive to other antiviral therapies –
Adults: 40 mg P.O. q 12 hours.

*Liquid form contains alcohol.
**May contain tartrazine.

Common reactions are in italics; ***life-threatening,*** in bold italics.

ADVERSE REACTIONS
CNS: *peripheral neuropathy.*
Hematologic: bone marrow suppression.
Other: myalgia, hepatotoxicity.

INTERACTIONS
Myelosuppressants: additive myelosuppression. Avoid concomitant use.

CONTRAINDICATIONS
• Contraindicated in patients hypersensitive to the drug and in patients who have experienced peripheral neuropathy while taking other nucleoside analogues. Also contraindicated in patients with preexisting moderate to severe peripheral neuropathy, and in pregnant or breast-feeding patients.
• Use cautiously and with close monitoring in patients with advanced symptomatic HIV infection.

NURSING CONSIDERATIONS
• Information is based on current literature and may change with further clinical experience.
• Tell the patient that the drug may be taken without regard to meals.
• Periodically monitor CBC, serum levels of creatinine, AST, ALT, and alkaline phosphatase.
• Peripheral neuropathy appears to be the major dose-limiting adverse effect of stavudine. It may or may not resolve after drug is discontinued. Teach the patient signs and symptoms of peripheral neuropathy – pain, burning, aching, weakness, or pins and needles in the extremities – and tell him to report these immediately.
• Warn the patient not to take any other drugs for HIV or AIDS (especially from the "street") unless the doctor has approved them.
• Advise the patient that he cannot receive stavudine if he experienced peripheral neuropathy while receiving any other nucleoside analogue or if his treatment plan includes a cytotoxic antineoplastic agent.

tolrestat
Alderase

ACTION
Mechanism: Blocks the enzyme aldose reductase, preventing the intracellular formation of sorbitol from glucose and galactitol from galactose. This metabolic pathway is active in patients with diabetes and may be responsible for late diabetic complications.

INDICATIONS & DOSAGE
Prevention of late complications of diabetes, including diabetic retinopathy and neuropathy –
Adults: dosage not clearly established. Early studies have used 50 to 200 mg P.O. once or twice daily.

ADVERSE REACTIONS
CNS: dizziness.
Hepatic: elevated liver enzyme levels.
Skin: rash.

INTERACTIONS
Salicylates, tolbutamide: increased plasma levels of active tolrestat by displacing the drug from protein-binding sites. Avoid concomitant use.

CONTRAINDICATIONS
• Contraindicated in patients hypersensitive to the drug.

NURSING CONSIDERATIONS
• Information is based on current literature and may change with further clinical experience.
• Aldose reductase inhibitors have no effect on blood glucose, and patients must continue antidiabetic agents as instructed. The purpose of therapy is to prevent late complications of diabetes that may be secondary to chronic elevation of blood glucose levels.
• The benefits of tolrestat therapy

have been difficult to establish because of the slow onset of complications of diabetes. The drug was well tolerated in clinical trials.

trimebutine maleate

Modulon†

HOW SUPPLIED

Tablets: 100 mg†
Injection: 50 mg/5 ml†

ACTION

Mechanism: Acts on intestinal opiate and serotonin receptors to regulate normal intestinal motility.

INDICATIONS & DOSAGE

Symptomatic relief of irritable bowel syndrome –
Adults: 100 to 200 mg P.O. t.i.d. before meals.
Postoperative paralytic ileus –
Adults: 50 to 100 mg I.M. t.i.d. May also be given by slow I.V. push, or infused I.V. over 1 hour.

ADVERSE REACTIONS

CNS: dizziness, syncope, drowsiness, tiredness, headache.
CV: hypotension.
GI: constipation, diarrhea, nausea, vomiting, abdominal pain.

INTERACTIONS

Antihypertensives: possible excessive hypotension. Use together cautiously.
Tubocurarine: animal studies indicated that trimebutine maleate may prolong neuromuscular blockade of tubocurarine.

CONTRAINDICATIONS

- Contraindicated in patients hypersensitive to the drug.

NURSING CONSIDERATIONS

- Information is based upon current literature and may change with further clinical experience.
- **I.V. use:** Rapid I.V. injection may cause hypotension. Inject drug over 1 minute. I.V. infusions may be mixed with 0.9% sodium chloride solution or D_5W.

varicella vaccine

Varivax

Pregnancy risk category: X

ACTION

Mechanism: Prevents chickenpox by inducing the production of antibodies to varicella-zoster virus.
Onset: within 6 weeks. **Duration:** protective antibody levels persist for at least 6 years.

INDICATIONS & DOSAGE

Prevention of varicella-zoster (chickenpox) infections –
Adults and children: 0.5 ml S.C.

ADVERSE REACTIONS

Other: fever, injection site reactions (swelling, redness, pain, rash), varicella-like rash.

INTERACTIONS

Blood products, immune globulin: may inactivate vaccine. Avoid using these products 2 to 4 weeks before or 6 to 8 weeks after vaccination.
Immunosuppressants: risk of severe reactions to live-virus vaccines. Postpone routine vaccination.

CONTRAINDICATIONS

- Contraindicated in patients hypersensitive to the drug.
- Use cautiously in immunocompromised patients because they are at greater risk for varicella-related complications.

NURSING CONSIDERATIONS

- Information is based on current literature and may change with further clinical experience.
- Although this drug has been safely

and effectively used in combination with measles, mumps, and rubella vaccine, check with the manufacturer for current recommendations.

- In clinical trials, the vaccine was less effective in adults as compared to children.
- Studies are underway to determine the incidence of herpes zoster, which may occur following a latent period.
- The vaccine contains a live attenuated virus. There is some evidence that children who develop a rash may be capable of transmitting the virus.
- A Safety Study protocol program is available for children and adolescents (ages 12 to 17 years) with acute lymphocytic leukemia (ALL). Doctors can enroll patients in this program by contacting Biopharm Clinical Services at (215) 283-0897.

vindesine sulfate

Eldisine†

HOW SUPPLIED

Injection: 5-mg vials†

ACTION

Mechanism: Arrests mitosis in metaphase, blocking cell division.

INDICATIONS & DOSAGE

Acute lymphoblastic leukemia, breast cancer, malignant melanoma, lymphosarcoma, non-small-cell lung carcinoma –

Adults: 3 to 4 mg/m² I.V. q 7 to 14 days, or continuous I.V. infusion of 1.2 to 1.5 mg/m²/day for 5 days q 3 weeks.

ADVERSE REACTIONS

CNS: *paresthesia, decreased deep tendon reflex, muscle weakness.*

GI: *constipation, abdominal cramping,* nausea, vomiting.

Hematologic: *leukopenia, thrombocytopenia.*

Other: ***acute bronchospasm,*** *reversible alopecia,* jaw pain, fever with continuous infusions, *phlebitis,* necrosis on extravasation.

CONTRAINDICATIONS

- Contraindicated in patients hypersensitive to the drug.

NURSING CONSIDERATIONS

- **I.V. use:** Do not give as a continuous infusion unless patient has a central I.V. line.
- Avoid extravasation. Drug is a painful vesicant. Give 10 ml of 0.9% sodium chloride solution flush before administering drug to test vein patency and after giving drug to flush tubing.
- When reconstituted with the 10 ml of diluent provided or 0.9% sodium chloride solution, the drug is stable for 30 days if refrigerated.
- Do not mix vindesine with other drugs; compatibility with other drugs has not yet been determined.
- After administering, monitor the patient for life-threatening acute bronchospasm. If this occurs, notify the doctor immediately. Reaction most likely to occur in patients who are also receiving mitomycin.
- To prevent paralytic ileus, encourage the patient to drink fluids, increase ambulation, and use stool softeners.
- Instruct the patient to report any symptoms of neurotoxicity: numbness and tingling of extremities, jaw pain, constipation (may be an early symptom).
- Assess for depression of Achilles tendon reflex, footdrop or wristdrop, and slapping gait (late signs of neurotoxicity).
- To detect neuropathy, record the patient's signature before each course of therapy and observe for deterioration of handwriting.
- Monitor CBC.

Appendices and Index

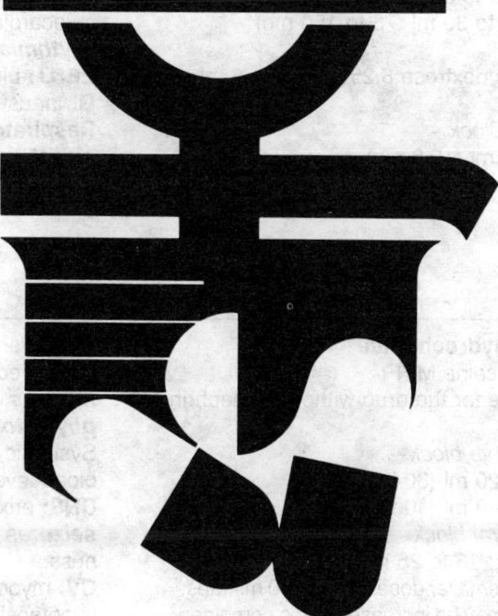

Anesthetics: Local, general, and topical ophthalmic

DRUG, INDICATIONS, DOSAGE	ADVERSE REACTIONS
Local	
bupivacaine HCl (Marcain‡, Marcaine, Sensorcaine) Dosages given are for the drug without epinephrine and for adults. *Epidural block–* 0.25% solution: 10 to 20 ml (25 to 50 mg) 0.5% solution: 10 to 20 ml (50 to 100 mg) 0.75% solution: 10 to 20 ml (75 to 150 mg) *Caudal block–* 0.25% solution: 15 to 30 ml (37.5 to 75 mg) 0.5% solution: 15 to 30 ml (75 to 150 mg) *Spinal block–* 0.75% solution (in dextrose 8.25%): 1 to 1.6 ml (7.5 to 12 mg) *Peripheral nerve block–* 0.25% solution: 5 ml (12.5 mg) 0.5% solution: 5 ml (25 mg)	**Skin:** dermatologic reactions. **Other:** edema, ***status asthmaticus, anaphylaxis, anaphylactoid reactions.*** Systemic effects from high blood levels of the drug– **CNS:** anxiety, nervousness, ***seizures*** followed by drowsiness. **CV:** bradycardia, hypotension, myocardial depression, ***arrhythmias, cardiac arrest.*** **EENT:** blurred vision, tinnitus. **GI:** nausea, vomiting. **Respiratory:** ***respiratory arrest.***
chloroprocaine hydrochloride (Nesacaine, Nesacaine MPF) Dosages given are for the drug without epinephrine and for adults. *Infiltration and nerve block–* 1% solution: 3 to 20 ml (30 to 200 mg) 2% solution: 2 to 40 ml (40 to 800 mg) *Caudal and epidural block–* 2% to 3% solution: 15 to 25 ml (300 to 750 mg). May repeat with smaller doses q 40 to 50 minutes. Dose and interval may be increased when combined with epinephrine. Maximum adult dosage is 800 mg or 11 mg/kg; when combined with epinephrine, maximum dosage is 1 g.	**Skin:** dermatologic reactions. **Other:** edema, ***status asthmaticus, anaphylaxis, anaphylactoid reactions.*** Systemic effects from high blood levels of the drug– **CNS:** anxiety, nervousness, ***seizures*** followed by drowsiness. **CV:** myocardial depression, hypotension, ***arrhythmias, cardiac arrest.*** **EENT:** blurred vision, tinnitus. **GI:** nausea, vomiting. **Respiratory:** ***respiratory arrest.***
etidocaine hydrochloride (Duranest) Dosages given are for the drug without epinephrine and for adults. Dose limit is 4 mg/kg or 300 mg per injection. When combined with epinephrine, dose limit is 5.5 mg/kg or 400 mg per injection. May be repeated q 2 to 3 hours. *Peripheral nerve block–* 0.5% solution: 5 to 40 ml (25 to 200 mg) 1% solution: 5 to 40 ml (50 to 400 mg)	**Skin:** dermatologic reactions. **Other:** edema, ***status asthmaticus, anaphylaxis, anaphylactoid reactions.*** Systemic effects from high blood levels of the drug– **CNS:** anxiety, apprehension, nervousness, ***seizures*** followed by drowsiness.

INTERACTIONS	NURSING CONSIDERATIONS
Beta-adrenergic blockers: enhanced sympathomimetic effects. Avoid concomitant use. *Chloroprocaine:* may lessen bupivacaine's action. Don't use together. *Cyclic antidepressants, MAO inhibitors:* severe, sustained hypertension when used with bupivacaine with epinephrine. Use with extreme caution. *Enflurane, halothane, isoflurane, related drugs:* arrhythmias when used with bupivacaine with epinephrine. Use with extreme caution.	• Contraindicated in children under 12 years and for spinal or topical anesthesia or paracervical block. Some solutions contain sulfites and should be avoided in patients with sulfite hypersensitivity. • Use cautiously in debilitated, elderly, or acutely ill patients and in patients with severe hepatic disease or drug allergies. • Should not be used for I.V. regional anesthesia (Bier's anesthesia). • The 0.75% solution should not be used for obstetrical surgery; lower concentrations are effective and less hazardous. • Use solutions with epinephrine cautiously in patients with CV disorders and in body areas with limited blood supply (ears, nose, fingers, toes). • Keep resuscitation equipment and drugs available. • Don't use solution with preservatives for caudal or epidural block. • Discard partially used vials without preservatives. • Check solution for particles. • Protect solutions containing epinephrine from light.
None significant.	• Contraindicated in patients with hypersensitivity to procaine, tetracaine, or other PABA derivatives, and for spinal or topical anesthesia. Epidural and caudal blocks are contraindicated in patients with CNS disease. • Use cautiously in debilitated, elderly, or acutely ill patients; in children; and in patients with drug allergies, paracervical block, or CV disease. • Keep resuscitation equipment and drugs available. • Don't use solution with preservatives for caudal or epidural block. • Don't use discolored solution. • Check solution for particles. • Discard partially used vials without preservatives.
Cyclic antidepressants, MAO inhibitors, phenothiazines: severe, sustained hypertension or hypotension when used with etidocaine with epinephrine. Use with extreme caution. *Enflurane, halothane, isoflurane, related drugs:* arrhythmias when used with etidocaine with epinephrine. Use with extreme caution.	• Contraindicated in patients with inflammation or infection in puncture region, septicemia, severe hypertension, spinal deformities, or neurologic disorders; in children under 14 years; and for spinal anesthesia. Some solutions contain sulfites and should be avoided in patients with sulfite hypersensitivity. • Use cautiously in debilitated, elderly, or acutely ill patients; in patients with severe shock, heart block, general drug allergies, or hepatic and renal disease; and as epidural block in obstetric patients.

(continued)

Anesthetics: Local, general, and topical ophthalmic *(continued)*

DRUG, INDICATIONS, DOSAGE	ADVERSE REACTIONS
Local *(continued)*	
etidocaine hydrochloride *(continued)* *Central neural block (lower limbs, cesarean section, lumbar, epidural)–* 1% solution: 10 to 30 ml (100 to 300 mg) 1.5% solution: 10 to 20 ml (150 to 300 mg) *Transvaginal block–* 1% solution: 5 to 20 ml (50 to 200 mg) *Caudal block–* 1% solution: 10 to 30 ml (100 to 300 mg)	**CV:** myocardial depression, hypotension, ***arrhythmias, cardiac arrest.*** **EENT:** blurred vision, tinnitus. **GI:** nausea, vomiting. **Respiratory: *respiratory arrest.***
lidocaine hydrochloride **[lignocaine hydrochloride]** (L-Caine, Lidoject-1, Lidoject-2, LidoPen, Truxacaine, Uad-Caine, Xylocaine) Dosages given are for the drug without epinephrine and for adults. *For anesthesia other than spinal–* Maximum single dose is 4.5 mg/kg or 300 mg. When used with epinephrine, the maximum dose is 7 mg/kg or 500 mg. *Caudal (obstetric) or epidural (thoracic) block–* 1% solution: 20 to 30 ml (200 to 300 mg) *Epidural (lumbar anesthesia) block–* 1.5% solution: 15 to 20 ml (225 to 300 mg) 2% solution: 10 to 15 ml (200 to 300 mg) *Spinal surgical anesthesia–* 5% (with 7.5% dextrose): 1.5 to 2 ml (75 to 100 mg) *Caudal (surgery) block–* 1.5% solution: 15 to 20 ml (225 to 300 mg)	**Skin:** dermatologic reactions. **Other:** edema, ***status asthmaticus, anaphylaxis, anaphylactoid reactions.*** Systemic effects from high blood levels of the drug– **CNS:** anxiety, nervousness, ***seizures*** followed by drowsiness. **CV:** myocardial depression, hypotension, ***arrhythmias, cardiac arrest.*** **EENT:** blurred vision, tinnitus. **GI:** nausea, vomiting. **Respiratory: *respiratory arrest.***
mepivacaine hydrochloride (Carbocaine, Polocaine) Dosages given are for the drug without levonordefrin. Dose and interval may be increased with levonordefrin. **Adults:** maximum single dose is 7 mg/kg up to 550 mg. Don't repeat more often than q 90 minutes. Maximum dosage is 1,000 mg daily. **Children:** maximum dose is 6 mg/kg. In children under 3 years or weighing less than 14 kg, use 0.5% or 1.5% solution only. *Nerve block–* 1% solution: 5 to 20 ml (50 to 200 mg) 2% solution: 5 to 20 ml (100 to 400 mg) *Transvaginal block or infiltration (maximum dose)–* 1% solution: 20 ml (200 mg) *Paracervical block (obstetric)–* 1% solution: 10 ml (100 mg). Give on each side (200 mg total) per 90-minute period.	**Skin:** dermatologic reactions. **Other:** edema, ***status asthmaticus, anaphylaxis, anaphylactoid reactions.*** Systemic effects from high blood levels of the drug– **CNS:** anxiety, nervousness, ***seizures*** followed by drowsiness. **CV:** myocardial depression, hypotension, ***arrhythmias, cardiac arrest.*** **EENT:** blurred vision, tinnitus. **GI:** nausea, vomiting. **Respiratory: *respiratory arrest.***

*Liquid form contains alcohol.
**May contain tartrazine.

Common reactions are in italics; ***life-threatening,*** in bold italics.

INTERACTIONS	NURSING CONSIDERATIONS
	• Use solutions with epinephrine cautiously in patients with CV disease and in body areas with limited blood supply (ears, nose, fingers, toes). • Don't use solution with preservatives for caudal or epidural block. • Keep resuscitation equipment and drugs available. • Check solution for particles.
Cyclic antidepressants, MAO inhibitors: severe, sustained hypertension when used with lidocaine with epinephrine. Use with extreme caution. *Enflurane, halothane, isoflurane, related drugs:* arrhythmias when used with lidocaine with epinephrine. Use with extreme caution.	• Contraindicated in patients with inflammation or infection in puncture region, septicemia, severe hypertension, spinal deformities, and neurologic disorders. • Use cautiously in debilitated, elderly, or acutely ill patients; in patients with severe shock, heart block, general drug allergies, or in obstetric patients; and for paracervical block. • Dosage and interval are increased with epinephrine. • Use solutions with epinephrine cautiously in patients with CV disorders and in body areas with limited blood supply (ears, nose, fingers, toes). • Do not use solutions with preservatives for spinal, epidural, or caudal block. • Keep resuscitation equipment and drugs available. • Discard partially used vials without preservatives. • Check solution for particles.
Cyclic antidepressants, MAO inhibitors: severe, sustained hypertension when used with mepivacaine with levonordefrin. *Enflurane, halothane, isoflurane, related drugs:* arrhythmias when used with mepivacaine with levonordefrin. Use with extreme caution.	• Contraindicated in patients with sensitivity to methylparaben, or heart block, or for spinal anesthesia. • Use cautiously in debilitated, elderly, or acutely ill patients, and for paracervical block. • Use solutions with levonordefrin cautiously in patients with CV disease and in body areas with limited blood supply (ears, nose, fingers, toes). • Monitor fetal heart rate when paracervical block is used in delivery. • Keep resuscitation equipment and drugs available.

(continued)

Anesthetics: Local, general, and topical ophthalmic *(continued)*

DRUG, INDICATIONS, DOSAGE	ADVERSE REACTIONS
Local *(continued)*	
mepivacaine hydrochloride *(continued)* *Caudal and epidural block–* 1% solution: 15 to 30 ml (150 to 300 mg) 1.5% solution: 10 to 25 ml (150 to 375 mg) 2% solution: 10 to 20 ml (200 to 400 mg) *Peripheral nerve block–* 1% solution: 1 to 5 ml (10 to 50 mg) 2% solution: 1 to 5 ml (20 to 100 mg)	
procaine hydrochloride (Novocain) *Spinal anesthesia–* **Adults:** maximum dose is 11 mg/kg, or 14 mg/kg when combined with epinephrine. Dose and interval may be increased with epinephrine. Before using, dilute 10% solution with 0.9% sodium chloride injection, sterile distilled water, or CSF. For hyperbaric technique, use dextrose solution. *Perineum:* use 0.5 ml 10% solution and 0.5 ml diluent injected at the L4 interspace. *Perineum and lower extremities:* use 1 ml 10% solution and 1 ml diluent injected at the L3 or L4 interspace. *Up to costal margin:* use 2 ml 10% solution and 1 ml diluent injected at the L2, L3, or L4 interspace. *Epidural block–* 1.5% solution: 25 ml (375 mg) *Peripheral nerve block–* 1% solution: 50 ml (500 mg) 2% solution: 25 ml (500 mg) *Infiltration–* 250 to 600 mg in a 0.25% to 0.5% solution. Maximum initial dose is 1 g.	**Skin:** dermatologic reactions. **Other:** edema, ***status asthmaticus, anaphylaxis, anaphylactoid reactions.*** Systemic effects from high blood levels of the drug– **CNS:** anxiety, nervousness, ***seizures*** followed by drowsiness. **CV:** myocardial depression, hypotension, ***arrhythmias, cardiac arrest.*** **EENT:** blurred vision, tinnitus. **GI:** nausea, vomiting. **Respiratory:** ***respiratory arrest.***
tetracaine hydrochloride (Pontocaine) Dosage for adults varies according to the extent of the block as follows. *Low spinal (saddle) block in vaginal delivery–* 2 to 5 mg as hyperbaric solution (in 10% dextrose). *Perineum and lower extremities:* 5 to 10 mg. *Up to costal margin:* 15 to 20 mg.	**Skin:** dermatologic reactions. **Other:** edema, ***status asthmaticus, anaphylaxis, anaphylactoid reactions.*** Systemic effects from high blood levels of the drug– **CNS:** anxiety, nervousness, ***seizures*** followed by drowsiness. **CV:** myocardial depression, hypotension, ***arrhythmias, cardiac arrest.*** **EENT:** blurred vision, tinnitus. **GI:** nausea, vomiting. **Respiratory:** ***respiratory arrest.***

INTERACTIONS	NURSING CONSIDERATIONS
	• Don't use solutions with preservatives for caudal or epidural block. • Discard partially used vials without preservatives. • Check solution for particles.
Echothiophate iodide: reduced hydrolysis of procaine. Use together cautiously. *Succinylcholine:* prolonged neuromuscular blockade. Use together cautiously.	• Contraindicated in patients with traumatized urethras and in those with hypersensitivity to chloroprocaine, tetracaine, or other PABA derivatives. • Use cautiously in hyperexcitable patients and in those with CNS diseases, infection at puncture site, shock, profound anemia, cachexia, sepsis, hypertension, hypotension, GI hemorrhage, bowel perforation or strangulation, peritonitis, cardiac decompensation, massive pleural effusions, or increased intra-abdominal pressure, and in obstetric patients. • Contraindicated for obstetric use in patients with cephalopelvic disproportion, placenta previa, abruptio placentae, floating fetal head, and intrauterine manipulation. • Keep resuscitation equipment and drugs available. • Use solution without preservatives for epidural block. • Discard partially used vials without preservatives. • Check solution for particles.
None significant.	• Contraindicated in patients with infection at injection site or CNS diseases and in those with hypersensitivity to procaine or related agents. • Saddle block is contraindicated in patients with cephalopelvic disproportion, placenta previa, abruptio placentae, intrauterine manipulation, and floating fetal head. • Use cautiously in patients with shock, profound anemia, cachexia, hypertension, hypotension, peritonitis, cardiac decompensation, massive pleural effusion, increased intracranial pressure, and infection. • Keep resuscitation equipment and drugs available. • When CSF is added to powdered drug or drug solution during spinal anesthesia, solution may be cloudy. Don't use discolored or crystallized solutions. • Protect from light; store in refrigerator.

(continued)

Anesthetics: Local, general, and topical ophthalmic *(continued)*

DRUG, INDICATIONS, DOSAGE	ADVERSE REACTIONS
General	
droperidol (Droleptan‡, Inapsine) *Preoperative medication—* **Adults and children over 12 years:** 2.5 to 10 mg I.M. 30 to 60 minutes before surgery. **Children 2 to 12 years:** 0.088 to 0.165 mg/kg I.M. *As an induction agent—* **Adults and children over 12 years:** 0.22 to 0.275 mg/kg I.V. with analgesic or general anesthetic. **Children 2 to 12 years:** 0.088 to 0.165 mg/kg I.V. Titrate dosage. *To suppress nystagmus, nausea, vomiting, and vertigo associated with an acute attack of Ménière's disease—* **Adults:** 5 mg I.M. as a single dose. *Management of severe agitation of psychotic disorders‡—* **Adults:** 10 to 25 mg P.O. daily in divided doses. *Maintenance dosage in general anesthesia—* **Adults:** 1.25 to 2.5 mg I.V.	**CNS:** extrapyramidal reactions (dystonia, akathisia), upward rotation of eyes and oculogyric crises, extended neck, flexed arms, fine tremor of limbs, dizziness, chills or shivering, facial diaphoresis, restlessness, decreased seizure threshold. **CV:** *hypotension,* tachycardia. **Hematologic:** ***agranulocytosis.*** **Respiratory:** ***laryngospasm, bronchospasm.***
etomidate (Amidate) *Induction of general anesthesia—* **Adults and children over 10 years:** 0.2 to 0.6 mg/kg I.V. over 30 to 60 seconds.	**CNS:** myoclonic movements, averting movements, tonic movements. **CV:** hypertension, hypotension, tachycardia, bradycardia. **EENT:** *eye movements,* ***laryngospasm.*** **GI:** nausea or vomiting. **Respiratory:** transient apnea, hyperventilation, hypoventilation. **Other:** hiccups, snoring, inhibition of adrenal steroid production, *transient venous pain.*
fentanyl citrate with droperidol (Innovar) *Anesthesia—* **Adults:** 0.5 to 2 ml I.M. 45 to 60 minutes before surgery. **Children:** 0.25 ml/20 lb body weight I.M. 45 to 60 minutes before surgery. *Adjunct to general anesthesia—* **Adults:** induction with 0.1 ml/kg or 1 ml/20 to 25 lb body weight by slow I.V. to produce neuroleptanalgesia; not indicated as sole agent for maintaining surgical anesthesia. **Children:** 0.05 ml/kg or 0.5 ml/20 lb body weight I.V. (total combined dose for induction and maintenance).	**CNS:** emergence delirium and hallucinations, postoperative drowsiness. **CV:** vasodilation, *hypotension,* decreased pulmonary arterial pressure, bradycardia, tachycardia. **EENT:** blurred vision, ***laryngospasm.*** **GI:** *nausea, vomiting.* **Respiratory:** ***respiratory depression, apnea, or arrest.*** **Other:** drug dependence, muscle rigidity, chills, *shivering,* diaphoresis.

*Liquid form contains alcohol. *Common* reactions are in italics; ***life-threatening,*** in bold italics.
**May contain tartrazine.

INTERACTIONS	NURSING CONSIDERATIONS
Epinephrine: may cause hypotension. Avoid concomitant use.	• Use cautiously in elderly or debilitated patients and in patients with hypotension or other CV disease, impaired hepatic or renal function, and Parkinson's disease. • Watch for extrapyramidal reactions. Call the doctor immediately if any occur. • Has greater tendency to cause extrapyramidal reactions than other antipsychotics. • Has been used as an I.V. antiemetic in cancer chemotherapy. • Give I.V. injections slowly. • Keep I.V. fluids and vasopressors available for treatment of hypotension. • Do not place patient in Trendelenburg's position; severe hypotension and deeper anesthesia may result, causing respiratory arrest. • If hypotension occurs, do not treat with epinephrine; it may worsen hypotension.
None significant.	• Contraindicated during labor and delivery, including cesarean sections. • Smaller increments of I.V. etomidate may be administered to adults during short operations to supplement subpotent anesthetic agents, such as nitrous oxide. • Transient muscle movements can be decreased by first administering 0.1 mg of fentanyl. • Have resuscitation equipment and drugs available. Maintain airway.
CNS depressants, such as barbiturates, tranquilizers, narcotics, and general anesthetics: additive effect. Reduce dosage. *Epinephrine:* may worsen hypotension. Avoid concomitant use. *MAO inhibitors:* increased adverse effects. Do not use within 2 weeks of MAO inhibitor therapy.	• Contraindicated in patients with intolerance to either component. • Use cautiously in patients with head injuries and increased intracranial pressure, COPD, hepatic and renal dysfunction, or bradyarrhythmias, and in elderly or debilitated patients. • Hypotension is a common adverse reaction. However, if blood pressure drops, also consider hypovolemia as a possible cause. Use appropriate parenteral fluids to help restore blood pressure. Do not treat with epinephrine; it may worsen hypotension. • Safe use in children under 2 years has not been established.

(continued)

Anesthetics: Local, general, and topical ophthalmic *(continued)*

DRUG, INDICATIONS, DOSAGE	ADVERSE REACTIONS
General *(continued)*	
fentanyl citrate with droperidol *(continued)* *Adjunct in regional anesthesia–* **Adults:** 1 to 2 ml I.M. or slow I.V. *Diagnostic procedures–* **Adults:** 0.5 to 2 ml I.M. 45 to 60 minutes before procedure. In prolonged procedure, give 0.5 to 1 ml I.V. cautiously and without a general anesthetic.	
ketamine hydrochloride (Ketalar) *Induction of anesthesia for procedures, especially short-term diagnostic or surgical, not requiring skeletal muscle relaxation; before giving other general anesthetics or to supplement low-potency agents, such as nitrous oxide–* **Adults and children:** 1 to 4.5 mg/kg I.V., administered over 60 seconds; or 6.5 to 13 mg/kg I.M. To maintain anesthesia, repeat in increments of half to full initial dose.	**CNS:** *tonic and clonic movements resembling seizures, dreamlike states, hallucinations, confusion, excitement,* irrational behavior, psychic abnormalities, *emergence delirium.* **CV:** *increased blood pressure and pulse rate,* hypotension, bradycardia. **EENT:** diplopia, nystagmus, slight increase in intraocular pressure, ***laryngospasm,*** *salivation.* **GI:** mild anorexia, nausea, vomiting. **Respiratory:** ***respiratory depression and apnea with rapid administration.*** **Skin:** transient erythema, measleslike rash.
methohexital sodium [methohexitone sodium] (Brevital Sodium, Brietal Sodium†‡) *Anesthesia for short-term procedures (oral surgery, gynecologic and GU examinations); reduction of fractures; before electroconvulsive therapy; for prolonged anesthesia when used with gaseous anesthetics–* **Adults and children:** 5 to 12 ml of 1% solution (50 to 120 mg) I.V. at 1 ml/5 seconds. Induction dose may vary from 50 to 120 mg or more, averages about 70 mg, and provides anesthesia for 5 to 7 minutes.	**CNS:** *muscular twitching,* headache, emergence delirium. **CV:** *transient hypotension, tachycardia,* circulatory depression, ***peripheral vascular collapse.*** **GI:** excessive salivation, *nausea, vomiting.* **Respiratory:** ***laryngospasm, bronchospasm, respiratory depression, apnea.***

*Liquid form contains alcohol. *Common* reactions are in italics; ***life-threatening,*** in bold italics.
**May contain tartrazine.

INTERACTIONS	NURSING CONSIDERATIONS
	• Respiratory depression, rigidity of respiratory muscles, and respiratory arrest can occur. Have narcotic antagonist and resuscitation equipment available. Maintain airway. • Postoperative electroencephalographic pattern may return to normal slowly. • If narcotic analgesics are required postoperatively, give one-third to one-quarter the typical dose.
Barbiturates, opiates, other CNS depressants: may prolong recovery time. Monitor closely. *Halothane:* increased risk of adverse cardiac effects. Monitor closely. *Thyroid hormones:* may elevate blood pressure and cause tachycardia. Give together cautiously.	• Contraindicated in patients with history of CVA or those threatened by a significant rise in blood pressure (including those with increased intracranial pressure or intraocular pressure), and those with severe hypertension or cardiac decompensation, or those undergoing surgery of the pharynx, larynx, or bronchial tree (unless used with muscle relaxants). • Use cautiously in chronic alcoholics, alcohol-intoxicated patients, and those with elevated CSF pressure before anesthesia. • Because of rapid induction, physically support patient during administration. • For continuous infusion, infuse diluted drug at a rate of 1 to 2 mg/minute. • Chemically incompatible with barbiturates. • Have resuscitation equipment available. Maintain airway. • Start supportive respiration if respiratory depression occurs. Use mechanical support rather than administering analeptics. • Minimize verbal, tactile, and visual stimulation during recovery phase to reduce incidence of emergent reactions. • Control hallucinations and excitement after anesthesia with diazepam. • Dissociative effect and hallucinatory adverse reactions have made this a popular drug of abuse.
None significant.	• Contraindicated in patients with severe hepatic dysfunction, hypersensitivity to barbiturates, or porphyria; in shock or impending shock; and in those for whom general anesthetics would be hazardous. • Use cautiously in debilitated patients; in patients with asthma, respiratory obstruction, severe hypertension or hypotension, myocardial disease, CHF, severe anemia, and in obese patients. • Have resuscitation equipment and drugs ready. Maintain pulmonary ventilation.

(continued)

Anesthetics: Local, general, and topical ophthalmic *(continued)*

DRUG, INDICATIONS, DOSAGE	ADVERSE REACTIONS
General *(continued)*	
methohexital sodium *(continued)* *Maintenance–* Intermittent injection: 2 to 4 ml 1% solution (20 to 40 mg) q 4 to 7 minutes. Continuous I.V. drip: administer 0.2% solution (1 drop/second). Rate of flow must be individualized for each patient.	**Skin:** tissue necrosis with extravasation. **Other:** hiccups, coughing, acute allergic reactions, thrombophlebitis, pain at injection site, injury to nerves adjacent to injection site. Extended use may cause cumulative effect.
propofol (Diprivan) *Induction–* **Adults:** individualize doses according to patient's condition and age. Most patients classified as American Society of Anesthesiologists (ASA) Physical Status category (PS) I or II under 55 years require 2 to 2.5 mg/kg I.V. The drug is usually administered in 40-mg boluses q 10 seconds until the desired response is obtained. Elderly, debilitated, or hypovolemic patients, or patients in ASA PS III or IV should receive half of the usual induction dose (20 mg-boluses q 10 seconds). *Maintenance–* **Adults:** may be given as a variable-rate infusion, titrated to clinical effect. Most patients may be maintained with 0.1 to 0.2 mg/kg/minute (6 to 12 mg/kg/hr). Elderly, debilitated, or hypovolemic patients, or patients in ASA PS III or IV should receive half of the usual maintenance dose (0.05 to 0.1 mg/kg/minute, or 3 to 6 mg/kg/hr).	**CNS:** headache, dizziness, twitching, clonic or myoclonic movement. **CV:** *hypotension, bradycardia,* hypertension. **GI:** nausea, vomiting, abdominal cramping. **Respiratory:** ***apnea,*** cough. **Skin:** flushing. **Other:** fever; hiccups; burning or stinging, pain, tingling or numbness, and coldness at injection site.

*Liquid form contains alcohol. *Common* reactions are in italics; ***life-threatening,*** in bold italics.
**May contain tartrazine.

INTERACTIONS	NURSING CONSIDERATIONS
	• Reduce postoperative nausea by having patient fast before administration. • Discontinue immediately if extravasation occurs. • Incompatible with lactated Ringer's solution. Do not mix with acid solutions, such as atropine sulfate. • Do not use distilled water or diluents that contain bacteriostatic agents. Alternative diluents are 5% dextrose solution or 0.9% sodium chloride solution. • Solutions may be stored and used as long as they remain clear and colorless. Solutions can't be sterilized. • Incompatible with silicone; avoid contact with rubber stoppers or silicone-treated syringes.
Inhalation anesthetics (such as enflurane, isoflurane, and halothane) or supplemental anesthetics (such as nitrous oxide and opiates): enhanced anesthetic and CV actions of propofol. *Opiate analgesics, sedatives:* may cause pronounced drop in systolic, diastolic, and mean arterial pressures and cardiac output; may also decrease induction dose requirements.	• Contraindicated in patients hypersensitive to propofol or any components of the emulsion, including soybean oil, egg, lecithin, and glycerol. • Use cautiously in patients with a history of lipid metabolism disorders, such as pancreatitis or primary hyperlipoproteinemia and diabetic hyperlipidemia. Also use cautiously in elderly or debilitated patients and those with circulatory disorders. Cardiac output may be markedly depressed in patients undergoing assisted or controlled positive-pressure ventilation. • Not recommended for obstetric anesthesia, in patients with increased intracranial pressure or impaired cerebral circulation, or in breast-feeding patients. • Monitor patients for signs of significant hypotension or bradycardia. Apnea, which may occur during induction, may persist for longer than 60 seconds and require ventilatory support. • Prepare under strict aseptic technique. Postoperative fevers have been linked to the use of contaminated solutions. Unused solution should be discarded after the procedure. • Do not mix with other drugs or blood products. If diluted before infusion, use only D_5W and not in a concentration of less than 2 mg/ml. • When administered into a running I.V. catheter, propofol emulsion is compatible with D_5W, lactated Ringer's injection, lactated Ringer's in dextrose 5% solution, dextrose 5% in 0.45% sodium chloride solution, and dextrose 5% in 0.2% sodium chloride solution. • Store emulsion between 40° F (4° C) and 72° F (22° C). Do not refrigerate.

(continued)

Anesthetics: Local, general, and topical ophthalmic *(continued)*

DRUG, INDICATIONS, DOSAGE	ADVERSE REACTIONS
General *(continued)*	
thiopental sodium [thiopentone sodium] (Intraval Sodium‡, Pentothal Sodium) *Induction of anesthesia –* **Adults:** administer a test dose of 25 to 75 mg I.V. to assess for hypersensitivity. Then give 210 to 280 mg (3 to 4 ml/kg) I.V., which is usually required for average adult (70 kg). *General anesthetic for short-term procedures –* **Adults:** 2 to 3 ml 2.5% solution (50 to 75 mg) administered I.V. at intervals of 20 to 40 seconds. Repeat dose with caution, if necessary. *Seizures following anesthesia –* **Adults:** 75 to 125 mg (3 to 5 ml of 2.5% solution) immediately. *Psychiatric disorders (narcoanalysis, narcosynthesis) –* **Adults:** 100 mg/minute (4 ml/minute 2.5% solution) until confusion occurs and before sleep. *Basal anesthesia –* **Adults and children:** administer up to 1 g/22.5 kg (50 lb) body weight P.R. or 0.5 ml 10% solution/kg body weight P.R. Maximum dose is 1 to 1.5 g for children ≥ 34 kg, 3 to 4 g for adults ≥ 91 kg.	**CNS:** *prolonged somnolence,* retrograde amnesia, emergence delirium. **CV:** myocardial depression, ***arrhythmias.*** **Skin:** tissue necrosis with extravasation. **Respiratory:** ***respiratory depression*** *(momentary apnea following each injection is typical),* ***bronchospasm, laryngospasm.*** **Other:** sneezing, coughing, *shivering,* pain at injection site.
Topical ophthalmic	
proparacaine hydrochloride (Alcaine, Ophthaine, Ophthetic) *Anesthesia for tonometry, gonioscopy; removal of sutures or foreign bodies from cornea –* **Adults and children:** instill 1 to 2 drops of 0.5% solution in eye just before procedure. *Anesthesia for cataract extraction, glaucoma surgery –* **Adults and children:** instill 1 drop of 0.5% solution in eye q 5 to 10 minutes for five to seven doses.	**EENT:** conjunctival redness, transient eye pain. **Other:** hypersensitivity reactions.
tetracaine (Pontocaine Eye Ointment) **tetracaine hydrochloride** (Pontocaine) *Anesthesia for tonometry, gonioscopy; removal of corneal foreign bodies, suture removal from cornea; other diagnostic and minor surgical procedures –* **Adults and children:** instill 1 to 2 drops of 0.5% solution or a small strip of ointment in eye just before procedure.	**EENT:** transient stinging in eye 30 seconds after initial instillation, epithelial damage in excessive or long-term use. **Other:** sensitization with repeated use (allergic skin rash, urticaria).

*Liquid form contains alcohol.
**May contain tartrazine.

Common reactions are in italics; ***life-threatening,*** in bold italics.

INTERACTIONS	NURSING CONSIDERATIONS
None significant.	• Contraindicated in absence of suitable veins for I.V. administration, and in patients with hypersensitivity to barbiturates, status asthmaticus, porphyria, respiratory depression or obstruction, decompensated cardiac disease, severe anemia, hepatic cirrhosis, shock, renal dysfunction, and myxedema. • For general anesthesia, give atropine sulfate as premedication to diminish laryngeal reflexes and to prevent laryngospasm. • Have resuscitation equipment and oxygen available. Maintain airway. • Avoid extravasation. • Monitor vital signs before, during, and after anesthesia. • Thiopental is rarely administered rectally for basal sedation or anesthesia because of variable absorption from the rectum. • Solutions of atropine sulfate, *d*-tubocurarine, or succinylcholine may be given concurrently. • Do not heat solutions for sterilization. Solutions should be used within 24 hours.
None significant.	• Use cautiously in patients with cardiac disease and hyperthyroidism. • Not for long-term use; may delay wound healing. • Warn patients not to rub or touch eye while cornea is anesthetized. This may cause corneal abrasion and greater discomfort when anesthesia wears off. • Warn patients with corneal abrasion that pain is relieved only temporarily. • Don't use discolored solution. • Store in tightly closed container. Refrigerate opened containers.
Cholinesterase inhibitors: prolonged ocular anesthesia and increased risk of toxicity. *Sulfonamides:* interference with sulfonamide antibacterial activity. Wait ½ hour after anesthesia before instilling sulfonamide.	• Contraindicated in patients hypersensitive to the drug. • Avoid long-term use. • Does not dilate the pupil, paralyze accommodation, or increase intraocular pressure. • Don't use discolored solution. Keep container tightly closed. • Warn patient not to touch or rub the eye while the cornea is anesthetized. This may cause corneal abrasion and greater discomfort when the anesthetic wears off.

Topical agents

DRUG	INDICATIONS & DOSAGE
Antibacterials and antifungals	
alcohol, ethyl and isopropyl	*To disinfect skin, instruments, and ampules:* disinfect as needed. Isopropyl alcohol is superior to ethyl alcohol as an anti-infective (70%). *Antipyresis:* apply 25% solution. *Anhidrosis:* apply 50% solution p.r.n.
hydrogen peroxide	*Cleaning wounds:* use 1.5% to 3% solution, p.r.n. *Mouthwash for necrotizing ulcerative gingivitis:* gargle with 3% solution, p.r.n. *Cleaning douche:* use 2% solution q.i.d., p.r.n.
Antiseptics and germicidals	
benzalkonium chloride (Benza, Germicin, Spensomide, Zephiran)	*Preoperative disinfection of unbroken skin:* apply 1:750 tincture or spray. *Disinfection of mucous membranes and denuded skin:* apply 1:10,000 to 1:5,000 aqueous solution. *Irrigation of vagina:* instill 1:5,000 to 1:2,000 aqueous solution. *Irrigation of deep infected wounds:* instill 1:20,000 to 1:3,000 aqueous solution. *Preservation of metallic instruments, ampules, thermometers, and rubber articles:* wipe with or soak objects in 1:5,000 to 1:750 solution. *Disinfection of operating room equipment:* wipe with 1:5,000 solution.
chlorhexidine gluconate (Hibiclens, Hibistat, Peridex)	*Surgical hand scrub, hand wash, hand rinse, skin wound cleanser:* use p.r.n. *Gingivitis:* use 0.12% strength (Peridex oral rinse), p.r.n.
hexachlorophene (pHisoHex, pHisoScrub, Septisol, Septsoft)	*Surgical scrub, bacteriostatic skin cleanser:* use 0.25% to 3% concentrations p.r.n.
iodine (Sepp)	*Preoperative disinfection of skin (small wounds and abraded areas):* apply p.r.n.

*Available in Canada only.

ACTION	SPECIAL CONSIDERATIONS
Antibacterial effect through reduction of surface tension of bacterial cell walls, inhibiting bacterial growth. Also antipyretic and astringent effects.	• Avoid contact with eyes and mucous membranes. • Contraindicated in patients taking disulfiram if used over large surface area. • Do not apply to open wounds.
Antibacterial effect through oxidation.	• Do not instill into closed body cavities or abscesses because released gas cannot escape. • Store in tightly capped, dark container in cool, dry place. • Do not confuse with peroxide (6% to 20%) used for bleaching hair.
Cationic surface action producing bacteriostatic or bactericidal effect, depending on the concentration used.	• Do not use with occlusive dressings or packs. • Use only in proper diluted strength for each use. • Inactivated by anionic compounds such as soap. • Rinse area thoroughly after each application. • Skin inflammation and irritation may require lower concentration or discontinuation.
Persistent antimicrobial effect against gram-negative and gram-positive bacteria.	• Avoid contact with eyes, ears, and mucous membranes. Rinse well if drug enters eyes or ears. • May cause deafness if drug enters middle ear.
Bacteriostatic effect against staphylococci and other gram-positive bacteria, probably due to inhibition of bacterial membrane-bound enzymes.	• To prevent increased absorption and neurotoxicity, do not use on broken skin, skin lesions, burns, wounds, or under occlusive dressings. • Do not use around eyes or mucous membranes. • Use for at least 3 days preoperatively for optimal effect. • Rinse thoroughly after use. • Do not use in infants; use cautiously in children. • May be toxic if ingested.
Germicidal effect against bacteria, fungi, and viruses, probably due to disruption of microorganism proteins.	• Clean area before applying. • Do not cover after application to avoid irritation. • Iodine stains skin and clothing. • Do not use near eyes or on mucous membranes. • Toxic if ingested; sodium thiosulfate is antidote.

(continued)

Topical agents *(continued)*

DRUG	INDICATIONS & DOSAGE
Antiseptics and germicidals *(continued)*	
povidone-iodine (Acu-dyne, Betadine, Biodine, Efodine, Frepp, Iodex, Isodine, Operand, Pharmadine, Polydine, Proviodine*, Sepp)	*Preoperative skin preparation and scrub; germicide for surface wounds; postoperative application to incisions; prophylactic application to urinary meatus of catheterized patients; miscellaneous disinfection:* apply p.r.n., or use as scrub p.r.n.
Astringents	
calamine	*Astringent and protectant; pruritus, poison ivy and poison oak, nonpoisonous insect bites, mild sunburn, minor skin irritations:* apply p.r.n., t.i.d., or q.i.d.
hamamelis water, witch hazel (Mediconet, Tucks)	*Anal discomfort, pruritus, burning, minor external hemorrhoidal or outer vaginal discomfort, diaper rash:* apply t.i.d. or q.i.d.
Emollients	
petrolatum (Vaseline)	*Dry rough skin; temporary relief of discomfort due to sunburn, windburn, or any drying of epithelial tissue:* for topical protection and emollience, use alone or with other drugs and apply p.r.n.
Keratolytics	
podophyllum resin (Pod-Ben 25, Podoben, Pudofin)	*Venereal warts:* apply podophyllum resin preparation to the lesion, cover with waxed paper, and bandage. Keep covered for 4 to 6 hours; then wash lesion to remove medication. Repeat at weekly intervals, if indicated. *Multiple superficial epitheliomatosis and keratosis:* apply daily with applicator and allow to dry. Remove necrotic tissue before each application.
salicylic acid (Calicylic, Compound W, Derma-Soft Creme, Freezone, Gordofilm, Hydrisalic, Keralyt, Occlusal, Off-Ezy, Salacid, Salonil, Wart-Off)	*Scaling dermatoses, hyperkeratosis, calluses, warts:* apply to affected area and cover with occlusive dressing at night.
Protectants	
collodion, flexible collodion	*Protectant; vehicle for other medicinal agents; sealant for small wounds:* apply to dry skin, p.r.n., or use flexible collodion when a flexible film is desired.

*Available in Canada only.

ACTION	SPECIAL CONSIDERATIONS
Germicidal effect against bacteria, fungi, and viruses; has same action as iodine without its irritating effects.	• Contraindicated in patients with known sensitivity to iodine. • Do not use around eyes; do not use full-strength solution on mucous membranes. • May stain skin and mucous membranes.
Antipruritic and astringent activity through drying effect.	• Avoid use on eyes and mucous membranes. • Do not apply to raw, oozing areas. • Clean and dry area before each application.
Soothing, cooling effect on superficial irritation through astringent action.	• Avoid use around eyes. • Clean area before use.
Protective and emollient effect through formation of moisture barrier, increasing the natural retention of moisture.	• Avoid use in eyes. • May stain clothing. • May cause body surfaces to become slippery. • Apply sparingly; is not absorbed, so coating is all that is necessary.
Caustic and erosive action from disruption of epithelial cell division.	• Avoid eye contact. • May be toxic if applied to large surface area or applied too frequently. • Should not be used in pregnant patients. • Wash hands thoroughly after applying. • Protect surrounding area with petrolatum. • Wash off thoroughly with soap and water after prescribed time. • May cause abnormal pigmentation.
Causes desquamation of cornified epithelium by increasing hydration.	• Avoid use on eyes and mucous membranes. • Do not use in aspirin-sensitive patients. • Apply emollient to surrounding skin for protection. • Do not use on birthmarks, moles, or areas with hair follicle involvement. • Wash off thoroughly after overnight use.
Protects wounds from the environment by forming an occlusive seal and excluding air.	• Do not use on deep or puncture wounds; may promote growth of anaerobic bacteria. • Avoid use on eyes and mucous membranes. • May be painful on application or cause dry skin. • Use alcohol or acetone as solvent for removal.

(continued)

Topical agents *(continued)*

DRUG	INDICATIONS & DOSAGE
Protectants *(continued)*	
compound benzoin tincture	*Demulcent and protectant (cutaneous ulcers, bedsores, cracked nipples, fissures of lips and anus):* apply locally once daily or b.i.d.
zinc gelatin (Dome-Paste, Unna's Boot, Unna's Powder)	*Protectant (lesions or injuries of lower legs or arms):* wrap the wet bandage in place and retain for about 1 week. Dome-Paste, in 3″ to 4″ (8 to 10 cm) bandages, can be applied directly to arm or leg.
Wet dressings, soaks	
aluminum acetate, aluminum sulfate (Bluboro Powder, Burow's solution, Domeboro powder, Pedi-Boro Soak Paks)	*Mild skin irritation from exposure to soaps, chemicals, diaper rash, acne, eczema:* apply p.r.n. *Skin inflammation, contact dermatoses:* mix powder or tablet with 1 pint of lukewarm water. Apply to loose dressing q 15 to 30 minutes for 4 to 8 hours.
Miscellaneous agents	
hydroquinone (Eldoquin, Esoterica, Porcelana, Solaquin Forte)	*Treatment of hyperpigmentation in conditions such as freckling, inactive chloasma, lentigo, photosensitization:* apply uniformly to desired area b.i.d., until desired depigmentation occurs, then as needed to maintain depigmentation.
methyl salicylate (Ben-Gay, Icy Hot Balm/ Cream, Deep Heating Rub)	*Counterirritant (minor pains of osteoarthritis, rheumatism, sprains, muscle and tendon soreness and tightness, lumbago, sciatica):* apply with gentle massage several times daily for adults.
para-aminobenzoic acid (PABA) (Pabanol)	*Topical protectant; sunburn protection, sun-sensitive skin, slow tanning:* apply evenly to dry skin indoors before exposure to sun. Reapply after swimming.
selenium sulfide (Exsel, Head and Shoulders, Selsun, Selsun Blue)	*Tinea versicolor:* massage into affected area; rinse after 10 minutes. Apply daily for 7 days. *Dandruff, seborrheic scalp dermatitis:* massage 1 to 2 teaspoonfuls into wet scalp. After 2 to 3 minutes, rinse thoroughly, and repeat application.

*Available in Canada only.

ACTION	SPECIAL CONSIDERATIONS
Protects skin from external environment by coating action.	• Avoid contact with eyes and mucous membranes. • Clean and dry area before applying. • Useful in protection of skin from adhesive.
Protects skin by forming occlusive barrier.	• Avoid contact with eyes and mucous membranes. • Watch for signs of infection. • Warn patient not to shower or bathe with gel on. • Remove by soaking in warm water. Remove all of previous application before reapplying. • Apply with nap of hair to avoid folliculitis. • Do not use with constrictive bandage.
Reduces friction and provides soothing relief through astringent action.	• Avoid use around eyes and mucous membranes. • Do not use with occlusive dressings. • Discontinue if irritation occurs.
Depigmenting action.	• Avoid use near eyes and on broken skin. • Sunscreen and protective clothing should be used during and after use to prevent repigmentation. • Should not be used in children or pregnant patients. • May be toxic if ingested.
Acts as counterirritant, replacing pain perception with another sensation that blocks pain temporarily.	• Avoid use around eyes, on mucous membranes, or on broken skin; in patients allergic to salicylates; and in children. • May be toxic if ingested. • Do not use with heating pad or hot water.
Provides sun-screening action by absorbing ultraviolet rays.	• Avoid use in eyes and on mucous membranes. • May discolor clothing. • Not recommended for infants.
Antiseborrheic effect through cytostatic action on epithelial cells, which inhibits corneocyte production.	• Avoid use in eyes and on mucous membranes or inflamed areas. • May damage jewelry. • Should not be used in pregnant patients. • May discolor hair or cause increased hair loss.

Cancer chemotherapy: Acronyms and protocols

Combination chemotherapy is well established for treatment of cancer. The chart below lists commonly used acronyms and protocols, including standard dosages for specific cancers.

ACRONYM & INDICATION	DRUG		DOSAGE
	Generic name	**Trade name**	
AA (Leukemia – AML, induction)	cytarabine (ara-C)	Cytosar-U	100 mg/m² daily by continuous I.V. infusion for 7 to 10 days
	doxorubicin	Adriamycin	30 mg/m² I.V., days 1 to 3
ABVD (Hodgkin's lymphoma)	doxorubicin	Adriamycin	25 mg/m² I.V., days 1 and 15
	bleomycin	Blenoxane	10 units/m² I.V., days 1 and 15
	vinblastine	Velban	6 mg/m² I.V., days 1 and 15
	dacarbazine	DTIC-Dome	375 mg/m² I.V., days 1 and 15 *Repeat cycle q 28 days.*
AC (Multiple myeloma)	doxorubicin	Adriamycin	30 mg/m² I.V., day 1
	carmustine	BiCNU	30 mg/m² I.V., day 1 *Repeat cycle q 21 to 28 days.*
AC (Bony sarcoma)	doxorubicin	Adriamycin	75 to 90 mg/m² by 96-hour continuous I.V. infusion
	cisplatin	Platinol	90 to 120 mg/m² IA or I.V., day 6 *Repeat cycle q 28 days.*
AFM (Breast cancer)	doxorubicin	Adriamycin	25 mg/m² by continuous I.V. infusion, days 1 to 3
	fluorouracil (5-FU)	Adrucil	400 mg/m² I.V., days 1 to 5
	methotrexate	Folex	250 mg/m² I.V., day 18
	leucovorin calcium	Wellcovorin	15 mg/m² P.O. q 6 hours, days 19 to 20 *Repeat cycle q 21 days for four cycles.*
AP (Ovarian cancer, epithelial)	doxorubicin	Adriamycin	50 to 60 mg/m² I.V., day 1
	cisplatin	Platinol	50 to 60 mg/m² I.V., day 1 *Repeat cycle q 21 days.*
APE (EAP) (Gastric cancer)	doxorubicin	Adriamycin	20 mg/m² I.V. daily, days 1 and 7
	cisplatin	Platinol	40 mg/m² I.V. daily, days 2 and 8
	etoposide (VP-16)	VePesid	120 mg/m² I.V. daily, days 4, 5, and 6 *Repeat cycle q 8 weeks.*
ASHAP (Non-Hodgkin's lymphoma)	doxorubicin	Adriamycin	10 mg/m² daily by continuous I.V. infusion, days 1 to 4
	cisplatin	Platinol	25 mg/m² daily by continuous I.V. infusion days 1 to 4
	cytarabine (ara-C)	Cytosar-U	1,500 mg/m² I.V. immediately after completion of doxorubicin and cisplatin therapy
	methylprednisolone	Solu-Medrol	500 mg I.V. daily, days 1 to 5 *Repeat cycle q 21 to 25 days.*

Cancer chemotherapy: Acronyms and protocols *(continued)*

ACRONYM & INDICATION	DRUG		DOSAGE
	Generic name	Trade name	
BACON (Non-small-cell lung cancer)	bleomycin	Blenoxane	30 units I.V. q 6 weeks, day 2
	doxorubicin	Adriamycin	40 mg/m² I.V. q 4 weeks, day 1
	lomustine (CCNU)	CeeNU	65 mg/m² P.O. q 8 weeks, day 1
	vincristine	Oncovin	0.75 to 1 mg/m² I.V. q 6 weeks, day 2
	mechlorethamine (nitrogen mustard)	Mustargen	8 mg/m² I.V. q 4 weeks, day 1
BACOP (Non-Hodgkin's lymphoma)	bleomycin	Blenoxane	5 units/m² I.V. daily, days 15 and 22
	doxorubicin	Adriamycin	25 mg/m² I.V., days 1 and 8
	cyclophosphamide	Cytoxan	650 mg/m² I.V., days 1 and 8
	vincristine	Oncovin	1.4 mg/m² (2 mg maximum) I.V., days 1 and 8
	prednisone	Deltasone	60 mg/m² P.O., days 15 to 28 *Repeat cycle q 28 days.*
BCP (Multiple myeloma)	carmustine	BiCNU	75 mg/m² I.V., day 1
	cyclophosphamide	Cytoxan	400 mg/m² I.V., day 1
	prednisone	Deltasone	75 mg P.O., days 1 to 7 *Repeat cycle q 28 days.*
BEP (Genitourinary cancer)	bleomycin	Blenoxane	30 units I.V., days 2, 9, and 16
	etoposide (VP-16)	VePesid	100 mg/m², days 1 to 5
	cisplatin	Platinol	20 mg/m² I.V., days 1 to 5
BHD (Malignant melanoma)	carmustine	BiCNU	100 to 150 mg/m² I.V. q 6 weeks
	hydroxyurea	Hydrea	1,480 mg/m² P.O. q 3 weeks, days 1 to 5
	dacarbazine	DTIC-Dome	100 to 150 mg/m² I.V. q 3 weeks, days 1 to 5
CA (Breast cancer)	cyclophosphamide	Cytoxan	200 mg/m² P.O., days 3 to 6
	doxorubicin	Adriamycin	40 mg/m² I.V., day 1 *Repeat cycle q 21 to 28 days.*
CAE (ACE) (Small-cell lung cancer)	cyclophosphamide	Cytoxan	1 g/m² I.V., day 1
	doxorubicin	Adriamycin	50 mg/m² I.V., day 1
	etoposide (VP-16)	VePesid	80 to 120 mg/m² I.V., day 1 *Repeat cycle q 21 days.*
CAF (FAC) (Breast cancer)	cyclophosphamide	Cytoxan	100 mg/m² P.O., days 1 to 14
	doxorubicin	Adriamycin	30 mg/m² I.V., days 1 and 8
	fluorouracil (5-FU)	Adrucil	400 to 500 mg/m² I.V., days 1 and 8 *Repeat cycle q 28 days.*
or	cyclophosphamide	Cytoxan	500 mg/m² I.V., day 1
	doxorubicin	Adriamycin	50 mg/m² I.V., day 1
	fluorouracil (5-FU)	Adrucil	500 mg/m² I.V., day 1 *Repeat cycle q 21 days.*

(continued)

Cancer chemotherapy: Acronyms and protocols *(continued)*

ACRONYM & INDICATION	DRUG		DOSAGE
	Generic name	Trade name	
CAMP (Non-small-cell lung cancer)	cyclophosphamide	Cytoxan	300 mg/m² I.V., days 1 and 8
	doxorubicin	Adriamycin	20 mg/m² I.V., days 1 and 8
	methotrexate sodium	Folex	15 mg/m² I.V., days 1 and 8
	procarbazine	Matulane	100 mg/m² P.O., days 1 to 10 *Repeat cycle q 28 days.*
CAP (Genitourinary cancer)	cisplatin	Platinol	60 mg/m² I.V., day 1
	doxorubicin	Adriamycin	40 mg/m² I.V., day 1
	cyclophosphamide	Cytoxan	400 mg/m² I.V., day 1 *Repeat cycle q 21 days.*
CAP (Non-small-cell lung cancer)	cyclophosphamide	Cytoxan	400 mg/m² I.V., day 1
	doxorubicin	Adriamycin	40 mg/m² I.V., day 1
	cisplatin	Platinol	60 mg/m² I.V., day 1 *Repeat cycle q 28 days.*
CAP (PAC) (Ovarian cancer, epithelial)	cisplatin	Platinol	50 mg/m² I.V., day 1
	doxorubicin	Adriamycin	50 mg/m² I.V., day 1
	cyclophosphamide	Cytoxan	500 mg/m² I.V., day 1 *Repeat cycle q 21 days for eight cycles.*
CAV (Small-cell lung cancer)	cyclophosphamide	Cytoxan	750 mg/m² I.V., day 1
	doxorubicin	Adriamycin	50 mg/m² I.V., day 1
	vincristine	Oncovin	2 mg/m² I.V., day 1 *Repeat cycle q 3 weeks.*
CAVe (Hodgkin's lymphoma)	lomustine (CCNU)	CeeNU	100 mg/m² I.V., day 1
	doxorubicin	Adriamycin	60 mg/m² I.V., day 1
	vinblastine	Velban	5 mg/m² I.V., day 1 *Repeat cycle q 6 weeks.*
CC (Ovarian cancer, epithelial)	carboplatin	Paraplatin	300 mg/m² I.V., day 1
	cyclophosphamide	Cytoxan	600 mg/m² I.V., day 1 *Repeat cycle q 20 days.*
CD (DC) (Leukemia – ANLL, consolidation)	cytarabine (ara-C)	Cytosar-U	3,000 mg/m² I.V. q 12 hours for 6 days
	daunorubicin	Cerubidine	30 mg/m² I.V. daily for 3 days, after cytarabine therapy

Cancer chemotherapy: Acronyms and protocols *(continued)*

ACRONYM & INDICATION	DRUG Generic name	Trade name	DOSAGE
CDC (Ovarian cancer, epithelial)	carboplatin	Paraplatin	300 mg/m² I.V., day 1
	doxorubicin	Adriamycin	40 mg/m² I.V., day 1
	cyclophosphamide	Cytoxan	500 mg/m² I.V., day 1 *Repeat cycle q 28 days.*
CF (Head and neck cancer)	cisplatin	Platinol	100 mg/m² I.V., day 1
	fluorouracil (5-FU)	Adrucil	1,000 mg/m² daily by continuous I.V. infusion, days 1 to 5 *Repeat cycle q 21 to 28 days.*
or	carboplatin	Paraplatin	400 mg/m² I.V., day 1
	fluorouracil (5-FU)	Adrucil	1,000 mg/m² daily by continuous I.V. infusion, days 1 to 5 *Repeat cycle q 21 to 28 days.*
CFL (Head and neck cancer)	cisplatin	Platinol	100 mg/m² I.V., day 1
	fluorouracil (5-FU)	Adrucil	600 to 800 mg/m² daily by continuous I.V. infusion, days 1 to 5
	leucovorin calcium	Wellcovorin	200 to 300 mg/m² I.V. daily, days 1 to 5 *Repeat cycle q 21 days.*
CFM (Breast cancer)	cyclophosphamide	Cytoxan	500 mg/m² I.V., day 1
	fluorouracil (5-FU)	Adrucil	500 mg/m² I.V., day 1
	mitoxantrone	Novantrone	10 mg/m² I.V., day 1 *Repeat cycle q 21 days.*
CFPT (Breast cancer)	cyclophosphamide	Cytoxan	150 mg/m² I.V., days 1 to 5
	fluorouracil (5-FU)	Adrucil	300 mg/m² I.V., days 1 to 5
	prednisone	Deltasone	10 mg P.O. t.i.d. for first 7 days of each course
	tamoxifen	Nolvadex	10 mg P.O. b.i.d. (daily through each course) *Repeat cycle q 6 weeks.*
CHAP (Ovarian cancer, epithelial)	cyclophosphamide	Cytoxan	300 to 500 mg/m² I.V., day 1
	altretamine	Hexalen	150 mg/m² P.O., days 1 to 7
	doxorubicin	Adriamycin	30 to 50 mg/m² I.V., day 1
	cisplatin	Platinol	50 mg/m² I.V., day 1 *Repeat cycle q 28 days.*
ChIVPP (Hodgkin's lymphoma)	chlorambucil	Leukeran	6 mg/m² P.O., days 1 to 14 (10 mg/day maximum)
	vinblastine	Velban	6 mg/m² I.V., days 1 to 8 (10 mg/day maximum)
	procarbazine	Matulane	50 mg P.O., days 1 to 14 (150 mg/day maximum)
	prednisone	Deltasone	40 mg/m² P.O., days 1 to 14 (25 mg/m² for child)

(continued)

Cancer chemotherapy: Acronyms and protocols *(continued)*

ACRONYM & INDICATION	DRUG		DOSAGE
	Generic name	Trade name	
CHOP (Non-Hodgkin's lymphoma)	cyclophosphamide	Cytoxan	750 mg/m² I.V., day 1
	doxorubicin	Adriamycin	50 mg/m² I.V., day 1
	vincristine	Oncovin	1.4 mg/m² (2 mg maximum) I.V., day 1
	prednisone	Deltasone	100 mg/m² P.O., days 1 to 5 *Repeat cycle q 21 days.*
CHOP-Bleo (Non-Hodgkin's lymphoma)	cyclophosphamide	Cytoxan	750 mg/m² I.V., day 1
	doxorubicin	Adriamycin	50 mg/m² I.V., day 1
	vincristine	Oncovin	2 mg I.V., days 1 and 5
	prednisone	Deltasone	100 mg P.O., days 1 to 5
	bleomycin	Blenoxane	15 units I.V., days 1 and 5 *Repeat cycle q 21 days.*
CISCA (Genitourinary cancer)	cyclophosphamide	Cytoxan	650 mg/m² I.V., day 1
	doxorubicin	Adriamycin	50 mg/m² I.V., day 1
	cisplatin	Platinol	70 to 100 mg/m² I.V., day 2 *Repeat cycle q 21 to 28 days.*
CMF (Breast cancer)	cyclophosphamide	Cytoxan	100 mg/m² P.O., days 1 to 14, or 400 to 600 mg/m² I.V., day 1
	methotrexate	Folex	40 to 60 mg/m² I.V., days 1 and 8
	fluorouracil (5-FU)	Adrucil	400 to 600 mg/m² I.V., days 1 and 8 *Repeat cycle q 28 days.*
CMFVP (Cooper's) (Breast cancer)	cyclophosphamide	Cytoxan	2 to 2.5 mg/kg P.O. daily for 9 months
	methotrexate	Folex	0.7 mg/kg/week I.V. for 8 weeks, then every other week for 7 months
	fluorouracil (5-FU)	Adrucil	12 mg/kg/week I.V. for 8 weeks, then weekly for 7 months
	vincristine	Oncovin	0.035 mg/kg (2 mg/week maximum) I.V. for 5 weeks, then once monthly
	prednisone	Deltasone	0.75 mg/kg P.O. daily, days 1 to 10, then taper over next 40 days and discontinue
CMFVP (SWOG) (Breast cancer)	cyclophosphamide	Cytoxan	60 mg/m² P.O. daily for 1 year
	methotrexate	Folex	15 mg/m² I.V. weekly for 1 year
	fluorouracil (5-FU)	Adrucil	300 mg/m² I.V. weekly for 1 year
	vincristine	Oncovin	0.625 mg/m² I.V. weekly for 1 year
	prednisone	Deltasone	30 mg/m² P.O., days 1 to 14; 20 mg/m², days 15 to 28; 10 mg/m², days 29 to 42 *Repeat cycle q 42 days.*

Cancer chemotherapy: Acronyms and protocols *(continued)*

ACRONYM & INDICATION	DRUG: Generic name	DRUG: Trade name	DOSAGE
COAP (Leukemia – AML, induction)	cyclophosphamide	Cytoxan	100 mg/m² I.V. or P.O., days 1 to 5
	vincristine	Oncovin	2 mg/m² I.V., day 1
	cytarabine (ara-C)	Cytosar-U	100 mg/m² I.V., days 1 to 5
	prednisone	Deltasone	100 mg P.O., days 1 to 5
COB (Head and neck cancer	cisplatin	Platinol	100 mg/m² I.V., day 1
	vincristine	Oncovin	1 mg I.V., days 2 and 5
	bleomycin	Blenoxane	30 units by continuous I.V. infusion, days 2 to 5 *Repeat cycle q 21 days.*
COMLA (Non-Hodgkin's lymphoma)	cyclophosphamide	Cytoxan	1,500 mg/m² I.V., day 1
	vincristine	Oncovin	1.4 mg/m² (2.5 mg maximum) I.V., days 1, 8, and 15
	methotrexate	Folex	120 mg/m² I.V., days 22, 29, 36, 43, 50, 57, 64, and 71
	leucovorin calcium	Wellcovorin	25 mg/m² P.O. q 6 hours for four doses, beginning 24 hours after methotrexate dose
	cytarabine (ara-C)	Cytosar-U	300 mg/m² I.V., days 22, 29, 36, 43, 50, 57, 64, and 71 *Repeat cycle q 21 days.*
COP (Non-Hodgkin's lymphoma)	cyclophosphamide	Cytoxan	800 to 1,000 mg/m² I.V., day 1
	vincristine	Oncovin	1.4 mg/m² (2 mg maximum) I.V., day 1
	prednisone	Deltasone	60 mg/m² P.O., days 1 to 5 *Repeat cycle q 21 days.*
COP-BLAM (Non-Hodgkin's lymphoma)	cyclophosphamide	Cytoxan	400 mg/m² I.V., day 1
	vincristine	Oncovin	1 mg/m² I.V., day 1
	prednisone	Deltasone	40 mg/m² P.O., days 1 to 10
	bleomycin	Blenoxane	15 mg I.V., day 14
	doxorubicin	Adriamycin	40 mg/m², day 1
	procarbazine	Matulane	100 mg/m², days 1 to 10
COPE (Small-cell lung cancer)	cyclophosphamide	Cytoxan	750 mg/m² I.V., day 1
	cisplatin	Platinol	20 mg/m² I.V., days 1 to 3
	etoposide (VP-16)	VePesid	100 mg/m² I.V., days 1 to 3
	vincristine	Oncovin	2 mg/m² I.V., day 3 *Repeat cycle q 21 days.*
COPP (Non-Hodgkin's lymphoma)	cyclophosphamide	Cytoxan	400 to 650 mg/m² I.V., days 1 and 8
	vincristine	Oncovin	1.4 to 1.5 mg/m² (2 mg maximum) I.V., days 1 and 8
	procarbazine	Matulane	100 mg/m² P.O., days 1 to 10 or 1 to 14
	prednisone	Deltasone	40 mg/m² P.O., days 1 to 14 *Repeat cycle q 28 days.*

(continued)

Cancer chemotherapy: Acronyms and protocols *(continued)*

ACRONYM & INDICATION	DRUG: Generic name	DRUG: Trade name	DOSAGE
CP (Ovarian cancer, epithelial)	cyclophosphamide	Cytoxan	1,000 mg/m² I.V., day 1
	cisplatin	Platinol	50 to 60 mg/m² I.V., day 1 *Repeat cycle q 21 days.*
CV (Small-cell lung cancer)	cisplatin	Platinol	50 mg/m² I.V., day 1
	etoposide (VP-16)	VePesid	60 mg/m² I.V., days 1 to 5 *Repeat cycle q 21 to 28 days.*
CV (Non-small-cell lung cancer)	cisplatin	Platinol	60 to 80 mg/m² I.V., day 1
	etoposide (VP-16)	VePesid	120 mg/m² I.V., days 4, 6, and 8 *Repeat cycle q 21 to 28 days.*
CVEB (Genitourinary cancer)	cisplatin	Platinol	40 mg/m² I.V., days 1 to 5
	vinblastine	Velban	7.5 mg/m² I.V., day 1
	etoposide (VP-16)	VePesid	100 mg/m² I.V., days 1 to 5
	bleomycin	Blenoxane	30 units I.V. weekly *Repeat cycle q 21 days.*
CVI (VIC) (Non-small-cell lung cancer)	carboplatin	Paraplatin	300 mg/m² I.V., day 1
	etoposide (VP-16)	VePesid	60 to 100 mg/m² I.V., day 1
	ifosfamide	Ifex	1.5 g/m² I.V., days 1, 3, and 5
	mesna	Mesnex	Dosage is 20% of ifosfamide dose, given immediately before and at 4 and 8 hours after ifosfamide infusion *Repeat cycle q 28 days.*
CVP (Leukemia – CLL, blast crisis)	cyclophosphamide	Cytoxan	300 mg/m² P.O., days 1 to 5
	vincristine	Oncovin	1.4 mg/m² (2 mg maximum) I.V., day 1
	prednisone	Deltasone	100 mg/m² P.O., days 1 to 5 *Repeat cycle q 21 days.*
CVP (Non-Hodgkin's lymphoma)	cyclophosphamide	Cytoxan	400 mg/m² P.O., days 1 to 5
	vincristine	Oncovin	1.4 mg/m² (2 mg maximum) I.V., day 1
	prednisone	Deltasone	100 mg/m² P.O., days 1 to 5 *Repeat cycle q 21 days.*
CVPP (Hodgkin's lymphoma)	lomustine (CCNU)	CeeNU	75 mg/m² P.O., day 1
	vinblastine	Velban	4 mg/m² I.V., days 1 and 8
	procarbazine	Matulane	100 mg/m² P.O., days 1 to 14
	prednisone	Deltasone	30 mg/m² P.O., days 1 to 14 (cycles 1 and 4 only) *Repeat cycle q 28 days.*
CYADIC (Soft-tissue sarcoma)	cyclophosphamide	Cytoxan	600 mg/m² I.V., day 1
	doxorubicin	Adriamycin	15 mg/m² by continuous I.V. infusion, days 1 to 4
	dacarbazine	DTIC-Dome	250 mg/m² by continuous I.V. infusion, days 1 to 4

Cancer chemotherapy: Acronyms and protocols *(continued)*

ACRONYM & INDICATION	DRUG: Generic name	DRUG: Trade name	DOSAGE
CYVADIC (Bony sarcoma)	cyclophosphamide	Cytoxan	600 mg/m² I.V., day 1
	vincristine	Oncovin	1.4 mg/m² (2 mg maximum) I.V. weekly for 6 weeks, then on day 1 of future cycles
	doxorubicin	Adriamycin	15 mg/m² by continuous I.V. infusion, days 1 to 4
	dacarbazine	DTIC-Dome	250 mg/m² by continuous I.V. infusion, days 1 to 4 *Repeat cycle q 21 to 28 days.*
CYVADIC (Soft-tissue sarcoma)	cyclophosphamide	Cytoxan	500 mg/m² I.V., day 1
	vincristine	Oncovin	1.4 mg/m² (2 mg maximum) I.V., days 1 and 5
	doxorubicin	Adriamycin	50 mg/m² I.V., day 1
	dacarbazine	DTIC-Dome	250 mg/m² I.V., days 1 to 5 *Repeat cycle q 21 days.*
DC (Leukemia – pediatric AML, induction)	daunorubicin	Cerubidine	45 to 60 mg/m² I.V., days 1 to 3
	cytarabine (ara-C)	Cytosar-U	100 mg/m² I.V. or S.C. q 12 hours for 5 to 7 days
DCPM (Leukemia – pediatric AML, induction)	daunorubicin	Cerubidine	25 mg/m² I.V., day 1
	cytarabine (ara-C)	Cytosar-U	80 mg/m² I.V., days 1 to 3
	prednisone	Deltasone	40 mg/m² P.O. daily
	mercaptopurine (6-MP)	Purinethol	100 mg/m² P.O. daily
DCT (Leukemia – ANLL, induction)	daunorubicin	Cerubidine	60 mg/m² I.V., days 1 to 3
	cytarabine (ara-C)	Cytosar-U	200 mg/m² daily by continuous I.V. infusion, days 1 to 5
	thioguanine (6-TG)		100 mg/m² P.O. q 12 hours, days 1 to 5
DHAP (Hodgkin's lymphoma)	dexamethasone	Decadron	40 mg P.O. or I.V., days 1 to 4
	cisplatin	Platinol	100 mg/m² by continuous I.V. infusion, day 1
	cytarabine (ara-C)	Cytosar-U	2 g/m² I.V. q 12 hours for two doses, day 2 *Repeat cycle q 3 to 4 weeks.*
DTIC-ACTD (Malignant melanoma)	dacarbazine	DTIC-Dome	750 mg/m² I.V., day 1
	dactinomycin (actinomycin D)	Cosmegen	1 mg/m² I.V., day 1 *Repeat cycle q 28 days.*
DVP (Leukemia – ALL, induction)	daunorubicin	Cerubidine	45 mg/m² I.V., days 1 to 4
	vincristine	Oncovin	2 mg/m² (2 mg maximum) I.V. weekly for 4 weeks
	prednisone	Deltasone	45 mg/m² P.O., for 28 to 35 days

(continued)

Cancer chemotherapy: Acronyms and protocols *(continued)*

ACRONYM & INDICATION	DRUG		DOSAGE
	Generic name	Trade name	
EP (Small-cell or non-small-cell lung cancer)	cisplatin	Platinol	75 to 100 mg/m² I.V., day 1
	etoposide (VP-16)	VePesid	75 to 100 mg/m² I.V., days 1 to 3 *Repeat cycle q 21 to 28 days.*
ESHAP (Non-Hodgkin's lymphoma)	etoposide (VP-16)	VePesid	40 mg/m² I.V. over 30 to 60 minutes, days 1 to 4
	cisplatin	Platinol	25 mg/m² daily by continuous I.V. infusion, days 1 to 4
	cytarabine (ara-C)	Cytosar-U	2 g/m² I.V. immediately after completion of etoposide and cisplatin therapy
	methylprednisolone	Solu-Medrol	500 mg I.V. daily, days 1 to 4 *Repeat cycle q 21 to 28 days.*
EVA (Hodgkin's lymphoma)	etoposide (VP-16)	VePesid	100 mg/m² I.V., days 1 to 3
	vinblastine	Velban	6 mg/m² I.V., day 1
	doxorubicin	Adriamycin	50 mg/m² I.V., day 1 *Repeat cycle q 28 days.*
FAC (CAF) (Breast cancer)	fluorouracil (5-FU)	Adrucil	500 mg/m² I.V., days 1 and 8
	doxorubicin	Adriamycin	50 mg/m² I.V., day 1
	cyclophosphamide	Cytoxan	500 mg/m² I.V., day 1 *Repeat cycle q 21 days.*
FAM (Colon cancer; gastric cancer)	fluorouracil (5-FU)	Adrucil	600 mg/m² I.V., days 1, 8, 29, and 36
	doxorubicin	Adriamycin	30 mg/m² I.V., days 1 and 29
	mitomycin	Mutamycin	10 mg/m² I.V., day 1 *Repeat cycle q 8 weeks.*
FAM (Non-small-cell lung cancer)	fluorouracil (5-FU)	Adrucil	600 mg/m² I.V., days 1, 8, 28, and 36
	doxorubicin	Adriamycin	30 mg/m² I.V., days 1 and 28
	mitomycin	Mutamycin	10 mg/m² I.V., day 1 *Repeat cycle q 8 weeks.*
FAM (Pancreatic cancer)	fluorouracil (5-FU)	Adrucil	600 mg/m² I.V., days 1, 8, 29, and 36
	doxorubicin	Adriamycin	30 mg/m² I.V., days 1 and 29
	mitomycin	Mutamycin	10 mg/m² I.V., day 1 *Repeat cycle q 8 weeks.*
FAME (Gastric cancer)	fluorouracil (5-FU)	Adrucil	350 mg/m² I.V., days 1 to 5 and 36 to 40
	doxorubicin	Adriamycin	40 mg/m² I.V., days 1 and 36
	semustine (methyl CCNU)		150 mg/m² P.O., day 1 *Repeat cycle q 10 weeks.*
FCE (Gastric cancer)	fluorouracil (5-FU)	Adrucil	900 mg/m² by continuous I.V. infusion, days 1 to 5
	cisplatin	Platinol	20 mg/m² I.V., days 1 to 5
	etoposide (VP-16)	VePesid	90 mg/m² I.V., days 1, 3, and 5 *Repeat cycle q 21 days.*

Cancer chemotherapy: Acronyms and protocols *(continued)*

ACRONYM & INDICATION	DRUG: Generic name	DRUG: Trade name	DOSAGE
F-CL (Colon cancer)	fluorouracil (5-FU)	Adrucil	370 to 400 mg/m² I.V., days 1 to 5
	leucovorin calcium	Wellcovorin	200 mg/m² daily I.V., days 1 to 5, begun 15 minutes before fluorouracil infusion *Repeat cycle q 21 days.*
5+2 (Leukemia–ANLL, consolidation)	cytarabine (ara-C)	Cytosar-U	100 mg/m² I.V. q 12 hours for 6 days
	daunorubicin	Cerubidine	45 mg/m² I.V., days 1 and 2
FL (Genitourinary cancer) *or*	flutamide	Eulexin	250 mg P.O. t.i.d.
	leuprolide acetate	Lupron	1 mg S.C. daily
	flutamide	Eulexin	250 mg P.O. t.i.d.
	leuprolide acetate	Lupron Depot	7.5 mg I.M. q 28 days
FLe (Colon cancer)	levamisole	Ergamisol	50 mg P.O. t.i.d. for 3 days, repeated q 2 weeks for 1 year
	fluorouracil (5-FU)	Adrucil	450 mg/m² I.V. for 5 days, then, after a pause of 4 weeks, 450 mg/m² I.V. weekly for 48 weeks
FMS (Pancreatic cancer)	fluorouracil (5-FU)	Adrucil	600 mg/m² I.V., days 1, 8, 29, and 36
	mitomycin	Mutamycin	10 mg/m² I.V., day 1
	streptozocin	Zanosar	1 g/m² I.V., days 1, 8, 29, and 36 *Repeat cycle q 8 weeks.*
FMV (Colon cancer)	fluorouracil (5-FU)	Adrucil	10 mg/kg I.V., days 1 to 5
	semustine (methyl CCNU)		175 mg/m² P.O., day 1
	vincristine	Oncovin	1 mg/m² (2 mg maximum) I.V., day 1 *Repeat cycle q 35 days.*
FZ (Genitourinary cancer)	flutamide	Eulexin	250 P.O. t.i.d.
	goserelin acetate	Zoladex	3.6 mg implant S.C. q 28 days
HDMTX (high-dose methotrexate) (Bony sarcoma)	methotrexate	Folex	12 g/m² I.V. (20 g maximum)
	leucovorin calcium	Wellcovorin	15 mg I.V. or P.O. q 6 hours for 10 doses, beginning 24 hours after methotrexate dose (serum methotrexate levels must be monitored) *Repeat cycle q 4 to 16 weeks.*
Hexa-CAF (Ovarian cancer, epithelial)	altretamine	Hexalen	150 mg/m² P.O., days 1 to 14
	cyclophosphamide	Cytoxan	150 mg/m² P.O., days 1 to 14
	methotrexate	Folex	40 mg/m², days 1 and 8
	fluorouracil (5-FU)	Adrucil	600 mg/m² I.V., days 1 and 8 *Repeat cycle q 28 days.*
HiDAC (Leukemia–ANLL, consolidation)	cytarabine (ara-C)	Cytosar-U	3,000 mg/m² I.V. q 12 hours, days 1 to 6

(continued)

Cancer chemotherapy: Acronyms and protocols *(continued)*

ACRONYM & INDICATION	DRUG: Generic name	DRUG: Trade name	DOSAGE
IMF (Breast cancer)	ifosfamide	Ifex	1.5 g/m² I.V., days 1 and 8
	mesna	Mesnex	Dosage is 20% of ifosfamide dose, given immediately before and at 4 and 8 hours after ifosfamide infusion
	methotrexate	Folex	40 mg/m² I.V., days 1 and 8
	fluorouracil (5-FU)	Adrucil	600 mg/m² I.V., days 1 and 8 *Repeat cycle q 28 days.*
L-VAM (Genitourinary cancer)	leuprolide acetate	Lupron	1 mg S.C. daily
	vinblastine	Velban	1.5 mg/m² by continuous I.V. infusion, days 2 to 7
	doxorubicin	Adriamycin	50 mg/m² by 24-hour continuous I.V. infusion, day 1
	mitomycin	Mutamycin	10 mg/m² I.V., day 2 *Repeat VAM cycle q 28 days.*
MACC (Non-small-cell lung cancer)	methotrexate	Folex	30 to 40 mg/m² I.V., day 1
	doxorubicin	Adriamycin	30 to 40 mg/m² I.V., day 1
	cyclophospamide	Cytoxan	400 to 600 mg/m² I.V., day 1
	lomustine (CCNU)	CeeNU	30 to 40 mg/m² P.O., day 1 *Repeat cycle q 21 to 28 days.*
MACOP-B (Non-Hodgkin's lymphoma)	methotrexate	Folex	100 mg/m² I.V., weeks 2, 6, and 10; then 300 mg/m² I.V. for 4 hours, weeks 2, 6, and 10
	leucovorin calcium	Wellcovorin	15 mg P.O.q 6 hours for 6 doses, beginning 24 hours after methotrexate
	doxorubicin	Adriamycin	50 mg/m² I.V., weeks 1, 3, 5, 7, 9, and 11
	cyclophospamide	Cytoxan	350 mg/m² I.V., weeks 1, 3, 5, 7, 9, and 11
	vincristine	Oncovin	1.4 mg/m² I.V. (2 mg maximum), weeks 2, 4, 8, 10, and 12
	bleomycin	Blenoxane	10 mg/m² I.V., weeks 4, 8, and 12
	prednisone	Deltasone	75 mg P.O. daily
MAID (Bony sarcoma)	mesna	Mesnex	Uroprotection 1.5 g/m² by continuous I.V. infusion, days 1 to 4
	doxorubicin	Adriamycin	15 mg/m² by continuous I.V. infusion, days 1 to 3
	ifosfamide	Ifex	1.5 g/m² by continuous I.V. infusion, days 1 to 3
	dacarbazine	DTIC-Dome	250 mg/m² by continuous I.V. infusion, days 1 to 3 *Repeat cycle q 21 to 28 days.*
MAID (Soft-tissue sarcoma)	mesna	Mesnex	1.5 g/m² by continuous I.V. infusion, days 1 to 4
	doxorubicin	Adriamycin	15 mg/m² by continuous I.V. infusion, days 1 to 3
	ifosfamide	Ifex	1.5 g/m² by continuous I.V. infusion, days 1 to 3
	dacarbazine	DTIC-Dome	250 mg/m² by continuous I.V. infusion, days 1 to 3 *Repeat cycle q 21 to 28 days.*

Cancer chemotherapy: Acronyms and protocols *(continued)*

ACRONYM & INDICATION	DRUG Generic name	Trade name	DOSAGE
MAP (Head and neck cancer)	mitomycin	Mutamycin	8 mg/m² I.V., day 1
	doxorubicin	Adriamycin	40 mg/m² I.V., day 1
	cisplatin	Platinol	60 mg/m² I.V., day 1 *Repeat cycle q 28 days.*
m-BACOD (Non-Hodgkin's lymphoma)	bleomycin	Blenoxane	4 units/m² I.V., day 1
	doxorubicin	Adriamycin	45 mg/m² I.V., day 1
	cyclophosphamide	Cytoxan	600 mg/m² I.V., day 1
	vincristine	Oncovin	1 mg/m² I.V., day 1
	dexamethasone	Decadron	6 mg/m² I.V., days 1 to 5
	methotrexate	Folex	200 mg/m² I.V., days 8 and 15
	leucovorin calcium	Wellcovorin	10 mg/m² P.O. q 6 hours for 8 doses, beginning 24 hours after methotrexate dose *Repeat cycle q 21 days.*
m-BACOS (Non-Hodgkin's lymphoma)	doxorubicin	Adriamycin	50 mg/m² by 24-hour continuous I.V. infusion, day 1
	vincristine	Oncovin	1.4 mg/m² (2 mg maximum) I.V., day 1
	bleomycin	Blenoxane	10 units/m² I.V., day 1
	cyclophosphamide	Cytoxan	750 mg/m² I.V., day 1
	methotrexate	Folex	1 g/m² I.V., day 2
	leucovorin calcium	Wellcovorin	15 mg P.O. q 6 hours for 8 doses starting 24 hours after methotrexate dose *Repeat cycle q 21 to 25 days.*
MBC (Head and neck cancer)	methotrexate	Folex	40 mg/m² I.M. or I.V., days 1 and 15
	bleomycin	Blenoxane	10 units I.M. or I.V. weekly
	cisplatin	Platinol	50 mg/m² I.V., day 1 *Repeat cycle q 21 days.*
MC (Leukemia – ANLL, consolidation)	mitoxantrone	Novantrone	12 mg/m² I.V. daily, days 1 and 2
	cytarabine (ara-C)	Cytosar-U	100 mg/m² daily by continuous I.V. infusion, days 1 to 5 *Repeat cycle.*
MC (Leukemia – ANLL, induction)	mitoxantrone	Novantrone	12 mg/m² I.V., days 1 to 3 and 17 to 18
	cytarabine (ara-C)	Cytosar-U	100 mg/m² daily by continuous I.V. infusion, days 1 to 7 and 17 to 21
MF (Head and neck cancer)	methotrexate	Folex	125 to 150 mg/m² I.V., day 1
	fluorouracil (5-FU)	Adrucil	600 mg/m² I.V., beginning 1 hour after methotrexate dose
	leucovorin calcium	Wellcovorin	10 mg/m² I.V. or P.O. q 6 hours for 5 doses, beginning 24 hours after methotrexate dose *Repeat cycle weekly.*

(continued)

Cancer chemotherapy: Acronyms and protocols *(continued)*

ACRONYM & INDICATION	DRUG: Generic name	DRUG: Trade name	DOSAGE
MICE (ICE) (Small-cell and non-small-cell lung cancer)	mesna	Mesnex	Dosage is 20% of ifosfamide doses given I.V. immediately before and at 4 and 8 hours after ifosfamide infusion
	ifosfamide	Ifex	2,000 mg/m² I.V., days 1 to 3
	carboplatin	Paraplatin	300 to 350 mg/m² I.V., day 1
	etoposide (VP-16)	VePesid	60 to 100 mg/m² I.V., days 1 to 3
MINE (Non-Hodgkin's lymphoma)	mesna	Mesnex	1.3 to 1.5 g/m² I.V., days 1 to 3
	ifosfamide	Ifex	1.3 to 1.5 g/m² I.V., days 1 to 3
	mitoxantrone	Novantrone	8 to 10 mg/m² I.V., day 1
	etoposide (VP-16)	VePesid	65 to 80 mg/m² I.V., days 1 to 3
MM (Leukemia – ALL, maintenance)	mercaptopurine (6-MP)	Purinethol	50 mg/m² P.O. daily
	methotrexate	Folex	20 mg/m² P.O. or I.V. weekly
MOF (Colon cancer)	fluorouracil (5-FU)	Adrucil	10 mg/kg/day I.V., days 1 to 5
	semustine (methyl CCNU)		175 mg/m² P.O., day 1
	vincristine	Oncovin	1 mg/m² (2 mg maximum) I.V., day 1 *Repeat cycle q 35 days.*
MOP (Pediatric brain tumors)	mechlorethamine (nitrogen mustard)	Mustargen	6 mg/m² I.V., days 1 and 8
	vincristine	Oncovin	1.4 mg/m² (2 mg maximum) I.V., days 1 and 8
	procarbazine	Matulane	100 mg/m² P.O., days 1 to 14 *Repeat cycle q 28 days.*
MOPP (Hodgkin's lymphoma)	mechlorethamine (nitrogen mustard)	Mustargen	6 mg/m² I.V., days 1 and 8
	vincristine	Oncovin	1.4 mg/m² (2 mg maximum) I.V., days 1 and 8
	procarbazine	Matulane	100 mg/m² P.O., days 1 to 14
	prednisone	Deltasone	40 mg/m² P.O., days 1 to 14 *Repeat cycle q 28 days.*
MP (Multiple myeloma)	melphalan (L-phenylalanine mustard)	Alkeran	8 mg/m² P.O., days 1 to 4
	prednisone	Deltasone	40 mg/m² P.O., days 1 to 7 *Repeat cycle q 28 days.*
m-PFL (Genitourinary cancer)	methotrexate	Folex	60 mg/m², day 1
	cisplatin	Platinol	25 mg/m² by continuous I.V. infusion, days 2 to 6
	fluorouracil (5-FU)	Adrucil	800 mg/m² by continuous I.V. infusion, days 2 to 6
	leucovorin calcium	Wellcovorin	500 mg/m² by continuous I.V. infusion, days 2 to 6 *Repeat cycle q 28 days for four cycles.*

Cancer chemotherapy: Acronyms and protocols *(continued)*

ACRONYM & INDICATION	DRUG: Generic name	DRUG: Trade name	DOSAGE
M-2 (Multiple myeloma)	vincristine	Oncovin	0.03 mg/kg (2 mg maximum) I.V., day 1
	carmustine	BiCNU	0.5 mg/kg I.V., day 1
	cyclophosphamide	Cytoxan	10 mg/kg I.V, day 1
	melphalan (L-phenylalanine mustard)	Alkeran	0.25 mg/kg P.O., days 1 to 14
	prednisone	Deltasone	1 mg/kg, days 1 to 7, then taper over next 14 days *Repeat cycle q 35 days.*
MV (Leukemia – AML, induction)	mitoxantrone	Novantrone	10 mg/m² I.V., days 1 to 5
	etoposide (VP-16)	VePesid	100 mg/m² I.V., days 1 to 3
MVAC (Genitourinary cancer)	methotrexate	Folex	30 mg/m² I.V., days 1, 15, and 22
	vinblastine	Velban	3 mg/m² I.V., days 2, 15, and 22
	doxorubicin	Adriamycin	30 mg/m² I.V., day 2
	cisplatin	Platinol	70 mg/m² I.V., day 2 *Repeat cycle q 28 days.*
MVP (Non-small-cell lung cancer)	mitomycin	Mutamycin	8 mg/m² I.V., days 1, 29, and 71
	vinblastine	Velban	4.5 mg/m² I.V., days 15, 22, and 29, then q 2 weeks
	cisplatin	Platinol	120 mg/m² I.V., days 1 and 29, then q 6 weeks
MVPP (Hodgkin's lymphoma)	mechlorethamine (nitrogen mustard)	Mustargen	6 mg/m² I.V., days 1 and 8
	vinblastine	Velban	6 mg/m² I.V., days 1 and 8
	procarbazine	Matulane	100 mg/m² P.O., days 1 to 14
	prednisone	Deltasone	40 mg/m² P.O., days 1 to 14 *Repeat cycle q 42 days for six cycles.*
OPEN (Non-Hodgkin's lymphoma)	vincristine	Oncovin	2 mg I.V., day 1
	prednisone	Deltasone	100 mg P.O. daily for 5 days
	etoposide (VP-16)	VePesid	100 mg/m² I.V. daily for 3 days
	mitoxantrone	Novantrone	10 mg/m² I.V., day 1
PCV (Pediatric brain tumors)	procarbazine	Matulane	60 mg/m² P.O., days 18 to 21
	lomustine (CCNU)	CeeNU	110 mg/m² P.O., day 1
	vincristine	Oncovin	1.4 mg/m² (2 mg maximum), days 8 and 29 *Repeat cycle q 6 to 8 weeks.*
PFL (Head and neck cancer)	cisplatin	Platinol	25 mg/m² by continuous I.V. infusion, days 1 to 5
	5-fluorouracil (5-FU)	Adrucil	800 mg/m² by continuous I.V. infusion, days 2 to 6
	leucovorin calcium	Wellcovorin	500 mg/m² by continuous I.V. infusion, days 1 to 6 *Repeat cycle q 28 days.*

(continued)

Cancer chemotherapy: Acronyms and protocols *(continued)*

ACRONYM & INDICATION	DRUG: Generic name	DRUG: Trade name	DOSAGE
PFL (Non-small-cell lung cancer)	cisplatin	Platinol	25 mg/m² I.V., days 1 and 15
	fluorouracil (5-FU)	Adrucil	800 mg/m² by continuous I.V. infusion, days 1 to 5
	leucovorin calcium	Wellcovorin	500 mg/m² by continuous I.V. infusion, days 1 to 5 *Repeat cycle q 28 days.*
ProMACE (Non-Hodgkin's lymphoma)	prednisone	Deltasone	60 mg/m² P.O., days 1 to 14
	methotrexate	Folex	1.5 g/m² I.V., day 14
	leucovorin calcium	Wellcovorin	50 mg/m² I.V. q 6 hours for 5 doses, beginning 24 hours after methotrexate dose
	doxorubicin	Adriamycin	25 mg/m² I.V., days 1 and 8
	cyclophosphamide	Cytoxan	650 mg/m² I.V., days 1 and 8
	etoposide (VP-16)	VePesid	120 mg/m² I.V., days 1 and 8 *Repeat cycle q 28 days; MOPP therapy to begin after the required number of ProMACE cycles are completed.*
ProMACE/ cytaBOM (Non-Hodgkin's lymphoma)	cyclophosphamide	Cytoxan	650 mg/m² I.V., day 1
	doxorubicin	Adriamycin	25 mg/m² I.V., day 1
	etoposide (VP-16)	VePesid	120 mg/m² I.V., day 1
	prednisone	Deltasone	60 mg/m² P.O., days 1 to 14
	cytarabine (ara-C)	Cytosar-U	300 mg/m² I.V., day 8
	bleomycin	Blenoxane	5 mg/m² I.V., day 8
	vincristine	Oncovin	1.4 mg/m² I.V., day 8
	methotrexate	Folex	120 mg/m² I.V., day 8
	leucovorin calcium	Wellcovorin	25 mg/m² P.O. q 6 hours for 4 doses *Repeat cycle q 28 days.*
(pulse) VAC (Soft-tissue sarcoma)	vincristine	Oncovin	1.5 g/m² (2 mg maximum) I.V., day 1 or weekly, starting on day 1
	dactinomycin (actinomycin D)	Cosmegen	0.4 mg/m² I.V., day 1
	cyclophosphamide	Cytoxan	1,000 mg/m² I.V., day 1 *Repeat cycle q 3 to 4 weeks.*
7 + 3 (A + D) (Leukemia – AML, induction)	cytarabine (ara-C)	Cytosar-U	100 or 200 mg/m² by continuous I.V. infusion, days 1 to 7
	daunorubicin	Cerubidine	45 mg/m² I.V., days 1 to 3
TC (Leukemia – ANLL, maintenance)	thioguanine (6-TG)		40 mg/m² P.O. q 12 hours for 8 doses, days 1 to 4
	cytarabine (ara-C)	Cytosar-U	60 mg/m² S.C. day 5 *Repeat cycle weekly.*

Cancer chemotherapy: Acronyms and protocols *(continued)*

ACRONYM & INDICATION	DRUG: Generic name	DRUG: Trade name	DOSAGE
T-10 (Pediatric bony sarcoma)	methotrexate	Folex	12 g/m² I.V. for 12 or 16 doses
	leucovorin calcium	Wellcovorin	15 mg I.V. or P.O. q 6 hours for 10 doses, each starting 20 hours after methotrexate dose
	doxorubicin	Adriamycin	30 mg/m² I.V. for 2 to 3 days
	cisplatin	Platinol	120 mg/m² I.V. for 1 day
	bleomycin	Blenoxane	15 units/m² I.V. for 2 days
	cyclophosphamide	Cytoxan	600 mg/m² I.V. for 2 days
	dactinomycin (actinomycin D)	Cosmegen	0.6 mg/m² I.V. for 2 days
VA (Wilms' tumor)	vincristine	Oncovin	1.5 mg/m² (2 mg maximum) weekly
	dactinomycin (actinomycin D)	Cosmegen	0.4 mg/m² q 2 weeks
VAB (Genitourinary cancer)	vinblastine	Velban	4 mg/m² I.V., day 1
	dactinomycin (actinomycin D)	Cosmegen	1 mg/m² I.V., day 1
	bleomycin	Blenoxane	30 units I.V. push, then 20 units/m² by continuous I.V. infusion, days 1 to 3
	cisplatin	Platinol	120 mg/m² I.V., day 4
	cyclophosphamide	Cytoxan	600 mg/m² I.V., day 1 *Repeat cycle q 21 days.*
VAC (Small-cell lung cancer)	vincristine	Oncovin	2 mg I.V., day 1
	doxorubicin	Adriamycin	50 mg/m² I.V., day 1
	cyclophosphamide	Cytoxan	750 mg/m² I.V., day 1 *Repeat cycle q 21 days for four cycles.*
VAC (Ovarian cancer, germ-cell)	vincristine	Oncovin	1.2 to 1.5 mg/m² (2 mg maximum) I.V. weekly for 10 to 12 weeks, or q 2 weeks for 12 doses
	dactinomycin (actinomycin D)	Cosmegen	0.3 to 0.4 mg/m² I.V., days 1 to 5
	cyclophosphamide	Cytoxan	150 mg/m² I.V., days 1 to 5 *Repeat cycle q 28 days.*
VAC (Wilms' tumor)	vincristine	Oncovin	1.5 mg/m² (2 mg maximum) weekly
	dactinomycin (actinomycin D)	Cosmegen	1.25 g/m² q 3 weeks
	cyclophosphamide	Cytoxan	1,000 mg/m² q 3 weeks
VAD (Multiple myeloma)	vincristine	Oncovin	0.4 mg by continuous I.V. infusion, days 1 to 4
	doxorubicin	Adriamycin	9 to 10 mg/m² by continuous I.V. infusion, days 1 to 4
	dexamethasone	Decadron	40 mg P.O. on days 1 to 4, 9 to 12, and 17 to 20 *Repeat cycle q 25 to 35 days.*

(continued)

Cancer chemotherapy: Acronyms and protocols *(continued)*

ACRONYM & INDICATION	DRUG		DOSAGE
	Generic name	**Trade name**	
VAP (VP + A) (Leukemia – pediatric ALL, induction)	vincristine	Oncovin	1.5 to 2 mg/m² (2 mg maximum) I.V. weekly for 4 weeks
	asparaginase	Elspar	10,000 units I.M., days 1 and 8 (other doses include 6,000 units/m² I.M. for 3 days/week or 25,000 units/m²)
	prednisone	Deltasone	40 mg/m² P.O., days 1 to 28, then taper over 7 days
VATH (Breast cancer)	vinblastine	Velban	4.5 mg/m² I.V., day 1
	doxorubicin	Adriamycin	45 mg/m² I.V., day 1
	thiotepa	Thiotepa	12 mg/m² I.V., day 1
	fluoxymesterone	Halotestin	30 mg P.O. (daily through each course) *Repeat cycle q 21 days.*
VB (Genitourinary cancer)	vinblastine	Velban	3 to 4 mg/m² I.V., day 1
	methotrexate	Folex	30 to 40 mg/m² I.V., day 1 *Repeat cycle weekly.*
VBAP (Multiple myeloma)	vincristine	Oncovin	1 mg I.V., day 1
	carmustine	BiCNU	30 mg/m² I.V., day 1
	doxorubicin	Adriamycin	30 mg/m² I.V., day 1
	prednisone	Deltasone	100 mg P.O., days 1 to 4 *Repeat cycle q 21 days.*
VBC (Malignant melanoma)	vinblastine	Velban	6 mg/m² I.V., days 1 and 2
	bleomycin	Blenoxane	15 units/m² by continuous I.V. infusion, days 1 to 5
	cisplatin	Platinol	50 mg/m² I.V., day 5 *Repeat cycle q 28 days.*
VBP (Genitourinary cancer)	vinblastine	Velban	6 mg/m² I.V., days 1 and 2
	bleomycin	Blenoxane	30 units I.V. weekly
	cisplatin	Platinol	20 mg/m² I.V., days 1 to 5 *Repeat cycle q 21 to 28 days.*
VC (Small-cell lung cancer)	etoposide (VP-16)	VePesid	100 to 200 mg/m² I.V., days 1 to 3
	carboplatin	Paraplatin	50 to 125 mg/m² I.V., days 1 to 3 *Repeat cycle q 28 days.*
VCAP (Multiple myeloma)	vincristine	Oncovin	1 mg I.V., day 1
	cyclophosphamide	Cytoxan	100 mg/m² P.O., days 1 to 4
	doxorubicin	Adriamycin	25 mg/m² I.V., day 2
	prednisone	Deltasone	60 mg/m² P.O., days 1 to 4 *Repeat cycle q 28 days.*

Cancer chemotherapy: Acronyms and protocols *(continued)*

ACRONYM & INDICATION	DRUG: Generic name	DRUG: Trade name	DOSAGE
VDP (Malignant melanoma)	vinblastine	Velban	5 mg/m² I.V., days 1 and 2
	dacarbazine	DTIC-Dome	150 mg/m² I.V., days 1 to 5
	cisplatin	Platinol	75 mg/m² I.V., day 5 *Repeat cycle q 21 to 28 days.*
VIP (Genitourinary cancer)	vinblastine	Velban	0.11 mg/kg I.V., days 1 and 2
	ifosfamide	Ifex	1.2 g/m² I.V., days 1 to 5
	cisplatin	Platinol	20 mg/m², days 1 to 5
	mesna	Mesnex	400 mg I.V., 15 minutes before ifosfamide, then 1.2 g by continuous I.V. infusion, days 1 to 5 *Repeat cycle q 3 weeks for four cycles.*
or	etoposide (VP-16)	VePesid	75 mg/m² I.V., days 1 to 5
	ifosfamide	Ifex	1.2 g/m² I.V., days 1 to 5
	cisplatin	Platinol	20 mg/m², days 1 to 5
	mesna	Mesnex	400 mg I.V., 15 minutes before ifosfamide, then 1.2 g by continuous I.V. infusion, days 1 to 5 *Repeat cycle q 3 weeks for four cycles.*

Orphan drugs and biologicals

As defined by the Orphan Drug Act, an orphan drug is one that is useful for the diagnosis, treatment, or prevention of a rare disease or disorder. This act defines a rare disease as one that affects fewer than 200,000 persons in the United States, or one for which the expected sales will not recover the cost of developing and making the drug available. The following list includes the drugs and biologicals that have received orphan drug designation.

GENERIC NAME	TRADE NAME	DESIGNATED USE
Drugs		
aconiazide	Not established	Treatment of tuberculosis.
adenosine	Not established	Treatment of brain tumors.
AI-RSA	Not established	Treatment of autoimmune uveitis.
allopurinol	Zyloprim	For use in the ex vivo preservation of cadaveric kidneys for transplantation.
allopurinol riboside	Not established	Treatment of cutaneous and visceral leishmaniasis and Chagas' disease.
aminosidine	Gabbromicina	Treatment of tuberculosis.
anagrelide	Not established	Treatment of polycythemia vera, thrombocytosis in chronic myelogenous leukemia, and essential thrombocythemia.
ananain (comosain)	Vianain	Enzymatic debridement of severe burns.
anaritide acetate	Auriculin	Early improvement of kidney function following kidney transplantation.
antiepilepsirine	Not established	Treatment of refractory generalized tonic-clonic seizures.
antipyrine	Not established	Antipyrine test as an index of hepatic drug-metabolizing capacity.
apomorphine hydrochloride	Not established	Treatment of on-off phenomenon associated with late-stage Parkinson's disease.
arginine butyrate	Not established	Treatment of beta-thalassemia and beta-hemoglobinopathies.
AS-101	Not established	Treatment of AIDS.
3′ azido-2, 3′dideoxyuridine	Not established	Treatment of AIDS.
bacitracin zinc	Altracin	Treatment of antibiotic-associated pseudomembranous enterocolitis caused by toxins A and B from *Clostridium difficile.*

Orphan drugs and biologicals *(continued)*

GENERIC NAME	TRADE NAME	DESIGNATED USE
Drugs *(continued)*		
bethanidine sulfate	Not established	Prevention or treatment of primary ventricular fibrillation.
BMY-45622	Not established	Treatment of ovarian cancer.
bromhexine	Not established	Treatment of keratoconjunctivitis sicca in patients with Sjögren's syndrome.
BW B759U	Not established	Treatment of severe human CMV infections in specific immunosuppressed patient populations (for example, bone marrow transplantation, AIDS).
BW 12C	Not established	Treatment of sickle cell disease crisis.
C1-esterase-inhibitor, human	Not established	Prevention and treatment of acute attacks of hereditary angioedema.
calcium gluconate gel	H-F Gel	Emergency topical treatment of hydrogen fluoride (hydrofluoric acid) burns.
carbovir	Not established	Treatment of AIDS and symptomatic HIV infection.
ceramide trihexosidase/alpha-galactosidase A	Not established	Treatment of Fabry's disease.
cetiedil citrate	Not established	Treatment of sickle cell crisis.
2-chlorodeoxyadenosine	Not established	Treatment of chronic lymphocytic leukemia and hairy-cell leukemia.
2-chloro-2′-deoxyadenosine	Not established	Treatment of acute myeloid leukemia.
9-cis retinoic acid	Not established	Treatment of acute promyelocytic leukemia.
citric acid, glucono-delta-lactone, and magnesium carbonate	Renacidin	Treatment of apatite or struvite renal or bladder calculi.
copolymer 1 (COP 1)	Not established	Treatment of multiple sclerosis.
cyproterone acetate	Androcur, Cyproteron	Treatment of severe hirsutism.
cysteamine hydrochloride (2-aminoethanethiol)	Not established	Treatment of nephropathic cystinosis.

(continued)

Orphan drugs and biologicals *(continued)*

GENERIC NAME	TRADE NAME	DESIGNATED USE
Drugs *(continued)*		
cystic fibrosis transmembrane conductance regulator gene	Not established	Treatment of cystic fibrosis.
decitabine (5-AZA-2′-deoxycytidine; DAC)	Not established	Treatment of acute leukemia.
defibrotide	Not established	Treatment of thrombotic thrombocytopenic purpura.
deslorelin	Somagard	Treatment of central precocious puberty.
dexrazoxane	Zinecard	Prevention of doxorubicin-induced cardiomyopathy.
dextran and deferoxamine	Bio-Rescue	Treatment of acute iron poisoning.
dextran sulfate aerosol inhalation	Uendex	Adjunctive treatment of cystic fibrosis.
dextran sulfate sodium (UA001)	Not established	Treatment of AIDS.
3,4-diaminopyridine	Not established	Treatment of Eaton-Lambert (myasthenic) syndrome.
dianeal PD-2 peritoneal dialysis solution	Nutrineal	Nutritional supplementation in patients undergoing continuous ambulatory peritoneal dialysis.
diaziquone	Not established	Treatment of primary brain malignancies (grades III to IV astrocytomas).
2′-3′-dideoxy-adenosine	Not established	Treatment of AIDS.
2′-3′-dideoxycytidine	Not established	Treatment of AIDS.
2′-3′-dideoxyinosine	Not established	Treatment of AIDS.
diethyldithiocarbamate (DTC)	Imuthiol	Treatment of AIDS.
dihematoporphyrin ethers	Photofrin II	Photodynamic treatment of primary or recurrent obstructive esophageal carcinoma; treatment of transitional cell carcinoma of the bladder.
2,3-dimercaptosuccinic acid (DMSA)	Not established	Treatment of lead poisoning in children.
dimethyl sulfoxide (DMSO)	Sclerosol	Treatment of cutaneous manifestations of scleroderma.

Orphan drugs and biologicals *(continued)*

GENERIC NAME	TRADE NAME	DESIGNATED USE
Drugs *(continued)*		
disodium clodronate tetrahydrate	Bonefos	Treatment of bone resorption caused by malignant tumors.
disodium silibinin dihemisuccinate	Legalon Sil	Treatment of hepatic intoxication by *Amanita phalloides* (mushroom poisoning).
dynamine	Not established	Treatment of Eaton-Lambert (myasthenic) syndrome and Charcot-Marie-Tooth disease.
enisoprost	Not established	Adjunctive treatment (with cyclosporine) to reduce rejection and decrease cyclosporine nephrotoxicity in transplant recipients.
epoprostenol	Cyclo-Prostin	Replacement of heparin in patients requiring hemodialysis who are at increased risk for hemorrhage.
ethiofos	Ethyol	Adjunctive therapy (chemoprotective agent) with cisplatin or cyclophosphamide in the treatment of cancer.
fatty acid solution, short chain	Not established	Treatment of ulcerative colitis (active phase) with involvement restricted to the left side of the colon.
flumecinol	Zixoryn	Hyberbilirubinemia in neonates unresponsive to phototherapy.
flunarizine	Sibelium	Treatment of alternating hemiplegia.
fosphenytoin	Not established	Acute treatment of status epilepticus.
gentamicin-impregnated PMMA beads on surgical wire	Septopal	Treatment of chronic osteomyelitis.
gentamicin liposome injection	Not established	Treatment of disseminated *Mycobacterium avium-intracellulare* infection.
GM 6001	Not established	Treatment of corneal ulcers.
gossypol	Not established	Treatment of adrenal cortex cancer.
herpes simplex virus gene	Not established	Treatment of primary and metastatic brain tumors.
HPA-23	Not established	Treatment of AIDS.
human growth hormone-releasing factor	Not established	Treatment of children with growth failure caused by lack of endogenous growth hormone secretion.

(continued)

Orphan drugs and biologicals *(continued)*

GENERIC NAME	TRADE NAME	DESIGNATED USE
Drugs *(continued)*		
humanized anti-TAC	Not established	Prevention of acute renal allograft rejection and acute graft-versus-host disease after bone marrow transplantation.
4-hydroperoxycyclo-phosphamide (4-HC)	Not established	Ex vivo treatment of bone marrow in patients with acute myelogenous leukemia undergoing autologous bone marrow transplantation.
hydroxycobalamin/ sodium thiosulfate	Not established	Treatment of severe acute cyanide poisoning.
iloprost	Not established	Treatment of heparin-induced thrombocytopenia and Raynaud's phenomenon secondary to systemic sclerosis.
inosine pranobex	Isoprinosine	Treatment of subacute sclerosing panencephalitis.
interleukin-1 receptor antagonist, human recombinant	Antril	Prevention and treatment of graft-versus-host disease in transplant recipients; treatment of juvenile rheumatoid arthritis.
iodine ^{131}I 6B-iodomethyl-19-norcholesterol	Not established	Adrenocortical imaging.
iodine ^{131}I meta-iodobenzyl-guanidine	Not established	Diagnostic adjunct in patients with pheochromocytoma.
isobutyramide	Not established	Treatment of beta-hemoglobinopathies and beta-thalassemia.
leupeptin	Not established	Adjunctive treatment of microsurgical nerve repair.
levocabastine hydrochloride	Not established	Treatment of vernal keratoconjunctivitis.
LHRH [(des-gly^{10})-d-trp^{6}-Pro^{9}-N-ethylamide]	Not established	Treatment of central precocious puberty.
L-5 hydroxytryptophan (L-5-HTP)	Not established	Treatment of postanoxic intention myoclonus.
L-leucine, L-isoleucine, and L-valine	Not established	Treatment of amyotrophic lateral sclerosis.
L-leucovorin	Isovorin	Palliative treatment (with fluorouracil) of metastatic adenocarcinoma of the colon and rectum.

Orphan drugs and biologicals *(continued)*

GENERIC NAME	TRADE NAME	DESIGNATED USE
Drugs *(continued)*		
loxoribine	Not established	Treatment of common variable immunodeficiency.
L-threonine	Threostat	Treatment of amyotropic lateral sclerosis.
lysine acetylsalicylate	Aspegic	Treatment of pain and fever associated with sickle cell crisis.
methotrexate with laurocapram	Not established	Treatment of mycosis fungoides.
4-methylpyrazole (4-MP)	Not established	Treatment of poisoning from methanol, ethylene glycol, 2-methoxy-ethanol, or 2-butoxyethanol.
mitodrine hydrochloride	Midamine	Treatment of idiopathic orthostatic hypotension.
mitolactol (dibromodulcitol, DBD)	Not established	Treatment of invasive cervical cancer.
modafinil	Not established	Treatment of narcolepsy.
N-acetylprocainamide (NAPA)	Not established	Adjunctive treatment of ventricular fibrillation in patients with automatic implantable cardioverter defibrillators.
NG-29	Somatrel	Assessment of pituitary function in children with suspected growth hormone deficiency.
ovine corticotropin-releasing hormone (oCRH)	Not established	To differentiate pituitary and ectopic production of corticotropin in patients with corticotropin-dependent Cushing's syndrome.
oxaliplatin	Not established	Treatment of ovarian cancer.
PEG-adenosine deaminase (PEG-ADA)	Imudon	Enzyme replacement therapy for ADA deficiency in patients with severe combined immunodeficiency.
phosphocysteamine	Not established	Treatment of cystinosis.
piracetam	Nootropil	Treatment of myoclonus.
piritrexim isethionate	Not established	Treatment of infections caused by *Pneumocystis carinii, Toxoplasma gondii,* and *Mycobacterium avium-intracellulare.*
poloxamer 188	Rheoth Rx Copolymer	Treatment of sickle cell crisis and severe burns.

(continued)

Orphan drugs and biologicals *(continued)*

GENERIC NAME	TRADE NAME	DESIGNATED USE
Drugs *(continued)*		
poloxamer 331	Protox	Initial treatment of toxoplasmosis in patients with AIDS.
polymer implant containing carmustine	Biodel	Localized treatment of recurrent malignant melanoma in the brain.
potassium citrate and citric acid	Polycitra-K	Dissolution and control of uric acid and cystine calculi in the urinary tract.
PPI-002	Not established	Treatment of malignant mesothelioma.
PR-122 (redox-phenytoin)	Not established	Emergency treatment of status epilepticus.
PR-225 (redox acyclovir)	Not established	Treatment of herpes simplex encephalitis in patients with AIDS.
PR-239 (redox penicillin G)	Not established	Treatment of neurosyphilis associated with AIDS.
PR-320 (molecusol-carbamazepine)	Not established	Emergency treatment of status epilepticus.
pramiracetam sulfate	Not established	Treatment of cognitive dysfunction and enhancement of antidepressant activity associated with electroconvulsive therapy.
prednimustine	Sterecyt	Treatment of non-Hodgkin's lymphomas.
propamidine isethionate 0.1%	Brolene Eye Drops	Treatment of *Acanthamoeba* keratitis.
protirelin (TRH)	Thymone	Treatment of amyotrophic lateral sclerosis.
rifampin, isoniazid, pyrazinamide	Rifater	Short-course treatment of tuberculosis.
riluzole	Not established	Treatment of amyotrophic lateral sclerosis.
roquinimex	Linomide	Stimulation of immunologic response in patients with chronic myelocytic leukemia who have undergone autologous bone marrow transplantation.
SDZ MSL-109	Not established	Prevention of CMV disease in transplant recipients; treatment of CMV retinitis in patients with AIDS.
secalciferol (24, 25 dihydroxycholecalciferol)	Osteo-D	Treatment of uremic osteodystrophy and familial hypophosphatemic rickets.

Orphan drugs and biologicals *(continued)*

GENERIC NAME	TRADE NAME	DESIGNATED USE
Drugs *(continued)*		
sodium dichloroacetate	Not established	Treatment of homozygous familial hypercholesterolemia and congenital lactic acidosis.
sodium monomercaptoundecahydro-closo-dodecaborate	Borolife	Treatment of glioblastoma multiforme as an alternative to conventional photon therapy.
sodium oxybate (sodium gammahydroxybutyrate)	Not established	Treatment of narcolepsy and the auxiliary symptoms of cataplexy, sleep paralysis, hypnagogic hallucinations, and automatic behavior.
sodium tetradecyl sulfate	Sotradecol	Treatment of bleeding esophageal varices.
spiramycin	Rovamycine	Symptomatic relief and parasitic cure of chronic cryptosporidiosis in immunosuppressed pateints.
superoxide dismutase (recombinant, human)	Not established	Protection of donor organ tissue from damage or injury mediated by oxygen-derived free radicals generated during the necessary periods of ischemia (hypoxia), and especially reperfusion, anoxia associated with the operative procedure; prevention of bronchopulmonary dysplasia in premature neonates (under 1,500 g).
T4 endonuclease V, liposome encapsulated	T4N5 Liposomes	Prevention of skin abnormalities such as cutaneous neoplasms in patients with xeroderma pigmentosum.
teriparatide	Parathar	To aid diagnosis in patients with clinical and laboratory evidence of hypocalcemia from either hypoparathyroidism or pseudohypoparathyroidism.
terlipressin	Glypressin	Treatment of bleeding esophageal varices.
thalidomide	Not established	Prevention and treatment of graft-versus-host disease in patients receiving bone marrow transplantation; treatment and maintenance of reactional lepromatous leprosy; treatment of clinical signs of mycobacterial infection.

(continued)

Orphan drugs and biologicals *(continued)*

GENERIC NAME	TRADE NAME	DESIGNATED USE
Drugs *(continued)*		
thymoxamine hydrochloride	Not established	Reversal of phenylephrine-induced mydriasis in patients who have narrow anterior angles and are at risk for developing acute angle-closure glaucoma after mydriasis.
titratricol	Triacana	To suppress thyroid-stimulating hormone production in patients with thyroid cancer.
tocophersolan oral solution (vitamin E, d-alpha tocopheryl polylene glycol-1000 succinate, TPGS)	Not established	Treatment of vitamin E deficiency in patients with malabsorption caused by prolonged cholestatic hepatobiliary disease.
topiramate	Topimax	Treatment of Lennox-Gastaut syndrome.
tranexamic acid	Cyklokapron	Treatment of hereditary angioedema, patients undergoing prostatectomy when there is hemorrhage or risk of hemorrhage from increased fibrinolysis or fibrinogenolysis, and patients with congenital coagulopathies who are undergoing surgical procedures, such as dental extractions.
transforming growth factor beta-2	Not established	Treatment of full-thickness macular hole disease.
tretinoin	Not established	Treatment of squamous metaplasia of the ocular surface epithelia (conjunctiva or cornea) with mucus deficiency and keratinization.
triptorelin pamoate	Decapeptyl Injection	Palliative treatment of advanced ovarian cancer of epithelial origin.
troleandomycin	Not established	Adjunctive treatment of severe steroid-dependent asthma.
tumor necrosis factor-binding protein I	Not established	Treatment of AIDS.
tumor necrosis factor-binding protein II	Not established	Treatment of AIDS.
urofollitropin	Metrodin	Induction of ovulation in patients with polycystic ovarian disease who have an elevated luteinizing hormone to follicle-stimulating hormone ratio and who have failed to respond to adequate clomiphene therapy.

Orphan drugs and biologicals *(continued)*

GENERIC NAME	TRADE NAME	DESIGNATED USE
Drugs *(continued)*		
viloxazine hydrochloride	Catatrol	Treatment of narcolepsy and cataplexy.
zinc acetate	Not established	Treatment of Wilson's disease.
Biologicals		
aerosolized pooled immune globulin	Not established	Treatment of respiratory syncytial virus.
alpha-1-antitrypsin (recombinant DNA origin)	Not established	Supplementation therapy for alpha-1-antitrypsin deficiency in the ZZ phenotype population.
alpha-galactosidase A	CC-Galactosidase	Treatment of Fabray's disease.
alpha-galactoside A	FABRase	Treatment of Fabray's disease.
ancrod	Arvin	Treatment of heparin-induced thrombosis or thrombocytopenia.
anticytomegalovirus monoclonal antibodies	Not established	Prevention or treatment of CMV infection in patients with AIDS, and in organ transplantation or bone marrow transplant recipients.
antihemophilic factor (recombinant DNA origin)	Kogenate	Prophylaxis and treatment of bleeding in patients with hemophilia A.
antimelanoma antibody XMMME-001-RTA	Not established	Treatment of Stage III melanoma not amenable to surgical resection.
anti-TAP-72 immunotoxin	Xomazyme-791	Treatment of metastatic colorectal adenocarcinoma.
benzylpenicillin, benzylpenicilloic acid, and benzylpenilloic acid	Pre-Pen/MDM	For assessing the risk of administering penicillin when it is the drug of choice in adults with a history of clinical hypersensitivity.
beta-glucocerberocidase, recombinant	Not established	Replacement therapy in patients with Type I, II, or III Gaucher's disease.
botulism immune globulin	Not established.	Treatment of infant botulism.
bovine colostrum	Not established	Treatment of AIDS-related diarrhea.
butyrylcholinesterase	Not established	Treatment of cocaine overdose and postoperative apnea.
CD4, human recombinant soluble	Receptin	Treatment of AIDS.

(continued)

Orphan drugs and biologicals *(continued)*

GENERIC NAME	TRADE NAME	DESIGNATED USE
Biologicals *(continued)*		
CD4, human truncated-369 AA polypeptide (recombinant CHO cells)	Soluble T4	Treatment of AIDS.
CD4 immunoglobulin G (recombinant human)	Not established	Treatment of AIDS.
CD-45 monoclonal antibodies	Not established	Prevention of rejection of human organ transplantation.
CD5-T lymphocyte Immunotoxin	Xomazyme-H65	Ex vivo treatment to eliminate mature T cells from potential bone marrow grafts, in vivo treatment of bone marrow recipients to prevent graft rejection and graft-versus-host disease (GVHD), and treatment of GVHD or rejection in patients who have received bone marrow transplantation.
chimeric M-T412 (human-murine) IgG monoclonal anti-CD4	Not established	Treatment of multiple sclerosis.
ciliary neurotrophic factor	Not established	Treatment of amyotrophic lateral sclerosis.
C1-inhibitor	C1-inhibitor (human) vapor treated, Immuno	Prevention or treatment of acute attacks of angioedema.
cryptosporidium hyperimmune bovine colostrum IgG concentrate	Not established	Treatment of *Cryptosporidium parvum*-induced diarrhea in patients with AIDS.
deoxyribonuclease, recombinant human (rhDNase)	Not established	To reduce the viscosity of mucus secretions and enhance airway clearance in patients with cystic fibrosis.
disaccharide tripeptide glycerol dipalmitoyl	Immther	Treatment of hepatic and pulmonary metastases in patients with colorectal adenocarcinoma.
epidermal growth factor (human)	Not established	Acceleration of corneal epithelial regeneration and healing of stromal tissue in patients with nonhealing corneal defects or after corneal transplantation, and promotion of cutaneous wound healing in extreme burn treatment protocols.

Orphan drugs and biologicals *(continued)*

GENERIC NAME	TRADE NAME	DESIGNATED USE
Biologicals *(continued)*		
epoetin beta (recombinant-human)	Marogen	Treatment of anemia associated with end-stage renal disease.
factor VIIa (recombinant, DNA origin)	Not established	Treatment of von Willebrand's disease and of patients with hemophilia A and B with and without antibodies against factors VIII and IX.
factor XIII	Fibrogammin	Congenital factor XIII deficiency.
fibronectin (human plasma derived)	Not established	Treatment of epithelial defects or nonhealing corneal ulcers unresponsive to conventional therapy.
fire ant venom, allergenic extract	Not established	Skin testing or immunotherapy for victims of fire ant stings.
gangliosides as sodium salts	Cronaissal	Treatment of retinitis pigmentosa.
glucocerbrosidase/ beta glucosidase (placenta-derived)	Not established	Treatment of type 1 Gaucher's disease.
group B streptococcus immune globulin	Not established	Treatment of disseminated group B streptococcal infection in neonates.
heme arginate	Normosang	Treatment of acute, symptomatic porphyria.
hemin	Panhematin	Amelioration of recurrent attacks of acute intermittent porphyria temporally related to the menstrual cycle in susceptible women and similar symptoms that occur in other patients with acute intermittent porphyria, porphyria variegata, and hereditary coproporphyria.
HIV-neutralizing antibodies	Immupath	Treatment of AIDS.
human IgM monoclonal antibody (C-58) to CMV	Centovir	Prophylaxis and treatment of CMV infections in bone marrow transplant recipients.
human immunodeficiency virus (HIV-1) immune globulin (human) I.V.	Not established	Treatment of AIDS.
human monoclonal antibody against hepatitis B virus	Not established	Prophylaxis against reinfection with hepatitis B in patients undergoing liver transplant secondary to end-stage chronic hepatitis B infection.

(continued)

Orphan drugs and biologicals *(continued)*

GENERIC NAME	TRADE NAME	DESIGNATED USE
Biologicals *(continued)*		
human T-lymphotropic virus type III gp160 antigens, recombinant vaccine, alum absorbed	VaxSyn HIV-1	Treatment of AIDS.
interferon beta (recombinant, human)	Betaseron	Treatment of AIDS and multiple sclerosis.
interleukin-1 alpha (recombinant, human)	Not established	Promotion of graft acceptance in patients undergoing bone marrow transplantation.
interleukin-2, recombinant, liposome-encapsulated	Not established	Treatment of brain tumors.
interleukin-3 (recombinant, human)	Not established	Promotion of erythropoiesis in patients with congenital pure cell aplasia (Diamond-Blackfan anemia).
iodine ^{131}I Lym-1 monoclonal antibody	Not established	Treatment of B-cell lymphoma.
iodine ^{131}I murine monoclonal antibody to human alpha-fetoprotein	ImmuRAIT, AFP-I 131	Treatment of hepatocellular carcinoma, hepatoblastoma, and alpha-fetoprotein-producing germ-cell tumors.
iodine ^{131}I murine monoclonal antibody to human chorionic gonadotropin (HcG)	ImmuRAIT, hCG-I 131 human	Treatment of HcG-producing tumors, including germ-cell and trophoblastic cell tumors.
iodine ^{131}I murine monoclonal antibody IgG_{2a} to B cell	ImmuRAIT, LL-2-I 131	Treatment of B-cell leukemia and B-cell lymphoma.
lactobin	Lactobin	Treatment of refractory diarrhea associated with AIDS.
melanoma vaccine	Melaccine	Treatment of melanoma (stage III or IV).
monoclonal antibodies (murine or human) recognizing B-cell lymphoma idiotypes	Not established	Treatment of B-cell lymphoma.
monoclonal antibodies PM-81 and AML-2-23	Not established	Treatment of patients with acute myelogenous leukemia undergoing bone marrow transplantation.
monoclonal antibody 17-1A	Panorex	Treatment of pancreatic cancer.

Orphan drugs and biologicals *(continued)*

GENERIC NAME	TRADE NAME	DESIGNATED USE
Biologicals *(continued)*		
monoclonal antibody PM-81	Not established	Adjunctive treatment of acute myelogenous leukemia.
monoclonal antibody for immunization against lupus nephritis	Not established	Treatment of lupus nephritis.
monoclonal factor IX	Not established	Treatment of hemophilia B.
mucoid exopolysaccharide *Pseudomonas* hyperimmune globulin	MEPIG	Prevention or treatment of *Pseudomonas aeruginosa* pulmonary infections in patients with cystic fibrosis.
myelin	Not established	Treatment of multiple sclerosis.
PEG-interleukin 2	Not established	Treatment of immunodeficiencies associated with T-cell defects.
PEG-L-asparaginase	Not established	Treatment of acute lymphocytic leukemia.
pentastarch	Pentaspan	Adjunctive use in leukapheresis, to improve the harvesting and increase the yield of leukocytes by centrifugal means.
poly I:poly C12U	Ampligen	Treatment of renal cell carcinoma.
polyribonucleotide	Ampligen	Treatment of AIDS.
respiratory syncytial virus (RSV) immune globulin (human)	Hyperimmune RSV	Prophylaxis and treatment of RSV infections in hospitalized infants and children.
ricin (blocked) conjugated murine monoclonal antibody (anti-B4) to B cell (CD19)	Not established	Treatment of B-cell leukemia and B-cell lymphoma.
ricin (blocked) conjugated murine monoclonal antibody (anti-My^9) to myeloid cells (CD-33)	Anti-My^9-bR	Treatment of myeloid leukemias.
ricin (blocked) conjugated murine monoclonal antibody (N901)	Not established	Treatment of small-cell lung cancer.
secretory leukocyte protease inhibitor, recombinant	Not established	Treatment of congenital alpha-1-antitrypsin deficiency; treatment of cystic fibrosis.

(continued)

Orphan drugs and biologicals *(continued)*

GENERIC NAME	TRADE NAME	DESIGNATED USE
Biologicals *(continued)*		
Serratia marcescens extract (ribosomes and lipid vesicles)	ImuVert	Treatment of primary malignant brain tumors.
SK&F 110679	Not established	Treatment of growth failure in children, caused by a lack of endogenous growth hormone.
ST1-RTA immunotoxin (SR 44163)	Not established	Prevention of acute graft-versus-host disease in allogenic bone marrow transplantation and treatment of patients with B-chronic lymphocytic leukemia.
teceleukin	Not established	Treatment of metastatic malignant melanoma (with interferon alfa-2a).
thymosin alpha-1	Not established	Adjunctive treatment of active chronic hepatitis B.
trisaccharides A and B	Not established	Treatment of moderate to severe hemolytic disease in neonates, caused by placental transfer of antibodies against blood group substances A and B; use in ABO-incompatible solid organ transplantation, including kidney, heart, liver, and pancreas; and treatment of moderate to severe transfusion reactions arising from transfusion of ABO-incompatible blood, blood products, and blood derivatives.
vasoactive intestinal polypeptide	Not established	Treatment of acute esophageal food impaction.

Index

A

Abbocillin VK, 94
Abbokinase, 868
Abenol, 297
Abitrate, 286
absorbable gelatin sponge, 853
A.C.&C., 335
Accupril, 269
Accurbron, 605
Accutane, 1193
acebutolol, 234-235
Acel-Imune, 946
Aceon, 1217
Acetaco, 335
Aceta Elixir, 297
Acet-Am, 605
acetaminophen, 297-299
Acetaminophen Uniserts, 297
Aceta Tablets, 297
Aceta with Codeine, 335
Acetazolam, 792
acetazolamide, 792-794
acetazolamide sodium, 792-794
acetic acid, 1044
acetohexamide, 750-751
acetohydroxamic acid, 1181-1182
acetophenazine maleate, 440-441
acetylcholine chloride, 1012
acetylcysteine, 608-609
acetylsalicylic acid, 299-302
Aches-N-Pain, 316
Achromycin, 1076
Achromycin Ophthalmic, 1002
Achromycin V, 135
acidifier, 836-837
Aclin, 332
Acne-10, 1185
Acne-Aid, 1185
Acon, 1107
aconiazide, 1262t
ACT-3, 316
Actamin, 297
Actamin Extra, 297
ACTH, 778-779
Acthar, 778
Acticort, 1101
Actidose-Aqua, 1160
Actifed, 584
Actigall, 636
Actilyse, 863
Actimmune, 987
Actimol, 297
Actinex, 1196
actinomycin D, 904-905
Activase, 863
activated charcoal, 1160-1161
Actraphane HM, 757
Actraphane HM Penfill, 757
Actraphane MC, 757
Actrapid HM, 757
Actrapid HM Penfill, 757
Actrapid MC, 757
Actrapid MC Penfill, 757
Acu-dyne, 1240t
Acular, 1008
acyclovir, 1056-1057
acyclovir sodium, 154-155
Adalat, 223
Adalat CC, 223
Adalat FT, 223
Adalat P.A., 223
adenine arabinoside, 162-163
Adenocard, 193
adenosine, 193-194, 1262t
ADH, 784-785
Adipex-P, 479
Adipost, 478
Adrenalin, 592
Adrenalin Chloride, 592, 1050
adrenaline, 592-594
adrenergic blockers, 537-540
adrenergics, 527-536
adrenocorticotropic hormone, 778-779
Adriamycin, 907
Adriamycin PFS, 907
Adriamycin RDF, 907
Adrucil, 895
adsorbents, 624-631
Adsorbocarpine, 1018
Adsorbonac Ophthalmic Solution, 1041
Adsorbotear, 1032
adverse reactions, 9-10
Advil, 316
AeroBid, 621
Aerolone, 597
Aeroseb-Dex, 1092
Aeroseb-HC, 1101
aerosolized pooled immune globulin, 1271t
Aerosporin, 182
Afko-Lube, 649
Afrin, 1052
Afrin Children's Strength Nose Drops, 1052

t refers to a table.

Afrinol Repetabs, 535, 536
Aftate for Athlete's Foot, 1078
Aftate for Jock Itch, 1078
Agon, 247
Agon SR, 247
Agoral, 645
Agoral Plain, 653
AHF, 857-858
A-HydroCort, 687
Airbron, 608
AK-Chlor, 993
AK-Con, 1028
Ak-Dex, 684
AK-Dilate, 1024
Akineton, 482
Akineton Lactate, 482
AK-Nefrin Ophthalmic, 1024
Akne-mycin, 1064
AK-Pentolate, 1022
AK-Pred, 1010
Ala-Quin, 1066
Albalon-A Liquifilm, 1028
Albalon Liquifilm, 1028
albumin 5%, 856-857
albumin 25%, 856-857
Albuminar 5%, 856
Albuminar, 25%, 856
Albumisol 25%, 856
Albutein, 5%, 856
albuterol, 585-586
albuterol sulfate, 585-586
Alcaine, 1236t
alclometasone diproprionate, 1085-1086
Alclovate, 1085
Alclox, 82
alcohol, ethyl, 1238-1239t
alcohol, isopropyl, 1238-1239t
alcohol content, 3-4
Alconefrin 12, 1053
Alconefrin 25, 1053
Alconefrin 50, 1053
Aldactazide, 792
Aldactazide 50/50, 792
Aldactone, 816
Aldazine, 461
Aldecin Aqueous Nasal Spray, 1047
Aldecin Inhaler, 613
Alderase, 1219
aldesleukin, 977-979
Aldoclor-150, 232
Aldoclor-250, 232
Aldomet, 258
Aldomet Ester Injection, 258
Aldomet M, 258
Aldoril-15, 232
Aldoril-25, 232
Aldoril D30, 232
Aldoril D50, 232
Alepam, 438
Aleve, 326
Alexan, 891
Alfenta, 337
alfentanil hydrochloride, 337-338
Alferon N, 986
Algam, 941
alglucerase, 1182-1183
Alkaban-AQ, 933
alkalinizers, 837-839
Alka-Mints, 627
Alka-Seltzer, 624
Alka-Seltzer without Aspirin, 624
Alkeran, 884
alkylating agents, 870-889
Allay, 335
Allegron, 415
Alleract, 583
Aller-Chlor, 572
Allerdryl, 575
Allerest, 1028
Allerest No Drowsiness Tablets, 296
Allerest Tablets, 568
Allerest 12-Hour Nasal, 1052
Allergesic, 568
Allergex, 572
Allerid, 535
AllerMax Caplets, 575
Aller-med, 575
allopurinol, 1135-1136, 1262t
allopurinol riboside, 1262t
Alloremed, 1135
Alomide, 1040
Alophen Pills, 654
alpha-galactosidase A, 1271t
alpha-galactoside A, 1271t
Alphamox, 76
Alphamul, 648
AlphaNine, 859
AlphaNine-SD, 859
alpha-1-antitrypsin (recombinant DNA origin), 1271t
alpha-1 proteinase inhibitor (human), 613
Alphapress, 253
Alpha-Ruvite, 1109
Alpha-Tamoxifen, 920
Alphatrex, 1087
alprazolam, 427-428
Alprin, 184
alprostadil, 1183
Alramucil, 656
Al-RSA, 1262t
Altace, 271

t refers to a table.

alteplase, 863-864
ALternaGEL, 626
Altracin, 1262t
altretamine, 923-924
Alu-Cap, 626
Aludrox Suspension, 624
aluminum acetate, 1242-1243t
aluminum carbonate, 625
aluminum hydroxide, 626
aluminum-magnesium complex, 629
aluminum phosphate, 627
aluminum sulfate, 1242-1243t
Alupent, 599
Alurate, 362
Alu-Tab, 626
Alzapam, 435
Amacodone, 335
amantadine hydrochloride, 155-156
Amaphen, 296
ambenonium chloride, 501-502
Ambien, 378
Amcill, 78
amcinonide, 1086-1087
Amcort, 697
amebicides, 25-30
Amen, 736
Amersol, 316
A-Metha-pred, 689
Amicar, 1161
Amidate, 1230t
Amigesic, 307
amikacin sulfate, 65-66
Amikin, 65
amiloride hydrochloride, 794
Aminess, 1127
amino acid infusions, crystalline, 1127-1129
amino acid infusions for hepatic failure, 1127-1129
amino acid infusions for high metabolic stress, 1127-1129
amino acid infusions for renal failure, 1127-1129
amino acid infusions in dextrose, 1127-1129
amino acid infusions with electrolytes, 1127-1129
amino acid infusions with electrolytes in dextrose, 1127-1129
aminocaproic acid, 1161-1162
Aminofen, 297
Aminofen Max, 297
aminoglutethimide, 914-915
aminoglycosides, 65-74
Aminophyllin, 587
aminophylline, 587-589
aminosalicylate sodium, 55-56
aminosidine, 1262t
Aminosyn, 1127
Aminosyn-HBC, 1127
Aminosyn II, 1127
Aminosyn II with dextrose, 1127
Aminosyn II with electrolytes, 1127
Aminosyn II with electrolytes in dextrose, 1127
Aminosyn-PF, 1127
Aminosyn-RF, 1127
Aminosyn with electrolytes, 1127
amiodarone hydrochloride, 194-196
amiodipine besylate, 215-216
Amitone, 627
amitriptyline hydrochloride, 402-403
amitriptyline pamoate, 402-403
ammonia, 1162
ammonium chloride, 836-837
amobarbital, 360-362
amobarbital sodium, 360-362
amoxapine, 403-405
amoxicillin/clavulanate potassium, 75-76
amoxicillin trihydrate, 76-77
Amoxil, 76
amoxycillin/clavulanate potassium, 75-76
amoxycillin trihydrate, 76-77
amphetamine sulfate, 467-468
Amphojel, 626
amphotericin B, 37-38, 1057-1058
ampicillin, 78-79
ampicillin sodium, 78-79
ampicillin sodium/sulbactam sodium, 79-80
ampicillin trihydrate, 78-79
Ampicin, 78
Ampicyn Injection, 78
Ampicyn Oral, 78
Ampligen, 1275t
Amprace, 246
amrinone lactate, 187-188
amsacrine, 1209-1210
Amsidyl, 1209
amyl nitrite, 278-279
Amytal, 360
Amytal Sodium, 360
anabolic steroids, 700-713
Anabolin IM, 704
Anabolin LA, 704
Anacin-3, 297
Anacin-3 Children's Elixir, 297
Anacin-3 Children's Tablets, 297
Anacin-3 Extra Strength, 297
Anacin-3 Infants', 297

t refers to a table.

Anacin-3 Maximum Strength Caplets, 297
Anacin with Codeine, 335
Anacobin, 1109
Anadrol, 708
Anafranil, 406
anagrelide, 1262t
ananain, 1262t
Anapolon 50, 708
Anaprox, 326
Anaprox DS, 326
anaritide acetate, 1262t
Anaspaz, 515
Anatensol, 448
Anavar, 706
Ancalixir, 393
Ancasal, 299
Ancasal 8, 335
Ancasal 15, 335
Ancasal 30, 335
Ancef, 103
Ancobon, 40
Ancolan, 665
Ancotil, 40
ancrod, 1271t
Andro-100, 711
Androcur, 1263t
Andro-Cyp 100, 711
Andro-Cyp 200, 711
Andro-Estro 90-4, 700
androgens, 700-713
Androgyn L.A., 700
Android, 703
Android F, 701
Andro-LA, 711
Androlone, 704
Androlone-D, 704
Andronaq-50, 711
Andronaq-LA, 711
Andronate 100, 711
Andronate 200, 711
Andropository 100, 711
Andrumin, 662
Andryl 200, 711
Anectine, 563
Anectine Flo-Pack, 563
Anergan 25, 578
Anergan 50, 578
anesthetics, 1224-1237t
Anexsia 5/500, 335
Anexsia 7.5/650, 335
Angijen No. 1, 215
Anginine, 224
anisoylated plasminogen-streptokinase activator complex, 864-866
anistreplase, 864-866
Anodynos DHC, 335
Anolor DH5, 335
Anoquan, 296
Anorex, 478
Anpec, 230
Ansaid, 315
Anspor, 126
Antabuse, 492
antacids, 624-631
Antadine, 155
antagonists, 1160-1180
Anthel, 35
anthelmintics, 31-36
antianginals, 215-231
antianxiety agents, 427-439
antiarrhythmics, 193-214
antibacterials, 1238-1239t
anticholinergics, 510-526
anticoagulants, 845-852
anticonvulsants, 380-400
anticytomegalovirus monoclonal antibodies, 1271t
antidepressants, 402-426
antidiabetic agents, 750-763
antidiarrheals, 638-644
antidotes, 1160-1180
antiemetics, 660-671
antiepilepsirine, 1262t
antiflatulents, 624-631
Antiflux, 629
antifungals, 37-46, 1238-1239t
antigout agents, 1135-1140
antihemophilic factor, 857-858, 1271t
antihistamines, 568-583
antihypertensives, 232-277
anti-infectives
  local, 1056-1079
  miscellaneous, 167-186
  ophthalmic, 991-1005
anti-inflammatory agents,
  ophthalmic, 1006-1011
antileprotics, 55-64
antilipemics, 285-295
Antilirium, 507
antimalarials, 47-54
antimelanoma antibody XMMME-001-RTA, 1271t
antimetabolites, 890-902
Antiminth, 35
Anti-My9-bR, 1275t
Anti-Naus, 668
antineoplastics
  antibiotic, 903-913
  hormone balance-altering, 914-922
  miscellaneous, 923-936
antiparkinsonian agents, 481-491

t refers to a table.

antiprotozoals, 25-30
antipsychotics, 440-466
antipyrine, 1262t
antiseptics, 1238-1241
Antispas, 513
anti-TAP-72 immunotoxin, 1271t
antithrombin III, human, 858-859
antithymocyte globulin (equine), 941-942
antitoxins, 966-969
antituberculars, 55-64
Anti-Tuss, 611
Anti-Tuss DM Expectorant, 610
antitussives, 608-612
antiulcer agents, 672-679
Antivenin *(Latrodectus mactans)*, 966
antivenins, 966-969
Antivert, 665
Antivert/25, 665
Antivert/50, 665
antivirals, 154-166
Antril, 1266t
Anturan, 1139
Anturane, 1139
Anxanil, 434
Apacet Capsules, 297
Apacet Elixir, 297
Apacet Extra Strength Caplets, 297
Apacet Extra Strength Tablets, 297
Apacet Infants', 297
Apacet Regular Strength Tablets, 297
APAP, 297-299
Aparkane, 491
Apatate Drops, 1116
A.P.L., 745
Aplisol, 1157
Aplitest, 1158
Apo-Acetaminophen, 297
Apo-Acetazolamide, 792
Apo-Alpraz, 427
Apo-Amitriptyline, 402
Apo-Amoxi, 76
Apo-Ampi, 78
Apo-Atenolol, 235
Apo-Benztropine, 481
Apo-Cal, 822
Apo-Capto, 240
Apo-Carbamazepine, 380
Apo-Cephalex, 122
Apo-Chlordiazepoxide, 429
Apo-Chlorpropamide, 751
Apo-Chlorthalidone, 800
Apo-Clorazepate, 430
Apo-Cloxi, 82
Apo-Diazepam, 431
Apo-Dimenhydrinate, 662
Apo-Dipyridamole, 279
Apo-Doxy, 130
Apo-Erythro, 174
Apo-Erythro-ES, 174
Apo-Erythro-S, 174
Apo-Ferrous Sulfate, 842
Apo-Fluphenazine, 448
Apo-Flurazepam, 367
Apo-Flurbiprofen, 315
Apo-Furosemide, 803
Apo-Guanethidine, 252
Apo-Haloperidol, 450
Apo-Hydro, 805
Apo-Hydroxyzine, 434
Apo-Ibuprofen, 316
Apo-Imipramine, 411
Apo-Indomethacin, 318
Apo-ISDN, 219
Apo-Keto, 320
Apo-Keto-E, 320
Apo-Lorazepam, 435
Apo-Meprobamate, 437
Apo-Methyldopa, 258
Apo-Metoclop, 665
Apo-Metoprolol, 260
Apo-Metoprolol (Type L), 260
Apo-Metronidazole, 27
apomorphine hydrochloride, 1262t
Apo-Napro-Na, 326
Apo-Naproxen, 326
Apo-Nifed, 223
Apo-Nitrofurantoin, 180
Apo-Oxazepam, 438
Apo-Pen-VK, 94
Apo-Perphenazine, 455
Apo-Phenylbutazone, 330
Apo-Piroxicam, 331
Apo-Prednisone, 696
Apo-Primidone, 398
Apo-Propranolol, 228
Apo-Quinidine, 210
Apo-Ranitidine, 677
Apo-Sulfamethoxazole, 141
Apo-Sulfatrim, 138
Apo-Sulfatrim DS, 138
Apo-Sulin, 332
Apo-Tetra, 135
Apo-Thioridazine, 461
Apo-Timol, 275
Apo-Tolbutamide, 762
Apo-Triazo, 377
Apo-Trifluoperazine, 464
Apo-Trihex, 491
Apo-Trimip, 424
Apo-Verap, 230
Apo-Zidovudine, 165
Appecon, 478

t refers to a table.

apraclonidine hydrochloride, 1031
Apresazide 25/25, 232
Apresazide 50/50, 232
Apresazide 100/50, 232
Apresodex, 232
Apresoline, 253
Apresoline-Esidrix, 232
Aprinox, 795
Aprinox-M, 795
aprobarbital, 362-363
aprotinin, 1183-1184
APSAC, 864-866
A-200 Pyrinate, 1083
Aquachloral Supprettes, 364
AquaMEPHYTON, 1122
Aquamox, 814
Aquaphyllin, 605
Aquasol A, 1107
Aquasol E, 1120
Aquatensen, 811
ara-A, 162-163
ara-C, 891-892
Aralen HCl, 47
Aralen Phosphate, 47
Aralen Phosphate with Primaquine Phosphate, 47
Aramine, 531
Aratac, 194
Arcotrate No. 3, 215
Arduan, 560
Aredia, 1200
Arfonad, 276
Argesic-SA, 307
arginine butyrate, 1262t
Aristocort, 697, 1104
Aristocort Forte, 697
Aristocort Intralesional, 697
Aristospan Intra-articular, 697
Aristospan Intralesional, 697
Arm-a-Med Isoetharine, 596
Arm-A-Med Metaproterenol, 599
Arm and Hammer Pure Baking Soda, 837
Armour Thyroid, 769
aromatic spirits, 1162
Arrestin, 670
Artane, 491
Artane Sequels, 491
Arterioflexin, 286
Arthra-G, 307
Arthrexin, 318
Arthrinol, 299
Arthritis Pain Formula Aspirin Free, 297
Arthropan, 303
Articulose-50, 693
Articulose-L.A., 697
artificial tears, 1032
Artria SR, 299
Arvin, 1271t
ASA, 299
ASA Enseals, 299
ascorbic acid, 1118-1119
Ascorbicap, 1118
Ascriptin, 296
Ascriptin A/D, 296
Asendin, 403
Asig, 269
Asmalix, 605
Asmol, 585
AS-101, 1262t
asparaginase, 924-925
A-Spas, 513
Aspegic, 1267t
Aspergum, 299
aspirin, 299-302
Aspro, 299
astemizole, 569-570
AsthmalHaler, 592
Astramorph PF, 350
Astrin, 299
astringents, 1240-1241t
Atarax, 434
Atasol Caplets, 297
Atasol Drops, 297
Atasol Elixir, 297
Atasol Forte Caplets, 297
Atasol Forte Tablets, 297
Atasol Tablets, 297
Atenex, 431
atenolol, 235-236
ATG, 941-942
AT-10, 789
AT-III, 858-859
Ativan, 435
ATnativ, 858
Atolone, 697
atovaquone, 167-168
Atozine, 434
atracurium besylate, 550-551
Atromid-S, 286
atropine sulfate, 196-197, 1021-1022
Atropisol, 1021
Atropt, 1021
Atrovent, 595
A/T/S, 1064
Attenuvax, 955
Augmentin, 75
auranofin, 1152-1153
Aureomycin 3%, 1060
Auriculin, 1262t
Aurocaine 2, 1044
Auro-Dri, 1044

t refers to a table.

aurothioglucose, 1153-1154
Austramycin V, 135
Austrastaph, 82
Aventyl, 415
Avitene, 853
Avlosulfon, 58
Avomine, 578
Axicillin, 76
Axid, 675
Axotal, 296
Axsain, 1186
Ayercillin, 91
Aygestin, 737
Aygestin Cycle Pack, 737
Azactam, 169
azacytidine, 1210
5-azacytidine, 1210
azatadine maleate, 570-571
azathioprine, 937-938
Azide, 798
azidothymidine, 165-166
3′azido-2, 3′dideoxyuridine, 1262t
azithromycin, 168-169
Azmacort, 623
Azo Gantanol, 138
Azo Gantrisin, 138
Azolid, 330
Azo-Standard, 306
Azo Sulfamethoxazole, 138
Azo Sulfisoxazole, 138, 143
AZT, 165-166
aztreonam, 169-170
Azulfidine, 142
Azulfidine EN-Tabs, 142

B

bacampicillin hydrochloride, 80-81
Baciguent, 1058
bacillus Calmette-Guérin, live intravesical, 925-927
Bacitin, 1058
bacitracin, 170-171, 992, 1058
bacitracin zinc, 1262t
baclofen, 541-542
Bactine HC, 1101
Bactocill, 88
Bactrim, 138
Bactrim DS, 138
Bactrim I.V. Infusion, 138
Bactroban, 1070
BAL in Oil, 1164
Balminil D.M., 610
Balminil Expectorant, 611
Bancap-HC, 335
Banesin, 297
Banflex, 548
Banophen, 575
Banophen Caplets, 575
Banthine, 520
Barbidonna Elixir, 510
Barbidonna No. 2 Tablets, 510
Barbidonna Tablets, 510
Barbita, 393
Barbloc, 267
Barc, 1083
Baridium, 306
Basaljel, 625, 626
Bayer Aspirin, 299
Baytussin, 611
Baytussin DM, 610
BCG, 925-927
BCG vaccine, 943-944
BCNU, 872
Bebulin VH Immuno, 859
Beclodisk, 613
Becloforte Inhaler, 613
beclomethasone dipropionate, 613-614, 1047-1048
Beclovent, 613
Beclovent Rotacaps, 613
Beconase AQ Nasal Spray, 1047
Beconase Nasal Inhaler, 1047
Bedoce, 1109
Bedoz, 1109
Beepen-VK, 94
Beesix, 1114
Beldin, 575
Belix, 575
belladonna leaf, 510-511
Belladonna Tincture USP, 510
Bellafoline, 518
Bell/ans, 837
Bellaspaz, 515
Bellergal-S, 537
Bel-phen-ergot S, 537
Bena-D 10, 575
Bena-D 50, 575
Benadryl, 575
Benadryl 25, 575
Benadryl Kapseals, 575
Benahist 10, 575
Benahist 50, 575
Ben-Allergin-50, 575
Ben-Aqua 5, 1185
Ben-Aqua 10, 1185
benazepril hydrochloride, 237-238
bendrofluazide, 795-796
bendroflumethiazide, 795-796
Benemid, 1138
Ben-Gay, 1242t
Benisone, 1087
Benn, 1138

t refers to a table.

Benoject-10, 575
Benoject-50, 575
Benoxyl 5, 1185
Benoxyl 10, 1185
Bensylate, 481
Bentyl, 513
Bentylol, 513
Benuryl, 1138
Benylin Cough, 575
Benylin DM, 610
Benylin Expectorant Cough Formula, 610
Benza, 1238t
Benzac 5, 1185
Benzacot, 670
Benzac W 2½, 1185
Benzac W 5, 1185
Benzac W 10, 1185
Benzac W Wash 5, 1185
Benzac W Wash 10, 1185
5 Benzagel, 1185
10 Benzagel, 1185
benzalkonium chloride, 1238-1239t
Benzamycin Gel, 1056
Benzide, 795
benzonatate, 609-610
benzoyl peroxide cleansers, 1185
benzoyl peroxide creams, 1185
benzoyl peroxide gels, 1185
benzoyl peroxide lotions, 1185
benzphetamine hydrochloride, 468-469
benzquinamide hydrochloride, 660-661
benzthiazide, 796-797
benztropine mesylate, 481-482
benzyl benzoate lotion, 1080-1081
benzylpenicillin, benzylpenicilloic acid, and benzylpenilloic acid, 1271t
benzylpenicillin benzathine, 89-90
benzylpenicillin potassium, 90-91
benzylpenicillin procaine, 91-92
benzylpenicillin sodium, 92-93
Bepadin, 216
bepridil hydrochloride, 216
beractant, 614-616
Betachron E-R, 228
Betadine, 1240t
Betagan, 1038
beta-glucocerberocidase, recombinant, 1271t
Betaloc, 260
Betaloc Durules, 260
betamethasone, 680-682
betamethasone acetate and betamethasone sodium phosphate, 680-682
betamethasone benzoate, 1087-1088
betamethasone dipropionate, 1087-1088
betamethasone sodium phosphate, 680-682
betamethasone valerate, 1087-1088
Betamin, 1116
Betapace, 212
Betapen-VK, 94
Betaseron, 986, 1274t
Beta-Sol, 1116
Betatrex, 1087
Beta-Val, 1087
betaxolol hydrochloride, 238-239, 1032-1033
bethanecol chloride, 502-503
bethanidine sulfate, 1263t
Betnelan, 680
Betnesol, 680
Betnovate, 1087
Betoptic, 1032
Bex, 299
Bexophene, 335
Biamine, 1116
Biavax II, 962
Biaxin Filmtabs, 172
Bi-Chinine, 53
Bicillin L-A, 89
Bicitra, 836
BiCNU, 872
Bilron, 632
Biltricide, 34
BioCal, 822
Biodel, 872, 1268t
Biodine, 1240t
Bio-Gan, 670
Bioglan B_{12} Plus, 1109
Bioglan Panazyme, 633
biological response modifiers, 977-990
Bio-Rescue, 1264t
biperiden hydrochloride, 482-483
biperiden lactate, 482-483
Biquinate, 53
Biquin Durules, 210
Bisac-Evac, 645
bisacodyl, 645-646
Bisacolax, 645
Bisalax, 645
Bisco-Lax, 645
bishydroxycoumarin, 845-846
bismuth subgallate, 638-639
bismuth subsalicylate, 638-639
bisoprolol fumarate, 239-240
bitolterol mesylate, 589
Bitrate, 215
Black-Draught, 657
black widow spider antivenin, 966
Blenoxane, 903

t refers to a table.

bleomycin sulfate, 903-904
Blephamide Liquifilm Suspension, 1028
Blephamide S.O.P. Sterile Ophthalmic Ointment, 991
Bleph-10 Liquifilm Ophthalmic, 1001
Blinx, 992, 1036
Blocadren, 275
blood derivatives, 856-862
Bluboro Powder, 1242t
Blue Gel, 1083
BMY-45622, 1263t
Bonamine, 665
Bonefos, 1265t
Bonine, 665
Bontril PDM, 478
Bontril Slow Release, 478
boric acid, 992-993, 1044-1045
Borofair Otic, 1044
Borolife, 1269t
Botox, 1033
botulinum toxin type A, 1033-1034
botulism antitoxin, bivalent equine, 966-967
botulism immune globulin, 1271t
bovine colostrum, 1271t
BranchAmin, 1127
Breonesin, 611
Brethaire, 603
Brethine, 603
Bretylate, 197
bretylium tosylate, 197-198
Bretylol, 197
Brevibloc, 200
Brevicon, 730
Brevital Sodium, 1232t
Bricanyl, 603
Brietal Sodium, 1232t
Brolene Eye Drops, 1268t
Bromfed-AT, 568
bromhexine, 1263t
bromocriptine mesylate, 483-484
Bromphen, 571
brompheniramine maleate, 571-572
Bronchial Capsules, 584
Bronchobid Capsules, 584
bronchodilators, 584-607
Broncho-Grippol-DM, 610
Brondecon Tablets, 584
Broniten Mist, 592
Bronkaid Mist, 592
Bronkaid Mistometer, 592
Bronkaid Mist Suspension, 592
Bronkephrine, 594
Bronkodyl, 605
Bronkometer, 596
Bronkosol, 596
Brufen, 316
Bucladin-S, 661
buclizine hydrochloride, 661
budesonide, 1048-1049
Buff-A-Comp No. 3, 336
BufOpto Atropine, 1021
Bufopto Zinc Sulfate, 1029
Buf-Oxal 10, 1185
bumetanide, 797-798
Bumex, 797
Buminate 5%, 856
Buminate 25%, 856
bupivacaine HCL, 1224-1225t
Buprenex, 338
buprenorphine hydrochloride, 338-339
bupropion hydrochloride, 405-406
Burinex, 797
Burow's solution, 1242t
Buscospan, 524
Busodium, 363
BuSpar, 428
buspirone hydrochloride, 428-429
busulfan, 870-871
butabarbital sodium, 363-364
butabarbitone sodium, 363-364
Butace, 296
Butalan, 363
Butatab, 330
Butazolidin, 330
Butazone, 330
Butisol, 363
butoconazole nitrate, 1058-1059
butorphanol tartrate, 339-340
butyrylcholinesterase, 1271t
BW B795U, 1263t
BW 12C, 1263t
Bydramine Cough, 575

C

Cafergot, 537
Cafergot-PB Suppositories, 537
Cafergot Suppositories, 537
Caffedrine Caplets, 469
caffeine, 469-470
calamine, 1240-1241t
Calan, 230
Calan SR, 230
Calcarb 600, 822
Calcibind, 1176
Calci-Chew, 822
Calciday 667, 822
calcifediol, 786
Calciferol, 1119
Calciject, 822
Calcilac, 627, 822
Calcilean, 847

t refers to a table.

Calcimar, 787
Calcimax, 627
Calciparine, 847
calcipotriene, 1186
Calcite 500, 822
calcitonin (human), 786-788
calcitonin (salmon), 787-788
calcitriol, 788-789
Calcium 500, 822
Calcium 600, 822
calcium acetate, 822-825
calcium carbonate, 627-628, 822-825
calcium chloride, 822-825
calcium citrate, 822-825
Calcium Disodium Versenate, 1167
Calcium EDTA, 1167
calcium glubionate, 822-825
calcium gluceptate, 822-825
calcium gluconate, 822-825
calcium gluconate gel, 1263t
calcium lactate, 822-825
calcium phosphate, dibasic, 822-825
calcium phosphate, tribasic, 822-825
calcium polycarbophil, 646-647
Calcium-Sandoz, 822
CaldeCort, 1101
Calderol, 786
Calglycine, 627, 822
Calicylic, 1240t
Calmazine, 464
Calm X, 662
calorics, 1127-1134
Calsan, 822
Cal-Sup, 627
Caltrate 300, 822
Caltrate 600, 822
Caltrate Chewable, 822
Cama, Arthritis Strength, 296
Camalox Tablets, 624
Cam-ap-es, 232
cancer chemotherapy, 1244-1261t
Canesten, 1062
Cantil, 519
Capastat Sulfate, 56
Capital with Codeine, 336
Capoten, 240
Capozide 25/15, 233
Capozide 25/25, 233
Capozide 50/15, 233
Capozide 50/25, 233
capreomycin sulfate, 56-57
Caprin, 847
capsaicin, 1186-1187
captopril, 240-241
Capurate, 1135
Carafate, 678
Carbacel, 1012
carbachol (intraocular), 1012-1013
carbachol (topical), 1012-1013
carbamazepine, 380-382
carbamide, 820-821
carbamide peroxide, 1045
carbenicillin indanyl sodium, 82
carbidopa-levodopa, 484-486
Carbocaine, 1226t
carbol-fuchsin solution, 1059-1060
Carbolith, 493
carboplatin, 871-872
carboprost tromethamine, 1144
carbovir, 1263t
Carbrital, 372
Cardene, 222
Cardene SR, 222
Cardilate, 218
Cardioquin, 210
Cardizem, 216
Cardizem CD, 216
Cardizem SR, 216
Cardophyllin, 587
Cardura, 245
carisoprodol, 542-543
Carmol HC, 1101
carmustine, 872-874
Carnitor, 1194
carteolol, 242-243
Carter's Little Pills, 645
Cartrol, 242
cascara sagrada, 646-648
cascara sagrada aromatic fluidextract, 647-648
cascara sagrada fluidextract, 647-648
Castaderm, 1059
Castellani's paint, 1059-1060
castor oil, 648-649
Catapres, 243
Catapres-TTS, 243
Catatrol, 1271t
CC-Galactosidase, 1271t
CCNU, 881-882
CD4, human recombinant soluble, 1271t
CD4, human truncated-369 AA polypeptide (recombinant CHO cells), 1272t
CD4, immunoglobulin G (recombinant human), 1272t
CD-45 monoclonal antibodies, 1272t
CD5-T lymphocyte immunotoxin, 1272t
Cebid Timecelles, 1118
Ceclor, 100
Cecon, 1118
Cedocard-SR, 219
CeeNU, 881

Cee-1000 T.D., 1118
cefaclor, 100-101
cefadroxil monohydrate, 101-102
Cefadyl, 124
cefamandole nafate, 102-103
Cefanex, 122
cefazolin sodium, 103-105
cefixime, 105-106
Cefizox, 117
cefmetazole sodium, 106-107
cefmetazone, 106-107
Cefobid, 108
cefonicid sodium, 107-108
cefoperazone sodium, 108-110
Cefotan, 111
cefotaxime sodium, 110-111
cefotetan disodium, 111-112
cefoxitin sodium, 112-114
cefpodoxime proxetil, 114-115
cefprozil, 115-116
ceftazidime, 116-117
ceftizoxime sodium, 117-119
ceftriaxone sodium, 119-120
cefuroxime axetil, 120-122
cefuroxime sodium, 120-122
Cefzil, 115
Celestone, 680
Celestone Chronodose, 680
Celestone Phosphate, 680
Celestone Soluspan, 680
Celontin, 390
Cenafed, 535
Cena-K, 831
Cenocort A-40, 697
Cenocort Forte, 697
Cenolate, 1118
Centovir, 1273t
Centrax, 438
cephalexin hydrochloride, 122-123
cephalexin monohydrate, 122-123
cephalosporins, 100-128
cephalothin sodium, 123-124
cephapirin sodium, 124-126
cephradine, 126-127
Cephulac, 651
Ceporacin, 123
Ceporex, 122
Ceptaz, 116
ceramide trihexosidase/alpha-galactosidase A, 1263t
cerebral stimulants, 467-480
Ceredase, 1182
Cerespan, 282
Cerubidin, 905
Cerubidine, 905
Cerumenex, 1046
C.E.S., 723
Cetacort, 1101
Cetamide Ophthalmic, 1001
Cetapred Ointment, 991
cetiedil citrate, 1263t
Cevalin, 1118
Cevi-Bid, 1118
Ce-Vi-Sol, 1118
Cevita, 1118
Charcoaide, 1160
Charcocaps, 1160
Chardonna-2, 510
Chemet, 1178
Chenix, 632
chenodeoxycholic acid, 632-633
chenodiol, 632-633
Cheracol D Cough, 610
Cherapas, 233
Chibroxin, 998
Children's Advil, 316
Children's Dramamine, 662
Children's Hold, 610
Children's Sudafed Liquid, 535
chimeric M-T412 (human-murine) IgG monoclonal anti-CD4, 1272A
Chinine, 53
Chlo-Amine, 572
Chlor-100, 572
chloral hydrate, 364-365
chlorambucil, 874-875
chloramphenicol, 171-172, 993-994, 1045-1046, 1060
chloramphenicol palmitate, 171-172
chloramphenicol sodium succinate, 172-172
Chlorate, 572
chlordiazepoxide, 429-430
chlordiazepoxide hydrochloride, 429-430
chlorhexidine gluconate, 1238-1239t
Chlor-Niramine, 572
2-chlorodeoxyadenosine, 890-891, 1263t
2-chloro-2′-deoxyadenosine, 1263t
Chloromycetin, 171, 1060
Chloromycetin-Hydrocortisone Ophthalmic, 991
Chloromycetin Ophthalmic, 993
Chloromycetin Otic, 1045
Chloromycetin Palmitate, 171
Chloromycetin Sodium Succinate, 171
chloroprocaine hydrochloride, 1224-1225t
Chloroptic, 993
Chloroptic S.O.P., 993
chloroquine hydrochloride, 47-48
chloroquine phosphate, 47-48

t refers to a table.

chloroquine sulphate, 47-48
chlorothiazide, 798-800
chlorothiazide sodium, 798-800
chlorotrianisene, 714-716
Chlorpazine, 668
Chlorphed, 571
Chlorphed-LA, 1052
chlorphenesin carbamate, 543-544
chlorpheniramine maleate, 572-573
Chlor-Pro, 572
Chlor-Pro 10, 572
Chlorpromanyl-5, 442
Chlorpromanyl-20, 442
Chlorpromanyl-40, 442
chlorpromazine hydrochloride, 442-444
chlorpropamide, 751-753
chlorprothixene, 444-446
Chlorquin, 47
Chlorsig, 993
Chlorspan-12, 572
Chlortab-4, 572
Chlortab-8, 572
chlortetracycline hydrochloride, 1060-1061
chlorthalidone, 800-801
Chlor-Trimeton, 572
Chlor-Trimeton Decongestant, 568
Chlor-Trimeton Non-Drowsy Formula, 535
Chlor-Trimeton 12-Hour Allergy, 572
Chlor-Tripolon, 572
chlorzoxazone, 544-545
Chlotride, 798
Cholac, 651
cholecalciferol, 1119-1120
Choledyl, 600
cholera vaccine, 944-945
cholestyramine, 285-286
choline magnesium trisalicylate, 302-303
cholinergics, 501-509
choline salicylate, 303-304
choline salicylate and magnesium salicylate, 302-303
choline theophyllinate, 600-602
Choloxin, 288
Cholybar, 285
Chooz, 627, 822
Chrometrace, 1125
chromic chloride, 1125-1126
chromium, 1125-1126
Chronulac, 651
Chymodiactin, 1141
chymopapain, 1141-1142
Chymoral-100, 1141
Cibacalcin, 786
Cibalith-S, 493
ciclopirox olamine, 1061
Cidomycin, 66
Cilamox, 76
ciliary neurotrophic factor, 1272t
Cilicane VK, 94
Cillium, 656
Ciloxan, 994
cimetidine, 672-673
Cinalone-40, 697
Cinobac, 145
Cinonide-40, 697
cinoxacin, 145
Cin-Quin, 210
Cipro, 146
ciprofloxacin, 146-147
ciprofloxacin hydrochloride, 994-995
Cipro I.V., 146
Ciproxin, 146
cisapride, 1187
cisplatin, 875-877
cis-platinum, 875-877
9-cis retinoic acid, 1263t
citrate of magnesia, 652-653
citric acid, gluconodelta-lactone, and magnesium carbonate, 1263t
Citrical, 822
Citrical Liquitabs, 822
Citrocarbonate, 837
Citroma, 652
Citro-Mag, 652
citrovorum factor, 1112-1113
Citrucel, 653
cladribine, 890-891
Claforan, 110
Claratyne, 577
Claripex, 286
clarithromycin, 172-173
Claritin, 577
Clavulin, 75
Clearasil 10, 1185
Clearasil Maximum Strength, 1185
Clear by Design, 1185
Clear Eyes, 1028
clemastine fumarate, 573-574
Cleocin HCl, 173
Cleocin Pediatric, 173
Cleocin Phosphate, 173
Cleocin T Gel, Lotion, Solution, 1061
Cleocin Vaginal Cream, 1061
C-Lexin, 122
clidinium bromide, 511-512
clindamycin hydrochloride, 173-174
clindamycin palmitate hydrochloride, 173-174
clindamycin phosphate, 173-174, 1061-1062

t refers to a table.

Clinoril, 332
clioquinol, 1066-1067
clobetasol propionate, 1088-1089
clocortolone pivalate, 1089-1090
Cloderm, 1089
clofazimine, 57
Clofen, 541
clofibrate, 286-287
Clomid, 1187
clomiphene citrate, 1187-1188
clomipramine hydrochloride, 406-407
clonazepam, 382-383
clonidine hydrochloride, 243-244
Clopra, 665
clorazepate dipotassium, 430-431
clotrimazole, 1062-1063
cloxacillin sodium, 82-83
Cloxapen, 82
clozapine, 446-448
Clozaril, 446
CMV-IGIV, 970-971
CNS agents, miscellaneous, 492-500
Co Advil Sinus, 311
coccidioidin, 1155-1156
Codalan No. 1, 336
Codalan No. 2, 336
Codalan No. 3, 336
Codaminophen, 336
codeine phosphate, 340-341
codeine sulfate, 340-341
Codimal-A, 571
Codimal DH, 568
Codistan No. 1, 610
Codroxomin, 1109
Cogentin, 481
Co-Gesic, 335
Cognex, 499
Col, 286
Colace, 649
ColBENEMID, 1135
colchicine, 1136-1138
Colchicine MR, 1136
Coldrine, 296
Colestid, 287
colestipol hydrochloride, 287-288
colfosceril palmitate, 616-618
Colgout, 1136
collodion, 1240-1241t
Collyrium, 992, 1036
Cologel, 653
Colovage, 655
Coloxyl, 649
Coloxyl Enema Concentrate, 649
Colsalide, 1136
Coly-Mycin S Otic, 1044
CoLyte, 655
Combantrin, 35
Combipres 0.1, 233
Combipres 0.2, 233
comosain, 1262t
Compa-Z, 668
Compazine, 668
Compazine Spansule, 668
compound benzoin tincture, 1242-1243t
Compound W, 1240t
Compoz, 575
Condrin-LA, 568
Condylox, 1073
C1-esterase-inhibitor, human, 1263t
C1-inhibitor, 1272t
C1-inhibitor (human) vapor treated, 1272t
Congespirin, 584
Congestac N.D. caplets, 535
Conjec-B, 571
Constant-T, 605
Constilac, 651
Contac Capsules, 568
Contac 12-Hour Caplets, 568
controlled substance schedules, 1-2
Cope, 296
Cophene-B, 571
copolymer 1 (COP 1), 1263t
copper, 1125-1126
Coppertrace, 1125
Coradur, 219
Cordarone, 194
Cordarone X, 194
Cordilox, 230
Cordilox SR, 230
Cordran, 1097
Cordran-N Cream, Ointment, 1056
Cordran SP, 1097
Cordran Tape, 1097
Corgard, 221
Coricidin Nasal Mist, 1052
Coricidin Tablets, 568
corn oil, 1129-1130
Coronex, 219
Corophyllin, 587
Corque, 1066
CortaGel, 1102
Cortaid, 1102
Cortamed, 1102
Cortate, 682
Cort-Dome, 1101
Cortef, 687, 1101, 1102
Cortenema, 687, 1101
Corticaine, 1102
corticosteroids, 680-699
  topical, 1085-1105
corticotropin, 778-779

t refers to a table.

Corticreme, 1102
Cortifoam, 687, 1102
Cortin, 1066
Cortinal, 1101
cortisone acetate, 682-684
Cortisporin Ophthalmic Ointment, 991
Cortisporin Ophthalmic Suspension, 991
Cortisporin Otic, 1044
Cortizone 5, 1101
Cortone Acetate, 682
Cortril, 1101
Cortrosyn, 779
Coryphen, 299
Corzide, 233
Cosmegen, 904
cosyntropin, 779-780
Cotanal-65, 335
Cotazym Capsules, 635
Cotazym-S Capsules, 635
Cotranzine, 668
Cotrim, 138
Cotrim D.S., 138
co-trimoxazole, 138-140
Cotylbutazone, 330
Coumadin, 850
Cremacoat 2, 611
Cremesone, 1101
Creon, 633
Creon 25, 633
Creon 10 Capsules, 635
Critifib, 197
cromolyn sodium, 618-619
Cronaissal, 1273t
Cronetal, 492
crotaline antivenin, polyvalent, 967-968
crotamiton, 1081
Cruex, 1078
cryptosporidium hyperimmune bovine colostrum, IgG concentrate, 1272t
crystalline zinc insulin, 757-760
crystal violet, 1065-1066
Crystamine, 1109
Crystapen, 92
Crysti-12, 1109
Crysticillin-300 A.S., 91
Crystodigin, 188
C-Span, 1118
cupric chloride, 1125-1126
cupric sulfate, 1125-1126
Cuprid, 1179
Cuprimine, 1166
Curretab, 736
Cuticura Acne, 1185
Cutivate, 1098
C2 with Codeine, 335
Cyanabin, 1109
cyanocobalamin, 1109-1111
Cyanocobalamin, 1109
Cyano-Gel, 1109
Cyanoject, 1109
cyclandelate, 279
Cyclidox, 130
cyclizine hydrochloride, 661-662
cyclizine lactate, 661-662
cyclobenzaprine, 545-546
Cycloblastin, 877
Cyclocort, 1086
Cyclogyl, 1022
Cyclomen, 700
Cyclomydril Ophthalmic, 1021
cyclopentolate hydrochloride, 1022
cyclophosphamide, 877-878
Cyclo-Prostin, 1265t
cycloserine, 57-58
Cyclospasmol, 279
cyclosporin, 938-939
cyclosporine, 938-939
Cycrin, 736
CyKloKapron, 1270t
Cylert, 477
Cylert Chewable, 477
Cyomin, 1109
cyproheptadine hydrochloride, 574
Cyproteron, 1263t
cyproterone acetate, 1263t
Cyronine, 765
cysteamine hydrochloride (2-aminoethanethiol), 1263t
Cystex, 167
cystic fibrosis transmembrane conductance regulator gel, 1264t
Cystospaz, 515
Cystospaz-M, 515
Cytadren, 914
cytarabine, 891-892
CytoGam, 970
cytomegalovirus immune globulin, intravenous, 970-971
Cytomel, 765
Cytosar, 891
Cytosar-U, 891
cytosine arabinoside, 891-892
Cytotec, 675
Cytovene, 160
Cytoxan, 877
Cytoxan Lyophilized, 877

D

dacarbazine, 878-880
Dacodyl, 645
Dacriose, 1036

t refers to a table.

dactinomycin, 904-905
Dalacin C, 173
Dalacin C Palmitate, 173
Dalacin C Phosphate, 173
Dalalone, 684
Dalalone D.P., 684
Dalalone L.A., 684
Dalgan, 341
Dalmane, 367
D-Amp, 78
danazol, 700-701
Danocrine, 700
Dantrium, 546
Dantrium I.V., 546
dantrolene sodium, 546-547
Dapa, 297
Dapa XS, 297
dapiprazole hydrochloride, 1035
dapsone, 58-59
Dapsone 100, 58
Daranide, 801
Daraprim, 52
Darbid, 517
Daricon, 522
Darvocet-N, 357
Darvocet-N 50, 336
Darvocet-N 100, 336
Darvon, 357
Darvon Compound, 336
Darvon Compound-65, 335
Darvon-N, 357
Darvon-N Compound, 336
Darvon-N with ASA, 336
Darvon with ASA, 336
daunorubicin hydrochloride, 905-906
Daypro, 327
Dazamide, 792
DCF, 931-932
DDAVP, 780
ddC, 163-165
ddI, 156-158
Debrox, 1045
Decaderm, 1092
Decadrol, 684
Decadron, 684
Decadron L.A., 684
Decadron Phosphate, 684, 1092
Decadron Phosphate Ophthalmic, 1006
Decadron Phosphate Turbinaire, 1049
Decadron Respihaler, 619
Decadron with Xylocaine, 680
Deca-Durabolin, 704
Decaject, 684
Decaject-L.A., 684
Decapeptyl injection, 1270t
Decaspray, 1092
decitabine (5-AZA-2′-deoxycytidine; DAC), 1264t
Declomycin, 129
Decofed, 535
Decolone, 704
Deconade, 568
Deconamine, 568
Deep Heating Rub, 1242t
De Fed-60, 535
deferoxamine mesylate, 1162-1163
defibrotide, 1264t
Deficol, 645
Degest 2, 1028
Dehist, 571
Delacort, 1101
Deladumone, 700
Delaprem, 1214
Del Aqua 5, 1185
Del Aqua 10, 1185
Delatest, 711
Delatestryl, 711
Delaxin, 547
Delcid Suspension, 624
Delestrogen, 720
Del-Mycin, 1064
Delta-Cortef, 693
Delta-D, 1119
Delta-Lutin, 734
Deltasolone, 693
Deltasone, 696
Del-Vi-A, 1107
Demadex, 817
demeclocycline hydrochloride, 129-130
Demerol, 347
Demerol-APAP, 336
Demi-Regroton, 233
Demser, 261
Demulen 1/35, 730
Demulen 1/50, 730
2′-deoxycoformycin, 931-932
deoxyribonuclease recombinant human (rh DNase), 1272t
Depakene, 400
Depakene Syrup, 400
Depakote, 400
Depakote Sprinkle, 400
dep Andro 100, 711
dep Andro 200, 711
DepAndrogen, 700
Depen, 1166
depGynogen, 720
depMedalone-40, 689
depMedalone-80, 689
Depo-Estradiol, 720
Depoject-40, 689
Depoject-80, 689

t refers to a table.

Depo-Medrol, 689
Deponit, 224
Depopred-40, 689
Depopred-80, 689
Depo-Predate 40, 689
Depo-Predate 80, 689
Depo-Provera, 736
Depotest, 711
Depotestadiol, 700
Depotestogen, 700
Depo-Testosterone, 711
Deptran, 408
Deralin, 228
DermaCort, 1101
Dermacort, 1102
Dermacort Ointment, 1102
Derma-Soft Creme, 1240t
Dermolate, 1101
Dermovate, 1088
Dermtex HC, 1101
Deronil, 684
DES, 717
Desenex, 1078
Desenex Aerosol, 1078
Deseril, 539
Desferal, 1162
desipramine hydrochloride, 407-408
deslorein, 1264t
desmopressin acetate, 780-781
Desogen, 730
desonide, 1090-1091
DesOwen, 1090
deslorein, 1264t
desmopressin acetate, 780-781
Desogen, 730
desonide, 1090-1091
DesOwen, 1090
desoximetasone, 1091-1092
Desoxyn, 474
Desoxyn Gradumet, 474
Desquam-E, 1185
Desquam-X 2.5, 1185
Desquam-X 5, 1185
Desquam-X 10, 1185
Desquam-X 5 Wash, 1185
Desquam-X 10 Wash, 1185
Desyrel, 423
Detensol, 228
Devrom, 638
Dexacen-4, 684
Dexacen LA-8, 684
dexamethasone, 684-686, 1006-1007, 1092-1094
dexamethasone sodium phosphate inhalation, 619-620
Dexasone, 684
Dexasone-LA, 684
Dexchlor, 575
dexchlorpheniramine maleate, 575
Dexedrine, 470
Dexedrine Spansule, 470
Dexitac, 469
Dexone, 684
Dexone 0.5, 684
Dexone 0.75, 684
Dexone 1.5, 684
Dexone 4, 684
Dexone LA, 684
dexrazoxane, 1264t
Dextran 40, 825
dextran 40, 825-826
dextran 70, 826
Dextran 75, 826
dextran 75, 826
dextran and deferoxamine, 1264t
dextran, high molecular weight, 826-827
dextran, low molecular weight, 825-826
dextran sulfate aerosol inhalation, 1264t
dextran sulfate sodium (UA001), 1264t
dextroamphetamine sulfate, 470-472
dextromethorphan hydrobromide, 610-611
dextropropoxyphene hydrochloride, 357-358
dextropropoxyphene napsylate, 357-358
dextrose, 1130-1131
dextrothyroxine sodium, 288-289
Dey-Dose Isoetharine, 596
Dey-Dose Isoetharine S/F, 596
Dey-Dose Isoproterenol, 597
Dey-Dose Metaproterenol, 599
Dey-Lute Isoetharine, 596
Dey-Lute Metaproterenol, 599
dezocine, 341-342
DFMO, 25-26
D-glucose, 1130-1131
D.H.E. 45, 537
DHT Intensol, 789
DiaBeta, 755
Diabinese, 751
Diachlor, 798
diagnostic skin tests, 1155-1159
Dialose-Plus, 645
Dialume, 626
Diamine TD, 571
3,4-diaminopyridine, 1264t
Diamox, 792
Diamox Parenteral, 792
Diamox Sequels, 792
Diamox Sodium, 792

t refers to a table.

dianeal PD-2 peritoneal dialysis solution, 1264t
Diapid, 781
Diazemuls, 431
diazepam, 431-433
Diazepam Intensol, 431
diaziquone, 1264t
Di-Azo, 306
diazoxide, 244-245
diazoxide, oral, 1188-1189
Dibenyline, 265
Dibenzyline, 265
Dicarbosil, 627, 822
dichlorphenamide, 801-802
Dichlotride, 805
diclofenac sodium, 311-312
dicloxacillin sodium, 83-84
dicumarol, 845-846
dicyclomine hydrochloride, 513-514
didanosine, 156-158
2,3 didehydro-3-deoxythymidine, 1218-1219
2′-3′-dideoxyadenosine, 1264t
dideoxycytidine, 163-165
2′-3′-dideoxycytidine, 1264t
2′-3′-dideoxyinosine, 1264t
Didrex, 468
Didronel, 790
dienestrol, 716-717
dienoestrol, 716-717
diethyldithiocarbamate (DTC), 1264t
diethylpropion hydrochloride, 472-473
diethylstilbestrol, 717-719
diethylstilbestrol diphosphate, 717-719
difenoxin hydrochloride and atropine sulfate, 639-640
diflorasone diacetate, 1094-1095
Diflucan, 39
diflunisal, 304-305
Di-Gel Liquid, 624
digestants, 632-637
Digibind, 1163
Digitaline, 188
digitoxin, 188-190
digoxin, 190-192
digoxin immune FAB (ovine), 1163-1164
dihematoporphyrin ethers, 1264t
Dihydergot, 537
dihydroergotamine mesylate, 537-538
Dihydroergotamine-Sandoz, 537
dihydromorphinone hydrochloride, 345-346
dihydrotachysterol, 789-790
dihydroxyaluminum sodium carbonate, 628-629
1,25-dihydroxycholecalciferol, 788-789
diiodohydroxyquin, 26-27
Dilacor XR, 216
Dilantin, 396
Dilantin-125, 396
Dilantin Infatabs, 396
Dilantin Kapseals, 396-398
Dilantin-30 Pediatric, 396
Dilantin with Phenobarbital, 380
Dilar, 227
Dilatrate-SR, 219
Dilaudid, 345
Dilaudid HP, 345
Dilor, 590
Dilor-400, 590
Dilor-G Tablets, 584
Dilosyn, 577
diltiazem hydrochloride, 216-218
Dimelor, 750
dimenhydrinate, 662-663
dimercaprol, 1164-1165
2, 3-dimercaptosuccinic acid (DMAS), 1264t
Dimetabs, 662
Dimetane, 571
Dimetane Extentabs, 571
Dimetane-Ten, 571
Dimetapp Extentabs, 568
dimethyl sulfoxide (DMSO), 1264t
Dimycor, 215
Dinate, 662
dinoprostone, 1144-1145
Diocto, 649
dioctyl calcium sulfosuccinate, 649-650
dioctyl potassium sulfosuccinate, 649-650
dioctyl sodium sulfosuccinate, 649-650
Diodoquin, 26
Dioeze, 649
Diolax, 645
Diosuccin, 649
Dio-Sul, 649
Dioval, 720
Dipentum, 1200
Diphenacen-50, 575
Diphenadryl, 575
Diphenatol, 640
Diphen Cough, 575
Diphenhist, 575
Diphenhist Captabs, 575
diphenhydramine hydrochloride, 575-577
diphenidol hydrochloride, 663-664
diphenoxylate hydrochloride and atropine sulfate, 640-641
diphenylhydantoin, 396-398

t refers to a table.

diphtheria and tetanus toxoids, adsorbed, 945-946
diphtheria and tetanus toxoids and acellular pertussis vaccine, 946-947
diphtheria and tetanus toxoids and pertussis vaccine, 946-947
diphtheria antitoxin, equine, 968
dipivefrin, 1035-1036
Dipridacot, 279
Diprivan, 1234t
Diprolene, 1087
Diprolene AF, 1087
Diprosone, 1087
dipyridamole, 279-280
Diquinol, 26
disaccharide tripeptide glycerol dipalmitoyl, 1272t
Disalcid, 307
disalicylic acid, 307-308
Discase, 1141
disodium clodronate tetrahydrate, 1265t
Disodium EDTA, 1168
disodium silibinin dihemisuccinate, 1265t
Disonate, 649
Disophrol Chronotabs, 568
disopyramide, 198-200
disopyramide phosphate, 199-200
Di-Sosul, 649
Disotate, 1168
Di-Spaz, 513
Dispos-a-Med Isoetharine, 596
Dispos-a-Med Isoproterenol, 597
disulfiram, 492-493
Ditropan, 1150
Diucardin, 807
Diuchlor H, 805
Diulo, 812
Diupres-250, 233
Diupres-500, 233
Diurel, 798
Diurese-R, 233
diuretics, 792-821
Diurigen, 798
Diurigen with reserpine, 233
Diuril, 798
Diuril Sodium, 798
Diutensen, 233
Diutensen-R, 233
divalproex sodium, 400-401
Dixarit, 243
Dizmiss, 665
Dizymes Tablets, 633
DM Syrup, 610
DNR, 905-906
dobutamine hydrochloride, 527-528
Dobutrex, 527
docetaxel, 1211
docusate calcium, 649-650
docusate potassium, 649-650
docusate sodium, 649-650
Dodex, 1109
DOK-250, 649
DOK Liquid, 649
Doktors, 1053
Dolacet, 335
Dolanex, 297
Dolene, 357
Dolene-AP-65, 336
Dolobid, 304
Dolophine, 349
Doloxene, 357
Doloxene Co, 357
Domeboro Otic, 1044
Domeboro powder, 1242t
Dome-Paste, 1242t
Dommanate, 662
domperidone, 1211-1212
Donnagel-MB, 641
Donnagel-PG, 638
Donnagel Suspension, 638
Donnatal Elixir, 510
Donnatal Extentabs, 510
Donnatal No. 2 Tablets, 510
Donnatal Tablets and Capsules, 510
Donnazyme, 633
Donnazyme Tablets, 632
Dopamet, 258
dopamine hydrochloride, 528-529
Dopar, 486
Dopastat, 528
Dopram, 1165
Doral, 374
Doraphen, 357
Doraphen Compound-65, 335
Dorcol Children's Decongestant, 535
Dorcol Children's Fever and Pain Reducer, 297
Doriglute, 368
Dormarex 2, 575
Dormel, 364
dornase alfa, 620-621
Doryx, 130
Doss, 649
Doss 300, 649
Dovonex, 1186
doxacurium chloride, 551-553
Doxapap-N, 336
Doxaphene, 357
Doxaphene Compound, 335
doxapram hydrochloride, 1165-1166
doxazosin mesylate, 245-246

t refers to a table.

doxepin hydrocloride, 408
Doxidan, 645
Doxinate, 649
doxorubicin hydrochloride, 907-908
Doxy-Caps, 130
Doxycin, 130
doxycycline, 130-132
doxycycline hyclate, 130-132
doxycycline hydrochloride, 130-132
Doxylin, 130
Doxy-Tabs, 130
D-Penamine, 1166
D-penicillamine, 1166-1167
DPT, 946-947
Dramamine, 662
Dramamine Chewable, 662
Dramamine Liquid, 662
Dramanate, 662
Dramocen, 662
Dramoject, 662
Drenison, 1097
Drenison 1/4, 1097
Drenison Tape, 1097
D-Rex-65, 336
Dri/Ear, 1044
Drisdol, 1119
Dristan, 584
Dristan Long Lasting, 1052
Dristan Sinus Caplets, 311
Drixine Nasal, 1052
Drixoral, 536, 568
Drixoral Non-Drowsy Formula, 535
Drize, 568
Droleptan, 1230t
dronabinol, 664
droperidol, 1230-1231t
Droxomin, 1109
Dr. Scholl's Athlete's Foot Powder, 1078
Dr. Scholl's Athlete's Foot Spray, 1078
drug action, factors that modify, 6-7
drug administration, considerations for, 8
drug interactions, 8-9
drug therapy
in children, 13-17
in elderly patients, 18-20
nursing process and, 21-24
D-S-S, 649
D-S-S Plus, 645
d4T, 1218-1219
D-thyroxine sodium, 288-289
DTIC, 878-880
DTIC-Dome, 878
DTP, 946-947
Ducene, 431
Dulcolax, 645
Dull-C, 1118
Duocet, 335
Duo-Cyp, 700
Duo-Medihaler, 584
Duosol, 649
Duotrate, 227
Duphalac, 651
Durabolin, 704
Duradyne DHC, 335
Dura-Estrin, 720
Duragen 10, 720
Duragen 20, 720
Duragen 40, 720
Duragesic-25, 342
Duragesic-50, 342
Duragesic-75, 342
Duragesic-100, 342
Duralith, 493
Duralone-40, 689
Duralone-80, 689
Duralutin, 734
Duramist Plus, 1052
Duramorph, 350
Duramorph PF, 350
Duranest, 1224
Durapam, 367
Duraphyl, 605
Duraquin, 210
Duratest-100, 711
Duratest-200, 711
Duratestrin, 700
Durathate-200, 711
Duration, 1052, 1053
Durel-Cort, 1101
Duretic, 811
Duricef, 101
Durolax, 645
Duromine, 479
Durrax, 434
Duvoid, 502
DV, 716
D-Vert 15, 665
D-Vert 30, 665
Dyazide, 792
Dycill, 83
Dyflex, 590
Dyflex-400, 590
Dyflex-G Tablets, 584
Dyline-GG Tablets, 584
Dymadon, 297
Dymadon P, 297
Dymelor, 750
Dymenate, 662
DynaCirc, 254
dynamine, 1265t
Dynapen, 83

t refers to a table.

dyphylline, 590
Dyrenium, 818
Dyrexan OD, 478
Dytac, 818

E

Ear-Dry, 1044
Early Bird, 35
Easprin, 299
echothiophate iodide, 1015-1016
econazole nitrate, 1063-1064
Econopred Ophthalmic, 1010
Econopred Plus Ophthalmic, 1010
Ecosone, 1101
Ecostatin, 1063
ecothiopate iodide, 1015-1016
Ecotrin, 299
E-Cypionate, 720
Edecril, 802
Edecrin, 802
Edecrin Sodium, 802
edetate calcium disodium, 1167-1168
edetate disodium, 1168-1169
edrophonium chloride, 503-505
EDTA, 1028
EEG Dulcets, 174
E.E.S., 174
EES-400, 174
EES granules, 174
Effercal-600, 627
Effexor, 425
Efficol Cough Whip, 610
Efidac/24, 535
eflornithine hydrochloride, 25-26
Efodine, 1240t
Efudex, 895
Elase, 1142
Elavil, 402
Eldepryl, 490
Eldisine, 1221
Eldoquin, 1242t
electrolytes, 822-835
Elimite, 1081
Elixicon, 605
Elixomin, 605
Elixophyllin, 605
Elixophyllin SR, 605
Elocon, 1103
E-Lor, 336
Elspar, 924
Eltor 120, 535
Eltroxin, 764
Emcodeine No. 2, 336
Emcodeine No. 3, 336
Emcodeine No. 4, 336
Emcyt, 915
Emete-Con, 660
Emex, 665
Eminase, 864
Emitrip, 402
emollients, 1240-1241t
Empirin, 299
Empirin with Codeine No. 2, 336
Empirin with Codeine No. 3, 336
Empirin with Codeine No. 4, 336
Empracet-30, 335
Empracet-60, 336
Emtec-30, 335
Emulsoil, 648
EMU-V, 174
E-Mycin, 174
enalaprilat, 246-247
enalapril maleate, 246-247
Endep, 402
Endocan, 336
Endocet, 336
Endolor, 296
Endone, 353
Endoxan-Asta, 877
Endrate, 1168
Enduron, 811
Enduron M, 811
Enduronyl, 233
Enduronyl-Forte, 233
Ener-B, 1109
Engerix-B, 948
enisoprost, 1265t
Enlon, 503
Enovil, 402
enoxacin, 147-148
enoxaparin sodium, 846-847
Entacyl, 33
Entex, 527
Entex LA, 584
Entex Liquid, 527
Entozyme, 633
Entozyme Tablets, 632
Entrophen, 299
Enulose, 651
enzymes, 1141-1143
Ephed II, 591
ephedrine sulfate, 591-592, 1050
epidermal growth factor (human), 1272t
Epifoam, 1102
Epifrin, 1023
Epilim, 400
E-Pilo, 1012
Epimorph, 350
Epinal, 1023
epinephrine, 592-594
epinephrine bitartrate, 592-594

t refers to a table.

epinephrine hydrochloride, 592-594, 1023-1024, 1050
epinephryl borate, 1023-1024
Epi-Pen, 592
Epi-Pen Jr., 592
Epitol, 380
Epival, 400
epoetin alfa, 979-980
epoetin beta (recombinant human), 1273t
Epogen, 979
epoprostenol, 1265t
Eppy/N, 1023
Eprolin, 1120
epsom salts, 652-653
Equagesic, 427
Equalactin, 646
Equanil, 437
Equilet, 627
Ercaf, 537
Ergamisol, 939
Ergo-Caff PB, 537
ergocalciferol, 1119-1120
Ergodryl Mono, 538
Ergomar, 538
ergometrine maleate, 1145-1146
ergonovine maleate, 1145-1146
Ergostat, 538
ergotamine tartrate, 538-539
Ergotrate Maleate, 1145
Eridium, 306
Erwinia asparaginase, 924-925
Erybid, 174
ERYC, 174
ERYC-125, 174
ERYC-250, 174
Erycette, 1064
EryDerm, 1064
EryGel, 1064
EryPed, 174
Ery-Sol, 1064
Ery-Tab, 174
erythrityl tetranitrate, 218-219
Erythro, 174
Erythrocin, 174
Erythrocot, 174
Erythromid, 174
erythromycin, 995-996, 1064
erythromycin base, 174-176
erythromycin estolate, 174-176
erythromycin ethylsuccinate, 174-176
erythromycin gluceptate, 174-176
erythromycin lactobionate, 174-176
erythromycin stearate, 174-176
erythropoietin, 979-980
Erythrozone, 174
eserine salicylate, 507-508
Eserine Sulfate, 1018
Esgic, 296
Esidrix, 805
Esimil, 233
Eskalith, 493
Eskalith CR, 493
esmolol hydrochloride, 200-201
Esoterica, 1242t
Espotabs, 654
estazolam, 365-366
esterified estrogens, 719-720
Estinyl, 728
Estivin II, 1028
Estrace, 720
Estrace Vaginal Cream, 720
Estracyst, 915
Estraderm, 720
estradiol, 720-723
estradiol cypionate, 720-723
Estradiol L.A., 720
estradiol valerate, 720-723
Estra-L 20, 720
Estra-L 40, 720
estramustine phosphate sodium, 915-916
Estratab, 719
Estratest, 700
Estratest H.S., 700
Estraval, 720
Estraval P.A., 720
Estro-Cyp, 720
Estrofem, 720
estrogenic substances, conjugated, 723-725
estrogens, 714-742
estrogens, conjugated, 723-725
Estroject-2, 725
Estroject-L.A., 720
estrone, 725-726
Estrone A, 725
Estrone "5", 725
estropipate, 727-728
Estrovis, 740
ethacrynate sodium, 802-803
ethacrynic acid, 802-803
ethambutol hydrochloride, 60
Ethaquin, 280
Ethatab, 280
ethaverine hydrochloride, 280-281
Ethavex-100, 280
ethchlorvynol, 366-367
ethinyl estradiol, 728-730
ethinyl estradiol and levonorgestrel, 730-734

t refers to a table.

ethinyl estradiol and norethindrone, 730-734
ethinyl estradiol and norethindrone acetate, 730-734
ethinyl estradiol and norgestimate, 730-734
ethinyl estradiol and desogestrel, 730-734
ethinyl estradiol and ethynodiol diacetate, 730-734
ethinyl estradiol and norgestrel, 730-734
ethinyl estradiol, norethindrone acetate, and ferrous fumarate, 730-734
ethinyloestradiol, 728-730
ethiofos, 1265t
ethionamide, 60-61
Ethmozine, 205
ethosuximide, 383-384
ethotoin, 384-385
ethylnorepinephrine hydrochloride, 594
Ethyol, 1265t
Etibi, 60
etidocaine hydrochloride, 1224-1225t
etidronate disodium, 790-791
etodolac, 312-314
etomidate, 1230-1231t
etoposide, 928-929
Etrafon, 402
Etrafon-A, 402, 440
Etrafon-Forte, 402, 440
Etrafon 2-10, 402, 440
etretinate, 1189-1191
ETS, 1064
Euflex, 916
Euglucon, 755
Euhypnos 10, 376
Euhypnos 20, 376
Eulexin, 916
Eurax, 1081
Euthroid, 767
Evac-U-Gen, 654
Evac-U-Lax, 654
Everone, 711
E-Vista, 434
Excedrin Extra Strength, 296
Excedrin-IB Caplets, 316
Excedrin-IB Tablets, 316
Excedrin P.M., 296
Exdol, 297
Exdol Strong, 297
Exelderm, 1075
Ex-Lax, 654
Ex-Lax Maximum Relief Formula, 654
Ex-Lax Pills, 654
Exna, 796
Exna-R Tablets, 233
Exosurf Neonatal, 614
expectorants, 608-612
Exsel, 1242t
Extra Action Cough, 610
Extra-Strength Doan's, 305
Extra Strength Doan's P.M., 296
Extra Strength Gas-X, 630
Extra Strength Maalox Tablets, 624
eye irrigation solutions, 1036
Eye-Sed Ophthalmic, 1029
Eye-Stream, 1036

F

FABRase, 1271t
factor VIIa (recombinant, DNA origin), 1273t
factor IX complex, 859-860
factor IX (human), 859-860
factor XIII, 1273t
Factrel, 744
famciclovir, 1212
famotidine, 673-674
Famvir, 1212
Fansidar, 52
Fastin, 479
fat emulsions, 1131-1132
fatty acid solution, short chain, 1265t
5-FC, 40-41
Fedahist, 568
Feen-A-Mint, 654
Feen-A-Mint Gum, 654
felbamate, 385-386
Felbatal, 385
Feldene, 331
felodipine, 247-249
Femcet, 296
Feminate, 720
Feminone, 728
Femiron, 840
Femogen Forte, 725
Femogex, 720
Femstat, 1058
Fenac, 311
fenfluramine hydrochloride, 473-474
Fenicol, 993
fenoprofen calcium, 314-315
fentanyl citrate, 342-345
fentanyl citrate with droperidol, 1230-1231t
Fentanyl Oralet, 342
fentanyl transdermal system, 342-345
fentanyl transmucosal, 342-345
Feosol, 842
Feostat, 840
Feostat Drops, 840

t refers to a table.

Fergon, 841
Fergon Plus, 840
Fer-In-Sol, 842
Fer-In-Sol Drops, 842
Fer-In-Sol Syrup, 842
Fer-Iron Drops, 842
Feritard, 842
Fermalox, 840
Ferocyl, 840
Fero-Grad, 842
Fero-Gradumet, 842
Ferospace, 842
Ferralet, 841
Ferralyn Lanacaps, 842
Ferra-TD, 842
Ferro-Docusate-T.R., 840
Ferro-Dok TR, 840
Ferro-Dss S.R.., 840
Ferro-Sequels, 840
ferrous fumarate, 840-841
ferrous gluconate, 841-842
ferrous sulfate, 842-843
ferrous sulfate, dried, 842-843
Fertinic, 841
Feverall Children's, 297
Feverall Junior Strength, 297
Feverall Sprinkle Caps, Children's, 297
Feverall Sprinkle Caps, Junior Strength, 297
Fiberall, 646, 656
FiberCon, 646
FiberLax, 646
FiberNorm, 646
Fibrepur, 656
fibrinolysin and desoxyribonuclease, 1142-1143
Fibrogammin, 1273t
fibronectin (human plasma derived), 1273t
filgrastim, 980-981
finasteride, 1191-1192
Fioricet, 296
Fioricet with Codeine, 296
Fiorinal, 296
fire ant venom, allergenic extract, 1273t
Flagyl, 27
Flagyl I.V. RTU, 27
Flamazine, 1074
Flatulex, 624
Flavettes, 1118
flavoxate hydrochloride, 1150
Flaxedil, 553
flecainide acetate, 201-203
Fleet Babylax, 650
Fleet Bisacodyl, 645
Fleet Bisacodyl Prep, 645
Fleet Flavored Castor Oil, 648
Fleet Laxative, 645
Fleet Mineral Oil, 653
Fleet Phospho-Soda, 658
Fletcher's Castoria, 657
Flexeril, 545
flexible collodion, 1240-1241t
Flexoject, 548
Flexon, 548
Flint SSD, 1074
Florinef, 686
Florone, 1094
Floropryl, 1016
Floxin, 152
floxuridine, 892-893
fluconazole, 39-40
flucytosine, 40-41
Fludara, 893
fludarabine phosphate, 893-894
fludrocortisone acetate, 686-687
Flu-Imune, 950
Flumadine, 162
flumazenil, 1169-1170
flumecinol, 1265t
flunarizine, 1265t
flunarizine hydrochloride, 1212-1213
flunisolide, 621-622, 1050-1051
Fluocet, 1095
fluocinolone acetonide, 1095-1096
fluocinonide, 1096-1097
Fluogen Split, 950
Fluonid, 1095
Fluor-A-Day, 1124
fluorescein sodium, 1036
Fluorescite, 1036
Fluor-I-Strip, 1036
Fluor-I-Strip A.T., 1036
Fluoritab, 1124
5-fluorocytosine, 40-41
Fluorodex, 1124
fluorometholone, 1007-1008
Fluoroplex, 895
fluorouracil, 895-896
5-fluorouracil, 895-896
Fluosol, 860
Fluotic, 1124
fluoxetine hydrochloride, 410-411
fluoxymesterone, 701-703
fluphenazine decanoate, 448-450
fluphenazine enanthate, 448-450
fluphenazine hydrochloride, 448-450
Flura, 1124
Flura-Drops, 1124
Flura-Loz, 1124
flurandrenolide, 1097-1098
flurazepam hydrochloride, 367-368

t refers to a table.

flurbiprofen, 315-316
flurbiprofen sodium, 1008
Fluress, 1031
Flurosyn, 1095
Flu-Shield, 950
flutamide, 916
Flutex, 1104
fluticasone propionate, 1098-1099
Flutone, 1094
fluvastatin sodium, 289-290
fluvoxamine, 1213-1214
Fluzone Split, 950
Fluzone (Whole), 950
FML Liquifilm Ophthalmic, 1007
FML S.O.P., 1007
Foldan, 35
Folex PFS, 898
folic acid, 1111-1112
folinic acid, 1112-1113
Folvite, 1111
Footwork, 1078
Formulex, 513
Fortaz, 116
Fortral, 355, 356
foscarnet sodium, 158-160
Foscavir, 158
fosinopril sodium, 249-250
fosphenytoin, 1265t
Fostex 5% BPO, 1185
Fostex 10% BPO, 1185
Fostex 10% BPO Cleansing, 1185
Fostex 10% BPO Tinted, 1185
Fostex 10% BPO Wash, 1185
4-Way Long Acting, 1054
4-Way Long-Acting Nasal, 1052
4-Way Nasal Spray, 1047
FreAmine HBC, 1127
FreAmine III, 1127
FreAmine III with electrolytes, 1127
Freezone, 1240t
Frepp, 1240t
Froben, 315
Froben SR, 315
fructose, 1132-1133
frusemide, 803-805
5-FU, 895-896
FUDR, 892
Fulcin, 41
Ful-Glo, 1036
Fulvicin P/G, 41
Fulvicin-U/F, 41
Fumasorb, 840
Fumerin, 840
Funduscein Injections, 1036
Fungatin, 1078
Fungilin Oral, 37
Fungizone, 1057
Fungizone Intravenous, 37
Furacin, 1071
Furadantin, 180
Furan, 180
Furanite, 180
furosemide, 803-805
Furoside, 803
Fynex, 575

G

gabapentin, 386-387
Gabbromicina, 1262t
gallamine triethiodide, 553-555
gallium nitrate, 1192-1193
Gamastan, 972
Gamimune N, 972
Gamma Benzene, 1081
Gammagard S/D, 972
gamma globulin, 972-973
Gammar, 972
Gammar-IV, 972
Gamulin Rh, 974
ganciclovir, 160-161
gangliosides as sodium salts, 1273t
Ganite, 1192
Gantanol, 141
Gantanol DS, 141
Gantrisin, 143
Garamycin, 66, 1064
Garamycin Ophthalmic, 996
Gas-Relief, 630
Gastrocrom, 618
Gastrosed, 515
Gaviscon, 624
gBh, 1081
G-CSF, 980-981
2/G DM Cough, 610
Gee-Gee, 611
Gelfoam, 853
Gelusil, 624
Gelusil-II, 624
gemfibrozil, 290-291
Genabid, 282
Genagesic, 336
Genahist, 575
Genalac, 627
Genallerate, 572
Genapap Children's Elixir, 297
Genapap Children's Tablets, 297
Genapap Extra Strength Caplets, 297
Genapap Extra Strength Tablets, 297
Genapap Infants', 297
Genapap Regular Strength Tablets, 297
Genapax, 1065
Genaphed, 535

t refers to a table.

Genasal Spray, 1052
Genasoft, 649
Genaspor, 1078
Gencalc, 822
Gen-D-phen, 575
Genebs Extra Strength Caplets, 297
Genebs Regular Strength Tablets, 297
Genebs X-Tra, 297
Generlac, 651
Genoptic, 996
Genora 0.5/35, 730
Genora 1/35, 730
Genora 1/50, 730
Genpril Caplets, 316
Genpril Tablets, 316
Gentacidin, 996
Gentafair, 66
Gentak, 996
gentamicin, 996-997
gentamicin-impregnated PMMA beads on surgical wire, 1265t
gentamicin liposome injection, 1265t
gentamicin sulfate, 66-68, 996-997, 1064-1065
gentian violet, 1065-1066
Gentran 40, 825
Gentran 75, 826
Gen-Xene, 430
Geocillin, 82
Geopen Oral, 82
Geref, 782
Geridium, 306
germicidals, 1238-1241t
Germicin, 1238t
Gesterol 50, 740
Gesterol L.A. 250, 734
GG-CEN, 611
Glaucon, 1023
glibenclamide, 755-756
glipizide, 753-754
glucagon, 754-755
Glucamide, 751
glucocerebrosidase, 1182-1183
glucocerebrosidase-beta-glucosidase, 1182-1183, 1273t
Glucophage, 1215
glucosylceramidase, 1182-1183
Glucotrol, 753
Glu-K, 832
glutethimide, 368-369
Glyate, 611
glyburide, 755-756
glycerin, 650-651
glycerin, anhydrous, 1037-1038
glyceryl guaiacolate, 611
Glyceryl-T Capsules, 584
glyceryl trinitrate, 224-227
Glycoprep, 655
glycopyrrolate, 514-515
Glycotuss, 611
Glycotuss dM, 610
Glynase, 755
Glypressin, 1269t
Glytuss, 611
GM-CSF, 988-990
GM 6001, 1265t
G-Myticin, 1064
GnRH, 744-745
Gold-50, 1153
gold salts, 1152-1154
gold sodium thiomalate, 1153-1154
GoLYTELY, 655
gonadorelin acetate, 743-744
gonadorelin hydrochloride, 744-745
gonadotropin, chorionic, 745-746
gonadotropin releasing hormone, 744-745
gonadotropins, 743-749
Gordofilm, 1240t
goserelin acetate, 916-917
gossypol, 1265t
granisetron hydrochloride, 665
Granulex Aerosol, 1141
granulocyte colony-stimulating factor, 980-981
granulocyte-macrophage colony-stimulating factor, 988-990
Gravol, 662
Gravol L/A, 662
Grifulvin V, 41
Grisactin, 41
Grisactin Ultra, 41
griseofulvin microsize, 41-42
griseofulvin ultramicrosize, 41-42
Griseostatin, 41
Grisovin, 41
Grisovin 500, 41
Grisovin-FP, 41
Gris-PEG, 41
group B streptococcus immune globulin, 1273t
GTN-Pohl, 224
guaifenesin, 611
guanabenz acetate, 250-251
guanadrel sulfate, 251
guanethidine monosulfate, 252
guanfacine hydrochloride, 252-253
Guiamid D.M. Liquid, 610
Guiatuss, 611
Guiatuss-DM, 610
Gynecort, 1102
Gyne-Lotrimin, 1062

t refers to a table.

Gynergen, 538
Gynogen, 725
Gynogen L.A., 720

H

Habitrol, 496
Haemophilus b conjugate vaccine, diphtheria CRM_{197} protein conjugate, 947-948
Haemophilus b conjugate vaccine, diphtheria toxoid conjugate, 947-948
Haemophilus b conjugate vaccine, meningococcal protein conjugate, 947-948
Haemophilus b conjugate vaccines, 947-948
halazepam, 433-434
Halciderm, 1099
halcinonide, 1099-1100
Halcion, 377
Haldol, 450
Haldol Decanoate, 450
Haldol LA, 450
Haldrone, 692
Halenol Elixir, 297
Haley's M-O, 645
Halfan, 1214
halobetasol proprionate, 1100-1101
Halodrin, 700
halofantrine, 1214
Halofed, 535
Halofed Adult Strength, 535
Halog, 1099
haloperidol, 450-451
haloperidol decanoate, 450-451
haloperidol lactate, 450-451
haloprogin, 1066
Halotestin, 701
Halotex, 1066
Halotussin, 611
Halotussin DM Expectorant, 610
Halperon, 450
Haltran, 316
hamamelis water, 1240-1241t
Hartmann's solution, 834
H-BIG, 971
HbOC, 947-948
HC Cream, 1101
HCG, 745-746
HDCV, 961
Head and Shoulders, 1242t
Hemabate, 1144
hematinics, 840-844
heme arginate, 1273t
hemin, 1273t
Hemocyte, 840
Hemofil M, 857
hemostatics, 853-855
Hepalean, 847
heparin calcium, 847-850
heparin cofactor I, 858-859
Heparin Leo, 847
Heparin Lock Flush Solution (Tubex), 847
heparin sodium, 847-850
HepatAmine, 1127
hepatitis B immune globulin, human, 971
hepatitis B vaccine, recombinant, 948-950
Hep-B-Gammagee, 971
Hep Lock, 847
herpes simplex virus gene, 1265t
Herplex, 997
Hespan, 827
hetastarch, 827
Hexa-Betalin, 1114
hexachlorophene, 1238-1239t
Hexacrest, 1114
Hexadrol, 684
Hexadrol Phosphate, 684
Hexalen, 923
Hexalol, 167
hexamethylmelamine, 923-924
hexoprenaline sulfate, 1214-1215
H-F Gel, 1263t
H.H.R., 233
Hibiclens, 1238t
Hibistat, 1238t
HibTITER, 947
HI-Cor-2.5, 1101
Hiprex, 179
Hip-Rex, 179
Hismanal, 569
Histabid Duracaps, 568
Histaject Modified, 571
Histanil, 578
Histaspan-D, 568
Histaspan-Plus, 584
Histerone-50, 711
Histerone-100, 711
Histolyn-CYL, 1156
histoplasmin, 1156
histrelin acetate, 746-747
Hi-Vegi-Lip Tablets, 633
Hivid, 163
HIV-neutralizing antibodies, 1273t
HMM, 923-924
HMS Liquifilm Ophthalmic, 1009
Hold, 610
Homatrine, 1024

t refers to a table.

Homatropine, 1024
homatropine hydrobromide, 1024
Homo-Tet, 975
Honvol, 717
Hostacycline P, 135
HPA-23, 1265t
human growth hormone-releasing factor, 1265t
human IgM monoclonal antibody (C-58) to CMV, 1273t
human immunodeficiency virus (HIV-1) immune globulin (human) I.V., 1273t
humanized anti-TAC, 1266t
human monoclonal antibody against hepatitis B virus, 1273t
human T-lymphotropic virus type III gp 160, antigens, recombinant vaccine, alum absorbed, 1274t
Humate P, 857
Humatin, 28
Humibid L.A., 611
Humorsol, 1012
Humulin 50/50, 750, 757
Humulin 70/30, 750, 757
Humulin L, 757
Humulin N, 757
Humulin NPH, 757
Humulin R, 757
Hu-Tet, 975
Hy-5, 335
hyaluronidase, 1143
Hyate:C, 857
Hybolin Decanoate, 704
Hybolin Improved, 704
Hycodan, 336
Hycomed, 335
Hycopap, 335
Hyco-Pap, 335
Hycortole, 1101
Hycotuss, 336
Hydeltrasol, 693
Hydeltrasol Ophthalmic, 1010
Hydeltra-TBA, 694
Hydergine, 537
Hydextran, 843
Hydopa, 258
hydralazine hydrochloride, 253-254
Hydramine, 575
Hydramine Cough, 575
Hydramyn, 575
Hydrate, 662
Hydrea, 896
Hydrex, 796
Hydril, 575
Hydrisalic, 1240t
Hydrobexan, 1109
Hydrocet, 335
Hydro-chlor, 805
hydrochlorothiazide, 805-807
Hydrocil Instant, 656
Hydro-Cobex, 1109
Hydrocortex, 1101
hydrocortisone, 687-689, 1101-1103
hydrocortisone acetate, 687-689, 1102-1103
Hydrocortisone Acetate, 1102
hydrocortisone butyrate, 1102-1103
hydrocortisone cypionate, 687-689
hydrocortisone sodium phosphate, 687-689
hydrocortisone sodium succinate, 687-689
hydrocortisone valerate, 1102-1103
Hydrocortone, 687
Hydrocortone Acetate, 687
Hydrocortone Phosphate, 687
Hydro-Crysti-12, 1109
Hydro-D, 805
HydroDIURIL, 805
hydroflumethiazide, 807-808
hydrogen peroxide, 1238-1239t
Hydrogesic, 335
hydromorphone hydrochloride, 345-346
Hydromox, 814
Hydromox-R, 233
4-hydroperoxycyclophosphamide (4-HC), 1266t
Hydropine, 233
Hydropine HP, 233
Hydropres-25, 233
hydroquinone, 1242-1243t
Hydro-Reserp, 233
Hydro-Serp, 233
Hydroserpine, 233
Hydrotensin-25 Tablets, 233
HydroTex, 1101
Hydroxacen, 434
hydroxychloroquine sulfate, 48-50
hydroxyocobalamin, 1109-1111
hydroxycobalamin/sodium thiosulfate, 1266t
hydroxyprogesterone caproate, 734-735
hydroxyurea, 896-897
hydroxyzine embonate, 434-435
hydroxyzine hydrochloride, 434-435
hydroxyzine pamoate, 434-435
Hy/Gesterone, 734
Hygroton, 800
Hylorel, 251
Hylutin, 734
hyoscine butylbromide, 524-526
hyoscine hydrobromide, 524-526

t refers to a table.

hyoscyamine, 515-516
hyoscyamine sulfate, 515-516
Hy-Pam, 434
Hyperab, 973
HyperHep, 971
Hyperimmune RSV, 1275t
Hyperstat, 244
Hyper-Tet, 975
Hy-phen, 335
hypnotics, 360-379
Hypnovel, 371
Hypotears, 1032
HypRho-D, 974
Hyprogest 250, 734
Hypurin Isophane, 757
Hypurin Neutral, 757
Hyrexin-50, 575
Hytakerol, 789
Hytone, 1101
Hytrin, 275
Hytuss, 611
Hytuss-2X, 611
Hyzine-50, 434

I

Ibiamox, 76
Ibu-Cream, 316
Ibuprin, 316
ibuprofen, 316-317
Ibuprohm Caplets, 316
Ibuprohm Tablets, 316
Ibu-Tabs, 316
Icy Hot Balm/Cream, 1242t
Idamycin, 908
idarubicin hydrochloride, 908-910
idoxuridine, 997-998
IDU, 997-998
IFEX, 880
IFN-alpha 2, 983-986
ifosfamide, 880-881
IG, 972-973
IGIM, 972-973
IGIV, 972-973
IL-2, 977-979
I-Lite Eye Drops, 1036
iloprost, 1266t
Ilosone, 174
Ilotycin, 174
Ilotycin Ophthalmic, 995
Ilozyme Tablets, 635
Imdur, 219
Imferon, 843
imipenem/cilastatin sodium, 176-177
imipramine hydrochloride, 411-412
imipramine pamoate, 411-412
Imiprin, 411
Imitrex, 498
Immther, 1272t
ImmuCyst, 925
immune globulin intramuscular, 972-973
immune globulin intravenous, 972-973
immune serums, 970-976
Immuno, 1272t
immunosuppressants, 937-942
Immupath, 1273t
ImmuRAIT, AFP-I 131, 1274t
ImmuRAIT, hCG-I 131 human, 1274t
ImmuRAIT, LL-2-I 131, 1274t
Imodium, 642
Imodium A-D, 642
Imogam, 973
Imovax, 961
Impril, 411
Imudon, 1267t
Imuran, 937
ImuVert, 1276t
Inapsine, 1230t
Indameth, 318
indapamide, 808-809
Inderal, 228
Inderal L.A., 228
Inderide 40/25, 233
Inderide 80/25, 233
Inderide LA 80/50, 233
Indochron E-R, 318
Indocid, 318
Indocid PDA, 318
Indocid SR, 318
Indocin, 318
Indocin I.V., 318
Indocin SR, 318
indomethacin, 318-320
indomethacin sodium trihydrate, 318-320
InFeD, 843
Inflam, 316
Inflamase Forte, 1010
Inflamase Ophthalmic, 1010
influenza virus vaccine, 1994-1995
  trivalent types A & B (purified surface antigen), 950-952
influenza virus vaccine, 1994-1995
  trivalent types A & B (subvirion or split virion), 950-952
influenza virus vaccine, 1994-1995
  trivalent types A & B (whole virion), 950-952
Infumorph 200, 350
Infumorph 500, 350
INH, 61-62
Innovar Injection, 336, 1230t
Inocor, 187

t refers to a table.

inosine pranobex, 1266t
inotropics, 187-192
Insomnal, 575
Insulatard, 757
Insulatard Human, 757
Insulin 2, 757
insulin injection, 757-760
insulins, 757-760
insulin zinc suspension, extended (ultralente), 757-760
insulin zinc suspension (lente), 757-760
insulin zinc suspension, prompt, (semilente), 757-760
Intal, 618
Intal Inhaler, 618
Intal Spincaps, 618
interferon alfa-2a, recombinant, 981-983
interferon alfa-2b, recombinant, 983-986
interferon alfa-n3, 986
interferon beta (recombinant, human), 1274t
interferon beta-1b, recombinant, 986-987
interferon gamma-1b, 987-988
interleukin-1 alpha (recombinant, human), 1274t
interleukin-1 receptor antagonist, human recombinant, 1266t
interleukin-2, 977-979
interleukin-2, recombinant, liposome-encapsulated, 1274t
interleukin-3 (recombinant, human), 1274t
Intrabutazone, 330
Intralipid 10%, 1131
Intralipid 20%, 1131
Intraval Sodium, 1236t
intravascular perfluorochemical emulsion, 860-861
Intron A, 983
Intropin, 528
Inversine, 257
invert sugar, 1133-1134
investigational drugs, 1209-1221
Inza-250, 326
Inza-500, 326
Iodex, 1240t
iodine, 1125-1126, 1238-1239t
iodine ^{131}I 6B-iodomethyl-19-norcholesterol 1266t
iodine ^{131}I Lym-1 monoclonal antibody, 1274t
iodine ^{131}I metaiodobenzyl-guanidine, 1266t
iodine ^{131}I murine monoclonal antibody to human alphafetoprotein, 1274t
iodine ^{131}I murine monoclonal antibody to human chorionic gonadotropin (HcG), 1274t
iodine ^{131}I murine monoclonal antibody IgG2a to B cell, 1274t
iodochlorhydroxyquin, 1066-1067
Iodopen, 1125
iodoquinol, 26-27
Iodotope Therapeutic, 775
Iopidine, 1031
Iostat, 773
ipecac syrup, 1170-1171
I-Phrine 2.5%, 1924
IPOL, 959
ipratropium bromide, 594-596
IPV, 959-961
Ircon, 840
iron dextran, 843-844
Ismelin, 252
Ismo, 219
Ismotic, 1038
Iso-Bid, 219
isobutyramide, 1266t
isocarboxazid, 412-414
Isodine, 1240t
isoetharine hydrochloride, 596-597
isoetharine mesylate, 596-597
isoflurophate, 1016-1018
Isollyl Improved, 296
Isonate, 219
isoniazid, 61-62
isonicotinic acid hydride, 61-62
Isopap, 296
isophane insulin suspension, 757-760
isophane insulin suspension with insulin injection, 757-760
isoprenaline, 597-599
isopropamide iodide, 517-518
isoproterenol, 597-599
isoproterenol hydrochloride, 597-599
isoproterenol sulfate, 597-599
Isoptin, 230
Isoptin SR, 230
Isopto Alkaline, 1032
Isopto Atropine, 1021
Isopto Carbachol, 1012
Isopto Carpine, 1018
Isopto Cetamide Ophthalmic, 1001
Isopto Cetapred, 991
Isopto-Eserine, 1018
Isopto Fenicol, 993
Isopto Frin, 1024
Isopto Homatropine, 1024
Isopto Hyoscine, 1026

t refers to a table.

Isopto P-ES, 1012
Isopto Plain, 1032
Isopto Tears, 1032
Isorbid, 219
Isordil, 219
isosorbide, 1038
isosorbide dinitrate, 219-221
isosorbide mononitrate, 219-221
Isotamine, 61
Isotard MC, 757
Isotrate, 219
isotretinoin, 1193-1194
Isovex, 280
Isovorin, 1266t
isradipine, 254-255
Isuprel, 597
Isuprel Glossets, 597
Isuprel Mistometer, 597
itraconazole, 42-43
Ivocort, 1101
I.V. Persantine, 279

J

Janimine, 411
Japanese encephalitis virus vaccine, inactivated, 952-953
Jenamicin, 66
Je-Vax, 952

K

Kabikinase, 866
Kabolin, 704
Kalcinate, 822
Kaluril, 794
kanamycin sulfate, 68-69
Kanasig, 68
Kantrex, 68
Kaochlor 10%, 831
Kaochlor S-F 10%, 831
Kao-Con, 641
kaolin and pectin mixtures, 641-642
Kaon-Cl, 831
Kaon-Cl 20%, 831
Kaon Liquid, 832
Kaon Tablets, 832
Kaopectate, 641
Kaopectate Concentrate, 641
Kao-tin, 641
Kapectolin, 641
Karacil, 656
Karidium, 1124
Kato Powder, 831
Kaybovite, 1109
Kay Ciel, 831
Kayexalate, 1176
Kaylixer, 832
K + Care, 831
K + Care ET, 830
K + 10, 831
K-Dur, 831
Keflet, 122
Keflex, 122
Keflin, 123
Keftab, 122
Kefurox, 120
Kellogg's Castor Oil, 648
Kemadrin, 489
Kenacort, 697
Kenacort Diacetate, 697
Kenaject-40, 697
Kenalog, 697, 1104
Kenalog-40, 697
Kenalone, 1104
Keralyt, 1240t
keratolytics, 1240-1241t
Kerlone, 238
Kestrin Aqueous, 725
Kestrone-5, 725
Ketalar, 1232t
ketamine hydrochloride, 1232-1233t
ketoconazole, 43-44, 1067
ketoprofen, 320-321
ketorolac tromethamine, 321-322
ketorolac tromethamine, 1008-1009
ketotifen fumarate, 1215
Ketzol, 103
Key-Pred 25, 693
Key-Pred 50, 693
Key-Pred-SP, 693
K-FeRON, 843
K-Flex, 548
K-G Elixir, 832
K-Ide, 830
Kidrolase, 924
Kildane, 1081
Kinesed Tablets, 510
Kinidin Durules, 210
Klavikordal, 224
K-Lease, 831
Klonopin, 382
K-Lor, 831
Klor-Con, 831
Klor-Con/EF, 830
Klor-10%, 831
Klorvess, 822, 831
Klotrix, 831
K-Lyte, 830
Klyte-CL, 822
K-Lyte/Cl, 831
K-Norm, 831
Koate-HP, 857
Koate-HS, 857

t refers to a table.

Koffex, 610
Kogenate, 1271t
Kolephrin GG/DM, 610
Konakion, 1122
Kondremul, 653
Kondremul Plain, 653
Kondremul with Cascara, 645
Kondremul with Phenolphthalein, 645
Konsyl, 656
Konyne-80, 859
K-P, 641
K-Pek, 641
K-Tab, 831
Ku-Zyme HP Capsules, 635
Kwell, 1081
Kwellada, 1081
Kytril, 594

L

LA-12, 1109
labetalol hydrochloride, 255-256
Lacril, 1032
Lacrisert, 1032
lactation, drugs and, 11-12
lactobin, 1274t
Lactobin, 1274t
Lactulax, 651
lactulose, 651-652
L.A.E., 720
Lamisil, 1075
Lamprene, 57
Lanabiotic, 1056
Lanacort, 1102
Lanatrate, 537
Laniazid, 61
Laniroif, 296
Lanophyllin, 605
Lanophyllin-GG Capsules, 584
Lanorinal, 296
Lanoxicaps, 190
Lanoxin, 190
Lansoyl, 653
Lanvis, 900
Largactil, 442
Lariam, 50
Larodopa, 486
Larotid, 76
Lasix, 803
Lasix Special, 803
L-asparaginase, 924-925
Lauro Eye Wash, 1036
Lavoptik Eye Wash, 1036
laxatives, 645-659
Laxinate 100, 649
Laxit, 645
Lax-Pills, 654
Lax-Senna, 657
L-Caine, 1226t
L-carnitine, 1194-1195
Lcet 10/650, 336
L-deprenyl hydrochloride, 490-491
Ledercillin VK, 94
Ledermycin, 129
Legalon Sil, 1265t
Legatrin, 53
Lenoltec with Codeine No. 1, 336
Lente Insulin, 757
Lente MC, 757
Lente Purified Pork Insulin, 757
Lescol, 289
leucovorin calcium, 1112-1113
Leukeran, 874
Leukine, 988
leupeptin, 1266t
leuprolide acetate, 917-918
Leustatin, 890
levamisole hydrochloride, 939-940
levarterenol bitartrate, 532-534
Levate, 402
Levatol, 264
Levlen, 730
levobunolol hydrochloride, 1038-1039
levocabastine hydrochloride, 1039, 1266t
levocarnitine, 1194-1195
levodopa, 486-488
Levo-Dromoran, 346
Levoid, 764
levomepromazine hydrochloride, 369-371
levomethadyl acetate hydrochloride, 1195-1196
levonorgestrel, 735-736
Levophed, 532
Levoprome, 369
levorotatory alkaloids of belladonna, 518-519
levorphanol tartrate, 346-347
Levothroid, 764
levothyroxine sodium, 764-765
Levoxine, 764
Levsin, 515
Levsinex Timecaps, 515
Levsin S/L, 515
levulose, 1132-1133
LHRH, 744-745
LHRH [(des-gly[10]) d-trp [6]-Pro [9]-N-ethylamide], 1266t
L-5 hydroxytryptophan (L-5-HTP), 1266t
Librax Capsules, 427, 510
Libritabs, 429
Librium, 429

t refers to a table.

Lidemol, 1096
Lidex, 1096
Lidex-E, 1096
lidocaine hydrochloride, 203-204, 1226-1227t
Lidoject-1, 1226t
Lidoject-2, 1226t
Lido Pen Auto-Injector, 203, 1226t
lignocaine hydrochloride, 203-204, 1226-1227t
Limbitrol 5-12.5, 402, 427
Limbitrol 10-25, 402, 427
Lincocin, 177
lincomycin hydrochloride, 177-179
lindane, 1081-1082
LInomide, 1268t
Lioresal, 541
Lioresal Intrathecal, 541
liothyronine sodium, 765-767
liotrix, 767-769
Lipex, 294
Lipomul, 1129
Liposyn II 10%, 1131
Liposyn II 20%, 1131
Liposyn III 10%, 1131
Liposyn III 20%, 1131
Lipoxide, 429
Liquaemin Sodium, 847
Liqui-Char, 1160
Liqui-Doss, 653
liquid petrolatum, 653-654
Liquid Pred, 696
Liquifilm Forte, 1032
Liquifilm Tears, 1032
Liquiprin Infants' Drops, 297
lisinopril, 256-257
Lithane, 493
Lithicarb, 493
lithium carbonate, 493-495
lithium citrate, 493-495
Lithizine, 493
Lithonate, 493
Lithostat, 1181
Lithotabs, 493
Livostin, 1039
Lixolin, 605
L-leucine, L-isoleucine, and L-valine, 1266t
L-leucovorin, 1266t
10% LMD, 825
Locoid, 1102
Lodine, 312
lodoxamide tromethamine, 1040
Loestrin 21 1/20, 730
Loestrin 21 1.5/30, 730
Loestrin Fe 1/20, 730
Loestrin Fe 1.5/30, 730
Lofene, 640
Logen, 640
Logoderm, 1085
Lomanate, 640
lomefloxacin hydrochloride, 148-150
Lomine, 513
Lomotil, 640
lomustine, 881-882
Lonavar, 706
Loniten, 262
Lonox, 640
Lo/Ovral, 730
loperamide, 642-643
Lopid, 290
Lopresor, 260
Lopresor SR, 260
Lopressor, 260
Lopressor HCT 50/25, 233
Lopressor HCT 100/25, 233
Loprox, 1061
Lopurin, 1135
Lorabid, 127
loracarbef, 127-128
loratadine, 577
lorazepam, 435-436
Lorazepam Intensol, 435
Lorcet-HD, 335
Lorcet Plus, 335
Lorelco, 293
Loroxide, 1185
Lortab 2.5/500, 336
Lortab 5/500, 335
Lortab 7.5/500, 336
Lortab Oral Solution, 336
Losec, 676
Lotensin, 237
Lotrimin, 1062
Lotrisone Cream, 1056
Lo-Trol, 640
lovastatin, 291-292
Lovenox, 846
Lowsium, 629
Loxapac, 451
loxapine hydrochloride, 451-452
loxapine succinate, 451-452
Loxitane, 451
loxoribine, 1267t
Loxitane C, 451
Loxitane I.M., 451
loxoribine, 1267t
Lozide, 808
Lozol, 808
L-phenylalanine mustard, 884-885
L-threonine, 1267t

t refers to a table.

L-thyroxine sodium, 764-765
Lucrin, 917
Ludiomil, 414
Lufyllin, 590
Lufyllin-400, 590
Lugol's solution, 773-774
Luminal Sodium, 393
Lupron, 917
Lupron Depot, 917
Luride, 1124
Luride Lozi-Tabs, 1124
Luride-SF, 1124
Luride-SF Lozi-Tabs, 1124
Lurselle, 293
luteinizing hormone-releasing hormone, 744-745
Lutrepulse, 743
Luvox, 1213
lymphocyte immune globulin, 941-942
lypressin, 781-782
lysine acetylsalicylate, 1267t
Lysodren, 919
Lyspafen, 639
Lyteers, 1032

M

Maalox No. 1, 624
Maalox Plus Tablets, 624
Maalox TC Tablets, 624
Macrobid, 167
Macrodantin, 180
Macrodex, 826
Madopar, 481
Madopar HBS, 481
Madopar Q, 481
mafenide acetate, 1068-1069
magaldrate, 629
Magan, 305
Magenta paint, 1059-1060
Magnacef, 116
Magnatril, 624
magnesium chloride, 827-829
magnesium citrate, 652-653
magnesium hydroxide, 652-653
magnesium oxide, 629
magnesium salicylate, 305-306
magnesium sulfate, 387-388, 652-653, 827-829
Mag-Ox 400, 629
Malibar A, 478
Mallamint, 627
Malogen, 711
Malogex, 711
m-AMSA, 1209-1210
Mandameth, 179
Mandelamine, 179
Mandol, 102
manganese, 1125-1126
manganese chloride, 1125-1126
manganese sulfate, 1125-1126
Mangatrace, 1125
mannitol, 809-810
Maolate, 543
Maox, 629
maprotiline hydrochloride, 414-415
Marax, 584
Marbaxin-750, 547
Marcain, 1224t
Marcaine, 1224t
Marezine, 661
Marflex, 548
Margesic A-C, 335
Marinol, 664
Marmine, 662
Marnal, 296
Marogen, 1273t
Marplan, 412
Marzine, 661
Maso-Cort, 1101
masoprocol, 1196-1197
Matulane, 912
Maxair, 602
Maxaquin, 148
Maxenal, 535
Maxeran, 665
Maxidex Ophthalmic, 1006
Maxidex Ophthalmic Suspension, 1006
Maxiflor, 1094
Maximum Strength Pepto-Bismol Liquid, 638
Maximum Strength Phazyme, 630
Maxitrol Ointment/Ophthalmic Suspension, 991
Maxivate, 1087
Maxolon, 665
Maxolon High Dose, 665
Maxzide, 233, 792
Maxzide-25 mg, 792
Mazanor, 474
Mazepine, 380
mazindol, 474
M.C.T., 1134
measles, mumps, and rubella virus vaccine, live, 953-955
measles (rubeola) and rubella virus vaccine, live attenuated, 955
measles (rubeola) virus vaccine, live attenuated, 955-957
Measurin, 299
Mebaral, 389
Mebendacin, 31
mebendazole, 31

t refers to a table.

Mebutar, 31
mecamylamine hydrochloride, 257-258
mechlorethamine hydrochloride, 882-884
meclizine hydrochloride, 665-666
Meclofen, 322
meclofenamate, 322-324
Meclomen, 322
meclozine hydrochloride, 665-666
Meda Cap, 297
Mediconet, 1240t
Medigesic, 296
Medihaler-Epi, 592
Medihaler-Iso, 597
Medilax, 654
Medipren Caplets, 316
Medipren Tablets, 316
Mediquell, 610
Medi-Seltzer, 624
medium-chain triglycerides, 1134
Medralone-40, 689
Medralone-80, 689
Medrol, 689
Medrol Enpak, 689
medroxyprogesterone acetate, 736-737
medrysone, 1009-1010
mefenamic acid, 324-325
Mefic, 324
mefloquine hydrochloride, 50-51
Mefoxin, 112
Mega-Cal, 822
Megace, 918
Megacillin, 89, 90
Megagesic, 335
megestrol acetate, 918-919
Megostat, 918
Melaccine, 1274t
melanoma vaccine, 1274t
Melfiat 105 Unicelles, 478
Melipramine, 411
Mellamint, 822
Mellaril, 461
Mellaril Concentrate, 461
melphalan, 884-885
menadiol sodium diphosphate, 1121-1122
menadione, 1121-1122
Menaval, 720
Menest, 719
Meni-D, 665
meningitis vaccine, 957
Menoject-LA, 700
Menomune-A/C, 957
Menomune-A/C/Y/W-135, 957
menotropins, 747-748
Menrium 5-2, 427, 714
Menrium 5-4, 427, 714
Menrium 10-4, 427, 714
mepenzolate bromide, 519-520
meperidine hydrochloride, 347-349
Mephaquin, 50
mephentermine sulfate, 529-531
mephenytoin, 388-389
mephobarbital, 389-390
Mephyton, 1122
MEPIG, 1275t
mepivacaine hydrochloride, 1226-1227t
meprobamate, 437
Meprolone, 689
Mepron, 167
Meprospan-200, 437
Meprospan-400, 437
Merbentyl, 513
mercaptopurine, 897-898
6-mercaptopurine, 897-898
Meruvax II, 962
mesalamine, 1197
Mesantoin, 388
mesna, 1197-1198
Mesnex, 1197
mesoridazine besylate, 452-454
Mestinon, 508
Mestinon Supraspan, 508
Mestinon Timespan, 508
mestranol and norethindrone, 730-734
mesuximide, 390-391
Metahydrin, 819
Metamucil, 656
Metamucil Instant Mix, 656
Metamucil Sugar Free, 656
Metandren, 703
Metandren Linguets, 703
Metaprel, 599
metaproterenol sulfate, 599-600
metaraminol bitartrate, 531-532
Metastron, 1204
Metatensin Tablets #2/#4, 233
metformin, 1215-1216
methadone hydrochloride, 349-350
Methadose, 349
methamphetamine hydrochloride, 474-476
methantheline bromide, 520-521
methazolamide, 810-811
methdilazine hydrochloride, 577-578
methenamine hippurate, 179-180
methenamine mandelate, 179-180
Methergine, 1146
methicillin sodium, 84-85
methimazole, 772-773
methocarbamol, 547-548
methohexital sodium, 1232-1233t

t refers to a table.

methohexitone sodium, 1232-1233t
methotrexate, 898-900
methotrexate sodium, 898-900
methotrexate with laurocapram, 1267t
methotrimeprazine hydrochloride, 369-371
methotrimeprazine maleate, 369-371
methoxsalen (topical), 1198-1199
methscopolamine bromide, 521-522
methsuximide, 390-391
Methulose, 1032
methyclothiazide, 811-812
methyl CCNU, 1218
methylcellulose, 653
methyldopa, 258-260
methyldopate hydrochloride, 258-260
methylene blue, 180
methylergonovine maleate, 1146-1147
methylphenidate hydrochloride, 476-477
methylprednisolone, 689-692
methylprednisolone acetate, 689-692
methylprednisolone sodium succinate, 689-692
4-methylpyrazole (4-MP), 1267t
methylrosaniline chloride, 1065-1066
methyl salicylate, 1242-1243t
methyltestosterone, 703-704
methysergide maleate, 539-540
Meticorten, 696
Metimyd Ophthalmic Ointment/ Suspension, 991
Metin, 84
metipranolol hydrochloride, 1040-1041
metoclopramide hydrochloride, 666-667
metocurine iodide, 555-556
metolazone, 812-813
metoprolol succinate, 260-261
metoprolol tartrate, 260-261
Metra, 478
Metric-21, 27
Metrodin, 1270t
MetroGel, 1068
MetroGel-Vaginal, 1068
Metrogyl, 27
Metro I.V., 27
metronidazole, 27-28
metronidazole hydrochloride, 27-28
metronidazole (topical), 1068-1069
Metrozine, 27
Metubine, 555
metyrosine, 261-262
Mevacor, 291
mevinolin, 291-292
Mexate AQ, 898
mexiletine hydrochloride, 204-205
Mexitil, 204
Mezlin, 85
mezlocillin sodium, 85-87
M-G Pyregesic-C, 335
Miacalcin, 787
Micatin, 1069
miconazole, 44-45
miconazole nitrate, 1069-1070
MICRhoGAM, 974
Microcort, 1101
microfibrillar collagen hemostat, 853-854
Micro-K Extencaps, 831
Micronase, 755
Micronor, 737
Microsulfon, 140
Micrurus fulvius antivenin, 968-969
Midamine, 1267t
Midamor, 794
midazolam hydrochloride, 371-372
Midol-200, 316
Midrin, 296
Mifegyne, 1216
mifepristone, 1216-1217
Migral, 537
Milkinol, 653
milk of magnesia, 652-653
Milontin, 395
Milprem-200, 427
Milprem-400, 427
milrinone lactate, 192
Miltown-200, 437
Miltown-400, 437
Miltown-600, 437
Minax, 260
mineral oil, 653-654
minerals, 1106-1126
Minidiab, 753
Mini-Gamulin Rh, 974
Minims Castor Oil, 648
Minipress, 268
Minirin, 780
Minizide 1, 233
Minizide 2, 233
Minizide 5, 233
Minocin, 132
minocycline hydrochloride, 132-134
Minodyl, 262
Minomycin, 132
Minomycin IV, 132
minoxidil, 262-263
minoxidil (topical), 1199-1200
Mintezol, 35
Minzolum, 35
Miocarpine, 1018
Miochol, 1012
Miostat, 1012

t refers to a table.

miotics, 1012-1020
misoprostol, 675
Mithracin, 911
mithramycin, 911-912
mitodrine hydrochloride, 1267t
mitolactol (dibromodulcitol, DBD), 1267t
mitomycin, 910-911
mitomycin-C, 910-911
mitotane, 919-920
mitoxantrone hydrochloride, 929-930
Mitrolan, 646
Mivacron, 556
mivacurium chloride, 556-558
Mixtard Human, 750
M-kya, 47
M-M-RII, 953
Moban, 454
Mobenol, 762
Mobidin, 305
Moctanin, 633
modafinil, 1267t
Modane, 654, 656
Modane Mild, 654
Modane Plus, 645
Modane Soft, 649
Modecate, 448
Modecate Concentrate, 448
Moderil, 273
Modicon, 730
Moditen Enanthate, 448
Moditen HCl, 448
Moditen HCl-HP, 448
Modrastane, 921
Modulon, 1220
Moduretic, 792
Moisture Drops, 1032
Molatoc, 649
molindone hydrochloride, 454-455
Mol-Iron, 842
M.O.M., 652
mometasone furoate, 1103-1104
Monistat-Derm Cream and Lotion, 1069
Monistat I.V., 44
Monistat 3 Vaginal Suppository, 1069
Monistat 7 Vaginal Cream, 1069
Monistat 7 Vaginal Suppository, 1069
Monitan, 234
Monocid, 107
Monoclate, 857
Monoclate P, 857
monoclonal antibodies (murine or human) recognizing B-cell lymphoma idiotypes, 1274t
monoclonal antibodies PM-81 and AML-2-23, 1274t
monoclonal antibody 17-1A, 1274t
monoclonal antibody PM-81, 1275t
monoclonal antibody for immunization against lupus nephritis, 1275t
monoclonal factor IX, 1275t
monoctanoin, 633
Monodox, 130
Mono-Gesic, 307
Monoket, 219
Mononine, 859
Monopril, 249
Monotard HM, 757
Monotard MC, 757
Mono-Vacc Test, 1158
M-Orexic, 472
moricizine hydrochloride, 205-207
Morphine H.P., 350
morphine hydrochloride, 350-352
morphine sulfate, 350-352
morphine tartrate, 350-352
Morphitec, 350
M.O.S., 350
M.O.S.-S.R., 350
Motilium, 1211
Motofen, 639
Motrin, 316
Motrin IB Caplets, 316
Motrin IB Tablets, 316
Moxacin, 76
6-MP, 897-898
M-R-Vax II, 955
MS Contin, 350
MSIR, 350
MSTA, 1156
M.T.E.-4, 1106
M.T.E.-5, 1106
M.T.E.-6, 1106
M.T.E.-7, 1106
M.T.E.-4 Concentrated, 1106
M.T.E.-5 Concentrated, 1106
M.T.E.-6 Concentrated, 1106
mucoid exopolysaccharide *Pseudomonas* hyperimmune globulin, 1275t
Mucomyst, 608
Mucosol, 608
Multipax, 434
Multiple Trace Element, 1106
Multiple Trace Element Concentrated, 1106
Multitrace, 1106
Multitrace 5, 1106
Multitrace Concentrate, 1106
Multitrace Pediatric, 1107
mumps skin test antigen, 1156-1157
Mumpsvax, 957

t refers to a table.

mumps virus vaccine, live, 957-958
mupirocin, 1070
Murelax, 438
Murine Eye Drops, 1036
Murine Plus, 1029
muromonab-CD3, 942
Muro-128 Ointment, 1041
Mustargen, 882
Mutamycin, 910
Myambutol, 60
Myapap Elixir, 297
Myapap, Infants', 297
Myapap with Codeine, 336
Mycelex, 1062
Mycelex-7, 1062
Mycelex-G, 1062
Mycelex-OTC, 1062
Mycifradin, 69, 1071
Myciguent, 1071
Mycitracin Ointment, 1056
Mycitracin Ophthalmic Ointment, 991
Mycobutin, 183
Mycolog II Cream, Ointment, 1056
MyCort Lotion, 1102
Mycostatin, 45, 1072
Mydfrin, 1024
Mydriacyl, 1026
mydriatics, 1021-1027
My-E, 174
myelin, 1275t
Myfredine, 535
Myidone, 398
Myidyl, 583
Mykrox, 812
Mylanta Gas Maximum Strength, 630
Mylanta Gas Regular Strength, 630
Mylanta-II Tablets, 624
Mylanta Tablets, 624
Myleran, 870
Mylicon-80, 630
Mylicon-125, 630
Mymethasone, 684
Myochrysine, 1153
Myolin, 548
Myoquin, 53
Myproic Acid, 400
Myproic Acid Syrup, 400
Myrosemide, 803
Mysoline, 398
Mytelase, 501
Mytussin DM, 610

N

nabumetone, 325-326
N-acetylprocainamide (NAPA), 1267t
nadolol, 221-222
Nadopen-V-200, 94
Nadopen-V-400, 94
Nadopen-VK, 94
Nadostine, 1072
Nadostrine, 45
nafarelin acetate, 748-749
Nafcil, 87
nafcillin sodium, 87-88
naftifine, 1070-1071
Naftin, 1070
nalbuphine hydrochloride, 352-353
Nalcrom, 618
Naldecon, 568, 585
Naldecon Senior DX, 610
Naldecon Senior EX, 611
Nalfon, 314
Nalfon-200, 314
nalidixic acid, 150-151
Nallpen, 87
naloxone hydrochloride, 1171-1172
naltrexone hydrochloride, 1172-1173
Nandrobolic, 704
Nandrobolic L.A., 704
nandrolone decanoate, 704-706
nandrolone phenpropionate, 704-706
Napamide, 199
naphazoline hydrochloride, 1028-1029, 1051-1052
Naphcon, 1028
Naphcon Forte, 1028
Naprogesic, 326
Naprosyn, 326
Naprosyn-E, 326
Naprosyn SR, 326
naproxen, 326-327
naproxen sodium, 326-327
Naptrate, 227
Naqua, 819
Naquival, 233
Narcan, 1171
narcotic analgesics, 335-359
Nardil, 418
Nasahist B, 571
nasal agents, 1047-1055
Nasalcrom, 618
Nasalide, 1050
Natacyn, 998
natamycin, 998
Natrilix, 808
Natulan, 912
Naturacil, 656
natural lung surfactant, 614-616
Naturetin, 795
Naturetin W/K 2.5 mg, 233
Naturetin W/K 5 mg, 233
Nauseatol, 662

t refers to a table.

Navane, 462
Naxen, 326
ND-Stat Revised, 571
Nebcin, 73
NebuPent, 29
nedocromil sodium, 622-623
N.E.E. 1/35, 730
NegGram, 150
Nelova 0.5/35 E, 730
Nelova 1/35 E, 730
Nelova 1/50 M, 730
Nelova 10/11, 730
Nemasole, 31
Nemasol Sodium, 55
Nembutal, 372
Nembutal Sodium, 372
Neo-Calglucon, 822
Neo-Codema, 805
Neo-Cortef Ointment, 1056
Neo-Cultol, 653
Neocurb, 478
Neocyten, 548
NeoDecadron Cream, 1056
NeoDecadron Ophthalmic Ointment, 991
Neo-DM, 610
Neo-Durabolic, 704
Neo-Estrone, 719
NeoFed, 535
Neo-Fer, 840
Neo-Flo, 992, 1036
Neoloid, 648
Neo-Metric, 27
neomycin sulfate, 69-70, 1071
Neopap, 297
Neo-Polycin Ointment, 1056
Neoquess, 515
Neoquess Injection, 513
Neo-Rx, 1071
Neosar, 877
Neo-Spec, 611
Neosporin Cream, 1056
Neosporin G.U. Irrigant, 65
Neosporin Ophthalmic, 991
neostigmine bromide, 505-506
neostigmine methylsulfate, 505-506
Neosulf, 69
Neo-Synephrine, 534, 1024, 1053
Neo-Synephrine 12 Hour, 1052
Neo-Synephrine II, 1054
Neotal, 991
Neo-Tears, 1032
Neothyline, 590
Neothylline-GG Tablets, 584
Neotrace-4, 1107
NephrAmine, 1127
Nephro-Calci, 822
Nephronex, 180
Nephrox, 626
Neptazane, 810
Nervine Nighttime Sleep Aid, 575
Nesacaine, 1224t
Nesacaine MPF, 1224t
Nestrex, 1114
netilmicin sulfate, 70-72
Netromycin, 70
Neupogen, 980
neuromuscular blockers, 550-567
Neurontin, 386
neutral protamine Hagedorn insulin, 757-760
Neutra-phos, 822
Neutrexin, 901
NG-29,1267t
Niac, 1113
niacin, 1113-1114
niacinamide, 1113-1114
Niacor, 1113
nicardipine, 222-223
Niclocide, 31
niclosamide, 31-32
Nico-400, 1113
Nicobid, 1113
Nicoderm, 496
Nicolar, 1113
Nicorette, 495
Nicorette DS, 495
nicotinamide, 1113-1114
nicotine polacrilex, 495-496
nicotine resin complex, 495-496
nicotine transdermal system, 496-498
Nicotinex, 1113
nicotinic acid, 1113-1114
Nico-Vert, 662
Nidryl, 575
nifedipine, 223-224
Nilstat, 45, 1072
nimodipine, 281-282
Nimotop, 281
Niong, 224
Nipent, 931
Nipride, 263
Nitradisc, 224
Nitro-Bid, 224
Nitro-Bid I.V., 224
Nitrocap, 224
Nitrocap T.D., 224
Nitrocine, 224
Nitrodisc, 224
Nitro-Dur, 224
Nitro-Dur II, 224
Nitrofan, 180

t refers to a table.

nitrofurantoin macrocrystals, 180-182
nitrofurantoin microcrystals, 180-182
nitrofurazone, 1071-1072
Nitrogard, 224
Nitrogard SR, 224
nitrogen mustard, 882-884
nitroglycerin, 224-227
Nitroglyn, 224
Nitroject, 224
Nitrol, 224
Nitrolin, 224
Nitrolingual, 224
Nitronet, 224
Nitrong, 224
Nitrong S.R., 224
Nitropress, 263
nitroprusside sodium, 263-264
Nitrospan, 224
Nitro-Spray, 219
Nitrostat, 224
Nitrostat I.V., 224
Nitrotym-plus, 215
Nivaquine, 47
Nix, 1081
nizatidine, 675-676
Nizoral, 43, 1067
Nobesine, 472
Nobesine-75, 472
No Doz, 469
Nolamine, 568
Nolvadex, 920
Nolvadex-D, 920
nonnarcotic analgesics, 296-310
nonnarcotic antipyretics, 296-310
nonsteroidal anti-inflammatory drugs, 311-334
Nootropil, 1267t
Noradex, 548
noradrenaline acid tartrate, 532-534
Noradryl, 575
Norcept-E 1/35, 730
Norcet, 335
Norcet 7.5, 335
Norcuron, 566
Nordette, 730
Nordryl, 575
Nordryl Cough, 576
norepinephrine bitartrate, 532-534
norethindrone, 737-738
norethindrone acetate, 737-738
Norethin 1/35 E, 730
Norethin 1/50 M, 730
Norflex, 548
norfloxacin, 151-152, 998-999
Norfranil, 411
Norgesic, 541
Norgesic Forte, 541
norgestrel, 738-739
Norinyl 1 + 35, 730
Norinyl 1 + 50, 730
Norisodrine Aerotrol, 597
Norlestrin 21 1/50, 730
Norlestrin 21 2.5/50, 730
Norlestrin Fe 1/50, 730
Norlestrin Fe 2.5/50, 730
Norlutate, 737
Norlutin, 737
Nor-Mil, 640
Normison, 376
Normodyne, 255
Normosang, 1273t
Normozide 100/25, 233
Normozide 200/25, 233-234
Normozide 300/25, 234
Noroxin, 151
Norpace, 199
Norpace CR, 199
Norpanth, 523
Norplant System, 735
Norpramin, 407
Nor-Pred TBA, 694
Nor-Q.D., 737
Nortab, 415
Nor-Tet, 135
nortriptyline hydrochloride, 415-416
Nortussin, 611
Norvasc, 215
Norwich Aspirin Extra Strength, 299
Norzine, 670
Nostril, 1053
Nostrilla, 1052
Noten, 235
Novafed, 535
Novafed A, 569
Novagesic C8, 336
Novahistine Elixir, 569
Novamine, 1127
Novamoxin, 76
Novantrone, 929
Nova Rectal, 372
Novasen, 299
Novo-Alprazol, 427
Novo Ampicillin, 78
Novo-AZT, 165
Novobutazone, 330
Novocain, 1228t
Novo-Captopril, 240
Novocarbamaz, 380
Novochlorhydrate, 364
Novochlorocap, 171
Novo-Chlorpromazine, 442

t refers to a table.

Novoclopate, 430
Novocloxin, 82
Novocolchicine, 1136
Novodigoxin, 190
Novodimenate, 662
Novodipam, 431
Novodipiradol, 279
Novo-Doxepin, 408
Novodoxylin, 130
Novoferrogluc, 841
Novoferrosulfa, 842
Novofibrate, 286
Novoflupam, 367
Novo-Flurazine, 464
Novofolacid, 1111
Novofumar, 840
Novofuran, 180
Novohexidyl, 491
Novo-Hydrazide, 805
Novohydroxyzin, 434
Novo-Hylazin, 253
Novo-Keto-EC, 320
Novolexin, 122
Novolin 70/30, 750, 757
Novolin L, 757
Novolin N, 757
Novolin R, 757
Novolin R Penfill, 757
Novolorazem, 435
Novomedopa, 258
Novomethacin, 318
Novometoprol, 260
Novonaprox, 326
Novonaprox Sodium, 326
Novonidazol, 27
Novo-Nifedin, 223
Novopentobarb, 372
NovoPen-VK, 94
Novoperidol, 450
Novopheniram, 572
Novo-Pindol, 267
Novopirocam, 331
Novopoxide, 429
Novo-Pramine, 411
Novopranol, 228
Novoprednisone, 696
Novoprofen, 316
Novopropamide, 751
Novopropoxyn, 357
Novopropoxyn Compound, 336
Novoquindin, 210
Novoquinine, 53
Novoreserpine, 274
Novoridazine, 461
Novorythro, 174
Novosecobarb, 374
Novosemide, 803
Novosorbide, 219
Novosoxazole, 143
Novospiroton, 816
Novo-Sundac, 332
Novo-Tamoxifen, 920
Novotetra, 135
Novo-Thalidone, 800
Novotrimel, 138
Novotrimel DS, 138
Novotriolam, 377
Novo-Triptamine, 424
Novo-Triptyn, 402
Novo-Veramil, 230
Novoxapam, 438
Nozinan, 369
Nozinan Liquid, 369
Nozinan Oral Drops, 369
NP-27, 1078
NPH, 757-760
NPH Insulin, 757
NPH Purified Pork, 757
NTS, 224
NTZ Long Acting Nasal, 1052
Nu-Alpraz, 427
Nu-Amoxil, 76
Nu-Ampi, 78
Nu-Atenol, 235
Nubain, 352
Nu-Cal, 822
Nu-Cephalex, 122
Nu-Cloxi, 82
Nuelin, 605
Nuelin-SR, 605
Nu-Loraz, 435
NuLYTELY, 655
Nu-Medopa, 258
Nu-Metop, 260
Numorphan, 354
Numorphan HP, 354
Nu-Naprox, 326
Nu-Nifed, 223
Nu-Pen VK, 94
Nuprin Caplets, 316
Nuprin Tablets, 316
Nurofen, 316
Nuromax, 551
Nutracort, 1101
Nu-Triazo, 377
Nutrineal, 1264t
Nu-Verap, 230
Nydrazid, 61
nystatin, 45-46, 1072
Nystex, 45
Nytol Maximum Strength, 576
Nytol with DPH, 576

t refers to a table.

O

Obalan, 478
Obe-Del, 478
Obe-Mar, 479
Obe-Nix, 479
Obephen, 479
Obezine, 478
Oby-Trim, 479
Occlusal, 1240t
OCL, 655
Octamide, 665
Octamide PFS, 665
octreotide acetate, 643
Ocufen Liquifilm, 1008
Ocu-Gent, 996
Ocu-Pred, 1010
Ocusert Pilo, 1018, 1019
oestradiol, 720-723
oestradiol valerate, 720-723
oestrogens, conjugated, 723-725
oestrone, 725-726
Off-Ezy, 1240t
O-Flex, 548
ofloxacin, 152-153
Ogen, 727
olsalazine sodium, 1200
omeprazole, 676-677
Omnipen, 78
Omnipen-N, 78
Oncovin, 935
ondansetron hydrochloride, 667-668
Open-Cath, 868
Operand, 1240t
Ophthaine, 1236t
Ophthalgan, 1037
ophthalmic anti-infectives, 991-1005
ophthalmic anti-inflammatory agents, 1006-1011
ophthalmics, miscellaneous, 1031-1043
ophthalmic vasoconstrictors, 1028-1030
Ophtha P/S Ophthalmic Suspension, 991
Ophthetic, 1236t
Ophthoclor Ophthalmic, 993
Ophthocort, 991
opioid analgesics, 335-359
opium tincture, 643-644
  camphorated, 644
Optazine, 1028
Op-Thal-Zin, 1029
Opticrom, 618
Optigene, 1029
Optimine, 570
Optimyd, 991
OptiPranolol, 1040
Orabase HCA, 1101
Orahist, 569
Oraminic II, 571
Oramorph SR, 350
Orap, 457
Oraphen-PD, 297
Orasone, 696
Orbenin, 82
Orbenin Injection, 82
Orenzyme Bitabs Enteric-Coated Tablets, 1141
Oretic, 805
Oreticyl 25, 234
Oreticyl 50, 234
Oreticyl Forte, 234
Oreton Methyl, 703
Orflagen, 548
Original Doan's, 305
Orimune, 959
ORLAAM, 1195
Ormazine, 442
Ornade Spansules, 569
Ornex, 585
Ornex Cold, 535
Ornex-DM 15, 610
Ornex No Drowsiness Caplets, 296
Ornidyl, 25
Oroxine, 764
orphan drugs and biologicals, 1262-1276t
orphenadrine citrate, 548-549
Orphenate, 548
Orthoclone OKT 3, 942
Ortho Cyclen, 730
Ortho Dienestrol, 716
OrthoEST, 727
Ortho-Novum 1/35, 730
Ortho-Novum 1/50, 730
Ortho-Novum 7/7/7, 730
Ortho-Novum 10/11, 730
Or-Tyl, 513
Orudis, 320
Orudis E, 320
Orudis SR, 320
Oruvail, 320
Os-Cal, 822
Os-Cal 500, 822
Os-Cal Chewable, 822
Osmitrol, 809
Osteo-D, 1268t
otics, 1044-1046
Otocort, 1044
Otrivin, 535, 1054
Ovcon-35, 730

t refers to a table.

Ovcon-50, 730
ovine corticotropin-releasing hormone (oCRH), 1267t
Ovol, 630
Ovol-40, 630
Ovol-80, 630
Ovral, 730
Ovrette, 738
oxacillin sodium, 88-89
oxaliplatin, 1267t
oxamniquine, 32-33
Oxandrin, 706
oxandrolone, 706-708
oxaprozin, 327-328
oxazepam, 438
oxiconazole nitrate, 1073
oxidized cellulose, 854-855
Oxistat, 1073
Ox-Pam, 438
Oxsoralen-Ultra, 1198
oxtriphylline, 600-601
Oxy 5, 1185
Oxy 10, 1185
Oxy 10 Cover, 1185
Oxy-10 Wash, 1185
oxybutynin chloride, 1150-1151
Oxycel, 854
Oxycocet, 336
Oxycodan, 336
oxycodone hydrochloride, 353-354
oxycodone pectinate, 353-354
Oxydess II, 470
oxymetazoline hydrochloride, 1052-1053
oxymetholone, 708-709
oxymorphone hydrochloride, 354-355
oxyphenbutazone, 328-330
oxyphencyclimine hydrochloride, 522-523
oxytetracycline hydrochloride, 134-135
oxytocics, 1144-1149
Oxytocin, 1147
oxytocin, synthetic injection, 1147-1149
oxytocin, synthetic nasal solution, 1149
Oysco, 822
Oysco 500 Chewable, 822
Oyst-Cal 500, 822
Oyst-Cal 500 Chewable, 822
Oystercal 500, 822

P

PABA, 1242-1243t
Pabanol, 1242t
Pacaps, 296
paclitaxel, 930-931
PAC Revised Formula, 296
Palafer, 840
Palafer Pediatric Drops, 840
Palmiron, 840
2-PAM, 1173-1175
Pamelor, 415
pamidronate sodium, 1200-1201
Pamine, 521
Panadol, 297
Panadol Children's, 297
Panadol Extra Strength, 297
Panadol Infants', 297
Panadol Junior Strength Caplets, 297
Panadol Maximum Strength Caplets, 297
Panadol Maximum Strength Tablets, 297
Panafcort, 696
Panafcortelone, 693
Panamax, 297
Panasol, 696
Pancrease Capsules, 632, 635
Pancrease MT4, 635
Pancrease MT10, 635
Pancrease MT16, 635
pancreatin, 633-635
pancrelipase, 635-636
Pancrelipase Capsules, 635
Pancrezyme 4X Tablets, 633
pancuronium bromide, 558-560
Panectyl, 581
Panex, 297
Panex-500, 297
Panhematin, 1273t
Panmycin, 135
Panmycin P, 135
Panorex, 1274t
PanOxyl 5, 1185
PanOxyl 10, 1185
PanOxyl AQ 2 1/2, 1185
PanOxyl AQ 5, 1185
PanOxyl AQ 10, 1185
Panrexin M, 478
Panrexin MTP, 478
Panshape, 479
Pantheline, 523
papaverine hydrochloride, 282-283
para-aminobenzoic acid, 1242-1243t
para-amino salicylate, 55-56
paracetamol, 297-299
Paradione, 391
Paraflex, 544
Parafon Forte DSC, 544
Paralgin, 297
paramethadione, 391-392
paramethasone acetate, 692-693

t refers to a table.

Paraplatin, 871
Paraplatin-AQ, 871
Paraspen, 297
parasympathomimetics, 501-509
Parathar, 1269t
parathyroid-like agents, 786-791
paregoric, 644
Parepectolin, 638
Parlodel, 483
Par-Mag, 629
Parnate, 421
paromomycin sulfate, 28-29
paroxetine hydrochloride, 416-417
Parvolex, 608
Parzine, 478
PAS, 55-56
Pathocil, 83
patient teaching, drug use and, 12
Pavabid, 282
Pavabid HP Capsulets, 282
Pavabid Plateau Caps, 282
Pavacels, 282
Pavacot, 282
Pavagen, 282
Pavarine Spancaps, 282
Pavased, 282
Pavatine, 282
Pavatym, 282
Paveral, 340
Paverolan Lanacaps, 282
Pavulon, 558
Paxil, 416
Paxipam, 433
PBZ, 582
PBZ-SR, 582
PCE Disperstab, 174
P_1E_1, 1012
P_2E_1, 1012
P_3E_1, 1012
P_4E_1, 1012
P_6E_1, 1012
Pediacare Infant's Oral Decongestant Drops, 535
Pediaflor, 1124
Pediapred, 693
PediaProfen, 316
Pediatric Multiple Trace Element, 1107
Pediazole, 138
Pedi-Boro Soak Paks, 1242t
pediculicides, 1080-1084
Pedi-Dent, 1124
Pedtrace-4, 1107
PedvaxHIB, 947
PEG-adenosine deaminase (PEG-ADA), 1267t
PEG-interleukin 2, 1275t
PEG-L-asparaginase, 1275t
Peganone, 384
Pelamine, 582
pemoline, 477-478
Penamp-250, 78
Penamp-500, 78
Penbritin, 78
penbutolol sulfate, 264-265
Penecort, 1101
Penetrex, 147
Penglobe, 80
penicillin G benzathine, 89-90
penicillin G potassium, 90-91
penicillin G procaine, 91-92
penicillin G sodium, 92-93
penicillins, 75-99
penicillin V, 93-95
penicillin V potassium, 94-95
Pentacarinal, 29
Pentacef, 116
pentaerythritol tetranitrate, 227-228
Pentam 300, 29
pentamidine isethionate, 29-30
Pentamycetin, 171, 993
Pentasa, 1197
Pentaspan, 1275t
pentastarch, 1275t
Pentazine, 578
pentazocine hydrochloride, 355-357
pentazocine hydrochloride and naloxone hydrochloride, 355-357
pentazocine lactate, 356-357
pentobarbital, 372-374
pentobarbital sodium, 372-374
pentobarbitone, 372-374
pentostatin, 931-932
Pentothal Sodium, 1236t
pentoxifylline, 1201-1202
Pentritol, 227
Pentylan, 227
Pen Vee, 94
Pen Vee K, 94
Pepcid, 673
Pepcidine, 673
Pepto-Bismol, 638
Perbuzem, 215
Percocet, 336
Percodan, 336
Percodan-Demi, 336
Perdiem Plain, 656
pergolide mesylate, 488-489
Pergonal, 747
Periactin, 574
Peri-Colace, 645
Peridex, 1238t
Peridol, 450

t refers to a table.

perindopril, 1217
Peritrate, 227
Peritrate Forte, 227
Peritrate SA, 227
Permax, 488
permethrin, 1081-1083
Permitil, 448
Permitil Concentrate, 448
perphenazine, 455-457
Persa-Gel, 1185
Persa-Gel W 5%, 1185
Persa-Gel W 10%, 1185
Persantin, 279
Persantin 100, 279
Persantine, 279
Pertofran, 407
Pertofrane, 407
Pertropin, 1120
Pertussin Cough Suppressant, 610
Pertussin CS, 610
Pertussin ES, 610
pethidine hydrochloride, 347-349
PETN, 227
Petrogalar Plain, 653
petrolatum, 1240-1241t
Pfeiffer's Allergy, 572
Pfizerpen, 90
Pfizerpen-AS, 91
Pharmadine, 1240t
Pharmaflur, 1124
Pharmaflur df, 1124
Pharmaflur 1.1, 1124
Phazyme, 630
Phazyme 55, 630
Phazyme 95, 630
phenacemide, 392-393
phenacetylcarbamide, 392-393
Phenameth, 578
Phenaphen-650 with Codeine, 336-337
Phenaphen with Codeine No. 2, 337
Phenaphen with Codeine No. 3, 337
Phenaphen with Codeine No. 4, 337
Phenazine 25, 578
Phenazine 50, 578
Phenazo, 306
Phenazodine, 306
phenazopyridine hydrochloride, 306-307
Phencen-50, 578
Phendiet, 478
Phendiet-105, 478
Phendimet, 478
phendimetrazine tartrate, 478-479
Phendry, 576
Phendry Children's Allergy Medicine, 576
phenelzine sulfate, 418-419
Phenerbel-S, 537
Phenergan, 578
Phenergan-D, 585
Phenergan-Fortis, 578
Phenergan-Plain, 578
Phenetron, 572
phenobarbital, 393-395
phenobarbital sodium, 393-395
phenobarbitone, 393-395
phenobarbitone sodium, 393-395
Phenoject-50, 578
Phenolax Wafers, 654
phenolphthalein, white, 654-655
phenolphthalein, yellow, 654-655
phenoxybenzamine hydrochloride, 265-266
phenoxymethyl penicillin, 93-95
phenoxymethylpenicillin potassium, 94-95
phensuximide, 395-396
phenteramine hydrochloride, 479-480
Phentercot, 479
phentolamine mesylate, 266-267
Phentra, 478
Phentride, 479
Phentride Caplets, 479
Phentrol, 479
Phentrol-2, 479
Phentrol-4, 479
Phentrol-5, 479
Phenurone, 392
phenylazo diamino pyridine hydrochloride, 306-307
phenylbutazone, 330-331
phenylephrine hydrochloride, 534-535, 1024-1025, 1053
Phenylzin, 1028
Phenytex, 396
phenytoin, 396-398
phenytoin sodium, 396-398
Phenzine, 478
pHisoHex, 1238t
pHisoScrub, 1238t
Phos-Ex, 822
Phos-Flur, 1124
Phos-Lo, 822
Phosphaljel, 627
phosphocysteamine, 1267t
Phospholine Iodide, 1015
phosphonoformic acid, 158-160
Phrenilin, 296
Phrenilin Forte, 296
Phyllocontin, 587
Phyllocontin-350, 587
Physeptone, 349
physostigmine salicylate, 507-508, 1018

t refers to a table.

physostigmine sulfate, 1018
phytonadione, 1122-1124
Pilocar, 1018
pilocarpine, 1018-1020
pilocarpine hydrochloride, 1018-1020
pilocarpine nitrate, 1019-1020
Pilocel, 1018
Pilomiotin, 1018
Pilopine HS, 1018
Pilopt, 1018
Pima, 773
pimozide, 457-458
pindolol, 267-268
pipecuronium bromide, 560-561
piperacillin sodium, 95-96
piperacillin sodium and tazobactam sodium, 96-97
piperazine adipate, 33-34
piperazine citrate, 33-34
piperazine estrone sulfate, 727-728
pipobroman, 885-886
Pipracil, 95
Pipril, 95
piracetam, 1267t
pirbuterol, 601-602
Piriton, 572
piritrexim isethionate, 1267t
piroxicam, 331-332
Pitocin, 1147
Pitressin, 784
pituitary hormones, 778-785
Placidyl, 366
Plaquenil, 48
plague vaccine, 958-959
Plasbumin 5%, 856
Plasbumin 25%, 856
Plasmanate, 861
Plasma-Plex, 861
plasma protein fraction, 861-862
Plasmatein, 861
Platamine, 875
Platinol, 875
Platinol AQ, 875
Plendil, 247
Plendil ER, 247
plicamycin, 911-912
PMB 200, 427, 714
PMB 400, 427
PMS-Amitriptyline, 402
PMS Benztropine, 481
PMS-Carbamazepine, 380
PMS Diazepam, 431
PMS-Dimenhydrinate, 662
PMS Ferrous Sulfate, 842
PMS-Isoniazid, 61
PMS-Methylphenidate, 476
PMS Metronidazole, 27
PMS-Perphenazine, 455
PMS-Primidone, 398
PMS-Prochlorperazine, 668
PMS Procyclidine, 489
PMS-Promethazine, 578
pms-Propranolol, 228
PMS Pyrazinamide, 63
PMS Sulfasalazine E.C., 142
PMS Thioridazine, 461
PMS-Trifluoperazine, 464
pneumococcal vaccine, polyvalent, 959
Pneumopent, 29
Pneumovax 23, 959
Pnu-Imune 23, 959
Pod-Ben 25, 1240t
Podoben, 1240t
podofilox, 1073-1074
podophyllum resin, 1240-1241t
Poladex TD, 575
Polaramine, 575
Polaramine Repetabs, 575
poliovirus vaccine, inactivated, 959-961
poliovirus vaccine, live, oral, trivalent, 959-961
Polivax, 959
Polocaine, 1226t
poloxamer 188, 1267t
poloxamer 331, 1268t
Polycillin, 78
Polycillin-N, 78
Polycillin-PRB, 75
Polycitra-K, 1268t
Polydine, 1240t
polyethylene glycol-electrolyte solution, 655-656
Polygesic, 335
poly 1: poly C12U, 1275t
polymer implant containing carmustine, 1268t
Polymox, 76
polymyxin B sulfate, 182-183, 999-1000
polyribonucleotide, 1275t
Polysporin Ointment, 1056
Polysporin Ophthalmic Ointment, 991
polythiazide, 813-814
Polytrim Ophthalmic, 991
Ponderal, 473
Ponderal Pacaps, 473
Ponderax, 473
Ponderax Pacaps, 473
Pondimin, 473
Pondimin Extentabs, 473
Ponstan, 324
Ponstel, 324
Pontocaine, 1228t, 1236t

t refers to a table.

Pontocaine Eye Ointment, 1236t
Porcelana, 1242t
Pork NPH Iletin II, 757
Pork Regular Iletin II, 757
Portalac, 651
porton asparaginase, 924-925
Posture, 822
potassium acetate, 829-830
potassium bicarbonate, 830-831
potassium citrate and citric acid, 1268t
potassium chloride, 831-832
potassium gluconate, 832-833
potassium iodide, 773-774
  saturated solution, 773-774
Potassium Rougier, 832
povidone-iodine, 1240-1241t
Poyamin, 1109
PPD, 1157-1158
PPD-stabilized Solution (Mantoux test), 1157
PP1-002, 1268t
PR-122 (redox phenytoin), 1268t
PR-225 (redox acyclovir), 1268t
PR-239 (redox penicillin G), 1268t
PR-320 (molecusol-carbamazepine), 1268t
pralidoxime chloride, 1173-1175
Pramin, 665
pramiracetam sulfate, 1268t
Pravachol, 292
pravastatin sodium, 292-293
prazepam, 438-439
praziquantel, 34-35
prazosin hydrochloride, 268-269
Predaject-50, 693
Predalone-50, 693
Predalone TBA, 694
Predate-50, 693
Predate-S, 693
Predate TBA, 694
Predcor-50, 693
Predcor TBA, 694
Pred-Forte, 1010
Pred G, 991
Predicort-50, 693
Predicort RP, 693
Pred Mild Ophthalmic, 1010
Prednicen-M, 696
prednimustine, 1268t
prednisolone, 693-695
prednisolone acetate, 693-695
  suspension, 1010-1011
prednisolone acetate and prednisolone sodium phosphate, 693-695
prednisolone sodium phosphate, 693-695
  solution, 1010-1011
prednisolone steaglate, 693-695
prednisolone tebutate, 694-695
prednisone, 696-697
Prednisone Intensol, 696
Predsol Eye Drops, 1010
Predsol Retention Enema, 693
Predsol Suppositories, 693
Prefrin-A, 1028
Prefrin Liquifilm, 1024
pregnancy, drugs and, 10-11
pregnancy risk categories, 2
Pregnyl, 745
Prelone, 693
Prelu-2, 478
Premarin, 723
Premarin Intravenous, 723
Premarin with Methyltestosterone, 700
Pre-Pen/MDM, 1271t
Prepidil, 1144
Presolol, 255
Prestab, 755
Priadel, 493
Prilosec, 676
Primacor, 192
primaquine phosphate, 51-52
Primatene Mist, 592
Primatene Mist Suspension, 592
Primaxin, 176
Primazine, 458
primidone, 398-399
Primogyn Depot, 720
Principen, 78
Principen-250, 78
Principen-500, 78
Principen with Probenecid, 75
Prinivil, 256
Priscoline, 283
Privine, 1051
Pro-50, 578
Probalan, 1138
Pro-Banthine, 523
Probate, 437
Proben-C, 1135
probenecid, 1138-1139
Probenecid with Colchicine, 1135
probucol, 293-294
Procainamide Durules, 207
procainamide hydrochloride, 207-209
procaine hydrochloride, 1228-1229t
ProcalAmine with electrolytes, 1127
Procan SR, 207
procarbazine hydrochloride, 912-913
Procardia, 223
Procardia XL, 223
prochlorperazine, 668-670
prochlorperazine edisylate, 668-670

t refers to a table.

prochlorperazine maleate, 668-670
Procrit, 979
Proctocort, 1101
Proctofoam-HC, 1102
Procyclid, 489
procyclidine hydrochloride, 489-490
Procytox, 877
Pro-Depo, 734
Prodiem, 656
Prodrox, 734
Profasi, 745
Profasi HP, 745
Profenal, 1011
Proferdex, 843
Profilate SD, 857
progesterone, 739
Progestilin, 740
progestins, 714-742
Proglycem, 1188
ProHIBIT, 947
Proladone, 353
Prolastin, 613
Pro-Lax, 656
Proleukin, 977
Prolixin, 448
Prolixin Concentrate, 448
Prolixin Decanoate, 448
Prolixin Enanthate, 448
Proloprim, 184
promazine hydrochloride, 458-459
Prometh-25, 578
Prometh-50, 578
promethazine hydrochloride, 578-580
promethazine theoclate, 578-580
Promethegan, 578
Promine, 207
Pronestyl, 207
Pronestyl-SR, 207
Pronto, 1083
Propacet 100, 336
propafenone hydrochloride, 209-210
Pro-Pain-HC, 335
propamidine isethionate 0.1%, 1268t
Propanthel, 523
propantheline bromide, 523-524
proparacaine hydrochloride, 1236-1237t
Propine, 1035
Propion, 472
Proplex T, 859
propofol, 1234-1235t
Pro-Pox, 357
Pro Pox Plus, 335
Pro Pox with APAP, 336
Propoxycon, 357
propoxyphene hydrochloride, 357-358
propoxyphene napsylate, 357-358
propranolol hydrochloride, 228-230
Propulsid, 1187
propylthiouracil, 774-775
Propyl-Thyracil, 774
Prorazin, 668
Prorex-25, 578
Prorex-50, 578
Proscar, 1191
Pro-Sof, 649
Pro-Sof Liquid Concentrate, 649
Pro-Sof Liquid Plus, 649
ProSom, 365
Pro-Span, 734
Prostaphlin, 88
Prostep, 496
Prostigmin, 505
Prostigmin Bromide, 505
Prostin E_2, 1144
Prostin VR Pediatric, 1183
protamine sulfate, 1175
Protamine Zinc Insulin MC, 757
protamine zinc suspension, 757-760
Protaphane HM, 757
Protaphane MC, 757
protectants, 1240-1243t
Protenate, 861
Prothazine, 578
Prothazine Plain, 578
Protilase Capsules, 635
protirelin (TRH), 1268t
Protopam Chloride, 1173
Protophyline, 590
Protostat, 27
Protox, 1268t
Protrin, 138
Protrin DF, 138
protriptyline hydrochloride, 419-420
Protropin, 783
Proventil, 585
Proventil Repetabs, 585
Provera, 736
Providine, 1240t
Prozac, 410
Prozac-20, 410
Prozine-50, 458
PRP-D, 947-948
PRP-OMP, 947-948
Prulet, 654
Pseudo, 535
pseudoephedrine hydrochloride, 535-536
Pseudofrin, 535
Pseudogest, 535
Psorcon, 1094
Psorion, 1087

t refers to a table.

psyllium, 656-657
PT-105, 478
P.T.E.-4, 1107
P.T.E.-5, 1107
PTU, 774-775
Pudofin, 1240t
Pulmozyme, 620
Purge, 648
Purinethol, 897
P.V. Carpine Liquifilm, 1019
PVK, 94
PVF K, 94
P-V Tussin, 569
Pyranistan, 572
pyrantel embonate, 35
pyrantel pamoate, 35
pyrazinamide, 63
Pyrazodine, 306
pyrethrins, 1083-1084
Pyribenzamine, 582
Pyridiate, 306
Pyridin, 306
pyridine-2-aldoxime methochloride, 1173-1175
Pyridium, 306
pyridostigmine bromide, 508-509
pyridoxine hydrochloride, 1114-1116
pyrimethamine, 52-53
pyrimethamine with sulfadoxine, 52-53
Pyrinyl, 1083
Pyronium, 306
PZI, 757-760

Q

Quadrinal, 584
Quarzan, 511
quazepam, 374
Quektuss, 610
Quelicin, 563
Questran, 285
Questran Light, 285
Questran Lite, 285
Quibron Capsules, 584
Quibron Plus, 584
Quibron-T/SR, 605
Quick Pep, 469
Quiess, 434
Quin-260, 53
Quinaglute Dura-Tabs, 210
Quinalan, 210
Quin-amino, 53
Quinamm, 53
quinapril hydrochloride, 269-270
Quinate, 53, 210
Quinbisul, 53
Quindan, 53
Quine, 210
quinestrol, 740-742
quinethazone, 814-815
Quinidex Extentabs, 210
quinidine bisulfate, 210-212
quinidine gluconate, 210-212
quinidine polygalacturonate, 210-212
quinidine sulfate, 210-212
quinine bisulfate, 53-54
quinine bisulphate, 53-54
quinine sulfate, 53-54
quinine sulphate, 53-54
Quinoctal, 53
quinolones, 145-153
Quinora, 210
Quinsana Plus, 1078
Quiphile, 53
Q-vel, 47, 53

R

RA 27/3, 962-963
rabies immune globulin, human, 973-974
rabies vaccine, human diploid cell, 961
Racet Cream, 1056
radioactive iodine ^{131}I, 775-777
Radiostol, 1119
Radiostol Forte, 1119
Rafen, 316
Ramace, 271
ramipril, 271-272
ranitidine hydrochloride, 677-678
Raudixin, 272
Rauval, 272
Rauverid, 272
rauwolfia serpentina, 272-273
Rauzide, 234
Razepam, 376
R&C, 1083
Receptin, 1271t
Reclomide, 665
Recombivax HB, 948
Redoxon, 1118
Redutemp, 297
Reese's Pinworm Medicine, 35
Refresh, 1032
Regitine, 266
Reglan, 665
Regonol, 508
Regroton, 234
Regular (Concentrated) Iletin II, 757
Regular Iletin I, 757
regular insulin, 757-760
Regular Purified Pork Insulin, 757
Regulax SS, 649
Regulex, 649

t refers to a table.

Reguloid, 656
Regutol, 649
Rela, 542
Relafen, 325
Renacidin, 1263t
RenAmin, 1127
Renedil, 247
Renese, 813
Renese-R, 234
Renitec, 246
Repan, 296
replacement solutions, 822-835
rescinnamine, 273-274
reserpine, 274-275
Resonium A, 1176
Respbid, 605
respiratory agents, miscellaneous, 613-623
respiratory syncytial virus (RSV) immune globulin (human), 1275t
Respolin, 585
Respolin Autohaler Inhalation Device, 585
Respolin Inhaler, 585
Respolin Respirator Solution, 585
Resprim, 138
Restoril, 376
Resyl, 611
Retin-A, 1207
retinoic acid, 1207-1208
retinol, 1107-1109
Retrovir, 165
Reversol, 503
Revimine, 528
Rexigen, 478
Rexigen Forte, 478
Rexolate, 309
Rēv-Eyes, 1035
Rezide, 234
R-HCTZ-H, 234
Rh_o(D) immune globulin, human, 974-975
Rheomacrodex LMD, 825
Rheoth Rx copolymer, 1267t
Rhesonativ, 974
Rheumacin, 318
Rheumatrex, 898
Rhinalar Nasal Mist, 1050
Rhinall, 1053
Rhinall-10, 1053
Rhinex D-Lay, 569
Rhinocort, 1048
Rhinosyn-DMX Expectorant, 610
Rhodis, 320
Rhodis-E, 320
Rhodis-EC, 320
RhoGAM, 974
Rhotrimine, 424
Rhus Tox HC, 1101
ribavirin, 161-162
riboflavin, 1116
ricin (blocked) conjugated murine monoclonal antibody (anti-B4) to B cell (CD19), 1275t
ricin (blocked) conjugated murine monoclonal antibody (anti-My^9) to myeloid cells (CD-33), 1275t
ricin (blocked) conjugated murine monoclonal antibody (N901), 1275t
RID, 1083
Ridaura, 1152
Ridenol Caplets, 297
rifabutin, 183-184
Rifadin, 63
Rifadin IV, 63
Rifamate, 55
rifampicin, 63-64
rifampin, 63-64
rifampin, isoniazid, pyrazinamide, 1268t
Rifater, 1268t
rIFN-A, 981-983
riluzole, 1217-1218, 1268t
Rimactane, 63
Rimactane/INH Dual Pack, 55
rimantadine, 162
Rimycin, 63
Ringer's injection, 833-834
Ringer's injection, lactated, 834
Ringer's lactate solution, 834
Riopan, 629
Riopan Plus Chew Tablets, 624
Riopan Plus Suspension, 624
Riphen-10, 299
Risperdal, 459
risperidone, 459-461
Ritalin, 476
Ritalin-SR, 476
ritodrine hydrochloride, 1202-1203
Rivotril, 382
RMS Uniserts, 350
Roaccutane, 1193
Robafen, 611
Robaxin, 547
Robaxisal, 541
Robenecid, 1138
Robese, 470
Robicillin VK, 94
Robidex, 610
Robidrine, 535
Robigesic, 297
Robimycin, 174
Robinul, 514

t refers to a table.

Robinul Forte, 514
Robinul Forte Tablets, 510
Robinul Tablets, 510
Robitet, 135
Robitussin, 611
Robitussin DM, 610
Robitussin Pediatric, 610
Robomol-500, 547
Robomol-750, 547
Rocaltrol, 788
Rocephin, 119
Rocort, 1101
rocuronium bromide, 561-563
Rodex, 1114
Rofact, 63
Roferon-A, 981
Rogaine, 1199
Rogesic, 296
Rogesic No. 3, 335
Rogitine, 266
Rolaids, 628
Rolaids Calcium Rich, 627, 822
Romazicon, 1169
Rondec, 569
roquinimex, 1268t
Ro-Sulfiram-500, 492
Roubac, 138
Roubac DS, 138
Rounox, 297
Rounox and Codeine 15, 337
Rounox and Codeine 30, 337
Rounox and Codeine 60, 337
Rovamycine, 1269t
Rowawa, 1197
Roxanol, 350
Roxanol 100, 350
Roxanol Rescudose, 350
Roxanol SR, 350
Roxanol UD, 350
Roxicet, 336
Roxicet 5/500, 337
Roxicet Oral Solution, 337
Roxicodone, 353
Roxicodone Intensol, 353
Roxiprin, 336
RU 486, 1216-1217
rubella and mumps virus vaccine, live, 962
rubella virus vaccine, live attenuated, 962-963
Rubesol-1000, 1109
Rubesol-L.A., 1109
Rubex, 907
Rubion, 1109
Rubramin, 1109
Ru-Est-Span 20, 720
Ru-Est-Span 40, 720
Rufen, 316
Rum-K, 831
Ru-Vert M, 665
Rynacrom, 618
Rythmodan, 198
Rythmodan LA, 199
Rythmol, 209

S

Salacid, 1240t
Sal-Adult, 299
Salazopyrin, 142
Salazopyrin EN-Tabs, 142
salazosulfapyridine, 142-143
salbutamol, 585-586
salbutamol sulphate, 585-586
Saleto-200, 316
Saleto-400, 316
Saleto-600, 316
Saleto-800, 316
Salflex, 307
Salgesic, 307
salicylic acid, 1240-1241t
salicylsalicylic acid, 307-308
Sal-Infant, 299
salmeterol xinafoate, 602-603
Salonil, 1240t
salsalate, 307-308
Salsitab, 307
Saluron, 807
Salutensin, 234
Salutensin Demi, 234
Sandimmun, 938
Sandimmune, 938
Sandoglobulin, 972
Sandostatin, 643
Saneryl, 363
Sani-Supp, 650
Sanorex, 474
Sans-Acne, 1064
Sansert, 539
sargramostim, 988-990
Sarisol No. 2, 363
S.A.S., 142
S.A.S.-Enteric, 142
Scabanca, 1080
Scabene, 1081
scabicides, 1080-1084
SCF, 678
Sclavo Test, 1158
Scoline, 563
Scop, 524
scopolamine, 524-526
scopolamine butylbromide, 524-526
scopolamine hydrobromide, 524-526, 1026

t refers to a table.

SDZ MSL-109, 1268t
secalciferol (24, 25 dihydroxycholecalciferol), 1268t
secobarbital sodium, 374-376
Seconal Sodium, 374
secretory leukocyte protease inhibitor, recombinant, 1275t
Sectral, 234
sedatives, 360-379
Sedatuss, 610
Seldane, 580
Seldane Caplets, 580
Seldane-D, 569
selegiline hydrochloride, 490-491
selenious acid, 1125-1126
Selenitrace, 1125
selenium, 1125-1126
selenium sulfide, 1242-1243t
Selestoject, 680
Selsun, 1242t
Selsun Blue, 1242t
Semilente MC, 757
Semilente Purified Pork, 757
Semprex-D, 569
semustine, 1218
Senefen III, 335
Senexon, 657
senna, 657-658
Senokot, 657
Senokot-S, 645
Senolax, 657
Sensorcaine, 1224t
Sepp, 1238t, 1240t
Septisol, 1238t
Septopal, 1265t
Septra, 138
Septra DS, 138
Septra I.V. Infusion, 138
Septrin, 138
Septsoft, 1238t
Ser-A-Gen, 234
Seralazide, 234
Ser-Ap-Es, 234
Serax, 438
Serenace, 450
Serentil, 452
Serentil Concentrate, 452
Serepax, 438
Serevent, 602
sermorelin acetate, 782-783
Seromycin, 57-58
Serpalan, 274
Serpasil, 274
Serpasil-Apresoline #1, 234
Serpasil-Apresoline #2, 234
Serpasil-Esidrix #1, 234
Serpasil Esidrix #2, 234
Serpazide, 234
Serratia marcescens extract (ribosomes and lipid vesicles), 1276t
sertaline hydrochloride, 420-421
Sertan, 398
Serutan, 656
Setamol-500, 297
Sibelium, 1212, 1265t
Siblin, 656
Sigamine, 1109
Silexin Cough, 610
Silvadene, 1074
silver nitrate 1%, 1000-1001
silver sulfadiazine, 1074
simethicone, 630-631
simvastatin, 294-295
Sinarest 12-Hour, 1052
Sinemet, 484
Sinemet 10/100, 481
Sinemet 25/100, 481
Sinemet 25/250, 481
Sinemet CR, 481, 484
Sine-Off Nasal Spray, 1054
Sinequan, 408
Sinex, 1053
Sinex-L.A., 1054
Sinex Long-Acting, 1052
Sintisone, 693
Sinufed, 535
Sinus Excedrin No Drowsiness, 296
Sinus Relief Tablets, 296
Sinustat, 535
Sinutab, 296
Sinutab Maximum Strength, 296
Sinutab Maximum Strength without Drowsiness, 296,
642, 357
692, 335
SK&F 110679, 1276t
skeletal muscle relaxants, 541-549
Sleep-Eze 3, 576
Slo-bid Gyrocaps, 605
Slo-Phyllin, 605
Slow-Fe, 842
Slow-K, 831
Slow-Mag, 827
SMZ-TMP, 138
Snaplets-FR, 297
soaks, 1242-1243t
Soda Mint, 837
sodium benzoate and sodium phenylacetate, 1203-1204
sodium bicarbonate, 837-838
sodium cellulose phosphate, 1176-1177

t refers to a table.

sodium chloride, 834-835
sodium chloride, hypertonic, 1041-1042
Sodium Chloride Ointment 5%, 1041
sodium cromoglycate, 618-619
sodium dichloroacetate, 1269t
sodium fluoride, 1124-1125
sodium iodide, 1125-1126
sodium iodide ^{131}I, 775-777
Sodium Iodide ^{131}I Therapeutic, 775
sodium lactate, 838
sodium monomercaptoundecahydro-closododecaborate, 1269t
sodium oxybate (sodium gammahydroxybutyrate), 1269t
Sodium P.A.S., 55
sodium phosphates, 658-659
sodium polystyrene sulfonate, 1176-1178
sodium salicylate, 308-309
Sodium Sulamyd 10% Ophthalmic, 1001
Sodium Sulamyd 30% Ophthalmic, 1001
sodium tetradecyl sulfate, 1269t
sodium thiosalicylate, 309-310
Sodol, 542
Sofarin, 850
Solaquin Forte, 1242t
Solazine, 464
Solfoton, 393
Solganal, 1153
Solium, 429
Solone, 693
Solprin, 299
Soluble T4, 1272t
Solucap C, 1118
Solucap E, 1120
Solu-Cortef, 687
Solu-Flur, 1124
Solu-Medrol, 689
Solurex, 684
Solurex-LA, 684
Soma, 542
Soma Compound, 541
Soma Compound with Codeine, 541
Somagard, 1264t
Somatrel, 1267t
somatrem, 783-784
Sominex Formula 2, 576
Somophyllin, 587
Somophyllin-CRT, 605
Somophyllin-DF, 587
Somophyllin-T, 605
Sone, 696
Soothe, 1029
Sopamycin, 1045
Soprodol, 542
Sorbitrate, 219
Sorbitrate SA, 219
Soridol, 542
Sotacor, 212
sotalol, 212-213
Sotradecol, 1269t
Spancap #1, 470
Span-FF, 840
Sparine, 458
Spasmoban, 513
Spasmoject, 513
spasmolytics, 1150-1151
Spectazole, 1063
spectinomycin dihydrochloride, 184
Spectrobid, 80
Spensomide, 1238t
Spherulin, 1155
spiramycin, 1269t
spironolactone, 816-817
Spirotone, 816
Spirozide, 792
Sporanox, 42
SPS, 1176
S-P-T, 769
Squibb-HC, 1101
^{89}Sr chloride, 1204
SSD-Af, 1074
SSKI, 773-774
Stadol, 339
Stadol NS, 339
stanozolol, 709-711
Staphcillin, 84
Statex, 350
Staticin, 1064
Statrol, 991
stavudine, 1218-1219
Stelazine, 464
Stelazine Concentrate, 464
Stemetic, 670
Stemetil, 668
Sterapred, 696
Sterecyt, 1268t
Sterile 0.9% sodium chloride, 1036
Sterine, 179
S-T Expectorant, 611
StieVAA, 1207
stilboestrol, 717-719
Stilphostrol, 717
Stimate, 780
Stimate, 780
St. Joseph Aspirin-Free Fever Reducer for Children, 297
St. Joseph for Children, 610
St. Joseph Measured Dose Nasal Decongestant, 1053

t refers to a table.

ST1-RTA immunotoxin (SR 44163), 1276t
Storzolamide, 792
Stoxil, 997
Streptase, 866
streptokinase, 866-867
streptomycin sulfate, 72-73
streptozocin, 886-887
Strifon Forte DSC, 544
strong iodine solution, 773-774
strontium-89 chloride, 1204
Stulex, 649
Sublimaze, 342
succimer, 1178-1179
succinylcholine chloride, 563-565
Sucostrin, 563
sucralfate, 678-679
Sucrets Cough Control Formula, 610
Sudafed, 535
Sudafed Plus, 569
Sudafed-60, 535
Sudafed 12-Hour, 535
Sudrin, 535
Sufedrin, 535
Sufenta, 358
sufentanil citrate, 358-359
sulconazole nitrate, 1075
Sulcrate, 678
Suldiazo, 138
Sulfacel-15 Ophthalmic, 1001
sulfacetamide sodium 10%, 1001-1002
sulfacetamide sodium 15%, 1001-1002
sulfacetamide sodium 30%, 1001-1002
Sulfacet-R Lotion, 1056
sulfadiazine, 140-141
sulfafurazole, 143-144
Sulfamethoprim, 138
Sulfamethoprim DS, 138
sulfamethoxazole, 141-142
sulfamethoxazole-trimethoprim, 138-140
Sulfamylon, 1068
Sulfapred, 991
sulfasalazine, 142-143
sulfinpyrazone, 1139-1140
sulfisoxazole, 143-144
sulfonamides, 138-144
Sulf-10 Ophthalmic, 1001
sulindac, 332-333
Sulmeprim, 138
sulphafurazole, 143-144
sulphamethoxazole, 141-142
sulphasalazine, 142-143
Sulquin, 53
sumatriptan succinate, 498-499
Sumycin, 135
Supasa, 299
Super Calcium 1200, 822
Superchar, 1160
Supeudol, 353
superoxide dismutase (recombinant, human), 1269t
Suppap-120, 297
Suppap-325, 297
Suppap-650, 297
Supprelin, 746
Suprax, 105
suprofen, 1011
Surgicel, 854
Surmontil, 424
Survanta, 614
Sus-Phrine, 592
Sustaire, 605
suxamethonium chloride, 563-565
Syllact, 656
Symadine, 155
Symmetrel, 155
sympatholytics, 537-540
sympathomimetics, 527-536
Synacort, 1101
Synalar, 1095
Synarel, 748
Syn-Captopril, 240
Synemol, 1095
Synflex, 326
Synkavite, 1121
Synkayvite, 1121
Syn-Nadolol, 221
Synophylate, 605
Syn-Pindolol, 267
Synthroid, 764
Syntocinon, 1147, 1149
syvinolin, 294-295

T

T_3, 765-767
T_4, 764-765
Tac-3, 697
Tacaryl, 577
TACE, 714
tacrine hydrochloride, 499-500
Tagamet, 672
Talacen, 337
Talwin, 355, 356
Talwin Compound, 337
Talwin Nx, 355
Tambocor, 201
Tamofen, 920
Tamone, 920
Tamoplex, 920
tamoxifen citrate, 920-921
Tapanol Extra Strength Caplets, 297

t refers to a table.

Tapanol Extra Strength Tablets, 297
Tapazole, 772
Taractan, 444
Tarasan, 444
tartrazine dye content, 4
Tavist, 573
Tavist-1, 573
Tavist-D, 569
Taxol, 930
Taxotere, 1211
Tazac, 675
Tazicef, 116
Tazidime, 116
T-Cypionate, 711
T-Diet, 479
Tearisol, 1032
Tears Naturale, 1032
Tears Plus, 1032
Tebamide, 670
Tebrazid, 63
T.E.C., 1107
teceleukin, 1276t
Tecnal, 296
Tedral, 584
Tedral SA, 584
Teejel, 303
Tegamide, 670
Tega-Nil, 478
Tega-Vert, 662
Tegison, 1189
Tegopen, 82
Tegretol, 380
Tegretol Chew-Tabs, 380
Tegretol CR, 380
Telachlor, 572
Teldane, 580
Teldrin, 572
Temaril, 581
Temaze, 376
temazepam, 376-377
Temgesic Injection, 338
Temovate, 1088
Tempra, 297
Tempra Caplets, 297
Tempra Chewable Tablets, 297
Tempra Drops, 297
Tempra D.S., 297
Tencet, 296
Tenex, 252
teniposide, 932-933
Ten-K, 831
Tenol, 297
Tenoretic 50, 234
Tenoretic 100, 234
Tenormin, 235
Tensilon, 503
Tenuate, 472
Tenuate Dospan, 472
Tepanil, 472
Tepanil Ten-Tab, 472
Teramin, 479
Terazol 3 Vaginal Suppositories, 1076
Terazol 7 Vaginal Cream, 1076
terazosin hydrochloride, 275
terbinafine hydrochloride, 1075-1076
terbutaline sulfate, 603-604
terconazole, 1076
terfenadine, 580-581
Terfluzine, 464
Terfluzine Concentrate, 464
Teril, 380
teriparatide, 1269t
terlipressin, 1269t
terpin hydrate, 611-612
Terramycin, 134
Tertroxin, 765
Teslac, 921
Tessalon, 609
Testa-C, 711
Testamone 100, 711
Testaqua, 711
Test Est Cyp (oil), 700
Testex, 711
Testoderm, 713
Testoject-50, 711
Testoject-LA, 711
testolactone, 921
Testomet, 703
Testone L.A. 200, 711
testosterone, 711-713
testosterone cypionate, 711-713
testosterone enanthate, 711-713
testosterone propionate, 711-713
testosterone transdermal system, 713
Testred, 703
Testred Cypionate 200, 711
Testrin-P.A., 711
tetanus immune globulin, human, 975
tetanus toxoid, adsorbed, 963-964
tetanus toxoid, fluid, 963-964
tetracaine, 1236-1237t
tetracaine hydrochloride, 1228-1229t, 1236-1237t
Tetracap, 135
tetracycline hydrochloride, 135-137, 1002-1003, 1076-1077
tetracyclines, 129-137
tetrahydrocannabinol, 664-665
tetrahydrozoline hydrochloride, 1029, 1054
Tetralan, 135
Tetralean, 135
Tetramune, 943
Tetrasine, 1029

t refers to a table.

T4 endonuclease V, liposome encapsulated, 1269t
T4N5 Liposomes, 1269t
6-TG, 900-901
T-Gen, 670
Thalfed, 584
thalidomide, 1269t
Thalitone, 800
Tham, 838
Theelin Aqueous, 725
Theo-24, 605
Theobid Duracaps, 605
Theobid Jr. Duracaps, 605
Theochron, 605
Theo-Dur, 605
Theo-Dur Sprinkle, 605
Theolair, 605
Theolair-SR, 605
Theon, 605
theophylline, 604-607
theophylline ethylenediamine, 587-589
theophylline sodium glycinate, 604-607
Theospan SR, 605
Theo-Time, 605
Theovent Long-acting, 605
TheraCys, 925
Theralax, 645
Therevac Plus, 649
Therevac-SB, 649
Thermazene, 1074
Thia, 1116
thiabendazole, 35-36
Thiacide, 167
thiamine hydrochloride, 1116-1118
thiethylperazine maleate, 670-671
thioguanine, 900-901
6-thioguanine, 900-901
Thiola, 1206
thiopental sodium, 1236-1237t
thiopentone sodium, 1236-1237t
Thioprine, 937
thioridazine hydrochloride, 461-462
Thiotepa, 887
thiotepa, 887-888
thiothixene, 462-464
thiothixene hydrochloride, 462-464
Thorazine, 442
Thor-Prom, 442
Threostat, 1267t
thrombin, 855
Thrombinar, 855
thrombolytic enzymes, 863-869
Thrombostat, 855
Thyline, 590
Thymone, 1268t
thymosin alpha-1, 1276t
thymoxamine hydrochloride, 1270t
Thyrar, 769
Thyro-Block, 773
thyroid, 769-770
thyroid hormone antagonists, 772-777
thyroid hormones, 764-771
thyroid-stimulating hormone, 770-771
Thyroid Strong, 769
Thyroid USP, 769
Thyrolar, 767
thyrotropin, 770-771
Thytropar, 770
Ticar, 97
ticarcillin disodium, 97-98
ticarcillin disodium/clavulanate potassium, 99
TICE BCG, 925
Ticillin, 97
Ticlid, 1205
ticlopidine hydrochloride, 1205-1206
Ticon, 670
Tigan, 670
Tija, 134
Tilade, 622
Timentin, 99
Timentin injection, 75
Timolide 10/25, 234
timolol maleate, 275-276, 1042-1043
Timoptic Solution, 1042
Tinactin, 1078
Tindal, 440
Tine Test, 1158
Ting, 1078
tioconazole, 1077-1078
tiopronin, 1206-1207
Tipramine, 411
TISIT, 1083
tissue plasminogen activator, recombinant, 863
Titracid, 627
Titralac, 627, 822
Titralac Extra Strength, 627
Titralac Liquid, 624
Titralac Plus, 627
Titralac Tablets, 624
titratricol, 1270t
Tobradex, 991
tobramycin, 1003-1004
tobramycin sulfate, 73-74
Tobrex, 1003
tocainide hydrochloride, 213-214
Tocopher, 1120
tocopherol, 1120-1121
tocophersolan oral solution (vitamin E, d-alpha tocopheryl polylene glycol-1000 succinate, TPGS), 1270t
Tofranil, 411

t refers to a table.

Tofranil-PM, 411
Tolamide, 761
tolazamide, 761-762
tolazoline hydrochloride, 283-284
tolbutamide, 762-763
Tolectin, 333
Tolectin-200, 333
Tolectin-400, 333
Tolectin-600, 333
Tolectin DS, 333
Tolinase, 761
tolmetin sodium, 333-334
tolnaftate, 1078
tolrestat, 1219
Tolu-Sed DM Cough, 610
Tonocard, 213
topical agents, 1238-1243t
Topicort, 1091
Topicycline, 1076
Topimax, 1270t
topiramate, 1270t
Toprol XL, 260
Topsyn, 1096
TOPV, 959-961
Toradol, 321
Torecan, 670
Tornalate, 589
Torofor, 1066
torsemide, 817-818
Totacillin, 78
Totacillin-N, 78
toxic reactions, 10
toxoids, 943-965
t-PA, 863
T-Quil, 431
trace elements, 1125-1126
Trace Metals Additive, 1107
Tracrium, 550
Trac Tabs 2X, 167
Trancot, 437
Trandate, 255
tranexamic acid, 1270t
Transderm-Nitro, 224
Transderm-Scōp, 524
Transderm-V, 524
transforming growth factor beta-2, 1270t
Transiderm-Nitro, 224
Tranxene, 430
Tranxene-SD, 430
Tranxene-T-Tab, 430
tranylcypromine sulfate, 421-423
Trasylol, 1183
Travamine, 662
Travasol, 1127
Travasol with electrolytes, 1127
Travert, 1133
Travs, 662
trazodone hydrochloride, 423-424
Trazon, 423
Trecator-SC, 60
Trendar, 316
Trental, 1201
tretinoin, 1207-1208, 1270t
Trexan, 1172
Triacana, 1270t
Triacet, 1104
Triad, 296
Triadapin, 408
Trialodine, 423
Triam-A, 697
triamcinolone, 697-699
triamcinolone acetonide, 623, 697-699, 1104-1105
triamcinolone diacetate, 697-699
triamcinolone hexacetonide, 697-699
Triam-Forte, 697
Triaminic-12, 569
Triaminic Extended-Release Tablets, 569
Triamolone-40, 697
Triamonide-40, 697
triamterene, 818-819
Triaphen-10, 299
Triasox, 35
Triavil 2-10, 402, 440
Triavil 4-10, 402, 440
Triavil 2-25, 402, 440
Triavil 4-25, 402
Triavil 4-50, 402, 440
triazolam, 377-378
Trib, 138
Triban, 670
Tri-Barbs Capsules, 360
Tribenzagan, 670
Trichlorex, 819
trichlormethiazide, 819-820
Tricusal, 302
Tridesilon, 1090
Tridil, 224
Tridione, 399
Tridone Dulcets, 399
trientine hydrochloride, 1179-1180
triethanolamine polypeptide oleate-condensate, 1046
trifluoperazine hydrochloride, 464-466
trifluridine, 1004
Trihexane, 491
Trihexy-2, 491
Trihexy-5, 491
trihexyphenidyl hydrochloride, 491
Tri-Hydroserpine, 234
Tri-Immunol, 946
Tri-Kort, 697

t refers to a table.

Trikoside, 27
Trilafon, 455
Trilafon Concentrate, 455
Tri-Levlen, 730
Trilisate, 302
Trilog, 697
Trilone, 697
trilostane, 921-922
Trimcaps, 478
trimebutine maleate, 1220
trimeprazine tartrate, 581-582
trimethadione, 399-400
trimethaphan camsylate, 276-277
trimethobenzamide hydrochloride, 671
trimethoprim, 184-185
trimetrexate glucuronate, 901-902
trimipramine maleate, 424-425
Trimox, 76
Trimpex, 184
Trimstat, 478
Trinalin Repetabs, 569
Tri-Norinyl, 730
Tri-Otic, 1044
tripelennamine citrate, 582-583
tripelennamine hydrochloride, 582-583
Triphasil, 730
Triple Sulfa, 138
Triple X, 1083
Triprim, 184
triprolidine hydrochloride, 583
Triptil, 419
Triptone Caplets, 662
triptorelin pamoate, 1270t
trisaccharides A and B, 1276t
Tristoject, 697
Tritace, 271
Trobicin, 184
Trocal, 610
troleandomycin, 1270t
tromethamine, 838-839
TrophAmine, 1127
Tropicacyl, 1026
tropicamide, 1026-1027
Truxacaine, 1226t
Trymegen, 572
Tryptanol, 402
T/Scalp, 1101
TSH, 770-771
T-Stat, 1064
Tubarine, 565
Tubasal, 55
tuberculin purified protein derivative, 1157-1158
tuberculosis multiple-puncture tests, 1158-1159
Tubersol, 1157
Tubizid, 61
tubocurarine chloride, 565-566
Tucks, 1240t
Tuinal 200 mg Pulvules, 360
tumor necrosis factor-binding protein I, 1270t
tumor necrosis factor-binding protein II, 1270t
Tums, 627, 822
Tums E-X, 627, 822
Tums Liquid Extra Strength, 627
Tusal, 309
Tuss-DM, 610
Tusstat, 576
Twice-A-Day Nasal, 1052
Twilite Caplets, 576
Twin-K, 822
222, 335
222 Forte, 335
282, 335
292, 335
293, 335
Two-Dyne, 296
Tylaprin with Codeine, 335
Tylenol Caplets, 297
Tylenol Chewable Tablets, 297
Tylenol Children's Elixir, 297
Tylenol Drops, 297
Tylenol Elixir, 297
Tylenol Extra Strength Adult Liquid Pain Reliever, 297
Tylenol Extra Strength Caplets, 297
Tylenol Extra Strength Gelcaps, 297
Tylenol Extra Strength Tablets, 297
Tylenol Infants', 297
Tylenol Junior Strength Caplets, 297
Tylenol Junior Strength Tablets, 297
Tylenol Regular Strength Caplets, 297
Tylenol Regular Strength Tablets, 297
Tylenol Tablets, 297
Tylenol with Codeine Elixir, 336
Tylenol with Codeine No. 1, 337
Tylenol with Codeine No. 2, 337
Tylenol with Codeine No. 3, 337
Tylenol with Codeine No. 4, 337
Tylox, 337
Ty-Pap, 297
Ty-Pap Infants', 297
Ty-Pap Syrup, 297
Ty-Pap with Codeine Elixir, 336
typhoid vaccine, 964-965
typhoid vaccine, oral, 964-965
Tyrimide, 517
Ty-Tab Caplets, 297
Ty-Tab Capsules, 297
Ty-Tab Children's, 297
Ty-Tab Tablets, 297

t refers to a table.

Ty-Tab with Codeine No. 2, 337
Ty-Tab with Codeine No. 3, 337
Ty-Tab with Codeine No. 4, 337
Tyzine Drops, 1054
Tyzine Pediatric Drops, 1054

U

Uad-Caine, 1226t
Ucephan, 1203
Uendex, 1264t
Ukidan, 868
Ultracef, 101
ultradol, 312-314
Ultragesic, 335
Ultralente Insulin, 757
Ultralente Purified Beef, 757
Ultrase MT 12, 635
Ultrase MT 16, 635
Ultrase MT 24, 635
Ultratard HM, 757
Ultratard MC, 757
Ultra Tears, 1032
Ultravate, 1100
Ultrazine-10, 668
Unasyn, 79
Unasyn injection, 75
uncategorized drugs, 1181-1208
undecylenic acid and zinc
    undecylenate, 1078-1079
Uni-Bent Cough, 576
Unicort, 1101
Unigen, 725
Unilax, 645
Uniparin, 847
Uniparin-Ca, 847
Unipen, 87
Uniphyl, 605
Unipres, 234
Univol, 624
Unna's Boot, 1242t
Unna's Powder, 1242t
Unproco, 610
Urabeth, 502
uracil mustard, 888-889
Uracil Mustard Capsules, 888
urea, 820-821
Ureaphil, 820
Urecholine, 502
Urex, 179, 803
Urex-M, 803
Uridon, 800
Urisedamine, 167
Urispas, 1150
Uritol, 803
Urobiotic-250, 129
Urocarb Liquid, 502
Urocarb Tablets, 502
Urodine, 306
urofollitropin, 1270t
Uro Gantanol, 138
Urogesic, 306
urokinase, 868-869
Urolene Blue, 180
Uro-Mag, 629
Uro-Phosphate, 167
Uroplus DS, 138
Uroplus SS, 138
Uroquid-Acid, 167
Uroquid-Acid No. 2, 167
Urozide, 805
ursodiol, 636-637
Uticort, 1087

V

vaccines, 943-965
Vagistat, 1077
Valcote, 400
Valergen 10, 720
Valergen 20, 720
Valergen 40, 720
Valertest No. 1, 700
Valertest No. 2, 700
Valisone, 1087
Valium, 431
Vallergan, 581
Valorin, 297
Valorin Extra, 297
valproate sodium, 400-401
valproic acid, 400-401
Valrelease, 431
Vamate, 434
Vancenase AQ Nasal Spray, 1047
Vancenase Nasal Inhaler, 1047
Vanceril, 613
Vancocin, 185
Vancoled, 185
vancomycin hydrochloride, 185-186
Vanoxide, 1185
Vanquish, 296
Vansil, 32
Vantin, 114
Vapocet, 335
Vapo-Iso, 597
varicella vaccine, 1220-1221
varicella-zoster immune globulin,
    975-976
Varivax, 1220
Vascor, 216
Vaseline, 1240t
Vaseretic, 234
vasoactive intestinal polypeptide, 1276t
Vasocardol SR, 216
Vasocidin Ophthalmic Ointment, 991
Vasocidin Ophthalmic Solution, 991,
    1028

t refers to a table.

Vasoclear, 1028
Vasocon-A Ophthalmic Solution, 1028
Vasocon Regular, 1028
vasoconstrictors, ophthalmic, 1028-1038
vasodilators, 278-284
vasopressin, 784-785
Vasosulf, 991
Vasotec, 246
Vasotec I.V., 246
VaxSyn HIV-1, 1274t
Vazepam, 431
V-Cillin K, 94
VC-K, 94
vecuronium bromide, 566-567
Veetids, 94
Velban, 933
Velbe, 933
Velosef, 126
Velosulin Human, 757
Velosulin Insuject, 757
Veltane, 571
venlafaxine hydrochloride, 425-426
Venoglobulin-I, 972
Ventolin, 585
Ventolin Obstetric Injection, 585
Ventolin Rotacaps, 585
VePesid, 928
Veracaps SR, 230
verapamil, 230-231
verapamil hydrochloride, 230-231
Vercyte, 885
Verelan, 230
Vermox, 31
Versabran, 656
Versed, 371
Vertab, 662
V-Gan-25, 578
V-Gan-50, 578
Vianain, 1262t
Vibramycin, 130
Vibramycin IV, 130
Vibra-Tabs, 130
Vibra-Tabs 50, 130
Vicks Children's Cough, 610
Vicks Formula 44 Pediatric Formula, 610
Vicks Vatronol Nose Drops, 1050
Vicodin, 335, 337
Vicodin ES, 337
vidarabine, 1004-1005
vidarabine monohydrate, 162-163
Videx, 156
viloxazine hydrochloride, 1271t
vinblastine sulfate, 933-935
Vincasar PFS, 935
Vincent's Powders, 299
vincristine sulfate, 935-936
vindesine sulfate, 1221
Vioform, 1066
Vioform-Hydrocortisone Mild Cream, 1056
Viokase Powder, 635
Viokase Tablets, 635
Vira-A, 162
Vira-A Ophthalmic, 1004
Virazole, 161
Viridium, 306
Virilon, 703
Virilon IM, 711
Viroptic Ophthalmic Solution 1%, 1004
Visculose, 1032
Visine, 1029
Visken, 267
Vistacon, 434
Vistaject, 434
Vistaquel, 434
Vistaril, 434
Vistazine, 434
Vitacarn, 1194
Vita C Crystals, 1118
vitamin A, 1107-1109
vitamin A acid, 1207-1208
vitamin B_1, 1116-1118
vitamin B_2, 1116
vitamin B_3, 1113-1114
vitamin B_6, 1114-1116
vitamin B_9, 1111-1112
vitamin B_{12}, 1109-1111
vitamin B_{12a}, 1109-1111
vitamin C, 1118-1119
Vitamin D, 1119
vitamin D, 1119-1120
vitamin D_2, 1119-1120
Vitamin D_3, 1119
vitamin D_3, 1119-1120
vitamin E, 1120-1121
vitamin K_1, 1122-1124
vitamin K_3, 1121-1122
vitamins, 1106-1126
Vivactil, 419
Vivarin, 469
Vivol, 431
Vivotif Berna Vaccine, 964
V-Lax, 656
VLB, 933-935
VM-26, 932-933
Volmax, 585
Voltaren, 311
Voltaren SR, 311
Vontrol, 663
VoSol Otic, 1044

t refers to a table.

VP-16, 928-929
Vumon, 932
Vytone Cream, 1056
VZIG, 975-976

W

warfarin sodium, 850-852
Warfilone Sodium, 850
Wart-Off, 1240t
Wehdryl-10, 576
Wehdryl-50, 576
Wehgen, 725
Wehless, 478
Weightrol, 478
Wellbutrin, 405
Wellcovorin, 1112
Wescoid, 478
Westcort Cream, 1102
wet dressings, soaks, 1242-1243t
Wigraine, 537
Wigraine Suppositories, 537
Wilpowr, 479
WinGel, 624
Win-Kinase, 868
Winpred, 696
Winsprin Capsules, 299
Winstrol, 709
Wintrocin, 174
witch hazel, 1240-1241t
Wyamine, 529
Wyamycin S, 174
Wycillin, 91
Wydase, 1143
Wygesic, 336
Wymox, 76
Wytensin, 250

X

Xanax, 427
Xerac BP5, 1185
Xerac BP10, 1185
Xomazyme-H65, 1272t
Xomazyme-791, 1271t
4X Pancreatin 600 mg, 633
8X Pancreatin 900 mg, 633
X-Prep Liquid, 657
X-Trozine, 478
X-Trozine LA, 478
Xylocaine, 203
Xylocard, 203
xylometazoline hydrochloride, 1054-1055

Y

yellow fever vaccine, 965
YF-Vax, 965
Yodoxin, 26
Yomesan, 31
Yutopar, 1202

Z

Zadine, 570
Zaditen, 1215
zalcitabine, 163-165
Zanosar, 886
Zantac, 677
Zantac-C, 677
Zantryl, 479
Zapex, 438
Zarontin, 383
Zaroxolyn, 812
Zeasorb-Af, 1078
Zebeta, 239
Zefazone, 106
Zemuron, 561
Zephiran, 1238t
Zerit, 1218
Zeroxin-5, 1185
Zeroxin-10, 1185
Zestril, 256
Zetran, 431
Ziac, 234
Ziac 2.5, 792
Ziac 5, 792
Ziac 10, 792
zidovudine, 165-166
Zinacef, 120
Zinamide, 63
zinc, 1125-1126
zinc acetate, 1271t
zinc chloride, 1125-1126
Zincfrin, 1028
zinc gelatin, 1242-1243t
zinc sulfate, 1029-1030, 1125-1126
Zinctrace, 1125
Zinecard, 1264t
Zithromax, 168
Zixoryn, 1265t
Zocor, 294
Zofran, 667
Zoladex, 916
Zolicef, 103
Zoloft, 420
zolpidem tartrate, 378-379
ZORprin, 299
Zostrix, 1186
Zosyn, 96
Zovirax, 154, 1056
Zydone, 335
Zyloprim, 1135, 1262t
Zymase Capsules, 635
Zymenol, 653

t refers to a table.